Russell, Hugo & Ayliffe's
Principles and Practice of Disinfection, Preservation and Sterilization

Russell, Hugo & Ayliffe's

Principles and Practice of Disinfection, Preservation and Sterilization

EDITED BY

ADAM P. FRAISE MB, BS, FRCPath

Consultant Medical Microbiologist
Microbiology Department
Queen Elizabeth Medical Centre
Pathology – University Hospitals Birmingham NHS Foundation Trust
Queen Elizabeth Hospital
Birmingham, United Kingdom

JEAN-YVES MAILLARD Bsc, PhD, DSc

Reader in Pharmaceutical Microbiology
Cardiff School of Pharmacy and Pharmaceutical Sciences
Cardiff University
Cardiff, United Kingdom

SYED A. SATTAR PhD

Professor Emeritus of Microbiology and Director
Centre for Research on Environmental Microbiology
Faculty of Medicine
University of Ottawa
Ottawa
Ontario, Canada

5TH EDITION

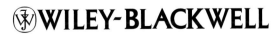
WILEY-BLACKWELL

A John Wiley & Sons, Ltd., Publication

This edition first published 2013 © 1982, 1992, 1999, 2004, 2013 by Blackwell Publishing Ltd.

Blackwell Publishing was acquired by John Wiley & Sons in February 2007. Blackwell's publishing program has been merged with Wiley's global Scientific, Technical and Medical business to form Wiley-Blackwell.

Registered office: John Wiley & Sons, Ltd, The Atrium, Southern Gate, Chichester, West Sussex, PO19 8SQ, UK

Editorial offices: 9600 Garsington Road, Oxford, OX4 2DQ, UK
The Atrium, Southern Gate, Chichester, West Sussex, PO19 8SQ, UK
111 River Street, Hoboken, NJ 07030-5774, USA

For details of our global editorial offices, for customer services and for information about how to apply for permission to reuse the copyright material in this book please see our website at www.wiley.com/wiley-blackwell

Library of Congress Cataloging-in-Publication Data
Principles and practice of disinfection, preservation, and sterilization. – 5th ed. / edited by Adam P. Fraise, Jean-Yves Maillard, Syed A. Sattar.
       p. ; cm.
    Rev. ed. of: Russell, Hugo & Ayliffe's principles and practice of disinfection, preservation & sterilization, c2004.
    Includes bibliographical references and index.
    ISBN 978-1-4443-3325-1 (hardback : alk. paper)
    I. Fraise, Adam P.   II. Maillard, J.-Y.   III. Sattar, Syed.
    [DNLM: 1. Disinfection–methods.   2. Sterilization–methods.   3. Anti-Infective Agents.
4. Decontamination.   5. Drug Resistance, Microbial.   6. Preservatives, Pharmaceutical. WA 240]

    614.4'8–dc23
                                          2012014816

A catalogue record for this book is available from the British Library.

Wiley also publishes its books in a variety of electronic formats. Some content that appears in print may not be available in electronic books.

Cover images: Left to right: (1) Cluster of *E. coli* bacteria. Courtesy of USDA/ARS. Photo by Eric Erbe, digital colorization by Christopher Pooley. (2) A scientist examining a petri dish containing bacterial cultures. © iStockphoto/Loran Nicolas. (3) *Actinomyces bovis* bacterial microcolony. Courtesy of CDC/ Dr. Lucille K. Georg

Cover design by Steve Thompson

Set in 9.25/12pt Minion by Toppan Best-set Premedia Limited
Printed and bound in Singapore by Markono Print Media Pte Ltd

01   2013

Contents

Contents

List of Contributors

Ibrahim Al-Adham
Associate Professor
Faculty of Pharmacy and Medical Sciences
Univeristy of Petra
Amman, Jordan

Michelle J. Alfa
Professor
Department of Medical Microbiology
University of Mantitoba;
Medical Director, Clinical Microbiology
Diagnostic Services of Manitoba
St. Boniface General Hospital
Winnipeg
Manitoba, Canada

Benedetta Allegranzi
World Health Organization Patient Safety
World Health Organization
Geneva, Switzerland

Peter D. Askew
Industrial Microbiological Services Ltd
Hartley Wintney, UK

Les Baillie
Professor of Microbiology
Cardiff School of Pharmacy and Pharmaceutical
Sciences
Cardiff University
Cardiff, Wales, UK

Richard Bancroft
Director of Development and Technical Services
Albert Browne Ltd
Leicester, UK

Christina Bradley
Laboratory Manager
Hospital Infection Research Laboratory
Queen Elizabeth Hospital
Birmingham, UK

Peter A. Burke
Senior Vice President and Chief Technology Officer
STERIS Corporation
Mentor, Ohio, USA

Jonathan L.S. Caplin
Senior Lecturer in Microbiology
School of Environment and Technology
University of Brighton
Brighton, UK

Ian A. Chisholm
Assessment Officer
AIDS and Viral Diseases Division
Bureau of Gastroentrerology
Infection and Viral Diseases
Therapeutic Products Directorate
Health Canada
Ottawa, Ontario, Canada

Phillip Collier
Senior Lecturer in Microbiology
School of Contemporary Sciences
University of Abertay
Dundee, Scotland, UK

Rose Cooper
Professor of Microbiology
Centre for Biomedical Sciences
Department of Applied Sciences
Cardiff School of Health Sciences
Cardiff Metropolitan University
Cardiff, Wales, UK

Andre G. Craan
Scientific Evaluator
Biotechnology Section
Marketed Biologicals
Biotechnology and Natural Health Products
Bureau
Marketed Health Products Directorate
Health Canada
Ottawa, Ontario, Canada

John V. Dadswell
Former Director
Reading Public Health Laboratory
Reading, UK

Anne Davin-Regli
UMR-MD1
Transporteurs Membranaires
Chimiorésistance et Drug-Design
Facultés de Médecine et de Pharmacie
Marseille, France

Stephen P. Denyer
Professor
Deputy Pro Vice-Chancellor
Education and Students
Cardiff School of Pharmacy and Pharmaceutical
Sciences
Cardiff University
Cardiff, Wales, UK

Nicolina Dias
Assistant Professor
IBB-Institute for Biotechnology and
Bioengineering
Centre of Biological Engineering
Micoteca da Universidade do Minho
Braga, Portugal

Patrick Duroselle
Retired
Sète, France

Jean-Yves Dusseau
Unité d'Hygiène
CHI Annemasse-Bonneville
Annemasse; Unité d'Hygiène
Hôpitaux du Léman
Thonon-les-Bains, France

List of Contributors

Valerie Edwards-Jones
Professor of Medical Microbiology
School of Research, Enterprise and Innovation
Faculty of Science and Engineering
Manchester Metropolitan University
Manchester, UK

Sara Fernandes
Post-Doc Researcher
Institute for Molecular and Cell Biology
Porto, Portugal

Adam P. Fraise
Microbiology Department
Queen Elizabeth Medical Centre
Pathology – University Hospitals Birmingham
NHS Foundation Trust
Birmingham, UK

Jean Freney
Institut des Sciences Pharmaceutiques et
Biologiques
UMR 5557 – CNRS Ecologie Microbienne
Bactéries pathogènes Opportunistes et
Environnement
Université Lyon 1
Lyon, France

Brendan F. Gilmore
Senior Lecturer in Pharmaceutical Microbiology
School of Pharmacy
Faculty of Medicine
Health and Life Sciences
Queen's University Belfast
Belfast, Northern Ireland, UK

Darla M. Goeres
Assistant Research Professor of Chemical and
Biological Engineering
Center for Biofilm Engineering
Montana State University
Bozeman, Montana, USA

Sean P. Gorman
Professor of Pharmaceutical Microbiology
School of Pharmacy
Faculty of Medicine
Health and Life Sciences
Queen's University Belfast
Belfast, Northern Ireland, UK

Randa Haddadin
Assistant Professor
Faculty of Pharmacy
University of Jordan
Amman, Jordan

Charles O. Hancock
Medical Sterilization Consultant
Charles O. Hancock Associates Inc.
Fairport
New York, USA

Geoffrey W. Hanlon
School of Pharmacy and Biomolecular Sciences
University of Brighton
Brighton, UK

Philippe Hartemann
Professor of Public Health
Department of Environment and Public Health
Nancy School of Medicine
Lorraine University
Vandoeuvre-Nancy, France

Sally Hayes
Senior Consultant and Co-Owner
Scientific & Regulatory Consultants, Inc.
Columbia City, Indiana, USA

Sarah J. Hiom
All Wales Specialist Pharmacist
Research and Development
St. Marys Pharmaceutical Unit
Cardiff and Vale University Health Board
Cardiff, Wales, UK

Peter Hoffman
Consultant Clinical Scientist
Laboratory of Healthcare-associated Infection
Health Protection Agency
London, UK

Jennifer A. Hopkins
European Regulatory Strategy and Advocacy
Manager
Bayer SAS Environmental Science
Lyon, France

James J. Kaiser
Principal Scientist
Microbiology and Sterilization Sciences
Bausch and Lomb
Rochester
New York, USA

Peter A. Lambert
Professor of Microbiology
School of Life and Health Sciences
Aston University
Birmingham, UK

Nelson Lima
Professor
IBB-Institute for Biotechnology and
Bioengineering
Centre of Biological Engineering
Micoteca da Universidade do Minho
Braga, Portugal

Jean-Yves Maillard
Cardiff School of Pharmacy and Pharmaceutical
Sciences
Cardiff University
Cardiff, Wales, UK

Andrew J. McBain
Senior Lecturer
School of Pharmacy and Pharmaceutical Sciences
The University of Manchester
Manchester, UK

Patrick J. McCormick
Research Fellow
Microbiology and Sterilization Sciences
Bausch and Lomb
Rochester
New York, USA

Gerald McDonnell
Vice President
Research and Technical Affairs
STERIS Ltd
Basingstoke, UK

Robert A. Monticello
International Antimicrobial Council
Washington, DC, USA

Susan E. Norton
Senior Director
Microbiology and Sterilization Sciences
Bausch and Lomb
Rochester
New York, USA

Jean-Marie Pagès
UMR-MD1
Transporteurs Membranaires
Chimiorésistance et Drug-Design
Facultés de Médecine et de Pharmacie
Marseille, France

Federica Pinto
Cardiff School of Pharmacy and Pharmaceutical
Sciences
Cardiff University
Cardiff, Wales, UK

Didier Pittet
Infection Control Program and WHO
Collaborating Centre on Patient Safety
University of Geneva Hospitals and Faculty of
Medicine
Geneva, Switzerland

Alexander H. Rickard
Assistant Professor
Department of Epidemiology
School of Public Health
University of Michigan
Ann Arbor, Michigan, USA

Cledir Santos
Scientist Researcher
IBB-Institute for Biotechnology and
Bioengineering
Centre of Biological Engineering
Micoteca da Universidade do Minho
Braga, Portugal

Syed A. Sattar
Professor Emeritus of Microbiology and Director
Centre for Research on Environmental
Microbiology (CREM)
Faculty of Medicine
University of Ottawa
Ottawa, Ontario, Canada

Peter Setlow
Professor
Department of Molecular,
Microbial and Structural Biology
University of Connecticut Health Center
Farmington, Connecticut, USA

Albert T. Sheldon
President
Antibiotic and Antiseptic Consultants Inc.
Cypress, Texas, USA

Marta Simões
IBB-Institute for Biotechnology and
Bioengineering
Centre of Biological Engineering
Micoteca da Universidade do Minho
Braga, Portugal

Susan Springthorpe
Centre for Research on Environmental
Microbiology
University of Ottawa
Ottawa, Ontario, Canada

Lawrence Staniforth
Campden BRI
Chipping Campden, UK

Najib Sufya
Assistant Professor
Microbiology and Immunology Department
Faculty of Pharmacy
University of Tripoli
Tripoli, Libya

Steven Theriault
Public Health Agency of Canada National
Microbiology Laboratory
Winnipeg, Canada

Vincent Thomas
Research Group Leader
STERIS SA
Research and Development
Fontenay-aux-Roses, France

Susannah E. Walsh
Senior Lecturer in Microbiology
School of Pharmacy
De Montfort University
Leicester, UK

Gareth J. Williams
Microbiologist
ECHA Microbiology Ltd
Willowbrook Technology Park
Cardiff, Wales, UK

Shannon C. Wright
Assessment Officer
Disinfectants Unit
Bureau of Gastroenterology
Infection and Viral Diseases
Therapeutic Products Directorate
Health Canada
Ottawa, Ontario, Canada

Preface to the Fifth Edition

It has been a particular privilege to be editors of this fifth edition, which has been substantially revised. Thirty-six of its 40 chapters are new and those from the previous edition have undergone major revisions/updates. Every attempt also has been made to cover the subject matter in all chapters from a global perspective.

Putting this edition together has been a daunting task in view of the rapidly expanding significance and scope of the subject matter covered while also considering the wide acceptance and utility of its previous editions. We thank the authors for their contributions and the publisher's staff for coordinating all dealings between the contributors and the editors.

We are most grateful to our respective families for allowing us to devote the long hours needed to edit this book.

Adam P. Fraise
Jean-Yves Maillard
Syed A. Sattar
November 2012

Preface to the First Edition

Sterilization, disinfection and preservation, all designed to eliminate, prevent or frustrate the growth of microorganisms in a wide variety of products, were incepted empirically from the time of man's emergence and remain a problem today. The fact that this is so is due to the incredible ability of the first inhabitants of the biosphere to survive and adapt to almost any challenge. This ability must in turn have been laid down in their genomes during their long and successful sojourn on this planet.

It is true to say that, of these three processes, sterilization is a surer process than disinfection, which in turn is a surer process than preservation. It is in the last field that we find the greatest interactive play between challenger and challenged. The microbial spoilage of wood, paper, textiles, paints, stonework, stored foodstuffs, to mention only a few categories at constant risk, costs the world many billions of pounds each year, and if it were not for considerable success in the preservative field, this figure would rapidly become astronomical. Disinfection processes do not suffer quite the same failure rate and one is left with the view that failure here is due more to uninformed use and naïve interpretation of biocidal data. Sterilization is an infinitely more secure process and, provided that the procedural protocol is followed, controlled and monitored, it remains the most successful of the three processes.

In the field of communicable bacterial diseases and some virus infections, there is no doubt that these have been considerably reduced, especially in the wealthier industrial societies, by improved hygiene, more extensive immunization and possibly by availability of antibiotics. However, hospital-acquired infection remains an important problem and is often associated with surgical operations or instrumentation of the patient. Although heat sterilization processes at high temperatures are preferred whenever possible, medical equipment is often difficult to clean adequately, and components are sometimes heat-labile. Disposable equipment is useful and is widely used if relatively cheap but is obviously not practicable for the more expensive items. Ethylene oxide is often used in industry for sterilizing heat-labile products but has a limited use for reprocessing medical equipment. Low-temperature steam, with or without formaldehyde, has been developed as a possible alternative to ethylene oxide in the hospital.

Although aseptic methods are still used for surgical techniques, skin disinfection is still necesssary and a wider range of non-toxic antiseptic agents suitable for application to tissues is required. Older antibacterial agents have been reintroduced, e.g. silver nitrate for burns, alcohol for hand disinfection in the general wards and less corrosive hypochlorites for disinfection of medical equipment.

Nevertheless, excessive use of disinfectants in the environment is undesirable and may change the hospital flora, selecting naturally antibiotic-resistant organisms, such as *Pseudomonas aeruginosa*, which are potentially dangerous to highly susceptible patients. Chemical disinfection of the hospital environment is therefore reduced to a minimum and is replaced where applicable by good cleaning methods or by physical methods of disinfection or sterilization.

A.D.R.
W.B.H.
G.A.J.A.

1   Historical Introduction

Adam P. Fraise

Microbiology Department, Queen Elizabeth Medical Centre, Pathology – University Hospitals Birmingham NHS Foundation Trust, Birmingham, UK

Early concepts

Disinfection and hygiene are concepts that have been applied by humans for thousands of years. Examples may be found in ancient literature such as the Bible where disinfection using heat was recorded in the Book of Numbers; the passing of metal objects, especially cooking vessels, through fire was declared to cleanse them. It was also noted from early times that water stored in pottery vessels soon acquired a foul odor and taste and Aristotle recommended to Alexander the Great the practice of boiling the water to be drunk by his armies. It may be inferred that there was awareness that something more than mechanical cleanness was required.

Chemical disinfection of a sort was practiced at the time of Persian imperial expansion, c. 450 BC, when water was stored in vessels of copper or silver to keep it potable. Wine, vinegar and honey were used on dressings and as cleansing agents for wounds and it is interesting to note that diluted acetic acid has been recommended comparatively recently for the topical treatment of wounds and surgical lesions infected by *Pseudomonas aeruginosa*.

The art of mummification, which so obsessed the Egyptian civilization (although it owed its success largely to desiccation in the dry atmosphere of the region), employed a variety of balsams containing natural preservatives. Natron, a crude native sodium carbonate, was also used to preserve the bodies of human and animal alike.

Practical procedures involving chemical agents were also applied in the field of food preservation. Thus tribes who had not progressed beyond the status of hunter-gatherers discovered that meat and fish could be preserved by drying, salting or mixing with natural spices. As the great civilizations of the Mediterranean and Near and Middle East receded, and European cultures arose, so the precepts of empirical hygiene were also developed. There was, of course, ongoing contact between Europe and the Middle and Near East through the Arab and Ottoman incursions into Europe, but it is difficult to find early European writers acknowledging the heritage of these empires.

An early account of procedures to try and combat the episodic scourge of the plague may be found in the writings of the 14th century, where Joseph of Burgundy recommended the burning of juniper branches in rooms where plague sufferers had lain. Sulfur, too, was burned in the hope of removing the cause of this disease. The association of malodor with disease and the belief that matter floating in the air might be responsible for diseases, a Greek concept, led to these procedures. If success was achieved it may have been due to the elimination of rats, later to be shown as the bearers of the causative organism.

In Renaissance Italy at the turn of the 15th century, a poet, philosopher and physician, Girolamo Fracastoro, who was

Russell, Hugo & Ayliffe's: Principles and Practice of Disinfection, Preservation and Sterilization, Fifth Edition. Edited by Adam P. Fraise, Jean-Yves Maillard, and Syed A. Sattar.

professor of logic at the University of Padua, recognized possible causes of disease, mentioning contagion and airborne infection; he thought there must exist "seeds of disease". Robert Boyle, the skeptical chemist, writing in the mid-17th century, wrote of a possible relationship between fermentation and the disease process. In this he foreshadowed the views of Louis Pasteur. There is, however, no evidence in the literature that Pasteur even read the opinions of Robert Boyle or Fracastoro.

The next landmark in this history was the discovery by Antonie van Leeuwenhoek of small living creatures in a variety of habitats, such as tooth scrapings, pond water and vegetable infusions. His drawings, seen under his simple microscopes (×300), were published in the *Philosophical Transaction of the Royal Society of London* before and after this date. Some of his illustrations are thought to represent bacteria, although the greatest magnification he is said to have achieved was ×300. When considering Leeuwenhoek's great technical achievement in microscopy and his painstaking application of it to original investigation, it should be borne in mind that bacteria in colony form must have been seen from the beginning of human existence. A very early report of this was given by the Greek historian Siculus, who, writing of the siege of Tire in 332 BC, states how bread, distributed to the Macedonians, had a bloody look. This was probably attributable to contamination by pigmented strains of *Serratia marcescens* and this phenomenon must have been seen, if not recorded, from time immemorial.

Turning back to Europe, it is also possible to find other examples of workers who believed, but could not prove scientifically, that some diseases were caused by invisible living agents, *contagium animatum*. Among these workers were Kircher (1658), Lange (1659), Lancisi (1718) and Marten (1720).

By observation and intuition, therefore, we see that the practice of heat and chemical disinfection, the inhibitory effect of desiccation and the implication of invisible objects with the cause of some diseases were known or inferred from early times.

Before moving on to a more formally scientific period in history it is necessary to report on a remarkable quantification of chemical preservation published in 1775 by Joseph Pringle. Pringle was seeking to evaluate preservation by salting and he added pieces of lean meat to glass jars containing solutions of different salts; these he incubated, and judged his end-point by the presence or absence of smell. He regarded his standard "salt" as sea salt and expressed the results in terms of the relative efficiency as compared with sea salt; niter, for example, had a value of 4 by this method. Rideal and Walker, 153 years later, were to use a similar method to measure the activity of phenolic disinfectants against *Salmonella typhi*; their standard was phenol.

Although the concept of bacterial diseases and spoilage was not widespread before the 19th century, procedures to preserve food and drink were used early in history. It is only more recently, that is in the 1960s, that the importance of microorganisms in pharmaceuticals was appreciated [1] and the principles of preservation of medicines introduced.

Chemical disinfection

As the science of chemistry developed, newer and purer chemical disinfectants began to be used. Mercuric chloride, which had been used since the Middle Ages and was probably first used by Arab physicians, began to be used as a wound dressing. In 1798 bleaching powder was first made and a preparation of it was employed by Alcock in 1827 as a deodorant and disinfectant. Lefèvre introduced chlorine water in 1843, and in 1839 Davies had suggested iodine as a wound dressing. Semmelweis used chlorine water in his work on childbed fever occurring in the obstetrics division of the Vienna General Hospital, where he achieved a sensational reduction in the incidence of the infection by insisting that all attending the birth washed their hands initially in chlorine water and later (in 1847) in chlorinated lime.

Wood and coal tar were used as wound dressings in the early 19th century and, in a letter to the *Lancet*, Smith described the use of creosote (Gr. *kreas* flesh, *soter* savior) as a wound dressing [2]. In 1850 Le Beuf, a French pharmacist, prepared an extract of coal tar by using the natural saponin of quillaia bark as a dispersing agent. Le Beuf asked a well-known surgeon, Jules Lemair, to evaluate his product. It proved to be highly efficacious. Küchenmeister was to use pure phenol in solution as a wound dressing in 1860 and Joseph Lister also used phenol in his great studies on antiseptic surgery during the 1860s. It is also of interest to record that a number of chemicals were being used as wood preservatives. Wood tar had been used in the 1700s to preserve the timbers of ships, and mercuric chloride was used for the same purpose in 1705. Copper sulfate was introduced in 1767 and zinc chloride in 1815. Many of these products are still in use today.

Turning back to evaluation, Bucholtz in 1875 determined what is known today as the minimum inhibitory concentration of phenol, creosote and benzoic and salicylic acids against bacteria. Robert Koch made measurements of the inhibitory power of mercuric chloride against anthrax spores but overvalued the products as he failed to neutralize the substance carried over in his tests. This was pointed out by Geppert, who, in 1889, used ammonium sulfide as a neutralizing agent for mercuric chloride and obtained much more realistic values for the antimicrobial powers of mercuric chloride.

It will be apparent that, in parallel with these early studies, an important watershed had been passed; that is, the scientific identification of a microbial species with a specific disease. Credit for this should go to an Italian, Agostino Bassi, a lawyer from Lodi (a small town near Milan). Although not a scientist or physician, he performed exacting scientific experiments to equate a disease of silkworms with a fungus. Bassi identified plague and cholera as being of microbial origin and also experimented with heat and chemicals as antimicrobial agents. His work anticipated the great names of Pasteur and Koch in the implication of microbes with certain diseases, but because it was published locally in Lodi and in Italian it has not found the place it deserves in many textbooks.

Two other chemical disinfectants still in use today were early introductions. Hydrogen peroxide was first examined by Traugott in 1893, and Dakin reported on chlorine-releasing compounds in 1915. Quaternary ammonium compounds were introduced by Jacobs in 1916.

In 1897, Kronig and Paul, with the acknowledged help of the Japanese physical chemist Ikeda, introduced the science of disinfection dynamics; their pioneering publication [3] was to give rise to innumerable studies on the subject lasting through to the present day.

Since then other chemical microbicides, which are now widely used in hospital practice, have been introduced – such as chlorhexidine, an important cationic microbicide, whose activity was described in 1958 [4].

More recently, a better understanding of hygiene concepts has provided the basis for an explosion in the number of products containing chemicals. In particular, quaternary ammonium compounds are being developed with altered chemistry and improved activity. Peroxygen compounds are gaining popularity due to their good *in vitro* activity (including activity against spores), and mechanisms for preparing compounds that release hypochlorous acid are also being adopted widely in the healthcare, veterinary and food industries. This rise in microbicide-containing products has also sparked a major concern about the improper use of chemical disinfectants and a possible emergence of microbial resistance to these microbicides and possible cross-resistance to antibiotics. Among the most widely studied microbicides are chlorhexidine and triclosan. The bisphenol triclosan is unique, in the sense that it has been shown that at a low concentration it inhibits selectively an enoyl reductase carrier protein, which is also a target site for antibiotic chemotherapy in some microorganisms.

Sterilization

Heat has been known as a cleansing and purifying agent for centuries. In 1832, William Henry, a Manchester physician, studied the effect of heat on contaminated material, that is clothes worn by sufferers from typhus and scarlet fever. He placed the material in a pressure vessel and realized that he could achieve temperatures higher than 100°C by using a sealed vessel fitted with a safety valve. He found that garments so treated could be worn with impunity by others, who did not then contract the diseases. Louis Pasteur also used a pressure vessel with a safety valve for sterilization.

Sterilization by filtration has been observed from early times. Foul-tasting waters draining from ponds and percolating through soil or gravel were sometimes observed, on emerging at a lower part of the terrain, to be clear and potable (drinkable), and artificial filters of pebbles were constructed. Later, deliberately constructed tubes of unglazed porcelain or compressed kieselguhr, the so-called Chamberland or Berkefeld filters, made their appearance (in 1884 and 1891, respectively).

Although it was known that sunlight helped wound healing and in checking the spread of disease, it was Downes and Blunt in 1887 who first set up experiments to study the effect of light on bacteria and other organisms. Using *Bacillus subtilis* as the test organism, Ward, in 1892, attempted to investigate the connection between the wavelength of light and its antimicrobial activity; he found that blue light was more active than red.

In 1903, using a continuous arc current, Barnard and Morgan demonstrated that the maximum bactericidal effect resided in the range 226–328 nm, that is, light in the ultraviolet range. Ultraviolet light is now a well-established agent for water and air decontamination.

At the end of the 19th century, a wealth of pioneering work was being carried out in subatomic physics. In 1895, the German physicist Röntgen discovered X-rays, and 3 years later Rieder found these rays to be harmful to common pathogens. X-rays of a wavelength between 10^{-10} and 10^{-11} are emitted by ^{60}Co and are now used extensively in sterilization processes.

Another major field of research in the concluding years of the 19th century was that of natural radioactivity. In 1879, Becquerel found that, if left near a photographic plate, uranium compounds would cause the plate to fog. He suggested that rays, later named Becquerel rays, were being emitted. Rutherford, in 1899, showed that when the emission was exposed to a magnetic field three types of radiation (α, β and γ) were given off. The γ-rays were shown to have wavelengths of the same order as X-rays. Beta-rays were found to be electrons, and α-rays were helium nuclei. These emissions were demonstrated to be antimicrobial by Mink in 1896, and by Pancinotti and Porchelli 2 years later. High-speed electrons generated by electron accelerators are now used in sterilization processes.

Thus, within 3 years of the discovery of X-rays and natural radiation, their effect on the growth and viability of microorganisms had been investigated and published. Both were found to be lethal. Ultraviolet light was shown in 1993 to be the lethal component of sunlight.

For more information on this aspect of sterilization see Hugo [5].

Sterilization can also be achieved by chemicals, although their use for this purpose does not offer the same quality assurance as heat or radiation sterilization. The term "chemosterilizer" was first defined by Borick in 1968. This has now been replaced by the term "chemical sterilants", which is used to refer to those chemicals used in hospital for sterilizing reusable medical devices. Among the earliest used chemical sterilants were formaldehyde and ethylene oxide. Another aldehyde, glutaraldehyde, has been used for this purpose for almost 40 years [6]. Compounds such as peracetic acid, chlorine dioxide and *ortho*-phthalaldehyde (OPA) have been introduced as substitutes for the dialdehyde and these compounds have been widely adopted for the decontamination of flexible fiberoptic endoscopes.

In the latter half of the 20th century the science of sterilization and disinfection followed a more ordered pattern of evolution, culminating in new technologies such as radiation sterilization and gas plasma sterilization. However, no method is foolproof and human error will always occur. Therefore, whatever technologies are used, all staff working in the field of sterilization must be vigilant and maintain a critical approach where evaluation of methodologies is an integral part of the process.

Future developments for microbicides

This is a very interesting time for those involved in the use of microbicides. For the last 50 years, our knowledge of microbicides has increased, but so have our concerns about their extensive use in hospital and domiciliary environments. One encouraging sign is the apparent willingness of the industry to understand the mechanisms of action of chemical microbicides and the mechanisms of microbial resistance to microbicides. Although "new" microbicidal molecules might not be produced in the future, novel products might concentrate on synergistic effects between microbicides and the combination of microbicide and permeabilizer or other non-microbicidal chemicals, so that an increase in antimicrobial activity is achieved. The ways microbicides are delivered is also the subject of extensive investigations. For example, the use of polymers for the slow release of microbicidal molecules, the use of light-activated microbicides and the use of alcoholic rubs for antisepsis are all signs of current concerted efforts to adapt laboratory concepts to practical situations.

Although, this might be a "golden age" for microbicidal science, many questions remain unanswered, such as the significance of microbicide resistance, the fine mechanism of action of microbicides, the possibility of primary action sites within target microorganisms, and the effect of microbicides on emerging pathogens and microbial biofilms. Some of these concepts will be discussed further in following chapters.

References

1 Kallings, L.O. *et al.* (1966) Microbial contamination of medical preparations. *Acta Pharmaceutica Suecica*, **3**, 219–228.
2 Smith, F. Sir (1836–1837) External employment of creosote. *Lancet*, **ii**, 221–222.
3 Kronig, B. and Paul, T. (1897) Die chemischen Gundlagen der Lehr von der Giftwirkung und Desinfection. *Zeitschrift fur Hygiene und Infection*skrankheiten, **25**, 1–112.
4 Denton, W. (2001) Chlorhexidine, in *Sterilisation and Preservation*, 5th edn (ed. S.S. Block), Lippincott Williams & Wilkins, Philadelphia, pp. 321–336.
5 Hugo, W.B. (1996) A brief history of heat, chemical and radiation preservation and disinfection. *International Biodeterioration and Biodegradation*, **36**, 197–221.
6 Bruch, C.W. (1991) Role of glutaraldehyde and other chemical sterilants in the processing of new medical devices, in *Sterilization of Medical Products*, vol. 5 (eds R.F. Morrissey and Y.I. Prokopenko), Polyscience Publications, Morin Heights, Canada, pp. 377–396.

Further reading

Brock, T.D. (ed.) (1961) *Milestones in Microbiology*, Prentice Hall, London.
Bullock, W. (1938) *The History of Bacteriology*, Oxford University Press, Oxford.
Collard, P. (1976) *The Development of Microbiology*, Cambridge University Press, Cambridge.
Hugo, W.B. (1991) A brief history of heat and chemical preservation and disinfection. *Journal of Applied Bacteriology*, **71**, 9–18.
Reid, R. (1974) *Microbes and Men*, British Broadcasting Corporation, London.

2 Types of Microbicidal and Microbistatic Agents

Ibrahim Al-Adham[1], Randa Haddadin[2] and Phillip Collier[3]

[1] Faculty of Pharmacy & Medical Sciences, University of Petra, Amman, Jordan
[2] Faculty of Pharmacy, University of Jordan, Amman, Jordan
[3] School of Contemporary Sciences, University of Abertay, Dundee, UK

Introduction

This chapter serves as a source of reference for those interested in developing an initial or general understanding of the chemistry and mode of action of a particular group of microbicidal agents. It is not intended to provide a definitive description of individual agents, but rather to introduce the reader to the general concepts of those agents and to provide key references as a starting point for more thorough investigations. With this in mind, the authors have undertaken a "hard edit" of the previous version of this chapter, including the removal of dated information and updates to the chemical groups discussed. Given this approach, the authors wish to acknowledge those who have nurtured and developed this chapter in previous editions of the book: Barry Hugo and Denver Russell (first, second and third editions) and Suzanne Moore and David Payne (fourth edition).

Phenols

Hugo [1, 2] and Marouchoc [3] showed that phenols and natural product distillates containing phenols shared, with chlorine and iodine, an early place in the armory of antiseptics. Today, they are widely used as general disinfectants and as preservatives for a variety of manufactured products [4], except where there is risk of contamination of foods. As a result of their long history, a vast literature has accumulated dealing with phenol and its analogs and a comprehensive review of these compounds can be found in Goddard and McCue [5]. While many different parameters have been used to express their microbicidal and microbistatic power, the phenol coefficient is perhaps the most widely employed.

A reasonable assessment of the relationship between structure and activity in the phenol series was compiled by Suter [6]. The main conclusions from this survey were:

Russell, Hugo & Ayliffe's: Principles and Practice of Disinfection, Preservation and Sterilization, Fifth Edition. Edited by Adam P. Fraise, Jean-Yves Maillard, and Syed A. Sattar.
© 2013 Blackwell Publishing Ltd. Published 2013 by Blackwell Publishing Ltd.

1. *Para*-substitutions of an alkyl chain up to six carbon atoms in length increases the bactericidal action of phenols, presumably by increasing the surface activity and ability to orientate at an interface. Activity falls off after this due to decreased water solubility. Straight chain *para*-substituents confer greater activity than branched-chain substituents containing the same number of carbon atoms.

2. Halogenation increases the bactericidal activity of phenols. The combination of alkyl and halogen substitution, which confers the greatest bactericidal activity, is that where the alkyl group is *ortho*- to the phenolic group and the halogen *para*- to the phenolic group.

3. Nitration, while increasing the toxicity of phenols towards bacteria, also increases the systemic toxicity and confers specific biological properties on the molecule, enabling it to interfere with oxidative phosphorylation. This has now been shown to be due to the ability of nitrophenols to act as uncoupling agents. Studies [7] have shown that the nitro group is not a prerequisite for uncoupling, as ethylphenol is an uncoupler. Nitrophenols have now been largely superseded as plant protection chemicals, whereas at one time they were in vogue, although 4-nitrophenol is still used as a preservative in the leather industry.

4. In the bisphenol series, activity is found with a direct bond between the two C_6H_5 groups or if they are separated by $-CH_2-$, $-S-$ or $-O-$. If a $-CO-$, $-SO-$ or $-CH(OH)-$ group separates the phenyl groups, activity is low. In addition, maximum activity is found with the hydroxyl group at the 2,2′- position of the bisphenol. Halogenation of the bisphenols confers additional microbicidal activity.

Chemistry of phenols

The phenol parent compound C_6H_5OH (Figure 2.1) is a white crystalline solid (melting point (m.p.) 39–40°C), which becomes pink and finally black on long standing. It is soluble in water 1 : 13 and is a weak acid, pK_a 10. Its biological activity resides in the undissociated molecule. Phenol is effective against both Gram-positive and Gram-negative vegetative bacteria, but is only slowly effective against bacterial spores and acid-fast bacteria.

Phenols are the reference standard for the Rideal–Walker (RW) and Chick–Martin tests for disinfectant evaluations. They find limited application in medicine today, but are used as preservatives in such products as animal glues. Although first obtained from coal tar, they are now obtained largely by synthetic processes, which include the hydrolysis of chlorobenzene of the high-temperature interaction of benzene sulfonic acid and alkali.

Mode of action

At low concentrations, phenols interact with bacterial enzymes needed for cell wall synthesis, resulting in cell lysis. High concentrations of phenols cause general coagulation of the cytoplasm and act as general protoplasmic poisons. In addition, phenols can affect the cytoplasmic membrane [8, 9] resulting in leakage of potassium ions first, then the cytosol. Hexachlorophene was found to have additional activity as an inhibitor of the electron transport chain, thus inhibiting the metabolic activities in bacteria [10].

Sources of phenols: the coal-tar industry

Most of the phenols used to make disinfectants are a by-product of the destructive distillation of coal. Coal is heated in the absence of air and the volatile products, one of which is tar, are condensed. The tar is fractionated to yield a group of products that include phenols (called tar acids), organic bases and neutral products, such as alkyl naphthalenes, which are known in the industry as neutral oils.

The cresols consist of a mixture of 2-, 3- and 4-cresol. The "xylenols" consist of the six isomeric dimethylphenols plus ethylphenols. The combined fraction, cresols and xylenols, is also available as a commercial product known as cresylic acid. High-boiling tar acids consist of higher alkyl homologs of phenols: for example the diethylphenols, tetramethylphenols and methylethylphenols, together with methylindanols, naphthols and methylresorcinols, the latter being known as dihydrics. There may be traces of 2-phenylphenol. The chemical constituents of some of the phenolic components are shown in Figure 2.1.

Properties of phenolic fractions

The passage from phenol (boiling point (b.p.) 182°C) to the higher-boiling phenols (b.p. up to 310°C) is accompanied by a well-defined gradation in properties, as follows: water solubility decreases, tissue trauma decreases, bactericidal activity increases, inactivation by organic matter increases. However, the ratio of activity against Gram-negative to activity against Gram-positive organisms remains fairly constant, although in the case of pseudomonads, activity tends to decrease with decreasing water solubility (Table 2.1).

Formulation of coal-tar disinfectants

It is seen from the above data that the progressive increase in desirable biological properties of the coal-tar phenols with increasing boiling point is accompanied by a decrease in water solubility. This presents formulation problems and part of the story

Table 2.1 Phenol coefficients of coal-tar products against *Salmonella typhi* and *Staphylococcus aureus*.

Product and m.p. range	Phenol coefficient		Water solubility (g/100 ml)
	S. typhi	*S. aureus*	
Phenol (182°C)	1	1	6.6
Cresols (190–203°C)	2.5	2.0	2.0
4-Ethylphenol (195°C)	6	6	Slightly
Xylenols (210–230°C)	5	4.5	Slightly
High-boiling tar acids (230–270°C)	40	25	Insoluble
High-boiling tar acids (250–275°C)	60	40	Insoluble

m.p., melting point.

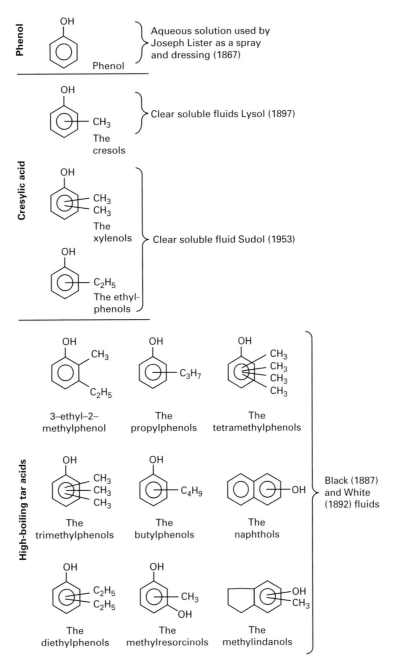

Figure 2.1 Phenol, cresols, xylenols, ethylphenols and high-boiling tar acids.

of the evolution of the present-day products is found in the evolution of formulation devices.

Modern range of solubilized and emulsified phenolic disinfectants

Black fluids are essential coal-tar fractions solubilized with soaps; white fluids are prepared by emulsifying tar fractions. Their composition as regards phenol content is shown in Figure 2.1. The term "clear soluble fluid" is also used to describe the solubilized products Lysol and Sudol.

Cresol and soap solution British Pharmacopoeia (BP) 1963 (Lysol)

This consists of cresol (a mixture of 2-, 3- and 4-cresols) solubilized with a soap prepared from linseed oil and potassium hydroxide. It forms a clear solution on dilution and is a broad-spectrum disinfectant showing activity against vegetative bacteria, mycobacteria, fungi and viruses [11]. Most vegetative pathogens, including mycobacteria, are killed in 15 min by dilutions of Lysol ranging from 0.3% to 0.6%. Bacterial spores are much more resistant, and there are reports of the spores of

Bacillus subtilis surviving in 2% Lysol for nearly 3 days. Even greater resistance has been encountered among clostridial spores. Lysol still retains the corrosive nature associated with the phenols and should be used with care. Both the method of manufacture and the nature of the soap used have been found to affect the microbicidal properties of the product [12]. RW coefficients (British Standard (BS) 541: 1985) are of the order of 2.

Black fluids

These consist of a solubilized crude phenol fraction prepared from tar acids, with a boiling range of 250–310°C (Figure 2.1). The solubilizing agents used to prepare the black fluids of commerce include soaps prepared from the interaction of sodium hydroxide with resins (which contain resin acids) and with the sulfate and sulfonate mixture prepared by heating castor oil with sulfuric acid (called sulfonated castor oil or Turkey red oil).

Additional stability is conferred by the presence of coal-tar hydrocarbon-neutral oils. The actual mechanism whereby they stabilize the black fluids has not been adequately elucidated; however, they do prevent crystallization of naphthalene present in the tar acid fraction. Mixtures of cresol and soap solution (Lysol type) of the *United States Pharmacopeia* have varying concentrations of neutral oil. Using a phenol coefficient-type test and *Salmonella typhi* as the test organism, a product containing 30% cresols and 20% neutral oil was found to be twice as active as a similar product containing 50% cresols alone. However, the replacement of cresol by neutral oil caused a progressive decrease in phenol coefficient when a hemolytic *Streptococcus* and *Mycobacterium tuberculosis* were used as test organisms. The results were further checked using a pure 2-methylnaphthalene in place of neutral oil and similar findings were obtained.

Black fluids give either clear solutions or emulsions on dilution with water, those containing greater proportions of higher phenol homologs giving emulsions. They are partially inactivated by the presence of electrolytes.

White fluids

These differ from the foregoing formulations in being emulsified, as distinct from solubilized, phenolic compounds. The emulsifying agents used include animal glue, casein and the carbohydrate extractable from seaweed called Irish moss. Products with a range of RW coefficients may be manufactured by the use of varying tar acid constituents.

As white fluids are already in the form of an oil-in-water emulsion, they are less liable to have their activity reduced on further dilution, as might happen with black fluids if dilution is carried out carelessly. They are much more stable in the presence of electrolytes. As might be expected from a metastable system, the emulsion, they are less stable on storage than black fluids, which are solubilized systems. As with the black fluids, products of varying RW coefficients may be obtained by varying the composition of the phenol. Neutral oils from coal tar may be included in the formulation.

Non-coal-tar phenols

The coal-tar (and to a lesser extent the petrochemical) industry yields a large array of phenolic products. However, phenol itself is now made in large quantities by a synthetic process, as are some of its derivatives. Three such phenols, which are used in a variety of roles, are 4-tertiary octylphenol, 2-phenylphenol and 4-hexylresorcinol (Figure 2.2).

4-Tertiary octylphenol

This phenol (often referred to as octylphenol) is a white crystalline substance, with a melting point of 83°C. The cardinal property in considering its application as a preservative is its insolubility in water, 1 in 60,000 (1.6×10^{-3}%). The sodium and potassium derivatives are more soluble. It is soluble in 1 in 1 of 95% ethanol and proportionally less soluble in ethanol containing varying proportions of water. It has been shown by animal feeding experiments to be less toxic than phenol or cresol.

Alcoholic solutions of the phenol are 400–500 times as effective as phenol against Gram-positive organisms, but against Gram-negative bacteria the factor is only one-fiftieth. Octylphenol is also fungistatic, and has been used as a preservative for proteinaceous products such as glues and non-food gelatins. Its activity is reduced in the presence of some emulgents, a property that might render it unsuitable for the preservation of soaps and cutting oils.

2-Phenylphenol (o-phenylphenol; 2-phenylphenoxide)

This occurs as a white crystalline powder, melting at 57°C. It is much more soluble than octylphenol, 1 part dissolving in 1000 parts of water, while the sodium salt is readily soluble in water. It is active against both bacteria and fungi and is used as a preservative, especially against fungi, in a wide variety of applications. Typical minimal inhibitory concentrations (MICs, µg/ml) for the sodium salt are: *Escherichia coli*, 32; *Staphylococcus aureus*, 32; *B. subtilis*, 16; *Pseudomonas fluorescens*, 16; *Aspergillus niger (brasiliensis)*, 4; *Epidermophyton* spp., 4; *Myrothecium verrucaria*, 2; and *Trichophyton interdigitale*, 8. Many strains of *Pseudomonas aeruginosa* are more resistant, requiring higher concentrations than those listed above for their inhibition.

Its main applications have been as ingredients in disinfectants of the pine type, as preservatives for cutting oils and as a general agricultural disinfectant. It has been particularly useful as a slimicide and fungicide in the paper and cardboard industry, and as an additive to paraffin wax in the preparation of waxed paper and liners for bottle and jar caps. In combination with *para*-tertiary amylphenol, phenylphenol is effective against *M. tuberculosis* and HIV [13].

Studies on *S. aureus* have revealed that *o*-phenylphenol inhibits anabolism of many amino acids and highly downregulates the genes that encode the enzymes involved in the diaminopimelate (DAP) pathway. Lysine and DAP are essential for building up the peptidoglycan in cell walls. It was suggested that the mode of action of *o*-phenylphenol is similar to the mechanism of action of some antibiotics [14].

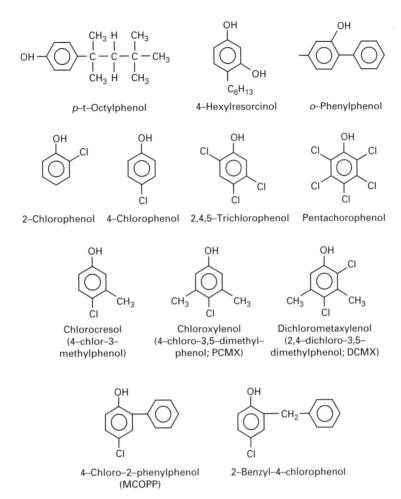

Figure 2.2 Examples of phenolic compounds.

4-Hexylresorcinol

This occurs as white crystalline needles (m.p. 67°C). It is soluble 0.5% in water, but freely soluble in organic solvents, glycerol and glycerides (fixed oils). It is of low oral toxicity, having been used for the treatment of roundworm and whipworm infections in humans. It is used as a 0.1% solution in 30% glycerol as a skin antiseptic and in lozenges and medicated sweets for the treatment of throat infections, where it has local anesthetic effect [15].

Halo and nitrophenols

The general effect of halogenation (see Figure 2.2) upon the microbicidal activity of phenols is to increase their activity – with the *para-* position being more effective than the *ortho-* position – but reduce their water solubility. There is also a tendency for them to be inactivated by organic matter.

In order to illustrate the effect of chlorination on the microbicidal activity of phenols, RW coefficients are as follows: 2-chlorophenol, 3.6; 4-chlorophenol, 4; 3-chlorophenol, 7.4; 2,4-dichlorophenol, 13; 2,4,6-trichlorophenol, 22; 4-chloro-3-methylphenol, 13; 4-chloro-3,5-dimethylphenol, 30.

Chlorophenols are made by the direct chlorination of the corresponding phenol or phenol mixture, using either chlorine or sulfuryl chloride.

2,4,6-Trichlorophenol

This is a white or off-white powder, which melts at 69.5°C and boils at 246°C. It is a stronger acid than phenol with a pK_a of 8.5 at 25°C. It is almost insoluble in water, but is soluble in alkali and organic solvents. This phenol has been used as a bactericidal, fungicidal and insecticidal agent. It has found application in textile and wood preservation, as a preservative for cutting oils and as an ingredient in some antiseptic formulations. Its phenol coefficient against *S. typhi* is 22 and against *S. aureus* 25.

Pentachlorophenol (2-phenylphenoxide, PCP)

A white to cream-colored powder (m.p. 174°C), it can crystallize with a proportion of water, and is almost insoluble in water, but is soluble in organic solvents. PCP and its sodium or potassium derivatives have micromicrobicidal, fungicidal and algicidal effects. Pentachlorophenol or its sodium derivative is used as a preservative for adhesives, textiles, wood, leather, paper and card-board. It has been used for the in-can preservation of paints, but it tends to discolor in sunlight. However, over the counter sales of PCP has been banned in the USA due to potential contamination to drinking water [16]. As with other phenols, the presence of iron in the products, which it is meant to preserve, can also cause discoloration.

4-Chloro-3-methylphenol (chlorocresol)

Chlorocresol is a colorless crystalline compound, which melts at 65°C and is volatile in steam. It is soluble in water at 3.8 g/l and readily soluble in ethanol, ether and terpenes. It is also soluble in alkaline solutions. Its pK_a at 25°C is 9.5. Chlorocresol is used as a preservative in pharmaceutical products and as an adjunct in a former UK pharmacopoeial sterilization process called "heating with a bactericide", in which a combination of heat (98–100°C) and a chemical microbicide enabled a sterilization process to be conducted at a lower temperature than the more usual 121°C (see Chapter 3). Its RW coefficient in aqueous solution is 13 and nearly double this value when solubilized with castor oil soap. It has been used as a preservative for industrial products, such as glues, paints, sizes, cutting oils and drilling muds and for pharmaceutical products such as topical preparations, injections and cosmetics.

4-Chloro-3,5-dimethylphenol (chloroxylenol, para-chloro-meta-xylenol, PCMX)

PCMX is a white crystalline substance. It has microbicidal activity against bacteria, fungi and algae [17]. It is used chiefly as a topical antiseptic and a disinfectant. In order to improve solubility, PCMX is often solubilized in a suitable soap solution and often in conjunction with terpineol or pine oil. The *British Pharmacopoeia* [18] contains a model antiseptic formulation for a chloroxylenol solution containing soap, terpineol and ethanol.

Phenol coefficients for the pure compound are: *S. typhi*, 30; *S. aureus*, 26; *Streptococcus pyogenes*, 28; *Trichophyton rosaceum*, 25; *P. aeruginosa*, 11. It is not sporicidal and has little activity against the tubercle bacillus. It is also inactivated in the presence of organic matter. Its properties have been re-evaluated [19].

2,4-Dichloro-3,5-dimethylphenol (dichloroxylenol, dichloro-meta-xylenol, DCMX)

This is a white powder with a melting point of 94°C. Although it is slightly less soluble than PCMX, it has similar properties and microbicidal spectrum. It is used as an ingredient in pine-type disinfectants and in medicated soaps and hand scrubs.

4-Chloro-3-methylphenol (para-chloro-meta-cresol, PCMC)

PCMC is more water soluble than other phenols with a solubility of 4 g/l at 20°C. It retains a reasonably broad spectrum of activity of microbicidal activity over a wide pH range due to its solubility. This makes it suitable as an industrial preservative for products such as thickeners, adhesives and pigments [5].

Monochloro-2-phenylphenol

This is obtained by the chlorination of 2-phenylphenol and the commercial product contains 80% of 4-chloro-2-phenylphenol and 20% of 6-chloro-2-phenylphenol. The mixture is a pale straw-colored liquid, which boils over the range 250–300°C. It is almost insoluble in water, but may be used in the formulation of pine disinfectants, where solubilization is effected by means of a suitable soap.

2-Benzyl-4-chlorophenol (chlorphen; ortho-benzyl-para-chlorophenol, OBPCP)

This occurs as a white to pink powder, which melts at 49°C. It has a slight phenolic odor and is almost insoluble in water (0.007 g/l at 20°C), but like PCMX is more soluble in alkaline solution and organic solvents. Suitably formulated by solubilization with vegetable-oil soaps or selected anionic detergents, it has a wide microbicidal spectrum, being active against Gram-positive and Gram-negative bacteria, *Mycobacterium tuberculosis*, viruses, protozoa and fungi. It is used as a sanitizer and disinfectant for cooling towers, poultry houses, food-processing plants and surfaces surrounding swimming pools [20]. However, OBPCP is more commonly used in combination with other phenolics in disinfectant formulations [5].

Mixed chlorinated xylenols

A mixed chlorinated xylenol preparation can be obtained for the manufacture of household disinfectants by chlorinating a mixed xylenol fraction from coal tar.

Formulated disinfectants containing chlorophenols

A formulation device, such as solubilization, can be used to prepare liquid antiseptics and disinfectants. This is based on the good activity and low level of systemic toxicity, and of the likelihood of tissue damage shown by chlorinated cresols and xylenols.

In 1933, Rapps [21] compared the RW coefficients of an aqueous solution and a castor oil soap-solubilized system of chlorocresol and chloroxylenol and found the solubilized system to be superior by a factor of almost 2. This particular disinfectant recipe received a major advance (also in 1933) when two gynecologists, seeking a safe and effective product for midwifery and having felt that Lysol, one of the few disinfectants available to medicine at the time, was too caustic, made an extensive evaluation of the chloroxylenol–castor oil product. Their recipe also contained terpineol [22]. It was fortunate that this preparation was active against β-hemolytic streptococci, which are a hazard in childbirth, giving rise to puerperal fever. A chloroxylenol–terpineol soap preparation is the subject of a monograph in the *British Pharmacopoeia* [18].

The bacteriology of this formulation has turned out to be controversial. The original appraisal indicated good activity against β-hemolytic streptococci and *E. coli*, with retained activity in the presence of pus, but subsequent bacteriological examinations by experienced workers gave divergent results. Thus, Colebrook in

1941 cast doubt upon the ability of solubilized chloroxylenolterpineol to destroy staphylococci on the skin, a finding which was refuted by Beath [23]. Ayliffe *et al.* [24] indicated that the product was more active against *P. aeruginosa* than *S. aureus*. As so often happens, however, *P. aeruginosa* was subsequently shown to be resistant and Lowbury [25] found that this organism would actually multiply in dilutions of chloroxylenol soap.

Although still an opportunistic organism, *P. aeruginosa* has become a dangerous pathogen, especially as more and more patients receive radiotherapy or radiomimetic drugs. Attempts have been made to potentiate chlorophenol disinfection and to widen its spectrum so as to embrace the pseudomonads. It is well known that ethylenediamine tetraacetic acid (EDTA) affected the permeability of pseudomonads and some enterobacteria to drugs to which they were normally resistant [26] and both Dankert and Schut [27] and Russell and Furr [28] were able to demonstrate that chloroxylenol solutions with EDTA were most active against pseudomonads. Hatch and Cooper [29] exhibited a similar potentiating effect with sodium hexametaphosphate. However, it is worth noting that the German industry trade association have undertaken to eliminate EDTA in products released to the aquatic environment, which would include disinfectants.

Pine disinfectants

As long ago as 1876, Kingzett took out a patent in Germany for a disinfectant deodorant made from oil of turpentine and camphor that had been allowed to undergo oxidation in the atmosphere. This was marketed under the trade name Sanitas. Later, Stevenson [30] described a fluid made from pine oil solubilized by a soap solution.

The chief constituent of turpentine is the cyclic hydrocarbon pinene (Figure 2.3), which has little or no microbicidal activity. The terpene alcohol terpineol (Figure 2.3) is another ingredient of pine disinfectants and had already been exploited as an ingredient of the Colebrook and Maxted [22] chloroxylenol formulation. Unlike pinene, it possesses microbicidal activity in its own right, and it shares with pinene the property of modifying the action of phenols in solubilized disinfectant formulations, although not in the same way for all microbial species.

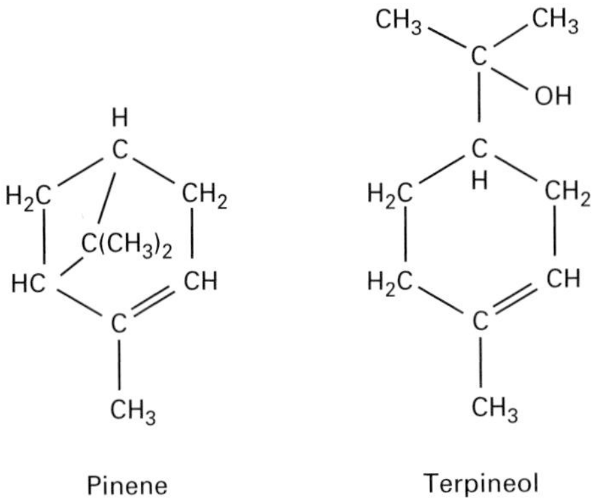

Terpineol is a colorless oil, which tends to darken on storing. It has a pleasant hyacinth odor and is used in perfumery, especially for soap products, as well as in disinfectant manufacture. Many solubilized products has been marketed, with "active" ingredients ranging from pine oil, pinene through terpineol to a mixture of pine oil and/or terpineol and a suitable phenol or chlorinated phenol. This gave rise to a range of products, extending from those which are really no more than deodorants to effective disinfectants.

Bisphenols

Hydroxy halogenated derivatives (Figure 2.4) of diphenyl methane, diphenyl ether and diphenyl sulfide have provided a number of useful microbicides active against bacteria, fungi and algae. In common with other phenolics they all seem to have low activity against *P. aeruginosa*; they also have low water solubility and share the property of the monophenols in that they are inactivated by non-ionic surfactants.

Ehrlich and co-workers were the first to investigate the microbicidal activity of the bisphenols and published their work in 1906. Klarmann and Dunning and colleagues described the preparation and properties of a number of these compounds [31, 32]. A useful summary of this early work has been made by Suter [6]. Later, Gump and Walter [33–35] and Walter and Gump [36]

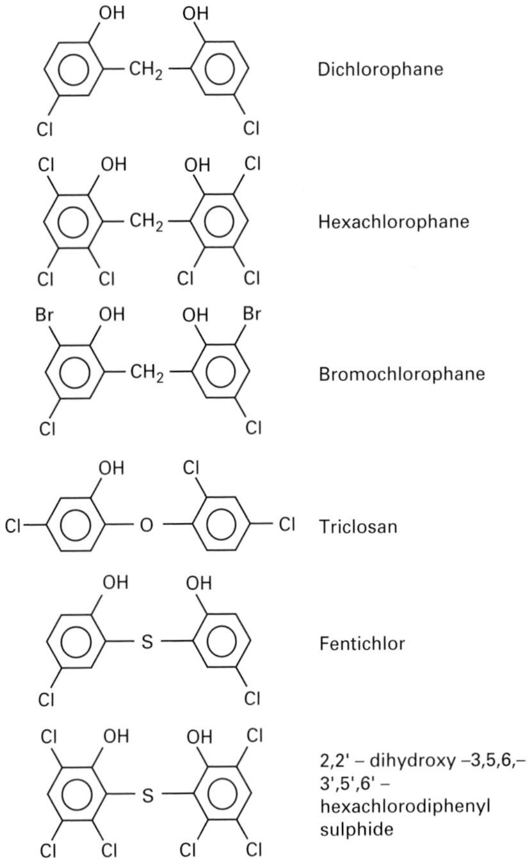

Figure 2.3 Pinene and terpineol.

Figure 2.4 Bisphenols.

made an exhaustive study of the microbicidal properties of many of these compounds, especially with a view to their use in cosmetic formulations.

Derivatives of dihydroxydiphenylmethane

Dichlorophen, G-4,5,5′-dichloro-2,2′-dihydroxydiphenylmethane (Panacide, Rotafix, Swansea, UK) is active to varying degrees against bacteria, fungi, helminths and algae. It is soluble in water at 30 μg/ml but more soluble (45–80 g/100 ml) in organic solvents. The pK_a values at 25°C for the two hydroxyl groups are 7.6 and 11.6, and it forms a very alkaline solution when diluted. It is typically used as an algicide, fungicide and at a dilution of 1 in 20 as a surface microbicide. It has found application as a preservative for toiletries, textiles and cutting oils and to prevent the growth of bacteria in water-cooling systems and humidifying plants. It is used as a slimicide in paper manufacture. It is used as antihelminthic in poultry, cats and dogs [37, 38]. It may be added to papers and other packing materials to prevent microbial growth and has been used to prevent algal growth in greenhouses.

Hexachlorophene, 2,2′-dihydroxy-3,5,6,3′,5′,6′-hexachlorodiphenylmethane, G11 is almost insoluble in water but soluble in ethanol, ether and acetone and in alkaline solutions. The pK_a values are 5.4 and 10.9. Its mode of action has been studied in detail by Gerhardt, Corner and colleagues [39–43]. It is used mainly for its bactericidal activity but it is much more active against Gram-positive than Gram-negative organisms. Typical MICs (bacteriostatic) in μg/ml are: *S. aureus*, 0.9; *B. subtilis*, 0.2; *Proteus vulgaris*, 4; *E. coli*, 28; and *P. aeruginosa*, 25. It has found chief application as an active ingredient in surgical scrubs and medicated soaps and has also been used to a limited extent as a preservative for cosmetics. Its use is limited by its insolubility in water, its somewhat narrow bactericidal spectrum, and by the fact that in the UK it is restricted by a control order made in 1973. In general, this order restricted the use of this product to 0.1% in human medicines and 0.75% in animal medicines. Its toxicity has restricted its use in cosmetic products, and the maximum concentration allowed is 0.1%, with the stipulation that it is not to be used in products for children or personal hygiene products.

Bromochlorophane, 3,3′-dibromo-5,5′-dichlor-2,2′-dihydroxydiphenylmethane is soluble in water at 100 μg/ml and is markedly more active against Gram-positive organisms than bacteria. Strains of *S. aureus* are inhibited at concentrations from 8 to 11 μg/ml, whereas 100 times these concentrations are required for *E. coli* and *P. aeruginosa*. It has been used as the active ingredient in deodorant preparations and toothpastes. It also has antiplaque activity [44].

Derivatives of hydroxydiphenylether

Triclosan, 2,4,4′-trichlor-2′-hydroxydiphenylether (Irgasan, registered Ciba Speciality Chemicals, Basle, Switzerland) is only sparingly soluble in water (10 mg/l) but is soluble in solutions of dilute alkalis and organic solvents. Its activity is not compromised by soaps, most surfactants, organic solvents, acids or alkalis.

However ethoxylated surfactants such as polysorbate 80 (Tween-80) entrap triclosan within micelles, thus preventing its action [45]. Triclosan is generally bacteriostatic against a broad range of Gram-positive and Gram-negative bacteria and also demonstrates some fungistatic activity. Triclosan has a wide range of activity. In general it is more active against Gram-positive bacteria than Gram-negative bacteria, particularly *Pseudomonas* spp. It is active against some fungi, *Plasmodium falciparum* and *Toxoplasma gondii* although bacterial spores are unaffected [46]. It inhibits staphylococci at concentrations ranging from 0.1 to 0.3 μg/ml. Paradoxically, a number of *E. coli* strains are inhibited over a similar concentration range. Most strains of *P. aeruginosa* require concentrations varying from 100 to 1000 μg/ml for inhibition. It inhibits the growth of several species of mold at concentrations from 1 to 30 μg/ml.

Triclosan is commonly found in a wide range of personal care products such as handwashes, shower foams, medicated soaps, deodorants and hand scrubs. It is also used in toothpastes and it has been suggested that it has antiplaque activity [44]. It is ideally suited to these applications as it has a low toxicity and irritancy and is substantive to the skin [45]. More recently it has been used in a range of other applications such as incorporation in plastics and fabrics to confer microbicidal activity. This, and the link made between triclosan-resistant bacteria and antibiotic resistance, has led to concerns about its use [47–49]. However, with the correct usage of this microbicidal, there is no direct evidence to suggest that a proliferation of antibiotic resistant bacteria will occur [50]. Some reports have shown that the inhibitory activity of triclosan results from blocking lipid synthesis by specifically inhibiting an NADH-dependent enoyl-acyl carrier protein (ACP) reductase, or FabI [46, 51]. Based on this mode of action, triclosan-based molecules are considered to be potential candidates for novel antituberculosis and antimalarial drugs [46, 52, 53].

Derivatives of diphenylsulfide

Fenticlor, 2,2′-dihydroxy-5,5′-dichlorodiphenylsulfide, is a white powder soluble in water at 30 μg/ml, but is much more soluble in organic solvents and oils. It shows more activity against Gram-positive organisms and a "*Pseudomonas* gap". Typical inhibitory concentrations (μg/ml) are: *S. aureus*, 2; *E. coli*, 100; and *P. aeruginosa*, 1000. Typical inhibitory concentrations (μg/ml) for some fungi are: *Candida* spp., 12; *Epidermophyton interdigitale*, 0.4; and *Trichophyton granulosum*, 0.4. Fenticlor has found chief application in the treatment of dermatophytic conditions. However, it can cause photosensitization and as such its use as a preservative is limited [5]. Its low water solubility and narrow spectrum are further disadvantages, but it has potential as a fungicide. Its mode of action has been described by Hugo and Bloomfield [54–56] and Bloomfield [57].

The chlorinated analog of fenticlor, 2,2′-dihydroxy-3,4,6,3′,4′,6′-hexachlorodiphenylsulfide or 2,2′-thiobis (3,4,6-trichlorophenol) is almost insoluble in water. In a field test, it proved to be an effective inhibitor of microbial growth in cutting-oil emulsions. An exhaustive study of the antifungal properties of hydroxydiphenyl-sulfides was made by Pflege *et al.* [58].

Organic and inorganic acids: esters and salts

A large family of organic acids (Figure 2.5), both aromatic and aliphatic, and one or two inorganic acids have found application as preservatives, especially in the food industry. Some, for example benzoic acid, are also used in the preservation of pharmaceutical products; others (salicylic, undecylenic and benzoic acids) have been used, suitably formulated, for the topical treatment of fungal infections of the skin.

Vinegar, containing acetic acid (ethanoic acid), has been found to act as a preservative. It was also used as a wound dressing. This application has been revived in the use of dilute solutions of acetic acid as a wound dressing where pseudomonal infections have occurred.

Hydrochloric and sulfuric acids are two mineral acids sometimes employed in veterinary disinfection. Hydrochloric acid at high concentrations is sporicidal and has been used for disinfecting hides and skin contaminated with anthrax spores. Sulfuric acid, even at high concentrations, is not sporicidal, but in some

Table 2.2 pK_a values of acids and esters used as microbicidal agents.

Acid or esters	pK_a
Acetic (ethanoic) acid	4.7
Propionic (propanoic acid)	4.8
Sorbic acid (2,4-hexadienoic acid)	4.8
Lactic acid	3.8
Benzoic acid	4.2
Salicylic acid	3.0
Dehydroacetic acid	5.4
Sulfurous acid	1.8, 6.9
Methyl-*p*-hydroxybenzoic acid	8.5
Propyl-*p*-hydroxybenzoic acid	8.1

countries it is used, usually in combination with phenol, for the decontamination of floors, feed boxes and troughs.

Citric acid is an approved disinfectant against foot-and-mouth disease virus. It also appears, by virtue of its chelating properties, to increase the permeability of the outer membrane of Gram-negative bacteria [59] when employed at alkaline pH. Malic acid and gluconic acid, but not tartaric acid, can also act as permeabilizers at alkaline pH [59].

Chemistry of organic and inorganic acids

If an acid is represented by the symbol AH, then its ionization will be represented by $A^- H^+$. Complete ionization, as seen in aqueous solutions of mineral acids, such as hydrogen chloride (where AH = ClH), is not found in the weaker organic acids and their solutions will contain three components: A^-, H^+ and AH. The ratio of the concentration of these three components is called the ionization constant of that acid, K_a, and $K_a = A^- \times H^+/AH$. By analogy with the mathematical device used to define the pH scale, if the negative logarithm of K_a is taken, a number is obtained, running from about 0 to about 14, called pK_a. Some typical pK_a values are shown in Table 2.2.

An inspection of the equation defining K_a shows that the ratio A^-/AH must depend on the pH of the solution in which it is dissolved, and Henderson and Hasselbalch derived a relationship between this ratio and pH as follows:

$$\mathrm{Log}\,(A^-/AH) = pH - pK_a$$

An inspection of the formula will also show that at the pH value equal to the pK_a value the product is 50% ionized. These data enable an evaluation to be made of the effect of pH on the toxicity of organic acids. Typically it has been found that a marked toxic effect is seen only when the conditions of pH ensure the presence of the un-ionized molecular species AH. As the pH increases, the concentration of AH falls and the toxicity of the system falls; this may be indicated by a higher MIC, longer death time or higher mean single-survivor time, depending on the criterion of toxicity (i.e. microbicidal activity) chosen.

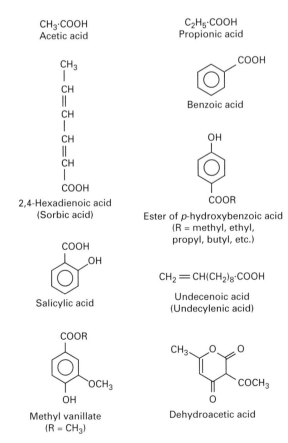

Figure 2.5 Organic acids and esters.

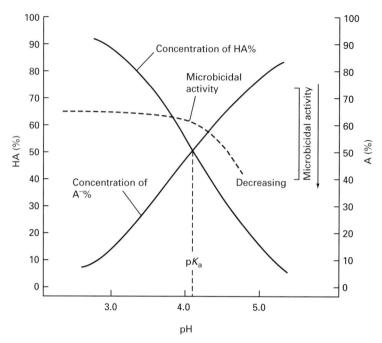

Figure 2.6 A generalized diagram of the effect of pH on the ionization and microbicidal activity of an acid (HA) of pK_a 4.1. A⁻ is the acid anion.

An inspection of Figure 2.6 would suggest that HA is more toxic than A⁻. However, an altering pH can alter the intrinsic toxicity of the environment. This is due to H⁺ alone, the ionization of the cell surface, the activity of transport and metabolizing enzymes, and the degree of ionization of the cell surface and hence sorption of the ionic species on the cell.

Predictions for the preservative ability of acids validated at one pH are rendered meaningless when such a preservative is added without further consideration to a formulation at a higher pH. The pK_a of the acid preservative should always be ascertained, and any pH shift of 1.5 units or more on the alkaline side of this can be expected to cause progressive loss of activity quite sufficient to invalidate the originally determined performance. That pH modifies the microbicidal effect of benzoic acid has been known for a long time [60]. For more detailed accounts of the effect of pH on the intensity of action of a large number of ionizable microbicides, the papers of Simon and Blackman [61] and Simon and Beevers [62, 63] should be consulted.

Mode of action

The mode of action of acids used as food preservatives has been reviewed by Eklund [64], Booth and Kroll [65] Cherrington *et al.* [66] and Russell [67]. Convincing evidence has been produced that many acid preservatives act by preventing the uptake of substrates, which depend on a proton-motive force for their entry into the cell; in other words, they act as uncoupling agents. In addition to acids such as benzoic, acetic and propionic, the esters of *p*-hydroxybenzoic acid (parabens) were also included in some of the above studies; they too acted as uncoupling agents, but also inhibited electron transport.

Equally interesting were experiments on the pH dependence of the substrate uptake effect. The intensity of uptake inhibition by propionate, sorbate and benzoate declined between pH 5 and 7, while that induced by propyl-*p*-hydroxybenzoic acid (pK_a 8.5) remained constant over the same pH range. The growth-inhibitory effect of ionizable microbicides shows pH dependence and this, as might be expected, is applicable to a biochemical effect upon which growth in turn depends.

Organic acids, such as benzoic acid and sorbic acid, are deliberately used as preservatives. Acids such as acetic, citric and lactic are often employed as acidulants, that is to lower artificially the pH of foods. However, a low pK_a value is not the only significant feature of acidulants, since: (i) sorbate and acetate have similar pK_a values but the latter is a less potent preservative; (ii) organic acids used as preservatives are more potent inhibitors than other weak acids of similar pH; and (iii) weak organic acid preservatives are more effective inhibitors of pH homeostasis than other acids of similar structure.

Individual compounds
Acetic acid (ethanoic acid)

This acid, as a diluted petrochemically produced compound or as the natural product vinegar, is used primarily as a preservative for vegetables. The toxicity of vinegars and diluted acetic acid must rely to an extent on the inhibitory activity of the molecule itself, as solutions of comparable pH made from mineral acid do not exhibit the same preservative activity. A 5% solution of acetic acid contains 4.997% CH₃COOH and 0.003% H⁺. As might be expected from the pK_a value, 4.7, the activity is rapidly lost at pH levels above this. This suggests that the acetate ion is less toxic than the undissociated molecule, although, as has been said, the concomitant reduction in hydrogen ion concentration must play some part in the reduction of toxicity. As has been stated, diluted 1–5% acetic acid has been used as a wound dressing where infection with *Pseudomonas* has occurred [68]. Acetic acid is also used as topical otological preparation [69].

Propionic acid

This acid is employed almost exclusively as the sodium, and to a lesser extent the calcium, salt in the baking industry, where it is used to inhibit mold and bacterial growth in breads and cakes. It is particularly useful in inhibiting the growth of the spore-forming aerobe *Bacillus macerans*, which gives rise to ropy bread. Manufacturers give explicit directions as to the amount to be used in different products, but in general 0.15–0.4% is added to the flour before processing. Other products that have been successfully preserved with propionates include cheeses and malt extract. In addition to foods, wrapping materials for foods have also been protected from microbial damage with propionates. It is added to poultry feed to protect from the growth of many bacteria like *E. coli*, *Salmonella* spp. and molds [70, 71].

Butyric acid

The sodium salt of butyric acid is commonly used as an additive to poultry feed to protect from *Salmonella* spp. infection and shedding [72, 73].

Caprylic acid

Caprylic acid is a natural eight-carbon fatty acid present in breast milk and bovine milk and is approved as generally recognizable as safe by the US Food and Drug Administration (FDA). It has microbicidal activity [74] and has been studied as a potential infant food additive to inhibit *Enterobacter (Cronobacter) sakazakii*, an emerging pathogen in dried infant formula that causes meningitis, bacteraemia, sepsis and necrotizing enterocolitis in neonates and children [75, 76].

Formic acid (methanoic acid)

Formic acid is an irritating, pungent liquid at room temperature. It is used mainly as an insecticide. It is used as a disinfectant against methicillin-resistant *S. aureus* (MRSA) at 55% w/w. It has shown good activity in the decontaminatation of meat surfaces contaminated with *E. coli* O157:H7 and *S. aureus*. Also, preparations containing a combination of formic acid and propionic acid have been used as feed additive to control *Salmonella* spp. in poultry [70].

Undecanoic acid (undecylenic acid)

This has been used either as such or as the calcium or zinc salt in the treatment of superficial dermatophytoses. It is usually applied in ointment form at concentrations of 2–15%. Undecanoic acid is rapidly being replaced as an antifungal agent by imidazole derivatives.

Sorbic acid (2,4-hexadienoic acid)

This unsaturated carboxylic acid is effective against a wide range of microorganisms and has been used as the acid itself, or its potassium salt, at concentrations of 0.01–0.1% to preserve bakery products, soft drinks, alcoholic beverages, cheeses, dried fruits, fish, pickles, wrapping materials and pharmaceutical products. As with all acids, there is a critical pH, in this case 6.5, above which activity begins to decline. The pK_a of sorbic acid is 4.8 and its activity decreases with increase in pH and ionization. It is most effective at pH 4 or less [77]. Again, it is the undissociated acid that is the active microbicidal species [78, 79]. Sorbic acid was believed to act by interfering with the functioning of the citric acid cycle [80, 81].

Sorbic acid is known to interfere with the uptake of amino and oxo acids in *E. coli* and *B. subtilis*. It affects the proton-motive force in *E. coli* and accelerates the movement of H^+ ions from low media pH into the cytoplasm. It probably acts overall by dissipating ΔpH across the membrane and inhibiting solute transport. The membrane potential ($\Delta \Psi$) is reduced but to a much smaller extent than ΔpH [26, 64, 75, 82]. Plumridge *et al.* [83] were able to demonstrate the gene responsible for decarobxylating sorbic acid in *Aspergillus niger (brasiliensis)*, thus playing a role in its resistance. A combination of sorbic acid with monolaurin has been shown to be often more active than parabens or sorbic acid alone [84].

Lactic acid

Lactic acid shares with some other hydroxy acids the interesting property of being able to destroy airborne microorganisms [85]. A careful study of hydroxyl acids, including lactic acid, as air disinfectants was made by Lovelock [86]. Lactic acid was found to be a cheap, efficient, aerial bactericide when sprayed into the area to be decontaminated. However, it has a slight irritant action on the nasal mucosa, which tends to limit its use. It could be used in emergencies for decontaminating glove boxes or hoods in the absence of other means.

Lactic acid in liquid form is less active than several other organic acids [64], but nevertheless is used as an acidulant for low pH foods and fruit juices [87, 88]. It has been shown to be an effective permeabilizer [89].

Benzoic acid

Benzoic acid, first shown to be antifungal in 1875, is a white crystalline powder, which is soluble 1:350 in water. It is used as a preservative for foods and pharmaceutical products, but is rapidly inactivated at pH values above 5.0 [64, 82, 88]. The pK_a of benzoic acid is 4.2, at which 50% of the acid is ionized, so it is advisable to limit the use of benzoic acid to preserve pharmaceuticals with a maximum pH of 5.0 and if possible <4.0. As with other preservatives, its activity may be modified by the milieu in which it acts [90, 91]. Resistance may develop and the acid may be metabolized by a contaminant it is meant to inhibit [92]. In addition to its use as a preservative, benzoic acid has been combined with other agents for the topical treatment of fungal infections. Benzoic acid, like many other compounds, inhibits the swarming of *Bacillus* spp. [93]. Studies with benzoic acid derivatives have demonstrated that lipophilicity and pK_a are the two most important parameters influencing activity [94]. A combination of sorbic acid and benzoic acid has been shown to exert additive effect against a number of yeasts [95].

Salicylic acid

This is often used, in combination with benzoic acid and other antifungal agents, for the topical treatment of fungal infections. Salicylic acid has keratinolytic activity and in addition affects metabolic processes. For an account of the action of benzoic and salicylic acids on the metabolism of microorganisms, see Freese *et al.* [96].

Dehydroacetic acid (DHA)

Dehydroacetic acid is a white or light yellow, odorless, crystalline compound, which is soluble at less than 0.1% in water; the sodium salt is soluble to the extent of 33%. Typical inhibitory concentrations (%) of the latter for selected microorganisms are: *Aerobacter aerogenes*, 0.3; *Bacillus cereus*, 0.3; *Lactobacillus plantarum*, 0.1; *S. aureus*, 0.3; *P. aeruginosa*, 0.4; *Aspergillus niger (brasiliensis)*, 0.05; *Penicillium expansum*, 0.01; *Rhizopus nigricans*, 0.05; *Trichophyton interdigitale*, 0.005; and *Saccharomyces cerevisiae*, 0.1. Extensive toxicological studies have indicated that the product is acceptable as a preservative for foods, cosmetics and medicines. The pK_a value of DHA is 5.4, but an inspection of pH/activity data suggests that activity loss above the pK_a value is not as great as with other preservative acids (propionic, benzoic). Indeed, in Wolf's 1950 paper [97], the MIC against *S. aureus* remained at 0.3% from pH 5 to 9. However, loss of activity at alkaline pH values was noted by Bandelin [98] in his detailed study of the effect of pH on the activity of antifungal compounds, as would be predicted by the pK_a value. Little was known about its mode of action, although Seevers *et al.* [99] produced evidence that DHA inhibited succinoxidase activity in mammalian tissue, while Wolf and Westveer [100] showed that it did not react with microbial –SH enzymes.

Sulfur dioxide, sulfites and bisulfites

The fumes of burning sulfur, generating sulfur dioxide, were used by the Greeks and Egyptians as fumigants for premises and food vessels to purify and deodorize. Lime sulfur, an aqueous suspension of elementary sulfur and calcium hydroxide, was introduced as a horticultural fungicide in 1803. Later, the salts, chiefly sodium, potassium and calcium, of sulfurous acid were used in wine and food preservation. In addition to their microbicidal properties, members of this group also act as antioxidants helping to preserve the color of food products, as enzyme inhibitors, as Maillard reaction inhibitors and as reducing agents [101]. Sulfur dioxide-releasing pads are packed with table grapes for storage [102].

A pH-dependent relationship exists in solution between the species SO_2, HSO_3^- and SO_3^{2-}. As the pH moves from acid to alkaline, the species predominance moves from SO_2, the toxic species, through HSO_3^- to SO_3^{2-}. Above pH 3.6, the concentration of SO_2 begins to fall, and with it the microbicidal power of the solution. It is postulated that SO_2 can penetrate cells much more readily than can the other two chemical species [103].

Yeasts and molds can grow at low pH values, hence the value of sulfites as inhibitors of fungal growth in acid environments such as fruit juices. For reviews on the microbicidal activity of sulfur dioxide, see Rose and Pilkington [103] and Gould and Russell [101].

Esters of p-Hydroxybenzoic acid (parabens)

The marked pH dependence of acids for their activity and the fact that the microbicidal activity lay in the undissociated form led to the notion that esterification of an aromatic hydroxycarboxylic acid might give rise to compounds in which the phenolic group was less easily ionized. Sabalitschka [104] prepared a series of alkyl esters of p-hydroxybenzoic acid and tested their microbicidal activity [105, 106]. This family of microbicides, which may be regarded as either phenols or esters of aromatic hydroxycarboxylic acids, is among the most widely used group of preservatives [107]. The esters usually used are the methyl, ethyl, propyl, butyl and benzyl compounds and are active over a wider pH range (4–8) than acid preservatives. They have low water solubility, which decreases in the order methyl to butyl (Table 2.3). A paper which gives extensive microbicidal data is that of Aalto *et al.* [108]. Again it can be seen that activity increases from the methyl to the butyl ester. The compounds show low systemic toxicity [109]. Russell and Furr [110–112] and Russell *et al.* [113, 114] studied the effects of parabens against wild-type and envelope mutants of *E. coli* and *Salmonella typhimurium*, and found that, as the homologous series was ascended, solubility decreased but activity became more pronounced, especially against the deep rough strains.

In summary, it can be said that the parabens are generally more active against Gram-positive bacteria and fungi, including yeasts, than against Gram-negative bacteria. In the latter group *P. aeruginosa* is, as is so often seen, more resistant, especially to the higher homologs.

Hugo and Foster [115] showed that a strain of *P. aeruginosa* isolated from a human eye lesion could metabolize the esters in dilute solution (0.0343%), a solution strength originally proposed as a preservative vehicle for medicinal eye drops. Beveridge and Hart [116] verified that the esters could serve as a carbon source for a number of Gram-negative bacterial species. Rosen *et al.* [117] studied the preservative action of a mixture of methyl (0.2%) and propyl (0.1%) p-hydroxybenzoic acid in a cosmetic lotion. Using a challenge test, they found that this concentration of esters failed to kill *P. aeruginosa*. This was part of their work indicating that these esters plus imidazolindyl urea were ideal to provide a broad-spectrum preservative system, with pseudomonads being successfully eliminated. Combinations of parabens have been found to have synergistic activity [118].

The rationale for the use of these esters in mixtures might be seen in the preservation of water-in-oil emulsion systems, where the more water-soluble methyl ester protects the aqueous phase while the propyl or butyl esters might preserve the oil phase [119]. The use of fennel oil in combination with methyl, ethyl, propyl and butyl parabens has been shown to be synergistic in terms of microbicidal activity [120]. Another factor that must be borne in mind when using parabens is that they share the property found with other preservatives containing a phenolic group of being inactivated by non-ionic surface agents. Hydrogen bonding between the phenolic hydrogen atom and oxygen residues in polyoxyethylated non-ionic surfactants is believed to be responsible for the phenomenon.

Various ways of quenching paraben activity, including the use of polysorbates, are considered by Sutton [121].

The mode of action of the parabens has been reviewed by Freese and Levin [122], Eklund [64] and Kabara and Eklund [82]. Haag and Loncrini [123] have produced a comprehensive report of their microbicidal properties. Several mechanisms of actions have been proposed for parabens and no one mechanism was proven to be dominant. These include: (i) interfering with the membrane proton-motive force [124]; (ii) partitioning into the membrane lipid affecting the mechano-sensitive channels, thus upsetting the osmotic gradient in the bacteria; and (iii) altering membrane permeability and causing efflux to cytoplasmic constituents like potassium ions [125–127].

Vanillic acid esters

The methyl, ethyl, propyl and butyl esters of vanillic acid (4-hydroxy-3-methoxy benzoic acid) possess antifungal properties when used at concentrations of 0.1–0.2%. These esters are not very soluble in water and are inactivated above pH 8. The ethyl ester has been shown to be less toxic than sodium benzoate and

it has been used in the preservation of foods and food-packing materials against fungal infestation.

Aromatic diamidines

Diamidines are a group of organic compounds of which a typical structure is shown in Figure 2.7. They were first introduced into medicine in the 1920s as possible insulin substitutes as they

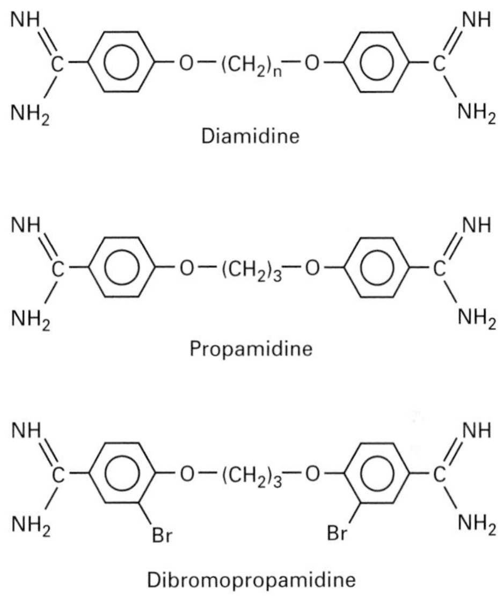

Figure 2.7 Typical structure of a diamidine, propamidine and dibromopropamidine.

Table 2.3 Chemical and microbiological properties of esters of *p*-hydroxybenzoic acid.

Property[a]	Ester			
	Methyl	**Ethyl**	**Propyl**	**Butyl**
Molecular weight	152	166	180	194
Solubility in water (g/100 g) at 15°C	0.16	0.08	0.023	0.005
K_{ow} (arachis oil)	2.4	13.4	38.1	239.6
Log P (octanol : water)	1.96	2.47	3.04	3.57
MIC values (molar basis)[b]				
Escherichia coli (wild-type)	3.95×10^{-3}	2.7×10^{-3}	1.58×10^{-3}	1.03×10^{-3}
Escherichia coli (deep rough)	2.63×10^{-3}	1.2×10^{-3}	2.78×10^{-4}	1.03×10^{-4}
MIC values (μg/ml)[c]				
Escherichia coli	800	560	350	160
Pseudomonas aeruginosa	1000	700	350	150
Concentration (mmol/l) giving 50% inhibition of growth and uptake process[d]				
Escherichia coli	5.5	2.2	1.1	0.4
Pseudomonas aeruginosa	3.6	2.8	>1.0	>1.0
Bacillus subtilis	4.3	1.3	0.9	0.46

[a] K_{ow}, partition coefficient, oil : water; P, partition coefficient, octanol : water.
[b] Russell *et al.* [113].
[c] El-Falaha *et al.* [632].
[d] Eklund [633].

lowered blood-sugar levels in humans. Later, they were found to possess an intrinsic trypanocidal activity and from this arose an investigation into their microbicidal activity [128, 129]. From these studies two compounds, propamidine and dibromopropamidine, emerged as useful microbicidal compounds, being active against both bacteria and fungi.

Mode of action

Diamidines have been shown to inhibit oxygen uptake and induce amino acid leakage [130]. In addition, marked damage to the cell envelope of some Gram-negative bacteria has been described [131]. Also, aromatic diamidines have been shown to bind to DNA and some of them are nucleoside sequence-selective binders [132].

Propamidine

Propamidine, 4,4′-diamidinophenoxypropane, is usually supplied as the di(2-hydroxyethane-sulfate), the isethionate, which has a better solubility. This product is a white hygroscopic powder, which is soluble in water, 1:5. Microbicidal activity and clinical applications are described by Thrower and Valentine [128]. A summary of its antibacterial and antifungal activity is given in Table 2.4. Its activity is reduced by serum, blood and by low pH values. Microorganisms exposed to propamidine quickly acquire a resistance to it by serial subculture in the presence of increasing doses. MRSA strains may show appreciable resistance to propamidine [133]. It is chiefly used in the form of a cream containing 0.15% as a topical application for wounds. Propamidine is considered the first line treatment for *Acanthamoeba* keratitis, a corneal disease associated with contact lens wear. Usually, it is used in combination with polyhexamethylene biguanide or neomycin to treat such eye infections [133–135].

Hexamidine diisethionate

Hexamidine diisethionate is used as preservative in cosmetics at concentrations from 0.03% to 0.1% w/v. It has greater cysticidal activity against *Acanthamoeba* than propamidine [136, 137].

Dibromopropamidine

Dibromopropamidine (2,2′-dibromo-4,4′-diamidinodiphenoxypropane), usually supplied as the isethionate, occurs as white crystals which are readily soluble in water. Dibromopropamidine is active against Gram-positive, non-spore-forming organisms; it is less active against Gram-negative organisms and spore formers, but is active against fungi (Table 2.4). Resistance can be acquired by serial subculture, and resistant organisms also show some resistance to propamidine. Russell and Furr [138, 139] found that Gram-negative bacteria present a permeability barrier to dibromopropamidine isethionate, and MRSA strains may be resistant to the diamidine. Its activity is reduced in acid environments and in the presence of blood and serum. It is usually applied as an oil-in-water cream emulsion containing 0.15% of the isethionate. More detailed reviews of this group of compounds can be found in Fleurette *et al.* [140].

Table 2.4 Microbicidal properties of propamidine and dibromopropamidine isethionates.

Microorganism	MIC (µg/ml) of propamidine isethionate[a]	Dibromopropamidine isethionate[b]
Staphylococcus aureus	1–16	1
Staphylococcus albus	6	
MRSA[c]	800/100	
MRSE[d]	250–800	
Streptococcus pyogenes	0.24–4	1
Streptococcus viridans	1–4	2
Streptococcus faecalis	25	
Pseudomonas aeruginosa	250–400	32 (64)
Proteus vulgaris	125–400	128 (256)
Escherichia coli	64–100	4 (32)
Clostridium perfringens	3–32	512
Clostridium histolyticum	256	256
Shigella flexneri	32	8
Salmonella enteriditis	256	65
Salmonella typhimurium	256	64
Actinomyces kimberi	100	10
Actinomyces madurae	100	50
Actinomyces hominis	1000	1000
Trichophyton tonsurans	100	25
Epidermophyton floccosum	250	
Achorion schoenleinii	3.5	
Blastomyces dermatitidis	3.5	
Geotrichum dermatitidis	3.5	200
Hormodendron langevonii		500

[a]Data from various sources, including Wien *et al.* [129].
[b]Data from Wien *et al.* [129]. Figures in parentheses denote bactericidal concentrations.
[c]MRSA, methicillin-resistant *S. aureus* carrying the *qac*A/*qac*B gene (data from Littlejohn *et al.* [634]).
[d]MRSE, methicillin-resistant *S. epidermidis* (data from Leelaporn *et al.* [305]).

Biguanides

Various biguanides show microbicidal activity, including chlorhexidine, alexidine and polymeric forms.

Mode of action

Various modes of action have been found for different biguanide compound as described below:

Chlorhexidine

Chlorhexidine (Figure 2.8a) is one of a family of N^1,N^5-substituted biguanides which has emerged from extensive synthetic and screening studies. It is available as a dihydrochloride, diacetate and gluconate. At 20°C the solubilities of the dihydrochloride and diacetate are 0.06 and 1.9% w/v, respectively; the gluconate is freely soluble. Chlorhexidine and its salts occur as white or faintly

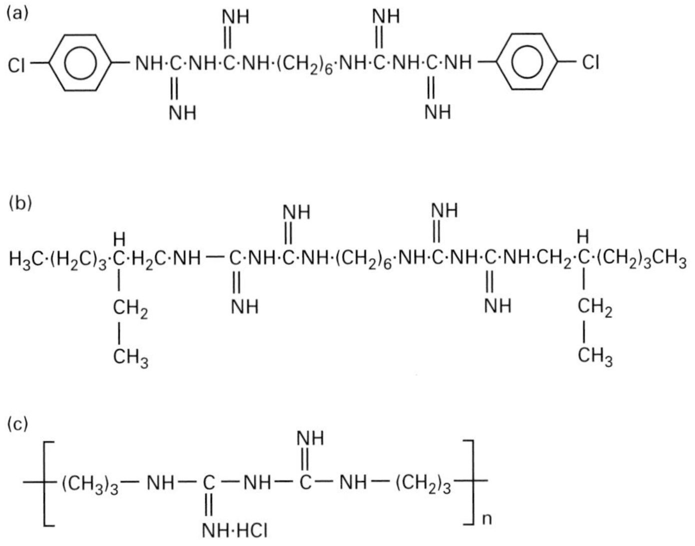

Figure 2.8 (a) Chlorhexidine, (b) alexidine and (c) Vantocil 1B, a polymeric biguanide in which mean *n* is 5.5.

Table 2.5 Bacteriostatic activity of chlorhexidine against various bacterial species.

Organism	Concentration of chlorhexidine (µg/ml) necessary for inhibition of growth
Streptococcus lactis	0.5
Streptococcus pyogenes	0.5
Streptococcus pneumoniae	1.0
Streptococcus faecalis	1.0
Staphylococcus aureus	1.0
Corynebacterium diphtheriae	1.0
Salmonella typhi	1.67
Salmonella pullorum	3.3
Salmonella dublin	3.3
Salmonella typhimurium	5.0
Proteus vulgaris	5.0
Pseudomonas aeruginosa (1)	5.0
Pseudomonas aeruginosa (2)	5.0
Pseudomonas aeruginosa (3)	12.5
Enterobacter aerogenes	10
Escherichia coli	10[a]
Vibrio cholerae	3.3
Bacillus subtilis	0.5
Clostridium welchii	10
Mycobacterium tuberculosis	0.5
Candida albicans[b]	5.0

Inoculum: one loopful of 24 h broth culture per 10 ml Difco heart–brain infusion medium. Incubation: 24 h at 37°C.
[a]Much higher than normally recorded.
[b]Yeast.

Table 2.6 Bactericidal activity of chlorhexidine against various bacterial species.

Organism	Concentration of chlorhexidine (µg/ml)		
	To effect 99% kill	To effect 99.9% kill	To effect 99.99% kill
Staphylococcus aureus	8	14	25
Streptococcus pyogenes	–	–	50
Escherichia coli	6.25	10	20
Pseudomonas aeruginosa	25	33	60
Salmonella typhi	5	–	8

Inoculum: 10[5] in distilled water. Contact time: 10 min at room temperature. Neutralizer: egg yolk medium.

cream-colored powders and are available in a number of pharmaceutical formulations. It is widely used combined with cetyltrimethylammonium bromide as a topical antiseptic (Savlon, Novartis Consumer Health, Basle, Switzerland).

Chlorhexidine has a wide spectrum of antibacterial activity against both Gram-positive and Gram-negative bacteria. Some bacteria, notably strains of *Proteus* and *Providencia* spp., may be highly resistant to the biguanide [141, 142]. It is not sporicidal at ambient temperatures [26, 143–146]. Chlorhexidine is not lethal to acid-fast organisms, although it shows a high degree of bacteriostasis [147–148] (Table 2.5). It is, however, tuberculocidal in ethanolic solutions and sporicidal at 98–100°C. A range of bacteriostatic and bactericidal values against a variety of bacterial species is shown in Tables 2.5 and 2.6, respectively.

Activity is reduced in the presence of serum, blood, pus and other organic matter. Because of its cationic nature, its activity is also reduced in the presence of soaps and other anionic compounds. Chlorhexidine exhibits the greatest microbicidal activity at pH 7 to 8 where it exists exclusively as di-cations. This pH dependency makes it compatible with quaternary ammonium compounds (QACs), which are most effective microbicidally at neutral and slightly alkaline pH, for example cetyltrimithyl ammonium bromide (cetrimide) as a topical microbicidal agent on skin and mucous membranes (e.g. Savlon). Since chlorhexidine possess a cationic nature, this results in its activity being reduced by anionic compounds, including soap, due to the formation of insoluble salts; anions such as bicarbonates, borates, carbonates, chloride, citrate, phosphate and hard water may partially or totally neutralize the charge and hence the activity. In the light of the above, users of chlorhexidine preparations are advised to use deionized or distilled water for dilution purposes.

Its main use is in medical and veterinary antisepsis [149]. An alcoholic solution is a very effective skin disinfectant [150, 151], in bladder irrigation and in obstetrics and gynecology. It is one of the recommended bactericides for inclusion in eye drops and is widely used in contact lens solutions [152]. In the veterinary context, chlorhexidine fulfils the major function of the application of a disinfectant of cows' teats after milking and can also be used as an antiseptic wound application. Chlorhexidine is also widely employed in the dental field due to its broad spectrum of activity, substantivity and low toxicity [153–155]. It has also been investigated in combination with sodium hypochlorite as an endodontic irrigant [156]. Chlorhexidine is a highly effective antibacterial agent as an antiseptic where a concentration of 1 : 2,000,000 prevents the growth of *S. aureus* and a 1 : 50,000 dilution prevents the growth of *P. aeruginosa*. However, some reports [157] indicating pseudomonal contamination of aqueous chlorhexidine solutions have promoted the inclusion of small amounts of ethanol or isopropanol into these preparations. The limited antifungal activity of chlorhexidine restricts its use as a general preservative.

Its mode of action has been studied by various authors [158–163]. ^{14}C-chlorhexidine gluconate is taken up very rapidly by bacterial [158] and fungal [164, 165] cells. At lower concentrations, up to 200 μg/ml, it inhibits membrane enzymes and promotes leakage of cellular constituents, which is probably associated with bacteriostasis. As the concentration increases above this value, cytoplasmic constituents are coagulated and a bactericidal effect is seen. In addition, high chlorhexidine concentrations inhibit adenosine triphosphatase (ATPase) and collapse membrane potentials, although this effect is not the primary cause of the lethal effect of biguanides [130]. Chlorhexidine has low oral toxicity and it may be administered for throat medication in the form of lozenges. Several infections have been reported due to the use of contaminated chlorhexidine solutions, the most common microorganisms isolated were *Pseudomonas* spp. [157].

Comprehensive surveys of its activity and uses have been published [145, 146, 166].

Alexidine

Alexidine (Figure 2.8b) is a bisbiguanide that possesses ethylhexyl end-groups as distinct from the chlorophenol end-groups found in chlorhexidine. Alexidine is considerably more active than chlorhexidine in inducing cell leakage from *E. coli*, and concentrations of alexidine (but not of chlorhexidine) above the MIC induce cell lysis [167, 168]. Alexidine has been recommended for use as an oral antiseptic and antiplaque compound [169]. It has amoebicidal activity against several pathogenic *Acanthamoeba* spp. and is used in contact lens disinfection solution [170, 171]. Unlike chlorhexidine, both alexidine and polyhexamethylene biguanide (PHMB) induce membrane lipid-phase separation and domain formation.

Polymeric biguanides

A polymer of hexamethylene biguanide (Figure 2.8c), with a molecular weight of approximately 3000 (weight average), has found particular use as a cleansing agent in the food industry. Its properties have been described by Davies *et al.* [172] under the trade name Vantocil 1B. PHMB is soluble in water and is usually supplied as a 20% aqueous solution. It inhibits the growth of most bacteria at between 5 and 25 μg/ml, but 100 μg/ml is required to inhibit *P. aeruginosa* while *Pseudomonas vulgaris* requires 250 μg/ml. It is less active against fungi; for example *Cladosporium resinae*, which has been implicated as a spoilage organism in pharmaceutical products, requires 1250 μg/ml to prevent growth.

PHMB is believed to gain access to Gram-negative bacteria by a mechanism of self-promotion through cation displacement from, predominantly, core lipopolysaccharides in the outer membrane [173]. Microbicidal activity of PHMB increases with increasing polymer length [174]. It is a membrane-active agent [175–178], inducing phospholipid phase separation [179]. A complete loss of membrane function ensues, with precipitation of intracellular constituents leading to a bactericidal effect. In addition, it has been shown that PHMB has broad spectrum interactions with nucleic acids, suggesting this as a partial cause of its antimicrobicidal activity [180, 181].

Because of the residual positive charges on the polymer, PHMB is precipitated from aqueous solutions by anionic compounds, which include soaps and detergents based on alkyl sulfates. It is also precipitated by detergent constituents, such as sodium hexametaphosphate, and in a strongly alkaline environment.

PHMB finds use as a general sterilizing agent in the food industry, provided the surfaces to which it is applied are free from occlusive debris, a stricture that applies in all disinfection procedures. Because it is not a surface-active agent, it can be used in the brewing industry, as it does not affect head retention on ales and beers. It has also been used very successfully for the disinfection of swimming pools. Apart from copper, which it tarnishes, this polymeric biguanide has no deleterious effect on most materials it might encounter in use.

PHMB has activity against both the trophozite and the cyst forms of *Acanthamoeba castellanii* [182–184]. More recently PHMB has been shown to have a beneficial effect in inhibiting plaque when used in mouthwashes [185]. Due to its broad spectrum of activity against Gram-positive and Gram-negative bacteria and its low toxicity, PHMB is used as an microbicidal agent in various ophthalmic products.

Surface-active agents

Surface-active agents (surfactants) have two regions in their molecular structure, one being a hydrocarbon water-repellent (hydrophobic) group and the other a water-attracting (hydrophilic or polar) group. Depending on the basis of the charge or absence of ionization of the hydrophilic group, surface-active agents are classified into cationic, anionic, non-ionic and amphoteric (ampholytic) compounds.

Cationic agents

Cationic surfactants possess strong bactericidal, but weak detergent, properties. The term "cationic detergent" usually signifies a quaternary ammonium compound (QAC, quat or onium).

Merianos [186] and Reverdy [187] have reviewed the surface-active quaternary ammonium germicides, and useful data about their properties and activity are provided by Wallhäusser [188] and about their uses by Gardner and Peel [189] and Denyer and Wallhäusser [190].

Chemistry of surface-active agents

The QACs may be considered as organically substituted ammonium compounds, in which the nitrogen atom has a valency of five, and four of the substituent radicals (R^1 to R^4) are alkyl or heterocyclic radicals and the fifth (X^-) is a small anion (Figure 2.9, general structure). Examples include compounds such as benzalkonium chloride, cetyltrimethylammonium bromide and cetylpyridinium chloride. The sum of the carbon atoms in the four R groups is more than 10. For a QAC to have a high microbicidal activity, at least one of the R groups must have a chain length in the range C_8 to C_{18}. Three of the four covalent links may be satisfied by nitrogen in a pyridine ring, as in the pyridinium compounds, such as cetylpyridinium chloride (Figure 2.9). QACs are most effective against most microorganisms at neutral or

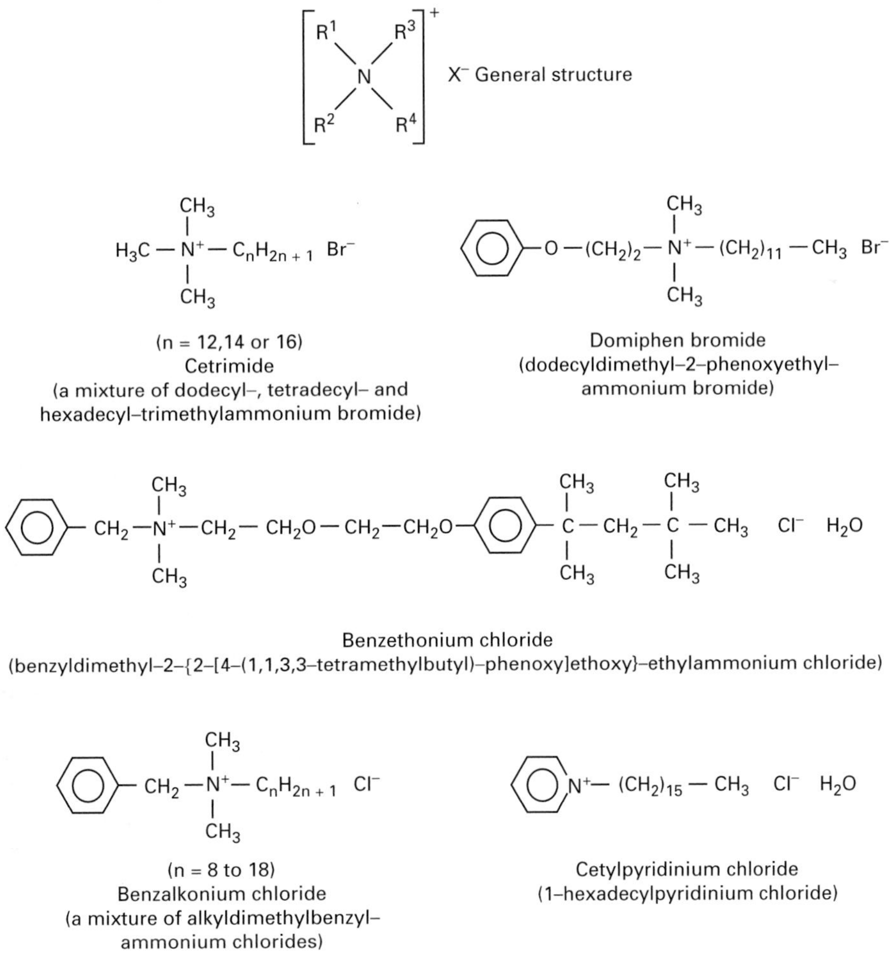

Figure 2.9 General structure and examples of quaternary ammonium compounds.

slightly alkaline pH and become virtually ineffective below pH 3.5. The cationic onium group may be a simple aliphatic ammonium, a pyridimum or piperidinium or other heterocyclic group.

Apart from the monoquaternary compounds, monoquaternary derivatives of 4-aminoquinaldine (e.g. laurolinium) are potent microbicidal agents, as are the bisquaternary compounds, such as hedaquinium chloride and dequalinium. In addition to the compounds mentioned above, polymeric QACs are used as industrial microbicides. One such compound is poly(oxyethylene (dimethylimino)ethylene) dichloride. Organosilicon-substituted (silicon-bonded) QACs, organic amines or amine salts have been introduced recently. Compounds with microbicidal activity in solution are also highly effective on surfaces. One such compound, 3-(trimethoxysily) propyloctadecyldimethyl ammonium chloride, demonstrates powerful microbicidal activity while chemically bonded to a variety of surfaces [191, 192]. Schaeufele [193] has pointed out that fatty alcohols and/or fatty acids, from both natural and synthetic sources, form the basis of the production of modern QACs, which have improved organic soil and increased hard-water tolerance. The newer QACs, referred to as twin chain or dialkyl quaternaries (e.g. didecyl dimethylammonium bromide and dioctyl dimethylammonium bromide), can retain activity in hard water and are tolerant of anionic residues [194].

Mode of action

The microbicidal properties of the QACs were first recognized in 1916, but they did not attain prominence until the work of Domagk [195]. Early workers claimed that the QACs were markedly sporicidal, but the fallacy of this hypothesis has been demonstrated by improved testing methods. The activity of QACs is attributed to their action on cytoplasmic membrane permeability causing leakage of chemical species, inactivation of energy-producing enzymes and denaturation of essential cell proteins.

The QACs are primarily active against Gram-positive bacteria, with concentrations as low as 1 in 200,000 (0.0005%) being lethal; higher concentrations (c. 1 in 30,000 or 0.0033%) are lethal to Gram-negative bacteria [196], although *P. aeruginosa* tends to be highly resistant. Nevertheless, cells of this organism, which are highly resistant to benzalkonium chloride (1 mg/ml, 0.1%), may still show ultrastructural changes when grown in its presence [197]. The QACs have a trypanocidal activity but are not mycobactericidal, presumably because of the lipid, waxy coat of these organisms. Gram-negative bacteria, such as *E. coli*, *P. aeruginosa* and *Salmonella typhimurium*, exclude QACs, but deep rough mutants are sensitive [26, 141]. Contamination of solutions of QACs with Gram-negative bacteria has been reported [198, 199].

Viruses are more resistant than bacteria or fungi to the QACs. This was clearly shown by Grossgebauer [200], who pointed out that the QACs have a high protein defect and that, whereas they are active against lipophilic viruses (such as herpes simplex, vaccinia, influenza and adenoviruses), they have only a poor effect against viruses that show hydrophilic properties (enteroviruses, e.g. poliovirus, coxsackievirus and echovirus).

The QACs possess antifungal properties, although they are fungistatic rather than fungicidal [201]. This applies not only to the monoquaternary compounds, but also to the bisonium compounds, such as hedaquinium and dequalinium.

Weiner *et al.* [202] studied the activity of three QACs (dodecyl trimethylammonium chloride, dodecyl dimethylammonium chloride and dodecyl pyridinium chloride) against *E. coli*, *S. aureus* and *Candida albicans*, and correlated these results with the surface properties of these agents. A clear relationship was found between the thermodynamic activity (expressed as a ratio of the surface concentration produced by a solution and the surface concentration at the critical micelle concentration (CMC)) and antibacterial activity.

Because most QACs are mixtures of homologs, Laycock and Mulley [203] studied the bactericidal activity of mono- and multicomponent solutions, using the homologous series *n*-dodecyl, *n*-tetradecyl and *n*-hexadecyl trimethylammonium bromides individually, binary systems containing C_{12}/C_{14} or C_{14}/C_{16} mixtures, and a ternary mixture (cetrimide) of the $C_{12}/C_{14}/C_{16}$ compounds. Bactericidal activity was measured as the concentrations needed to produce survivor levels of 1.0% and 0.01%; CMC was measured by the surface-tension method. In almost every instance, the thermodynamic activity (CMC/concentration to produce a particular survivor level) producing an equivalent biological response was reasonably constant, thereby supporting the Ferguson principle for these micelle-forming QACs.

QACs are incompatible with a wide range of chemical agents, including anionic surfactants, non-ionic surfactants, such as lubrols and Tweens, and phospholipids, such as lecithin and other fat-containing substances. Benzalkonium chloride has been found to be incompatible with the ingredients of some commercial rubber mixes, but not with silicone rubber; this is important when benzalkonium chloride is employed as a preservative in multiple dose eye drop formulations.

Although non-ionic surfactants are stated above to inactivate QACs, presumably as a consequence of micellar formation (see Elworthy [204] for a useful description of micelles), nevertheless potentiation of the antibacterial activity of the QACs by means of low concentrations of non-ionic agents has been reported [205], possibly as a result of increased cellular permeability induced by the non-ionic surfactant.

The microbicidal activity of the QACs is affected greatly by organic matter, including milk, serum and feces, which may limit their usefulness in practice. The uses of the QACs are considered below. They are more effective at alkaline and neutral pH than under acid conditions. The action of benzalkonium chloride on *P. aeruginosa* is potentiated by aromatic alcohols, especially 3-phenylpropanol [206].

Uses

The QACs have been recommended for use in food hygiene in hospitals and are frequently used in food-processing industries. Resistance to benzalkonium chloride among food-associated Gram-negative bacteria and *Enterococcus* spp. is not common, but if such disinfectants are used at sublethal concentrations resistance may occur [207]. Benzalkonium chloride has been employed for the preoperative disinfection of unbroken skin (0.1–0.2%), for application to mucous membranes (up to 0.1%) and for bladder and urethra irrigation (0.005%); creams are used in treating nappy (diaper) rash caused by ammonia-producing organisms and lozenges for the treatment of superficial mouth and throat infections. In the UK, benzalkonium chloride (0.01%) is one of four agents officially recognized as being suitable preservatives for inclusion in eye drop preparations [208]. Benzalkonium chloride is also widely used (at a concentration of 0.001–0.01%) in hard contact lens soaking (disinfecting) solutions. The QAC is too irritating to be used with hydrophilic soft (hydrogel) contact lenses because it can bind to the lens surface, be held within the water present in hydrogels and then be released into the eye [209]. Polyquad, a QAC used commercially in contact lens disinfectant solutions, has been shown to be active against the microorganisms associated with eye infections [210].

Benzethonium chloride is applied to wounds as an aqueous solution (0.1%) and as a solution (0.2%) in alcohol and acetone for preoperative skin disinfection and for controlling algal growth in swimming pools.

Cetrimide is used for cleaning and disinfecting burns and wounds and for preoperative cleansing of the skin. For general disinfecting purposes, a mixture (Savlon) of cetrimide with chlorhexidine is often employed. At pH 6, but not at pH 7.2, this product may be liable to contamination with *P. aeruginosa* [211]. Solutions containing 1–3% of cetrimide are employed as hair shampoos (e.g. Cetavlon P.C., a concentrate to be diluted with water before use) for seborrhea capitis and seborrheic dermatitis.

Cetylpyridinium chloride is employed pharmaceutically, for skin antisepsis and for antiseptic treatment of small wound surfaces (0.1–0.5% solutions), as an oral and pharyngeal antiseptic (e.g. lozenges containing 1–2 mg of the QAC) and as a preservative in emulsions. Cosmetically [212], it is used at a concentration of between 0.1% and 0.5% in hair preparations and in deodorants; lower concentrations (0.05–0.1%) are incorporated into face and shaving lotions.

In the veterinary context, the QACs have been used for the disinfection of automatic calf feeders and have been incorporated into sheep dips for controlling microbial growth in fleece and wool. However, QACs are not widely used on farm sites because of the large amount of organic debris they are likely to encounter.

In general, the QACs are very useful disinfectants and pharmaceutical and cosmetic preservatives. For further information on their uses and microbicidal properties see also BS 6471: 1984, BS EN 1276: 1997, BS 6424: 1984 and Reverdy [187].

Anionic agents

Anionic surface-active agents are compounds that, in aqueous solution, dissociate into a large complex anion (responsible for the surface activity) and a smaller cation. Examples of anionic surfactants are the alkali metal and metallic soaps, amine soaps, lauryl ether sulfates (e.g. sodium lauryl sulfate) and sulfated fatty alcohols.

Anionic surfactants have excellent detergent properties but have been generally considered to have little or no antibacterial action. However, this view is at odds with the literature, which reported the antibacterial potential of anionic and non-ionic surfactants as far back as the 1930s. Cowles [213] studied the bacteriostatic properties of a series of sodium alkyl sulfates and found that in general they inhibited the growth of Gram-positive bacteria, but not Gram-negative bacteria. Similar findings were published by Birkeland and Steinhaus [214] and Kabara [215]. Baker *et al.* [216] studied the bactericidal properties of a selection of anionic and cationic detergents and concluded that the anionics were much less effective than the cationics and were only effective against Gram-positive bacteria. Fatty acids have been shown to be active against Gram-positive but not Gram-negative bacteria [217, 218].

The benefits of anionic detergents in use are their stability and their lack of corrosive action. They also have wetting qualities resulting in a uniform film forming over the surface to be disinfected, thus producing a complete disinfecting action. Scales and Kemp [219] investigated the microbicidal properties of a range of anionic surfactants, including Triton 720, Aerosol OS, Aerosol OT, Aerosol DGA and various sulfonated oils. They concluded that solutions of such commercial surfactants possessed excellent microbicidal properties, particularly when the pH of the solution was acidic. Solutions of the surfactants at a pH of 4 possessed a germicidal action greater than that seen with sodium hypochlorite. At this pH they also found no difference in action of these anionic surfactants against Gram-positive and Gram-negative bacteria.

Non-ionic surface-active agents

These consist of a hydrocarbon chain attached to a non-polar water-attracting group, which is usually a chain of ethylene oxide units (e.g. cetomacrogols). The properties of non-ionic surfactants depend mainly on the proportions of hydrophilic and hydrophobic groups in the molecule. Other examples include the sorbitan derivatives, such as the polysorbates (Tweens).

The non-ionic surfactants are considered to have no microbicidal properties. However, low concentrations of polysorbates are believed to affect the permeability of the outer envelopes of Gram-negative cells, which are thus rendered more sensitive to various microbicidal agents. Non-ionic surfactants have also been shown to possess antifungal properties. The non-ionic surfactant Ag-98, which is 80% octyl phenoxypolyethoxyethanol, inhibited spore germination, germ tube growth and mycelial growth of *Botrytis cinerea*, *Mucor piriformis* and *Penicillium expansum*. It was also observed that Ag-98 had a potentiating effect on the antifungal activity of chlorine. The effect of alcohol ethoxylates on the green algae, *Chlamydomonas* spp., has also been demonstrated [220].

Pluronic F68 (polyoxyethylene-polyoxypropylene block co-polymer) has been shown to have an effect on membrane permeabilization and the enzyme activity of a batch culture of *Saccharomyces cerevisiae* [221]. Similar results were also seen with Triton X-100. These effects occurred at concentrations in excess of the CMC of the surfactants; no measurable effect was seen below these concentrations. More detailed information regarding the microbicidal activities of non-ionic (and anionic) surfactants, including structure–function relationships can be found in Moore [222].

High concentrations of Tweens overcome the activity of QACs, biguanides, parabens and phenolics. This is made use of in designing appropriate neutralizing agents [121, 223].

Amphoteric (ampholytic) agents

Amphoteric agents are compounds of mixed anionic–cationic character. They combine the detergent properties of anionic compounds with the bactericidal properties of the cationic ones. Their bactericidal activity remains virtually constant over a wide pH range and they are less readily inactivated than QACs by proteins. Examples of amphoteric agents include dodecyl-β-alanine, dodecyl-β-aminobutyric acid and dodecyl-di(aminoethyl)glycine. The last-named belongs to the Tego series of compounds, the name Tego being a trade name (Goldschmidt, Essen).

The Tego compounds are bactericidal to Gram-positive and Gram-negative bacteria, and, unlike the QACs and anionic and non-ionic agents, this includes the *Mycobacterium* spp. [224], although the rate of kill of these organisms is less than that of the others [225]. Compounds based on dodecyl-di(aminoethyl)glycine find use as disinfectants in the food industry [226].

Betaines are a group of amphoteric surfactants that have a similar structure to betaine or trimethylglycine, a natural constituent of beetroot and sugar beet obtained as a by-product of the sugar-beet industry. Such compounds are compatible with anionics and have high water solubility [227].

Analogs, in which one of the methyl groups is replaced by a long-chain alkyl residue (Figure 2.10), find application as detergents and as a basis for solubilizing or emulsifying phenolic microbicides. They have also been used in quaternary ammonium microbicides, but are not considered as microbicides per se.

Other chemical variants include the replacement of the –COOH group by –SO₃H (Figure 2.10) and of the two methyl groups by a ring system.

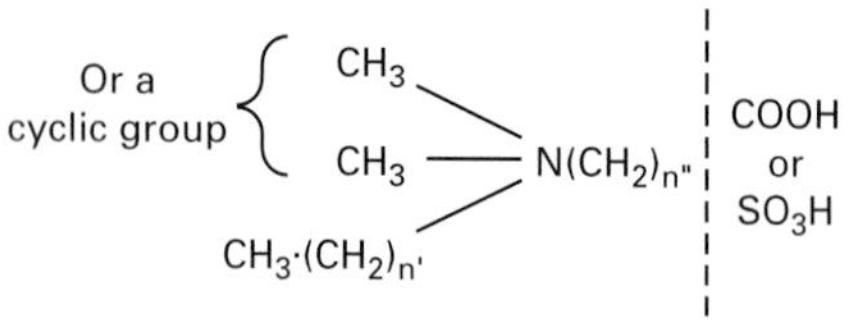

Aldehydes

Three aldehydes are of considerable importance as disinfectants, namely glutaraldehyde, formaldehyde and *ortho*-phthalaldehyde, although others have been studied and shown to possess microbicidal activity. Glyoxal (ethanedial), malonaldehyde (propanedial), succinaldehyde (butanedial) and adipaldehyde (hexanedial) all possess some sporicidal action, with aldehydes beyond adipaldehyde having virtually no sporicidal effects. This section on aldehydes will deal mainly with glutaraldehyde, formaldehyde and a "newer" aldehyde, *o*-phthalaldehyde.

Mode of action

Aldehydes act by alkylating various chemical groups associated with proteins and nucleic acids, which results in subsequent cross-linking of macromolecules.

Glutaraldehyde (pentanedial)
Chemistry of glutaraldehyde

Glutaraldehyde is a saturated five-carbon dialdehyde with an empirical formula of $C_5H_8O_2$ and a molecular weight of 100.12. Glutaraldehyde is usually obtained commercially as a 2%, 25% or 50% solution of acidic pH, although for disinfection purposes a 2% solution is normally supplied, which must be "activated" (made alkaline) before use.

The two aldehyde groups may react singly or together to form bisulfite complexes, oximes, cyanohydrins, acetals and hydrazones. Polymerization of the glutaraldehyde molecule occurs by means of the following possible mechanisms:

1. The dialdehyde exists as a monomer, with an equilibrium between the open-chain molecule and the hydrated ring structure (Figure 2.11a,b).

2. Ring formation occurs by an intramolecular mechanism, so that aqueous solutions of the aldehyde consist of free glutaraldehyde, the cyclic hemiacetal of its hydrate and oligomers of this in equilibrium (Figure 2.11c).

3. Different types of polymers may be formed at different pH values, and it is considered that polymers in the alkaline range are unable to revert to the monomer, whereas those in the neutral and acid range revert easily (Figure 2.12).

Polymerization increases with a rise in pH, and above pH 9 there is an extensive loss of aldehyde groups. Glutaraldehyde is more stable at acid than alkaline pH; solutions at pH 8 and above generally lose activity within 4 weeks. Novel formulations have

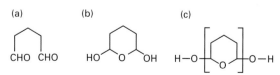

Figure 2.10 General structure of betaines ($n' = 14–16$, $n'' = 1$ or 2).

Figure 2.11 (a) Free glutaraldehyde, (b) hydrated ring structure (cyclic hemiacetal of its hydrate) and (c) oligomer.

been produced, and continue to be designed, to overcome the problems of loss of stability [228–230].

Interactions of glutaraldehyde

Glutaraldehyde is a highly reactive molecule. It reacts with various enzymes, but does not sterically alter them. The rate of reaction is pH dependent, increasing considerably over the pH range 4 to 9, and the reaction product is highly stable [231]. Glutaraldehyde prevents the dissociation of free ribosomes, but under the normal conditions of fixation little reaction appears to occur between nucleic acids and glutaraldehyde. There is little published information on the possible reactions of glutaraldehyde and lipids.

Mode of action

Glutaraldehyde possesses high microbicidal activity against bacteria and their spores, mycelial and spore forms of fungi and various types of viruses [232, 233]. Glutaraldehyde is considered to be an effective antimycobacterial agent [147, 234]. The mechanism of action of glutaraldehyde involves alkylation of hydroxyl, amino, carboxyl and sulfhydryl groups of microorganisms, which

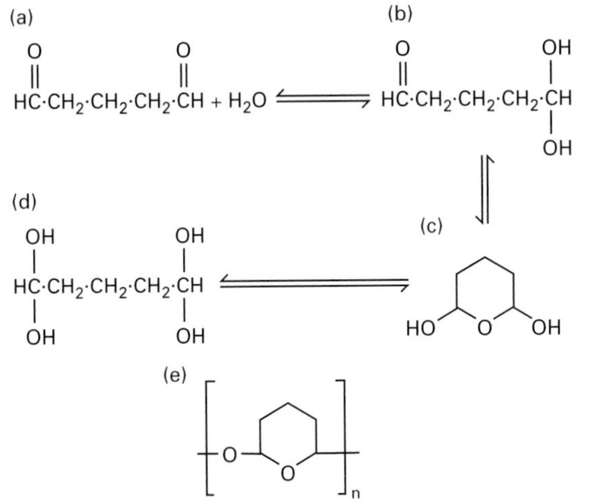

Figure 2.12 (a) Open-chain molecule of glutaraldehyde, (b–d) formation of several more stable "polymers" (hydrated) in aqueous alkaline solution, and (e) a polymer with an acetal-like structure, in neutral and acid ranges. (After Boucher [630])

affects RNA, DNA and protein synthesis [130]. Also, glutaraldehyde results in cross-linking of proteins and macromolecules in the cell envelope. The outer cell layers of spores, the cell wall of fungi (chitin) and the mycobacterial cell wall are believed to be the target sites for glutaraldehyde against bacterial spores, fungi and mycobacteria, respectively [130].

A summary of the microbicidal efficacy of glutaraldehyde is presented in Table 2.7, which demonstrates the effect of pH on its activity. However, acid-based products are also available commercially that claim to be of equal activity to potentiated alkaline glutaraldehyde. Acid glutaraldehyde is itself an effective microbicide provided that long contact periods are used. The fact that glutaraldehyde's rate of interaction with proteins and enzymes increases with increasing pH [231] is undoubtedly of importance. The cross-linking mechanism is also influenced by time, concentration and temperature [147, 148, 235, 236]. Acid glutaraldehyde is a markedly inferior disinfectant to alkaline glutaraldehyde, but this discrepancy disappears with increasing temperature. Resistance development to glutaraldehyde is a late event in sporulation [143, 147, 148, 237, 238] and sodium hydroxide-induced revival of spores of *Bacillus* spp. has been demonstrated [239–242].

Organic matter is considered to have no effect on the microbicidal activity of the aldehyde microbicidals. In view of the interaction of glutaraldehyde with the amino groups in proteins, this would appear to be a rather unusual finding. Dried spores are considerably more resistant to chemical disinfectants than are spores in suspension, and it would appear that glutaraldehyde is no exception. The use of the Association of Official Analytical Chemists (AOAC) test with dried spores of *B. subtilis* has shown that 2% alkaline glutaradehyde may require up to 10 h to meet sporicidal claims at 20°C [243]. The microbicidal activity of glutaraldehyde has been reviewed by Gorman *et al.* [229], Bruch [236], Russell [147], Ascenzi [244] and Power [230]. More recently reviews have tended to focus on the environmental and toxicological properties of glutaraldehyde [245, 246].

Uses of glutaraldehyde

Glutaraldehyde has been recommended for the disinfection/sterilization of certain types of medical equipment, notably cystoscopes and anesthetic equipment. Favero and Bond [247] have rightly drawn attention to the differences between physical

Table 2.7 Microbicidal activity of glutaraldehyde.[a]

Form of glutaraldehyde	Approximate pH value	Fungicidal activity[b]	Viricidal activity	Bactericidal activity[c]	Sporicidal activity
Acid	4–5	Low	Low to high	Low	Low to very high
Alkaline	8	High	High	High	Reasonable to very high

[a]See also Gorman *et al.* [229] and Russell [147].

[b]Use of low dialdehyde concentrations (0.01–0.02%); 2% solutions of acid and alkaline glutaraldehyde are both highly active against bacteria and probably viruses. A high-concentration (3.2%) glutaraldehyde solution is also available.

[c]Activity of acid glutaraldehyde increases markedly with temperature and at *c.* 37°C its activity approaches that of alkaline glutaraldehyde. Acid glutaraldehyde may also be sporicidal at ambient temperatures, provided that long periods of time (*c.* 10 h) are used.

methods of sterilization and liquid chemical microbicides and point out that 2% alkaline glutaraldehyde is capable of acting as a sporicidal agent, but only after prolonged periods of contact. Bearing this comment in mind, glutaraldehyde has long been used for the high-level disinfection of endoscopes, although problems have arisen because of its toxicity. Glutaraldehyde has also been employed for the disinfection of arthroscopes and laparoscopes. The US FDA has approved several commercial products containing glutaraldehyde in concentrations ranging from 2.4% to 3.5% w/v to be used as high-level disinfectants for the processing of reusable medical devices [248]. Glutaraldehyde has a broad spectrum of activity and rapid rate of killing, most vegetative bacteria being killed within a minute of exposure. Bacterial spores may require 3 h or more depending on the inherent resistance of spores.

Alkaline glutaraldehyde is more active, but less stable, than the acid form. However, 2% activated alkaline glutaraldehyde should not be used continuously to disinfect endoscopes for 14 days after activation, although it is effective over this period if not repeatedly reused [249, 250]. Babb and Bradley [249, 250] recommend reuse for endoscopes provided that the concentration does not fall appreciably below 1.5%. Glutaraldehyde possesses two aldehydic groups. The two groups are highly reactive and their presence is important for its microbicidal activity. The monomeric (active) molecule is in equilibrium with the polymeric (inactive) form. Physical conditions, such as temperature and pH, have a great effect on the equilibrium between these two forms. Accordingly, glutaraldehyde activity is much affected by pH of the solution, that is at pH 8 microbicidal activity is greatest, but stability is poor due to polymerization. In contrast acid solutions are more stable but they are less microbicidally effective and this is mainly due to polymerization. However, if temperature increases, there is a breakdown in the polymeric form, which exists in the acidic solution, and a concomitant increase in the free active monomeric dialdehyde (dial) and, hence, better microbicidal activity.

Problems in reusing glutaraldehyde are associated with accumulation of organic matter, dilution of disinfectant, change in product pH and difficulties in accurately assaying residual concentrations [251–253]. Color indicators are not always satisfactory [254]. Glutaraldehyde has been employed in the veterinary field for the disinfection of utensils and of premises [255], but its potential mutagenic and carcinogenic effects [255] make these uses hazardous to personnel. The main advantages claimed for glutaraldehyde are that it has a broad spectrum of activity with a rapid microbicidal action and that it is non-corrosive to metals, rubber and lenses. Its toxicity (see above) remains a problem and as such it is no longer used in some countries. In the market glutaraldehyde is mainly supplied as an acidic aqueous solution of 2% or more, which is stable for long-term storage. This acidic glutaraldehyde solution is "activated" before use by a suitable alkalinizing agent to bring the pH of the solution to its optimum activity, c. pH 8.0. The activated solution will have a shelf-life of about 2 weeks.

Ortho-phthaladehyde is also a suitable alternative to glutaraldehyde. It has been demonstrated to be an effective bactericidal agent [256], with activity also demonstrated against mycobacteria [257]; it is not an effective sporicide.

Formaldehyde (methanal)

Formaldehyde is used as a disinfectant as a liquid or vapor. The liquid form will be considered in this section. Formaldehyde vapor is not very active at temperatures below 20°C and requires a relative humidity (RH) of at least 70%.

The Health and Safety Executive of the UK previously indicated that the inhalation of formaldehyde vapor may be presumed to pose a carcinogenic risk to humans. This indication has had considerable impact on the role and use of formaldehyde and formaldehyde releasers in sterilization and disinfection processes.

Chemistry of formaldehyde

Formaldehyde occurs as formaldehyde solution (formalin), an aqueous solution containing c. 34–38% w/w CH_2O. Methyl alcohol is present to inhibit polymerization. Formaldehyde displays many typical chemical reactions, combining with amines to give methylolamines, carboxylic acids to give esters of methylene glycol, phenols to give methylphenols, and sulfides to produce thiomethylene glycols.

Interactions of formaldehyde

Formaldehyde interacts with protein molecules by attaching itself to the primary amide and amino groups, whereas phenolic moieties bind less well to the aldehyde. Subsequently, it has been shown that formaldehyde results in an intermolecular crosslinkage of protein or amino groups with phenolic or indole residues. In addition to interacting with many terminal groups in viral proteins, formaldehyde can also react extensively with the amino groups of nucleic acid bases, although it is much less reactive with deoxyribonucleic acid (DNA) than with ribonucleic acid (RNA).

Mode of action

Formaldehyde is a microbicidal agent, with lethal activity against bacteria and their spores, fungi and many viruses. Its first reported use as a disinfectant was in 1892. However, its sporicidal action is slower than that of glutaraldehyde [243]. Formaldehyde combines readily with proteins and is less effective in the presence of protein-containing matter. Plasmid-mediated resistance to formaldehyde has been described, presumably due to aldehyde degradation [258]. Formaldehyde vapor may be released by evaporating formalin solutions, by adding potassium permanganate to formalin or, alternatively, by heating, under controlled conditions, the polymer paraformaldehyde $(HO(CH_2O)_nH)$, urea formaldehyde or melamine formaldehyde. The activity of the vapor depends on aldehyde concentration, temperature and RH.

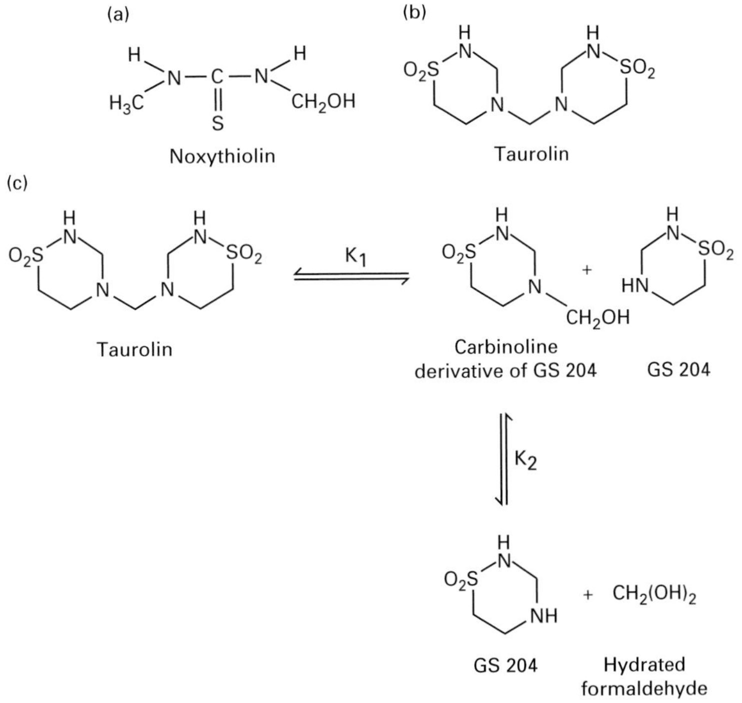

Figure 2.13 (a) Noxythiolin, (b) taurolin and (c) postulated equilibrium of taurolin in aqueous solution. (After Myers *et al.* [631])

Formaldehyde-releasing agents

Noxythiolin (oxymethylenethiourea; Figure 2.13a) is a bactericidal agent [259–261] that apparently owes its activity to the release of formaldehyde [259, 262, 263]. Noxythiolin has been found to protect animals from lethal doses of endotoxin [260, 264] and is claimed to be active against fungi and against all bacteria, including those resistant to other types of antibacterial agents [261].

Noxythiolin has been widely used both topically and in accessible body cavities, notably as an irrigation solution in the treatment of peritonitis [262]. Unfortunately, solutions are rather unstable (after preparation they should be stored at 10°C and used within 7 days). Commercially, noxythiolin is available as Noxyflex S and Noxyflex (Geistlich Ltd, Chester, UK), the latter containing amethocaine hydrochloride as well as noxythiolin. Solutions of Noxyflex (containing 1% or 2.5% noxythiolin) are employed where local discomfort is experienced.

The amino acid taurine was used as the starting point in the design of the novel antibacterial agent, taurolin (Figure 2.13b), which is a condensate of two molecules of taurine and three molecules of formaldehyde. Taurolin (bis(1,1-dioxoperhydro-1,2,4-thiazinyl-4)methane) is water soluble and is stable in aqueous solution. It has a wide spectrum of microbicidal activity *in vitro* and *in vivo* [265–268] and has been shown to be an effective antifungal agent [269].

Taurine is considered to act as a non-toxic formaldehyde carrier, donating methylol groups to bacterial protein and endotoxin [266]. According to Browne *et al.* [266], taurine has a lower

affinity for formaldehyde than bacterial protein, but a greater affinity than animal protein, the consequence of which is a selective lethal effect. Taurolin has been shown to protect experimental animals from the lethal effects of *E. coli* and *Bacteroides fragilis* endotoxin [270]

This viewpoint, that the activity of taurolin results from a release of formaldehyde, which is adsorbed by bacterial cells, is however no longer tenable. When taurolin is dissolved in water, an equilibrium is established (Figure 2.13c) to release two molecules of the monomer (1,1-dioxoperhydro-1,2,4-thiadizine (GS 204)) and its carbinolamine derivative. The antibacterial activity of taurolin is considerably greater than that of free formaldehyde [271] and Allwood and colleagues thus concluded that the activity of taurolin was not due entirely to bacterial adsorption of free formaldehyde, but also to a reaction with a masked (or latent) formaldehyde. Since GS 204 has only a low antibacterial effect, then the carbinolamine must obviously play an important role. Clinically, the intraperitoneal administration of taurolin has been shown to bring about a significant reduction of morbidity in peritonitis [268].

A third formaldehyde-releasing agent is hexamine (methenamine). Hexamine itself is inactive, but it breaks down by acid hydrolysis to release formaldehyde. It has been reviewed by Allwood and Myers [271].

Uses of formaldehyde

Formaldehyde is employed as a disinfectant in both the liquid and gaseous states. Vapor-phase formaldehyde is used in the disinfection of sealed rooms. The vapor can be produced as described above, or alternatively an equal volume of industrial methylated spirits (IMS) can be added to formaldehyde and the mixture used as a spray. Other uses of formaldehyde vapor have been summarized by Russell [272]. These include the following: low-temperature steam plus formaldehyde vapor (LTSF) for the disinfection/sterilization of heat-sensitive medical materials; hospital bedding and blankets; and fumigation of poultry houses, of considerable importance in hatchery hygiene [273].

Aerobic spores exposed to liquid formaldehyde can be revived by a sublethal post-heat treatment [274, 275]. Revival of LTSF-treated *Geobacillus stearothermophilus* spores can also be accomplished by such means [276], which casts considerable doubt on the efficacy of LTSF as a potential sterilizing process.

Formaldehyde in liquid form has been used as a virucidal agent in the production of certain types of viral vaccines, such as polio (inactivated) vaccine. Formaldehyde solution has also been employed for the treatment of warts, as an antiseptic mouthwash, for the disinfection of membranes in dialysis equipment and as a preservative in hair shampoos. Formaldehyde-releasing agents were considered in the previous section. Formaldehyde and formaldehyde-condensates have been reviewed in depth by Rossmore and Sondossi [277].

Ortho-phthalaldehyde
Chemistry of ortho-phthalaldehyde
Ortho-phthalaldehyde (OPA) (Figure 2.14) is an aromatic aldehyde. It is used as 0.55% 1,2-benzenedicarboxaldehyde solution. OPA solution is a clear, pale-blue liquid with a pH of 7.5 [194].

Interactions of ortho-phthalaldehyde
OPA has been shown to interact with amino acids, proteins and microorganisms, although not as effectively as glutaraldehyde. However, OPA is lipophilic, aiding uptake through the cell walls of Gram-negative bacteria and mycobacteria, compensating for its lower cross-linking ability compared with glutaraldehyde [278]. Its microbicidal activity has been shown to result from a sequence of events: binding to membrane receptors due to cross-linkage; impairing the membrane functions, allowing the microbicide to enter through the permeabilized membrane; and interacting with intracellular reactive molecules, such as RNA, compromising the growth cycle of the cells and, at last, with DNA [279].

Mode of action
OPA is a high-level disinfectant that received US FDA clearance in 1999 [194]. OPA has been shown to have potent bactericidal

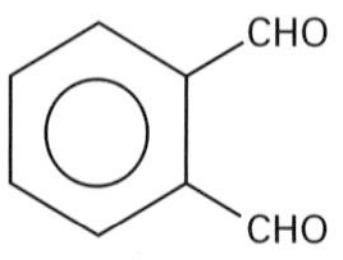

Figure 2.14 *Ortho*-phthalaldehyde (OPA).

and virucidal activity [256, 257, 280–284]. It is also active against mycobacteria, including glutaraldehyde-resistant strains [285].

Some sporicidal activity has also been reported for this agent, but activity is not nearly as good as that seen against vegetative cells. The spore coat appears to be a significant factor in this reduced activity but is not the only factor as OPA appears to demonstrate sporicidal activity by blocking the spore germination process [285, 286].

Uses of ortho-phthalaldehyde
OPA has several potential advantages over glutaraldehyde [283, 287] as follows: it does not irritate the eyes and nasal passages,; it does not require activation or exposure monitoring; it has excellent stability over a wide pH range (pH 3 to 9); it does not coagulate blood or fix tissues to surfaces; its odor is barely detectable; and a short exposure time is required to achieve high-level disinfection. However, it causes staining to environmental surfaces and clothing. OPA stains proteins gray, thus it stains skin and mucous membranes and therefore it should be handled carefully with protective gloves, and copious water rinsing is needed for instruments disinfected with it to prevent patient skin or mouth discoloration.

OPA solution is approved by the US FDA to be used as high-level disinfectant for endoscopes (manually and in automated systems) and for reprocessing heat-sensitive medical devices [248]. It has been shown to be compatible with instruments made from various materials [283]. A hundred cycles of high-level disinfection of a ureteroscope with OPA did not show significant adverse effect on its structure or function [288].

In April 2004, the manufacturer of OPA (DSM Gist, Netherlands) released information to users about patients who experienced an anaphylaxis-like reaction after cystoscopy where the scope had been reprocessed using OPA. Twenty-four cases out of approximately 1 million urological procedures performed using instruments reprocessed using OPA have reported anaphylaxis-like reactions after repeated cystoscopy (typically after four to nine treatments). Preventive measures suggested include the removal of OPA residues by thorough rinsing and not using OPA for reprocessing urological instrumentation used to treat patients with a history of bladder cancer [194]. Glycine (5 g/l) can be used to neutralize OPA to make it safe for disposal through the sanitary sewer system [194].

Other aldehydes
Other aldehydes have been studied, but results have sometimes been conflicting and they have thus been reinvestigated [289]. Sporicidin (containing 1.12% glutaraldehyde plus 1.93% phenol/phenate) and aldahol III (containing 3.4% glutaraldehyde plus 26% isopropanol) were approved by the FDA in 2009 for device sterilization and high-level disinfection [248]. Gigasept, containing butan-1,4-dial, dimethoxytetrahydrofuran and formaldehyde, and used at 5% and 10% v/v dilutions, is considerably less active [289]. Glyoxal (2%) is weakly sporicidal, and butyraldehyde has no activity. It is essential that adequate procedures are employed to remove residual glutaraldehyde (and phenol/

phenate, if present) or other aldehydes in determining survivor levels. The properties and uses of various aldehydes have been reviewed by Bartoli and Dusseau [290].

Microbicidal dyes

There are three main groups of dyes that find application as microbicidal agents: the acridines, the triphenylmethane group and the quinones. Halogenated fluorescein (hydroxyxanthene) dyes have also been demonstrated to possess microbicidal activity against *S. aureus* [291, 292].

Acridines
Chemistry of acridines
The acridines (Figure 2.15) are heterocyclic compounds that have proved to be of some value as microbicidal agents. Acridine itself is weakly basic, but two of the five possible monoaminoacridines are strong bases, and these (3-aminoacridine and 9-aminoacridine) exist as the resonance hybrid of two canonical formulae. Both these monoacridines are well ionized as the cation at pH 7.3 and this has an important bearing on their microbicidal activity (Table 2.8). Further information on the chemistry of the acridines can be found in Wainright's comprehensive review [293].

Mode of action
Acridines and their derivatives are known to be broad chemotherapeutic agents. They have antibacterial, antimalarial and antitumor activity [293–295]. These activities are related to the high affinity and interaction of acridines with DNA. The polycyclic planar structure of acridines is inserted between the base pairs of the DNA structure. This intercalation will interfere with the major metabolic processes. In addition, some acridine derivatives have been shown to interfere with critical enzymes such as topoisomerase and telomerase and to target multidrug resistance processes [296, 297].

The acridines are of considerable interest because they illustrate how small changes in the chemical structure of the molecule cause significant changes in antibacterial activity. The most important limiting factor governing this activity is the degree of ionization, although this must be cationic in nature (Table 2.8). Acridine derivatives that form anions or zwitterions are only poorly antibacterial in comparison with those that form cations.

Table 2.8 Dependence of antibacterial activity of acridines on cationic ionization (based on Albert [635]).

Substance	Predominant type (and percentage) of ionization at pH 3 and 37°C	Inhibitory activity
9-Aminoacridine	Cation (99%)	High
9-Aminoacridine-2-carboxylic acid	Zwitterion (99.8%)	Low
Acridine	Neutral molecule (99.7%)	Low
Acridine-9-carboxylic acid	Anion (99.3%)	Low

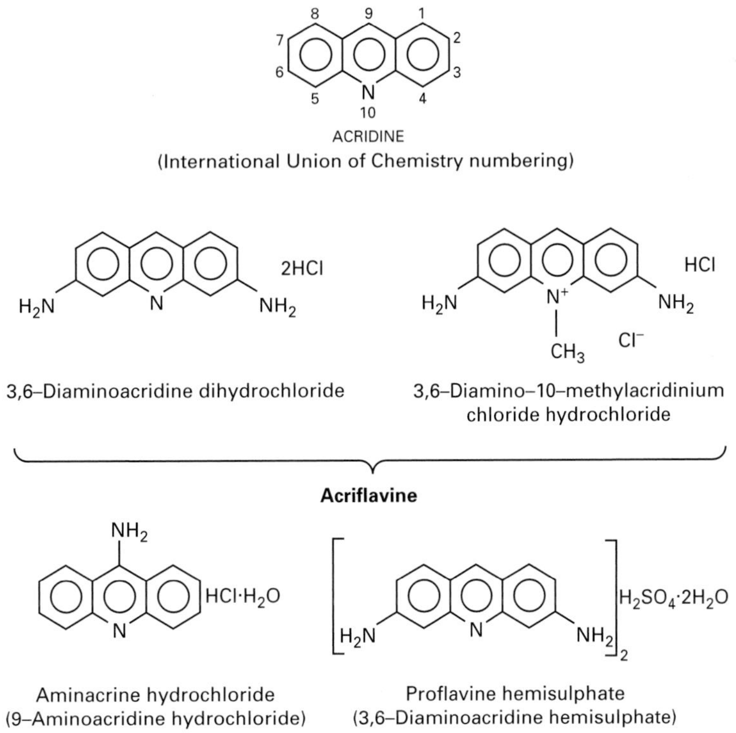

ACRIDINE
(International Union of Chemistry numbering)

3,6–Diaminoacridine dihydrochloride

3,6–Diamino–10–methylacridinium chloride hydrochloride

Acriflavine

Aminacrine hydrochloride
(9–Aminoacridine hydrochloride)

Proflavine hemisulphate
(3,6–Diaminoacridine hemisulphate)

Figure 2.15 Acridine compounds.

In general terms, if the degree of ionization is less than 33% there is only weak antibacterial activity, whereas above about 50% there is little further increase in activity. Acridines do not display a selective action against Gram-positive organisms, nor are they inactivated by serum. Acridines compete with H⁺ ions for anionic sites on the bacterial cell and are more effective at alkaline than acid pH. They are relatively slow in their action and are not sporicidal [298]. Resistance to the acridines develops as a result of mutation and indirect selection [299, 300]. Interestingly, acridines can eliminate resistance in R⁺ strains [301]. Viljanen and Boratynski [302] provide interesting information about plasmid curing. The microbicidal activity of aminoacridines has been shown to be increased on illumination with low-power white light [303, 304]. However, attempts at increasing the degree of bacterial DNA intercalation and, hence, microbicidal activity by synthesis of dimeric bis(aminoacridines) did not lead to increased activity [304]. MRSA and methicillin-resistant *Staphylococcus epidermidis* (MRSE) strains are more resistant to acridines than are antibiotic-sensitive strains, although this resistance depends on the presence of *qac* genes, especially *qac*A or *qac*B [305].

Uses of acridines

For many years, the acridines held a valuable place in medicine. However, with the advent of antibiotics and other chemotherapeutic agents, they are now used infrequently. Their major use has been the treatment of infected wounds. The first compound to be used medically was acriflavine (a mixture of 3,6-diaminoacridine hydrochloride and 3,6-diamino-10-methylacridinium hydrochloride, the former component being better known as proflavine). Proflavine hemisulfate and 9-aminoacridine (aminacrine) have found use in treating wounds; aminacrine is particularly useful as it is non-staining. Recently, and based on acridine's mechanism of action and affinity towards DNA, several acridine derivatives are being synthesized, which have shown potential

activity as anticancer agent. In addition, some have shown potential impact on Alzheimer's disease [295] and as antiviral drugs [295, 297, 306].

Triphenylmethane dyes

The most important members of this group are crystal violet, brilliant green and malachite green (Figure 2.16). These were used as local antiseptics for application to wounds and burns, but were limited in being effective against Gram-positive bacteria (inhibitory concentrations 1 in 750,000 to 1 in 5,000,000), but much less so against Gram-negative organisms, and in suffering a serious decrease in activity in the presence of serum. Their selective activity against Gram-positive bacteria has a practical application in the formulation of selective media for diagnostic purposes, for example crystal violet lactose broth in water filtration control work. The triphenylmethane dyes are fungistatic.

The activity of the triphenylmethane dyes is a property of the pseudobase, the formation that is established by equilibrium between the cation and the base; thus, both the ionization and the equilibrium constants will affect the activity. Microbicidal potency depends on external pH, being more pronounced at alkaline values [307].

MRSA and MRSE strains containing *qac* genes are more resistant to crystal violet than are plasmidless strains of *S. aureus* and *S. epidermidis*, respectively [305]. This is believed to be the result of an efficient efflux system in the resistant strains [308, 309]. However, crystal violet finds little, if any, use nowadays as an antibacterial agent, and the clinical relevance of this finding thus remains uncertain [26, 310].

Quinones

Quinones are natural dyes that give color to many forms of plant and animal life. Chemically (Figure 2.17), they are

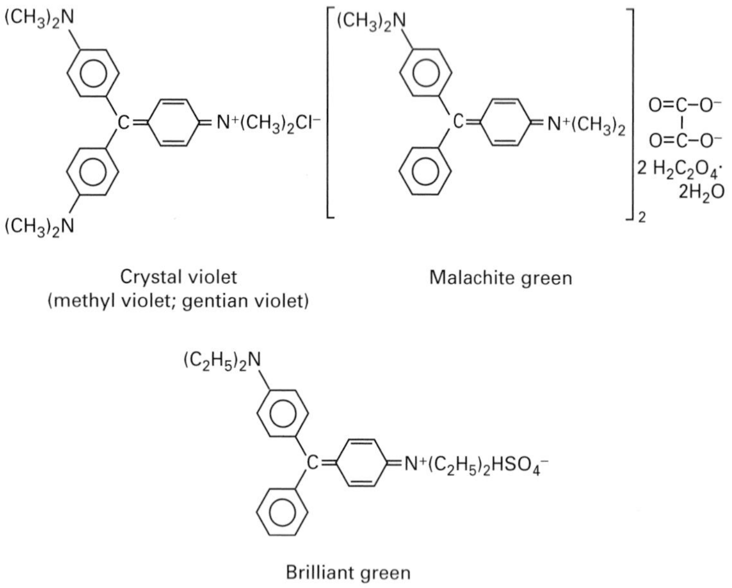

Crystal violet
(methyl violet; gentian violet)

Malachite green

Brilliant green

Figure 2.16 Triphenylmethane dyes.

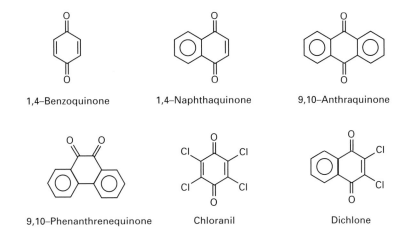

Figure 2.17 Quinones.

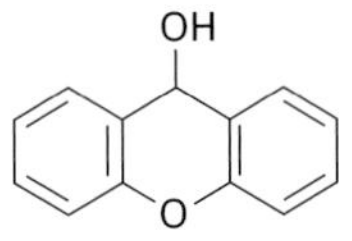

Figure 2.18 General structure of 9-hydroxyxanthene.

diketocyclohexadienes; the simplest member is 1,4-benzoquinone. In terms of toxicity to bacteria, molds and yeast, naphthaquinones are the most toxic, followed (in this order) by phenanthrenequinones, benzoquinones and anthraquinones.

Microbicidal activity is increased by halogenation, and two powerful agricultural fungicides are chloranil (tetrachloro-1,4-benzoquinone) and dichlone (2,3-dichloro-1,4-naphthaquinone); see D'Arcy [201] and Owens [311].

Halogenated fluorescein (hydroxyxanthene)

The hydroxyxanthenes (Figure 2.18) are primarily used as dyestuffs in the food, cosmetics and textile industries. However, they also have clinical applications due to their staining, fluorescent and microbicidal properties. The halogenated hydroxyxanthenes exhibit microbicidal properties that may be useful for reducing or eliminating bacterial pathogens from a variety of environments, including drinking water and food products. The mode of action of the hydroxyxanthenes is photo-oxidation, by which a variety of cytotoxic compounds are produced (e.g. singlet oxygen, superoxide anion and other radicals). Gram-positive bacteria exhibit species-specific sensitivity to the halogenated hydroxyxanthenes. Gram-negative bacteria are more tolerant to inactivation by these compounds due to the barrier properties of the outer membrane [292].

Halogens

The most important microbicidal halogens are iodine compounds, chlorine compounds and bromine. Fluorine is far too toxic, irritant and corrosive for use as a disinfectant [312], although, interestingly, fluoride ions have been shown to induce bacterial lysis [313]. This section will deal predominantly with iodine, iodophors and chlorine-releasing compounds (those which are bactericidal by virtue of "available chlorine"), but bromine, iodoform and chloroform will also be considered briefly. A more detailed treatment of the chemistry, bactericidal activity and uses of chlorine and chlorine-based microbicides can be found in Khanna and Naidu [314].

Iodine compounds
Free iodine

Iodine was first employed in the treatment of wounds some 140 years ago and has been shown to be an efficient microbicidal agent with rapid lethal effects against bacteria and their spores, molds, yeasts and viruses [315]. The active agent in elemental iodine (I_2) is only slightly soluble in water; iodide ions are needed to prepare an aqueous solution of iodine (Lugol's solution BP 1988, 5% iodine, 10% potassium iodide). Tincture of iodine (alcoholic solution of iodine) can be prepared by using 2.5% iodine, 2.5% potassium iodide and ethanol (90%) (weak solution of iodine BP 1988). Iodine is less reactive chemically than chlorine, and is less affected by the presence of organic matter than is the latter. However, whereas the activity of high concentrations of iodine is little affected by organic matter, that of low concentrations is significantly reduced. The activity of iodine is greater at acid than at alkaline pH (Table 2.9). Unfortunately, iodine

Table 2.9 Effect of pH on the microbicidal activity of iodine compounds (based on Trueman [312]).

pH	Active form	Comment
Acid and neutral	I_2 (diatomic iodine)	Highly bactericidal
	Hypo-iodous acid	Less bactericidal
Alkaline	Hypo-iodide ion	Even less bactericidal
	Iodate (IO_3^-), iodide	
	(I^-) and tri-iodide	
	(I_3^-) ions	All inactive

solutions stain skin and fabrics, sensitize skin and mucous membranes and tend to be toxic. The microbicidal activity of iodine covers Gram-positive and Gram-negative bacteria, bacterial spores, mycobacteria, fungi and viruses. Its activity is less dependent on temperature and pH.

The microbicidal activity of iodine incorporated in an enzyme-based disinfectant has been reported by Duan *et al.* [316]. This disinfectant is a powder concentrate composed of sodium iodide, horseradish peroxidase, citric acid and calcium peroxide. Horseradish peroxidase catalyses the oxidation of iodide to molecular iodine in the presence of water:

$$2H^+ + 2I^- + 2H_2O_2 \rightarrow I_2 + H_2O$$

This system is able to reoxidize reduced iodine giving the advantage of a controlled and continuous release of active iodine and demonstrates rapid bactericidal, fungicidal and virucidal activity.

Iodophors

Iodophors (iodine carriers) are complexes of iodine and compounds that act as carriers or solubilizers for iodine. They allow slow, sustained release of iodine from the complex. Iodophors were developed to eliminate the undesirable properties of iodine while maintaining its microbicidal activity. The complexing agent could be a cationic surfactant (quaternary ammonium) iodophor, non-ionic (ethoxylated) iodophor, polyoxymer (with propylene or ethylene oxide polymers) iodophor and polyvinylpyrrolidone iodophor (povidone-iodine (PVP-I)) [77, 143] (Figure 2.19). The surfactant iodophors combine microbicidal activity with detergency. In most iodophor preparations, the carrier is usually a non-ionic surfactant, in which the iodine is present as micellar aggregates. When an iodophor is diluted with water, dispersion of the micelles occurs and most (80–90%) of the iodine is slowly liberated. Dilution below the critical micelle concentration (CMC) of the non-ionic surface-active agent results in iodine being in simple aqueous solution. A paradoxical effect of dilution on the activity of povidone-iodine has been observed [317, 318]. As the degree of dilution increases, then beyond a certain point bactericidal activity also increases. An explanation of this arises from consideration of physicochemical studies, which demonstrate that, starting from a 10% commercially available povidone-iodine solution, the concentration of

non-complexed iodine (I_2) initially increases as dilution increases. This reaches a maximum value at about 0.1% and then falls. In contrast, the content of other iodine species (e.g. I^- and I_3^-) decreases continuously. These properties affect the sporicidal activity of iodine solutions [319].

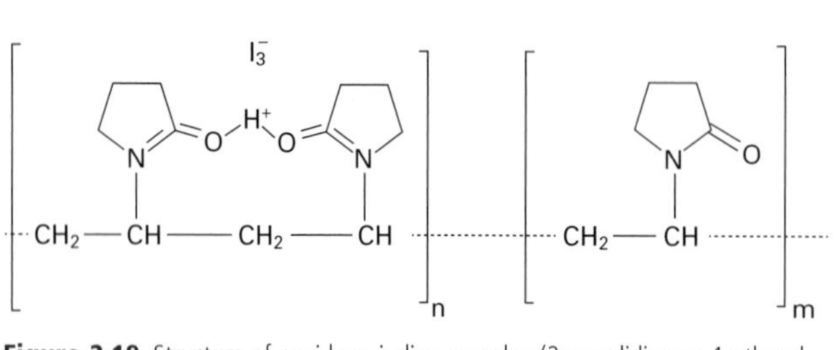

The iodophors, as stated above, are microbicidal, with activity over a wide pH range. The presence of a surface-active agent as carrier improves the wetting capacity. It must be noted that different concentrations of iodophors are used for antiseptic and disinfectant purposes, and that the lower concentrations employed in antisepsis are not claimed to be sporicidal [320].

Gershenfeld [321] has shown that povidone-iodine is sporicidal, and Lowbury *et al.* [322] found that povidone-iodine compresses reduced the numbers of viable spores of *Bacillus globigii* on the skin by >99% in 1 h, suggesting that this iodophor had a part to play in removing transient sporing organisms from operation sites. However, the US FDA has not approved any chemical sterilizing agent or high-level disinfectant with an iodophor as main ingredient, as there is no proven efficacy against bacterial spores, mycobacteria and some fungi [323, 324]. The importance of povidone-iodine in preventing wound infection was re-emphasized as a result of the studies of Galland *et al.* [325] and Lacey [326]. Povidone-iodine has been shown to be effective against a range of MRSA, *Chlamydia*, Herpes simplex, adenoviruses and enteroviruses [327] and produced significant reductions in skin microflora, demonstrating its suitability as a pre-surgical hand treatment [328]. More in-depth information regarding the physical properties and microbicidal activity of povidone-iodine can be found in Barabas and Brittain [329].

The concentration of free iodine in aqueous or alcoholic iodine solutions is responsible for microbicidal activity. Likewise, the concentration of free iodine in an iodophor is responsible for its activity.

Iodophors may be used in the dairy industry (when employed in the cleansing of dairy plant it is important to keep the pH on the acid side to ensure adequate removal of milkstone) and for skin and wound antisepsis. Iodophors, such as Betadine, in the form of alcoholic solutions are widely used in the USA for antisepsis of hands before invasive procedures such as operations and obstetrics. Leung *et al.* [330] demonstrated that warming povidone-iodine for use before amniocentesis to increase patient comfort still gives the desired level of microbicidal efficacy. Pseudobacteraemia (false-positive blood cultures) has been found to result from the use of contaminated antiseptics. Craven *et al.* [331] have described such an outbreak of pseudobacteraemia caused by a 10% povidone-iodine solution contaminated with *Burkholderia cepacia*.

Cadexomer-I_2 is an iodophor. It consists of spherical hydrophilic beads of dextrin and epichlorhydrin that contains iodine 0.9% w/w. It is highly absorbent and releases iodine slowly in the wound area. It is used for its absorbent and antiseptic properties in the management and healing of skin ulcers, venous leg ulcers and pressure sores [77, 332]. It has shown activity against *P. aeruginosa*, MRSA and *S. aureus* biofilms [333–335]. The mechanism

Figure 2.19 Structure of povidone-iodine complex (2-pyrrolidinone, 1-ethenyl-, homopolymer) compared with iodine.

by which it induces healing of wounds is believed to be related to the induction of proinflammatory cytokines and vascular endothelial growth factor [336].

Mode of action

Iodine can penetrate the cell wall of microorganisms quickly. It reacts with and oxidizes thiol groups that occur in the cytoplasm. Therefore, the lethal effects are believed to result from the disruption of protein and nucleic acid structure and synthesis [10].

Chlorine compounds
Chlorine-releasing compounds

Until the development of chlorinated soda solution (Dakin's surgical solution) in 1916, the commercial chlorine-releasing disinfectants then in use were not of constant composition and contained free alkali and sometimes free chlorine. The stability of free available chlorine in solution is dependent on a number of factors, especially: (i) chlorine concentration; (ii) pH of organic matter; and (iii) light [337].

The types of chlorine compounds that are most frequently used are the hypochlorites and *N*-chloro compounds [189, 247, 312, 337–340]. Chlorine compounds are commonly used as sanitizing agents in the food industry due to their high microbicidal efficacy, low toxicity to humans, range of applications and low cost, but suffer the disadvantages of being irritant and corrosive. The organochlorines are less irritating and corrosive than inorganic chlorines and have a greater stability, but are slower acting in terms of bactericidal efficacy by comparison.

Hypochlorites have a wide bactericidal spectrum, although they are less active against spores than against non-sporulating bacteria and have been stated to be of low activity against mycobacteria [224]. It has been suggested that chlorine compounds are among the most potent sporicidal agents [341]. The hypochlorites show activity against lipid and non-lipid viruses [340, 342].

Two factors that can affect quite markedly their microbicidal action are organic matter, since chlorine is a highly reactive chemical, and pH, the hypochlorites being more active at acid than at alkaline pH (Table 2.10). Acid pH promotes the hydro-

lysis of HOCl. The former problem can, to some extent, be overcome by increasing the hypochlorite concentration, and it has been shown that the sporicidal activity of sodium hypochlorite (200 parts/10^6 available chlorine) can be potentiated by 1.5–4% sodium hydroxide, notwithstanding the above comment about pH [315, 343]. The sporicidal activity can also be potentiated by low concentrations of ammonia and in the presence of bromine; chlorine-resistant bacteria have been found to be unaffected by bromine, but to be readily killed by chlorine–bromine solutions. Such mixtures could be of value in the disinfection of natural waters.

Organic chlorine compounds (*N*-chloro compounds), which contain the =N–Cl group, show microbicidal activity. Examples of such compounds, the chemical structures of which are shown in Figure 2.20, are chloramine-T, dichloramine-T, halazone, halane, dichloroisocyanuric acid, sodium and potassium dichloroisocyanurates and trichloroisocyanuric acid. All appear to hydrolyze in water to produce an imino (=NH) group. Their action is claimed to be slower than that of the hypochlorites, although this can be increased under acidic conditions. A series of imidazolidinone *N′,N′*-dihalamine disinfectants has been described [344–346]. The dibromo compound (Figure 2.20) was the most rapidly acting bactericide, particularly under halogen demand-free conditions, with the mixed bromo–chloro compound (Figure 2.20) occupying an intermediate position. However, when stability of the compounds in the series was also taken into account, it was concluded that the mixed product was the most useful as an aqueous disinfectant solution.

Coates [347] found that solutions of sodium hypochlorite (NaOCl) and sodium dichloroisocyanurate (NaDCC) containing the same levels of available chlorine had similar bactericidal activity despite significant differences in their pH. Solutions of NaDCC are less susceptible than NaOCl to inactivation by organic matter [347–349]. Hypochlorite- and monochloramine-based compounds have been shown to inactivate biofilm bacteria effectively [350, 351].

Uses of Chlorine-releasing compounds

Chlorinated soda solution (Dakin's solution), which contains 0.5–0.55% (5000–5500 ppm) available chlorine, and chlorinated lime and boric acid solution (Eusol), which contains 0.25% (2500 ppm) available chlorine, are chlorine disinfectants that contain chlorinated lime and boric acid. Dakin's solution is used as a wound antiseptic or, when appropriately diluted, as an irrigation solution for bladder and vaginal infections. Eusol is used as a wound antiseptic, but Morgan [352] has suggested that chlorinated solutions delay wound healing.

Chlorine gas has been employed to disinfect public water supplies. Sodium hypochlorite is normally used for the disinfection of swimming pools. Chloramine-T, dichloramine-T and halazone are used to disinfect contaminated drinking water [77, 353].

Blood spillages containing human immunodeficiency virus (HIV) or hepatitis B virus can be disinfected with NaOCl solutions containing 10,000 ppm available chlorine [354]. Added

Table 2.10 Factors influencing activity of hypochlorites.

Factor	Result
pH	Activity decreased by increasing pH (see text and use of NaOH also)
Concentration of hypochlorite (pH constant)	Activity depends on concentration of available chlorine
Organic matter	Microbicidal activity reduced considerably
Other agents	Potentiation may be achieved by: • addition of ammonia • 1.5–4% sodium hydroxide • addition of small amounts of bromide[a]

[a]In the presence of bromide, hypochlorite also has an enhanced effect in bleaching cellulosic fibres.

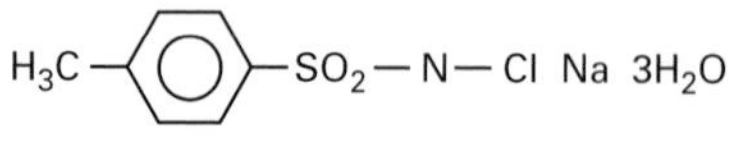

Chloramine T
(sodium-*p*-toluene-sulphonchloramide)

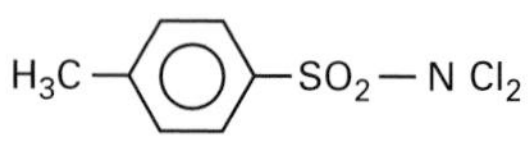

Dichloramine T
(*p*-toluene-sulphondichloramide)

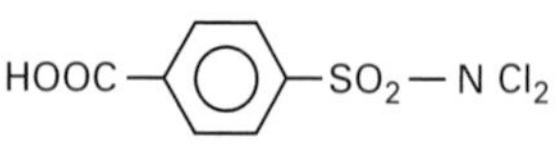

Halazone
(*p*-sulphondichloramide benzoic acid)

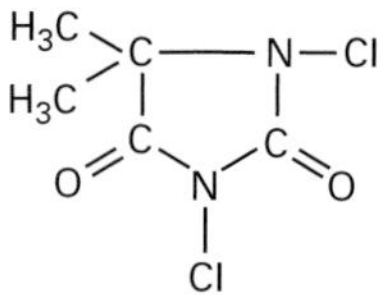

Halane

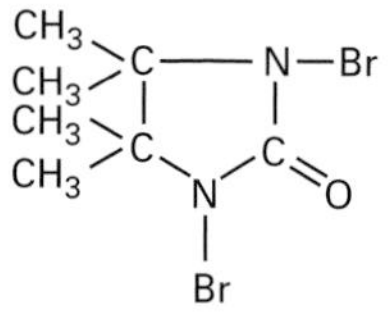

1,3-dibromo-4,4,5,5-
tetramethyl-2-imidazoldinone

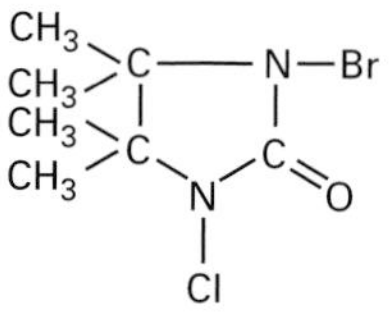

1-bromo-3-chloro-4,4,5,5-
tetramethyl-2-imidazolidinone

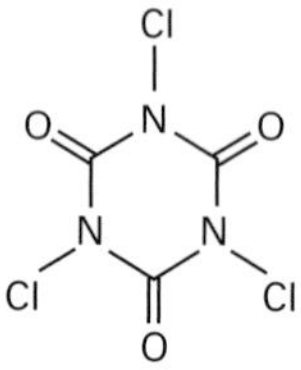

Trichloroisocyanuric acid

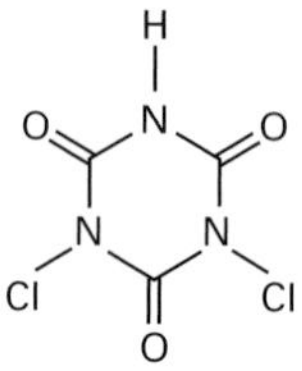

Dichloroisocyanuric acid

Figure 2.20 Organic chlorine compounds.

directly to the spillage as powder or granules, NaDCC is also effective, may give a larger margin of safety because a higher concentration of available chlorine is achieved, and is also less susceptible to inactivation by organic matter, as pointed out above [349]. Furthermore, only a very short contact time (2–3 min) is necessary before the spill can be removed safely [355]. Chlorine-releasing powder formulations with high available chlorine concentrations are particularly useful for this purpose [356, 357].

Chlorine dioxide, an alternative to sodium hypochlorite, retains its microbicidal activity over a wide pH range [358] and in the presence of organic matter and is more environmentally satisfactory. A low concentration of chlorine dioxide gas was shown to have a protective effect against influenza A virus [359]. Oxine (Bio-cide International Inc., USA) is a sodium chlorite solution that when acidified generates chlorine dioxide, giving a final solution which is a mixture of chlorite and chlorine dioxide. This product is an Environmental Protection Agency (EPA) registered disinfection compound and is more efficacious in controlling the growth of pathogenic bacteria compared with chlorine dioxide alone [360].

Chlorine-releasing agents continue to be widely studied. Their sporicidal activity has been described by Te Giffel *et al.* [361] and Coates [362], their antiviral efficacy by Bellamy [363], van Bueren [364], Bond [365] and Hernandez *et al.* [366, 367] and their usefulness in dental practice by Molinari [153], Cottone and Molinari [154] and Gurevich *et al.* [368].

Mode of action

The exact mechanism by which chlorine destroys microbial cells is still unknown. However, it is believed that chlorine activity against microorganisms involves several targets, such as oxidation of sulfhydryl enzymes and amino acids; ring chlorination of amino acids; cell wall and membrane disruption by attacking structural proteins, carbohydrates and lipids; loss of intracellular contents; decreased uptake of nutrients; inhibition of protein synthesis; decreased oxygen uptake; disruption of oxidative phosphorylation and other membrane-associated enzymes activities; direct protein degradation into smaller polypeptides and precipitation; decreased adenosine triphosphate production; and breaks in DNA and depressed DNA synthesis [369].

Chloroform

Chloroform ($CHCl_3$) has been used as a preservative in many pharmaceutical products intended for internal use, for more than a century. In recent years, with the object of minimizing microbial contamination, this use has been extended. Various authors, notably Westwood and Pin-Lim [370] and Lynch *et al.* [371] have shown chloroform to be a bactericidal agent, although it is not sporicidal and its high volatility means that a fall in concentration could result in microbial growth. For details of its antibacterial activity in aqueous solutions and in mixtures containing insoluble powders and the losses, through volatilization, under "in-use" conditions, see the paper by Lynch *et al.* [371].

Chloroform does not appear as an approved material in the latest version of *Cosmetics Directive* [372], but is still listed in the *British Pharmacopoeia* [18] as a general anesthetic and a preservative. It is totally banned in the USA.

Bromine

The microbicidal activity of bromine was first observed in the 1930s, but it was not until the 1960s that it was used commercially in water disinfection. The most commonly used oxidizing microbicide in recirculating waters is chlorine, but bromine has been put forward as an alternative [373].

Elemental bromine is not itself employed commercially. The two available methods [374] are: (i) activated bromide produced by reacting sodium bromide with a strong oxidizing agent, such as sodium hypochlorite or gaseous chlorine; and (ii) organic bromine-releasing agents, such as *N*-bromo-*N*-chlorodimethyl-hydantoin (BCDMH) (Figure 2.21a). When BCDMH hydrolyses in water, it liberates the microbicidal agents hypobromous acid (HOBr) and hypochlorous acid (HOCl), together with the carrier, dimethylhydantoin (DMH) (Figure 2.21b).

Both HOBr and HOCl would appear to contribute towards the overall microbicidal activity of BCDMH. However, Elsmore [373, 374] has pointed out that the primary agent present in water is HOBr. Hypochlorous acid is used up in regenerating "spent bromine" produced when HOBr reacts with organic materials and microorganisms:

$$HOCl + Br^- \rightarrow HOBr + Cl^-$$

Bromine is claimed to have a greater bactericidal activity than chlorine. It is effective against *Legionella pneumophila* in the laboratory and in field studies [375]. The pK_a for HOBr (8.69) is higher than that for HOCl (7.48) and thus, at the normal

alkaline pH values found in cooling towers, there is a significantly higher amount of active microbicide present with HOBr than with HOCl.

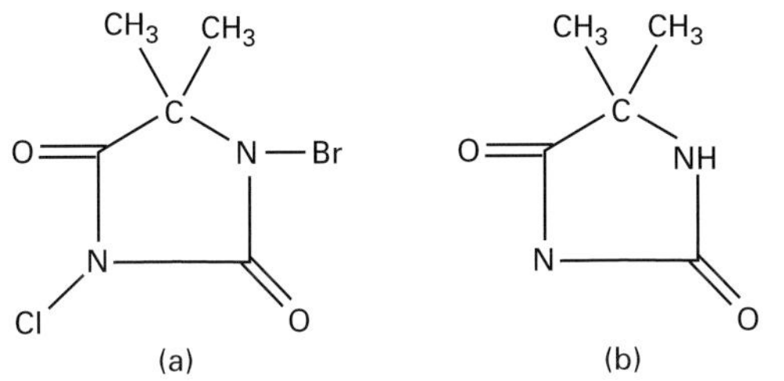

Quinoline and isoquinoline derivatives

There are three main groups of derivatives: 8-hydroxyquinoline derivatives, 4-aminoquinaldinium derivatives and isoquinoline derivatives. They are described in Figures 2.22 and 2.23. However, new quinoline derivatives such as hydrazinoquinolines [376], pyridazinoquinoline and spiroindoquinoline [377] have been shown to possess microbicidal activity.

8-Hydroxyquinoline Derivatives

8-Hydroxyquinoline (oxine) possesses antibacterial activity against Gram-positive bacteria, but much less against Gram-negative organisms. It actively disrupts the cell walls of *S. aureus* including MRSA and causes cell lysis [378]. It also has antifungal activity, although this occurs at a slower rate. Other useful compounds are depicted in Figure 2.22b. Like oxine, clioquinol, chlorquinandol and halquinol have very low water solubilities, and are generally employed as applications to the skin. An interesting feature of their activity is the fact that they are chelating agents, which are active only in the presence of certain metal ions. Currently, clioquinol is under extensive investigation, not for its antibacterial activity, rather for its activity as a potential anticancer agent and as a therapeutic agent for Alzheimer's disease. These effects depend on its ability to form stable complexes with different metals [379, 380].

4-Aminoquinaldinium derivatives

These are QACs (see Figure 2.23), which also fall into the quinoline group. The most important members are laurolinium acetate and dequalinium chloride (a bis-QAC). Both compounds possess antibacterial activity, especially against Gram-positive bacteria [381, 382], as well as significant activity against many species of yeasts and fungi [201, 383]. Dequalinium chloride is used for the treatment of vaginal infections and has been shown to have a broad spectrum of microbicidal activity against relevant organisms [384]. It is also used as lozenges or paint in the treatment of infections of the mouth and throat. Laurolinium has been used as a preoperative skin disinfectant, although this was never widely adopted. The activity of both agents is decreased in the presence of lecithin; serum decreases the effectiveness of laurolinium, but not of dequalinium.

Isoquinoline derivatives

The most important isoquinoline derivative is hedaquinium chloride (Figure 2.22c), a bisquaternary salt. This possesses antibacterial and antifungal activity [201, 381], and is regarded as one of the most active antifungal QAC agents [201].

Figure 2.21 (a) Bromochlorodimethylhydantoin (BCDMH) and (b) dimethylhydantoin (DMH).

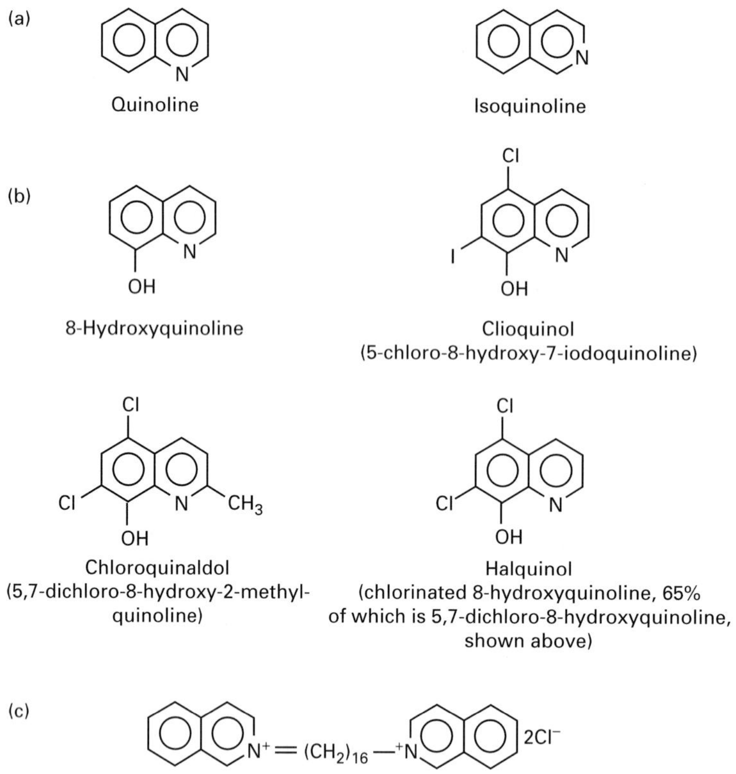

Figure 2.22 (a) Structures of quinoline and isoquinoline, (b) 8-hydroxyquinoline derivatives with antimicrobial properties and (c) hedaquinium chloride.

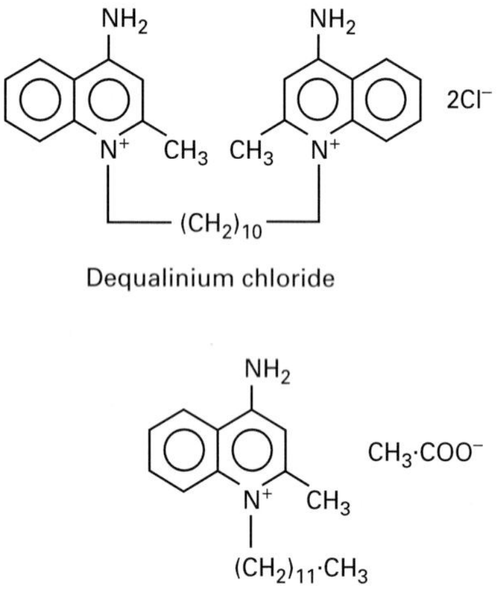

Figure 2.23 4-Aminoquinaldinium derivatives with antimicrobial properties.

Alcohols

Several alcohols have been shown to possess microbicidal properties. Generally, the alcohols have rapid bactericidal activity [385], including acid-fast bacilli, but are not sporicidal. They have low activity against some viruses, but are virucidal towards others. Their chemical structures are shown in Figure 2.24. Alcohols,

according to their chemical structure, are divided into aliphatic alcohol and aromatic alcohols. Most of the aliphatic alcohols (ethyl and isopropyl) are widely used as antiseptics and disinfectants. However, some aliphatic alcohols can be used as preservatives (chlorbutanol and bronopol). Aromatic alcohols are used mainly as preservatives (benzyl alcohol, phenylethanol and phenoxy ethanol). Aliphatic alcohols have good bactericidal activity against vegetative forms including *Mycobacterium* spp. and good virucidal activity, but no sporicidal activity at ambient temperature. The good microbicidal activity and volatility of alcohols make them ideal antiseptics for skin before injections, surgical procedures and hand hygiene in clinical situations. These properties also make the alcohols ideal disinfectants for mixing containers, filling lines, etc. in both food and pharmaceutical industries.

Mode of action

Based on the fact that the activity of alcohols increases in the presence of water (as mixtures of alcohols and water are more microbicidally active than absolute alcohol) and since protein denaturation occurs more rapidly in the presence of water, it is believed that alcohols act by damaging cell membranes, denaturing essential microbial proteins and consequently interfering with metabolism and resulting in cell lysis [130]. In addition, some reports have shown that alcohols cause denaturation of dehydrogenases in *E. coli* and an increase in the length of the lag phase of *Enterobacter aerogenes*, an event which has been attributed to inhibition of metabolic processes [130].

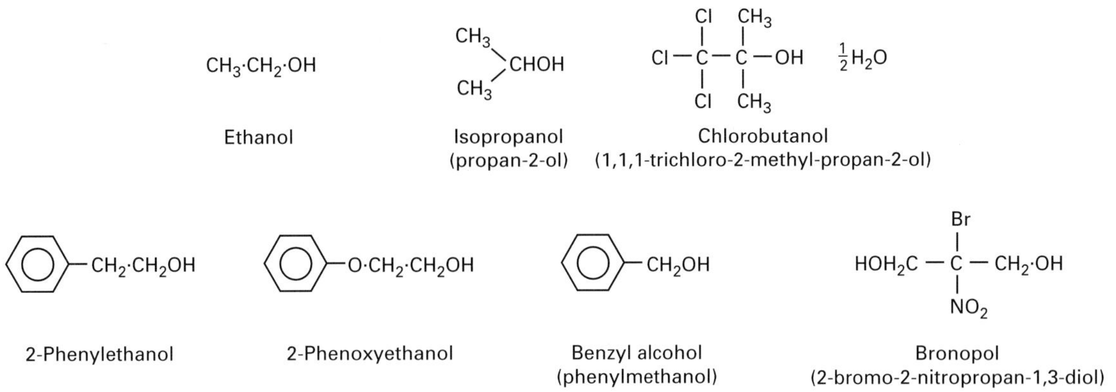

Figure 2.24 Alcohols.

Ethyl alcohol (ethanol)

Ethanol is rapidly lethal to non-sporulating bacteria and destroys mycobacteria [224], but is ineffective at all concentrations against bacterial spores [315]. Setlow *et al.* [386], showed that a reduction in the viability of *B. subtilis* spores can be achieved by treatment with ethanol at 65°C. The proposed mechanism of action of this killing is a disruption to the spore permeability barrier. The presence of water is essential for its activity, but concentrations below 30% have little or no action. Activity, in fact, drops sharply below 50% [387].

The most effective concentration is about 60–70% [388] for skin antisepsis, clean instruments and environmental surfaces. However, at higher concentrations (*c.* 90%) it is active against most viruses including HIV. Solutions of iodine or chlorhexidine in 70% alcohol may be employed for the preoperative disinfection of the skin. Ethanol is the alcohol of choice in cosmetic products because of its relative lack of odor and irritation [389]. Alcohol-based hand rubs are becoming increasingly popular for sanitizing hands. Hand hygiene is of particular importance in the healthcare professions to prevent nosocomial infections caused by cross transmission of microorganisms. Compliance with a hand-sanitizing regime has been shown to be improved by the introduction of an alcohol-based hand rub compared with soap and water [390]. However, there is some debate about the effectiveness of such products. While some studies report alcohol hand rubs to be more effective than hand washing with antiseptic soap and water [391, 392] other investigators have reported such products to be less effective [393].

Variable results have been reported about the effects of ethanol on HIV [394]. They showed that 70% ethanol in the presence of 2.5% serum produced a 3-log/ml reduction in virus titer after a 10 min contact period, as determined by plaque assay or immunofluorescence. In contrast, using a tissue culture infective dose 50% ($TCID_{50}$) assay, Resnick *et al.* [395] found that 70% alcohol after 1 min and in the presence of 50% plasma yielded a 7-log reduction in $TCID_{50}$/ml, again in a suspension test. Van Bueren *et al.* [396] also described a rapid inactivation of HIV-1 in suspension, irrespective of the protein load. The rate of inactivation decreased when high protein levels were present when a carrier test was employed. A notable feature of the experiments carried out by van Bueren *et al.* [396] was the care taken to ensure that residual alcohol was neutralized to prevent toxicity to the cell line employed in detecting residual active viral load. The non-enveloped poliovirus is more resistant to microbicides in general than the herpesvirus, and ethanol caused no inactivation of poliovirus in a suspension test [397].

Methyl alcohol (methanol)

Methyl alcohol has poor bactericidal activity and is not sporicidal [315, 389]. Furthermore, it is potentially toxic and is thus little used. However, freshly prepared mixtures of alcohols (especially methanol) and sodium hypochlorite are highly sporicidal. Although it was then considered that methanol was potentiating the activity of hypochlorites, it is, in fact, more likely that hypochlorites, by virtue of their effects on the outer spore layers [338], are aiding the penetration of methanol into the spore.

Isopropyl alcohol (isopropanol)

Isopropyl and *n*-propyl alcohols are more effective bactericides than ethanol, but are not sporicidal. Isopropyl alcohol has a slightly greater activity than ethanol, but is also twice as toxic. It is less active against viruses, particularly non-enveloped viruses, and should be considered a limited spectrum virucide [387]. They are miscible with water in all proportions, but isopropanol has a less objectionable odor than *n*-propanol and is considered as a suitable alternative to ethanol in various cosmetic products, either as a solvent or as a preservative [389, 398]. Van Bueren *et al.* [396] have demonstrated inactivation of HIV type 1 by isopropanol. For further information, the papers by Tyler *et al.* [397] and Sattar and Springthorpe [399] should be consulted.

Benzyl alcohol

In addition to having microbicidal properties, benzyl alcohol is a weak local anesthetic. It has activity against Gram-positive and Gram-negative bacteria and against molds [201]. Benzyl alcohol is incompatible with oxidizing agents and is inactivated by non-ionic surfactants; it is stable to autoclaving and is normally used at a concentration of 1% v/v [190].

Phenylethanol (phenylethyl alcohol)

Phenylethyl alcohol is a microbicidal agent with selective activity against various bacteria, especially Gram-negative ones and has been recommended for use as a preservative in ophthalmic solutions, often in conjunction with another microbicide. Because of its higher activity against Gram-negative bacteria, phenylethyl alcohol may be incorporated into culture media for isolating Gram-positive bacteria from mixed flora, for example phenylethyl alcohol agar. Phenylethanol is commonly used at a concentration of 0.3–0.5% v/v; it shows poor stability with oxidants and is partially inactivated by non-ionic surfactants [190].

Bronopol

Bronopol, 2-bromo-2-nitropropan-1,3-diol, is an aliphatic halogenonitro compound with potent antibacterial activity [400], including against pseudomonads, with some activity against bacterial biofilms [401] but limited activity against fungi [402]. Its activity is reduced somewhat by 10% serum and to a greater extent by sulfydryl compounds, but is unaffected by 1% polysorbate or 0.1% lecithin. It has a half-life of about 96 days at pH 8 and 25°C [403].

Bronopol is most stable under acid conditions; the initial decomposition appears to involve the liberation of formaldehyde and the formulation of bromonitroethanol (Figure 2.25a). A second-order reaction involving bronopol and formaldehyde occurs simultaneously to produce 2-hydroxymethyl-2-nitro-1,3-propanediol (Figure 2.25b), which itself decomposes with the loss of formaldehyde.

Bronopol has been employed extensively as a preservative for pharmaceutical and cosmetic products. However, its use to preserve products containing secondary amines should be avoided as the by-product of this reaction is nitrosoamine, which is carcinogenic. Details of the microbiological activity, chemical stability, toxicology and uses of bronopol are documented by Bryce et al. [404], Croshaw and Holland [405], Toler [403] and Rossmore and Sondossi [277]. Denyer and Wallhäusser [190] have provided useful information about bronopol, the typical in-use concentration of which is 0.01–0.1% w/v. Sulfhydryl compounds act as appropriate neutralizers in preservative efficacy tests.

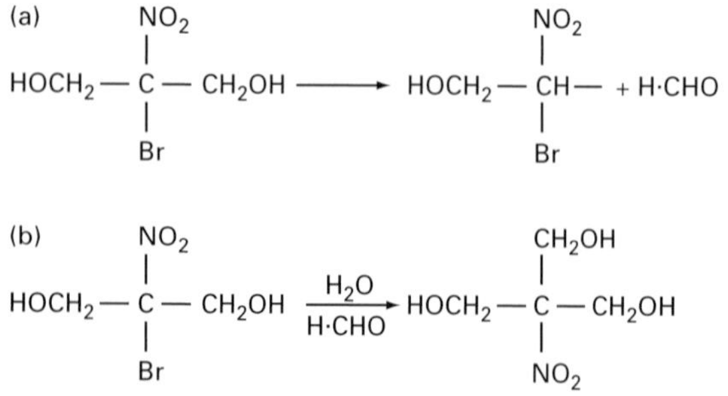

Figure 2.25 (a) Initial process in the decomposition of bronopol and (b) second-order reaction involving bronopol and formaldehyde.

Phenoxyethanol (phenoxetol)

The microbicidal activity of phenoxyethanol and other preservatives has been reviewed by Gucklhorn [263, 406]. Gilbert et al. elucidated its mode of action against E. coli [407–409] and against Bacillus megaterium [410]. Phenoxyethanol was shown by Berry [411] to possess significant activity against P. aeruginosa, but it has less activity against other Gram-negative organisms or against Gram-positive bacteria. Phenoxyethanol is stable to autoclaving and is compatible with anionic and cationic surfactants, but it shows reduced activity in the presence of polysorbate 80. It is used as a preservative, at a typical concentration of 1% [190].

Chlorbutanol (chlorbutol)

Chlorbutol is an antibacterial and antifungal agent. It has been used, at a concentration of 0.5% w/v, as a bactericide in injections. One drawback to its employment is its instability, since at acid pH it decomposes at the high temperature used in sterilization processes into hydrochloric acid, and at alkaline pH it is unstable at room temperature. Chlorbutanol is incompatible with some non-ionic surfactants. Its typical in-use concentration as a pharmaceutical preservative is 0.3–0.5% w/v [190].

2,4-Dichlorobenzyl alcohol

This substance is a white powder, soluble in water to 1% and readily soluble in alcohols. Its ionization is negligible for all practical purposes and it is thus active over a wide pH range. 2,4-Dichlorobenzyl alcohol has a broad spectrum of activity, but both pseudomonads and S. aureus show some resistance [403].

Peroxygens

Both hydrogen peroxide and peracetic acid are considered to be high-level disinfectants by virtue of their production of the highly reactive hydroxyl radicals. The advantage of this group over the other microbicidal groups is that their decomposition products are non-toxic and biodegradable.

Hydrogen peroxide

Hydrogen peroxide (H_2O_2) is a familiar household antiseptic. It was discovered in 1818 and was recognized as possessing bactericidal properties. These were extensively investigated in 1893 by Traugott. Hydrogen peroxide is available as a solution designated as 20- or 10-volume, a means of indicating its strength by describing the volume (20 or 10, respectively) of oxygen evolved from 1 volume of the peroxide solution. Strengths for industrial use of 35%, 50% or 90% are available. Hydrogen peroxide solutions are unstable, and benzoic acid or another suitable substance is added as a stabilizer.

Hydrogen peroxide solutions possess disinfectant, antiseptic and deodorant properties. It is a high-level disinfectant. Many products containing hydrogen peroxide are approved by the FDA as chemisterilants [248]. When in contact with living tissue and many metals they decompose, evolving oxygen. Hydrogen peroxide is bactericidal and sporicidal [143, 146, 343, 412–414]. It is believed to act as a generator of free hydroxyl radicals, which attack membrane lipids, essential cell components, [194] and can cause DNA strand breakage in growing bacteria. However, the mechanism of action of hydrogen peroxide on spores is dissimilar. The current hypothesis is that hydrogen peroxide treatment results in spores that cannot swell properly during spore germination [415]. Hydrogen peroxide is an oxidizing agent and reacts with oxidizable material. It is environmentally friendly, because its decomposition products are oxygen and water [416] and has been investigated as a potential sanitizing agent in the food industry [415, 417].

Hydrogen peroxide has been used in aseptic packaging technology and also for disinfecting contact lenses, as it has been shown to be effective against the opportunistic pathogen *Acanthameoba* spp, the causative agent of *Acanthameoba* keratitis. This is a potentially blinding infection that contact lens users are more susceptible to than others [418]. The use of hydrogen peroxide as a contact lens disinfectant has been reviewed [416].

Microbial inactivation is more rapid with liquid peroxide than with vapor generated from that liquid acting at the same temperature [419]. However, the vapor can be used for the purposes of sterilization, where, at a concentration of 1–5 mg/l, it generally shows good penetration.

Attention has been devoted to the development of a plasma-activated peroxide vapor process in which radiowaves produce the plasma. This is believed to be microbicidal by virtue of the hydroxyl ions and other free radicals that are generated [420, 421].

Peracetic acid

Peracetic acid, CH_3COOH, was introduced as a bactericidal agent in 1955. It is available commercially as a 15% aqueous solution, in which equilibrium exists between peracetic acid and its decomposition products acetic acid (CH_3COOH) and hydrogen peroxide.

Peracetic acid is a more potent microbicidal agent than hydrogen peroxide and it has a broad spectrum of activity, including that against mycobacteria, bacteria and their spores, molds, yeasts, algae and viruses. It is employed as a chemosterilant for medical equipment such as flexible endoscopes and other reusable medical and dental instruments [248]. It finds extensive use in the food industry and for disinfecting sewage sludge. It is a powerful oxidizing agent and in certain situations can be corrosive. The main advantage of peracetic acid is that its final decomposition products, oxygen and water, are innocuous. More comprehensive data on peracetic acid are provided by Baldry [413], Fraser [422], Baldry and Fraser [414], Coates [362] and Russell and Chopra [26]. The combination of peracetic acid with hydrogen peroxide is synergistic and many such products are approved by the FDA as cold sterilizing agents for dialysis machines [77, 248]. Peracetic acid is believed to act by denaturing proteins, disrupting cell wall permeability and oxidizing sulfhydryl and sulfur bonds in

proteins, enzymes and other metabolites [423]. Both hydrogen peroxide and peracetic acid are active in liquid and vapor phases and are active in the presence of organic matter.

Performic acid

Performic acid (HC(O)OOH) is prepared by mixing formic acid with hydrogen peroxide. It is unstable and should be prepared immediately prior to use. Performic acid is a well-known oxidizing agent and disinfectant in the medical field and food industry. It is active against bacteria, bacterial spores, viruses, mycobacteria and fungi [282]. It is used as a chemisterilant for endoscopes [282]. It has been studied as a potential wastewater disinfectant. The by-products of performic acid breakdown are environmentally safe (formic acid and hydrogen peroxide) [424].

Chelating agents

This section will deal briefly with chelating agents based on ethylenediamine tetraacetic acid (EDTA).

The chemical structures of EDTA, ethylenedioxybis(ethyliminodi(aceticacid))(EGTA),*N*-hydroxyethylethylenediamine-*NN′N′*-triacetic acid (HDTA), *trans*-1,2-diaminocyclohexane-*NNN′N′*-tetraacetic acid (CDTA), iminodiacetic acid (IDA) and nitrilotriacetic acid (NTA) are provided in Figure 2.26a–f, respectively. Table 2.11 lists their chelating and antibacterial activities.

Ethylendiamine tetraacetic acid

In medicine, EDTA is commonly employed as sodium or sodium-calcium salts. Sodium-calcium edetate is used in the treatment of chronic lead poisoning, and the sodium salts are used clinically to chelate calcium ions, thereby decreasing serum calcium. Also, EDTA is used as a stabilizing agent in certain injections and eye drop preparations [425].

The most important early findings, in a microbiological context, were made by Repaske [426, 427], who showed that certain Gram-negative bacteria became sensitive to the enzyme lysozyme in the presence of EDTA in tris buffer and that EDTA alone induced lysis of *P. aeruginosa*. The importance of tris itself has been recognized [428, 429], since it appears to affect the permeability of the wall of various Gram-negative bacteria, as well as the nucleotide pool and RNA, which may be degraded. A lysozyme–tris–EDTA system in the presence of sucrose is a standard technique for producing spheroplasts/protoplasts in Gram-negative bacteria. During this conversion, several enzymes are released into the surrounding medium. A technique known as "cold shock", which involves treating *E. coli* with EDTA with tris in hypertonic sucrose, followed by rapid dispersion in cold magnesium chloride, thus producing a sudden osmotic shift, again results in the release of enzymes but without destroying the viability of the cells.

In the context of disinfection, EDTA is most important in that it will potentiate the activity of many bactericidal agents against

Table 2.11 Properties of chelating agents.[a]

Property	EDTA	EGTA	HDTA	CDTA	IDA	NTA
Log stability constant						
Ba	7.76	8.41	5.54	7.99	1.67	4.82
Ca	10.70	11.0	8.0	12.5	2.59	6.41
Mg	8.69	5.21	5.2	10.32	2.94	5.41
Zn	16.26	14.5	14.5	18.67	7.03	10.45
Antibacterial activity						
Alone	Good	Good	Good	Low	Low	–
As a potentiating agent for disinfectants	Yes	–	Yes	Yes	Somewhat	Somewhat

[a]See text for abbreviated chelating agents in full.

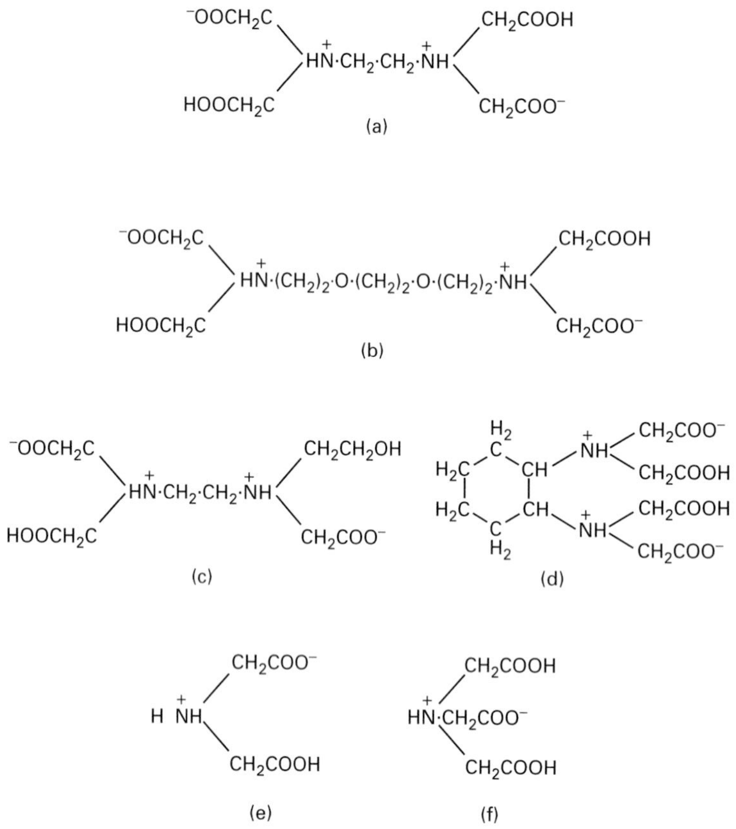

Figure 2.26 Chelating agents: (a) ethylenediamine tetraacetic acid (EDTA), (b) ethylenedioxybis(ethyliminodi(acetic acid)) (EGTA), (c) *N*-hydroxyethylenediamine-*NN′N′*-triacetic acid (HDTA), (d) *trans*-1,2-diaminocyclohexane-*NNN′N′*-tetra-acetic acid (CDTA), (e) iminodiacetic acid (IDA) and (f) nitrilotriacetic acid (NTA).

many types of Gram-negative but not Gram-positive bacteria. EDTA induces a non-specific increase in the permeability of the outer envelope of Gram-negative cells, thereby allowing more penetration of non-related agents. Ayres *et al.* [59] reported on the permeabilizing activity of EDTA and other agents against *P. aeruginosa* in a rapid test method, the principle of which was the rapid lysis induced in this organism on exposure to the presumed permeabilizing agent plus lysozyme, an enzyme normally excluded in whole cells from its peptidoglycan target.

Other chelating agents

Chelating agents other than EDTA are described chemically in Figure 2.26, and some of their properties are listed in Table 2.11. While EGTA forms a stronger complex with Ca than does EDTA, for most other metals, except Ba and Hg, it is a weaker complexing agent than EDTA. Notably, there is a divergency of 5.79-log K units between the stability constants of the Ca and Mg complexes with EGTA. Compared with EDTA, CDTA has superior complexing powers and it is better than all the other chelating agents listed in complexing Mg^{2+} ions. From a microbiological point of view, CDTA was found to be the most toxic compound to *P. aeruginosa* and other Gram-negative bacteria in terms of leakage, lysis and loss of viability and in extracting metal ions from isolated cell envelopes [430].

The chelating agent HDTA corresponds to EDTA, one acetic acid of the latter molecule being replaced by a hydroxyethyl group. Its complexes are invariably less stable than those of EDTA. In a microbiological context, HDTA was found [430] to be rather less effective than EDTA. Metal chelation of EDTA has also been shown to reduce its microbicidal activity [431].

N,N'-ethylenebis(2-(2-hydroxyphenyl)-glycine (EHPG), a chelating agent containing two phenyl groups, has been shown to exhibit microbicidal activity against a range of bacteria and fungi and was shown to be more active than EDTA [431].

Iminodiacetic acid forms weak complexes with most metal ions, whereas NTA is more reactive. Both have little activity against *P. aeruginosa*, although both, to some extent, potentiate the activity of other agents (disinfectants) against this organism.

Permeabilizers

Permeabilizers (permeabilizing agents) are chemicals that increase bacterial permeability to microbicides [432]. Such chemicals include chelating agents (described above), polycations, lactoferrin, transferrin and the salts of certain acids.

Polycations

Polycations such as poly-L-lysine (lysine$_{20}$; PLL) (Figure 2.27) induce lipopolysaccharide (LPS) release from the outer membrane of Gram-negative bacteria. Organisms treated with PLL show greatly increased sensitivity to hydrophobic antibiotics [433–435], but responses to microbicides do not appear to have been studied.

Lactoferrin

Lactoferrin is a natural microbicidal glycoprotein present in milk and other exocrine secretions [436]. It is an iron-binding protein that acts as a chelator, inducing partial LPS loss from the outer membrane of Gram-negative bacteria [437]. The resulting

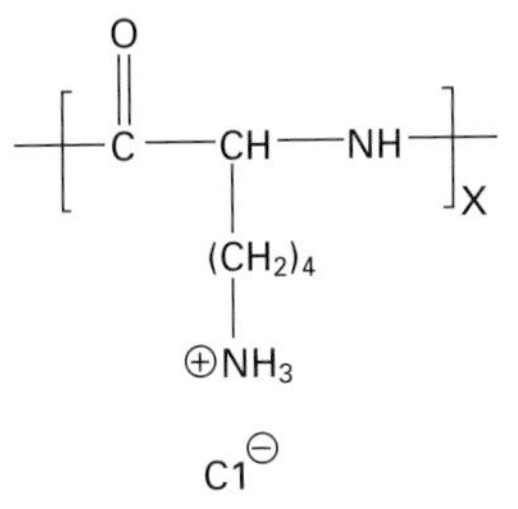

Figure 2.27 L-lysine repeating units used to form the backbone of the L-lysine polymer.

permeability alteration increases the susceptibility of bacteria to lysozyme [438] and antibiotics such as penicillin [439] resulting in synergistic combinations. This protein has applications in skin care products, oral hygiene products, animal feed supplements and as an active ingredient in infant formulae [436]. Lactoferricin B is a microbicidal β-hairpin peptide produced by gastric peptic digestion of bovine lactoferrin. It is a much more potent agent than lactoferrin, binds rapidly to the bacterial cell surface and damages the outer membrane, but has reduced activity in the presence of divalent cations [440]. Further information regarding lactoferrin can be found in the reviews of Chierici [441], Weinberg [442], Adlerova *et al.* [443] and Pierce and Legrand [444].

Transferrin

This iron-binding protein is believed to have a similar effect to lactoferrin [437]. All are worthy of further studies as potentially important permeabilizers. Transferrin is often considered in reviews alongside lactoferrin and hence the reviews of Adlerova *et al.* [443] and Pierce and Legrand [444] may be of interest on this topic.

Citric and other acids

Used at alkaline pH, citric, gluconic and malic acids all act as permeabilizers [59]. They perform as chelating agents and activity is reduced in the presence of divalent cations.

Lactic acid has also been demonstrated to permeabilize the outer membrane of Gram-negative bacteria but at low pH. The proposed mechanism of action for this agent is not as a chelator like citric, gluconic and malic acids, but as a protonator of anionic components such as phosphate and carbonyl groups resulting in weakening of the molecular interactions between outer membrane components [89].

Heavy metal derivatives

The early use of high concentrations of salt, employed empirically in the salting process as a preservative for meat, and the use of copper and silver vessels to prevent water from becoming fouled by microbial growth have been examined elsewhere. Salting is still used in some parts of the world as a meat preservative and salts of heavy metals, especially silver, mercury, copper and, more recently, organotin, are still used as microbicidal agents. The metal derivatives of copper, silver, mercury and tin, which find use as antiseptics and preservatives, will be discussed in this chapter. Kushner [445] reviewed the action of solutes other than heavy metal derivatives on microorganisms.

In addition to possessing microbicidal activity in their own right, many metal ions are necessary for the activity of other drugs. A typical example is 8-hydroxyquinoline, which needs Fe^{2+} for activity. The interesting relationship between microbicidal compounds and metal cations has been reviewed by Weinberg [446].

Copper compounds

Although the pharmacopoeias list a number of recipes containing copper salts (sulfate, acetate, citrate) as ingredients of antiseptic astringent lotions, the main microbicidal use of copper derivatives is in algicides and fungicides. The copper (II) ion Cu^{2+} is pre-eminently an algicidal ion, and at a final concentration of 0.5–2.9 µg/ml, as copper sulfate, it has been used to keep swimming pools free from algae. Copper is thought to act by the poisoning effect of the copper (II) ion on thiol enzymes (enzymes with thiol groups at the active or vicinal sites) and possibly other thiol groups in microbial cells (e.g. glutathione, etc.).

Copper ions have been shown to potentiate the microbicidal activity of two commonly used disinfectants, cetylpyridinium chloride and povidone-iodine, against hospital isolates of *S. aureus, P. aeruginosa* and *Candida albicans* [447].

Copper sulfate and copper sulfate mixed with lime (known as Bordeaux mixture, introduced in 1885) are used as fungicides in plant protection (especially vines). The latter formulation proved particularly efficacious as it formed a slow-release copper complex, which was not easily washed from foliage. It was said to be first used as a deterrent to human scavengers of the grape crop because of its bitter taste, and its antifungal properties emerged later. Copper metal in powder form finds an interesting application as a microbicidal additive to cements and concretes. Its function is to inhibit microbial attack on the ingredients of these products. These uses of copper metal, and as vessels for drinking water in the ancient world, illustrate a phenomenon that has been called the oligodynamic action of metals [448]. Metals are slightly soluble in water and in the case of copper and silver a sufficient concentration of ions in solution is achieved to inhibit microbial growth. Copper complexes, such as copper naphthenate and copper-7-hydroxyquinolate, have been particularly successful in the preservation of cotton fabrics. More recently, polyester fibers coated with copper sulfides have been demonstrated to possess some microbicidal activity [449]. Copper compounds are mainly used in the wood, paper and paint industries as preservatives, and have little, if any, use in the pharmaceutical and cosmetic industries.

Silver compounds

Silver and its compounds have found a place in microbicidal application from ancient times to the present day [450]. Apart from the use of silver vessels to maintain water in a potable state, the first systematic use of a silver compound in medicine was its use in the prophylaxis of ophthalmia neonatorum by the instillation of silver nitrate solution into the eyes of newborn infants. Silver compounds have been used in the prevention of infection in burns, with variable effectiveness. An organism frequently associated with such infections is *P. aeruginosa* and Brown and Anderson [451] discussed the effectiveness of Ag^+ in the killing of this organism. Among the Enterobacteriaceae, plasmids may carry genes specifying resistance to antibiotics and to metals. Plasmid-mediated resistance to silver salts is of particular importance in the hospital environment, because silver nitrate and silver

sulfadiazine (AgSu) may be used topically for preventing infections in severe burns [452].

Silver nitrate is an astringent compound and below 10^{-4} mol/l is a protein precipitant. Attempts to reduce this undesirable propensity while maintaining microbicidal potency have been made. A device much used in pharmaceutical formulation to promote slow release of a potent substance is to combine it with a high molecular weight polymer. By mixing silver oxide or silver nitrate with gelatin or albumen, a water-soluble adduct is obtained, which slowly releases silver ions but lacks the astringency of silver nitrate. A similar slow-release compound has been prepared by combining silver with disodium dinaphthylmethane disulfate [453]. Silver nitrate has also been investigated as a treatment for peridontitis. A concentration of 0.5 µg/ml was sufficient to produce a minimum of 3-log reductions against a range of peridontal pathogens. However, increasing the concentration of silver nitrate by 100-fold was not sufficient to kill oral streptococci [454].

Sustained release of silver nitrate from a subgingival drug delivery system has also shown to be active against a range of peridontal microorganisms over a period of 21 days [455]. The inclusion of silver ions in other surfaces with the aim of producing a microbicidal effect has been investigated further. Kim *et al.* [456] demonstrated the microbicidal effect of a ceramic composed of hydroxapatite and silver nitrate against *E. coli*, while the inclusion of silver and zinc ions on stainless steel pins has been shown to have microbicidal activity against *S. aureus* [457] and *Legionella pneumophilia* [458].

The oligodynamic action of silver [448] has been exploited in a water-purification system employing what is called katadyn silver. Here, metallic silver is coated on to sand used in filters for water purification. Silver-coated charcoal was used in a similar fashion [459]. The activity of a silver-releasing surgical dressing has been described by Furr *et al.* [460], who used a neutralization system to demonstrate that the Ag^+ ions released were responsible for its antibacterial effects.

Russell and Hugo [461] have reviewed the microbicidal activity and action of silver compounds. At a concentration of 10^{-9} to 10^{-6} mol/l, Ag^+ is an extremely active microbicide. Originally considered to act as a general protoplasmic poison, this is now seen as an oversimplification. Silver reacts strongly with structural and functional thiol groups in microbial cells, induces cytological changes and interacts with the bases in DNA. Silver ions cause the release of K^+ ions from the cell (indicating membrane leakage), inhibit cell division and damage the cell envelope of bacteria [130].

Silver sulfadiazine is essentially a combination of two antibacterial agents, Ag^+ and sulfadiazine. It has a broad spectrum of activity, produces surface and membrane blebs and binds to various cell components, especially DNA [461], although its precise mode of action has yet to be elucidated. Silver sulfadiazine has been reinvestigated by Hamilton-Miller *et al.* [462] and is often used in combination with chlorhexidine as an anti-biofilm agent in clinical situations [463].

Mercury compounds

Mercury, long a fascination for early technologists (alchemists, medical practitioners, etc.), was used in medicine by the Persian physician Ibn Sina (known in the west as Avicenna), in the early 11th century. In the 1850s, mercury salts comprised, with phenol, the hypochlorites and iodine – the complement of topical microbicidal drugs at the physician's disposal. Mercuric chloride was used and evaluated by Robert Koch and by Geppert. Nowadays its use in medicine has decreased, although a number of organic derivatives of mercury (Figure 2.28) are used as bacteriostatic and fungistatic agents and as preservatives and bactericides in injections; examples include mercurochrome, nitromersol, thiomersal and phenylmercuric nitrate (Figure 2.28). Salts such as the stearate, oleate and naphthenate were, until much more recently, extensively employed in the preservation of wood, textiles, paints and leather. The Minimata disaster in Japan in 1956, due to mercury waste leakage into the environment, has led to restrictions in the use of mercury in any form where it might pollute the environment and its continued use has met popular and governmental resistance. Hence, it is unlikely that the inclusion of mercury in any product where environmental pollution may ensue will be countenanced by regulatory authorities.

Mercury resistance is inducible and is not the result of training or tolerance. Plasmids conferring resistance are of two types: (i) "narrow spectrum", encoding resistance to Hg(II) and to a few specified organomercurials; and (ii) "broad spectrum", encoding resistance to those in (i) plus other organomercury compounds [464]. In (i) there is enzymatic reduction of mercury to Hg metal and its vaporization, and in (ii) there is enzymatic hydrolysis of an organomercurial to inorganic mercury and its subsequent reduction as in (i) [465]. Ono et al. [466] showed that the yeast cell wall acted as an adsorption filter for Hg^+ ions. Later, they demonstrated that methylmercury-resistant mutants of Saccharomyces cerevisiae overproduced hydrogen sulfide [467], with an accumulation of hydrosulfide (HS^-) ions intracellularly, which was responsible for the detoxification of methylmercury.

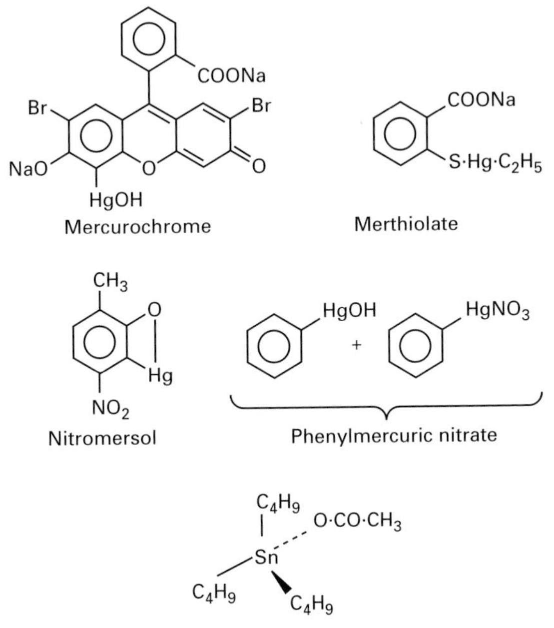

Mercurochrome (disodium-2,7-dibromo-4-hydroxymercurifluorescein)

This is now only of historical interest. It was the first organic mercurial to be used in medicine and an aqueous solution of it enjoyed a vogue as a substitute for iodine solutions as a skin disinfectant.

Nitromersol (anhydro-2-hydroxymercuri-6-methyl-3-nitrophenol)

A yellow powder, it is not very soluble in water or organic solvents but will dissolve in aqueous alkali, and is used as a solution of the sodium salt. It is active against vegetative microorganisms, but ineffective against spores and acid-fast bacteria. It is mostly used in the USA.

Thiomersal (merthiolate, sodium-o-(ethylmercurithio)-benzoate)

This derivative was used as a skin disinfectant, and is now employed as a fungicide and as a preservative (0.01–0.02%) for biological products, for example bacterial and viral vaccines and ophthalmic preparations. It possesses antifungal properties but has no action on spores. The use of thiomersal in vaccines for children is controversial, as it is suggested as a possible cause of autism and other psychoneurological disorders in children. It has been subjected to extensive study and debate where, so far, the scientific evidence is inconclusive [468–471]. However, various international committees recommend the elimination of thiomersal from pediatric vaccines as a precaution [468].

Solutions of thiomersal are stable when autoclaved, but less stable when exposed to light or to alkaline conditions, and they are incompatible with various chemicals, including heavy metal salts [190].

Phenylmercuric nitrate (PMN)

This organic derivative of mercury is used as a preservative in multidose containers of parenteral injections and eye-drops at a concentration of 0.001% and 0.002% w/v, respectively [451]. It was formerly employed in the UK as an adjunct to heat in the now discarded process of "heating with a bactericide".

Phenylmercuric nitrate (PMN) is incompatible with various compounds, including metals. Its activity is reduced by anionic emulsifying and suspending agents [190]. PMN is incompatible with some packaging materials, for example rubber and some plastics. Both PMN and phenylmercuric acetate (PMA) are

Figure 2.28 Mercurochrome, merthiolate (thiomersal, sodium ethylmercurithiosalicylate), nitromersol, phenylmercuric nitrate and tributyltin acetate.

absorbed from solutions by rubber closures and plastic containers to a significant extent. Sulfydryl agents are used as neutralizers in bactericidal studies and in sterility testing [121, 223]. PMN is a useful preservative and is also employed as a spermicide.

PMN solutions at room temperature are ineffective against bacterial spores, but they possess antifungal activity and are used as antifungal agents in the preservation of paper, textiles and leather. Voge [472] discussed PMN in a short review. A formulation of PMN with sodium dinaphthylmethane disulfonate has been described, in which enhanced activity and greater skin penetration is claimed [453].

Phenylmercuric acetate (PMA)

This has the same activity, properties and general uses as PMN [190] and finds application as a preservative in pharmaceutical and other fields. The use of both PMN and PMA has declined considerably due to concerns about mercury toxicity and risk of hypersensitivity or local irritation.

Tin and its compounds (organotins)

Tin, stannic or tin (IV) oxide was at one time used as an oral medicament in the treatment of superficial staphylococcal infections. Tin was claimed to be excreted via sebaceous glands and, thus, concentrated at sites of infection. More recently, organic tin derivatives (Figure 2.28) have been used as fungicides and bactericides and as textile and wood preservatives [473].

The organotin compounds that find use as microbicides are derivatives of tin (IV). They have the general structure R_3SnX, where R is butyl or phenyl and X is acetate, benzoate, fluoride, oxide or hydroxide. In structure–activity studies, activity has been shown to reside in the R group and the nature of X determines physical properties such as solubility and volatility [474]. The R_3SnX compounds combine high microbicidal activity with low mammalian toxicity. These compounds are used as microbicides in the paper and paint industry, and in agriculture as fungicides and pesticides. Tributyltin benzoate $((C_4H_9)_3SnOCOC_6H_5)$ is used as a germicide when combined with formaldehyde or a QAC and triphenyltin hydroxide $((C_6H_5)_3SnOH)$ as a disinfectant (as well as an agricultural pesticide). Examples of MICs of tributyltin oxide are shown in Table 2.12. Tin differs significantly from

Table 2.12 Minimum inhibitory concentrations (MICs) of tributyltin oxide towards a range of microorganisms.

Organism	MIC (μg/ml)
Aspergillus niger (brasiliensis)	0.5
Chaetomium globosum	1.0
Penicillium expansum	1.0
Aureobasidium pullulans	0.5
Trichoderma viride	1.0
Candida albicans	1.0
Bacillus mycoides	0.1
Staphylococcus aureus	1.0
Bacterium ammoniagenes	1.0
Pseudomonas aeruginosa	>500
Enterobacter aerogenes	>500

copper, silver and mercury salts in being intrinsically much less toxic. It is used to coat cans and vessels employed to prepare food or boil water. Organotin compounds have some effect on oxidative phosphorylation and act as ionophores for anions. Possible environmental toxicity should be borne in mind when tin compounds are used.

Titanium

The use of titanium as a microbicidal agent in the oral cavity has been investigated. Granules of titanium were examined for activity against oral bacteria, but showed very low antibacterial activity [475]. Titanium also has found use in medical implants including dental implants. Titanium surfaces implanted with fluorine ions demonstrated microbicidal activity. However, this was not found to be due to fluorine ion release but was hypothesized to be due to the formation of a titanium–fluorine complex on the implant surface [476].

Anilides

Anilides (Figure 2.29) have the general structure C_6H_5NHCOR. Two derivatives salicylanilide, where $R = C_6H_4OH$, and dipheny-

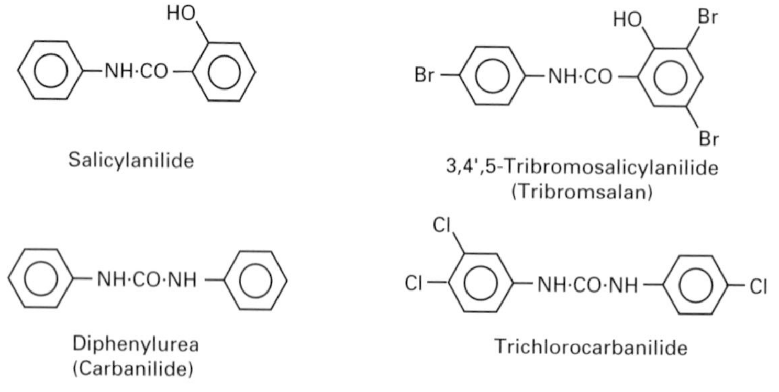

Salicylanilide

3,4',5-Tribromosalicylanilide
(Tribromsalan)

Diphenylurea
(Carbanilide)

Trichlorocarbanilide

Figure 2.29 Anilides.

lurea (carbanilide), where R = C$_6$H$_5$NH, have formed the basis for microbicidal compounds.

Mode of action
The compounds owe their bacteriostatic action to their ability to discharge part of the proton-motive force, thereby inhibiting processes dependent upon it – that is, active transport and energy metabolism. In addition, the anilides are thought to cause cell death by adsorbing to and destroying the semipermeability of the cytoplasmic membrane [130]. Some reports have shown the ability of salicylanilide derivatives to inhibit the two-component system of bacteria (the signal transduction device that plays a role in bacterial virulence) [477].

Salicylanilide
The parent compound, salicylanilide, was introduced in 1930 as a fungistat for use on textiles. It occurs as white or slightly pink crystals (m.p. 137°C), which are soluble in water and organic solvents. It has also been used in ointment form for the treatment of ringworm, but concentrations above 5% should not be used in medicinal products because of skin irritancy. Minimum inhibitory concentrations (μg/ml) for a number of fungi were: *Trichophyton mentagrophytes*, 12; *Trichophyton tonsurans*, 6; *Trichophyton rubrum*, 3; *Epidermophyton floccosum*, 6; and *Microsporum audovinii*, 1.5. Despite the effectiveness of the parent compound, attempts were made to improve on its performance by the usual device of adding substituents, notably halogens, to the benzene residues; these are considered below.

Lemaire *et al.* [478] investigated 92 derivatives of salicylanilide and related compounds, that is benzanilides and salicylaldehydes. The intrinsic microbicidal activity was obtained from literature values and was usefully summarized as follows. A one-ring substituent would give a MIC value for *S. aureus* of 2 μg/ml, but this value could be decreased to 1 μg/ml if substitution occurred in both rings.

The researchers were particularly interested in the role of these compounds as antiseptics for addition to soaps, and went on to evaluate them as such. They also investigated to what extent these compounds remained on the skin (skin substantivity) after washing with soaps containing them. They found that di- to pentachlorination or bromination with more or less equal distribution of the substituent halogen in both rings gave the best results both for microbicidal activity and skin substantivity. However, it was also found that skin photosensitization was caused by some analogs.

Of the many compounds tested, the 3,4′,5-tribromo, 2,3,5,3′- and 3,5,3′,4′-tetrachloro salicylanilides have been the most widely used as microbicidal agents. However, their photosensitizing properties have tended to restrict their use in any situation where they may come in contact with human skin.

Over and above this, many workers who have investigated germicidal soaps – that is, ordinary soap products with the addition of a halogenated salicylanilide, carbanilide or, for that matter, phenolic compounds such as hexachlorophene or DCMX – have doubted their value in this role. However, some may act as deodorants by destroying skin organisms, which react with sweat to produce body odor. Several derivatives have been synthesized that have antituberculosis activity and some of them were selected for preclinical studies [479–481].

Diphenylureas (carbanilides)
From an extensive study by Beaver *et al.* [482], 1,3,4,4′-trichlorocarbanilide (TCC, triclocarban) emerged as one of the most potent of this family of microbicides. It inhibits the growth of many Gram-positive bacteria including MRSA and vancomycin-resistant *Enterococcus* (VRE) [483], but is not active against Gram-negative organisms [484]. Typical growth inhibitory concentrations for Gram-positive organisms range from 0.1 to 1.0 μg/ml. Fungi were found to be more resistant, since 1000 μg/ml failed to inhibit *Aspergillus niger (brasiliensis)*, *Penicillium notatum*, *Candida albicans* and *Fusarium oxysporium*. *Trichophyton gypseum* and *Trichophyton inguinale* were inhibited at 50 μg/ml.

It occurs as a white powder, m.p. 250°C and is very slightly soluble in water. Like the salicylanilides, it has not found favor in products likely to come in contact with human skin, despite the fact that it had been extensively evaluated as the active ingredient of some disinfectant soaps.

Miscellaneous preservatives

Included in this section are those chemicals that are useful preservatives, but which do not form part of the microbicidal groups already considered above.

Derivatives of 1,3-dioxane
Dimethoxane (2,6-dimethyl-1,3-dioxan-4-ol acetate)
Dimethoxane (Figure 2.30) is a liquid, colorless when pure and soluble in water and organic solvents. It has a characteristic odor. Dimethoxane is not affected by changes in pH, but it is slowly hydrolyzed in aqueous solution, producing ethanal (acetaldehyde). It is compatible with non-ionic surface-active agents, but may cause discoloration in formulations that contain amines or amides. Dimethoxane finds application as a preservative for emulsions, water-based industrial processes, emulsion paints and cutting oils. In a bacteriological study, Woolfson [485] attributed the action of the commercial product partially to its aldehyde content and partially to the 1,3-dioxane components.

Bronidox (5-bromo-5-nitro-1,3-dioxane)
This nitro-bromo derivative of dioxane is available as a 10% solution in propylene glycol as Bronidox L. It is used as a preservative for toiletries and has been described in some detail by Potokar *et al.* [486] and Lorenz [487]. Its stability at various pH values is tabulated by Croshaw [488]. Bronidox (Figure 2.30) is active against bacteria and fungi and does not show a *Pseudomonas*-gap. Minimum inhibitory concentrations of the active ingredient (μg/ml) were: *E. coli*, 50; *P. aeruginosa*, 50;

Proteus vulgaris, 50; *Pseudomonas fluorescens*, 50; *S. typhi*, 50; *Serratia marcescens*, 25; *S. aureus*, 75; *Stretococcus faecalis*, 75; *Candida albicans*, 25; *Saccharomyces cerevisiae*, 10; and *Aspergillus niger (brasiliensis)*, 10.

Bronidox has broad-spectrum microbicidal activity that is similar to bronopol, but it is more stable [489]. Its activity is not affected between pH 5 and 9 and it probably acts as an oxidizing agent, oxidizing thiol to disulfhydryl groups in essential enzymes. It does not act as a formaldehyde releaser. It is suitable for the preservation of surfactant preparations, which are rinsed off after application and do not contain secondary amines.

Derivatives of imidazole

Imidazolines (Figure 2.31) are 2,3-dihydroimidazoles; 2-heptadecyl-2-imidazoline was introduced as an agricultural fungicide in 1946. Other derivatives containing the imidazole ring have recently found successful application as preservatives. Two are derivatives of 2,4-dioxotetrahydroimidazole, the imidazolidones; the parent diketone is hydantoin.

Dantoin (1,3-di(hydroxymethyl)-5,5-dimethyl-2,4-dioxoimidazole, 1,3-di-hydroxymethyl-5,5-dimethylhydantoin)

A 55% solution of this compound (Figure 2.31) is available commercially as Glydant (Lonza Group UK Ltd, Slough, UK). This product is water soluble, stable and non-corrosive, with a slight odor of formaldehyde. It is active over a wide range of pH and is compatible with most ingredients used in cosmetics. It has a wide spectrum of activity against bacteria and fungi, being active at concentrations of between 250 and 500 µg/ml. However, the molds *Microsporum gypseum* and *Trichophyton asteroides* are particularly susceptible, being inhibited at 32 µg/ml. The mode of action of dantoin is attributed to its ability to release formaldehyde, the rate of release of which is more rapid at high pH values (9 to 10.5) than low (3 to 5). Its optimum stability lies in the range pH 6 to 8. It has an acceptable level of toxicity and can be used as a preservative over a wide field of products. Glydant 2000 (launched in 2005), based on a patented process, is an ultra-low (<0.1%) free formaldehyde hydantoin for use in the personal care industry.

Germall (N,N′-methylene-bis-(5′(1-hydroxymethyl)-2,5-dioxo-4-imidazolidinyl urea))

In 1970 a family of imidazolidinyl ureas for use as preservatives was described [490]. One of these, under the name Germall 115 (Figure 2.31), was studied in the 1970s [491, 492]. Germall 115 is a white powder that is very soluble in water and hence tends to remain in the aqueous phase of emulsions. It is non-toxic, non-irritating and non-sensitizing. However, contact dermatitis caused by this product has been reported [493, 494]. It is compatible with emulsion ingredients and with proteins.

It has been claimed that Germall 115 has the ability to act synergistically with other preservatives [117, 495, 496]. Intrinsically it is more active against bacteria than fungi. Most of the microbiological data are based on challenge tests in cosmetic formulations, data which are of great value to the cosmetic microbiologist. An investigation of its activity against a series of *Pseudomonas* species and strains [492] showed that in a challenge test 0.3% of the compound cleared all species but *Pseudomona putida* and *Pseudomonas aureofaciens* in 24 h. The latter species were killed at between 3 and 7 days. In an agar cup-plate test, 1% solution gave the following size inhibition zones (mm): *S. aureus*, 7,6; *S. aureus*, penicillin sensitive, 15.5; *Staphylococcus albus*, 9.0; *B. subtilis*, 15.0; *Corynebacterium acne*, 5.0; *E. coli*, 3.6; and *Pseudomonas ovale*, 2.0.

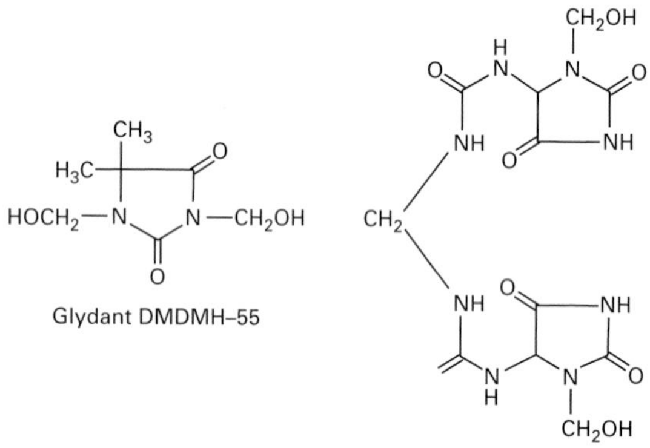

Figure 2.31 Dantoin or Glydant DMDMH-55 and Germall 115.

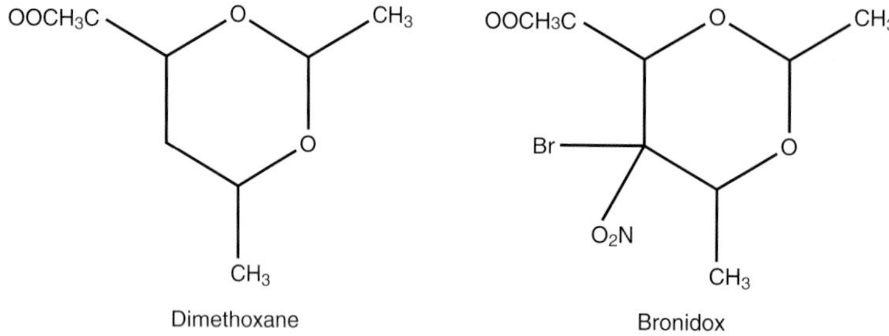

Figure 2.30 Dioxanes: dimethoxane and bronidox.

Diazolidinyl urea

Diazolidinyl urea (Figure 2.32) is a heterocyclic substituted urea produced by the reaction of allantoin and formaldehyde in a different ratio than that for imidazolidinyl urea. It is available as a powder commercially as Germall II (ISP, New Jersey, USA), and when used at 0.1–0.3% is stable at pH 2 to 9 providing broad-spectrum antibacterial activity with some activity against molds. It is twice as active as imidazolidinyl urea. It is often used in conjunction with methyl- and propyl-paraben to provide additional activity against mold. When combined with 3-iodo-2-propynylbutylcarbamate a synergistic action is achieved.

Isothiazolones

Ponci et al. [497] studied the antifungal activity of a series of 5-nitro-1,2-dibenzisothiazolones and found many of them to possess high activity. Since this publication a number of isothiazolones (Figure 2.33) have emerged as microbicidal preservatives. They are available commercially, usually as suspensions rather than as pure compounds, and find use in a variety of industrial situations. Nicoletti et al. [498] have described their activity.

Mode of action

The isothiazolones are thiol-interactive agents, which act by two steps: (i) rapid inhibition of metabolism and growth, which involves disruption of dehydrogense enzymes; and then (ii) irreversible cell damage. Therefore, growth, respiration and energy generation (ATP synthesis) are rapidly inhibted. Microbial death results from the destruction of protein thiols and production of free radicals [499]. At growth-inhibitory concentrations, 1,2-benzisothiazolin-3-one (BIT) has little effect on the membrane integrity of S. aureus, but significantly inhibits active transport and oxidation of glucose and has a marked effect on thiol-containing enzymes.

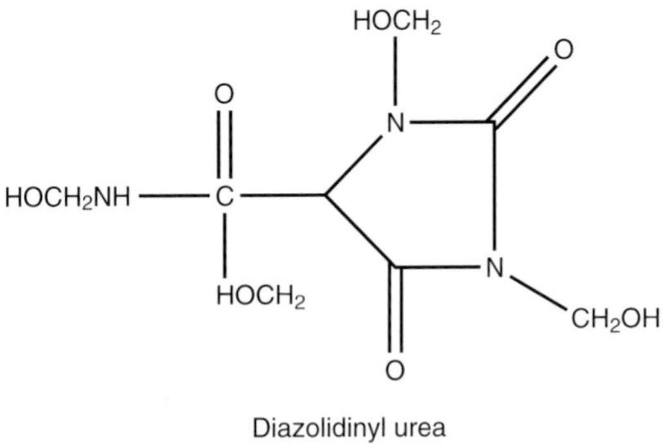

Thiol-containing compounds quench the activity of BIT, 5-chloro-2-methyl-4-isothiazolin-3-one (CMIT) and 2-methyl-4-isothiazolin-3-one (MIT) against E. coli, which suggests that these isothiazolones interact strongly with thiol groups. The activity of CMIT is also overcome by non-thiol amino acids, so that this compound might thus react with amines as well as with essential thiol groups [500, 501]. Collier et al. [501] showed that CMIT could tautomerize to form a thio-acyl-chloride compound, which is many fold more chemically reactive than its parent product (Figure 2.34). The tautomer may react with amines and hydroxyls in addition to thiols and, hence, is responsible for the greatly enhanced microbicidal activity of chlorinated isothiazolones.

5-Chloro-2-methyl-4-isothiazolin-3-one (CMIT) and 2-methyl-4-isothiazolin-3-one (MIT)

A mixture of these two derivatives (3 parts CMIT to 1 part MIT), known as Kathon 886 MW (Rohm and Haas (UK) Ltd, Coventry, UK), containing about 14% of active ingredients, is available as a preservative for cutting oils and as an in-can preservative for emulsion paints. This mixture is active at concentrations of 2.25–9 µg/ml active ingredients against a wide range of bacteria and fungi and does not show a Pseudomonas gap. It is also a potent algistat. It has major application in industrial water treatment to control microbial growth and biofouling [499].

Kathon CG, containing 1.5% active ingredients and magnesium salts, has been widely used in cosmetic products. The level of activity to be included in cosmetic rinse-off products is restricted to 15 ppm and for leave-on products 7.5 ppm because of irritancy issues primarily due to the CMIT element. It possesses the additional advantage of being biodegradable to non-toxic metabolites, water soluble and compatible with most emulsions. The stability of Kathon 886 at various pH values is described by Croshaw [488].

Methylisothiazolinone alone as 9.5% in water (commercially available as Neolane M-10 (Rohm and Haas)) is stable over a wide range of pH and temperature conditions and is compatible with a variety of surfactants. It has broad-spectrum activity and is said to be particularly useful for replacing formaldehyde in a wide range of applications at levels of 50–150 ppm active ingredient [502]. From August 2001, in the EC, any product containing CMIT/MIT in the ratio 3:1 in excess of 15 ppm must display an appropriate R phrase warning.

2-n-Octyl-4-isothiazolin-3-one (Skane)

This is available as a 45% solution in propylene glycol and is active against bacteria over a range of 400–500 µg/ml active ingredient.

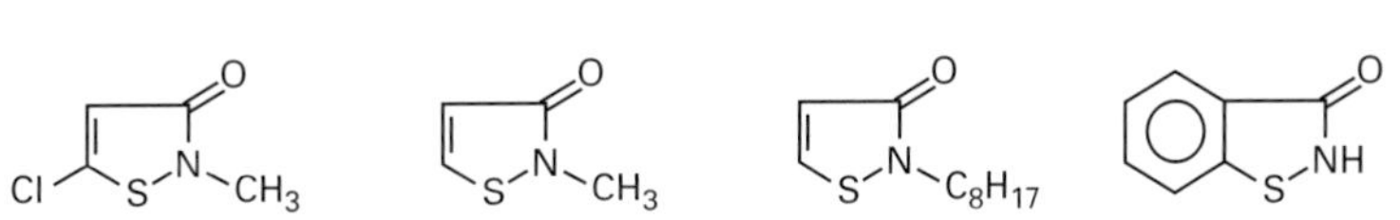

Diazolidinyl urea

Figure 2.32 Diazolidinyl urea.

Figure 2.33 Isothiazolones, from left to right: 5-chloro-2-methyl-4-isothiazolin-3-one (CMIT), 2-methyl-4-isothiazolin-3-one (MIT), 2-n-octyl-4-isothiazolin-3-one and 1,2-benzisothiazolin-3-one (BIT).

To inhibit the growth of one strain of *P. aeruginosa* required 500 µg/ml. Fungistatic activity was shown against a wide number of species over the range 0.3–8.0 µg/ml. It is also effective at preventing algal growth at concentrations of 0.5–5.0 µg/ml. It is biodegradable but shows skin and eye irritancy. As might be expected from its *n*-octyl side-chain, it is not soluble in water.

1,2-Benzisothiazolin-3-one (BIT)

This is available commercially in various formulations and is recommended as a preservative for industrial emulsions, adhesives, polishes, glues, household products and paper products. It possesses low mammalian toxicity but is not a permitted preservative for cosmetics.

Derivatives of hexamine

Hexamine (hexamethylene tetramine; 1,3,5,7-triaza-1-azonia-adamantane) has been used as a urinary antiseptic since 1894. Its activity is attributed to a slow release of formaldehyde. Wohl in 1886 was the first to quaternize hexamine, and in 1915/1916 Jacobs and co-workers attempted to extend the microbicidal range of hexamine by quaternizing one of its nitrogen atoms with halo-hydrocarbons [503, 504]. These workers did not consider that their compounds acted as formaldehyde releasers, but that activity resided in the whole molecule.

Scott and Wolf [505] re-examined quaternized hexamine derivatives with a view to using them as preservatives for toiletries, cutting oils and other products. They looked at 31 such

compounds and compared their activity with hexamine and formaldehyde. As well as determining their inhibitory activity towards *Staphylococcus* spp., an enterobacteria and a pseudomonad, they also assessed inhibitory activity towards *Desulfovibrio desulfuricans*, a common contaminant of cutting oils.

Polarographic and spectroscopic studies of formaldehyde release were made on some of the derivatives; this release varied with the substituent used in forming the quaternary salt. A typical set of data for the microbicidal activity (MIC) of one derivative compared with hexamine and formaldehyde is shown in Table 2.13. In general, the quaternized compounds were found to be more active w/w than hexamine, but less active than formaldehyde. Although chemically they contain a quaternized nitrogen atom, unlike the more familiar microbicidal quaternized compounds they are not inactivated by lecithin or protein. The compounds are not as surface active as conventional QACs. Thus an average figure for the surface tension (dyne/cm) for 0.1% solutions of the quaternized hexamines was 54; that for 0.1% cetrimide was 34.

One of these derivatives of hexamine, which quaternized with *cis*-1,3-dichloropropene, is being used as a preservative under the name Dowicil 200 (Dow Chemical Company). *Cis*-1-(3-cis-chloroallyl)-3,5,7-triaza-1-azonia-admantane chloride *N*-(3-chloroallyl) hexamine (Dowicil 200; Figure 2.35) is a highly water-soluble, hygroscopic, white powder; it has a low oil solubility. It is active against bacteria and fungi. Typical MICs (µg/ml) were: *E. coli*, 400; *Proteus vulgaris*, 100; *S. typhi*, 50; *Alcaligenes*

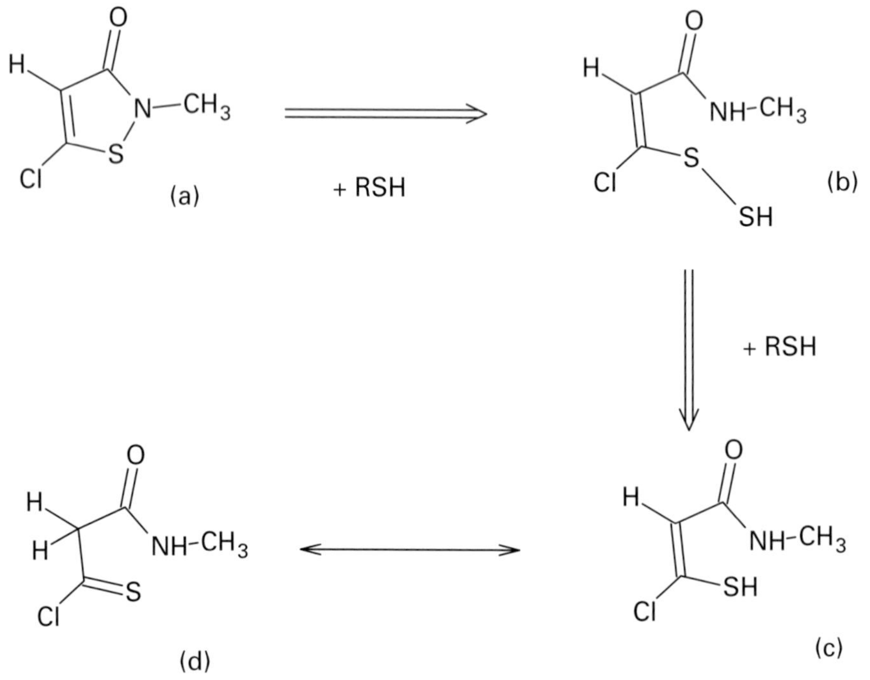

Figure 2.34 Pathway for the reaction of chloro-2-methyl-4-isothiazolin-3-one (CMIT) with thiol (RSH) (a) to give a mixed disulphide (b), and with excess thiol (RSH) a "ring-open" form (c). This latter form may then tautomerize to give a thio-acyl-chloride (d). (After Collier *et al.* [501].)

Table 2.13 Inhibitory concentrations for hexamine quaternized with –CH₂Cl=CHCl compared with values for hexamine and formaldehyde.

Inhibitor	MIC[a] against					
	S. aureus	*S. typhi*	*K. aerogenes*	*P. aeruginosa*	*B. subtilis*	*D. desulfuricans*
Hexamine quaternized with –CH₂-CH=CHCl	4×10^{-4} (100)	2×10^{-4} (50)	2×10^{-4} (50)	2×10^{-3} (500)	4×10^{-4} (100)	2.9×10^{-2} (7250)
Hexamine	3.5×10^{-2} (5000)	3.5×10^{-3} (500)	–	–	–	5.3×10^{-2} (7500)
Formaldehyde	1.6×10^{-3} (50)	3.3×10^{-3} (100)	1.6×10^{-3} (50)	–	–	–

[a] Molar values (in parentheses in µg/ml).

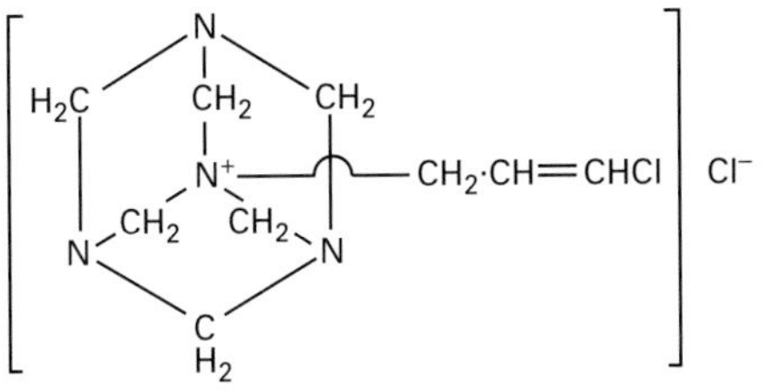

Figure 2.35 Dowicil 200 (*N*-(3-*cis*-chloroallyl)hexamine).

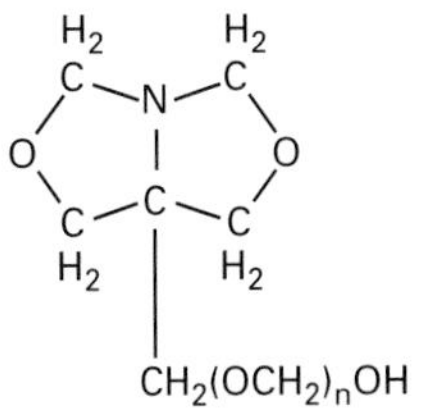

Figure 2.37 Nuosept 95 (*n* = 0–5).

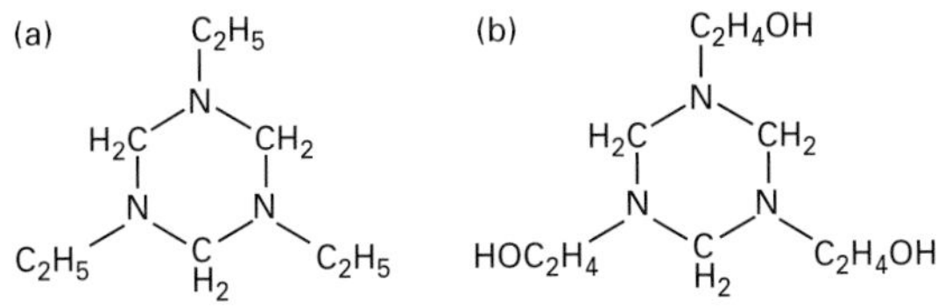

Figure 2.36 (a) Hexahydro-1,3,5-triethyl-*s*-triazine and (b) 1,3,5-tris(2-hydroxyethyl)-*s*-triazine (Grotan).

faecalis, 50; *P. aeruginosa*, 600; *S. aureus*, 200; *B. subtilis*, 200; *Aspergillus niger (brasiliensis)*, 1200; and *Trichophyton interdigitale*, 50.

It is recommended for use as a preservative for cosmetic preparations at concentrations from 0.05% to 0.2%. Because of its high solubility, it does not tend to concentrate in the oil phase of these products, but remains in the aqueous phase, where contamination is likely to arise. It is not inactivated by the usual ingredients used in cosmetic manufacture. Its activity is not affected over the usual pH ranges found in cosmetic or cutting oil formulations. For further information, see Rossmore and Sondossi [277].

Triazines

The product, theoretically from the condensation of three molecules of ethylamine with three of formaldehyde, is hexahydro-1,3,5-triethyl-*s*-triazine (Figure 2.36a). This is a clear white or slightly yellow viscous liquid, readily soluble in water, acetone, ethanol and ether. It is bactericidal and fungicidal and inhibits most bacteria, including *P. aeruginosa* and *Desulfovibrio desulfuricans* at concentrations of 0.3 mg/ml. Fungi, such as *Aspergillus niger (brasiliensis)*, *Penicillium glaucum* and *Penicillium notatum* are inhibited at 0.1 mg/ml, and *Saccharomyces cerevisiae* at

0.05 mg/ml. It owes its activity to a release of formaldehyde. It has been used as a preservative for cutting oils, for the preservation of emulsion paints, for proteinaceous adhesives and to control slime in paper and cardboard manufacture, and to prevent the growth of microorganisms in water-cooling systems. It has a low intrinsic toxicity and at use dilutions is not irritating to the skin.

If formaldehyde is reacted with ethanolamine, the compound 1,3,5-tris(2-hydroxyethyl)-*s*-triazine can be formed (Grotan: Troy Corporation, New Jersey, USA) (Figure 2.36b). This has both antibacterial and antifungal activity and is recommended as a preservative for cutting oils. Despite the figures for fungal inhibition, it is often found in practical preservation situations that, although this triazine will inhibit microbial growth, a fungal superinfection is often established; a total preservation system that includes a triazine might well have to contain an additional antifungal compound [506]. This situation may be compared with that found with imidazole derivatives. Rossmore [507] discussed the uses of heterocyclic compounds as industrial microbicides, and Rossmore and Sondossi [277] have reviewed formaldehyde condensates in general.

Oxazolo-oxazoles

By reacting formaldehyde with tris(hydroxymethyl)-methylamine, a series of derivatives is obtained. The commercial product (Nuosept 95: ISP, New Jersey, USA) (Figure 2.37) contains the molecule species: 5-hydroxymethoxymethyl-1-aza-3,7-dioxabicyclo (3.3.0) octane, 24.5%; 5-hydroxymethyl-1-aza-3,7-dioxabicyclo(3.3.0)octane, 17.7%; and 5-hydroxypolymethylenoxy (74% C₂, 21% C₃, 4% C₄, 1% C₅) methyl-1-aza-3,7-dioxabicyclo (3.3.0) octane, 7.8%. It acts as a biostat by virtue of being a formaldehyde releaser.

It is obtained as a clear, pale yellow liquid, which is miscible with water, methanol, ethanol, chloroform and acetone in all proportions, and is recommended as a preservative for cutting oils, water-treatment plants, emulsion (latex) paints, industrial slurries, and starch- and cellulose-based products. It is a slight irritant to intact and abraded skin and is a severe eye irritant.

Sodium hydroxymethylglycinate

A 50% aqueous solution of this compound (Figure 2.38) is available commercially as Suttocide A (ISP, New Jersey, USA). The solution is a clear alkaline liquid with a mild characteristic odor. It is active over a pH range of 3.5 to 12.0 and has a broad spectrum of activity against Gram-positive and Gram-negative bacteria, yeasts and molds at concentrations between 0.05% and 0.25%. Sodium hydroxymethylaglycinate is also used as preservative in personal care products.

Methylene bisthiocyanate

This is available commercially as a 10% solution and is recommended for the control of slime in paper manufacture, where it provides a useful alternative to mercurials. The compound (Figure 2.39) is a skin and eye irritant and thus care is required in its use. Its toxicity is low enough to enable it to be used in the manufacture of papers destined for the packaging of food. At in-use dilutions, it is unlikely to cause corrosion of materials used in the construction of paper-manufacturing equipment. It is used as a bactericide, fungicide, algicide and disinfectant [508].

Captan

Captan is N-(trichloromethylthio)cyclohex-4-ene-1,2-dicarboximide (Figure 2.40). It is a white crystalline solid, insoluble in

water and only slightly soluble in organic solvents. It is decomposed in alkaline solution. Despite its low solubility, it can be shown to be an active microbicide, being active against both Gram-negative and Gram-positive bacteria, yeasts and molds. It has been used as an agricultural fungicide, being primarily employed against diseases of fruit trees. It has also been used to prevent spoilage of stored fruit and in the treatment of skin infections due to fungi in humans and animals.

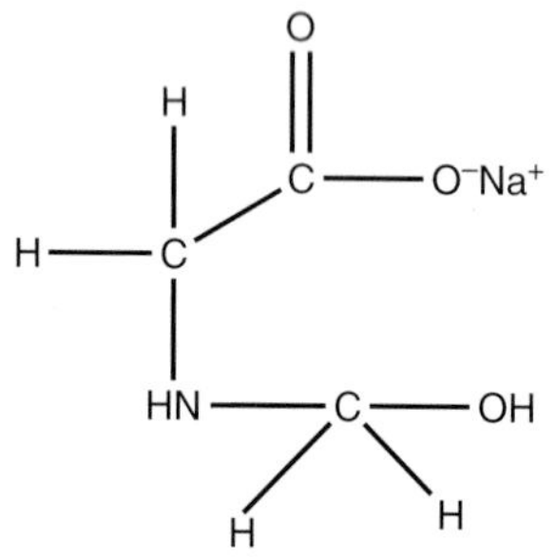

1,2-dibromo-2,4-dicyanobutane (Tektamer 38)

A halogenated aliphatic nitrile, 1,2-dibromo-2,4-dicyanobutane (Figure 2.41) is an off-white powder with a mildly pungent odor. It is available commercially as Tektamer 38 (Nalco Chemical Company, Illinois, USA). It is a broad-spectrum microbicide, being most active over the pH range 2.0 to 9.5, at an effective concentration of 0.025–0.15%. It is used in paints, joint cements, adhesives, pigments and metal-working fluids.

Glucoprotamin

Glucoprotamin, a new disinfectant, is based on a conversion product of L-glutamic acid and coco(C12/14)alkylpropylene-1,3-diamine. It is active *in vitro* against vegetative bacteria including mycobacteria, fungi and viruses [509, 510]. Undiluted glucoprotamin is also effective against bacterial spores. It is highly active against mycobacteria, which usually have a higher level of resistance to disinfectants. Glucoprotamin is non-corrosive to metals and compatible with most materials used in healthcare. It is licensed in Europe as a high-level disinfectant that is used for reprocessing medical instruments [511].

Essential oils

Essential oils have been used empirically throughout history as preservatives. Their re-examination as microbicidal agents has received attention from many workers, as their use as natural preservatives has contemporary appeal.

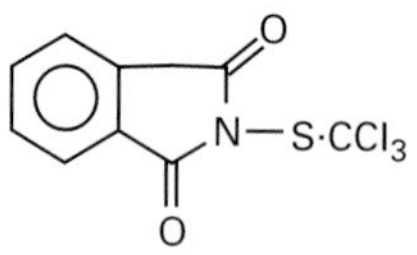

Sodium hydroxymethylglycinate

Figure 2.38 Sodium hydroxymethylglycinate.

Figure 2.40 Captan.

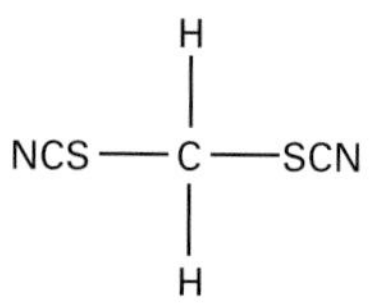

Figure 2.39 Methylene bisthiocyanate.

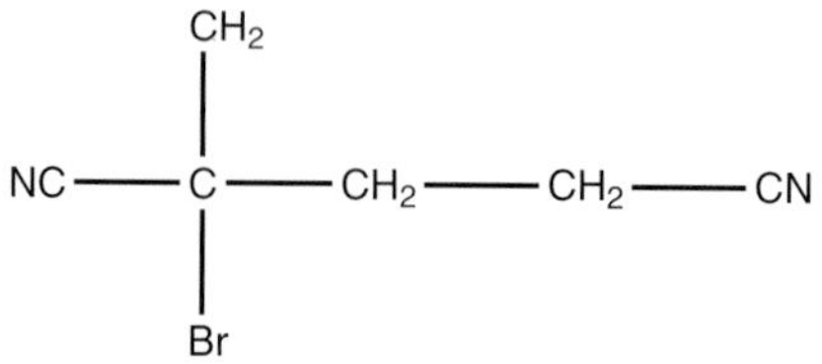

Figure 2.41 1,2-Dibromo-2,4-dicyanobutane (Tektamer 38).

Tea tree oil

Melaleuca alternifolia (tea tree) oil (TTO) has been included increasingly in consumer products as a microbicidal agent. Studies have shown that TTO is an effective microbicidal agent demonstrating activity against MRSA [512–514], yeasts [515–517] and herpes simplex virus [518]. TTO is active against most bacteria at concentrations of 1% or less. However, concentrations above 2% are required for *P. aeruginosa*, *Enterococcus faecalis* and *Staphylococcus* spp. Vaporized TTO can inhibit *Mycobacterium avium*, *E. coli*, *Haemophilus influenzae*, *S. pyogenes* and *Streptococcus pneumoniae*. TTO was found to cause loss of membrane integrity and function, leading to inhibition of glucose-dependent respiration, loss of viability and induction of lysis. Its effects are observed to be greater for bacteria in the exponential phase of growth than those at other phases [519].

Thymol and carvacrol

Thymol and carvacrol (an isomer of thymol) are believed to be the active ingredients of several essential oils and are found in plants such as thyme and oregano [520]. Oregano and thyme essential oils have been shown to be strongly microbicidal against Gram-positive and Gram-negative bacteria and fungi [520] and are very effective against *E. coli* O157:H7 [521]. Carvacrol is thought to exert its microbicidal activity by destabilizing the cytoplasmic membrane and acting as a proton exchanger [522]. Thymol has also found use as an active ingredient in mouthwashes. Listerine® Antiseptic (Johnson and Johnson), which contains thymol, menthol and eucalyptol essential oils, demonstrated microbicidal activity against oral microorganisms in dental plaque [523–525].

Clove oil

Clove oil obtained from *Syzygium aromaticum* has been used in many preparations for toothache, earache and topical antiseptics in addition to its use in the fragrance and flavoring industries. It contains carvacrol, cinnamaldehyde and thymol, but its main constituent is eugenol. It has antifungal activity against *Candida* spp., dermatophytes and *Aspergillus* spp. [526, 527]. Recent studies have shown that it has quorum-sensing inhibitory activity [528].

Eucalyptus oil

Eucalyptus oil is obtained by distillation of leaves of certain *Eucalyptus* tree leaves. The main component of the oil is 1,8-cineol (eucalyptol). Eucalyptus oil has wide applications as insect repellent, disinfectant, antiseptic and in many medical preparations such as an inhalation for colds and flu, lozenges and cough syrups [529, 530]. It was shown to have good bactericidal activity against some respiratory tract pathogens [531, 532], an anti-inflammatory effect [533] and in promoting periodontal health [534].

Essential oils have also been shown to act synergistically with other microbicidal agents [120, 535] and physical conditions [536, 537]. Many other essential oils have been isolated and investigated with varying degrees of microbicidal activity demonstrated. Activity has been shown to be influenced by factors such as the vapor activity of the oils [538] and the test method employed [539]. The antibacterial properties of essential oils have been reviewed by Deans and Ritchie [540] and Nakatsu *et al.* [520].

General statement

An ever-present problem with the preservation of cosmetics is that of contact sensitization. This is discussed in some detail by Marzulli and Maibach [541] and is a point which must be carefully checked before a preservative is committed to a product. Another hazard which may arise is that of an induced change in the skin microflora during long-term use of products containing microbicidal preservatives.

Vapor-phase disinfectants

It is only comparatively recently that a scientific basis for using vapors and gases as sterilizing or disinfecting agents has been established. Factors influencing the activity of gaseous formaldehyde were described by Nordgren [542] and later by the Committee on Formaldehyde Disinfection [543]. The possible uses of gaseous formaldehyde in the disinfection of hospital bedding and blankets and, in conjunction with low-temperature steam, for disinfection of heat-sensitive material, are considered below.

Phillips and Kaye [544] reviewed the earlier work on the bactericidal, mycobactericidal, sporicidal, fungicidal and virucidal activity of ethylene oxide [545]. A later review has been done by Richards *et al.* [546].

Other gases of possible value include propylene oxide, ozone, methyl bromide and glycidaldehyde [272]. Physical and chemical properties of these and the two most important ones (ethylene oxide and formaldehyde) are listed in Table 2.14 and their chemical structures given in Figure 2.42.

Ethylene oxide

Ethylene oxide's microbicidal activity is affected by concentration, temperature, relative humidity and the water content of the microorganisms. It acts, by virtue of its alkylating properties, on proteins and nucleic acids. A consideration of its microbicidal activity with compounds of a similar chemical structure (Figures 2.42 and 2.43) demonstrates that cyclopropane, which is not an alkylating agent, is not microbicidal, whereas those that have the ability to alkylate are potent microbicides. Useful reviews are those by Sintim-Damoa [419], Richards *et al.* [546], Burgess and Reich [547], Jorkasky [548] and Page [549].

Formaldehyde-releasing agents

Paraformaldehyde ($HO(CH_2O)_nH$, where $n = 8–100$) is a polymer of formaldehyde and is produced by evaporating aqueous

Table 2.14 Properties of the most commonly used gaseous disinfectants.

Gaseous disinfectant	Molecular weight	Boiling point (°C)	Solubility in water	Sterilizing concn (mg/l)	Relative humidity requirements (%)	Penetration of materials	Microbicidal activity[a]	Best application as gaseous disinfectant
Ethylene oxide	44	10.4	Complete	400–1000	Non-desiccated 30–50; large load 60	Moderate	Moderate	Sterilization of plastic medical supplies
Propylene oxide	58	34	Good	800–2000	Non-desiccated 30–60	Fair	Fair	Decontamination
Formaldehyde	30	90 (formalin)[b]	Good	3.10	75	Poor (surface sterilant)	Excellent	Surface sterilant for rooms
Methyl bromide	95	4.6	Slight	3500	30–50	Excellent	Poor	Decontamination

[a] Based on an equimolar comparison.
[b] Formalin contains formaldehyde plus methanol.

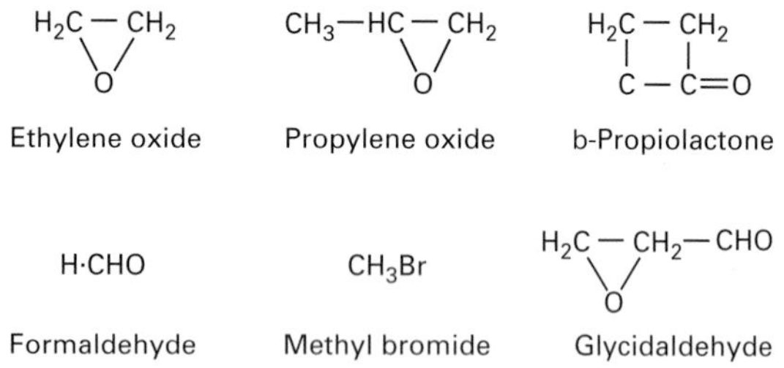

Figure 2.42 Chemical structures of gaseous disinfectants.

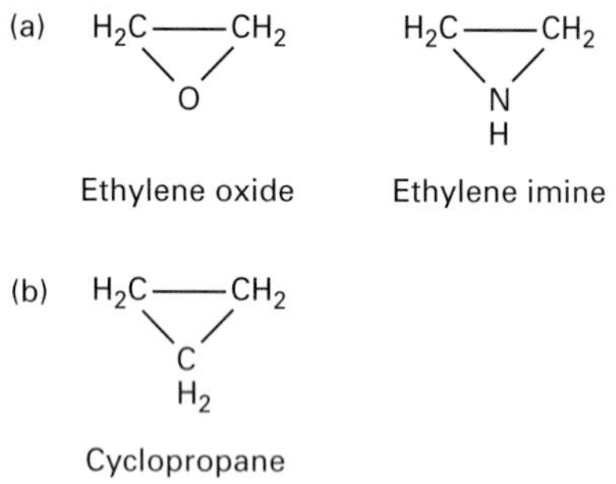

Figure 2.43 Compounds similar to ethylene oxide: (a) alkylating and antimicrobial compounds and (b) a non-alkylating, non-antimicrobial agent.

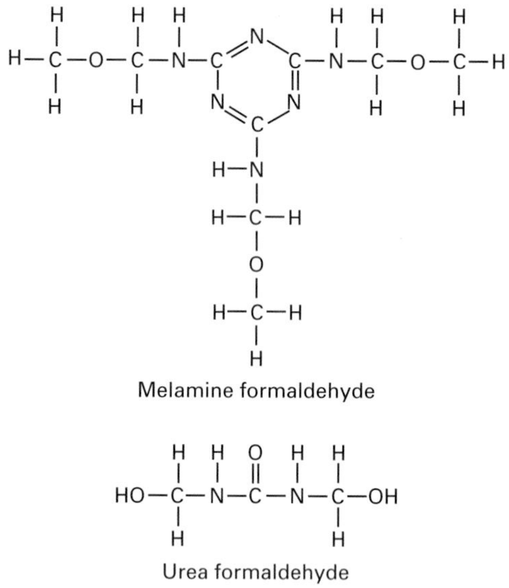

Figure 2.44 Melamine formaldehyde and urea formaldehyde.

solutions of formaldehyde. Although it was considered originally to be of little practical use [542] paraformaldehyde has since been shown to depolymerize rapidly when heated, to produce formaldehyde. Paraformaldehyde is considered to be an excellent source of monomeric formaldehyde gas because it can be produced in a temperature-controlled reaction and there are no contaminating residues (methanol and formic acid) produced during the evaporation of formalin solutions, in contrast to the method of evaporating formalin solutions containing 10% methanol to prevent polymerization.

Other formaldehyde-releasing agents are melamine formaldehyde and urea formaldehyde (Figure 2.44). The former is produced from formaldehyde and melamine under alkaline conditions and the latter is a mixture of monomethyloyl urea and dimethyloyl urea. When exposed to elevated temperatures these agents release potentially sterilizing amounts of gaseous formaldehyde, the rate of release being a function of time and temperature. However, these formaldehyde-releasing agents are much less effective as disinfecting or sterilizing agents than paraformaldehyde. The reason for this is that there is a much greater release of formaldehyde from paraformaldehyde than from the resins at various temperatures and the microbicidal process is strictly a function of the available formaldehyde gas.

Applications and mode of action of formaldehyde-condensate microbicides have been reviewed by Rossmore and Sondossi [277] and Rossmore [550]. Formaldehyde vapor has found use as a disinfectant in the following situations [272]:

1. In combination with low-temperature steam (70–90°C) as a method for disinfecting heat-sensitive materials [551].
2. Rarely, in the disinfection of hospital bedding and blankets, when formaldehyde solutions are used in the penultimate rinse

of laundering blankets to give a residual bactericidal activity because of the slow evolution of formaldehyde vapor [551].

3. In the terminal disinfection of premises, although this is considered to be of limited value [552].

4. As a fumigant in poultry houses after emptying and before new stock is introduced [273] and in the hatchery to prevent bacterial contamination of shell eggs [553].

5. In the disinfection of biological safety cabinets.

However, recently concerns have been expressed over the use of formaldehyde and glutaraldehyde due to their association with nasal cytotoxicity [554] and leukemia [555, 556].

Propylene oxide
Propylene oxide requires only mild heating to produce the vapor form and has a fair penetration of materials (see Table 2.14). It hydrolyzes slowly in the presence of only a small amount of moisture to give non-toxic propylene glycol and there is no need to remove it from exposed materials. Bactericidal activity decreases with an increase in relative humidity [557], although with desiccated organisms the reverse applies. Propylene oxide has been shown to be suitable for treating powdered or flaked foods [557].

Ozone
Ozone, O_3, is an allotropic form of oxygen. It has powerful oxidizing properties, inhibits bacterial growth [558] and is bactericidal, virucidal and sporicidal, although spores are 10^{15} times more resistant than non-sporing bacteria [559, 560]. In addition, ozone is considered the most effective protozoan cysticide [130]. Ozone is approved by the US FDA as alternate to ethylene oxide for sterilizing reusable medical equipment [194]. Gaseous ozone reacts with amino acids, RNA and DNA. It is unstable chemically in water, but activity persists because of the production of free radicals, including $HO^{\cdot}$. Synergistic effects have been shown with the simultaneous use of sonication [561] and ultraviolet [562] and negative air ions [563]. Ozone is used for water treatment in dialysis units or in industry [564]. In addition, it is used to wash and sanitize fruits and vegetables with intact surfaces [565]. Recent studies have shown that ozone has a promising potential in dentistry [566]. The use of ozone for enhancing food safety and quality has been reviewed by Kim *et al.* [567] and Khadre *et al.* [568]. Ozone generators have been proven to be effective in decontaminating surfaces and fields in healthcare settings [569, 570].

Carbon dioxide
Carbon dioxide in soft drinks inhibits the development of various types of bacteria [571]. The growth of psychrotolerant, slime-producing bacteria is markedly inhibited by CO_2 gas in the atmosphere [572].

Mode of action
For further information, the reader is referred to the reviews by Russell [272], Richards *et al.* [546] and Russell and Chopra [26]. As noted above (see also Figures 2.42 and 2.43), there is strong evidence that ethylene oxide acts by virtue of its alkylating properties. This gaseous agent reacts with proteins and amino acids, and with nucleic acid guanine (to give 7-(2'-hydroxyethyl) guanine), with alkylation of phosphated guanine possibly being responsible for its activity. Formaldehyde is an extremely reactive chemical that interacts with cellular proteins RNA and DNA.

Aerial disinfectants

An early procedure for aerial disinfection was the employment of sulfur dioxide, obtained by burning sulfur, or of chlorine for fumigating sickrooms. An effective aerial disinfectant should be capable of being dispersed in the air so that complete and rapid mixing of contaminated air and disinfectant ensues. Additionally, an effective concentration should be maintained in the air, and the disinfectant must be highly and rapidly effective against airborne microorganisms at different relative humidities. To these microbiological properties must be added the property of no toxicity or irritancy. The most important means of using aerial disinfectants is by aerosol production. Aerosols consist of a very fine dispersed liquid phase in a gaseous (air) disperse phase. The lethal action of aerosols is believed to be due to condensation of the disinfectant on to the microbial cell. Thus, the disinfectant must be nebulized in a fine spray to enable it to remain airborne and thereby come into contact, by random collision, with any microorganisms present in the air. Relative humidity has an important bearing on activity and at low RH inadequate condensation of disinfectant on to the microbial cell occurs. This means that dustborne organisms are less susceptible to aerial disinfectants than are those enclosed in droplets; the optimum RH is usually 40–70%. In practice, chemical aerosols may be generated by spraying liquid chemicals into the air from an atomizer; solids may be vaporized by heat from a thermostatically controlled hotplate or dissolved in an appropriate solid and atomized. Various chemicals have been employed for disinfecting air, including the following:

1. Hexylresorcinol: this phenolic substance is active against a wide range of bacteria, but not spores, in air. It is vaporized from a thermostatically controlled hotplate, and the vapor is odorless.

2. Lactic acid: this is an effective bactericidal aerial agent, but is irritating at high concentrations.

3. Propylene glycol: this may be employed as a solvent for dissolving a solid disinfectant prior to atomization, but is also a fairly effective and non-irritating microbicidal agent in its own right [558].

4. Formaldehyde: in summary of previous information, formaldehyde gas may be generated by:
   a. evaporating commercial formaldehyde solution (formalin);
   b. adding formalin to potassium permanganate;

c. volatilizing paraformaldehyde;

d. exposing certain organic resins or polymers, such as melamine formaldehyde or urea formaldehyde, to elevated temperatures [272].

Fumigation by formaldehyde has found considerable use in poultry science [273].

Engineering control technologies are applied in order to control bioaerosols in indoor settings. These include air cleaners that are combined with upper room ultraviolet germicidal irradiation (UVGI), which emit non-ionizing electromagnetic radiation UVC light (250 nm). UV light damages microbial DNA sufficiently to interfere with microbial replication. UV lamps must be placed so as to maximize microbial exposure to the radiation while minimizing any harm to the personnel in the room [573–575].

Other recent approaches for in-door disinfection include heterogenous photocatalysis or plasma-based disinfection. Heterogenous photocatalysis is based on the UV irradiation of a solid catalyst, usually titanium dioxide (TiO_2), to generate pairs of electrons and holes (electron vacancy in valence band) that diffuse and are trapped on or near the TiO_2 surface. These excited electrons and holes have strong reducing and oxidizing activity and react with atmospheric water and oxygen to yield reactive species such as hydroxyl radicals ($^{\cdot}OH$), superoxide anions (O_2^{-}) and hydrogen peroxide (H_2O_2). These radicals can induce complete oxidation of microbial cells and organic compounds to CO_2 in addition to their ability to attack polyunsaturated phospholipids [576] resulting in significant damage to cell membranes [577]. However, attempts are now underway at replacing UV light with visible light [576, 578, 579].

Low-temperature plasma is a gas or vapor produced by exposing a gas to a magnetic or electric field that will cause a major proportion of the gas to become ionized [580]. Therefore, gas plasmas are composed of ions, electrons, uncharged particles such as atoms, molecules (e.g. O_3), radicals (OH^{-}, NO^{-}, etc.) and UV photons. Plasmas may be generated from many substances such as chlorine, glutaraldehyde, hydrogen peroxide and oxygen [580, 581]. The resulting ions and uncharged particles can be in an excited state that can return to a normal state by emitting a photon or through collisions with surfaces. These events can erode microorganisms atom by atom through intrinsic photodesorption or etching. Sometimes, etching is further activated by UV photons, which contributes to microbial elimination [582].

Inactivation of prions

Prions are abnormal, misfolded pathogenic forms of proteins that propagate themselves by imposing their conformation on to the cellular prion proteins (PrPC) of the host. Hence, prions are the converted form of normal proteins. Prions cause transmissible spongiform encephalopathy (TSE), a group of neurodegenerative diseases of humans and a variety of animals [583]. Prions are protease resistant and resist inactivation by conventional procedures such as irradiation, boiling, dry heat and chemicals (formalin, β-propiolactone, alcohol). Autoclaving alone does not produce complete inactivation of prions. Current recommendations for their inactivation include immersion in 1N NaOH (as final concentration) or 20,000 ppm sodium hypochlorite for 1 h followed by autoclaving (gravity displacement) for 1 h at 121°C. Surfaces or heat-sensitive materials can be treated by 2N NaOH or 20,000 ppm sodium hypochlorite for 1 h [137]. Prions were found to become protease sensitive after exposure to branched polyamines, including polyamidoamine and polypropyleneimine dendrimers, in acetic acid [584]. Exposure to enzymatic cleaners followed by autoclaving can reduce prion infectivity to undetectable levels [585]. Similar results were obtained from a combination of proteinase K, pronase with sodium dodecyl sulfate [586]. Treatment with acidic sodium dodecyl sulfate followed by autoclaving has also been found to eliminate human prions [587].

Other uses of microbicidal and microbistatic agents

Microbicidal agents are used widely as disinfectants and antiseptics in the hospital and domestic environments, as preservatives or bactericides in sterile or non-sterile pharmaceutical or cosmetic products [588], and as preservatives in certain foodstuffs. Additionally, they are employed in certain specialized areas, such as cutting oils, fuels, paper, wood, paint, textiles and the construction industry.

Use in the food, dairy, pharmaceutical and cosmetic industries

The effectiveness of many microbicides is reduced in the presence of organic/inorganic matter ("soil") in its various forms, such as blood, serum, pus, dirt, milkstone, food residues and fecal material. This decreased activity has an important bearing on the field use of such chemicals in the cosmetic [589], pharmaceutical [590], food [226, 339, 591] and dairy [592] industries. The principle in all cases is the same, namely, either adequate pre-cleaning or the addition of a suitable detergent.

In the presence of soil, the activity of a given chemical may become neutralized to varying degrees and/or the target microorganism may be physically shielded from attack.

Disinfectants in recreational waters

Various microorganisms have been associated with infections arising from hydrotherapy pools, swimming pools and whirlpools, but the most frequently implicated organism is *P. aeruginosa*, the source of which is often the pool pumps [593, 594]. Chlorine-based microbicides are commonly used as a sanitary control measure. Iodine-based formulations, though less expensive and more stable than chlorine for treating swimming pool waters, are not active against algae [595, 596]. Another useful agent used for the disinfection of swimming pools is the polymeric biguanide, Baquacil SB (Avecia, Blackley, Manchester, UK). Warren *et al.* [597] have published a comparative assessment of swimming pool disinfectants. Problems arising from the increasing use of whirlpools are referred to in the *Report of the Expert Advisory Committee on Biocides* [598].

Which microbicidal or microbistatic agent?

Regulatory requirements
The US FDA, the EU for the European Community (Directive 98/8/EC of the European Parliament and of the Council of 16 February 1998 concerning the placing of microbicidal products on the market) and most other countries publish information on the permitted use and concentration of preservatives. Current regulations should be consulted and complied with when manufacturing in these countries and exporting to them.

Cosmetic preservatives allowed in the EU are prescribed in Annex VI of the Cosmetics Directive, which includes details of concentration limits and restrictions for certain product types. In the UK, the Food Standards Agency publishes information on food additives and E numbers.

Which preservative?
Because of the many variables that affect the activity of microbistatic agents, it is almost impossible from a mere scrutiny of the literature to select a preservative that will be optimal in a particular product. Legislation passed in the USA by the FDA requires the manufacturers of cosmetics to declare the ingredients in their products and to state their function or purpose.

As regards combinations, an appraisal of the literature seems to suggest that a combination of one of the more water-soluble esters of *p*-hydroxybenzoic acid, probably the methyl ester, together with one of the water-soluble urea derivatives or a sulphydryl reactive compound, might be a good combination to start with. Denyer *et al.* [599] have discussed synergy in preservative combinations.

If the product is a water-in-oil emulsion, and it is felt that the oily phase needs protection, especially from mold growth, then a third component, one of the oil-soluble esters of *p*-hydroxybenzoic acid, for example the butyl ester, or an oil-soluble phenol, such as *o*-phenylphenol, might well be added. Over and above this, there remains the question-begging proviso "providing other criteria such as compatibility, stability, toxicity and regulatory requirements are satisfied".

Other concepts

In recent years, "natural agents" have increasingly been considered as potential preservatives for food products. These agents may be associated with immune systems and have been examined in mammals, insects and amphibians. As pointed out by Board [600], an agent active against prokaryotic but not mammalian cells is of obvious interest. Although Board [600] was discussing natural agents from animals as potential food preservatives, their possible use in other areas should also be investigated.

Likewise, the potential of natural food ingredients for the inhibition of microorganism growth has been investigated [601]. Such ingredients include plant extracts, essential oils, citrus fruits (such as grapefruit peel extracts) [602] and honey, shown to be active against Gram-positive cocci [603].

Bacteria such as lactic acid bacteria produce peptides (bacteriocins), which have been shown to have microbicidal activity. Cleveland *et al.* [604] have reviewed the bacteriocins produced by lactic acid bacteria such as nisin and pediocin and has shown them to be safe and have potential as natural food preservatives. While these agents themselves are not new, consumer focus is increasingly moving towards "natural" or "naturally produced" food additives. Further information about their microbicidal/ microbitatic spectrum, mode of action and physiochemical properties can be found in Ennahar *et al.* [605], Nes and Holo [606], Cintas *et al.* [607] and Cleveland *et al.* [604].

Microbicidal peptides can also be isolated from plants, insects, fish and mammals and have been shown to have antifungal activity [608–610]. The use of light-activated microbicides (or photodynamic therapy) has received a lot of attention recently. This approach uses compounds which, when activated by a light source, will generate free radicals and reactive oxygen species and damage the target cells. Applications such as in dentistry, for the treatment of periodontal disease, require the target cells to be killed without causing damage to human tissue. Poly-L-lysine-chlorine 6 activated by red light has been demonstrated to be effective at killing oral bacteria without any adverse effects to epithelial cells [611]. This technology can also be applied to wound sites. Griffiths and co-workers [612] have demonstrated that aluminum disulphonated phthalocyanine when activated by red light killed a range of strains of MRSA.

Light-activated TiO_2 systems may also have applications in water sanitization although activity is reduced in the presence of organic materials and inorganic radical scavengers [613]. In addition to bactericidal activity, photocatalyzed TiO_2 has also been demonstrated to have activity against endotoxins [614] and viruses [615, 616]. Lee and co-workers [615], using bacteriophage Q as a model virus, proposed the mechanism of virucidal action to be due to nucleic acid damage generated by photocatalysis.

Other photosensitive compounds and wavelengths of light have been investigated for use as photodynamic therapy systems and are discussed in the comprehensive review of Wainwright [617].

Superoxidized water is a disinfectant that is based on the concept of electrolyzing a saline solution to produce hypochlorous acid (e.g. at a concentration of about 144 mg/l) and chlorine. The end-product of this process (water) does not damage the environment. One method of generating the disinfectant at the point of use is by passing a saline solution over titanium-coated electrodes at 9 amp. In October 2002, the FDA cleared superoxidized water as a high-level disinfectant. In the absence of organic material, freshly produced superoxidized water is rapidly effective (<2 min) in achieving a 5-log reduction of pathogenic microorganisms (*M. tuberculosis*, *Mycobacterium chelonae*, poliovirus, HIV, MRSA, *E. coli*, *Candida albicans*, *Enterococcus faecalis*, *P. aeruginosa*). However, the activity of this disinfectant is reduced in the presence of organic load [424]. Its mode of action is not well understood, but is probably related to the activity of oxidizing species. Superoxidized water is recently under investigation for use in the food industry and wound treatment [618–620].

Another future avenue for microbicides may lie, not with new agents, but with novel delivery systems to ensure that the microbicide reaches its target. One such delivery system is the use of biodegradable lactic acid polymers for delivery of antibiotics in chronic bone infections [621]. The aim of the delivery system is to obtain high levels of the antibiotic at the site of the infection. The use of pH-sensitive liposomes to deliver gentamicin has the same rationale. Gentamicin has a poor penetration through biological membranes and use of this delivery system was shown to increase gentamicin accumulation to the disease site [622, 623]. It is foreseeable that such techniques will be used for the delivery of microbicides in the future.

Surfacine is a persistent microbicidal agent that may be used on animate or inanimate surfaces by rinsing, spraying or washing. It includes a water-insoluble microbicidal compound (silver iodide) in a surface-immobilized coating (a modified polyhexamethylenebiguanide). Silver iodide will chemically recognize and interact with the lipid bilayer of the bacterial outer cell membrane by electrostatic attraction. When a microbe contacts the surface, the microbicidal agent (silver) will be transferred from the coating to the organism. Microorganisms in contact with the surface will accumulate silver until the toxicity threshold is exceeded, when they lyse and detach from the surface. Therefore, whenever there is a contact with an organism the coating acts "on demand" to release the microbicide (silver) directly to the microorganism without releasing any silver into solution. This mechanism of silver release differs from that of topically applied silver compounds (e.g. silver nitrate). In the conventional way, silver ions are released into solution and a bactericidal ion concentration is generated in the solution. Surfacine is effective for several days, depending on the microbial load and the amount of silver present. The coating contains low levels of silver iodide ($c.\ 10\,\mu g/cm^2$ of coated surface), and coated surfaces are resistant to biofilm formation. It is active against bacteria, fungi, yeast and viruses [424].

Additional considerations

With the introduction of the Biocidal Products Directive in Europe [624], the cost to manufacturers of registering even existing microbicides has resulted in some being removed from the market, and the incentive to research and develop new microbicides is severely restricted. New combinations of existing microbicides are likely to be the focus of attention.

With the emergence of "new" pathogenic entities, such as prions, glycopeptide-resistant enterococci and multidrug-resistant mycobacteria, as well as microbicide-resistant mycobacteria, it is clear that better usage of existing microbicides is necessary. This has been discussed by Russell and Chopra [26]. In brief, future policies might well examine combinations of microbicides, or of a microbicide with a permeabilizer, to re-evaluate older, perhaps discarded, molecules, to consider whether physical procedures can enhance microbicidal activity and, where relevant, to determine how natural microbicidal systems can be better utilized.

A long-term goal should be the achievement of a better understanding of the ways in which microorganisms are inactivated and of the mechanisms whereby they circumvent the action of a microbicide.

Nanotechnology

Recent developments in nanotechnology have led to the generation of microbicides with remarkable and unusual physicochemical characteristics and biological activity. In this technology, the material is engineered into ultrafine nanoscale particles resulting in novel morphology and properties. Mesoporous silica is a development of nanotechnology where an organic silica derivative is formed into nano-sized spheres or rods that are filled with a regular arrangement of pores. These spheres can be loaded with various agents, such as microbicides, that can be targeted toward microorganisms. Recent studies have shown the potential of using mesoporous silica as implantable material or a coating for implants [625]; the silver-loaded spheres were shown to have promising effects as antibacterial and hemostatic agents [626].

Silver nanoparticles (nanosilver) are another area of nanotechnology showing promise as microbicidal agents. They have remarkable microbicidal activity and have applications in the medical field, such as in contraceptive devices, surgical instrument cleansers and bone prostheses, which can all be coated or embedded with nanosilver [627]. Many commercial products containing nanosilver have been approved by the FDA or the European Food and Safety Authority for wound dressings and antibacterial application. In addition nanosilver coatings are used on various textiles and are marketed as a water disinfectant and room spray. Silver nanoparticles have improved antibacterial properties compared with bulk silver due to high surface area and high fraction of surface atoms, leading to more nanoparticles being incorporated inside the bacteria. Silver nanoparticles are effective at nano concentrations and are even more effective than silver ions at microconcentrations [628, 629]. Work on microemulsions as pharmaceutical delivery systems has also yielded some interesting findings, indicating that they are antimicrobial in their own right. Al-Adham *et al.* [636, 637] have shown that they are active against both planktonic and biofilm cells of a selection of test bacteria and fungi.

References

1 Hugo, W.B. (1979) Phenols: a review of their history and development as antimicrobial agents. *Microbios*, **23**, 83–85.

2 Hugo, W.B. (1991) The degradation of preservatives by micro-organisms. *International Biodeterioration and Biodegradation*, **27**, 185–194.

3 Marouchoc, S.R. (1979) Classical phenol derivatives and their uses. *Developments in Industrial Microbiology*, **20**, 15–24.

4 Freney, J. (1995) Composés phénoliques, in *Antisepsie et Désinfection* (eds J. Fleurette *et al.*), Editions ESKA, Paris, pp. 90–134.

5 Goddard, P.A. and McCue, K.A. (2001) Phenolic compounds, in *Disinfection, Sterilization, and Preservation*, 5th edn (ed. S.S. Block), Lippincott Williams & Wilkins, Philadelphia, pp. 255–281.

6 Suter, G.M. (1941) Relationships between the structure and bactericidal properties of phenols. *Chemical Reviews*, **28**, 269–299.

7 Hugo, W.B. and Bowen, J.G. (1973) Studies on the mode of action of 4-ethylphenol. *Microbios*, **8**, 189–197.

8 Judis, J. (1965) Mechanism of action of phenolic disinfectants IV. Effects on induction of and accessibility of substrate to b-galactosidase in *Escherichia coli*. *Journal of Pharmaceutical Sciences*, **54** (3), 417–420.

9 Judis, J. (1965) Mechanism of action of phenolic disinfectants V. Effect of 2,4-dichlorophenol on the incorporation of labeled substrates by *Escherichia coli*. *Journal of Pharmaceutical Sciences*, **54** (4), 541–544.

10 Denyer, S. and Russel, D. (2004), Non-antibiotic antibacterial agents: mode of action and resistance, in *Hugo and Russell's Pharmaceutical Microbiology*, 7th edn (eds S. Dennyer *et al.*), Blackwell Publishing, Oxford, pp. 306–322.

11 British Association of Chemical Specialties (1998) *Guide to the Choice of Disinfectant*, BACS, Lancaster.

12 Berry, H. and Stenlake, J.B. (1942) Variations in the bactericidal value of Lysol BP. *Pharmaceutical Journal*, **148**, 112–113.

13 http://www.epa.gov/oppad001/list_b_tuberculocide.pdf; accession 01/06/12).

14 Jang, H. *et al.* (2008) Microarray analysis of toxicogenomic effects of ortho-phenylphenol in *Staphylococcus aureus*. *BMC Genomics*, **9**, 411.

15 Buchholz, V. *et al.* (2009) Topical antiseptics for the treatment of sore throat block voltage-gated neuronal sodium channels in a local anaesthetic-like manner. *Naunyn-Schmiedeberg's Archives of Pharmacology*, **380** (2), 161–168.

16 Factsheet: http://www.epa.gov/ogwdw/pdfs/factsheets/soc/pentachl.pdf (accessed June 1, 2012).

17 Factsheet: http://www.epa.gov/oppsrrd1/REDs/factsheets/3045fact.pdf (accessed June 1, 2012).

18 British Pharmacopoeia (2012) *British Pharmacopoeia*, HMSO, London.

19 Bruch, M.K. (1996) Chloroxylenol: an old–new antimicrobial, in *Handbook of Disinfectants and Antiseptics* (ed. J.M. Ascenzi), Marcel Dekker, New York, pp. 265–294.

20 Factsheet: http://www.epa.gov/oppsrrd1/REDs/factsheets/2045fact.pdf (accessed June 1, 2012).

21 Rapps, N.F. (1933) The bactericidal efficiency of chlorocresol and chloroxylenol. *Journal of the Society of Chemical Industry*, **52**, 175T–176T.

22 Colebrook, L. and Maxted, W.R. (1933) Antiseptics in midwifery. *Journal of Obstetrics and Gynaecology of the British Empire*, **40**, 966–990.

23 Beath, T. (1943) The suppression of infection in recent wounds by the use of antiseptics. *Surgery*, **13**, 667–676.

24 Ayliffe, G.A.J. *et al.* (1966) Cleansing and disinfection of hospital floors. *British Medical Journal*, **ii**, 442–445.

25 Lowbury, E.J.L. (1951) Contamination of cetrimide and other fluids with *Pseudomonas aeruginosa*. *British Journal of Industrial Medicine*, **8**, 22–25.

26 Russell, A.D. and Chopra, I. (1996) *Understanding Antibacterial Action and Resistance*, 2nd edn, Ellis Horwood, Chichester.

27 Dankert, J. and Schut, I.K. (1976) The antibacterial activity of chloroxylenol in combination with ethylenediamine tetraacetic acid. *Journal of Hygiene, Cambridge*, **76**, 11–22.

28 Russell, A.D. and Furr, J.R. (1977) The antibacterial activity of a new chloroxylenol preparation containing ethylenediamine tetraacetic acid. *Journal of Applied Bacteriology*, **43**, 253–260.

29 Hatch, E. and Cooper, P. (1948) Sodium hexametaphosphate in emulsions of Dettol for obstetric use. *Pharmaceutical Journal*, **161**, 198–199.

30 Stevenson, A.F. (1915) *An Efficient Liquid Disinfectant*, Public Health Reports 30, US Public Health Service, Washington, DC, pp. 3003–3008.

31 Klarmann, E.G. and von Wowern, J. (1929) The preparation of certain chloro- and bromo-derivatives of 2,4-dihydroxydiphenylmethane and ethane and their germicidal action. *Journal of the American Chemical Society*, **51**, 605–610.

32 Dunning, F. *et al.* (1931) Preparation and bacteriological study of some symmetrical organic sulphides. *Journal of the American Chemical Society*, **53**, 3466–3469.

33 Gump, W.S. and Walter, G.R. (1960) Chemical and antimicrobial activity of his phenols. *Journal of the Society of Cosmetic Chemists*, **11**, 307–314.

34 Gump, W.S. and Walter, G.R. (1963) Chemical structure and antimicrobial activity of his phenols. III. Broad spectrum evaluation of hexachlorophane and its isomers. *Journal of the Society of Cosmetic Chemists*, **14**, 269–276.

35 Gump, W.S. and Walter, G.R. (1964) Chemical structure and antimicrobial activity of his phenols. IV Broad spectrum evaluation of 2,2′-methylene bis (dichlorophenols). *Journal of the Society of Cosmetic Chemists*, **15**, 717–725.

36 Walter, G.R. and Gump, W.S. (1962) Chemical structure and antimicrobial activity of bis-phenols. II. Bactericidal activity in the presence of an anionic surfactant. *Journal of the Society of Cosmetic Chemists*, **13**, 477–482.

37 Fischer, M. (2001) Endoparasites in the dog and cat 1. Helminths. *In Practice*, **23**, 462–471.

38 Skallerup, P. *et al.* (2005) The impact of natural helminth infections and supplementary protein on growth performance of free-range chickens on small holder farms in El Sauce, Nicaragua. *Preventive Veterinary Medicine*, **69** (3–4), 229–244.

39 Corner, T.R. *et al.* (1971) Antimicrobial actions of hexachlorophane: lysis and fixation of bacterial protoplases. *Journal of Bacteriology*, **108**, 501–507.

40 Joswick, H.L. *et al.* (1971) Antimicrobial actions of hexachlorophane: release of cytoplasmic materials. *Journal of Bacteriology*, **168**, 492–500.

41 Silvernale, J.N. *et al.* (1971) Antimicrobial action of hexachlorophene: cytological manifestations. *Journal of Bacteriology*, **108**, 482–491.

42 Frederick, J.F. *et al.* (1974) Antimicrobial actions of hexachlorophane: inhibition of respiration in *Bacillus megaterium*. *Antimicrobial Agents and Chemotherapy*, **6**, 712–721.

43 Lee, C.R. and Corner, T.R. (1975) Antimicrobial actions of hexachlorophane: iron salts do not reverse inhibition. *Journal of Pharmacy and Pharmacology*, **27**, 694–696.

44 Hioe, K.P. and van der Weijden, G.A. (2005) The effectiveness of self-performed mechanical plaque control with triclosan containing dentifrices. *International Journal of Dental Hygiene*, **3** (4), 192–204.

45 Bhargava, H.N. and Leonard, P.A. (1996) Triclosan: applications and safety. *American Journal of Infection Control*, **24**, 209–218.

46 Russell, A.D. (2004) Whither triclosan? *Journal of Antimicrobial Chemotherapy*, **53**, 693–695.

47 McMurry, L.M. *et al.* (1998) Triclosan targets lipid synthesis. *Nature*, **394**, 531–532.

48 McMurry, L.M. *et al.* (1998) Overexpression of *marA*, *soxS*, or *acrAB* produces resistance to triclosan in laboratory and clinical strains of *Escherichia coli*. *FEMS Microbiology Letters*, **166**, 305–309.

49 McMurry, L.M. *et al.* (1999) Genetic evidence that InhA of *Mycobacterium smegmatis* is a target for triclosan. *Antimicrobial Agents and Chemotherapy*, **43**, 711–713.

50 Ochs, D. (1999) Biocide resistance. *Household and Personal Products Industry (HAPPI)*, **36** (4), 130–135.

51 Aiello, A.E. *et al.* (2007) Consumer antibacterial soaps: effective or just risky? *Clinical Infectious Diseases*, **45**, S137–S147.

52 Perozzo, R. *et al.* (2002) Structural elucidation of the specificity of the antibacterial agent triclosan for malarial enoyl acyl carrier protein reductase. *Journal of Biological Chemistry*, **277** (15), 13106–13114.

53 Heath, R.J. *et al.* (2002) Inhibitors of fatty acid synthesis as antimicrobial chemotherapeutics. *Applied Microbiology and Biotechnology*, **58** (6), 695–703.

54 Hugo, W.B. and Bloomfield, S.F. (1971) Studies on the mode of action of the phenolic antibacterial agent Fentichlor against *Staphylococcus aureus* and *Escherichia coli*. I. The absorption of Fentichlor by the bacterial cell and its antibacterial activity. *Journal of Applied Bacteriology*, **34**, 557–567.

55 Hugo, W.B. and Bloomfield, S.F. (1971) Studies on the mode of action of the phenolic antimicrobial agent Fentichlor against *Staphylococcus aureus* and *Escherichia coli*. II. The effects of Fentichlor on the bacterial membrane and the cytoplasmic constituents of the cell. *Journal of Applied Bacteriology*, **34**, 569–578.

56 Hugo, W.B. and Bloomfield, S.F. (1971) Studies on the mode of action on the antibacterial agent Fentichlor on *Staphylococcus aureus* and *Escherichia coli*. III. The effect of Fentichlor on the metabolic activities of *Staphylococcus aureus* and *Escherichia coli*. *Journal of Applied Bacteriology*, **34**, 579–591.

57 Bloomfield, S.F. (1974) The effect of the antibacterial agent Fentichlor on energy coupling in *Staphylococcus aureus*. *Journal of Applied Bacteriology*, **37**, 117–131.

58 Pflege, R. *et al.* (1949) Zur Chemotherapie der Pilzimfektionen. I. Mitteilung: *in vitro* untersuchungen aromatischer sulphide. *Zeitschrift für Naturforschung*, **4b**, 344–350.

59 Ayres, H.M. *et al.* (1993) A rapid method of evaluating permeabilizing activity against *Pseudomonas aeruginosa*. *Letters in Applied Microbiology*, **17**, 149–151.

60 Cruess, W.V. and Richert, P. (1929) Effects of hydrogen ion concentration on the toxicity of sodium benzoate to micro-organisms. *Journal of Bacteriology*, **17**, 363–371.

61 Simon, E.W. and Blackman, G.E. (1949) *The Significance of Hydrogen Ion Concentration in the Study of Toxicity*, Symposium of the Society of Experimental Biology No. 3, Cambridge University Press, Cambridge, pp. 253–265.

62 Simon, E.W. and Beevers, H. (1952) The effect of pH on the biological activities of weak acids and bases. I. The most usual relationship between pH and activity. *New Phytologist*, **51**, 163–190.

63 Simon, E.W. and Beevers, H. (1952) The effect of pH on the biological activities of weak acids and bases. II. Other relationships between pH and activity. *New Phytologist*, **51**, 191–197.

64 Eklund, T. (1989) Organic acids and esters, in *Mechanisms of Action of Food Preservation Procedure* (ed. G.W. Gould), Elsevier Applied Science, London, pp. 161–200.

65 Booth, I.R. and Kroll, R.G. (1989) The preservation of foods by low pH, in *Mechanisms of Action of Food Preservation Procedures* (ed. G.W. Gould), Elsevier Applied Science, London, pp. 119–160.

66 Cherrington, C.A. *et al.* (1991) Organic acids: chemistry, antibacterial activity and practical applications. *Advances in Microbial Physiology*, **32**, 87–108.

67 Russell, J.B. (1992) Another explanation for the toxicity of fermentation acids at low pH: anion accumulation versus uncoupling. *Journal of Applied Bacteriology*, **73**, 363–370.

68 Phillips, I. *et al.* (1968) Acetic acid in the treatment of superficial wounds infected by *Pseudomonas aeruginosa*. *Lancet*, **i**, 11–12.

69 Thorp, M.A. *et al.* (1998) The antibacterial activity of acetic acid and Burow's solution as topical otological preparations. *Journal of Laryngology and Otology*, **112** (10), 925–928.

70 Iba, A.M. and Berchieri, A. Jr. (1995) Studies on the use of a formic acid-propionic acid mixture (Bio-add) to control experimental *Salmonella* infection in broiler chickens. *Avian Pathology*, **24** (2), 303–311.

71 Roy, R.D. *et al.* (2002) Influence of a propionic acid feed additive on performance of turkey poults with experimentally induced poult enteritis and mortality syndrome. *Poultry Science*, **81** (7), 951–957.

72 Van Immersel, F. *et al.* (2005) Supplementation of coated butyric acid in the feed reduces colonization and shedding of *Salmonella* in poultry. *Poultry Science*, **84** (12), 1851–1856.

73 Fernandez-Rubio, C. *et al.* (2009) Butyric acid-based feed additives help protect broiler chickens from *Salmonella enteritidis* infection. *Poultry Science*, **88**, 943–948.

74 De los Santos, F.S. *et al.* (2009) The natural feed additive caprylic acid decreases *Campylobacter jejuni* colonization in market-aged broiler chickens. *Poultry Science*, **88**, 61–64.

75 Nair, M.K. *et al.* (2004) Inactivation of *Enterobacter sakazakii* in reconstituted infant formula by monocaprylin. *Journal of Food Protection*, **67** (12), 2815–2819.

76 Jang, H.I. and Rhee, M.S. (2009) Inhibitory effect of caprylic acid and mild heat on *Cronobacter* spp. (*Enterobacter sakazakii*) in reconstituted infant formula and determination of injury by flow cytometry. *International Journal of Food Microbiology*, **133** (1–2), 113–120.

77 Gorman, S.P. and Scott, E.M. (2004) Chemical disinfectants, antiseptics and preservatives, in *Hugo and Russell's Pharmaceutical Microbiology*, 7th edn (eds S. Dennyer *et al.*), Blackwell Publishing, pp. 285–305.

78 Beneke, E.S. and Fabian, F.W. (1955) Sorbic acid as a fungistatic agent at different pH levels for moulds isolated from strawberries and tomatoes. *Food Technology*, **9**, 486–488.

79 Gooding, C.M. *et al.* (1955) Sorbic acid as a fungistatic agent for foods. IX. Physico-chemical considerations in using sorbic acid to protect foods. *Food Research*, **20**, 639–648.

80 York, G.K. and Vaughan, R.H. (1955) Site of microbial inhibition by sorbic acid. *Bacteriological Proceedings*, **55**, 20.

81 Palleroni, N.J. and de Prinz, M.J.R. (1960) Influence of sorbic acid on acetate oxidation by *Saccharomyces cerevisae* var. *ellipsoideus*. *Nature, London*, **185**, 688–689.

82 Kabara, J.J. and Eklund, T. (1991) Organic acids and esters, in *Food Preservatives* (eds N.J. Russell and G.W. Gould), Blackie, Glasgow, pp. 44–71.

83 Plumridge, A. *et al.* (2008) The weak-acid preservative sorbic acid is decarboxylated and detoxified by a phenylacrylic acid decarboxylase, PadA1, in the spoilage mold *Aspergillus niger*. *Applied and Environmental Microbiology*, **74** (2), 550–552.

84 Kabara, J.J. (1980) GRAS antimicrobial agents for cosmetic products. *Journal of the Society of Cosmetic Chemists*, **31**, 1–10.

85 Lovelock, J.E. *et al.* (1944) Aerial disinfection. *Nature, London*, **153**, 20–21.

86 Lovelock, J.E. (1948) Aliphatic-hydroxycarboxylic acids as air disinfectants, in *Studies in Air Hygiene*, Medical Research Council Special Report Series No. 262 (eds R.B. Bourdillon *et al.*), HMSO, London, pp. 89–104.

87 Russell, N.J. and Gould, G.W. (1991) *Food Preservatives*, Blackie, Glasgow.

88 Russell, N.J. and Gould, G.W. (1991) Factors affecting growth and survival, in *Food Preservatives* (eds N.J. Russell and G.W. Gould), Blackie, Glasgow, pp. 13–21.

89 Alakomi, H.-L. *et al.* (2001) Lactic acid permeabilizes Gram-negative bacteria by disrupting the outer membrane. *Applied and Environmental Microbiology*, **66**, 2001–2005.

90 Anderson, R.A. and Chow, C.E. (1967) The distribution and activity of benzoic acid in some emulsified systems. *Journal of the Society of Cosmetic Chemists*, **18**, 207–214.

91 Beveridge, E.G. and Hope, I.A. (1967) Inactivation of benzoic acid in sulphadimidine mixture for infants B.P.C. *Pharmaceutical Journal*, **198**, 457–458.

92 Stanier, R.Y. and Orston, L.N. (1973) The ketoadipic pathway, in *Advances in Microbial Physiology*, Vol. 9 (eds A.H. Rose and D.W. Tempest), Academic Press, London, pp. 89–151.

93 Thampuran, N. and Surendran, P.K. (1996) Effect of chemical agents on swarming of *Bacillus* species. *Journal of Applied Bacteriology*, **80**, 296–302.

94 Ramos-Nino, M.E. *et al.* (1996) Quantitative structure activity relationship for the effect of benzoic acids, cinnamic acids and benzaldehydes on *Listeria monocytogenes*. *Journal of Applied Bacteriology*, **80**, 303–310.

95 Arroyo-Lopez, F.N. *et al.* (2008) Modelling the inhibition of sorbic and benzoic acids on a native yeast cocktail from table olives. *Food Microbiology*, **25** (4), 566–574.

96 Freese, E. *et al.* (1973) Function of lipophilic acids as antimicrobial food additives. *Nature, London*, **241**, 321–325.

97 Wolf, P.A. (1950) Dehydroacetic acid, a new microbiological inhibitor. *Food Technology*, **4**, 294–297.

98 Bandelin, F.J. (1950) The effects of pH on the efficiency of various mould inhibiting compounds. *Journal of the American Pharmaceutical Association, Scientific Edition*, **47**, 691–694.

99 Seevers, H.M. *et al.* (1950) Dehydroactic acid (DHA). II. General pharmacology and mechanism of action. *Journal of Pharmacology and Experimental Therapeutics*, **99**, 69–83.

100 Wolf, P.A. and Westveer, W.M. (1950) The antimicrobial activity of serveral substituted pyrones. *Archives of Biochemistry*, **28**, 201–206.

101 Gould, G.W. and Russell, N.J. (1991) Sulphite, in *Food Preservatives* (eds N.J. Russell and G.W. Gould), Blackie, Glasgow, pp. 72–88.

102 Lichter, A. *et al.* (2008) Evaluation of table grape storage in boxes with sulfur dioxide-releasing pads with either an internal plastic liner or external wrap. *HortTechnology*, **18**, 206–214.

103 Rose, A.H. and Pilkington, B.J. (1989) Sulphite, in *Mechanisms of Action of Food Preservation Procedures* (ed. G.W. Gould), Elsevier Applied Science, London, pp. 201–223.

104 Sabalitschka, T. (1924) Chemische konstitution and *Konservierungsvermögen*. *Pharmazeutisch Monatsblatten*, **5**, 235–327.

105 Sabalitschka, T. and Dietrich, R.K. (1926) Chemical constitution and preservative properties. *Disinfection*, **11**, 67–71.

106 Sabalitschka, T. *et al.* (1926) Influence of esterification of carboxyclic acids on inhibitive action with respect to micro-organisms. *Pharmazeutische Zeitung*, **71**, 834–836.

107 Richardson, E.L. (1981) Update: frequency of preservative use in cosmetic formulas as disclosed to FDA. *Cosmetics and Toiletries*, **96**, 91–92.

108 Aalto, T.R. *et al.* (1953) *p*-Hydroxybenzoic acid esters as preservatives. 1. Uses, antibacterial and antifungal studies, properties and determination. *Journal of the American Pharmaceutical Association*, **42**, 449–457.

109 Mathews, C. *et al.* (1956) *p*-Hydroxybenzoic acid esters as preservatives. II. Acute and chronic toxicity in dogs, rats and mice. *Journal of the American Pharmaceutical Association*, **45**, 260–267.

110 Russell, A.D. and Furr, J.R. (1986) The effects of antiseptics, disinfectants and preservatives on smooth, rough and deep rough strains of *Salmonella typhimurium*. *International Journal of Pharmaceutics*, **34**, 115–123.

111 Russell, A.D. and Furr, J.R. (1986) Susceptibility of porin- and lipopolysaccharide-deficient strains of *Escherichia coli* to some antiseptics and disinfectants. *Journal of Hospital Infection*, **8**, 47–56.

112 Russell, A.D. and Furr, J.R. (1987) Comparative sensitivity of smooth, rough and deep rough strains of *Escherichia coli* to chlorhexidine, quaternary ammonium compounds and dibromopropamide isethionate. *International Journal of Pharmaceutics*, **36**, 191–197.

113 Russell, A.D. *et al.* (1985) Susceptibility of porin- and lipopolysaccharide-deficient mutants of *Escherichia coli* to a homologous series of esters of *p*-hydroxybenzoic acid. *International Journal of Pharmaceutics*, **27**, 163–173.

114 Russell, A.D. *et al.* (1987) Sequential loss of outer membrane lipopolysaccharide and sensitivity of *Escherichia coli* to antibacterial agents. *International Journal of Pharmaceutics*, **35**, 227–232.

115 Hugo, W.B. and Foster, J.H.S. (1964) Growth of *Pseudomonas aeruginosa* in solutions of esters of *p*-hydroxy benzoic acid. *Journal of Pharmacy and Pharmacology*, **16**, 209.

116 Beveridge, E.G. and Hart, A. (1970) The utilisation for growth and the degradation of *p*-hydroxybenzoate esters by bacteria. *International Biodeterioration Bulletin*, **6**, 9–12.

117 Rosen, W.E. *et al.* (1977) Preservation of cosmetic lotions with imidazolidinyl urea plus parabens. *Journal of the Society of Cosmetic Chemists*, **28**, 83–87.

118 Charnock, C. and Finsrud, T. (2007) Combining esters of para-hydroxy benzoic acid (parabens) to achieve increased antimicrobial activity. *Journal of Clinical Pharmacy and Therapeutics*, **32** (6), 567–572.

119 O'Neill, J.J. *et al.* (1979) Selection of parabens as preservatives for cosmetics and toiletries. *Journal of the Society of Cosmetic Chemists*, **30**, 25–39.

120 Hodgson, I. *et al.* (1995) Synergistic antimicrobial properties of plant essential oils and parabens: potential for the preservation of food. *International Biodeterioration and Biodegradation*, **36**, 465.

121 Sutton, S.V.W. (1996) Neutralizer evaluations as control experiments for antimicrobial efficacy tests, in *Handbook of Disinfectants and Antiseptics* (ed. J.M. Ascenzi), Marcel Dekker, New York, pp. 43–62.

122 Freese, E. and Levin, B.C. (1978) Action mechanisms of preservatives and antiseptics. *Developments in Industrial Microbiology*, **19**, 207–227.

123 Haag, T.E. and Loncrini, D.F. (1984) Esters of parahydroxybenzoic acid, in *Cosmetic and Drug Preservation. Principles and Practice* (ed. J.J. Kabara), Marcel Dekker, New York, pp. 63–77.

124 Eklund, T. (1985) Inhibition of microbial growth at different pH levels by benzoic and propionic acids and esters of *p*-hydroxybenzoic acid. *International Journal of Food Microbiology*, **2**, 159–167.

125 Bredin, J. *et al.* (2005) Propyl paraben induces potassium efflux in *Escherichia coli*. *Journal of Antimicrobial Chemotherapy*, **55** (6), 1013–1015.

126 Nguyen, T. *et al.* (2005) The effects of parabens on the mechanosensitive channels of *E. coli*. *European Biophysics Journal*, **34** (5), 389–395.

127 Kamaraju, K. and Sukharev, S. (2008) The membrane lateral pressure-perturbing capacity of parabens and their effects on the mechanosensitive channel directly correlate with hydrophobicity. *Biochemistry*, **47** (40), 10540–10550.

128 Thrower, W.R. and Valentine, F.C.O. (1943) Propamidine in chronic wound sepsis. *Lancet*, **i**, 133.

129 Wien, R. *et al.* (1948) Diamidines as antibacterial compounds. *British Journal of Pharmacology*, **3**, 211–218.

130 McDonnell, G. and Russell, A.D. (1999) Antiseptics and disinfectants: activity, action, and resistance. *Clinical Microbiology Reviews*, **12**, 147–179.

131 Richards, R.M. *et al.* (1993) Investigation of cell envelope damage to *Pseudomonas aeruginosa* and *Enterobacter cloacae* by dibromopropamidine isethionate. *Journal of Pharmaceutical Science*, **82** (9), 975–977.

132 Bailly, C. *et al.* (1997) Sequence-selective binding to DNA of bis(amidinophenoxy) alkanes related to propamidine and pentamidine. *Biochemical Journal*, **323** (1), 23–31.

133 Al-Masaudi, S.B. *et al.* (1991) Comparative sensitivity to antibiotics and biocides of methicillin-resistant *Staphylococcus aureus* strains isolated from Saudi Arabia and Great Britain. *Journal of Applied Bacteriology*, **71**, 331–338.

134 Seal, D. (2003) Treatment of *Acanthamoeba keratitis*. *Expert Review of Anti-infective Therapy*, **1** (2), 205–208.

135 Walochnik, J. *et al.* (2003) Treatment of *Acanthamoeba keratitis*: possibilities, problems, and new approaches. *Wiener Klinische Wochenschrift*, **115** (3), 10–17.

136 Lindsay, R.G. *et al.* (2007) *Acanthamoeba keratitis* and contact lens wear. *Clinical and Experimental Optometry*, **90** (5), 351–360.

137 Anon. (2007) Final report on the safety assessment of hexamidine and hexamidine diisethionate. *International Journal of Toxicology*, **26** (Suppl. 3), 79–88.

138 Russell, A.D. and Furr, J.R. (1986) Susceptibility of porin- and lipopolysaccharide-deficient strains of *Escherichia coli* to some antiseptics and disinfectants. *Journal of Hospital Infection*, **8**, 47–56.

139 Russell, A.D. and Furr, J.R. (1987) Comparative sensitivity of smooth, rough and deep rough strains of *Escherichia coli* to chlorhexidine, quaternary ammonium compounds and dibromopropamide isethionate. *International Journal of Pharmaceutics*, **36**, 191–197.

140 Fleurette, J. *et al.* (1995) *Antisepsie et Désinfection*, Editions ESKA, Paris.

141 Russell, A.D. (1986) Chlorhexidine: antibacterial action and bacterial resistance. *Infection*, **14**, 212–215.

142 Baillie, L. (1987) Chlorhexidine resistance among bacteria isolated from urine of catheterized patients. *Journal of Hospital Infection*, **10**, 83–86.

143 Russell, A.D. (1990) The bacterial spore and chemical sporicides. *Clinical Microbiology Reviews*, **3**, 99–119.

144 Russell, A.D. (1991) Chemical sporicidal and sporistatic agents, in *Disinfection, Sterilization and Preservation*, 4th edn (ed. S.S. Block), Lea & Febiger, Philadelphia, pp. 365–376.

145 Russell, A.D. and Day, M.J. (1993) Antibacterial activity of chlorhexidine. *Journal of Hospital Infection*, **25**, 229–238.

146 Ranganathan, N.S. (1996) Chlorhexidine, in *Handbook of Disinfectant and Antiseptics* (ed. J.M. Ascenzi), Marcel Dekker, New York, pp. 235–264.

147 Russell, A.D. (1995) Mechanisms of microbial resistance to disinfectant and antiseptic agents, in *Chemical Germicides in Health Care* (ed. W.A. Rutala), Polyscience, Morin Heights, Canada, pp. 256–269.

148 Russell, A.D. (1996) Activity of biocides against mycobacteria. *Journal of Applied Bacteriology, Symposium Supplement*, **81**, 87S–101S.

149 Holloway, P.M. *et al.* (1986) The effects of sub-lethal concentrations of chlorhexidine on bacterial pathogenicity. *Journal of Hospital Infection*, **8**, 39–46.

150 Lowbury, E.J.L. and Lilley, H.A. (1960) Disinfection of the hands of surgeons and nurses. *British Medical Journal*, **i**, 1445–1450.

151 Traore, O. *et al.* (2000) Comparison of *in-vivo* antibacterial activity of two skin disinfection procedures for insertion of peripheral catheters: povidone iodine versus chlorhexidine. *Journal of Hospital Infection*, **44**, 147–150.

152 Gavin, J. *et al.* (1996) Efficacy of standard disinfectant test methods for contact lens-care solutions. *International Biodeterioration and Biodegradation*, **36**, 431–440.

153 Molinari, J.A. (1995) Disinfection and sterilization strategies for dental instruments, in *Chemical Germicides in Health Care* (ed. W. Rutala), Polyscience Publications, Morin Heights, Canada, pp. 129–134.

154 Cottone, J.A. and Molinari, J.A. (1996) Disinfectant use in dentistry, in *Handbook of Disinfectants and Antiseptics* (ed. J.M. Ascenzi), Marcel Dekker, New York, pp. 73–82.

155 Gomes, P.F.A. *et al.* (2001) *In vitro* antimicrobial activity of several concentrations of sodium hypochlorite and chlorhexidine gluconate in the elimination of *Enterococcus faecalis*. *International Journal of Endodontics*, **34**, 424–428.

156 Kuruvilla, J.R. and Kamath, M.P. (1998) Antimicrobial activity of 2.5% sodium hypochlorite and 0.2% chlorhexidine gluconate separately and combined, as endodontic irrigants. *Journal of Endodontics*, **24**, 472–476.

157 Weber, D.J. *et al.* (2007) Outbreaks associated with contaminated antiseptics and disinfectants. *Antimicrobial Agents and Chemotherapy*, **51** (12), 4217–4224.

158 Fitzgerald, K.A. *et al.* (1989) Uptake of ^{14}C-chlorhexidine diacetate to *Escherichia coli* and *Pseudomonas aeruginosa* and its release by azolectin. *FEMS Microbiology Letters*, **60**, 327–332.

159 Fitzgerald, K.A. *et al.* (1992) Sensitivity and resistance of *Escherichia coli* and *Staphylococcus aureus* to chlorhexidine. *Letters in Applied Microbiology*, **14**, 33–36.

160 Fitzgerald, K.A. *et al.* (1992) Effect of chlorhexidine and phenoxyethanol on cell surface hydrophobicity of Gram-positive and Gram-negative bacteria. *Letters in Applied Microbiology*, **14**, 91–95.

161 Kuyyakanond, T. and Quesnel, L.B. (1992) The mechanism of action of chlorhexidine. *FEMS Microbiology Letters*, **100**, 211–216.

162 Barrett-Bee, K. *et al.* (1994) The membrane destabilising action of the antibacterial agent chlorhexidine. *FEMS Microbiology Letters*, **119**, 249–254.

163 Russell, A.D. and Day, M.J. (1996) Antibiotic and biocide resistance in bacteria. *Microbios*, **85**, 45–65.

164 Hiom, S.J. *et al.* (1995) X-ray microanalysis of chlorhexidine-treated cells of *Saccharomyces cerevisiae*. *Letters in Applied Microbiology*, **20**, 353–356.

165 Hiom, S.J. *et al.* (1995) Uptake of ^{14}C-chlorhexidine gluconate by *Saccharomyces cerevisiae*, *Candida albicans* and *Candida glabrata*. *Letters in Applied Microbiology*, **21**, 20–22.

166 Reverdy, M.-E. (1995) La chlorhexidine, in *Antisepsie et Désinfection* (eds J. Fleurette *et al.*), Editions ESKA, Paris, pp. 135–168.

167 Chawner, J.A. and Gilbert, P. (1989) A comparative study of the bactericidal and growth inhibitory activities of the bisbiguanides, alexidine and chlorhexidine. *Journal of Applied Bacteriology*, **66**, 243–252.

168 Chawner, J.A. and Gilbert, P. (1989) Interaction of the bisbiguanides chlorhexidine and alexidine with phospholipid vesicles: evidence for separate modes of action. *Journal of Applied Bacteriology*, **66**, 253–258.

169 Gjermo, P. *et al.* (1973) The effect on dental plaque formation and some *in vitro* properties of 12 bis-biguanides. *Journal of Periodontology*, **8**, 81–88.

170 Rosenthal, R.A. *et al.* (2006) Biocide uptake in contact lenses and loss of fungicidal activity during storage of contact lenses. *Eye and Contact Lens*, **32** (6), 262–266.

171 Alizadeh, H. *et al.* (2009) Amoebicidal activities of alexidine against 3 pathogenic strains of acanthamoeba. *Eye and Contact Lens*, **35** (1), 1–5.

172 Davies, A. *et al.* (1968) Comparison of the action of Vantocil, cetrimide and chlorhexidine on *Escherichia coli* and the protoplasts of Gram-positive bacteria. *Journal of Applied Bacteriology*, **31**, 448–461.

173 Gilbert, P. *et al.* (1990) Barrier properties of the Gram-negative cell envelope towards high molecular weight polyhexamethylene biguanides. *Journal of Applied Bacteriology*, **69**, 585–592.

174 Gilbert, P. *et al.* (1990) Synergism within polyhexamethylene biguanide biocide formulations. *Journal of Applied Bacteriology*, **69**, 593–598.

175 Broxton, P. *et al.* (1983) A study of the antibacterial activity of some polyhexamethylene biguanides towards *Escherichia coli* ATCC 8739. *Journal of Applied Bacteriology*, **54**, 345–353.

176 Broxton, P. *et al.* (1984) Interaction of some polyhexamethylene biguanides and membrane phospholipids in *Escherichia coli*. *Journal of Applied Bacteriology*, **57**, 115–124.

177 Broxton, P. *et al.* (1984) Binding of some polyhexamethylene biguanides to the cell envelope of *Escherichia coli* ATCC 8739. *Microbios*, **41**, 15–22.

178 Woodcock, P.M. (1988) Biguanides as industrial biocide, in *Industrial Biocides* (ed. K.R. Payne), Wiley, Chichester, pp. 19–36.

179 Ikeda, T. *et al.* (1984) Interaction of a polymeric biguanide biocide with phospholipid membranes. *Biochimica et Biophysica Acta*, **769**, 57–66.

180 Allen, M.J. *et al.* (2004) Cooperativity in the binding of the cationic biocide polyhexamethylene biguanide to nucleic acids. *Biochemical and Biophysical Research Communications*, **318** (2), 397–404.

181 Allen, M.J. *et al.* (2006) The response of *Escherichia coli* to exposure to the biocide polyhexamethylene biguanide. *Microbiology*, **152**, 989–1000.

182 Khunkitti, W. *et al.* (1996) The lethal effects of biguanides on cysts and trophozoites of *Acanthamoeba castellanii*. *Journal of Applied Bacteriology*, **81**, 73–77.

183 Khunkitti, W. *et al.* (1997) Aspects of the mechanisms of action of biguanides: on trophozoites and cysts of *Acanthamoeba castellanii*. *Journal of Applied Microbiology*, **82**, 107–114.

184 Khunkitti, W. *et al.* (1998) *Acanthamoeba castellanii*: growth, encystment, excystment and biocide susceptibility. *Journal of Infection*, **36**, 43–48.

185 Rosin, M. *et al.* (2002) The effect of a polyhexamethylene biguanide mouthrinse compared to an essential oil rinse and a chlorhexidine rinse on bacterial counts and 4-day plaque regrowth. *Journal of Clinical Periodontology*, **29**, 392–399.

186 Merianos, J.J. (1991) Quaternary ammonium compounds, in *Disinfection, Sterilisation and Preservation*, 4th edn (ed. S.S. Block), Lea & Febiger, Philadelphia, pp. 225–255.

187 Reverdy, M.-E. (1995) Les ammonium quaternaires, in *Antisepsie et Désinfection* (eds J. Fleurette *et al.*), Editions ESKA, Paris, pp. 174–198.

188 Wallhäusser, K.H. (1984) Antimicrobial preservatives used by the cosmetic industry, in *Cosmetic and Drug Preservation: Principles and Practice* (ed. J.J. Kabara), Marcel Dekker, New York, pp. 605–745.

189 Gardner, J.F. and Peel, M.M. (1991) *Introduction to Sterilization, Disinfection and Infection Control*, Churchill Livingstone, Edinburgh.

190 Denyer, S.P. and Wallhäusser, K.H. (1990) Antimicrobial preservatives and their properties, in *Guide to Microbial Control in Pharmaceuticals* (eds S.P. Denyer and R.M. Baird), Ellis Horwood, Chichester, pp. 251–273.

191 Malek, J.R. and Speier, J.L. (1982) Development of an organosilicone antimicrobial agent for the treatment of surfaces. *Journal of Coated Fabrics*, **12**, 38–45.

192 Speier, J.L. and Malek, J.R. (1982) Destruction of micro-organisms by contact with solid surfaces. *Journal of Colloid and Interfacial Science*, **89**, 68–76.

193 Schaeufele, P.J. (1986) Advances in quaternary ammonium biocides, in *Proceedings of the 3rd Conference on Progress in Chemical Disinfection*, Binghamton, New York, pp. 508–519.

194 Rutala, W.A., Weber, D.J. and the Healthcare Infection Control Practices Advisory Committee (HICPAC) (2008) *Guideline for Disinfection and Sterilization in Healthcare Facilities, 2008*, CDC Department of Health and Human Services, Atlanta, GA.

195 Domagk, G. (1935) Eine neue Klasse von Disinfektionsmitteln. *Deutsche Medizinische Wochenschrift*, **61**, 829–932.

196 Hamilton, W.A. (1971) Membrane-active antibacterial compounds, in *Inhibition and Destruction of the Microbial Cell* (ed. W.B. Hugo), Academic Press, London, pp. 77–106.

197 Hoffman, H. *et al.* (1973) Ultrastructural alterations associated with the growth of resistant *Pseudomonas aeruginosa* in the presence of benzalkonium chloride. *Journal of Bacteriology*, **113**, 409–416.

198 Frank, M.J. and Schaffner, W. (1976) Contaminated aqueous benzalkonium chloride: an unnecessary hospital infection hazard. *Journal of the American Medical Association*, **236**, 2418–2419.

199 Kaslow, R.A. *et al.* (1976) Nosocomial pseudobacteraemia: positive blood cultures due to contaminated benzalkonium antiseptic. *Journal of the American Medical Association*, **236**, 2407–2409.

200 Grossgebauer, K. (1970) Virus disinfection, in *Disinfection* (ed. M. Benarde), Marcel Dekker, New York, pp. 103–148.

201 D'Arcy, P.F. (1971) Inhibition and destruction of moulds and yeasts, in *Inhibition and Destruction of the Microbial Cell* (ed. W.B. Hugo), Academic Press, London, pp. 613–686.

202 Weiner, N.D. *et al.* (1965) Application of the Ferguson principle to the antimicrobial activity of quaternary ammonium salts. *Journal of Pharmacy and Pharmacology*, **17**, 350–355.

203 Laycock, H.H. and Mulley, B.A. (1970) Application of the Ferguson principle to the antibacterial activity of mono- and multi-component solutions of quaternary ammonium surface-active agents. *Journal of Pharmacy and Pharmacology*, **22**, 157S–162S.

204 Elworthy, P.H. (1976) The increasingly clever micelle. *Pharmaceutical Journal*, **217**, 566–570.

205 Schmolka, I.R. (1973) The synergistic effects of non ionic surfactants upon cationic germicidal agents. *Journal of the Society of Cosmetic Chemists*, **24**, 577–592.

206 Richards, R.M.E. and McBride, R.J. (1973) Enhancement of benzalkonium chloride and chlorhexidine acetate activity against *Pseudomonas aeruginosa* by aromatic alcohols. *Journal of Pharmaceutical Sciences*, **62**, 2035–2037.

207 Singh, S.M. *et al.* (2002) Resistance to quaternary ammonium compounds in food-related bacteria. *Microbial Drug Resistance*, **8**, 393–399.

208 British Pharmacopoeia (2002), *British Pharmacopoeia*, HMSO, London.

209 Davies, D.J.G. (1980) Manufacture and supply of contact lens products. I. An academic's view. *Pharmaceutical Journal*, **225**, 343–345.

210 Codling, C.E. *et al.* (2003) Performance of contact lens disinfecting solutions against *Pseudomonas aeruginosa* in the presence of organic load. *Eye and Contact Lens*, **29**, 100–102.

211 Bassett, D.C.J. (1971) The effect of pH on the multiplication of a pseudomonad in chlorhexidine and cetrimide. *Journal of Clinical Pathology*, **24**, 708–711.

212 Quack, J.M. (1976) Quaternary ammonium compounds in cosmetics. *Cosmetics and Toiletries*, **91** (2), 35–52.

213 Cowles, P.B. (1938) Alkyl sulfates: their selective bacteriostatic action. *Yale Journal of Biological Medicine*, **11**, 33–38.

214 Birkeland, J.M. and Steinhaus, E.A. (1939) Selective bacteriostatic action of sodium lauryl sulfate and of "Dreft". *Proceedings of the Society of Experimental Biological Medicine*, **40**, 86–88.

215 Kabara, J.J. (1978) Structure–function relationships of surfactants as antimicrobial agents. *Journal of the Society of Cosmetic Chemists*, **29**, 733–741.

216 Baker, Z. *et al.* (1941) The bactericidal action of synthetic detergents. *Journal of Experimental Medicine*, **74**, 611–620.

217 Galbraith, H. *et al.* (1971) Antibacterial activity of long chain fatty acids and the reversal with calcium, magnesium, ergocalciferol and cholesterol. *Journal of Applied Bacteriology*, **34**, 803–813.

218 Kabara, J.J. (1984) Medium chain fatty acids and esters as antimicrobial agents, in *Cosmetic and Drug Preservation: Principles and Practice* (ed. J.J. Kabara), Marcel Dekker, New York, pp. 275–304.

219 Scales, F.M. and Kemp, M. (1941) A new group of sterilizing agents for the food industries and a treatment for chronic mastitis. *International Association of Milk Dealers*, **33**, 491–519.

220 Ernst, R.E. *et al.* (1983) Biological effects of surfactants: Part 6 – effects of anionic, non-ionic and amphoteric surfactants on a green alga (Chlamydomonas). *Environmental Pollution (Series A)*, **31**, 159–175.

221 Laouar, L. *et al.* (1996) Yeast response to non-ionic surfactants. *Enzyme and Microbial Technology*, **18**, 433–438.

222 Moore, S.L. (1997) *The mechanisms of antibacterial action of some non-ionic surfactants*. PhD thesis, University of Brighton, Brighton.

223 Russell, A.D. *et al.* (1979) Microbiological applications of the inactivation of antibiotics and other antimicrobial agents. *Journal of Applied Bacteriology*, **46**, 207–245.

224 Croshaw, B. (1971) The destruction of mycobacteria, in *Inhibition and Destruction of the Microbial Cell* (ed. W.B. Hugo), Academic Press, London, pp. 419–449.

225 Block, S.S. (1983) Surface-active agents: amphoteric compounds, in *Disinfection, Sterilisation and Preservation*, 3rd edn (ed. S.S. Block), Lea & Febiger, Philadelphia, pp. 335–345.

226 Kornfeld, F. (1966) Properties and techniques of application of biocidal ampholytic surfactants. *Food Manufacture*, **41**, 39–46.

227 Ernst, R. and Miller, E.J. (1982) Surface-active betaines, in *Amphoteric Surfactants* (eds B.R. Bluestein and C.L. Hilton), Marcel Dekker, New York, pp. 148–154.

228 Babb, J.R. *et al.* (1980) Sporicidal activity of glutaraldehyde and hypochlorites and other factors influencing their selection for the treatment of medical equipment. *Journal of Hospital Infection*, **1**, 63–75.

229 Gorman, S.P. *et al.* (1980) Antimicrobial activity, uses and mechanism of action of glutaraldehyde. *Journal of Applied Bacteriology*, **48**, 161–190.

230 Power, E.G.M. (1997) Aldehydes as biocides. *Progress in Medicinal Chemistry*, **34**, 149–201.

231 Hopwood, D. *et al.* (1970) The reactions between glutaraldehyde and various proteins. An investigation of their kinetics. *Histochemical Journal*, **2**, 137–150.

232 Borick, P.M. (1968) Chemical sterilizers (chemosterilizers). *Advances in Applied Microbiology*, **10**, 291–312.

233 Borick, P.M. and Pepper, R.E. (1970) The spore problem, in *Disinfection* (ed. M. Benarde), Marcel Dekker, New York, pp. 85–102.

234 Russell, A.D. (1994) Glutaraldehyde: its current status and uses. *Infection Control and Hospital Epidemiology*, **15**, 724–733.

235 Eager, R.C. *et al.* (1986) Glutaraldehyde: factors important for microbicidal efficacy, in *Proceedings of the 3rd Conference on Progress in Chemical Disinfection* (eds G.E. Janauer and W.C. Ghiorse), Binghamton, New York, pp. 32–49.

236 Bruch, C.W. (1991) Role of glutaraldehyde and other liquid chemical sterilants in the processing of new medical devices, in *Sterilization of Medical Products*, vol. V (eds R.F. Morrissey and Y.I. Prokopenko), Polyscience Publications Inc., Morin Heights, Canada, pp. 377–396.

237 Power, E.G.M. *et al.* (1988) Emergence of resistance to glutaraldehyde in spores of *Bacillus subtilis* 168. *FEMS Microbiology Letters*, **50**, 223–226.

238 Knott, A.G. *et al.* (1995) Development of resistance to biocides during sporulation of *Bacillus subtilis*. *Journal of Applied Bacteriology*, **79**, 492–498.

239 Dancer, B.N. *et al.* (1989) Alkali-induced revival of *Bacillus* spores after inactivation by glutaraldehyde. *FEMS Microbiology Letters*, **57**, 345–348.

240 Power, E.G.M. *et al.* (1989) Possible mechanisms for the revival of glutaraldehyde-treated spores of *Bacillus subtilis* NCTC 8236. *Journal of Applied Bacteriology*, **67**, 91–98.

241 Power, E.G.M. *et al.* (1990) Effect of sodium hydroxide and two proteases on the revival of aldehyde-treated spores of *Bacillus subtilis*. *Letters in Applied Microbiology*, **10**, 9–13.

242 Williams, N.D. and Russell, A.D. (1992) The nature and site of biocide-induced sublethal injury in *Bacillus subtilis* spores. *FEMS Microbiology Letters*, **99**, 277–280.

243 Rubbo, S.D. *et al.* (1967) Biocidal activities of glutaraldehyde and related compounds. *Journal of Applied Bacteriology*, **30**, 78–87.

244 Ascenzi, J.M. (1996) Glutaraldehyde-based disinfectants, in *Handbook of Disinfectants and Antiseptics* (ed. J.M. Ascenzi), Marcel Dekker, New York, pp. 111–132.

245 Zeiger, E. *et al.* (2005) Genetic toxicity and carcinogenicity studies of glutaraldehyde – a review. *Mutation Research/Reviews in Mutation Research*, **589** (2), 136–151.

246 Agin, J. *et al.* (2008) Committee on antimicrobial efficacy testing. *Journal of AOAC International*, **91** (1), 68B–72B.

247 Favero, M.S. and Bond, W.W. (1991) Chemical disinfection of medical and surgical materials, in *Disinfection, Sterilization and Preservation*, 4th edn (ed. S.S. Block), Lea & Febiger, Philadelphia, pp. 617–641.

248 Anon. (2009) *FDA-Cleared Sterilants and High Level Disinfectants with General Claims for Processing Reusable Medical and Dental Devices*, http://www.fda.gov/MedicalDevices/DeviceRegulationandGuidance/Reprocessingof Single-UseDevices/ucm133514.htm (accessed June 6, 2012).

249 Babb, J.R. (1993) Disinfection and sterilization of endoscopes. *Current Opinion in Infectious Diseases*, **6**, 532–537.

250 Babb, J.R. and Bradley, C.R. (1995) A review of glutaraldehyde alternatives. *British Journal of Theatre Nursing*, **5**, 20–24.

251 Mbithi, J.N. *et al.* (1993) Bactericidal, virucidal and mycobacterial activities of reused alkaline glutaraldehyde in an endoscopy unit. *Journal of Clinical Microbiology*, **31**, 2933–2995.

252 Rutala, W.A. and Weber, D.J. (1995) FDA labelling requirements for disinfection of endoscopes: a counterpoint. *Infection Control and Hospital Epidemiology*, **16**, 231–235.

253 Springthorpe, V.S. *et al.* (1995) Microbiocidal activity of chemical sterilants under reuse conditions, in *Chemical Germicides in Health Care* (ed. W.A. Rutala), Polyscience Publications, Morin Heights, Canada, pp. 181–202.

254 Power, E.G.M. and Russell, A.D. (1988) Studies with Cold Sterilog, a glutaraldehyde monitor. *Journal of Hospital Infection*, **11**, 376–380.

255 Quinn, P.J. (1987) Evaluation of veterinary disinfectants and disinfection processes, in *Disinfection in Veterinary and Farm Animal Practice* (eds A.H. Linton *et al.*), Blackwell Scientific Publications, Oxford, pp. 66–116.

256 Alfa, M.J. and Sitter, D.L. (1994) In-hospital evaluation of *ortho*-phthalaldehyde as a high level disinfectant for flexible endoscopes. *Journal of Hospital Infection*, **26**, 15–26.

257 Walsh, S.E. *et al.* (2001) Possible mechanisms for the relative efficacies of *ortho*-phthalaldehyde and glutaraldehyde against glutaraldehyde-resistant *Mycobacterium chelonae*. *Journal of Applied Microbiology*, **91**, 80–92.

258 Heinzel, M. (1988) The phenomena of resistance to disinfectants and preservatives, in *Industrial Biocides*, vol. 22, Critical Reports on Applied Chemistry (ed. K.R. Payne), John Wiley & Sons, Chichester, pp. 52–67.

259 Kingston, D. (1965) Release of formaldehyde from polynoxyline and noxythiolin. *Journal of Clinical Pathology*, **18**, 666–667.

260 Wright, C.J. and McAllister, T.A. (1967) Protective action of noxythiolin in experimental endotoxaemia. *Clinical Trials Journal*, **4**, 680–681.

261 Browne, M.K. and Stoller, J.L. (1970) Intraperitoneal noxythiolin in faecal peritonitis. *British Journal of Surgery*, **57**, 525–529.

262 Pickard, R.G. (1972) Treatment of peritonitis with per and post-operative irrigation of the peritoneal cavity with noxythiolin solution. *British Journal of Surgery*, **59**, 642–648.

263 Gucklhorn, I.R. (1970) Antimicrobials in cosmetics. Parts 1–7. *Manufacturing Chemist and Aerosol News*, **41** (6), 44–45; (7) 51–52; (8) 28–29; (10) 49–50; (11) 48–49; (12) 50–51.

264 Haler, D. (1974) The effect of "Noxyflex" (Noxythiolin), on the behaviour of animals which have been infected intraperitoneally with suspensions of faeces. *International Journal of Clinical Pharmacology*, **9**, 160–164.

265 Reeves, D.S. and Schweitzer, F.A.W. (1973) Experimental studies with an antibacterial substance, Taurolin, in *Proceedings of the 8th International Congress of Chemotherapy (Athens)*, Hellenic, Athens, pp. 583–586

266 Browne, M.K. *et al.* (1976) Taurolin, a new chemotherapeutic agent. *Journal of Applied Bacteriology*, **41**, 363–368.

267 Browne, M.K. *et al.* (1977) The *in vitro* and *in vivo* activity of Taurolin against anaerobic pathogenic organisms. *Surgery, Gynaecology and Obstetrics*, **145**, 842–846.

268 Browne, M.K. *et al.* (1978) A controlled trial of Taurolin in establishing bacterial peritonitis. *Surgery, Gynaecology and Obstetrics*, **146**, 721–724.

269 Nicholson, A. *et al.* (2008) *In vitro* activity of taurolin against filamentous fungi isolated from lung transplant patients. *Journal of Heart and Lung Transplantation*, **27** (2), S74–S74.

270 Pfirrman, R.W. and Leslie, G.B. (1979) The anti-endotoxic activity of Taurolin in experimental animals. *Journal of Applied Bacteriology*, **46**, 97–102.

271 Allwood, M.C. and Myers, E.R. (1981) *Formaldehyde-Releasing Agents*, Society for Applied Bacteriology Technical Series 16, Academic Press, London, pp. 69–76.

272 Russell, A.D. (1976) Inactivation of non-sporing bacteria by gases, in *Society for Applied Bacteriology Symposium No. 5: Inactivation of Vegetative Micro-Organisms* (eds F.A. Skinner and W.B. Hugo), Academic Press, London, pp. 61–88.

273 Anonymous (1970) *The Disinfection and Disinfestation of Poultry Houses*, Ministry of Agriculture, Fisheries and Food Advisory Leaflet 514, revised 1970, HMSO, London.

274 Spicher, G. and Peters, J. (1976) Microbial resistance to formaldehyde. I. Comparative quantitative studies in some selected species of vegetative bacteria, bacterial spores, fungi, bacteriophages and viruses. *Zentralblatt für Bakteriologie und Hygiene I, Abteilung Originale*, **B163**, 486–508.

275 Spicher, G. and Peters, J. (1981) Heat activation of bacterial spores after inactivation by formaldehyde: dependence of heat activation on temperature and duration of action. *Zentralblatt für Bakteriologie und Hygiene 1, Abteilung Originale*, **B173**, 188–196.

276 Wright, A.M. *et al.* (1996) Biological indicators for low temperature steam and formaldehyde sterilization: investigation of the effect of the change in temperature and formaldehyde concentration on spores of *Bacillus stearothermophilus* NCIMB 8224. *Journal of Applied Bacteriology*, **80**, 259–265.

277 Rossmore, H.W. and Sondossi, M. (1988) Applications and mode of action of formaldehyde condensate biocides. *Advances in Applied Microbiology*, **33**, 223–277.

278 Simons, C. *et al.* (2000) A note: *ortho*-phthalaldehyde: proposed mechanism of action of a new antimicrobial agent. *Letters in Applied Microbiology*, **31**, 299–302.

279 Simoes, M. *et al.* (2007) Antimicrobial mechanisms of ortho-phthalaldehyde action. *Journal of Basic Microbiology*, **47** (3), 230–242.

280 Gregory, G.W. *et al.* (1999) The mycobactericidal efficacy of *ortho*-phthalaldehyde and the comparative resistances of *Mycobacterium bovis*, *Mycobacterium terrae* and *Mycobacterium chelonae*. *Infection Control and Hospital Epidemiology*, **20**, 324–330.

281 Walsh, S.E. *et al.* (1999) Studies on the mechanisms of the antibacterial action of *ortho*-phthalaldehyde. *Journal of Applied Microbiology*, **87**, 702–710.

282 Rutala, W.A. and Weber, D.J. (2001) New disinfection and sterilization methods. *Emerging Infectious Diseases*, **7**, 348–353.

283 Akamatsu, T. *et al.* (2005) Evaluation of the antimicrobial activity and materials compatibility of orthophthalaldehyde as a high-level disinfectant. *Journal of International Medical Research*, **33** (2), 178–187.

284 Walsh, S.E. *et al.* (1999) *Ortho*-phthalaldehyde: a possible alternative to glutaraldehyde for high level disinfection. *Journal of Applied Microbiology*, **86** (6), 1039–1046.

285 Cabrera-Martinez, R.-M. *et al.* (2002) Studies on the mechanisms of the sporicidal action of *ortho*-phthalaldehyde. *Journal of Applied Microbiology*, **92**, 675–680.

286 Acosta-Gio, A.E. *et al.* (2005) Sporicidal activity in liquid chemical products to sterilize or high-level disinfect medical and dental instruments. *American Journal of Infection Control*, **33** (5), 307–309.

287 Cooke, R.P. *et al.* (2003) An evaluation of Cidex OPA (0.55% orthophthalaldehyde) as an alternative to 2% glutaraldehyde for high-level disinfection of endoscopes. *Journal of Hospital Infection*, **54** (3), 226–231.

288 Abraham, J.B. *et al.* (2007) Rapid communication: effects of Steris 1 sterilization and Cidex ortho-phthalaldehyde high-level disinfection on durability of new-generation flexible ureteroscopes. *Journal of Endourology*, **21** (9), 985–992.

289 Power, E.G.M. and Russell, A.D. (1990) Sporicidal action of alkaline glutaraldehyde: factors influencing activity and a comparison with other aldehydes. *Journal of Applied Bacteriology*, **69**, 261–268.

290 Bartoli, M. and Dusseau, J.-Y. (1995) Aldéhydes, in *Antisepsie et Désinfection* (eds J. Fleurette *et al.*), Editions ESKA, Paris, pp. 292–304.

291 Rasooly, A. and Weisz, A. (2002) *In vitro* antibacterial activities of Phloxine B and other halogenated fluoresceins against Methicillin-resistant *Staphylococcus aureus*. *Antimicrobial Agents and Chemotherapy*, **46**, 3650–3653.

292 Waite, J.G. and Yousef, A.E. (2009) Antimicrobial properties of hydroxyxanthenes. *Advances in Applied Microbiology*, **69**, 79–98.

293 Wainwright, M. (2001) Acridine – a neglected antibacterial chromophore. *Journal of Antimicrobial Chemotherapy*, **47**, 1–13.

294 Dheyongera, J.P. *et al.* (2005) Antimalarial activity of thioacridone compounds related to the acronycine alkaloid. *Bioorganic and Medicinal Chemistry*, **13** (5), 1653–1659.

295 Belmont, P. *et al.* (2007) Acridine and acridone derivatives, anticancer properties and synthetic methods: where are we now? *Anti-cancer Agents in Medicinal Chemistry*, **7** (2), 139–169.

296 Denny, W.A. (2002) Acridine derivatives as chemotherapeutic agents. *Current Medicinal Chemistry*, **9**, 1655–1665.

297 Goodell, J.R. *et al.* (2006) Synthesis and evaluation of acridine- and acridone-based anti-herpes agents with topoisomerase activity. *Bioorganic and Medicinal Chemistry*, **14** (16), 5467–5480.

298 Foster, J.H.S. and Russell, A.D. (1971) Antibacterial dyes and nitrofurans, in *Inhibition and Destruction of the Microbial Cell* (ed. W.B. Hugo), Academic Press, London, pp. 185–208.

299 Thornley, M.J. and Yudkin, J. (1959) The origin of bacterial resistance to proflavine. I. Training and reversion in *Escherichia coli*. *Journal of General Microbiology*, **20**, 355–364.

300 Thornley, M.J. and Yudkin, J. (1959) The origin of bacterial resistance to proflavine. 2. Spontaneous mutation to proflavine resistance in *Escherichia coli*. *Journal of General Microbiology*, **20**, 365–372.

301 Watanabe, T. (1963) Infective heredity of multiple drug resistance in bacteria. *Bacteriological Reviews*, **27**, 87–115.

302 Viljanen, P. and Borakynski, J. (1991) The susceptibility of conjugative resistance transfer in Gram-negative bacteria to physicochemical and biochemical agents. *FEMS Microbiology Reviews*, **88**, 43–54.

303 Wainwright, M. *et al.* (1997) *In vitro* photobactericidal activity of aminoacridines. *Journal of Antimicrobial Chemotherapy*, **40**, 587–589.

304 Wainwright, M. *et al.* (1998) A comparison of the bactericidal and photobactericidal activity of aminoacridines and bis(aminoacridines). *Letters in Applied Microbiology*, **26**, 404–406.

305 Leelaporn, A. *et al.* (1994) Multidrug resistance to antiseptics and disinfectants in coagulase-negative staphylococci. *Journal of Medical Microbiology*, **40**, 214–220.

306 Tabarrini, O. *et al.* (2006) Synthesis and anti-BVDV activity of acridones as new potential antiviral agents. *Journal of Medicinal Chemistry*, **49** (8), 2621–2627.

307 Moats, W.A. and Maddox, S.E. Jr. (1978) Effect of pH on the antimicrobial activity of some triphenylmethane dyes. *Canadian Journal of Microbiology*, **24**, 658–661.

308 Paulsen, I.T. *et al.* (1996) Multidrug resistance proteins qacA and qacB from *Staphylococcus aureus*. Membrane topology and identification of residues involved in substrate specificity. *Proceedings of the National Academy of Sciences of the United States of America*, **93**, 3630–3635.

309 Paulsen, I.T. *et al.* (1996) The SMR family: a novel family of multidrug efflux proteins involved with the efflux of lipophilic drugs. *Molecular Microbiology*, **19**, 1167–1175.

310 Russell, A.D. (1997) Plasmids and bacterial resistance to biocides. *Journal of Applied Microbiology*, **82**, 155–165.

311 Owens, R.G. (1969) Organic sulphur compounds, in *Fungicides*, vol. 2 (ed. D.C. Torgeson), Academic Press, New York, pp. 147–301.

312 Trueman, J.R. (1971) The halogens, in *Inhibition and Destruction of the Microbial Cell* (ed. W.B. Hugo), Academic Press, London, pp. 135–183.

313 Lesher, R.J. *et al.* (1977) Bacteriolytic action of fluoric ions. *Antimicrobial Agents and Chemotherapy*, **12**, 339–345.

314 Khanna, N. and Naidu, A.S. (2000) Chlorocides, in *Natural Food Antimicrobial Systems* (ed. A.S. Naido), CRC Press, Boca Raton, pp. 739–781.

315 Russell, A.D. (1971) The destruction of bacterial spores, in *Inhibition and Destruction of the Microbial Cell* (ed. W.B. Hugo), Academic Press, London, pp. 451–612.

316 Duan, Y. *et al.* (1999) Properties of an enzyme based low level iodine disinfectant. *Journal of Hospital Infection*, **43**, 219–229.

317 Gottardi, W. (1985) The influence of the chemical behaviour of iodine on the germicidal action of disinfection solutions containing iodine. *Journal of Hospital Infection*, **6** (Suppl. A), 1–11.

318 Rackur, H. (1985) New aspects of the mechanism of action of povidone-iodine. *Journal of Hospital Infection*, **6** (Suppl. A), 13–23.

319 Williams, N.D. and Russell, A.D. (1991) The effects of some halogen-containing compounds on *Bacillus subtilis* endospores. *Journal of Applied Bacteriology*, **70**, 427–436.

320 Favero, M.S. (1985) Sterilization, disinfection and antisepsis in the hospital, in *Manual of Clinical Microbiology*, 4th edn (eds E.H. Lennette *et al.*), American Society for Microbiology, Washington, DC, pp. 129–137.

321 Gershenfeld, L. (1962) Povidone-iodine as a sporicide. *American Journal of Pharmacy*, **134**, 78–81.

322 Lowbury, E.J.L. *et al.* (1964) Methods of disinfection of hands. *British Medical Journal*, **ii**, 531–536.

323 Terleckyj, B. and Axler, D.A. (1987) Quantitative neutralization assay of fungicidal activity of disinfectants. *Antimicrobial Agents and Chemotherapy*, **31** (5), 794–798.

324 Best, M. *et al.* (1990) Efficacies of selected disinfectants against *Mycobacterium tuberculosis*. *Journal of Clinical Microbiology*, **28** (10), 2234–2239.

325 Galland, R.B. *et al.* (1977) Prevention of wound infection in abdominal operations by per-operative antibiotics or povidone-iodine. *Lancet*, **ii**, 1043–1045.

326 Lacey, R.W. (1979) Antibacterial activity of povidone iodine towards non-sporing bacteria. *Journal of Applied Bacteriology*, **46**, 443–449.

327 Reimer, K. *et al.* (2002) Antimicrobial effectiveness of povidone-iodine and consequences for new application areas. *Dermatology*, **204**, 114–120.

328 Darwish, R.M. (2002) Immediate effects of local commercial formulations of chlorhexidine and povidone-iodine used for surgical scrub. *Journal of Pharmaceutical Science*, **16**, 15–18.

329 Barabas, E.S. and Brittain, H.G. (1998) Povidone-iodine. *Analytical Profiles of Drug Substances and Excipients*, **25**, 342–362.

330 Leung, M.P. *et al.* (2002) The effect of temperature on bactericidal properties of 10% povidone iodine solution. *American Journal of Obstetrics and Gynecology*, **186**, 869–871.

331 Craven, D.E. *et al.* (1981) Pseudobacteremia caused by povidone-iodine solution contaminated with *Pseudomonas cepacia*. *New England Journal of Medicine*, **305**, 621–623.

332 Steele, K. *et al.* (1986) Cadexomer iodine in the management of venous leg ulcers in general practice. *The Practitioner*, **230** (1411), 63–68.

333 Danielsen, L. *et al.* (1997) Cadexomer iodine in ulcers colonised by *Pseudomonas aeruginosa*. *Journal of Wound Care*, **6** (4), 169–172.

334 Mertz, P.M. *et al.* (1999) The evaluation of a cadexomer iodine wound dressing on methicillin resistant *Staphylococcus aureus* (MRSA) in acute wounds. *Dermatologic Surgery*, **25** (2), 89–93.

335 Akiyama, H. *et al.* (2004) Assessment of cadexomer iodine against *Staphylococcus aureus* biofilm *in vivo* and *in vitro* using confocal laser scanning microscopy. *Journal of Dermatology*, **31** (7), 529–534.

336 Ohtani, T. *et al.* (2007) Cadexomer as well as cadexomer iodine induces the production of proinflammatory cytokines and vascular endothelial growth factor by human macrophages. *Experimental Dermatology*, **16** (4), 318–323.

337 Dychdala, G.R. (1983) Chlorine and chlorine compounds, in *Disinfection, Sterilization and Preservation*, 3rd edn (ed. S.S. Block), Lea & Febiger, Philadelphia, pp. 157–182.

338 Bloomfield, S.F. and Arthur, M. (1994) Mechanisms of inactivation and resistance of spores to chemical biocides. *Journal of Applied Bacteriology Symposium Supplement*, **76**, 91S–104S.

339 Banner, M.J. (1995) The selection of disinfectants for use in food hygiene, in *Handbook of Biocide and Preservative Use* (ed. H.W. Rossmore), Blackie Academic & Professional, London, pp. 315–333.

340 Bloomfield, S.F. (1996) Chlorine and iodine formulations, in *Handbook of Disinfectants and Antiseptics* (ed. J.M. Ascenzi), Marcel Dekker, New York, pp. 133–158.

341 Coates, D. and Hutchinson, D.N. (1994) How to produce a hospital disinfection policy. *Journal of Hospital Infection*, **26**, 57–68.

342 Morris, E.J. and Darlow, H.M. (1971) Inactivation of viruses, in *Inhibition and Destruction of the Microbial Cell* (ed. W.B. Hugo), Academic Press, London, pp. 687–702.

343 Russell, A.D. (1982) *The Destruction of Bacterial Spores*, Academic Press, London.

344 Williams, D.E. *et al.* (1987) Bactericidal activities of selected organic *N*-halamines. *Applied and Environmental Microbiology*, **53**, 2082–2089.

345 Williams, D.E. *et al.* (1988) Is free halogen necessary for disinfection? *Applied and Environmental Microbiology*, **54**, 2583–2585.

346 Worley, S.D. *et al.* (1987) The stabilities of new *N*-halamine water disinfectants. *Water Research*, **21**, 983–988.

347 Coates, D. (1985) A comparison of sodium hypochlorite and sodium dichloroisocyanurate products. *Journal of Hospital Infection*, **6**, 31–40.

348 Bloomfield, S.F. and Uso, E.E. (1985) The antibacterial properties of sodium hypochlorite and sodium dichloroisocyanurate as hospital disinfectants. *Journal of Hospital Infection*, **6**, 20–30.

349 Coates, D. (1988) Comparison of sodium hypochlorine and sodium dichloroisocyanurate disinfectants: neutralization by serum. *Journal of Hospital Infection*, **11**, 60–67.

350 LeChevallier, M.W. *et al.* (1988) Inactivation of biofilm bacteria. *Applied and Environmental Microbiology*, **54** (10), 2492–2499.

351 Marion-Ferey, K. *et al.* (2003) Biofilm removal from silicone tubing: an assessment of the efficacy of dialysis machine decontamination procedures using an *in vitro* model. *Journal of Hospital Infection*, **53** (1), 64–71.

352 Morgan, D.A. (1989) Chlorinated solutions: E (useful) or (E) useless? *Pharmaceutical Journal*, **243**, 219–220.

353 Rose, L.J. *et al.* (2005) Chlorine inactivation of bacterial bioterrorism agents. *Applied and Environmental Microbiology*, **71** (1), 566–568.

354 Working Party of the Hospital Infection Society (1985) Acquired immune deficiency syndrome: recommendations of a Working Party of the Hospital Infection Society. *Journal of Hospital Infection*, **6** (Suppl. C), 67–80.

355 Coates, D. and Wilson, M. (1989) Use of sodium dichloroisocyanurate granules for spills of body fluids. *Journal of Hospital Infection*, **13**, 241–251.

356 Bloomfield, S.F. and Miller, E.A. (1989) A comparison of hypochlorite and phenolic disinfectants for disinfection of clean and soiled surfaces and blood spillages. *Journal of Hospital Infection*, **13**, 231–239.

357 Bloomfield, S.F. *et al.* (1990) Evaluation of hypochlorite-releasing agents against the human immunodeficiency virus (HIV). *Journal of Hospital Infection*, **15**, 273–278.

358 Simpson, G.D. *et al.* (2001) Chlorine dioxide: the "ideal" biocide. *Speciality Chemicals*, **20**, 358–359.

359 Ogata, N. and Shibata, T. (2008) Protective effect of low-concentration chlorine dioxide gas against influenza A virus infection. *Journal of General Virology*, **89** (1), 60–67.

360 Lin, W. *et al.* (1996) Bactericidal activity of aqueous chlorine and chlorine dioxide solutions in a fish model system. *Journal of Food Science*, **61**, 1030–1034.

361 Te Giffel, M.C. *et al.* (1996) Sporicidal effect of disinfectants on *Bacillus cereus* isolated from the milk processing environment. *International Biodeterioration and Biodegradation*, **36**, 421–430.

362 Coates, D. (1996) Sporicidal activity of sodium dichloroisocyanurate, peroxygen and glutaraldehyde disinfectants against *Bacillus subtilis*. *Journal of Hospital Infection*, **32**, 283–294.

363 Bellamy, K. (1995) A renew of the test methods used to establish virucidal activity. *Journal of Hospital Infection*, **30** (Suppl.), 389–396.

364 van Bueren, J. (1995) Methodology for HIV disinfectant testing. *Journal of Hospital Infection*, **30** (Suppl.), 383–388.

365 Bond, W.W. (1995) Activity of chemical germicides against certain pathogens: human immunodeficiency virus (HIV), hepatitis B virus (HBV) and *Mycobacterium tuberculosis* (MTB), in *Chemical Germicides in Health Care* (ed. W. Rutala), Polyscience Publications, Morin Heights, Canada, pp. 135–148.

366 Hernández, A. *et al.* (1996) Evaluation of the disinfectant effect of Solprogel against human immunodeficiency virus type 1 (HTV1). *Journal of Hospital Infection*, **34**, 223–228.

367 Hernández, A. *et al.* (1997) Inactivation of hepatitis B virus: evaluation of the efficacy of the disinfectant "Solprogel" using a DNA-polymerase assay. *Journal of Hospital Infection*, **36**, 305–312.

368 Gurevich, I. *et al.* (1996) Dental instrument and device sterilization and disinfection practices. *Journal of Hospital Infection*, **32**, 295–304.

369 McDonnell, G.E. (2007) Chemical disinfection, in *Antisepsis, Disinfection, and Sterilization: Types, Action, and Resistance* (G.E. McDonnell), ASM Press, Washington, DC, pp. 79–148.

370 Westwood, N. and Pin-Lim, B. (1972) Survival of *E. coli*, *S. aureus*, *Ps. aeruginosa* and spores of *B. subtitlis* in BPC mixtures. *Pharmaceutical Journal*, **208**, 153–154.

371 Lynch, M. *et al.* (1977) Chloroform as a preservative in aqueous systems. Losses under "in-use" conditions and antimicrobial effectiveness. *Pharmaceutical Journal*, **219**, 507–510.

372 Anon. (2002) *Cosmetics Directive 76/768/EEC*, as amended up to 14 March 2000, http://eur-lex.europa.eu/LexUriServ/LexUriServ.do?uri=CONSLEG:1976L0768:20100301:en:PDF (accessed June 6, 2012).

373 Elsmore, R. (1993) Practical experience of the use of bromine based biocides in cooling towers. *Biodeterioration and Biodegradation*, **9**, 114–122.

374 Elsmore, R. (1995) Development of bromine chemistry in controlling microbial growth in water systems. *International Biodeterioration and Biodegradation*, **36**, 245–253.

375 McCoy, W.F. and Wireman, J.W. (1989) Efficacy of bromochlorodimethylhydantoin against *Legionella pneumophila* in industrial cooling water. *Journal of Industrial Microbiology*, **4**, 403–408.

376 Naik, J. *et al.* (1998) Hydrazino di-methyl substituted quinolines as antitubercular/antibacterial agents. *Asian Journal of Chemistry*, **10**, 388–390.

377 El-Ahl, A.A. *et al.* (1996) Synthesis and antibacterial testing of some new quinolines, pyridazinoquinolines and spiroindoloquinolines. *Bollettino Chimico Farmaceutico*, **135**, 297–300.

378 Short, B.R. *et al.* (2005) *In vitro* activity of a novel compound, the metal ion chelating agent AQ+, against clinical isolates of *Staphylococcus aureus*. *Journal of Antimicrobial Chemotherapy*, **57** (1), 104–109.

379 Di, C. *et al.* (2007) Clioquinol, a therapeutic agent for Alzheimer's disease, has proteasome-inhibitory, androgen receptor-suppressing, apoptosis-inducing, and antitumor activities in human prostate cancer cells and xenografts. *Cancer Research*, **67** (4), 1636–1644.

380 Ding, W.Q. *et al.* (2008) Zinc-binding compounds induce cancer cell death via distinct modes of action. *Cancer Letters*, **271** (2), 251–259.

381 Collier, H.O.J. *et al.* (1959) Further observations on the biological properties of dequalinium (Dequadin) and hedaquinium (Teoquil). *Journal of Pharmacy and Pharmacology*, **11**, 671–680.

382 Cox, W.A. and D'Arcy, P.F. (1962) A new cationic antimicrobial agent. *N*-dodecyl-4-amino quinaldinium acetate (laurolinium acetate). *Journal of Pharmacy and Pharmacology*, **15**, 129–137.

383 Frier, M. (1971) Derivatives of 4-amino-quinaldinium and 8-hydroxyquinoline, in *Inhibition and Destruction of the Microbial Cell* (ed. W.B. Hugo), Academic Press, London, pp. 107–120.

384 Della Casa, V. *et al.* (2002) Antimicrobial activity of dequalinium chloride against leading germs of vaginal infections. *Arzneimittel-Forschung/Drug Research*, **52**, 699–705.

385 Morton, H.E. (1950) Relationship of concentration and germicidal efficiency of ethyl alcohol. *Annals of the New York Academy of Sciences*, **53**, 191–196.

386 Setlow, B. *et al.* (2002) Mechanisms of killing spores of *Bacillus subtilis* by acid, alkali and ethanol. *Journal of Applied Microbiology*, **92**, 362–375.

387 Rutala, W.A. (1990) APIC Guidelines for infection control practice. *American Journal of Infection Control*, **18**, 99–117.

388 Scott, E.M. and Gorman, S.P. (1987) Chemical disinfectants, antiseptics and preservatives, in *Pharmaceutical Microbiology*, 4th edn (eds W.B. Hugo and A.D. Russell), Blackwell Scientific Publications, Oxford, pp. 226–252.

389 Bandelin, F.J. (1977) Antibacterial and preservative properties of alcohols. *Cosmetics and Toiletries*, **92**, 59–70.

390 Bischoff, W.E. *et al.* (2000) Handwashing compliance by health-care workers. *Archives of Internal Medicine*, **160**, 1017–1021.

391 Zaragoza, M. *et al.* (1999) Handwashing with soap or alcoholic solutions? A randomized clinical trial of its effectiveness. *American Journal of Infection Control*, **27**, 258–261.

392 Girou, E. *et al.* (2002) Efficacy of handrubbing with alcohol based solution versus standard handwashing with antiseptic soap: randomised clinical trial. *British Medical Journal*, **325**, 362–365.

393 Moadab, A. *et al.* (2001) Effectiveness of a nonrinse, alcohol-free antiseptic hand wash. *Journal of the American Podiatric Medical Association*, **91**, 288–293.

394 Tjøtta, E. *et al.* (1991) Survival of HIV-1 activity after disinfection, temperature and pH changes, or drying. *Journal of Medical Virology*, **35**, 223–227.

395 Resnick, L. *et al.* (1986) Stability and inactivation of HTLV-III/LAV under clinical and laboratory conditions. *Journal of the American Medical Association*, **255**, 1887–1891.

396 van Bueren, J. *et al.* (1994) Inactivation of human immunodeficiency virus type 1 by alcohols. *Journal of Hospital Infection*, **28**, 137–148.

397 Tyler, R. *et al.* (1990) Virucidal activity of disinfectants: studies with the poliovirus. *Journal of Hospital Infection*, **15**, 339–345.

398 Hill, G. (1995) Preservation of cosmetics and toiletries, in *Handbook of Biocide and Preservative Use* (ed. H.W. Rossmore), Blackie Academic & Professional, London, pp. 349–415.

399 Sattar, S.A. and Springthorpe, V.S. (1991) Survival and disinfectant inactivation of the human immunodeficiency virus: a critical review. *Reviews of Infectious Diseases*, **13**, 430–447.

400 Shepherd, J.A. *et al.* (1988) Antibacterial action of 2-bromo-2-nitropropane-1,3-diol (bronopol). *Antimicrobial Agents and Chemotherapy*, **32** (11), 1693–1698.

401 MacLehose, H.G. *et al.* (2004) Biofilms, homoserine lactones and biocide susceptibility. *Journal of Antimicrobial Chemotherapy*, **53**, 180–184.

402 Guthrie, W.G. (1999) Bronopol – the answer to preservative problems. *SOFW Journal*, **125**, 67–71.

403 Toler, J.C. (1985) Preservative stability and preservative systems. *International Journal of Cosmetic Sciences*, **7**, 157–164.

404 Bryce, D.M. *et al.* (1978) The activity and safety of the antimicrobial agent bronopol (2-bromo-2-nitropropan-1,3-diol). *Journal of the Society of Cosmetic Chemists*, **29**, 3–24.

405 Croshaw, B. and Holland, V.R. (1984) Chemical preservatives: use of bronopol as a cosmetic preservative, in *Cosmetic and Drug Preservation. Principles and Practice* (ed. J.J. Kabara), Marcel Dekker, New York, pp. 31–62.

406 Gucklhorn, I.R. (1971) Antimicrobials in cosmetics. Parts 8 and 9. *Manufacturing Chemist and Aerosol News*, **42** (1), 35–37. (2) 35–39.

407 Gilbert, P. *et al.* (1977) The lethal action of 2-phenoxyethanol and its analogues upon *Escherichia coli* NCTC 5933. *Microbios*, **19** (76), 125–141.

408 Gilbert, P. *et al.* (1977) Inhibition of some respiration and dehydrogenase enzyme systems in *Escherichia coli* NCTC 5933 by phenoxyethanol. *Microbios*, **20** (79), 29–37.

409 Gilbert, P. *et al.* (1977) Effect of phenoxyethanol on the permeability of *Escherichia coli* NCTC 5933 to inorganic ions. *Microbios*, **19** (75), 17–26.

410 Gilbert, P. *et al.* (1980) Effect of 2-phenoxyethanol upon RNA, DNA and protein biosynthesis in *Escherichia coli* NCTC 5933. *Microbios*, **28** (111), 7–17.

411 Berry, H. (1944) Antibacterial values of ethylene glycol monophenyl ether (phenoxetol). *Lancet*, **ii**, 175–176.

412 Russell, A.D. (1991) Principles of antimicrobial activity, in *Disinfection, Sterilization and Preservation*, 4th edn (ed. S.S. Block), Lea & Febiger, Philadelphia, pp. 27–58.

413 Baldry, M.G.C. (1983) The bactericidal, fungicidal and sporicidal properties of hydrogen peroxide and peracetic acid. *Journal of Applied Bacteriology*, **54**, 417–423.

414 Baldry, M.G.C. and Fraser, J.A.L. (1988) Disinfection with peroxygens, in *Industrial Biocides*, vol. 22, Critical Reports on Applied Chemistry (ed. K.R. Payne), John Wiley & Sons, Chichester, pp. 91–116.

415 Melly, E. *et al.* (2002) Studies on the mechanism of killing of *Bacillus subtilis* spores by hydrogen peroxide. *Journal of Applied Microbiology*, **93**, 316–325.

416 Miller, M.J. (1996) Contact lens disinfectants, in *Handbook of Disinfectants and Antiseptics* (ed. J.M. Ascenzi), Marcel Dekker, New York, pp. 83–110.

417 Shin, S.Y. *et al.* (2001) Inhibition of *Campylobacter jejuni* in chicken by ethanol, hydrogen peroxide and organic acids. *Journal of Microbiology and Biotechnology*, **11**, 418–422.

418 Hughes, R. and Kilvington, S. (2001) Comparisn of hydrogen peroxide contact lens disinfection systems and solutions against *Acanthameoba polyphaga*. *Antimicrobial Agents and Chemotherapy*, **45**, 2038–2043.

419 Sintim-Damoa, K. (1993) Other gaseous sterilization methods, in *Sterilization Technology* (eds R.F. Morrissey and G.B. Phillips), Van Nostrand Reinhold, New York, pp. 335–347.

420 Groschel, D.H.M. (1995) Emerging technologies for disinfection and sterilization, in *Chemical Germicides in Health Care* (ed. W. Rutala), Polyscience Publications, Morin Heights, Canada, pp. 73–82.

421 Lever, A.M. and Sutton, S.V.W. (1996) Antimicrobial effects of hydrogen peroxide as an antiseptic and disinfectant, in *Handbook of Disinfectants and Antiseptics* (ed. J.M. Ascenzi), Marcel Dekker, New York, pp. 159–176.

422 Fraser, J.A.L. (1986) Novel applications of peracetic acid. *Chemspec '86: BACS Symposium*, pp. 65–69.

423 Gerald McDonnell, G. and Russell, A.D. (1999) Antiseptics and disinfectants: activity, action, and resistance. *Clinical Microbiology Reviews*, **12** (1), 147–179.

424 Gehr, R. *et al.* (2009) Performic acid (PFA): tests on an advanced primary effluent show promising disinfection performance. *Water Science and Technology*, **59** (1), 89–96.

425 Russell, A.D. *et al.* (1967) Inclusion of antimicrobial agents in pharmaceutical products. *Advances in Applied Microbiology*, **9**, 1–38.

426 Repaske, R. (1956) Lysis of Gram-negative bacteria by lysozyme. *Biochimica et Biophysica Acta*, **22**, 189–191.

427 Repaske, R. (1958) Lysis of Gram-negative organism and the role of versene. *Biochimica et Biophysica Acta*, **30**, 225–232.

428 Leive, L. and Kollin, V. (1967) Controlling EDTA treatment to produce permeable *E. coli* with normal metabolic process. *Biochemical and Biophysical Research Communications*, **28**, 229–236.

429 Neu, H.C. (1969) The role of amine buffers in EDTA toxicity and their effect on osmotic shock. *Journal of General Microbiology*, **57**, 215–220.

430 Haque, H. and Russell, A.D. (1976) Cell envelopes of Gram-negative bacteria: composition, response to chelating agents and susceptibility of whole cells to antibacterial agents. *Journal of Applied Bacteriology*, **40**, 89–99.

431 Bergan, T. *et al.* (2001) Chelating agents. *Chemotherapy*, **47**, 10–14.

432 Vaara, M. (1992) Agents increase the permeability of the outer membrane. *Microbiological Reviews*, **56**, 395–411.

433 Vaara, M. and Vaara, T. (1983) Polycations sensitise enteric bacteria to antibiotics. *Antimicrobial Agents and Chemotherapy*, **24**, 107–113.

434 Vaara, M. and Vaara, T. (1983) Polycations as outer membrane-disorganizing agents. *Antimicrobial Agents and Chemotherapy*, **24**, 114–122.

435 Viljanen, P. (1987) Polycations which disorganize the outer membrane inhibit conjugation in *Escherichia coli*. *Journal of Antibiotics*, **40**, 882–886.

436 Naidu, A.S. (2000) *Lactoferrin, Natural, Multifunctional, Antimicrobial*, CRC Press, Boca Raton, FL.

437 Ellison, R.T. *et al.* (1988) Damage of the outer membrane of enteric Gram-negative bacteria by lactoferrin and transferrin. *Infection and Immunity*, **56**, 2774–2781.

438 Leitch, E.C. and Willcox, M.D.P. (1998) Synergistic antistaphylococcal properties of lactoferrin and lysozyme. *Journal of Medical Microbiology*, **47**, 837–842.

439 Diarra, M.S. *et al.* (2002) Effect of lactoferrin in combination with penicillin on the morphology and the physiology of *Staphylococcus aureus* isolated from bovine mastitis. *Journal of Dairy Science*, **85**, 1141–1149.

440 Jones, E.M. *et al.* (1994) Lactoferricin, a new antimicrobial peptide. *Journal of Applied Bacteriology*, **77**, 208–214.

441 Chierici, R. (2001) Antimicrobial actions of lactoferrin. *Advances in Nutritional Research*, **10**, 247–269.

442 Weinberg, E.D. (2001) Human lactoferrin: a novel therapeutic with broad spectrum potential. *Journal of Pharmacy and Pharmacology*, **53**, 1303–1310.

443 Adlerova, L. *et al.* (2008) Lactoferrin: a review. *Veterinarni Medicina*, **53** (9), 457–468.

444 Pierce, A. and Legrand, D. (2009) Advances in lactoferrin research. *Biochimie*, **91** (1), 1–2.

445 Kushner, D.J. (1971) Influence of solutes and ions on micro-organisms, in *Inhibition and Destruction of the Microbial Cell* (ed. W.B. Hugo), Academic Press, London, pp. 259–283.

446 Weinberg, E.D. (1957) The mutual effect of antimicrobial compounds and metallic cations. *Bacteriological Reviews*, **21**, 46–68.

447 Zeelie, J.J. and McCarthy, T.J. (1998) Effects of copper and zinc ions on the germicidal properties of two popular pharmaceutical antiseptic agents cetylpyridinium chloride and povidone-iodine. *The Analyst*, **123**, 503–507.

448 Langwell, H. (1932) Oligodynamic action of metals. *Chemistry and Industry*, **51**, 701–702.

449 Grzybowski, J. and Trafny, E.A. (1999) Antimicrobial properties of copper-coated electroconductive polyester fibers. *Polymers in Medicine*, **29**, 27–33.

450 Weber, D.J. and Rutala, W.A. (1995) Use of metals as microbicides for the prevention of nosocomial infections, in *Chemical Germicides in Health Care* (ed. W. Rutala), Polyscience Publications, Morin Heights, Canada, pp. 271–286.

451 Brown, M.R.W. and Anderson, R.A. (1968) The bacterial effect of silver ions on *Pseudomonas aeruginosa*. *Journal of Pharmacy and Pharmacology*, **20**, 1S–3S.

452 Russell, A.D. (1985) The role of plasmids in bacterial resistance to antiseptics, disinfectants and preservatives. *Journal of Hospital Infection*, **6**, 9–19.

453 Goldberg, A.A. *et al.* (1950) Antibacterial colloidal electrolytes: the potentiation of the activities of mercuric, phenylmercuric and silver ions by a colloidal and sulphonic anion. *Journal of Pharmacy and Pharmacology*, **2**, 20–26.

454 Spacciapoli, P. *et al.* (2001) Antimicrobial activity of silver nitrate against periodontal pathogens. *Journal of Periodontal Research*, **36**, 108–113.

455 Bromberg, L.E. *et al.* (2000) Sustained release of silver from periodontal wafers for treatment of periodontitis. *Journal of Controlled Release*, **68**, 63–72.

456 Kim, T.N. *et al.* (1998) Antimicrobial effects of metal ions (Ag, Cu^2, Zn^2) in hydroxyapatite. *Journal of Materials Science: Materials in Medicine*, **9**, 129–134.

457 Bright, K.R. *et al.* (2002) Rapid reduction of *Staphylococcus aureus* populations on stainless steel surfaces by zeolite ceramic coatings containing silver and zinc ions. *Journal of Hospital Infection*, **52**, 307–309.

458 Rusin, P. *et al.* (2003) Rapid reduction of *Legionella pneumophila* on stainless steel with zeolite coatings containing silver and zinc ions. *Letters in Applied Microbiology*, **36**, 69–72.

459 Moiseev, S. (1934) Sterilization of water with silver coated sand. *Journal of the American Water Works Association*, **26**, 217–222.

460 Furr, J.R. *et al.* (1994) Antibacterial activity of Actisorb, Actisorb Plus and silver nitrate. *Journal of Hospital Infection*, **27**, 201–208.

461 Russell, A.D. and Hugo, W.B. (1994) Antibacterial action and activity of silver. *Progress in Medicinal Chemistry*, **31**, 351–371.

462 Hamilton-Miller, J.M.T. *et al.* (1993) Silver sulphadiazine: a comprehensive *in vitro* reassessment. *Chemotherapy*, **39**, 405–409.

463 Schuerer, D.J.E. *et al.* (2007) Effect of chlorhexidine/silver sulfadiazine-impregnated central venous catheters in an intensive care unit with a low blood stream infection rate after implementation of an educational program: a before–after trial. *Surgical Infections*, **8** (4), 445–454.

464 Foster, T.J. (1983) Plasmid-determined resistance to antimicrobial drugs and toxic metal ions in bacteria. *Microbiological Reviews*, **47**, 361–409.

465 Silver, S. and Misra, S. (1988) Plasmid-mediated heavy metal resistances. *Annual Review of Microbiology*, **42**, 717–743.

466 Ono, B.-I. *et al.* (1991) Role of hydrosulfide ions (HS) in methylmercury resistance in *Saccharomyces cerevisiae*. *Applied and Environmental Microbiology*, **57**, 3183–3186.

467 Ono, B. *et al.* (1988) Role of the cell wall in *Saccharomyces cerevisae* mutants resistant to Hg^2. *Journal of Bacteriology*, **170**, 5877–5882.

468 Weisser, K. *et al.* (2004) Thiomersal and immunisations. *Bundesgesundheitsblatt, Gesundheitsforschung, Gesundheitsschutz*, **47** (12), 1165–1174.

469 Bigham, M. and Copes, R. (2005) Thiomersal in vaccines: balancing the risk of adverse effects with the risk of vaccine-preventable disease. *Drug Safety*, **28** (2), 89–101.

470 Clements, C.J. and McIntyre, P.B. (2006) When science is not enough – a risk/benefit profile of thiomersal-containing vaccines. *Expert Opinion on Drug Safety*, **5** (1), 17–29.

471 Tozzi, A.E. *et al.* (2009) Neuropsychological performance 10 years after immunization in infancy with thimerosal-containing vaccines. *Pediatrics*, **123** (2), 475–482.

472 Voge, C.I.B. (1947) Phenylmercuric nitrate and related compounds. *Manufacturing Chemist and Manufacturing Perfumer*, **18**, 5–7.

473 Smith, P.J. and Smith, L. (1975) Organotin compounds and applications. *Chemistry in Britain*, **11**, 208–212. 226.

474 Rose, M.S. and Lock, E.A. (1970) The interaction of triethyltin with a component of guinea-pig liver supernatant. *Biochemical Journal*, **190**, 151–157.

475 Leonhardt, Å. and Dahlén, G. (1995) Effect of titanium on selected oral bacteria species *in vitro*. *European Journal of Oral Science*, **103**, 382–387.

476 Yoshinari, M. *et al.* (2001) Influence of surface modifications to titanium on antibacterial activity *in vitro*. *Biomaterials*, **22**, 2043–2048.

477 Macielag, M.J. *et al.* (1998) Substituted salicylanilides as inhibitors of two-component regulatory systems in bacteria. *Journal of Medicinal Chemistry*, **41** (16), 2939–2945.

478 Lemaire, H.C. *et al.* (1961) Synthesis and germicidal activity of halogenated salicylanilides and related compounds. *Journal of Pharmaceutical Sciences*, **50**, 831–837.

479 Waisser, K. *et al.* (2006) The oriented development of antituberculotics: salicylanilides. *Archiv der Pharmazie (Weinheim)*, **339** (11), 616–620.

480 Vinsova, J. *et al.* (2007) Salicylanilide acetates: synthesis and antibacterial evaluation. *Molecules*, **12** (1), 1–12.

481 Imramovsky, A. *et al.* (2008) Salicylanilide esters of N-protected amino acids as novel antimicrobial agents. *Bioorganic and Medicinal Chemistry Letters*, **19** (2), 348–351.

482 Beaver, D.J. *et al.* (1957) The preparation and bacteriostatic activity of substituted ureas. *Journal of the American Chemical Society*, **79**, 1236–1245.

483 Suller, M.T.E. and Russell, A.D. (1999) Antibiotic and biocide resistance in methicillin-resistant *Staphylococcus aureus* and vancomycin-resistant *Enterococcus*. *Journal of Hospital Infection*, **43**, 281–291.

484 Walsh, S.E. *et al.* (2003) Mechanisms of action of selected biocidal agents on Gram-positive and Gram-negative bacteria. *Journal of Applied Microbiology*, **94**, 240–247.

485 Woolfson, A.D. (1977) The antibacterial activity of dimethoxane. *Journal of Pharmacy and Pharmacology*, **29**, 73P.

486 Potokar, M. *et al.* (1976) Bronidox, ein neues Konservierungsmittel fur die Kosmetic Eigenschaften and toxikologisch-dermatologischen Prufergebnisse. *Fette, Seife, Anstrichmittel*, **78**, 269–276.

487 Lorenz, P. (1977) 5-Bromo-5-nitro-1, 3-dioxane: a preservative for cosmetics. *Cosmetics and Toiletries*, **92**, 89–91.

488 Croshaw, B. (1977) Preservatives for cosmetics and toiletries. *Journal of the Society of Cosmetic Chemists*, **28**, 3–16.

489 Ghannoum, M. *et al.* (1986) Mode of action of the antimicrobial compound 5-bromo-5-nitro-1,3-dioxane (Bronidox). *Folia Microbiologica*, **31** (1), 19–31.

490 Berke, P.A. and Rosen, W.E. (1970) Germall, a new family of antimicrobial preservatives for cosmetics. *American Perfumer and Cosmetics*, **85**, 55–60.

491 Rosen, W.E. and Berke, P.A. (1973) Modern concepts of cosmetic preservation. *Journal of the Society of Cosmetic Chemists*, **24**, 663–675.

492 Berke, P.A. and Rosen, W.E. (1978) Imidazolidinyl urea activity against *Pseudomonas*. *Journal of the Society of Cosmetic Chemists*, **29**, 757–766.

493 O'Brien, T.J. (2007) Imidazolidinyl urea (Germall 115) causing cosmetic dermatitis. *Australasian Journal of Dermatology*, **28** (1), 36–37.

494 Jong, C.T. *et al.* (2007) Contact sensitivity to preservatives in the UK, 2004–2005: results of multicentre study. *Contact Dermatitis*, **57** (3), 165–168.

495 Jacobs, G. *et al.* (1975) The influence of pH, emulsifier and accelerated ageing upon preservative requirements of o/w emulsions. *Journal of the Society of Cosmetic Chemists*, **26**, 105–117.

496 Berke, P.A. and Rosen, W.E. (1980) Are cosmetic emulsions adequately preserved against *Pseudomonas*? *Journal of the Society of Cosmetic Chemists*, **31**, 37–40.

497 Ponci, R. *et al.* (1964) Antifungal activity of 2′,2′-dicarbamino-4′,4-dinitrodiphenyldisulphides and 5-nitro-1,2-benzisothiazolones. *Farmaco, Edizione Scientifica*, **19**, 121–136.

498 Nicoletti, G. *et al.* (1993) The antimicrobial activity *in vitro* of chlorhexidine, a mixture of isothiazolines ("Kathon" CG) and cetyltrimethylammonium bromide (CTAB). *Journal of Hospital Infection*, **23**, 87–111.

499 Williams, T.M. (2007) The mechanism of action of isothiazolone biocide. *PowerPlant Chemistry*, **9**, 14–22.

500 Collier, P.J. *et al.* (1990) Growth inhibitory and biocidal activity of some isothiazolone biocides. *Journal of Applied Bacteriology*, **69**, 569–577.

501 Collier, P.J. *et al.* (1990) Chemical reactivity of some isothiazolone biocides. *Journal of Applied Bacteriology*, **69**, 578–584.

502 Diehl, M.A. (2002) A new preservative for high pH systems. *Household and Personal Products Industry (HAPPI)*, **39** (8), 72–74.

503 Jacobs, W.A. and Heidelberger, M. (1915) The quaternary salts of hexamethylenetetramine. I. Substituted benzyl halides and the hexamethylene tetramine salts derived therefrom. *Journal of Biological Chemistry*, **20**, 659–683.

504 Jacobs, W.A. and Heidelberger, M. (1915) The quaternary salts of hexamethylenetetramine. VIII. Miscellaneous substances containing aliphatically bound halogen and the hexamethylenetetramine salts derived therefrom. *Journal of Biological Chemistry*, **21**, 465–475.

505 Scott, C.R. and Wolf, P.A. (1962) The antibacterial activity of a series of quaternaries prepared from hexamethylene tetramine and halohydrocarbons. *Applied Microbiology*, **10**, 211–216.

506 Paulus, W. (1976) Problems encountered with formaldehyde-releasing compounds used as preservatives in aqueous systems, especially lubricoolants – possible solutions to the problems, in *Proceedings of the 3rd International Biodegradation Symposium* (eds J.M. Shaply and A.M. Kaplan), Applied Science Publishers, London, pp. 1075–1082.

507 Rossmore, H.W. (1979) Heterocyclic compounds as industrial biocides. *Developments in Industrial Microbiology*, **20**, 41–71.

508 Anon. (1997) *Methylene Bis(thiocyanate), R.E.D. Facts, United States Environmental Protection Agency, Prevention, Pesticides and Toxic Substances*, EPA-738-F-97-005, EPA, Washington, DC.

509 Disch, K. (1999) Glucoprotamine – a new antimicrobial substance. *Zentralblatt fur Hygiene Und Umweltmedizin*, **195** (5–6), 357–365.

510 Meyer, B. and Kluin, C. (1999) Efficacy of Glucoprotamin® containing disinfectants against different species of atypical mycobacteria. *Journal of Hospital Infection*, **42** (20), 151–154.

511 Widmer, A.F. and Frei, R. (2003) Antimicrobial activity of glucoprotamin: a clinical study of a new disinfectant for instruments. *Infection Control and Hospital Epidemiology*, **24**, 762–764.

512 Carson, C.F. *et al.* (1995) Susceptibility of methicillin-resistant *Staphylococcus aureus* to the essential oil of *Melaleuca alternifolia*. *Journal of Antimicrobial Chemotherapy*, **35**, 421–424.

513 Elsom, G.K.F. and Hide, D. (1999) Susceptibility of methicillin-resistant *Staphylococcus aureus* to tea tree oil and mupirocin. *Journal of Antimicrobial Chemotherapy*, **43**, 427–428.

514 May, J. *et al.* (2000) Time-kill studies of tea tree oils on clinical isolates. *Journal of Antimicrobial Chemotherapy*, **45**, 639–643.

515 Hammer, K.A. *et al.* (1998) *In-vitro* activity of essential oils, in particular *Melaleuca alternifolia* (tea tree) oil and tea tree oil products, against *Candida* spp. *Journal of Antimicrobial Chemotherapy*, **42**, 591–595.

516 Hammer, K.A. *et al.* (2000) *In vitro* activities of ketoconazole, econazole, iconazole, and *Melaleuca alternifolia* (tea tree) oil against *Malassezia* species. *Antimicrobial Agents and Chemotherapy*, **44**, 467–469.

517 Mondello, F. *et al.* (2003) *In vitro* and *in vivo* activity of tea tree oil against azole-susceptible and resistant human pathogenic yeasts. *Journal of Antimicrobial Chemotherapy*, **51**, 1223–1229.

518 Carson, C.F. *et al.* (2001) *Melaleuca alternifolia* (tea tree) oil gel (6%) for the treatment of recurrent herpes labialis. *Journal of Antimicrobial Chemotherapy*, **48**, 445–458.

519 Carson, C.F. *et al.* (2006) Melaleuca alternifolia (tea tree) oil: a review of antimicrobial and other medicinal properties. *Clinical Microbiology Reviews*, **19** (1), 50–62.

520 Nakatsu, T. *et al.* (2000) Biological activity of essential oils and their constituents. *Studies in Natural Products Chemistry*, **21**, 571–631.

521 Burt, S.A. and Reinders, R.D. (2003) Antibacterial activity of selected plant essential oils against *Escherichia coli* O157:H7. *Letters in Applied Microbiology*, **36**, 162–167.

522 Ultee, A. *et al.* (2002) The phenolic hydroxyl group of Carvacrol is essential for action against the food borne pathogen *Bacillus cereus*. *Applied and Environmental Microbiology*, **68**, 1561–1568.

523 Fine, D.H. *et al.* (2000) Effect of an essential oil containing antiseptic mouthrinse on plaque and salivary *Streptococcus mutans* levels. *Journal of Clinical Periodontology*, **27**, 157–161.

524 Fine, D.H. *et al.* (2001) Comparative antimicrobial activities of antiseptic mouthwashes against isogenic planktonic and biofilm forms of *Actinobacillus actinomycetemcomitans*. *Journal of Clinical Periodontology*, **28**, 697–700.

525 Pan, P. *et al.* (2000) Determination of the *in situ* bactericidal activity of an essential oil mouthrinse using a vital stain method. *Journal of Clinical Periodontology*, **27**, 256–261.

526 Chaieb, K. *et al.* (2007) The chemical composition and biological activity of clove essential oil, *Eugenia caryophyllata* (*Syzygium aromaticum* L. Myrtaceae). *Phytotherapy Research*, **21** (6), 501–506.

527 Pinto, E. *et al.* (2009) Antifungal activity of the clove essential oil from *Syzygium aromaticum* on Candida, Aspergillus and dermatophyte species. *Journal of Medical Microbiology*, **58**, 1454–1462.

528 Khan, M.S. *et al.* (2009) Inhibition of quorum sensing regulated bacterial functions by plant essential oils with special reference to clove oil. *Letters in Applied Microbiology*, **49** (3), 354–360.

529 Lu, X.Q. *et al.* (2004) Effect of *Eucalyptus globulus* oil on lipopolysaccharide-induced chronic bronchitis and mucin hypersecretion in rats. *Zhongguo Zhong Yao Za Zhi (China Journal of Chinese Materia Medica)*, **29** (2), 168–171.

530 Nerio, L.S. *et al.* (2010) Repellent activity of essential oils: a review. *Bioresource Technology*, **101** (1), 372–378.

531 Salari, M.H. *et al.* (2006) Antibacterial effects of *Eucalyptus globulus* leaf extract on pathogenic bacteria isolated from specimens of patients with respiratory tract disorders. *Clinical Microbiology and Infection*, **12** (2), 194–196.

532 Cermelli, C. *et al.* (2008) Effect of eucalyptus essential oil on respiratory bacteria and viruses. *Current Microbiology*, **56** (1), 89–92.

533 Juergens, U.R. *et al.* (2003) Anti-inflammatory activity of 1.8-cineol (eucalyptol) in bronchial asthma: a double-blind placebo-controlled trial. *Respiratory Medicine*, **97** (3), 250–256.

534 Nagata, H. *et al.* (2008) Effect of eucalyptus extract chewing gum on periodontal health: a double-masked, randomized trial. *Journal of Periodontology*, **79** (8), 1378–1385.

535 Shin, S. and Kang, C.-A. (2003) Antifungal activity of the essential oil of *Agastache rugosa* Kuntze and its synergism with ketoconazole. *Letters in Applied Microbiology*, **36**, 111–115.

536 Skandamis, P.N. and Nycas, G.-J.E. (2000) Development and evaluation of a model predicting the survival of *Escherichia coli* 0157:H7 NCTC 12900 in homemade eggplant salad at various temperatures, pHs and oregano essential oil concentrations. *Applied and Environmental Microbiology*, **66**, 1646–1653.

537 Karatzas, A.K. *et al.* (2001) The combined action of carvacrol and high hydrostatic pressure on *Listeria monocytogenes* Scott A. *Journal of Applied Microbiology*, **90**, 463–469.

538 Inouye, S. *et al.* (2001) Antibacterial activity of essential oils and their major constituents against respiratory tract pathogens by gaseous contact. *Journal of Antimicrobial Chemotherapy*, **47**, 565–573.

539 Suhr, K.I. and Nielsen, P.V. (2003) Antifungal activity of essential oils evaluated by two different application techniques against rye bread spoilage fungi. *Journal of Applied Microbiology*, **94**, 665–674.

540 Deans, S.G. and Ritchie, G. (1987) Antibacterial properties of plant essential oils. *International Journal of Food Microbiology*, **5**, 165–180.

541 Marzulli, F.N. and Maibach, H.J. (1973) Antimicrobials: experimental contact sensitization in man. *Journal of the Society of Cosmetic Chemists*, **24**, 399–421.

542 Nordgren, C. (1939) Investigations on the sterilising efficacy of gaseous formaldehyde. *Acta Pathologica et Microbiologica Scandinavica, Supplement*, **XL**, 1–165.

543 Anon. (1958) Disinfection of fabrics with gaseous formaldehyde. Committee on formaldehyde disinfection. *Journal of Hygiene, Cambridge*, **56**, 488–515.

544 Phillips, C.R. and Kaye, S. (1949) The sterilizing action of gaseous ethylene oxide. I. Review. *American Journal of Hygiene*, **50**, 270–279.

545 Ernst, R.R. (1974) Ethylene oxide sterilization kinetics. *Biotechnology and Bioengineering Symposium*, **4**, 865–878.

546 Richards, C. *et al.* (1984) Inactivation of micro-organisms by lethal gases, in *Cosmetic and Drug Preservation: Principles and Practice* (ed. J.J. Kabara), Marcel Dekker, New York, pp. 209–222.

547 Burgess, D.J. and Reich, R.R. (1993) Industrial ethylene oxide sterilization, in *Sterilization Technology. A Practical Guide for Manufacturers and Uses of Health Care Products* (eds R.F. Morrissey and G. B. Phillips), Van Nostrand Reinhold, New York, pp. 152–195.

548 Jorkasky, J.F. (1993) Special considerations for ethylene oxide: chlorofluorocarbons (CFCs), in *Sterilization Technology. A Practical Guide for Manufacturers and Users of Health Care Products* (eds R.F. Morrissey and G. B. Phillips), Van Nostrand Reinhold, New York, pp. 391–401.

549 Page, B.F.J. (1993) Special considerations for ethylene oxide: product residues, in *Sterilization Technology* (eds R.F. Morrissey and G.B. Phillips), Van Nostrand Reinhold, New York, pp. 402–420.

550 Rossmore, H.W. (1995) *Handbook of Biocide and Preservative Use*, Blackie, London.

551 Alder, V.G. *et al.* (1990) Disinfection of heat-sensitive material by low-temperature steam and formaldehyde. *Journal of Clinical Pathology*, **19**, 83–89.

552 Kelsey, J.C. (1967) Use of gaseous antimicrobial agents with special reference to ethylene oxide. *Journal of Applied Bacteriology*, **30**, 92–100.

553 Harry, E.G. (1963) The relationship between egg spoilage and the environment of the egg when laid. *British Poultry Science*, **4**, 91–100.

554 McGregor, D. *et al.* (2006) Formaldehyde and glutaraldehyde and nasal cytotoxicity: case study within the context of the 2006 IPCS human framework for the analysis of a cancer mode of action for humans. *Critical Reviews in Toxicology*, **36** (10), 821–835.

555 Collins, J.J. and Lineker, G.A. (2004) A review and meta-analysis of formaldehyde exposure and leukaemia. *Regulatory Toxicology and Pharmacology*, **40** (2), 81–91.

556 Golden, R. *et al.* (2006) Formaldehyde as a potential human leukemogen: an assessment of biological plausibility. *Critical Reviews in Toxicology*, **36** (2), 135–153.

557 Bruch, C.W. and Koesterer, M.G. (1961) The microbicidal activity of gaseous propylene oxide and its application to powdered or flaked foods. *Journal of Food Science*, **26**, 428–435.

558 Baird-Parker, A.C. and Holbrook, R. (1971) The inhibition and destruction of cocci, in *Inhibition and Destruction of the Microbial Cell* (ed. W.B. Hugo), Academic Press, London, pp. 369–397.

559 Gurley, B. (1985) Ozone: pharmaceutical sterilant of the future? *Journal of Parenteral Science and Technology*, **39**, 256–261.

560 Rickloff, J.R. (1985) An evaluation of the sporicidal activity of ozone. *Applied and Environmental Microbiology*, **53**, 683–686.

561 Burleson, G.R. *et al.* (1975) Inactivation of viruses and bacteria by ozone, with and without sonication. *Applied Microbiology*, **29**, 340–344.

562 Selma, M.V. *et al.* (2008) Disinfection potential of ozone, ultraviolet-C and their combination in wash water in the fresh-cut industry. *Food Microbiology*, **25**, 809–814.

563 Fan, L. *et al.* (2002) Interaction of ozone and negative air ions to control microorganisms. *Journal of Applied Microbiology*, **93**, 114–148.

564 Smeets, E. *et al.* (2003) Prevention of biofilm formation in dialysis water treatment systems. *Kidney International*, **63** (4), 1574–1576.

565 Kim, J.G. *et al.* (2003) Ozone and its current and future application in the food industry. *Advances in Food and Nutrition Research*, **45**, 167–218.

566 Azarpazhooh, A. and Limeback, H. (2008) The application of ozone in d entistry: a systematic review of literature. *Journal of Dentistry*, **36** (2), 104–116.

567 Kim, J.G. *et al.* (1999) Applications of ozone for enhancing the microbiological safety and quality of foods: a review. *Journal of Food Protection*, **62**, 1071–1087.

568 Khadre, M.A. *et al.* (2001) Microbiological aspects of ozone applications in food: a review. *Journal of Food Science*, **66**, 1242–1252.

569 Hudson, J.B. *et al.* (2007) Inactivation of Norovirus by ozone gas in conditions relevant to healthcare. *Journal of Hospital Infection*, **66** (1), 40–45.

570 Sharma, M. and Hudson, J.B. (2008) Ozone gas is an effective and practical antibacterial agent. *American Journal of Infection Control*, **36** (8), 559–563.

571 Dunn, C.G. (1968) Food preservatives, in *Disinfection, Sterilization and Preservation* (eds C.A. Lawrence and S.S. Block), Lea & Febiger, Philadelphia, pp. 632–651.

572 Clark, D.S. and Lentz, C.P. (1969) The effect of carbon dioxide on the growth of slime producing bacteria on fresh beef. *Canadian Institute of Food Technology Journal*, **2**, 72–75.

573 Peng, X. *et al.* (2005) Impact of environmental factors on efficacy of upper-room air ultraviolet germicidal irradiation for inactivating airborne mycobacteria. *Environmental Science and Technology*, **39**, 9656–9664.

574 Kujundzic, E. *et al.* (2006) UV air cleaners and upper-room air ultraviolet germicidal irradiation for controlling airborne bacteria and fungal spores. *Journal of Occupational and Environmental Hygiene*, **3** (10), 536–546.

575 McDevitt, J.J. *et al.* (2008) Inactivation of poxviruses by upper-room UVC light in a simulated hospital room environment. *PLoS ONE*, **3** (9), e3186.

576 Cheng, C. *et al.* (2009) The effects of the bacterial interaction with visible-light responsive titania photocatalyst on the bactericidal performance. *Journal of Biomedical Science*, **16** (1), 7.

577 Paschoalino, M.P. and Jardim, W.F. (2008) Indoor air disinfection using a polyester supported TiO2 photo-reactor. *Indoor Air*, **18** (6), 473–479.

578 Yu, J.C. *et al.* (2005) Efficient visible-light-induced photocatalytic disinfection on sulfur-doped nanocrystalline titania. *Environmental Science and Technology*, **39** (4), 1175–1179.

579 Hou, Y.D. *et al.* (2008) N-doped SiO₂/TiO₂ mesoporous nanoparticles with enhanced photocatalytic activity under visible-light irradiation. *Chemosphere*, **72** (3), 414–421.

580 Terrier, O. *et al.* (2009) Cold oxygen plasma technology efficiency against different airborne respiratory viruses. *Journal of Clinical Virology*, **45** (2), 119–124.

581 Denyer, S. and Hodges, N. (2004) Sterilization procedures and sterility assurance, in *Hugo and Russell's Pharmaceutical Microbiology*, 7th edn (eds S. Dennyer *et al.*), Blackwell Publishing, Oxford, pp. 346–375.

582 Moisan, M. *et al.* (2001) Low-temperature sterilization using gas plasmas: a review of the experiments and an analysis of the inactivation mechanisms. *International Journal of Pharmaceutics*, **226** (1–2), 1–21.

583 Aguzzi, A. and Calella, A.M. (2009) Prions: protein aggregation and infectious diseases. *Physiological Reviews*, **89**, 1105–1152.

584 Supattapone, S. *et al.* (2009) A protease-resistant 61-residue prion peptide causes neurodegeneration in transgenic mice. *Molecular and Cellular Biology*, **21** (7), 2608–2616.

585 Lawson, V.A. *et al.* (2007) Enzymatic detergent treatment protocol that reduces protease-resistant prion protein load and infectivity from surgical-steel monofilaments contaminated with a human-derived prion strain. *Journal of General Virology*, **88**, 2905–2914.

586 Jackson, G.S. *et al.* (2005) An enzyme–detergent method for effective prion decontamination of surgical steel. *Journal of General Virology*, **86**, 869–878.

587 Supattapone, S. *et al.* (2006) On the horizon: a blood test for prions. *Trends in Microbiology*, **14** (4), 149–151.

588 Hodges, N.A. and Denyer, S.P. (1996) Preservative testing, in *Encyclopedia of Pharmaceutical Technology* (eds J. Swarbrick and J.C. Boylen), Marcel Dekker, New York, pp. 21–37.

589 Davis, J.G. (1972) Fundamentals of microbiology in relation to cleansing in the cosmetics industry. *Journal of the Society of Cosmetic Chemists*, **23**, 45–71.

590 Bean, H.S. (1967) The microbiology of topical preparations in pharmaceutical practice. 2. Pharmaceutical aspects. *Pharmaceutical Journal*, **199**, 289–292.

591 Olivant, D.J. and Shapton, D.A. (1970) Disinfection in the food processing industry, in *Disinfection* (ed. M.A. Benarde), Marcel Dekker, New York, pp. 393–428.

592 Anon. (1977) *Recommendations for Sterilisation of Plant and Equipment Used in the Dairying Industry*, BS 5305, British Standards Institution, London.

593 Friend, P.A. and Newsom, S.W.B. (1986) Hygiene for hydrotherapy pools. *Journal of Hospital Infection*, **8**, 213–216.

594 Aspinall, S.T. and Graham, R. (1989) Two sources of contamination of a hydrotherapy pool by environmental organisms. *Journal of Hospital Infection*, **14**, 285–292.

595 Black, A.P. *et al.* (1970) The disinfection of swimming pool water. Part I. Comparison of iodine and chlorine as swimming pool disinfectants. *American Journal of Public Health*, **60**, 535–545.

596 Black, A.P. *et al.* (1970) The disinfection of swimming pool water. Part II. A field study of the disinfection of public swimming pools. *American Journal of Public Health*, **60**, 740–750.

597 Warren, I.C. *et al.* (1981) Comparative assessment of swimming pool disinfectants, in *Disinfectants: their Use and Evaluation of Effectiveness*, Society for Applied Bacteriology Technical Series No. 16 (eds C.H. Collins *et al.*), Academic Press, London, pp. 123–139.

598 Anon. (1989) *Report of the Expert Advisory Committee on Biocides*, HMSO, London, p. 32.

599 Denyer, S.P. *et al.* (1985) Synergy in preservative combinations. *International Journal of Pharmaceutics*, **25**, 245–253.

600 Board, R.G. (1995) Natural antimicrobials from animals, in *New Methods of Food Preservation* (ed. G.W. Gould), Blackie Academic & Professional, London, pp. 40–57.

601 Beales, N. (2002) *Food Ingredients as Natural Antimicrobial Agents*, Review No. 31, Campden & Chorleywood Food Research Association Group, Campden, UK.

602 Negi, P.S. and Jayaprakasha, G.K. (2001) Antibacterial activity of grapefruit (*Citrus paradisi*) peel extracts. *European Journal of Food Research Technology*, **213**, 484–487.

603 Cooper, R.A. *et al.* (2002) The sensitivity to honey of Gram-positive cocci of clinical significance isolated from wounds. *Journal of Applied Microbiology*, **93**, 857–863.

604 Cleveland, J. *et al.* (2001) Bacteriocins: natural antimicrobials for food preservation. *International Journal of Food Microbiology*, **71**, 1–20.

605 Ennahar, S. *et al.* (1999) Class IIa bacteriocins from lactic acid bacteria: antibacterial activity and food preservation. *Journal of Bioscience and Bioengineering*, **87**, 705–716.

606 Nes, I.F. and Holo, H. (2000) Class II antimicrobial peptides from lactic acid bacteria. *Biopolymers*, **55**, 50–61.

607 Cintas, L.M. *et al.* (2001) Review: bacteriocins of lactic acid bacteria. *Food Science and Technology International*, **7**, 281–305.

608 Müller, F.-M.C. *et al.* (1999) Antimicrobial peptides as potential new antifungals. *Mycoses*, **42**, 77–82.

609 Lupetti, A. *et al.* (2002) Antimicrobial peptides: therapeutic potential for the treatment of *Candida* infections. *Expert Opinion on Investigational Drugs*, **11**, 309–318.

610 Rose, W.M. and Ourth, D.D. (2009) Isolation of lysozyme and an antifungal peptide from sea lamprey (*Petromyzon marinus*) plasma. *Veterinary Immunology and Immunopathology*, **132** (2–4), 264–269.

611 Soukos, N.S. *et al.* (1998) Targeted antimicrobial chemotherapy. *Antimicrobial Agents and Chemotherapy*, **42**, 2595–2601.

612 Griffiths, M.A. *et al.* (1997) Killing of methicillin-resistant *Staphylococcus aureus in vitro* using aluminum disulphonated phthalocyanine, a light-activated antimicrobial agent. *Journal of Antimicrobial Chemotherapy*, **40**, 873–876.

613 Ireland, J.C. *et al.* (1993) Inactivation of *Escherichia coli* by titanium dioxide photocatalytic oxidation. *Applied and Environmental Microbiology*, **59**, 1668–1670.

614 Sunada, K. *et al.* (1998) Bactericidal and detoxification effects of TiO₂ thin film photocatalysts. *Environmental Science and Technology*, **32**, 726–728.

615 Lee, S. *et al.* (1998) Inactivation of phage Q, by 245nm UV light and titanium dioxide photocatalyst. *Journal of Environmental Science Health: Part A – Toxic/Hazardous Substances and Environmental Engineering*, **33**, 1643–1655.

616 Kashige, N. *et al.* (2001) Mechanism of the photocatalytic inactivation of *Lactobacillus casei* phage PL-1 by titania thin film. *Current Microbiology*, **42**, 184–189.

617 Wainwright, M. (1998) Photodynamic antimicrobial chemotherapy. *Journal of Antimicrobial Chemotherapy*, **42**, 13–28.

618 Hricová, A. *et al.* (2006) The *SCABRA3* nuclear gene encodes the plastid RpoTp RNA polymerase, which is required for chloroplast biogenesis and mesophyll cell proliferation in arabidopsis. *Plant Physiology*, **141**, 942–956.

619 Hricova, D. *et al.* (2008) Electrolyzed water and its application in the food industry. *Journal of Food Protection*, **71** (90), 1934–1947.

620 Maribel Abadias, M. *et al.* (2008) Efficacy of neutral electrolyzed water (NEW) for reducing microbial contamination on minimally-processed vegetables. *International Journal of Food Microbiology*, **123** (1–2), 151–158.

621 Kanellakopoulou, K. *et al.* (1999) Lactic acid polymers as biodegradable carriers of fluoroquinolones: an *in vitro* study. *Antimicrobial Agents and Chemotherapy*, **43**, 714–716.

622 Lutwyche, P. *et al.* (1998) Intracellular delivery and antibacterial activity of gentamicin encapsulated in pH-sensitive liposomes. *Antimicrobial Agents and Chemotherapy*, **42**, 2511–2520.

623 Cordeiro, C. *et al.* (2000) Antibacterial efficacy of gentamicin encapsulated in pH-sensitive liposomes against an *in vivo Salmonella enterica* serovar Typhimurium intracellular infection model. *Antimicrobial Agents and Chemotherapy*, **44**, 533–539.

624 Anon. (1998) Biocidal Products Directive 98/8/EC. *Official Journal of the European Communities*, **41** (April 24), L123.

625 Izquierdo-Barba, I. *et al.* (2009) Incorporation of antimicrobial compounds in mesoporous silica film monolith. *Biomaterials*, **30** (29), 5729–5736.

626 Dai, C. *et al.* (2009) Degradable, antibacterial silver exchanged mesoporous silica spheres for hemorrhage control. *Biomaterials*, **30** (29), 5364–5375.

627 Chen, X. and Schluesener, H.J. (2008) Nanosilver: a nanoproduct in medical application. *Toxicology Letters*, **176** (1), 1–12.

628 Bajpai, S.K. *et al.* (2007) Synthesis of polymer stabilized silver and gold nanostructures. *Journal of Nanoscience and Nanotechnology*, **7** (9), 2994–3010.

629 Vimala, K. *et al.* (2009) Controlled silver nanoparticles synthesis in semihydrogel networks of poly(acrylamide) and carbohydrates: a rational methodology for antibacterial application. *Carbohydrate Polymers*, **75** (3), 463–471.

630 Boucher, R.M.G. (1974) Potentiated acid 1.5-pentanedial solution – a new chemical sterilizing and disinfecting agent. *American Journal of Hospital Pharmacy*, **31**, 546–557.

631 Myers, J.A. *et al.* (1980) The relationship between structure and activity of Taurolin. *Journal of Applied Bacteriology*, **48**, 89–96.

632 El-Falaha, B.M.A. *et al.* (1983) Sensitivities of wild-type and envelope-defective strains of *Escherichia coli* and *Pseudomonas aeruginosa* to antibacterial agents. *Microbios*, **38**, 99–105.

633 Eklund, T. (1980) Inhibition of growth and uptake processes in bacteria by some chemical food preservatives. *Journal of Applied Bacteriology*, **48**, 423–432.

634 Littlejohn, T.G. *et al.* (1992) Substrate specificity and energetics of antiseptic and disinfectant resistance in *Staphylococcus aureus*. *FEMS Microbiology Letters*, **95**, 259–266.

635 Albert, A. (1966) *The Acridines: their Preparation, Properties and Uses*, 2nd edn, Edward Arnold, London.

636 Al-Adham, I.S.I. *et al.* (2000) Microemulsions are membrane-active, antimicrobial, self-preserving systems. *Journal of Applied Microbiology*, **89**, 32–39.

637 Al-Adham, I.S.I. *et al.* (2003) Microemulsions are highly effective anti-biofilm agents. *Letters in Applied Microbiology*, **36**, 97–100.

3 Factors Affecting the Activities of Microbicides

Jean-Yves Maillard

Cardiff School of Pharmacy and Pharmaceutical Sciences, Cardiff University, Cardiff, UK

Introduction

The activities of microbicides (antiseptics, disinfectants and preservatives) can be profoundly affected by a number of factors that are inherent to microorganisms and microbicide chemistry as well as the field use of such formulations. While these factors are considered in any efficacy test protocols for microbicidal activity, they need a wider awareness [1–3] to forestall failure of microbial control [2–4]. In addition, improper use of the widening array and applications of microbicidal products may increase the risk of emergence of microbicide resistance and also cross-resistance to antibiotics [5].

Overall, factors affecting the microbicidal action of chemicals can be grouped depending on the degree of their relevance to the initial development of a given formulation, its field use and in assessing the outcome of its actual field application. This chapter is a general review of the topic with references to other chapters where additional details are given.

The impact of factors such as concentration of the active(s), pH, temperature and the presence of soiling on microbicidal activity is more widely recognized. Much less is known on the synergistic and antagonistic influences of excipients in a given formulation [6–10]. Likewise, there is insufficient information on what influence different surface types have on disinfection of environmental surfaces. Differences in microbial susceptibility to microbicides are now generally better understood [11–13], except when it comes to protozoan cysts/oocysts, fungi and yeasts. The generally higher resistance of microbial biofilms to environmental surface and medical device disinfectants is now fully acknowledged [14–16].

It is also recognized that environmental isolates often show higher resistance to microbicides than their reference counterparts from culture collections [17], and that microorganisms in general are highly versatile in their ability to express and acquire protective mechanisms to overcome the detrimental effects of chemical and physical stresses (see Chapter 6).

Factors affecting microbicidal activity during the development of a given formulation

A key factor affecting the activity of a microbicide during its initial formulation is the way the target microorganism is maintained and cultured for testing, and the importance of producing standardized inocula is emphasized in commonly used efficacy tests (e.g. European Norms, International Organization for Standardization, ASTM International, AOAC International) with details required on microbial source, culture media, passage history and the conditions of culture and processing (see Chapter 12). In case of viruses, particulars are needed on the passage history and handling of host cells as well (see Chapter 9).

Russell, Hugo & Ayliffe's: Principles and Practice of Disinfection, Preservation and Sterilization, Fifth Edition. Edited by Adam P. Fraise, Jean-Yves Maillard, and Syed A. Sattar.
© 2013 Blackwell Publishing Ltd. Published 2013 by Blackwell Publishing Ltd.

Culturing microorganisms for test inocula

In standard test protocols, challenge microorganisms are normally grown as batch cultures with inevitable variations in the age and physiological state of individual cells in the population. Though continuous cultures from chemostats can be more uniform [18], they are rarely used as inocula. Composition of the culture medium and growth conditions can induce changes in the structure of the bacterial cell wall [19], thus influencing susceptibility to microbicides [20, 21]. However, such differences may depend on the type of microbicide. For example *Staphylococcus aureus* [22] and *Listeria monocytogenes* [23] in the exponential phase showed greater susceptibility to cationic and oxidizing microbicides than those in the decline phase of growth. However, Gomez-Escalada *et al.* [24] observed that high concentration of triclosan was bactericidal against *Escherichia coli, Pseudomonas aeruginosa* and *Enterococcus hirae* regardless of their phase of population growth, although bacterial populations in a stationary phase and, particularly, washed suspensions, were less susceptible to the microbicidal effect of the bisphenol.

An early study observed aerobic microorganisms to be more resistant to phenol than anaerobic ones, although facultative anaerobes were found to be less susceptible to phenol when grown under anaerobic conditions [25].

The age of the culture might also affect microbial susceptibility to microbicides, notably by affecting the cell wall composition. For example, the cell wall of yeasts, notably their glucan and mannoprotein composition, has been shown to act as a barrier to chlorhexidine [26]. The age of the culture was shown to affect the porosity of the cell wall [27], with older cultures being less susceptible to the biguanide [28, 29]. Bundgaard-Nielsen and Nielsen [30] noted that the resistance of ascospores to 70% (v/v) ethanol increased with age.

Composition of growth medium and physical parameters

The composition of the growth medium can markedly affect the susceptibility of microorganisms to antimicrobials. This is well recognized for antibiotics but with limited information with regard to microbicides [31–33]. "Fattening" of bacterial cells by culturing then in glycerol altered their susceptibility to phenols [34] and the parabens [35]. Culturing bacteria with different amino acids can also affect the cell structure and microbicide susceptibility. Adding L-alanine instead of L-cystine produced more permeable *E. coli* cells and increased their susceptibility to microbicides [36]. Magnesium limitation was shown to affect the structure of *P. aeruginosa* cells [37], subsequently affecting their susceptibility to ethylenediamine tetraacetic acid (EDTA) [38], to chloroxylenol [39] and to a combination of chloroxylenol and EDTA [40]. Gilbert and Wright [41] proposed that magnesium limitation caused the replacement of the Mg^{2+}-stabilizing bridge with polyamides, which effectively reduced bacterial cell sensitivity to ion chelators and microbicides.

Not surprisingly, the susceptibility of spores to microbicides has been shown to be affected by the composition of the medium used for sporulation [42]. Knott *et al.* [43] observed that the type of water used in preparing spore culture also had a profound influence on germination, outgrowth and sporulation of *Bacillus subtilis*. Rose *et al.* [33] observed that spores prepared in liquid- or agar-based media showed different susceptibility and germination patterns, with those prepared in a liquid medium being the most susceptible and prone to germination. These observations probably resulted from a difference in the composition of the spore inner membrane, since no difference in levels of dipicolinic acid, core water, small acid-soluble proteins (SASPs), coat protein and cross-linking of a coat protein were observed.

There is little information on the effect of pH change on the susceptibility of microorganisms to microbicides. It is well known that bacteria, for example, will change the pH of their environment when they grow [44, 45]. A change in pH has been shown to affect phospholipid content of batch-grown bacteria [46, 47], but there is little insight as to whether or not these changes would affect microbial response to microbicides.

A change in temperature was shown to affect spore composition and their response to heat and radiation [48]. An early investigation reported that the germination of *B. subtilis* spores produced at 37°C was more sensitive to chlorocresol-induced inhibition than spores produced at 50°C [49]. Melly *et al.* [50] showed that spores produced at different temperatures had different susceptibility to moist heat and a number of microbicides, with spores produced at a high temperature (48°C) being the most resistant.

Pretreatments

Pre-exposure to surface active agents can affect bacterial susceptibility to microbicides. Polysorbates are non-ionic surface active agents that find application in the formulation of certain pharmaceutical products. An early investigation showed that pretreatment of *P. aeruginosa* with polysorbate-80 produced bacteria more sensitive to benzalkonium chloride and chlorhexidine diacetate [51]. A possible explanation for such an observation is that polysorbate-80 increases the permeability of bacterial cells [52].

Pre-exposure of *P. aeruginosa* to benzalkonium chloride enhanced its susceptibility to polysorbate-80 and to phenethyl alcohol [53, 54]. This is not surprising as cationic agents are known to affect membrane permeability [55] and as such can be microbicidal in their own right.

The benefit of using permeabilizing agents to boost the activity of antimicrobials has been well documented with Gram-negative bacteria. Permeabilizers investigated include polycations, lactoferrin and transferrin, triethylene tetraamine and EDTA [8, 56–65]. The effect of EDTA on potentiating the activity of cationic microbicides has been particularly well studied [8, 65–67] and has found some important applications in the cosmetic industry [68]. EDTA is a chelating agent that removes cations, especially Mg^{2+} and Ca^{2+}, from the outer layers of Gram-negative bacteria, making the outer membrane more permeable through the loss of lipopolysaccharides (LPSs). At a high concentration EDTA can be toxic to bacteria. Likewise, citric and malic acids can chelate Mg^{2+} from the outer membrane of Gram-negative bacteria, while polycations displaced from the membrane release LPS. The iron-binding proteins, lactoferrin and transferrin, can cause a partial loss of LPSs. Ethambutol has been shown to increase the activity of microbicides against mycobacteria, presumably by affecting the arabinogalactan in cell wall structure [69].

There are also instances where an inappropriate pretreatment might interfere with microbicidal activity. Maruthamuthu *et al.* [70] observed that the pretreatment of a cooling tower with a combination of morpholine phosphate and zinc prevented corrosion, but the addition of zinc in particular abrogated the activity of the microbicides.

Factors affecting microbicidal activity during field use

Factors that can influence the activity of microbicides in their field use can be divided into those inherent to: (i) the microbicide formulation; (ii) the conditions of application; and (iii) the target microorganism(s) [1, 3, 71]. Failure to understand these factors may lead to ineffective microbial control and possibly in the spread of the microbial target over a wider area during decontamination along with an enhanced risk of human and environmental toxicity [72–80]. From a practical perspective, an appreciation of these factors is essential to avoid a false sense of security for the end-user. Additionally, using microbicides inappropriately may lead to the development of microbicide resistance and also cross-resistance to antibiotics and other microbicides [5, 79].

Factors inherent to microbicides
Concentration
The right concentration of the microbicide in the formulation as applied in the field is an important prerequisite [81]. This is particularly important nowadays with increasing restrictions on the environmental discharges of potentially harmful chemicals [82]. A given product may contain barely enough active(s) to make it price competitive and even slight deviations in dilution, storage and actual application may render it ineffective in the field [2, 75, 78, 83].

The influence of changing the concentration of the active(s) on microbicidal activity can be measured experimentally, with the determination of the kinetics of inactivation. Measuring the exposure times necessary to kill the same number of microorganisms at two different concentrations (all the other factors remaining constant) allows for the calculation of the concentration exponent η (sometimes named dilution coefficient). If C_1 and C_2 represent the two concentrations and t_1 and t_2 the respective times to reduce the viable population to a similar degree, then η can be calculated from the equation:

$$C_1^{\eta} t_1 = C_2^{\eta} t_2 \qquad (3.1)$$

or

$$\eta = (\log t_1 - \log t_2)/(\log C_1 - \log C_2) \qquad (3.2)$$

Equations 3.1 and 3.2 are based on the expected first-order kinetic obtained from the logarithmic plot of concentration versus time. However, it should be noted that a first-order kinetic is not always obtainable and adjustments may need to be made.

Practically, knowledge of the concentration exponent indicates the effect of dilution (or increase in concentration) on the activity of a microbicide against a given microorganism. Indeed, dilution of a microbicide with a high η-value will result in a marked increase in the time necessary to achieve a comparable kill (i.e. an overall decrease in activity) providing that other conditions remain constant. Microbicides with a low η-value will not be affected as much by dilution. Examples of η-values are given in Table 3.1.

The calculation of η-values allows the predictability of: (i) using a low concentration of a microbicide; (ii) excessive dilution of the microbicidal product; and (iii) increasing concentration of a microbicide on the overall microbicidal activity, particularly in the following applications:
1. The use of dilution to quench the microbicidal activity of a chemical using standard efficacy (see Chapters 12 and 13) and sterility tests [85].
2. Deciding what level(s) of dilution are reasonable for field use of a microbicidal product.
3. Deciding what is the lowest concentration of a microbicide that can be used in practice, notably for the preservation of pharmaceutical and cosmetic products, but also for microbicidal products containing a low concentration of a microbicide (e.g. antimicrobial surface, textile, etc.)

A knowledge of the η-value also provides some valuable information on the possible interactions between the microbicide and the microbial cell [55, 86] (Table 3.2). Concentration is also central to the definition of microbial resistance in practice (see Chapter 6.1). Hence the measurement of lethality rather than

Table 3.1 Examples of η-values (partly based on [84]).

Microbicides	η-Value	Increase in time factor to achieve a similar kill when the concentration is reduced to:	
		One-half	One-third
Alcohol	10	1024	59,000
Phenolics	6	64	729
Parabens	2.5	5.7	15.6
Chlorhexidine	2	4	8
Mercury compounds	1	2	3
Quaternary ammonium compounds	1	2	3
Formaldehyde	1	2	3

Table 3.2 Possible relationship between concentration exponents and mechanisms of action of microbicides (based on [86]]).

η-Value	Examples	Interactions
1–2	Chlorhexidine	Membrane disrupter
	Quaternary ammonium compounds	Membrane disrupter
	Mercury compounds	–SH reactors
	Glutaraldehyde	–NH$_2$ groups and nucleic acids
2–4	Parabens	Concentration-dependent effects: transport inhibited (low), membrane integrity affected (high)
	Sorbic acid	Transport inhibitor (effect on proton-motive force); other unidentified mechanisms?
>4	Aliphatic alcohols	Membrane disrupters
	Phenolics	

Table 3.3 Change in pH and antimicrobial activity.

Activity as environmental pH increases	Mechanisms
Decreased activity	
Phenols	Increase in degree of dissociation of the molecule
Organic acids (e.g. benzoic, sorbic)	
Hypochlorites	Undissociated hypochlorous acid is the active factor
Iodine	Most active form is diatomic iodine, I2
Increased activity	
Quaternary ammonium compounds	Increase in degree of ionization of bacterial surface groups leading to an increase in binding
Biguanides	
Diaminidines	
Acridines	Competition with H$^+$ ions leading to an increase in interaction with target such as nucleic acid
Triphenylmethane dyes	
Glutaraldehyde	Increased interaction with –NH$_2$ groups

inhibition is essential for microbicidal products. Unfortunately, there are many reports on microbicide activity solely based on the measurement of the minimum inhibitory concentration (MIC) [5]. Such a measurement does not provide information on the concentration exponent and fails to recognize that concentrations above the MIC level are usually used in practice [81]. In addition, there is evidence that microorganisms showing an elevated MIC are nevertheless susceptible to higher (in-use) concentration of a microbicide [87, 88].

The available concentration of one or more active(s) in a microbicidal product, often referred to as bioavailability or availability, is an important but complex concept that will be discussed in the sections on pH, formulations, soiling and biofilms below.

pH

The activity of a microbicide is affected by the pH of the formulation in two ways: (i) a change in the microbicide itself; and (ii) a change in the interaction between the microbicide and the microbial cell (Table 3.3). A change in pH has been shown to affect the activity of a number of alkylating and oxidizing microbicides [45, 89–97]. pH was recently shown to affect the level of injuries in *E. coli* following copper exposure [98].

A number of microbicides, mainly acids, such as benzoic acid, sorbic acid and dehydroacretic acid, but also phenol and hypochlorites are effective in their un-ionized form (see Chapter 2). Thus, an increase in pH will affect their degree of dissociation and will decrease their overall activity. The inhibitory activity of organic acids at different pH levels can be predicted. The relationship between pH and degree of dissociation is given by the Henderson and Haselbach equation where [A$^-$] is the concentration of ionized molecules and [AH] the concentration of the un-ionized molecule:

$$\log[A^-]/[AH] = pH - pKa \qquad (3.3)$$

The calculation of the proportion of ionized and un-ionized molecules at a specific pH allows the calculation of the change in activity based on the relationship between MIC and the level of dissociation of the molecule:

$$\text{MIC (at a given pH)} \times [AH] \text{ (at given pH)} = \text{MIC of } [AH] \qquad (3.4)$$

In contrast, for microbicides for which efficacy depends on the ionized molecule (e.g. dyes) an increase in pH will produce an increase in activity.

For other microbicides, a change in pH will affect the stability of the microbicide. For example glutaraldehyde (GTA) has been shown to be more stable at an acid pH, but more effective as a microbicide at an alkaline pH [89–93]. Practically, GTA stock solutions used, for example, in endoscope washer-disinfectors are usually acidic and GTA is "activated" before use (i.e. the pH of the in-use solution to be increased). Another aldehyde, *ortho*-phthalaldehyde has been shown to be less pH dependent but was found to become sporicidal at an alkaline pH [92, 93, 95].

A change in pH can also affect the charge on the cell surface. As pH increases, the number of negatively charged groups on the bacterial cell surface increases. Thus, positively charged molecules have an enhanced degree of binding, for example quaternary ammonium compounds (QACs) [99] and dyes, such as crystal violet and ethyl violet [100], which remain essentially in their ionized form over the pH range 5 to 9. Surface charge and isoelectric point (pI) have been shown to affect the susceptibility of *P. aeruginosa* exposed to QACs [101]. The effect of pH on activity is recognized in standard efficacy test, notably for microbicidal product used for cleaning in-place. A buffer solution providing a pH of 5.0 or 9.0 is recommended for use (see Chapter 12).

Formulation

The formulation of a microbicide has a profound effect on its microbicidal activity. This is actually an important issue when one considers the practical application of efficacy *in vitro* test results, which are often based on the non-formulated microbicide [3]. Various excipients can be found in microbicidal products including solvents (e.g. alcohols, urea, propylene glycol), emulsifiers/surfactants (e.g. lecithin, sodium lauryl sulfate, potassium laurate, non-ionic and other surfactants), thickeners (e.g. polyethylene glycol, pectin, alginates), chelating agents (e.g. EDTA), alkalis or acids, buffering agents (e.g. disodium phosphate), corrosion inhibitors (e.g. nitrates, phosphates), colors and flagrances (e.g. essential oils) [102–105]. Most of these excipients can interact with the microorganisms or the microbicide itself and ultimately affect the activity of the formulated product.

There is, however, relatively little information on the effect of different excipients on the activity of microbicides in the public domain. This is not surprising since the correct combination of excipients and microbicides is often a trade secret. Information available in the public domain is often derived from investigations performed in the 1960s and 1970s. In many cases it is not possible to develop a successful product without the use of one or more excipients.

Metal ions

Cations might have a profound effect on the activity of microbicide. For example, while Mn^{2+} reduces the activity of salicylaldehyde against *Pseudomonas* spp., Zn^{2+} reduces it. The activity of anionic surfactants against staphylococci increases with low concentrations of divalent cations, whereas that of long-chain fatty acids is diminished greatly in the presence of Mg^{2+}, Ca^{2+} or Ba^{2+} ions [106]. The presence of Mg^{2+} or Ca^{2+} reduces the activity of formulations containing EDTA [40], as presumably the addition of divalent cations counteracts the effect of the ion chelator. The activity of other microbicides such as chlorine dioxide is also affected by divalent cations [107] and such interference might be an issue in water and food industries, for example.

Bioavailability of microbicides

One of the problems with complex formulations is the decrease in activity of a microbicide, which on its own might have a good activity in an aqueous system. This is particularly the case where oil is present, for example in creams. Microorganisms are found in the aqueous phase of the cream, while the microbicide might be partitioned in the oil phase. Bean [108] derived the following equation whereby the concentration of a preservative in the aqueous phase may be obtained:

$$C_w = C(\varphi+1)/(K_{ow}\varphi+1) \tag{3.5}$$

where C_w represents the concentration of preservative in the aqueous phase, C the total preservative concentration and φ the oil:water ratio. The partition coefficient (K_{ow}) may vary widely for a single preservative, depending on the type of oil used. If K_{ow} is high, then an adequate aqueous-phase concentration of preservative can be achieved only by means of an excessive total concentration. The pH of the cream must be considered, since pH may affect K_{ow}, and cause dissociation of the preservative molecule.

Partitioning of the microbicide might also occur between a rubber closure and the aqueous product. The distribution between the rubber and the water for phenol is 25:75; for chlorocresol 85:15; for chlorbutanol 80–90:10–20; and for phenylmercuric nitrate 95:5 [109–113].

The available concentration of a microbicide can also be decreased by the addition of an inappropriate chemical. For example, the activity of the parabens (methyl and propyl *p*-hydroxybenzoates) and QAC is reduced by macromolecular polymers and by non-ionic agents such as polysorbates [114, 115]. The concentration of a microbicide bound to a non-ionic surfactant can be calculated with the following equation:

$$R = SC+1 \tag{3.6}$$

where R is the ratio of total to free preservative concentration, S is the surfactant concentration and C is a constant, which has a unique value for each surfactant – preservative mixture and which increases in value as the lipid solubility of the preservative increases. The interaction of microbicides with non-ionic surface active agents has important repercussions in the preservation of various types of pharmaceutical and cosmetic products, notably creams and emulsions.

However, the interaction between the non-ionic surfactants, the microbicides and the target microorganism can be more complex, whereby the non-ionic surfactants can increase the activity of the microbicides at certain concentrations. Indeed, at a lower concentration, the non-ionic surfactant affects the microbial cell surface, possibly increasing its permeability to the microbicide. At a higher concentration, the non-ionic surfactant will have some microbicidal activity of its own. However, the microbicide in the aqueous phase (and not bound to the non-ionic surfactant) provides the microbicidal activity.

Factors depending upon treatment conditions
Environmental temperature

Temperature can have a significant effect on the activity of nearly all microbicides, the relationship being directly proportional [116, 117]. For example, a decrease in environmental temperature from 30°C to 10°C resulted in a decrease in susceptibility of *E. coli* to benzalkonium chloride (BZC) [118]. Similar results were reported by Taylor *et al.* [119] for 18 disinfectants following a decrease in air temperature from 20 to 10°C. Recently, Pinto *et al.* [120] showed that a rise in air temperature dramatically increased the virucidal activity of polyhexamethylene biguanide (PHMB), although in this case the effect was due to preventing the formation of viral aggregates [120, 121].

Most standard efficacy tests for environmental surface disinfectants specify the air temperature of the test site to be around 20°C (see Chapter 12). Microbicides to be used in automatic

Table 3.4 Examples of Q_{10}-values and their applications.

Microbicides	Q_{10}-values
Phenols and cresols	3–5
Formaldehyde	1.5
Aliphatic alcohols	30–50
Ethylene oxide	2.7[a]
β-Propiolactone	2–3[a]

[a] Combination of these microbicides and heat is used for some sterilization processes.

endoscope reprocessors usually require testing at an elevated temperature as specified in label directions.

The effect of a 10°C change in environmental temperature on microbicidal activity can be measured by the Q_{10}. The Q_{10} is derived from the temperature coefficient (θ), which describes a change in activity (time to kill the same number of microorganisms) per 1°C rise [84], and is equivalent to $θ^{10}$. The formula used to measure a change in activity with a change in environmental temperature is:

$$θ(T_1 - T_2) = \text{Time needed to kill at } T_1/\text{time needed to kill at } T_2$$
(3.7)

where T_1 and T_2 are two different environmental temperatures in °C. Knowledge of the Q_{10} is useful for a number of applications such as the combination of a microbicide and heat (see Chapter 15), the storage of chemically preserved products (e.g. pharmaceuticals and medicine) at a low temperature, and the disinfection of surfaces at a low temperature. Examples of Q_{10}-values are given in Table 3.4.

Elevated air temperatures can also have a negative impact on microbicides either by accelerating the denaturation of the active or its enhanced evaporation, or both. For example, alkaline GTA formulation is less stable at 40°C [89, 91]. Landry et al. [122] recommended that the thermal instability of nanosilver formulations for antimicrobial dressing be evaluated.

Oxygenation

Oxygenation might also affect the bacterial susceptibility to microbicides. Langsrud and Sundheim [123] observed that aerobic conditions rendered E. coli more resistant towards BZC whereas S. aureus became more sensitive. Saby et al. [124] showed that both oxygenation and starvation produced E. coli cells less susceptible to chlorination. More recently, Bjergbæk et al. [118] reported that E. coli cells exposed to BZC were less susceptible in an aerobic condition at 30°C than in an anaerobic condition.

Type of surface

The type of surface to be treated has a profound influence on the activity of microbicides [125]. Porous surfaces may harbor microorganisms and are more difficult to clean and disinfect than hard, non-porous ones. Ideally, the types of surfaces common in field

settings should be used as substrates or carriers in tests for microbicidal activity (see Chapter 12). Since that is often not feasible for a variety of reasons, one or more materials are used as prototypes of those common in a given setting.

While the debate on the need for routine disinfection of environmental surfaces continues [126, 127], there is increasing recognition of the potential of many such surfaces in the spread of nosocomial pathogens [126–128]. Therefore, renewed efforts are needed not only to better understand the relative significance of environmental surfaces in the spread of infections in general but also to develop clearer criteria [129–131] for the need and procedures for their routine disinfection.

There is burgeoning interest in the development and marketing of "antimicrobial" surfaces that either contain or are coated with microbicides; the "self-sanitizing" ones mostly contain either silver or copper [132–135]. The potential benefits or drawbacks of the widespread use of such surfaces remain unknown at this point [136]. Chapter 20.1 is a more detailed treatment of this topic.

Soiling

Soiling is a well-recognized parameter that affects activity of the majority of microbicides. Indeed, standard efficacy tests describe the use of soiling, usually in the form of bovine serum albumin (3 g/l) when testing for activity in "dirty conditions". Other interfering substances can be used depending upon the final application of the microbicidal product; for example milk (1% v/v), yeast extract (10 g/l) and sucrose (10 g/l). Other types of soiling have been used [137–139]. In practice, soiling (also refer to as "soil load") can occur in various forms: serum, blood, pus, plasma, semen, vaginal charge, food residues, urine and fecal material. Soiling can affect microbicidal activity in three different ways: (i) it may interfere directly with the microbicide by reducing its "available" concentration; (ii) it may interact with the target microorganism, conferring protection from external damage; and (iii) it may promote the formation of microbial aggregates. Highly reactive microbicides (see Chapter 2) such as oxidizing and alkylating agents are affected by soiling, although for the latter there are conflicting reports [91, 140, 141]. There are numerous examples in the literature on the effect of soiling on the activity of microbicides against different types of microorganisms [1, 78, 142–147]. The limitation of microbicidal activity because of interference with organic material in certain applications is well established. Ionic silver (at a concentration of 10^{-9} to 10^{-6} mol/l) is an effective broad-spectrum antibacterial which finds application in wound dressing. However, silver ions adsorb rapidly to surfaces [148] and their "bioavailability" is further decreased by complexing with chlorides, sulfides and hard water to form insoluble inactive silver salts [149]. The maximum concentration of ionic silver in a physiological environment has been reported to be 1 µg/ml, presumably following interactions with proteinaceous fluids [150].

In the cosmetic industry, the continuous presence of soiling following usage of a product is a challenge for the preservative system. The strain put on the preservative system during usage can be tested somewhat with capacity tests that measure the efficacy of the microbicide following repeated challenges with a microorganism (see Chapter 12). In the food industry (notably the dairy industry) the presence of soiling is recognized as a problem for disinfection regimes [151, 152] so cleaning prior to disinfection is recommended. The use of pretreatment on surfaces is considered below. In the healthcare industry, cleaning should occur prior to surface disinfection or the disinfection of medical instruments such as endoscopes [153, 154]. For the latter application, enzymatic solutions are often used [138, 155].

Pretreatment of surfaces, especially when visibly soiled, is crucial to assuring or improving the microbicidal efficacy of their disinfection. The antagonistic and synergistic effects of non-ionic surfactants on the antibacterial activity of cationic surface active agents are well documented [156]. Below the critical micelle concentration (CMC) of the non-ionic agent, it is believed that potentiation occurs by an effect of this agent on the surface layers of the bacterial cell, resulting in an increased cellular permeability to the antimicrobial compound. Above the CMC of the non-ionic agent, the microbicide is distributed between the aqueous and micellar phases, or complexes with the non-ionic surfactant. However, it is only the "bioavailable" concentration of the microbicide in the aqueous phase that is interacting with microorganisms, producing an inhibitory or lethal effect.

Hard water must also be considered here as it is included in most standard microbicide efficacy tests (see Chapter 12). The presence of cations, for example, has been shown to decrease the activity of some microbicides [40, 157, 158].

Contact time

The microbicidal activity of chemicals usually increases with an increase in contact time. However, there is not a direct correlation between contact time and microbicidal activity, since first-order kinetic of inactivation is not often observed in practice [151, 159, 160]. The lack of correlation between concentration and contact time might reflect the effect of other factors on microbicidal activity [121]. Standard efficacy tests do not always reflect the exposure time on application. For example, the hygienic handwash protocol (CEN1499) [161] required demonstrating activity within a 1 min exposure time. In practice, this time is rarely achieved [162]. Likewise, for surface disinfection, the European Standard CEN1276 recommend a microbicide to achieve a 5-log_{10} reduction in bacterial viability within 5 min of exposure [163]. However, the relevance of such a contact time in practice is questionable [164]. This common disparity between the contact times in testing and label claims and those in actual field situations substantially increases the risk for ineffective microbial control [162].

Relative humidity

Relative humidity (RH) has a profound effect on the microbicidal activity of gaseous chemicals in particular and this is discussed further in Chapter 15.3. RH can influence the microbicidal action of ethylene oxide, β-propiolactone, formaldehyde [48, 165–167], chlorine dioxide [168] and vaporized hydrogen peroxide [12]. Pre-humidification and notably the state of hydration of the

microorganism are determining factors for their sensitivity to the antimicrobial processes (see Chapter 15.3). RH can also affect the activity of liquid microbicides applied on environmental surfaces by impacting on the rate of evaporation of water (see Chapter 20.1).

Factors inherent to microorganisms
Type of microorganisms

The well known and often extreme diversity of microorganisms can directly or indirectly influence their susceptibility to microbicides (Table 3.5). Such differences may be partly due to basic differences in the structures of microbial cells or virions [55]. The observed differences in the relative susceptibility/resistance of certain closely related and structurally similar organisms to a given microbicide are most likely due to differences in their metabolism and expression of "resistance" mechanisms (see Chapter 6). Such metabolic and resistance factors are better known in bacteria and bacterial endospores, but are still poorly understood for fungi, fungal spores, protozoa and viruses. Table 3.5 is an attempt at classifying the response of different types of microorganisms to microbicides. However, this table does not account for subtle differences within species or for some environmental isolates challenged with a specific microbicide. For example, Martin et al. [78] isolated some Gram-positive bacteria (*Micrococcus luteus*, *Streptococcus mutans*, *Streptococcus sanguis*, *Staphylococcus intermedius*) from endoscope washer disinfectors that survived an in-use concentration of chlorine dioxide.

Prions, the unconventional agents responsible for transmissible degenerative encephalopathies, are deemed to be the least susceptible to conventional chemical microbicides. However, their proteinaceous nature makes them more susceptible to enzyme inactivation and chemistry that denatures proteins, such as alkalis and possibly some oxidizing agents [169, 170]. More information on prions is provided in Chapter 10.

Bacterial endospores show relative resistance to many chemical and physical agents [170]. It is thus not surprising that they are used as biological indicators to validate many decontamination processes [85]. Endospores of *B. subtilis*, for example, are particularly well studied and certain factors behind their resistance to chemical and physical processes documented [171, 172]. The need for sporicides in healthcare settings is now evident with the mounting importance of *Clostridium difficile* (an anaerobic spore-former) as a nosocomial pathogen [128].

Aldehydes, such as glutaraldehyde and *ortho*-phthalaldehyde have a slow sporicidal activity (c. 6-log_{10} reduction in viability in hours) whereas halogen- and non-halogen-based oxidizers are more rapid as sporicides (c. 6-log_{10} reduction in viability in minutes) [128]. Other microbicides such as QACs, biguanides, alcohols, phenols and parabens can be sporistatic by inhibiting germination [173]. The structure of the spores, spore coats [174–177] and cortex and the presence of SASPs [178, 179] have been implicated in the lack of activity of many chemical microbicides (see Chapter 6.2 for more information). The presence of superdormant spores is of a particular concern for the food industry [180].

Table 3.5 Response of microorganisms to microbicide activity.

Microorganisms[a]	Examples	Comments	Further information
Prions	Scrapie, Creutzfeld–Jakob disease (CJD), new-variant CJD	Highly resistant to conventional microbicides due to their proteinaceous nature	See Chapter 10
Bacterial endospores	*Bacillus* spp., *Geobacillus* spp., *Clostridium difficile*	*Bacillus* used as biological indicators for sterilization processes due to their high intrinsic resistance	See Chapter 6.2
Protozoal oocysts	Cryptosporidium	Particularly challenging for water disinfection; associated with infection outbreaks	See Chapter 8
Mycobacteria	*M. chelonae*, *M. avium intracellulare*, *M. tuberculosis*, *M. terrae*	Environmental mycobacteria *M. chelonae*, *M. massiliense* might show a capacity to develop resistance to repeated microbicide exposure, and might become a challenge for high-level disinfection	See Chapter 6.3
Small non-enveloped viruses	Picornaviruses, noroviruses		See Chapter 9
Protozoal cysts	Giardia spp., *Acnathamoeba* spp.	Might harbor pathogenic bacteria and contribute to their survival when exposed to microbicides	See Chapter 8
Fungal spores	*Aspergillus* spp.	Very little information on microbicide activity against fungal spores	See Chapter 7
Gram-negative bacteria	*Pseudomonas* spp., *Burkholderia* spp., *Esherichia coli*, *Acinetobacter* spp.	*Pseudomonas* and *Burkholderia* are particularly challenging for preservative systems; pathogenic *E. coli* (e.g. O157) associated with surface contamination is often embedded with organic matter	See Chapter 6.1
Molds	*Aspergillus* spp.	Very little information on microbicide activity against molds	See Chapter 7
Yeasts	*Candida albicans*, *Saccharomyces cerevisiae*	Yeasts usually considered more susceptible than molds. Overall very little information available on yeast susceptibility to microbicides	See Chapter 7
Protozoa	*Acanthamoeba* spp., *Giardia* spp.	Important to control for water disinfection and contact lens disinfection	See Chapter 8
Large, non-enveloped viruses	Adenoviruses, rotaviruses	Certain rotaviruses more resilient, viruses often associated with soiling	See Chapter 9
Gram-positive bacteria	Staphylococci, streprotoccoci, enterococci		See Chapter 6.1
Enveloped viruses	HIV, HSV, influenza, RSV	Viruses on surfaces often associated with fomites	See Chapter 9

HIV, human immunodeficiency virus; HSV, herpes simplex virus; RSV, respiratory syncytial virus.
[a] Listed in order of resistance to microbicides from high to low.

Mycobacteria in general show a higher resistance to many microbicidal chemicals as compared with other types of vegetative bacteria. While many regard mycobacteria as a group to be more resistant than non-enveloped viruses [181, 182], this is not necessarily correct as such relative resistance may be formulation-specific and also related to the actual type of mycobacterium and virus involved.

The higher resistance of mycobacteria to microbicides is linked to their structure and particularly the high lipid content in their cell wall, which gives them higher hydrophobicity [183, 184] (see Chapter 6.3), although the composition of their cell wall arabinomannan/arabinogalactan might play a role against some microbicide such as glutaraldehyde [185]. Environmental isolates showing increased resistance to chemical disinfection with glutaraldehyde have been isolated [75, 94, 95]. Mycobacterial resistance to aldehydes has been associated with a change in cell wall structure [140] and enhanced hydrophobicity [94, 185] (see Chapter 6.1).

Gram-negative bacteria are often considered less susceptible to chemical microbicides than Gram-positive ones, and this view is mainly based on differences in cell permeability to antimicrobials [183, 186, 187]. Among the Gram-negative bacteria, *P. aeruginosa* and to some extent *Burkholderia cepacia* are of particular concern, notably for their resistance to preservative systems [119, 188–193]. It is interesting to note that environmental isolates might be less sensitive to microbicide activity than their reference counterpart from culture collections [194]. Among Gram-positive bacteria, differences in susceptibility occur when exposed to different microbicides, but there is generally no rule of thumb. However, an increase in resistance to microbicides in Gram-positive bacteria has been demonstrated, notably with the acquisition of new genetic determinants (see Chapter 6.1). The amount of cell wall lipid content has also been associated with microbicide susceptibility in staphylococci [34, 195, 196]. An increase in antibiotic resistance in clinical isolates of Gram-positive bacteria has, however, not been associated with an increase in resistance to microbicides [162, 164, 197].

Fungi are a diverse group of eukaryotic organisms comprising yeasts and molds, which are associated with many types of infections and also contamination of surfaces and spoilage of pharmaceutical, cosmetic and food products [198, 199]. The fungistatic and fungicidal activities of microbicides are overall poorly documented, although there is a renewed interest in these organisms because of their increasing resistance to available preservatives and mounting significance as nosocomial pathogens. Fungi are generally considered to be less susceptible to microbicides than non-sporulating bacteria [89, 200–203] and molds are less susceptible than yeasts (see Chapter 7). Although there is paucity of information on the mechanisms of action of microbicides against these organisms, especially molds, the differences in their susceptibility are believed to reside in the cell wall structure. Fungi also possess effective efflux systems and repair mechanisms. Surprisingly, there is little known about the susceptibility of fungal spores to microbicides, probably owing to the structural and size diversity of these spores. Jones *et al.* [204] observed that ascopores of *Saccharomyces cerevisiae* were significantly more resistant than vegetative cells to QACs and hypochlorite but not to peracetic acid. Likewise, it was found that ascospores were significantly more resistant to alcohols than vegetative cells [30].

Viruses can be separated into two main structural groups and their corresponding susceptibility to microbicides: enveloped viruses show higher susceptibility to even weaker microbicides, while the non-enveloped ones are comparatively more resistant but with a wider reaction range depending on the formulation and the specific type of virus under consideration (see Chapter 9). Among the non-enveloped viruses, the smaller ones (e.g. picornaviruses) normally show a higher degree of resistance to microbicides [205–209], with expected variations depending on the type of microbicide under consideration [210]. In comparison, medium-sized (e.g. adenoviruses) and larger-sized (e.g. rotaviruses) non-enveloped viruses possess a lower level of resistance to microbicides in general (see Chapter 9). The hierarchy of disinfectant resistance of non-enveloped viruses has been suggested as a predictor of activity against new and emerging viruses [211].

The relatively small size of viruses and their strict dependence on host cells limit our ability to know exactly how microbicides act on them. In very broad terms, essential lipids in enveloped viruses are the most likely targets for many actives, solvents and detergents in microbicidal products [55, 206, 210, 212, 213].

Because of their relatively simple structure and chemical composition, viruses as a group are less likely to develop the levels of microbicide resistance seen in certain types of bacteria [214]. In a recent study on the microbicidal activity of environmental surface disinfectants [215], there was incomplete inactivation of hepatitis A virus (a small, non-enveloped virus) while a mycobacterium, a vegetative bacterium and a bacterial spore-former in the test mixture were all rendered undetectable under identical conditions. This was most likely due to protection afforded to the virus by the uneven topography of the carrier surface, as well as the shielding by the soil load and the organisms in the mixture.

We now know a lot more about the susceptibility/resistance of protozoan trophozoites and their cysts to microbicides [216]. The renewed interest in free-living amoeba is due to the protection they give to intracellular bacterial and viral pathogens against damaging environmental factors including microbicides (see Chapter 9). The differences in microbicide sensitivity between trophozoites and cysts has been studied in a very few amoebal species such as *Acanthamoeba castellanii* [217–222]. Protozoan oocysts are known to be highly resistant to water disinfectants such as chlorine, although most of the available information is on *Cryptosporidium* spp. [216].

Number of microorganisms

The total number of microorganisms ("bioburden") on a given surface or object can also affect the activity of a microbicide by adding to the level of soiling and by providing protection to other organisms at the site. Most standard protocols for microbicidal activity employ a relatively large number of organisms in the test inoculum. Depending on the purpose of the test and the type of target organism, the level of viable organisms in the inoculum per tube or carrier may range from a minimum of 10^4 to a maximum of 10^8 viable units. Even though a microbicide may encounter much lower levels of the target organism(s) on a given unit surface area in the field, such high inocula are believed to represent the "worst case" scenario [3]. However, the relevance of using such high inocula has been questioned [162, 164, 223].

While it may not be necessary, or indeed feasible, to kill every single organism on an environmental surface for successful infection control in healthcare, the inability to do so in the case of cosmetics and pharmaceutical products can be quite detrimental, where the presence of even low levels of viable organisms could lead to rejection of a given lot [80]. Likewise, a given microbicide should be able to bring the levels of genetically modified microorganisms (GEMs) to undetectable levels [224] to forestall their accidental release into the environment. Similar considerations apply to infectious bioagents such as anthrax spores [215]

Microbial biofilm

Bacteria are frequently found in the environment in "biofilms", which are often complex microbial communities growing attached to submerged surfaces [225]. In the biofilm state bacteria are generally much more resistant to antimicrobials than their planktonic counterparts, thus presenting a major challenge for both antibiotics and microbicides in healthcare [14, 141, 226–232] as well as in the food and manufacturing industries [233–235] (see Chapter 4). Even though biofilm-associated contamination/infection is common, there are no standard efficacy protocols for testing microbicide activity against biofilms [236]. Several mechanisms have been identified for the decrease in susceptibility of biofilms to microbicides:

1. A reduction in the available concentration of microbicide due to the production of exopolysaccharides within the biofilm.
2. The presence of different environments caused by a reduction in oxygen and nutrients, allowing for different bacterial growth rates and the presence of dormant cells (persisters).
3. An increase in the production of degradative enzymes.
4. An increase in genetic exchange and cell-to-cell signaling.

Biofilm resistance to microbicides is given in more depth in Chapter 4.

Factors affecting recovery: microbial viability after microbicide exposure

A number of parameters will affect the recovery of microorganisms following exposure to microbicides. Understanding these factors is crucial, notably for the proper design and performance of microbicide tests as well as for the correct interpretation of the data generated. Indeed, standard efficacy tests describe in detail the neutralization solutions to be used for quenching the activity of microbicides as well as the recovery medium to be used (see Chapter 12).

Injury repair: viable but non-culturable microorganisms

Microorganisms are able to repair injuries following exposure to physical and chemical agents [237]. Bacteria are particularly efficient at repairing injuries caused to their genome following ultra-violet and ionizing radiations. Early studies on bacterial ability to repair injuries following exposure to a microbicide were based on plating treated bacteria and a culture medium that enhanced lethality to injured bacteria alone, but not to uninjured ones [238]. Such an approach was also used to study sublethal injuries to spores [239–242]. More recent approaches have made use of the difference in viability count between a traditional agar plate method and the use of the Bioscreen C Microbial Growth Analyzer that measures optical density/absorbance of bacterial growth in broth. Indeed, the difference in viable count between the two methods was deemed indicative of the extent of bacterial injury following treatment [9, 162, 243]. To date, the Bioscreen C Analyzer has, however, not been used to measure the repair capability of the treated bacteria.

Sterile distilled water, one-quarter strength Ringer's solution, 0.9% w/v saline, peptone water, tryptone sodium chloride and nutrient broth have been employed as diluents by various investigators. It should be noted that the use of an inappropriate diluent might enhance stress caused to injured bacteria.

Injuries caused to bacteria have been thought to produce viable-but-non-culturable s (VBNC) cells in normal recovery media [244]. The use of live – dead stain based on membrane permeability has indeed demonstrated that bacteria that could not form colonies on agar were actually viable [245]. The type of recovery medium is also important to consider. In standard efficacy tests, one common medium is tryptone soya agar. This medium allows for rapid growth and, when combined with optimal growth temperature, encourages rapid metabolism, which is unfavorable to injured bacteria. The formation of free radicals following rapid metabolism contributes to further injuries and results in bacterial commitment to cell death [245]. In short, the combination of a "rich" medium and optimal growth temperature enhances the lethal effect of the microbicide, by contributing to the killing of injured or stressed bacterial cells.

Neutralization of microbicidal activity

When tested for efficacy some microbicides can be transferred to the recovery medium at the same time as the microorganisms. Cationic agents and dyes in particular can bind strongly to the microbial cell surface (see Chapter 2). The microbicide concentration transferred can be inhibitory or microbicidal. It is thus crucial that the microbicide tested is neutralized effectively before recovering surviving microorganisms [246]. Failure to quench the activity of the test microbicide may overestimate the activity of the formulation being tested. Quenching of microbicidal activity can be achieved by adding a neutralizing chemical (inactivator, antidote) and/or by dilution for those actives with a high concentration exponent (see above). The neutralizer must itself be non-toxic to the test organisms and any reaction by-product of neutralization must likewise be harmless. Thus, the toxicity of the neutralizer and the efficacy of the neutralizer to quench the activity of a specific microbicide should be tested prior to the efficacy test. The use of neutralizers needs to be validated in standard efficacy tests (see Chapter 12).

In some instances, the use of a neutralizer is not possible. Microbicide removal by membrane filtration provides an alternative to quenching [247]. This offers a suitable alternative for a number of microbicides, but might be inefficient for those microbicides that attach strongly to microbial surface.

In tests for virucidal activity, any neutralizer used must also be non-toxic to the host cells and it also must neither suppress nor enhance the susceptibility of the host cells to the test virus [248]. Since membrane filtration to washout the test microbicide cannot be readily used in virucidal tests, gel filtration is often employed for the purpose [249]. Here, the virus – microbicide mixture is passed through a column of Sephadex or equivalent material to recover the virus while retaining any low molecular weight substances in the gel [248].

Recovery media

Several investigations have shown that the addition of specific compounds to the recovery media can reduce damage caused to microorganisms. Harris [250] showed that the addition of charcoal or various cations reduced both the rate and extent of damage of phenol-treated bacteria. Durant and Higdon [251] showed that the numbers of colonies from *P. aeruginosa* treated with bronopol were several-hundred-fold higher on recovery media containing catalase than on unsupplemented agar, presumably because of a better recovery of injured bacteria.

Incubation temperature

As mentioned above, bacteria exposed to a microbicide might recover better at a temperature below the optimum for undamaged bacteria. Harris [250] showed that the optimum temperature for phenol-damaged bacteria was 28°C. Williams and Russell [239–242] observed that the optimum incubation temperature was 30–37°C for spores exposed to halogen or glutaraldehyde. Spores exposed to a microbicide also required longer incubation periods before germination and growth [239].

Conclusions

The understanding of the factors affecting the activity of microbicides is vital to ensure an effective application in practice. In the healthcare environment, concentrations and exposure time for the application of a surface disinfectant do not always follow the manufacturer's recommendations or standard operating procedures [162, 164]. This might be, in particular, a concern for those organisms that are intrinsically resistant to many microbicides such as bacterial endospores. Indeed, for these microorganisms, an effective microbicide needs to be applied for several minutes to achieve an appropriate reduction in number, especially where soiling is present [128]. The inappropriate use of sporicides leads to spore survival and spore persistence, but it also can lead to an increase in sporulation [252] and increase in spore aggregation, the latter being associated with a further decrease in microbicide efficacy.

Factors affecting the efficacy of microbicides were mainly studied in the 1960s and 1970s, but some new information has been published more recently. A better understanding of these factors – but also of the use of chemicals to enhance microbicide activity – is paramount to ensure efficacy *in situ*, as well as improving microbicide efficacy in preservative applications in cosmetic, pharmaceutical and food products. This is particularly pertinent given the restrictions imposed by regulators on the microbicide to be used in certain applications (see Chapter 14).

Finally, within the last 10 years, a better understanding of the role of microbicides in emerging microbial resistance to these agents and to chemotherapeutic antibiotics, is adding pressure for microbicides to be used appropriately in a number of applications [5].

References

1 Maillard, J.-Y. (2005) Usage of antimicrobial biocides and products in the healthcare environment: efficacy, policies, management and perceived problems. *Therapeutics and Clinical Risk Management*, **1**, 340–370.

2 Maillard, J.-Y. (2007) Bacterial resistance to biocides in the healthcare environment: shall we be concerned? *Journal of Hospital Infection*, **65** (Suppl. 2), 60–72.

3 Maillard J.-Y. and Denyer S.P. (2009) Emerging bacterial resistance following biocide exposure: should we be concerned? *Chemica Oggi*, **27**, 26–28.

4 Poole, K. (2002) Mechanisms of bacterial biocide and antibiotic resistance. *Journal of Applied Microbiology*, **92** (Suppl.), 55–64.

5 SCENIHR (Scientific Committee on Emerging and Newly Identified Health Risks) (2009) The antibiotic resistance effect of biocides, adopted by the SCENIHR on January 19, 2009.

6 Denyer, S.P. *et al.* (1985) Synergy in preservative combinations. *International Journal of Pharmaceutics*, **25**, 245–253.

7 Lambert, R.J.W. *et al.* (2003) Theory of antimicrobial combinations: biocide mixtures – synergy or addition? *Journal of Applied Microbiology*, **94**, 747–759.

8 Lambert, R.J.W. *et al.* (2004) The synergistic effect of EDTA/antimicrobial combinations on *Pseudomonas aeruginosa*. *Journal of Applied Microbiology*, **96**, 244–253.

9 Johnston, M.D. *et al.* (2003) Membrane damage to bacteria caused by single and combined biocides. *Journal of Applied Microbiology*, **94**, 1015–1023.

10 Maillard, J.-Y. and Russell, A.D. (2001) Biocide activity: prospects for potentiation. *Chimica Oggi*, **12**, 33–36.

11 Spaulding, E.H. (1939) Chemical sterilization of surgical instruments. *Surgery Gynecology and Obstetrics*, **69**, 738–744.

12 McDonnell, G. and Russell, A.D. (1999) Antiseptics and disinfectants: activity, action and resistance. *Clinical Microbiology Reviews*, **12**, 147–179.

13 Maillard, J.-Y. (2005) Testing the effectiveness of disinfectants and sanitisers, in *Handbook of Hygiene Control in the Food Industry* (eds H.L.M. Lelieveld *et al.*), Woodhead Publishing, Cambridge, pp. 641–671.

14 Donlan, R.M. and Costerton, J.W. (2002) Biofilms; survival mechanisms of clinically relevant microorganisms. *Clinical Microbiology Reviews*, **15**, 167–193.

15 ASTM (2007) E2562. *Standard Test Method for Quantification of Pseudomonas aeruginosa Biofilm Grown with High Shear and Continuous Flow Using CDC Biofilm Reactor*, ASTM International, West Conshohocken, PA. doi: 10.1520/E2562-07

16 ASTM (2008) E2647, *Standard Test Method for Quantification of a Pseudomonas aeruginosa Biofilm Grown Using a Drip Flow Biofilm Reactor with Low Shear and Continuous Flow*, ASTM International, West Conshohocken, PA. doi: 10.1520/E2647-08

17 Lambert, R.J.W. *et al.* (2001) The relationships and susceptibilities of some industrial, laboratory and clinical isolates of *Pseudomonas aeruginosa* to some antibiotics and biocides. *Journal of Applied Microbiology*, **91**, 972–984.

18 Farewell, J.A. and Brown, M.R.W. (1971) The influence of inoculum history on the response of microorganisms to inhibitory and destructive agents, in *Inhibition and Destruction of the Microbial Cell* (ed. W.B. Hugo), Academic Press, London, pp. 703–752.

19 Ellwood, D.C. and Tempest, D.W. (1972) Effects of environment on bacterial wall content and composition. *Advances in Microbial Physiology*, **7**, 83–116.

20 Melling, J. *et al.* (1974) Effect of growth environment in a chemostat on the sensitivity of *Pseudomonas aeruginosa* to polymyxin B sulphate. *Proceedings of the Society for General Microbiology*, **1**, 61.

21 Dean, A.C.R. *et al.* (1976) The action of antibacterial agents on bacteria grown in continuous culture, in *Continuous Culture – Applications and New Techniques* (eds A.C.R. Dean *et al.*), Ellis Horwood, London, pp. 251–261.

22 Luppens, S.B.I. *et al.* (2002) The effect of growth phase on *Staphylococcus aureus* on resistance to disinfectants in a suspension test. *Journal of Food Science*, **65**, 124–129.

23 Luppens, S.B.I. *et al.* (2001) Effect of benzalkonium chloride on viability and energy metabolism in exponential- and stationary-growth-phase cells of *Listeria monocytogenes*. *Journal of Food Science*, **64**, 476–482.

24 Gomez Escalada, M. *et al.* (2005) Triclosan – bacteria interactions: single or multiple target sites? *Letters in Applied Microbiology*, **41**, 476–481.

25 Bennett, E.O. (1959) Factors affecting the antimicrobial activity of phenols. *Advances in Applied Microbiology*, **1**, 123–140.

26 Hiom, S.J. *et al.* (1992) Effects of chlorhexidine diacetate on *Candida albicans*, *C. glabrata* and *Saccharomyces cerevisiae*. *Journal of Applied Bacteriology*, **72**, 335–340.

27 Farkas, V. (1979) Biosynthesis of cell walls of fungi. *Microbiology Reviews*, **43**, 117–144.

28 Hiom, S.J. *et al.* (1995) Uptake of ^{14}C-chlorhexidine gluconate by *Saccharomyces cerevisiae*, *Candida albicans* and *Candida glabrata*. *Letters in Applied Microbiology*, **21**, 20–22.

29 Russell, A.D. and Furr, J.R. (1996) Microbicides: mechanisms of antifungal action and fungal resistance. *Science Progress*, **79**, 27–48.

30 Bungaard-Nielsen, K. and Nielsen, P.V. (1996) Fungicidal effect of 15 disinfectants against 25 fungal contaminants commonly found in bread and cheese manufacturing. *Journal of Food Protection*, **59**, 268–275.

31 Rodin, V.B. *et al.* (2000) Direct quantitative evaluation of the effects of biocides on *Pseudomonas fluorescens* in various nutrient media. *Applied Biochemistry and Microbiology*, **36**, 609–612.

32 Brill, F. *et al.* (2006) Influence of growth media on the sensitivity of *Staphylococcus aureus* and *Pseudomonas aeruginosa* to cationic biocides. *International Journal of Hygiene and Environmental Health*, **209**, 89–95.

33 Rose, R. *et al.* (2007) Comparison of the properties of *Bacillus subtilis* spores made in liquid or on agar plates. *Journal of Applied Microbiology*, **103**, 691–699.

34 Hugo, W.B. and Franklin, I. (1968) Cellular lipid and the antistaphylococcal activity of phenols. *Journal of General Microbiology*, **52**, 365–373.

35 Furr, J.R. and Russell, A.D. (1972) Uptake of esters of *p*-hydroxybenzoic acid by *Serratia marcescens* and by fattened and non-fattened cells of *Bacillus subtilis*. *Microbios*, **5**, 237–246.

36 Hugo, W.B. and Ellis, J.D. (1975) Cell composition and drug resistance in *Escherichia coli*, in *Resistance of Microorganisms to Disinfectants, 2nd International Symposium* (ed. W.B. Kedzia), Polish Academy of Sciences, Poznan, Poland, pp. 43–45.

37 Eagon, R.G. *et al.* (1975) Ultrastructure of *Pseudomonas aeruginosa* as related to resistance, in *Resistance of Pseudomonas aeruginosa* (ed. M.R.W. Brown), John Wiley & Sons, London, pp. 109–143.

38 Brown, M.R.W. and Melling, J. (1969) Loss of sensitivity to EDTA by *Pseudomonas aeruginosa* grown under conditions of Mg-limitation. *Journal of General Microbiology*, **54**, 439–444.

39 Cowen, R.A. (1974) Relative merits of "in use" and laboratory methods for the evaluation of antimicrobial products. *Journal of the Society of Cosmetic Chemists*, **25**, 307–323.

40 Dankert, J. and Schut, I.K. (1976) The antibacterial activity of chloroxylenol in combination with ethylenediamine tetraacetic acid. *Journal of Hygiene, Cambridge*, **76**, 11–22.

41 Gilbert, P. and Wright, N. (1987) Non-plasmidic resistance towards preservatives of pharmaceutical products, in *Preservatives in the Food, Pharmaceutical and Environmental Industries*, Society for Applied Bacteriology Technical Series No. 22 (eds R.G. Board *et al.*), Blackwell Scientific Publications, Oxford, pp. 255–279.

42 Hodges, N.A. *et al.* (1980) A comparison of chemically defined and complex media for the production of *Bacillus subtilis* spores having reproducible resistance and germination characteristics. *Journal of Pharmacy and Pharmacology*, **32**, 126–130.

43 Knott, A.G. *et al.* (1997) Non-variable sources of pure water and the germination and outgrowth of *Bacillus subtilis* spores. *Journal of Applied Microbiology*, **82**, 267–272.

44 Messager, S. *et al.* (2003) Assessment of skin viability: is it necessary to use different methodologies? *Skin Research and Technology*, **9**, 321–330.

45 Fraud, S. *et al.* (2005) Activity of amine oxide against biofilms of *Streptococcus mutans*: a potential biocide for oral care formulations. *Journal of Antimicrobial Chemotherapy*, **56**, 672–677.

46 Houtsmuller, U.M.T. and Van Deenen, L.L.M. (1964) Identification of a bacterial phospholipid as an *o*-ornithine ester of phosphatidyl glycerol. *Biochimica et Biophysica Acta*, **70**, 211–213.

47 Op den Kamp, J.A.E. *et al.* (1965) On the phospholipids of *Bacillus megaterium*. *Biochimica et Biophysica Acta*, **106**, 438–441.

48 Russell, A.D. (1982) *The Destruction of Bacterial Spores*, Academic Press, London.

49 Bell, N.D.S. and Parker, M.S. (1975) The effect of sporulation temperature on the resistance of *Bacillus subtilis* to a chemical inhibitor. *Journal of Applied Bacteriology*, **38**, 295–299.

50 Melly, E. *et al.* (2002) Analysis of the properties of spores of *Bacillus subtilis* prepared at different temperatures. *Journal of Applied Microbiology*, **92**, 1105–1115.

51 Brown, M.R.W. and Richards, R.M.E. (1964) Effect of polysorbate (Tween) 80 on the resistance of *Pseudomonas aeruginosa* to chemical inactivation. *Journal of Pharmacy and Pharmacology*, **16** (Suppl.), 51–55.

52 Brown, M.R.W. and Winsley, B.E. (1969) Effect of polysorbate 80 on cell leakage and viability of *Pseudomonas aeruginosa* exposed to rapid changes of pH, temperature and toxicity. *Journal of General Microbiology*, **56**, 99–107.

53 Hoffman, H.P. *et al.* (1973) Ultrastructural observations associated with the growth of resistant *Pseudomonas aeruginosa* in the presence of benzalkonium chloride. *Journal of Bacteriology*, **113**, 409–416.

54 Richards, R.M.E. and Cavill, R.H. (1976) Electron microscope study of effect of benzalkonium chloride and edentate disodium on cell envelope of *Pseudomonas aeruginosa*. *Journal of Pharmaceutical Sciences*, **65**, 76–80.

55 Maillard, J.-Y. (2002) Bacterial target sites for biocide action. *Journal of Applied Microbiology*, **92** (Suppl.), 16–27.

56 Smith, G. (1975) Triethylene tetramine, a new potentiator of antibiotic activity. *Experientia*, **31**, 84–85.

57 Vaara, M. and Vaara, T. (1983) Polycations sensitize enteric bacteria to antibiotics. *Antimicrobial Agents and Chemotherapy*, **24**, 107–113.

58 Vaara, M. and Vaara, T. (1983) Polycations as outer membrane disorganizing agents. *Antimicrobial Agents and Chemotherapy*, **24**, 114–122.

59 Hukari, R. *et al.* (1986) Chain length heterogencity of lipopolysaccharide released from *Salmonella typhimurium* by ethylene-diamine-tetraacetic acid or polycations. *Journal of Biological Chemistry*, **154**, 673–676.

60 Viljanen, P. (1987) Polycations which disorganize the outer membrane inhibit conjugation in *Escherichia coli*. *Journal of Antibiotics*, **40**, 882–886.

61 Ayres, H.M. *et al.* (1998) Use of the Malthus-AT system to assess the efficacy of permeabilizing agents on biocide activity against *Pseudomonas aeruginosa*. *Letters in Applied Microbiology*, **26**, 422–426.

62 Ayres, H.M. *et al.* (1998) Effect of permeabilizing agents on antibacterial activityagainst a simple *Pseudomonas aeruginosa* biofilm. *Letters in Applied Microbiology*, **27**, 79–82.

63 Ayres, H.M. *et al.* (1998) Effect of divalent cations on permeabilizer-induced lysozyme lysis of *Pseudomonas aeruginosa*. *Letters in Applied Microbiology*, **27**, 372–374.

64 Ayres, H.M. *et al.* (1999) Effect of permeabilizers on antibiotic sensitivity of *Pseudomonas aeruginosa*. *Letters in Applied Microbiology*, **28**, 13–18.

65 Wooley, R.E. *et al.* (2000) *In vitro* effect of ethylenediaminetetraacetic acid-tris on the efficacy of hatchery disinfectants. *Avian Diseases*, **44**, 901–906.

66 Russell, A.D. (1971) Ethylenediamine tetraacetic acid, in *Inhibition and Destruction of the Microbial Cell* (ed. W.B. Hugo), Academic Press, London, pp. 209–225.

67 Russell, A.D. (1990) The bacterial spore and chemical sporicidal agents. *Clinical Microbiology Reviews*, **3**, 99–119.

68 Hart, J.R. (1984) Chelating agents as preservative potentiators, in *Cosmetic and Drug Preservation: Principles and Practice* (ed. J.J. Kabara), Marcel Dekker, New York, pp. 323–337.

69 Broadley, S.J. *et al.* (1995) Potentiation of the effects of chlorhexidine diacetate and cetylpyridinium chloride on mycobacteria by ethambutol. *Journal of Medical Microbiology*, **43**, 458–460.

70 Maruthamuthu, S. *et al.* (2000) Interference between biocides and inhibitors in cooling water systems. *Bulletin of Electrochemistry*, **16**, 209–213.

71 Maillard, J.-Y. (2005) Biocides: health care application. *Pharmaceutical Journal*, **275**, 639–642.

72 Sanford, J.P. (1970) Disinfectants that don't. *Annals of Internal Medicine*, **72**, 282–283.

73 Prince, J. and Ayliffe, G.A.J. (1972) In-use testing of disinfectants in hospitals. *Journal of Clinical Pathology*, **25**, 586–589.

74 Centers for Disease Control (1974) Disinfectant or infectant: the label doesn't always say. *National Nosocomial Infections Study, Fourth Quarter*, **1973**, 18.

75 Griffiths, P.A. *et al.* (1997) Glutaraldehyde-resistant *Mycobacterium chelonae* from endoscope washer disinfectors. *Journal of Applied Microbiology*, **82**, 519–526.

76 Miyagi, F. *et al.* (2000) Evaluation of bacterial contamination in disinfectants for domestic use. *Revista de Saude Publica*, **34**, 444–448.

77 Russell, A.D. (2002) Introduction of biocides into clinical practice and the impact on antibiotic-resistant bacteria. *Journal of Applied Microbiology*, **92** (Suppl.), 121–135.

78 Martin, D.J.H. *et al.* (2008) Resistance and cross-resistance to oxidising agents of bacterial isolates from endoscope washer disinfectors. *Journal of Hospital Infection*, **69**, 377–383.

79 Duarte, R.S. *et al.* (2009) Epidemic of postsurgical infections caused by *Mycobacterium massiliense*. *Journal of Clinical Microbiology*, **47**, 2149–2155.

80 Lorenzen, K. (2005) Improving cleaning-in-place (CIP), in *Handbook of Hygiene Control in the Food Industry* (eds H.L.M. Lelieveld *et al.*), Woodhead Publishing, Cambridge, pp. 425–444.

81 Russell, A.D. and McDonnell, G. (2000) Concentration: a major factor in studying biocidal action. *Journal of Hospital Infection*, **44**, 1–3.

82 Anonymous (1998) *Biocidal Products Directive (BPD) 98/8/EC*, http://www. hse.gov.uk/biocides/bpd/ (accessed May 2, 2010).

83 Van Klingeren, B. and Pullen, W. (1993) Glutaraldehyde resistant mycobacteria from endoscope washers. *Journal of Hospital Infection*, **25**, 147–149.

84 Bean, H.S. (1967) Types and characteristics of disinfectants. *Journal of Applied Bacteriology*, **30**, 6–16.

85 British Pharmacopoeia Commission (2010) *British Pharmacopoeia*, The Stationery Office, London.

86 Denyer, S.P. and Stewart, G.S.A.B. (1998) Mechanisms of action of disinfectants. *International Biodeterioration and Biodegradation*, **41**, 261–268.

87 Thomas, L. *et al.* (2005) Antimicrobial activity of chlorhexidine diacetate and benzalkonium chloride against *Pseudomonas aeruginosa* and its response to biocide residues. *Journal of Applied Microbiology*, **98**, 533–543.

88 Lear, J.C. *et al.* (2006) Chloroxylenol- and triclosan-tolerant bacteria from industrial sources – susceptibility to antibiotics and other biocides. *International Biodeterioration and Biodegradation*, **57**, 51–56.

89 Gorman, S.P. *et al.* (1980) Antimicrobial activity, uses and mechanism of action of glutaraldehyde. *Journal of Applied Bacteriology*, **48**, 161–190.

90 Power, E.G.M. and Russell, A.D. (1990) Uptake of L(^{14}C)-alanine by glutaraldehyde-treated and untreated spores of *Bacillus subtilis*. *FEMS Microbiology Letters*, **66**, 271–276.

91 Russell, A.D. (1994) Glutaraldehyde: its current status and uses. *Infection Control and Hospital Epidemiology*, **15**, 724–733.

92 Walsh, S.E. *et al.* (1999) *Ortho*-phthalaldehyde: a possible alternative to glutaraldehyde for high level disinfection. *Journal of Applied Microbiology*, **86**, 1039–1046.

93 Walsh, S.E. *et al.* (1999) Studies on the mechanisms of the antibacterial action of *ortho*-phthalaldehyde. *Journal of Applied Microbiology*, **87**, 702–710.

94 Walsh, S.E. *et al.* (2001) Possible mechanisms for the relative efficacies of *ortho*-phthalaldehyde and glutaraldehyde against glutaraldehyde- resistant *Mycobacterium chelonae*. *Journal of Applied Microbiology*, **91**, 80–92.

95 Fraud, S. *et al.* (2001) Comparison of the mycobactericidal activity of *ortho*-phthalaldehyde, glutaraldehyde and other dialdehydes by a quantitative suspension test. *Journal of Hospital Infection*, **48**, 214–221.

96 Mercade, M. *et al.* (2009) Antimicrobial efficacy of 4.2% sodium hypochlorite adjusted to pH 12, 7.5, and 6.5 in infected human root canals. *Oral Surgery Oral Medicine Oral Pathology Oral Radiology and Endodontology*, **107**, 295–298.

97 Stopforth, J.D. *et al.* (2008) Effect of acidified sodium chlorite, chlorine, and acidic electrolyzed water on *Escherichia coli* O157: H7, *Salmonella*, and *Listeria monocytogenes* inoculated onto leafy greens. *Journal of Food Protection*, **71**, 625–628.

98 Sharan, R. *et al.* (2010) Inactivation and injury of *Escherichia coli* in a copper water storage vessel: effects of temperature and pH. *Antonie van Leeuwenhoek International Journal of General and Molecular Microbiology*, **97**, 91–97.

99 Hugo, W.B. (1965) Some aspects of the action of cationic surface-active agents on microbial cells with special reference to their action on enzymes, in *Surface Activity and the Microbial Cell*, Monograph 19, Society of Chemical Industry, London, pp. 67–82.

100 Moats, W. and Maddox, S.E. (1978) Effect of pH on the antimicrobial activity of some triphenylmethane dye. *Canadian Journal of Microbiology*, **24**, 658–661.

101 Bruinsma, G.M. *et al.* (2006) Resistance to a polyquaternium-1 lens care solution and isoelectric points of *Pseudomonas aeruginosa* strains. *Journal of Antimicrobial Chemotherapy*, **57**, 764–766.

102 Darwish, R.M. and Bloomfield, S.F. (1995) The effect of co-solvents on the antibacterial activity of paraben preservatives. *International Journal of Pharmaceutics*, **119**, 183–192.

103 Darwish, R.M. and Bloomfield, S.F. (1997) Effect of ethanol, propylene glycol and glycerol on the interaction of methyl and propyl p-hydroxybenzoate with *Staphylococcus aureus* and *Pseudomonas aeruginosa*. *International Journal of Pharmaceutics*, **147**, 51–60.

104 Gutierrez, J. *et al.* (2009) Antimicrobial activity of plant essential oils using food model media: efficacy, synergistic potential and interactions with food components. *Food Microbiology*, **26**, 142–150.

105 Papageorgiou, S. *et al.* (2010) New alternatives to cosmetics preservation. *Journal of Cosmetic Science*, **61**, 107–123.

106 Galbraith, H. and Miller, T.B. (1973) Effect of metal cations and pH on the antibacterial activity and uptake of long chain fatty acids. *Journal of Applied Bacteriology*, **36**, 635–646.

107 Valderrama, W.B. *et al.* (2009) Efficacy of chlorine dioxide against *Listeria monocytogenes* in brine chilling solutions. *Journal of Food Protection*, **72**, 2272–2277.

108 Bean, H.S. (1972) Preservatives for pharmaceuticals. *Journal of the Society of Cosmetic Chemists*, **23**, 703–720.

109 Wiener, S. (1955) The interference of rubber with the bacteriostatic action of thiomersalate. *Journal of Pharmacy and Pharmacology*, **7**, 118–125.

110 Wing, W.T. (1955) An examination of rubber used as a closure for containers of injectable solutions. Part I. Factors affecting the absorption of phenol. *Journal of Pharmacy and Pharmacology*, **7**, 648–658.

111 Wing, W.T. (1956) An examination of rubber used as a closure for containers of injectable solutions. Part II. The absorption of chlorocresol. *Journal of Pharmacy and Pharmacology*, **8**, 734–737.

112 Wing, W.T. (1956) An examination of rubber used as a closure for containers of injectable solutions. Part III. The effect of the chemical composition of the rubber mix on phenol and chlorocresol absorption. *Journal of Pharmacy and Pharmacology*, **7**, 738–743.

113 Allwood, M.C. (1978) Antimicrobial agents in single- and multi-dose injections. *Journal of Applied Bacteriology*, **44** (Suppl.), vii–xvii.

114 Patel, N.K. and Kostenbauder, H.B. (1958) Interaction of preservatives with macromolecules. I. *Journal of the American Pharmaceutical Association, Scientific Edition*, **47**, 289–293.

115 Kostenbauder, H.B. (1983) Physical factors influencing the activity of antimicrobial agents, in *Disinfection, Sterilization and Preservation*, 3rd edn (ed. S.S. Block), Lea & Febiger, Philadephia, pp. 811–828.

116 Mackey, B.M. and Seymour, D.A. (1990) The bactericidal effect of isoascorbic acid combined with mild heat. *Journal of Applied Bacteriology*, **67**, 629–638.

117 Wright, A.M. *et al.* (1997) Biological indicators for low temperature steam and formaldehyde sterilization: effect of variations in recovery conditions on the responses of spores of *Bacillus stearothemophilus* NCIB 8224 to low temperature steam and formaldehyde. *Journal of Applied Bacteriology*, **82**, 552–556.

118 Bjergbæk, L.A. *et al.* (2008) Effect of oxygen limitation and starvation on the benzalkonium chloride susceptibility of *Escherichia coli*. *Journal of Applied Microbiology*, **105**, 1310–1317.

119 Taylor, J.H. *et al.* (1999) A comparison of the bactericidal efficacy of 18 disinfectants used in the food industry against *Escherichia coli* O157:H7 and *Pseudomonas aeruginosa* at 10 and 20°C. *Journal of Applied Microbiology*, **87**, 718–725.

120 Pinto, F. *et al.* (2010) Effect of surfactants, temperature and sonication on the virucidal activity of polyhexamethylene biguanide against the bacteriophage MS2. *American Journal of Infection Control*, **38**, 393–398.

121 Pinto, F. *et al.* (2010) Polyhexamethylene biguanide exposure leads to viral aggregation. *Journal of Applied Microbiology*, **108**, 1080–1088.

122 Landry, B.K. *et al.* (2009) The kinetics of thermal instability in nanocrystalline silver and the effect of heat treatment on the antibacterial activity of nanocrystalline silver dressings. *Biomaterials*, **30**, 6929–6939.

123 Langsrud, S. and Sundheim, G. (1998) Factors influencing a suspension test method for antimicrobial activity of disinfectants. *Journal of Applied Microbiology*, **85**, 1006–1012.

124 Saby, S. *et al.* (1999) *Escherichia coli* resistance to chlorine and glutathione synthesis in response to oxygenation and starvation. *Applied and Environmental Microbiology*, **65**, 5600–5603.

125 Messager, S. *et al.* (2001) Determination of the antibacterial efficacy of several antiseptics tested on skin using the "ex-vivo" test. *Journal of Medical Microbiology*, **50**, 284–292.

126 Fraise, A. (2004) Decontamination of the environment and medical equipment in hospitals, in *Principles and Practice of Disinfection, Preservation and Sterilization*, 4th edn (eds A. Fraise *et al.*), Blackwell Science, Oxford, pp. 563–585.

127 Rutala, W.A. and Weber, D.J. (2004) The benefits of surface disinfection. *American Journal of Infection Control*, **32**, 226–231.

128 Maillard, J.-Y. (2011) Innate resistance to sporicides and potential failure to decontaminate. *Journal of Hospital Infection*, **77**, 204–209.

129 Griffith, C.J. *et al.* (2000) An evaluation of hospital cleaning regimes and standards. *Journal of Hospital Infection*, **45**, 19–28.

130 Dancer, S.J. (2004) How do we assess hospital cleaning? A proposal for micro-biological standards for surface hygiene in hospitals. *Journal of Hospital Infection*, **56**, 10–15.

131 Dettenkoffer, M. *et al.* (2004) Does disinfection of environmental surfaces influence nosocomial infection rates? A systematic review. *American Journal of Infection Control*, **32**, 84–89.

132 Noyce, J.O. *et al.* (2006) Potential use of copper surfaces to reduce survival of epidemic meticillin-resistant *Staphylococcus aureus* in the health care environment. *Journal of Hospital Infection*, **63**, 289–297.

133 Mehtar, S. *et al.* (2008) The antimicrobial activity of copper and copper alloys against nosocomial pathogens and *Mycobacterium tuberculosis* isolated from health care facilities in the Western Cape: an in-vitro study. *Journal of Hospital Infection*, **68**, 45–51.

134 Weaver, L. *et al.* (2008) Survival of *Clostridium difficile* on copper and steel: futuristic options for hospital hygiene. *Journal of Hospital Infection*, **68**, 145–151.

135 Santo, C.E. *et al.* (2008) Contribution of copper ion resistance to survival of *Escherichia coli* on metallic copper surfaces. *Applied and Environmental Microbiology*, **74**, 977–986.

136 Airey, P. and Verran, J. (2007) Potential use of copper as a hygienic surface; problems associated with cumulative soiling and cleaning. *Journal of Hospital Infection*, **67**, 271–277.

137 Sattar, S.A. *et al.* (1995) Mycobactericidal testing of disinfectants: an update. *Journal of Hospital Infection*, **30** (Suppl.), 372–382.

138 Bloß, R. and Kampf, G. (2004) Test models to determine cleaning efficacy with different types of bioburden and its clinical correlation. *Journal of Hospital Infection*, **56** (Suppl.), 44–48.

139 Perez, J. *et al.* (2005) Activity of selected oxidizing microbicides against the spores of *Clostridium difficile*: relevance to environmental control. *American Journal of Infection Control*, **33**, 320–325.

140 Fraud, S. *et al.* (2003) Effects of ortho-phthalaldehyde, glutaraldehyde and chlorhexidine diacetate on *Mycobacterium chelonae* and *M. abscessus* strains with modified permeability. *Journal of Antimicrobial Chemotherapy*, **51**, 575–584.

141 Shackelford, J.C.N. *et al.* (2006) Use of a new alginate film test to study the bactericidal efficacy of the high-level disinfectant *ortho*-phthalaldehyde. *Journal of Antimicrobial Chemotherapy*, **57**, 335–338.

142 Gélinas, P. and Goulet, J. (1983) Neutralization of the activity of eight disinfectants by organic matter. *Journal of Applied Bacteriology*, **54**, 243–247.

143 Sattar, S.A. and Springthorpe, V.S. (1991) Survival and disinfectant inactivation of the human immunodeficiency virus: a critical review. *Reviews in Infectious Diseases*, **13**, 430–447.

144 Sattar, S.A. *et al.* (2000) Foodborne spread of hepatitis A: recent studies on virus survival, transfer and inactivation. *Canadian Journal of Infectious Diseases*, **11**, 159–163.

145 Walsh, S.E. *et al.* (2003) Activity and mechanisms of action of some antibacterial agents on Gram-positive and -negative bacteria. *Journal of Applied Microbiology*, **94**, 240–247.

146 Wang, X.W. *et al.* (2005) Study on the resistance of severe acute respiratory syndrome-associated coronavirus. *Journal of Virological Methods*, **126**, 171–177.

147 Kawamura-Sato, K. *et al.* (2008) Reduction of disinfectant bactericidal activities in clinically isolated *Acinetobacter* species in the presence of organic material. *Journal of Antimicrobial Chemotherapy*, **61**, 568–576.

148 Richards, R.M. (1981) Antimicrobial action of silver nitrate. *Microbios*, **31**, 83–91.

149 Percival, S. *et al.* (2005) Bacterial resistance to silver in wound care. *Journal of Hospital Infection*, **60**, 1–7.

150 Walker, M. *et al.* (2006) Silver deposition and tissue staining associated with wound dressings containing silver. *Ostomy Wound Management*, **52**, 42–50.

151 Lambert, R.J.W. and Johnston, M.D. (2001) The effect of interfering substances on the disinfection process: a mathematical model. *Journal of Applied Microbiology*, **91**, 548–555.

152 Keener, L. (2005) Improving cleaning-out-of-place (COP), in *Handbook of Hygiene Control in the Food Industry* (eds H.L.M. Lelieveld *et al.*), Woodhead Publishing, Cambridge, pp. 445–467.

153 Alvarado, C.J. and Reichelderfer, M. (2000) APIC guideline for infection prevention and control in flexible endoscopy. *American Journal of Infection Control*, **28**, 138–155.

154 Banerjee, S. *et al.* (2008) ASGE Standards of Practice Committee. Infection control during GI endoscopy. *Gastrointestinal Endoscopy*, **67**, 781–790.

155 Shumway, R. and Broussard, J.D. (2003) Maintenance of gastrointestinal endoscopes. *Clinical Technique in Small Animal Practice*, **18**, 254–261.

156 Schmolka, I.R. (1973) The synergistic effects of non-ionic surfactants upon cationic germicidal agents. *Journal of the Society of Cosmetic Chemists*, **24**, 577–592.

157 Russell, A.D. and Furr, J.R. (1977) The antibacterial activity of a new chloroxylenol preparation containing ethylenediamine tetraacetic acid. *Journal of Applied Bacteriology*, **45**, 253–260.

158 Magarinos, M.C. *et al.* (2001) Effect of chlorhexidine upon hospital isolations of *Staphylococcus aureus* in different environmental conditions. *Revista Argentina de Microbiologia*, **33**, 241–246.

159 Lambert, R.J.W. and Johnston, M.D. (2000) Disinfection kinetics: a new hypothesis and model for the tailing of log-survivor/time curves. *Journal of Applied Microbiology*, **88**, 907–913.

160 Lambert, R.J.W. (2001) Advances in disinfection testing and modelling. *Journal of Applied Microbiology*, **91**, 351–363.

161 CEN (Comité Européen de Normalisation, European Committee for Standardization) (1997) *EN 1499. Chemical Disinfectants and Antiseptics – Hygienic Handwash – Test Method and Requirements (phase 2, step 2)*, CEN, Brussels.

162 Cheeseman, K.E. *et al.* (2009) Evaluation of the bactericidal efficacy of three different alcohol hand rubs against 57 clinical isolates of *Staphylococcus aureus*. *Journal of Hospital Infection*, **72**, 319–325.

163 CEN (Comité Européen de Normalisation, European Committee for Standardization) (1997) *EN 1276. Chemical Disinfectants and Antiseptics – Quantitative Suspension Test for the Evaluation of Bactericidal Activity of Chemical Disinfectants and Antiseptics for Use in Food, Industrial, Domestic and Institutional Areas – Test Method and Requirements (phase 2, step 1)*. CEN, Brussels.

164 Williams, G.J. *et al.* (2009) The use of sodium dichloroisocyanurate, NaDCC, in Welsh ITUs. *Journal of Hospital Infection*, **72**, 279–281.

165 Anonymous (1958) Disinfection of fabrics with gaseous formaldehyde. Committee on Formaldehyde Disinfection. *Journal of Hygiene, Cambridge*, **56**, 488–515.

166 Hoffman, R.K. (1971) Toxic gases, in *Inhibition and Destruction of the Microbial Cell* (ed. W.B. Hugo), Academic Press, London, pp. 225–258.

167 Richards, C. *et al.* (1984) Inactivation of micro-organisms by lethal gases, in *Cosmetic and Drug Preservation: Principles and Practice* (ed. J.J. Kabara), Marcel Dekker, New York, pp. 209–222.

168 Morino, H. *et al.* (2009) Inactivation of feline calicivirus, a norovirus surrogate, by chlorine dioxide gas. *Biocontrol Science*, **14**, 147–153.

169 Brown, P. *et al.* (1984) Sodium hydroxide decontamination of Creutzfeldt–Jakob disease virus. *New England Journal of Medicine*, **310**, 727.

170 McDonnell, G.E. (2007) Mechanisms of microbial resistance, in *Antisepsis, Disinfection, and Sterilization. Types, Action and Resistance*, ASM Press, Washington, DC, pp. 253–334.

171 Setlow, P. (2006) Spores of *Bacillus subtilis*: their resistance to and killing by radiation, heat and chemicals. *Journal of Applied Microbiology*, **101**, 514–525.

172 Setlow, P. (2007) I will survive: DNA protection in bacterial spores. *Trends in Microbiology*, **15**, 172–180.

173 Russell, A.D. *et al.* (1985) Reversal of the inhibition of bacterial spore germination and outgrowth by antibacterial agents. *International Journal of Pharmaceutics*, **25**, 105–112.

174 Knott, A.G. and Russell, A.D. (1995) Effects of chlorhexidine gluconate on the development of spores of *Bacillus subtilis*. *Letters in Applied Microbiology*, **21**, 117–120.

175 Knott, A.G. *et al.* (1995) Development of resistance to biocides during sporulation of *Bacillus subtilis*. *Journal of Applied Bacteriology*, **79**, 492–498.

176 Cabrera-Martinez, R.-M. *et al.* (2002) Studies on the mechanisms of the sporicidal action of *ortho*-phthalaldehyde. *Journal of Applied Microbiology*, **92**, 675–680.

177 Young, S.E. and Setlow, P. (2002) Mechanisms of killing of *Bacillus subtilis* spores by hypochlorite and chlorine dioxide. *Journal of Applied Microbiology*, **95**, 54–67.

178 Tennen, R. *et al.* (2000) Mechanisms of killing of spores of *Bacillus subtilis* by iodine, glutaraldehyde and nitrous acid. *Journal of Applied Microbiology*, **89**, 330–338.

179 Loshon, C.A. *et al.* (2001) Analysis of the killing of spores of *Bacillus subtilis* by a new disinfectant, Sterilox. *Journal of Applied Microbiology*, **91**, 1051–1058.

180 Ghosh, S. and Setlow, P. (2009) Isolation and characterization of superdormant spores of *Bacillus* species. *Journal of Bacteriology*, **191**, 1787–1797.

181 Favero, M.S. and Bond, W.W. (1991) Sterilization, disinfection and antisepsis in the hospital, in *Manual of Clinical Microbiology*, 5th edn (eds A. Balows *et al.*), American Society for Microbiology, Washington, DC, pp. 183–200.

182 Russell, A.D. (1996) Activity of biocides against mycobacteria. *Journal of Applied Bacteriology*, **81** (Suppl.), 87–101.

183 Lambert, P. (2002) Cellular impermeability and uptake of biocides and antibiotics in Gram-positive and mycobacteria. *Journal of Applied Microbiology*, **92** (Suppl.), 46–54.

184 Fraud, S. *et al.* (2003) Aromatic alcohols and their effect on Gram-negative bacteria, cocci and mycobacteria. *Journal of Antimicrobial Chemotherapy*, **51**, 1435–1436.

185 Manzoor, S.E. *et al.* (1999) Reduced glutaraldehyde susceptibility in *Mycobacterium chelonae* associated with altered cell wall polysaccharides. *Journal of Antimicrobial Chemotherapy*, **43**, 759–765.

186 Denyer, S.P. and Maillard, J.-Y. (2002) Cellular impermeability and uptake of biocides and antibiotics in Gram-negative bacteria. *Journal of Applied Microbiology*, **92**, 35–45.

187 Russell, A.D. (2002) Mechanisms of antimicrobial action of antiseptics and disinfectants: an increasingly important area of investigation. *Journal of Antimicrobial Chemotherapy*, **49**, 597–599.

188 Morrisson, A.J. and Wenzel, R.P. (1984) Epidemiology of infections due to *Pseudomonas aeruginosa*. *Reviews of Infectious Diseases*, **6** (Suppl. 3), 627–642.

189 Jones, M.W. *et al.* (1989) Resistance of *Pseudomonas aeruginosa* to amphoteric and quaternary ammonium biocides. *Microbios*, **58**, 49–61.

190 Na'was, T. and Alkofahi, A. (1994) Microbial contamination and preservative efficacy of topical creams. *Journal of Clinical Pharmacy and Therapeutics*, **19**, 41–46.

191 Schelenz, S. and French, G. (2000) An outbreak of multidrug-resistant *Pseudomonas aeruginosa* infection associated with contamination of bronchoscopes and an endoscope washer-disinfector. *Journal of Hospital Infection*, **46**, 23–30.

192 Ferrarese, L. *et al.* (2003) Bacterial resistance in cosmetics industrial plant: connected problems and their solution. *Annals of Microbiology*, **53**, 477–490.

193 Hutchinson, J. *et al.* (2004) *Burkholderia cepacia* infections associated with intrinsically contaminated ultrasound gel: the role of microbial degradation of parabens. *Infection Control and Hospital Epidemiology*, **25**, 291–296.

194 Russell, A.D. *et al.* (1986) Bacterial resistance to antiseptics and disinfectants. *Journal of Hospital Infection*, **7**, 213–225.

195 Hugo, W.B. and Davidson, J.R. (1973) Effect of cell lipid depletion in *Staphylococcus aureus* upon its resistance to antimicrobial agents. II. A comparison of the response of normal and lipid depleted cells of *S. aureus* to antibacterial drugs. *Microbios*, **8**, 63–72.

196 Fraise, A. (2002) Susceptibility of antibiotic-resistant bacteria to biocides. *Journal of Applied Microbiology*, **92** (Suppl.), 158–162.

197 Alqurashi, A.M. *et al.* (1996) Susceptibility of some strains of enterococci and staphylococci to antibiotics and biocides. *Journal of Antimicrobial Chemotherapy*, **38**, 745.

198 Pitt, J.I. and Hocking, A.D. (1997) *Fungi and Food Spoilage*, Blackie Academic & Professional, London.

199 Dupont, B. (2002) An epidemiological review of systemic fungal infections. *Journal de Mycologie Médicale*, **12**, 163–173.

200 Ellepola, A.N.B. and Samaranayake, L.P. (2001) Adjunctive use of chlorhexidine in oral candidoses: a review. *Oral Diseases*, **7**, 11–17.

201 Isman, M.B. (2000) Plant essential oils for pest and disease management. *Crop Protection*, **19**, 603–608.

202 Ferguson, J.W. *et al.* (2002) Effectiveness of intracanal irrigants and medications against the yeast *Candida albicans*. *Journal of Endodontics*, **28**, 68–71.

203 Sattar, S.A. *et al.* (2002) Combined application of simulated reuse and quantitative carrier test to assess high-level disinfection: experiments with an accelerated hydrogen peroxide-based formulation. *American Journal of Infection Control*, **30**, 449–457.

204 Jones, M.V. *et al.* (1991) Sensitivity of yeast vegetative cells and ascospores to biocides and environmental-stress. *Letters in Applied Microbiology*, **12**, 254–257.

205 Sattar, S.A. *et al.* (1989) Chemical disinfection of non-porous inanimate surfaces experimentally contaminated with four human pathogenic viruses. *Epidemiology and Infection*, **102**, 493–505.

206 Mbithi, J.N. *et al.* (1990) Chemical disinfection of hepatitis A virus on environmental surfaces. *Applied and Environmental Microbiology*, **56**, 3601–3604.

207 Mbithi, J.N. *et al.* (1993) Bactericidal, virucidal and mycobactericidal activity of alkaline glutaraldehyde under reuse in an endoscopy unit. *Journal of Clinical Microbiology*, **31**, 2988–2995.

208 Mbithi, J.N. *et al.* (1993) Comparative *in vivo* efficiency of hand-washing agents against hepatitis A virus (HM-175) and poliovirus type 1 (Sabin). *Applied and Environmental Microbiology*, **59**, 3463–3469.

209 Bigliardi, L. and Sansebastiano, G. (2006) Study on inactivation kinetics of hepatitis A virus and enteroviruses with peracetic acid and chlorine. New ICC/PCR method to assess disinfection effectiveness. *Journal of Preventive Medicine and Hygiene*, **47**, 56–63.

210 Maillard, J.-Y. (2001) Virus susceptibility to biocides: an understanding. *Reviews in Medical Microbiology*, **12**, 63–74.

211 Sattar, S.A. (2007) Hierarchy of susceptibility of viruses to environmental surface disinfectants: a predictor of activity against new and emerging viral pathogens. *Journal of AOAC International*, **90**, 1655–1658.

212 Wood, A. and Payne, D. (1998) The action of three antiseptics/disinfectants against enveloped and non-enveloped viruses. *Journal of Hospital Infection*, **38**, 283–295.

213 Howie, R. *et al.* (2008) Survival of enveloped and non-enveloped viruses on surfaces compared with other micro-organisms and impact of suboptimal disinfectant exposure. *Journal of Hospital Infection*, **69**, 368–376.

214 Maillard, J.-Y. *et al.* (1998) Resistance of the *Pseudomonas aeruginosa* F116 bacteriophage to sodium hypochlorite. *Journal of Applied Microbiology*, **85**, 799–806.

215 Sabbah, S. *et al.* (2010) A standard approach to assessing disinfection of environmental surfaces: experiments with a mixture of surrogates for infectious bioagents. *Applied and Environmental Microbiology*, **76**, 6020–6022.

216 Thomas, V. *et al.* (2010) Free-living amoebae and their intracellular pathogenic micro-organisms: risks for water quality. *FEMS Microbiology Review*, **34**, 231–259.

217 Khunkitti, W. *et al.* (1997) Aspects of the mechanisms of action of biguanides on trophozoites and cysts of *Acanthamoeba castellanii*. *Journal of Applied Microbiology*, **82**, 107–114.

218 Khunkitti, W. *et al.* (1998) *Acanthamoeba castellanii*: growth encystment, excystment and biocide susceptibility. *Journal of Infection*, **36**, 43–48.

219 Turner, N.A. *et al.* (1999) Acanthamoeba spp., antimicrobial agents and contact lenses. *Science Progress*, **82**, 1–8.

220 Turner, N.A. *et al.* (2000) Emergence of resistance to biocides during differentiation of *Acanthamoeba castellanii*. *Journal of Antimicrobial Chemotherapy*, **46**, 27–34.

221 Turner, N.A. *et al.* (2000) Microbial cell differentiation and changes in susceptibility to antimicrobial agents. *Journal of Applied Microbiology*, **89**, 751–759.

222 Lloyd, D. *et al.* (2001) Encystation in *Acanthamoeba castellanii*: development of biocide resistance. *Journal of Eukaryotic Microbiology*, **48**, 11–16.

223 Williams, G.J. *et al.* (2009) Limitations of the efficacy of surface disinfection in the healthcare settings. *Infection Control and Hospital Epidemiology*, **30**, 570–573.

224 Jackman, S.C. *et al.* (1992) Survival, detection and containment of bacteria. *Microbial Releases*, **1**, 125–154.

225 Hall-Stoodley, L. *et al.* (2004) Bacterial biofilms: from the natural environment to infectious diseases. *Nature Reviews Microbiology*, **2**, 95–108.

226 Dunne, W.M. (2002) Bacterial adhesion: seen any good biofilms recently? *Clinically Microbiology Reviews*, **15**, 155–166.

227 Pajkos, A. *et al.* (2004) Is biofilm accumulation on endoscope tubing a contributor to the failure of cleaning and decontamination? *Journal of Hospital Infection*, **58**, 224–229.

228 Sedlacek, M.J. and Walker, C. (2007) Antibiotic resistance in an *in vitro* subgingival biofilm model. *Oral Microbiology and Immunology*, **22**, 333.

229 Smith, K. and Hunter, I.S. (2008) Efficacy of common hospital biocides with biofilms of multi-drug resistant clinical isolates. *Journal of Medical Microbiology*, **57**, 966–973.

230 Lynch, A.S. and Robertson, G.T. (2008) Bacterial and fungal biofilm infections. *Annual Review of Medicine*, **59**, 415–428.

231 Williams, G.J. and Stickler, D.S. (2008) Effect of triclosan on the formation of crystalline biofilms by mixed communities of urinary tract pathogens on urinary catheters. *Journal of Medical Microbiology*, **57**, 1135–1140.

232 Stickler, D.J. and Jones, G.L. (2008) Reduced susceptibility of *Proteus mirabilis* to triclosan. *Antimicrobial Agents Chemotherapy*, **52**, 991–994.

233 Pan, Y. *et al.* (2006) Resistance of *Listeria monocytogenes* biofilms to sanitizing agents in a simulated food processing environment. *Applied and Environmental Microbiology*, **72**, 7711–7717.

234 Tabak, M. *et al.* (2007) Effect of triclosan on *Salmonella typhimurium* at different growth stages and in biofilms. *FEMS Microbiology Letters*, **267**, 200–206.

235 Kim, H. *et al.* (2007) Effectiveness of disinfectants in killing *Enterobacter sakazakii* in suspension, dried on the surface of stainless steel, and in a biofilm. *Applied and Environmental Microbiology*, **73**, 1256–1265.

236 Cookson, B. (2005) Clinical significance of emergence of bacterial antimicrobial resistance in the hospital environment. *Journal of Applied Microbiology*, **99**, 989–996.

237 Gilbert, P. (1984) The revival of micro-organisms sublethally injured by chemical inhibitors, in *The Revival of Injured Microbes*, Society for Applied Bacteriology Symposium Series No. 12 (eds M.H.E. Andrew and A.D. Russell), Academic Press, London, pp. 175–197.

238 Busta, F.F. (1978) Introduction to injury and repair of microbial cells. *Advances in Applied Microbiology*, **20**, 185–201.

239 Williams, N.D. and Russell, A.D. (1993) Injury and repair in biocide-treated spores of *Bacillus subtilis*. *FEMS Microbiology Letters*, **106**, 183–186.

240 Williams, N.D. and Russell, A.D. (1993) Revival of biocide treated spores of *Bacillus subtilis*. *Journal of Applied Bacteriology*, **75**, 69–75.

241 Williams, N.D. and Russell, A.D. (1993) Revival of *Bacillus subtilis* spores from biocide-induced injury in germination processes. *Journal of Applied Bacteriology*, **75**, 76–81.

242 Williams, N.D. and Russell, A.D. (1993) Conditions suitable for the recovery of biocide-treated spores of *Bacillus subtilis*. *Microbios*, **74**, 121–129.

243 Lambert, R.J.W. and van der Ouderaa, M.-L.H. (1999) An investigation into the differences between the bioscreen and the traditional plate count disinfectant test methods. *Journal of Applied Microbiology*, **86**, 689–694.

244 Dodd, C.E.R. *et al.* (1997) Inimical processes: bacterial self-destruction and sub-lethal injury. *Trends in Food Science and Technology*, **8**, 238–241.

245 Bloomfield, S.F. *et al.* (1998) The viable but non-culturable phenomenon explained? *Microbiology*, **144**, 1–4.

246 Russell, A.D. (1981) Neutralization procedures in the evaluation of bactericidal activity, in *Microbial Growth and Survival in Extreme Environments*, Society for Applied Bacteriology Technical Series No. 15 (eds G.W. Could and J.E.L. Corry), Academic Press, London, pp. 45–49.

247 Prince, J. *et al.* (1975) A membrane filter technique for testing disinfectants. *Journal of Clinical Pathology*, **28**, 71–76.

248 Sattar, S.A. *et al.* (2003) A disc-based quantitative carrier test method to assess the virucidal activity of chemical germicides. *Journal of Virology Methods*, **112**, 3–12.

249 Blackwell, J.H. and Chen, J.H.S. (1970) Effects of various germicidal chemicals on H. Ep.2 cell cultures and herpes simplex virus. *Journal of the Association of Official Analytical Chemists*, **53**, 1229.

250 Harris, N.D. (1963) The influence of recovery medium and incubation temperature on the survival of damaged bacteria. *Journal of Applied Bacteriology*, **26**, 387–397.

251 Durant, C. and Higdon, P. (1987) Preservation of cosmetic and toiletry products, in *Preservatives in the Food, Pharmaceutical and Environmental Industries*, Society for Applied Bacteriology Technical Series No. 22 (eds R.G. Board *et al.*), Blackwell Scientific Publications, Oxford, pp. 231–253.

252 Fawley, W.N. *et al.* (2007) Efficacy of hospital cleaning agents and germicides against epidemic *Clostridium difficile* strains. *Infection Control and Hospital Epidemiology*, **28**, 920–925.

4 Biofilm Recalcitrance: Theories and Mechanisms

Andrew J. McBain[1], Najib Sufya[2], and Alexander H. Rickard[3]

[1] School of Pharmacy and Pharmaceutical Sciences, The University of Manchester, Manchester, UK
[2] Microbiology and Immunology Department, Faculty of Pharmacy, University of Tripoli, Tripoli, Libya
[3] Department of Epidemiology, School of Public Health, University of Michigan, Ann Arbor, MI, USA

Introduction

It is now generally accepted that in the majority of non-sterile moist environments, bacterial populations develop in association with surfaces and form biofilms (for an overview see Costerton et al. [1]). Biofilms are functional consortia of microbial cells, enveloped within extracellular polymeric matrices, which bind the cells to the colonized surface and which further entrap microbial products such as enzymes and virulence factors [2, 3]. The biofilm matrix is visible in Figure 4.1 which shows a nascent *Pseudomonas aeruginosa* biofilm imaged using environmental scanning electron microscopy. Biofilms provide for a close proximity of individual cells in association with a surface, which might provide a nutrient source or may simply immobilize the community. Biofilms have been associated with many industrial, medical and environmental problems such as infections of indwelling medical devices, the fouling of pipe work and heat-exchange units, and in the bio-corrosion of materials. From a clinical perspective, they often represent the nidus of infection either to human and animal hosts or to manufactured products such as foods and pharmaceuticals. Biofilms are therefore most likely to be encountered in situations where their presence is undesirable, and where disinfection, preservation and chemical treatments are deployed to control or eradicate their presence. In this respect, it is particularly notable that the susceptibility of biofilms to chemical treatment agents bears little relationship to the susceptibility of the constituent organisms when in suspension (planktonic) or when simply dried onto a surface. Biofilms are often considerably less susceptible than planktonic cells and this phenomenon extends to a wide range of chemically unrelated microbicides, antimicrobials and antibiotics (for a review of biofilm resistance, see Gilbert et al. [4]).

Early reports connecting microbial recalcitrance to the formation of biofilms were published in the early 1980s [5–8]. This period was associated with increased use of implanted medical devices and presumably with correspondingly increased surgical site infection rates. In many instances, following implantation of the device, infections were reported that were apparently responsive to antibiotic treatment but which recurred after the treatment was stopped. Such infections could often only be resolved when the implanted devices were removed. This remains the case today. In a number of microbiological investigations, the removed devices were found to harbor the implicated pathogens growing as a biofilm [9, 10]. In the 1980s, examples of bacterial "resistance" towards microbicide treatments of inanimate surfaces were also being attributed to the biofilm mode of growth [11]. The range of antimicrobial molecules to which biofilm populations were (and still are) recalcitrant was considerable, and included all of

Russell, Hugo & Ayliffe's: Principles and Practice of Disinfection, Preservation and Sterilization, Fifth Edition. Edited by Adam P. Fraise, Jean-Yves Maillard, and Syed A. Sattar.

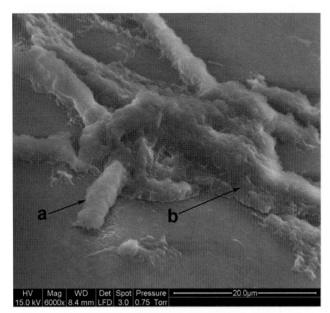

Figure 4.1 Early stages of biofilm formation of *Pseudomonas aeruginosa*. The biofilm was imaged using environmental scanning electron microscopy. Ruthenium red stain was used to improve the visualization of the biofilm matrix. The outline of individual cells can be seen (a), as can the enveloping matrix (b). A 20 μm scale bar is shown at the foot of the figure.

the clinically deployed antibiotics and microbicides such as the isothiazolones, halogens, quaternary ammonium compounds (QACs), biguanides and phenolic compounds. The breadth of treatment agents to which biofilms were resistant encouraged intuitively correct, but simplistic, explanations of the responsible mechanisms. Biofilms are enveloped within extensive extracellular polymeric matrices that cement the cells together and trap molecules and ions of environmental and microbial origin [12, 13]. It was thus not surprising that the original hypotheses implicated the matrix and suggested that biofilm communities were impervious because deep-lying cells that survived had evaded exposure.

The matrix

The matrix is heterogeneous, varying in hydration and chemical composition. Organisms within the matrix may be held in close proximity to their congeners. Adsorption sites within the matrices serve to anchor extracellular enzymes from the producer organisms, and will also actively concentrate metabolites from the community and ionic materials from the bulk fluid phase. Bound extracellular enzymes may mobilize complex nutrients captured from the fluid phase and may degrade antibacterial substances. The matrix is therefore able to moderate the microenvironments of each of the individual community members.

Biofilm matrix as a barrier to antibacterial agents

Many of the resistance characteristics of biofilm communities are lost when component cells are resuspended and separated from

their extracellular products. Indeed, early studies of antibiotic action against biofilms attributed their ineffectiveness to the presence of a diffusion barrier [2, 14]. Such explanations have since fallen out of favor because reductions in the diffusion coefficients of antibiotics such as tobramycin and cefsulodin, within biofilms or microcolonies, are insufficient to account for the observed changes in their activity [15]. Even if such changes in diffusivity were large, then they would only delay the achievement of an equilibrium. Ultimately, the concentration of antimicrobial in the bulk fluid phase would equal that at the biofilm – substratum interface. In order for the matrix to protect the enveloped cells, it would be necessary for it to interact with the treatment agent.

Biofilm matrix as an interactive barrier to antibacterial penetration

Retardation of the diffusion of antimicrobial agents therefore alone is insufficient to account for the reduced susceptibility of biofilms. For potent microbicides such as QACs and biguanides, however, or for chemically reactive compounds such as halogens and peroxygens, chemical quenching within the matrix during diffusion may occur. This can either be by adsorption to the charged matrix [16] or by chemical reactions that quench the agent [17, 18]. Whether or not the exopolymeric matrix constitutes a physical barrier to the antimicrobial depends upon the nature of the applied agent, the binding capacity of the polymeric matrix, the levels of agent deployed [19], the distribution of biomass and local hydrodynamics [20], together with the rate of turnover relative to antimicrobial diffusion rate [21]. This effect may be more pronounced for charged antibiotics such as the aminoglycosides [22] and cationic microbicides [23]. With chemically reactive agents such as halogens, aldehydes and peroxygens, the reaction capacity of the matrix is considerable [24]. If the underlying cells were to be protected through such adsorptive losses, the number of adsorption sites must however be sufficient to deplete the available microbicide within the treatment phase, which will often not be the case.

Enzyme-mediated reaction – diffusion resistance

In certain cases, the biofilm matrix can contain extracellular enzymes that are capable of degrading a diffusing antimicrobial. If this occurs, reaction – diffusion limitation will be enhanced. In this respect, enzymatic reaction may exacerbate antibiotic penetration failure [25], provided that the turnover of substrate by the enzyme is sufficiently rapid. In such respects it is significant that the expression of hydrolytic enzymes, such as β-lactamase, is reportedly induced in adherent populations and in those exposed to sublethal concentrations of β-lactam antibiotics [26]. These enzymes may become trapped and concentrated within the biofilm matrix and are able to further impede the penetration and action of susceptible antibiotics. In taxonomically diverse biofilms, the production of neutralizing enzymes by one species may confer protection upon the remainder [27, 28]. With respect to antibacterial agents used as disinfectants and preservatives, it is notable that the production of aldehyde lyase and aldehyde dehydrogenase enzymes can provide such protection against formaldehyde and glutaraldehyde [24, 29].

With the exception of the specific examples given above, which involve the presence of drug-inactivating enzymes, the invocation of matrix properties has generally proven to be insufficient to explain the whole panoply of resistance displayed by the biofilm communities [30, 31]. Accordingly, physiological changes in the biofilm cells – mediated through the induction of slow growth rates and starvation responses, together with the induction of separate attachment-specific, drug-resistant physiologies have been considered as further potential mediators of biofilm resistance [4].

Cellular phenotype in biofilm communities as a moderator of recalcitrance

Independent of the formation of a biofilm, the susceptibility of bacterial cells towards antibiotics and microbicides may be significantly affected by the physiological status of the individual cells, which together comprise the biofilm [30, 31]. Numerous phenotypes may be represented within a biofilm, reflecting the chemical heterogeneity of the matrix and the imposition, through cellular metabolism, of chemical, electrochemical, nutrient and gaseous gradients. Changes in antimicrobial susceptibility through alterations in phenotype may relate to growth rate-dependent changes in a variety of cellular components (including membrane fatty acids, phospholipids and envelope proteins) [32] and the production of extracellular enzymes [33] and polysaccharides [34]. Gradients of growth rate and the manifestation of phenotypic mosaics have been observed [35] and these contribute towards recalcitrance [31, 36, 37]. Within monoculture biofilms, the established physiological gradients are often non-uniform, with pockets of very slow-growing cells juxtaposed with relatively fast-growing areas [38].

A number of studies have associated the interdependence of growth rate and nutrient limitation in biofilms with their antimicrobial susceptibility [39]. These include calculated ratios of isoeffective concentration (growth inhibition and bactericidal activity) for biofilms and planktonic bacteria grown in broth or on catheter disks. In one such study, the calculated ratios correlated with those generated between non-growing and actively growing cultures. With the exception of ciprofloxacin, the antibiotic agents that were most effective against non-growing cultures (i.e. imipenem, meropenem) were also the most active against these biofilms. Other investigators have used perfused biofilm fermenters [40] to directly control and study the effects of growth rate within biofilms. Control populations of planktonic cells were generated in chemostats enabling the separate contributions of growth rate, and association within a biofilm, to be evaluated. Using this approach, decreased susceptibility of *Staphylococcus epidermidis* to ciprofloxacin [41] and *Escherichia coli* to cetrimide [36] and tobramycin [37] could be explained to a large extent in terms of specific growth rates, in that cells resuspended from

growth-rate controlled biofilms, and planktonic cells, grown at the same growth rate, possessed similar susceptibilities. In such instances, however, when intact biofilms were tested, the susceptibility was decreased from that of planktonic and resuspended biofilm cells. This strongly suggests that some resistance properties are associated with the organization of the cells within an exopolymeric matrix.

Neither the generation of chemical gradients nor physiological gradients provides a complete explanation of the observed resistance of biofilm communities. Stewart [42] has developed mathematical models that incorporate the concepts of metabolism-driven oxygen gradients, growth rate-dependent killing and reaction – diffusion properties of the matrix to explain the insusceptibility of *S. epidermidis* biofilms towards various antibiotics. His model predicted the reductions in susceptibility within thick biofilms through depletion of oxygen. Since nutrient and gaseous gradients increase in extent as biofilms thicken and mature, then growth rate effects become more evident in matured biofilms [43, 44]. This probably accounts for reports that aged biofilms are more recalcitrant to microbicide treatments than younger ones [43].

The contribution of reduced growth rate towards resistance is substantial within biofilm communities. As with reaction – diffusion limitation, however, this does not satisfactorily explain the totality of the observed resistance [45]. Physiological gradients depend upon growth and metabolism by cells on the periphery to deplete the nutrients and oxygen as they diffuse towards the more deeply located cells. Peripheral cells will therefore have growth rates and nutrient profiles that are similar to those in the planktonic phase. Consequently, these cells may be relatively sensitive to disinfectants and will quickly succumb. Lysis products from such cells will feed survivors within the depths of the biofilm which would, as a consequence, step up their metabolism and growth rate, adopt a more susceptible phenotype, and die [46]. This phenomenon could occur throughout the biofilm, proceeding inwards from the outside, until the biofilm was completely killed. Should the antimicrobial agent become depleted from the bulk phase, the biofilm could then re-establish almost as quickly as it was destroyed because of the local abundance of trapped nutrients. Growth rate-related processes might therefore delay the onset of killing in the recesses of a biofilm, but would not normally confer resistance against sustained exposure to antimicrobial agents.

Reaction – diffusion limitation of the access of agent and the existence of physiological gradients within biofilms therefore provide partial explanations for their reduced susceptibility, but neither explanation, separately or in combination, can fully explain the observation of sustained resistance towards a diverse array of treatment agents. In order for such resistance to be displayed, the biofilm population must either contain cells with uniquely insusceptible phenotypes, or the short-term survivors must adapt to a resistant phenotype during the window of opportunity provided by the buffering effects of diffusion and growth rate (i.e. a rapid response to sublethal treatment).

Drug-resistant phenotypes

The diversity of agents to which biofilms are recalcitrant, together with the long-term survival of biofilms in the face of vast excesses of treatment agent, make it likely that other processes are occurring in parallel to the establishment of chemical and physiological gradients. The long-term survival of biofilm populations is often associated with short-term losses in viability of several orders of magnitude. Survival might therefore be related to the presence of a small fraction of the population that expresses highly recalcitrant physiologies. The following sections will consider these, including the hyperexpression of efflux pumps and those induced by exposure to alarmone-signal molecules and dormant, quiescent or persister cells.

Efflux pumps

An increasingly studied resistance mechanism is the expression of multidrug efflux pumps [47]. In Gram-negative and Gram-positive bacteria the expression of such pumps may be induced through sublethal exposure to a broad range of agents [48]. These agents include antibiotics and other xenobiotics such as pine oil, salicylate and QACs [49]. Efflux pumps operate in many Gram-negative organisms and may be plasmid or chromosomally encoded [47]. In addition, multidrug efflux pumps such as QacA-G also contribute to microbicide tolerance in Gram-positive bacteria such as *Staphylococcus aureus* [50]. Sublethal exposure to many antimicrobials of *P. aeruginosa* MexAB efflux-deleted mutants can select for cells that hyperexpress the alternate efflux pump MexCD [51]. This highlights the multiple redundancies of efflux genes and their highly conserved nature.

Several attempts have been made to group efflux pumps into families [52] and to predict the structure and function of the proteins themselves [53]. Four superfamilies of efflux pumps have been recognized [54]. Although the families share no significant sequence identity, substrate specificity is often shared between them [55]. All the efflux superfamilies, however, contain pumps of varying specificity. An efflux pump may therefore primarily mediate the expulsion of endogenous metabolites or, alternatively, may primarily mediate the efflux of chemotherapeutic agents. Indeed, it is probable that these exporters were originally developed to expel endogenous metabolites.

Notable among the multidrug resistance operons is *mar* [48, 56]. The *mar* locus of *E. coli* regulates the AcrAB efflux pump and was the first mechanism found to be involved in the chromosomally encoded intrinsic resistance of Gram-negative bacteria to multiple drugs. Homologs have since been described in many Gram-negative bacteria. Moken *et al.* [57] and McMurry *et al.* [58] have shown that mutations causing overexpression of MarA or AcrAB are associated with exposure and reduced susceptibility towards a wide range of chemicals and antibiotics. If *mar* or other efflux systems were induced by growth as a biofilm per se, then this generalized efflux of toxic agents could provide an explanation of the ubiquitous observation of biofilm recalcitrance. Maira-Litran *et al.* [59], however, used perfused biofilm fermenters to grow *E. coli* strains for 48 h with various concentrations of ciprofloxacin and observed little or no difference between wild-type and *mar*-deleted strains [59, 60]. Similar experiments using biofilms constructed from strains in which the efflux pump gene *acrAB* was either deleted or constitutively expressed showed the *acrAB* deletion to not significantly affect susceptibility over that of the wild-type strain [61]. Constitutive expression of *acrAB* protected the biofilm against low concentrations of ciprofloxacin. Studies conducted in continuous culture with a *lacZ* reporter gene fused to *marOII*, showed *mar* expression to be inversely related to specific growth rate [61]. Thus, following exposure of biofilms to sublethal levels of β-lactams, tetracyclines and salicylates, *mar* expression will be greatest within the depths of the biofilm, where growth rates are suppressed, and might account for the long-term survival of the community when exposed to inducer molecules.

Another study of efflux in biofilms showed that expression of the major multidrug efflux pumps of *P. aeruginosa* actually decreased as the biofilm developed. Although expression was greatest in the depths of the biofilm, experiments with deletion mutants showed that none of the multidrug efflux pumps were contributing to the general increased resistance to antibiotics exhibited by the biofilm [61].

Quiescence and persistence

There has been much speculation concerning the ability of non-sporulating bacteria to adopt spore-like qualities while in a quiescent state. Specific growth rates of such cells approach zero [62] as they undergo reductive divisions in order to complete the segregation of initiated rounds of chromosome replication [62, 63]. Quiescence, as such, is commonly associated with populations that have undergone an extended period of starvation, and has most commonly been associated with bacteria found in oligotrophic marine environments [64, 65]. They are, however, also likely to be the dominant forms of bacteria within environments of naturally low nutrient availability. While mainly associated with aquatic Gram-negative bacteria, quiescence has been reported in Gram-positive species [66] and would appear to be a generically widespread response to extreme nutrient stress [67]. This has been termed the general stress response (GSR) and leads to populations of cells that synthesize the highly phosphorylated nucleotides ppApp and pppApp [68] and that, as a consequence, become resistant to a wide range of physical and chemical agents [69]. The GSR is now thought to account for much of the resistance observed in stationary phase cultures. Various terms have been adopted to describe such phenotypes, including "resting" [70], "quiescent" [71], "ultra-microbacteria" [63], "dormant" and "somnicells" [72]. It is also possible that the same or similar phenomenon describes the state of viable-but-non-culturable (VBNC) cells [73] since such bacterial cells often fail to produce colonies when transferred directly onto nutrient-rich agar. Indeed, when bacteria are collected and plated from oligotrophic environments then there is often a great disparity between the viable and total cell counts obtained [72, 74]. Even within biofilms that are in eutrophic environments, microenvironments exist where nutrients are scarce or even absent. Under such circumstances a small proportion of the cells present within a mature biofilm may be expressing the GSR regulator and will therefore be relatively recalcitrant to inimical treatments. Similar mechanisms have been proposed for the hostile take-over of batch cultures by killer phenotypes during the stationary phase [75] induced as part of the GSR in *E. coli*. This can lead to a phenotype that is not only more competitive in its growth than non-stressed cells, but which can also directly bring about the death of non-stressed ones [75].

The RpoS-encoded sigma factor sigma^s is a central regulator in a complex of network of genes moderating the stationary phase in *E. coli* [69]. In *Pseudomonas aeruginosa* it appears that two sigma factors, RpoS and AlgU, and the density-dependent cell–cell signaling systems orchestrate such responses [76]. Indeed, there is a hierarchical link between *n*-acyl homoserine lactones and RpoS expression [77] that might specifically induce the quiescent state at locations within a biofilm where signals accumulate and where nutrients are most scarce. In such respects it was demonstrated by Foley *et al.* [76] that the GSR response regulator RpoS was highly expressed in all of 19 *P. aeruginosa*-infected sputum samples taken from cystic fibrosis patients.

The persister hypothesis helps to fill some of the previously unexplained aspects of biofilm recalcitrance and is based on observations that were published over 60 years ago by Joseph Bigger in the *Lancet* [78]. Bigger demonstrated that although penicillin was bactericidal for *Staphylococcus pyogenes*, it did not eliminate *S. pyogenes* in the laboratory or in the patient's serum. This was described from the presence of "cocci which are called persisters at a frequency of approximately one per million of the staphylococci originally present and for which penicillin is bacteriostatic and only very slowly, if at all, bactericidal". It has subsequently been realized that persisters account for the tailing seen in many bacterial kill curves, which is often erroneously attributed to the antibiotic being expended. Bigger was ahead of his time (or alternatively, biofilm research has been slow off the mark) when he suggested that persisters were dormant forms (and thus indifferent to penicillin) and that they account for the fact that bacteria can be isolated from the pus of penicillin-treated patients, after treatment with penicillinase. Importantly, he suggested that failure to cure staphylococcal infections in man with penicillin could be due "to the presence in the body of persisters" [78]. Another important research article was published in the *Journal of General Microbiology* in 1964 by Gunnison *et al.* [79]. This made similar observations for *S. aureus*, again with penicillin, and discounted the possibility that persister cells were the result of stable genetic alteration. The recalcitrance of persisters was clearly demonstrated in this report where the proportion of survivors was not changed even by a 1000-fold increase in the dose of penicillin, or the addition of streptomycin. The Gunnison paper reported that persister cells were in a state unfavorable to the initiation of division or cell wall synthesis (i.e. they were drug indifferent).

Continued reports have appeared in the literature relating to bacterial persistence until a firm link between persistence and biofilm resistance was proposed. A paper by Spoering and Lewis

[80] presented susceptibility data for four different antimicrobial agents and *P. aeruginosa* (a very common test bacterium in biofilm studies) and suggested that biofilm recalcitrance is a function of slow growth rate and persister cells. This turned out to be a significant hypothesis and persisters now form an important part of most explanations of biofilm recalcitrance. The hypothesis suggests that biofilm recalcitrance often represents a Pyrrhic victory. This is because the majority of cells are inactivated, but the persister fraction remains to renew the biofilm once the inimical stress has been removed. It is proposed that the persisters represent a particularly effective survival mechanism when expressed within biofilms, since biofilms protect the persisters from phagocytes, predation, and physical/chemical stresses in other environments (Figure 4.2).

Biofilms as highly selective environments

Bacterial populations are genetically diverse and a sustained exposure to environmental stress will lead to an expansion of the most well-adapted genotype/phenotype. This is particularly the case for taxonomically diverse biofilms. The exposure of a population to sublethal concentrations of microbicides or antibiotics may therefore enrich the least susceptible clones. Equally, death and lysis of a subset of cells might lead to the transfer of resistance properties to the survivors.

It is known that pure cultures of bacteria can be "trained" to become less susceptible to antibiotics [81] and microbicides [82]. In such experiments, cultures are either grown in liquid media that contain concentrations of agent that are below the minimum inhibitory concentration (MIC) or they are streaked on to gradient plates that incorporate the agent. At each step in the process, the MIC is determined and the process repeated. Thus, it is relatively easy to select for populations of bacteria that have significantly reduced MIC values towards the selected agents. In some instances the changes in MIC are enough to render the cells resistant to normal treatment regimes. Where groups of agents have common biochemical targets, it is possible for selection by one agent to confer cross-resistance to a third party agent [83]. Such "resistance training" has for many years been regarded an artifact, since it is difficult to imagine a set of circumstances in the environment where bacteria will be exposed to gradually increasing concentrations of an inhibitory agent over a prolonged period (see Chapter 6.1). The repeated, sublethal treatment of biofilms in the environment and in infection, however, provides one situation where this might happen [46] as sublethal levels of agent will be sustained within the deeper recesses of the community.

As with any process involving changes in susceptibility to inimical agents, the nature of the genotype/phenotype selected reflects changes in the microbicidal/inhibitory targets, the adoption of alternate physiologies that circumvent the target, or to changes in drug access. The latter might be through modifications in the cell envelope [30, 31] or it might reflect active efflux mechanisms [84]. There may be a fitness cost associated with

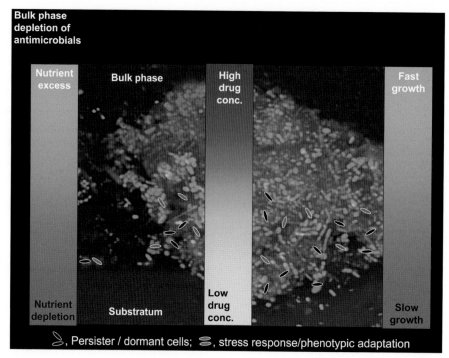

Figure 4.2 Major mechanisms of biofilm recalcitrance as currently understood, showing: (i) poor antimicrobial penetration; and (ii) gradients of nutrients and oxygen leading to variations in growth rate and other phenotypic variability (including stress-specific phenotypes and dormancy and persisters).

such adaptation, but this can decrease with continued exposure to the stress [85].

Mutations that increase the expression of multidrug efflux pumps can result in decreased susceptibility towards to a wide range of agents. For example, mutations in the *mar* operon increase the expression of the AcrAB efflux pump in *E. coli* [58] and mutations in the MexAB operon of *P. aeruginosa* leads to significant overexpression [86]. It should be borne in mind that the primary function of efflux is to defend the cell against naturally occurring environmental toxicants [49]. Efflux is often non-specific and equivalent to an emetic response. Cells that efflux permanently may therefore be poor competitors in heterogeneous communities, and may not prosper in the absence of the selection stress. Treatment with antimicrobials that act as substrates, but are not themselves inducers [59, 60], can lead to the clonal expansion of mutant cells that are constitutive in efflux pump expression. Treatment with agents that are both strong inducers and also substrates [57, 87] will confer no selective advantage upon the efflux mutants, but it must be borne in mind that induction of efflux by one agent may confer reductions in susceptibility to a range of chemically unrelated agents (see also Chapter 6.1).

Conclusions

The recalcitrance of microbial biofilms towards a wide variety of antimicrobial agents is clearly associated with the organization of cells within an exopolymer matrix that moderates the concentrations of antimicrobial and antibiotic to which the more deeply lying members of the biofilm community are exposed. These cells are typically starved or slow growing, and express stress-associated phenotypes that may include the expression or upregulation of efflux pumps. The phenotype of the deeply seated biofilm community reduces their susceptibility to the treatment agents and exacerbates the likelihood of being exposed to sublethal concentrations of antimicrobial agent. Deeper-lying cells will often outsurvive those at the surface and can proliferate once the bulk of the treatment agent is depleted or if the exposure is only transient. Thus, at the fringes of antimicrobial action, selection pressures may enrich the populations with the least susceptible genotype. It is possible under such conditions for repeated chronic exposure to sublethal treatments to select for a more resistant population. Alternative explanations for the recalcitrance of biofilm communities include the expression of biofilm-specific phenotypes that may be significantly less susceptible than planktonic cells, and the physical protection that the matrix confers on persister cells, which are recalcitrant through metabolic inactivity.

Acknowledgments

The authors would like to acknowledge the substantial contributions of their friend and colleague, Peter Gilbert (1951–2008).

References

1 Costerton, J.W. *et al.* (1994) Biofilms, the customized microniche. *Journal of Bacteriology*, **176** (8), 2137–2142.

2 Costerton, J.W. *et al.* (1987) Bacterial biofilms in nature and disease. *Annual Review of Microbiology*, **41**, 435–464.

3 Hall-Stoodley, L. *et al.* (2004) Bacterial biofilms: from the natural environment to infectious diseases. *Nature Reviews. Microbiology*, **2** (2), 95–108.

4 Gilbert, P. *et al.* (2002) The physiology and collective recalcitrance of microbial biofilm communities. *Advances in Microbial Physiology*, **46**, 202–256.

5 Gristina, A.G. *et al.* (1985) Bacterial colonization of percutaneous sutures. *Surgery*, **98** (1), 12–19.

6 Gristina, A.G. and Costerton, J.W. (1985) Bacterial adherence to biomaterials and tissue. The significance of its role in clinical sepsis. *Journal of Bone and Joint Surgery, American Volume*, **67** (2), 264–273.

7 Nickel, J.C. *et al.* (1985) Electron microscopic study of an infected Foley catheter. *Canadian Journal of Surgery*, **28** (1), 50–51. 54.

8 Sottile, F.D. *et al.* (1986) Nosocomial pulmonary infection: possible etiologic significance of bacterial adhesion to endotracheal tubes. *Critical Care Medicine*, **14** (4), 265–270.

9 Evans, R.C. and Holmes, C.J. (1987) Effect of vancomycin hydrochloride on *Staphylococcus epidermidis* biofilm associated with silicone elastomer. *Antimicrobial Agents and Chemotherapy*, **31** (6), 889–894.

10 Bisno, A.L. and Waldvogel, F.A. (2000) *Infections Associated with Indwelling Medical Devices*, ASM Press, Washington, DC.

11 Costerton, J.W. and Lashen, E.S. (1984) Influence of biofilm on the efficacy of biocides on corrosion-causing bacteria. *Materials Performance*, **23**, 34–37.

12 Sutherland, I.W. (2001) Exopolysaccharides in biofilms, flocs and related structures. *Water Science and Technology*, **43** (6), 77–86.

13 Flemming, H.C. *et al.* (2007) The EPS matrix: the "house of biofilm cells". *Journal of Bacteriology*, **189** (22), 7945–7947.

14 Slack, M.P. and Nichols, W.W. (1982) Antibiotic penetration through bacterial capsules and exopolysaccharides. *Journal of Antimicrobial Chemotherapy*, **10** (5), 368–372.

15 Gordon, C.A. *et al.* (1988) Antibiotic interaction and diffusion through alginate and exopolysaccharide of cystic fibrosis-derived *Pseudomonas aeruginosa*. *Journal of Antimicrobial Chemotherapy*, **22** (5), 667–674.

16 Hoyle, B.D. and Costerton, J.W. (1991) Bacterial resistance to antibiotics: the role of biofilms. *Progress in Drug Research*, **37**, 91–105.

17 Huang, C.T. *et al.* (1995) Nonuniform spatial patterns of respiratory activity within biofilms during disinfection. *Applied and Environmental Microbiology*, **61** (6), 2252–2256.

18 Stewart, P.S. *et al.* (1998) Analysis of biocide transport limitation in an artificial biofilm system. *Journal of Applied Microbiology*, **85** (3), 495–500.

19 Nichols, W.W. (1993) Biofilm permeability to antibacterial agents, in *Bacterial Biofilms and their Control in Medicine and Industry* (eds J. Wimpenny *et al.*), Bioline, Cardiff, pp. 141–149.

20 De Beer, D. *et al.* (1994) Direct measurement of chlorine penetration into biofilms during disinfection. *Applied and Environmental Microbiology*, **60** (12), 4339–4344.

21 Kumon, H. *et al.* (1994) A sandwich cup method for the penetration assay of antimicrobial agents through *Pseudomonas* exopolysaccharides. *Microbiology and Immunology*, **38** (8), 615–619.

22 Nichols, W.W. *et al.* (1988) Inhibition of tobramycin diffusion by binding to alginate. *Antimicrobial Agents and Chemotherapy*, **32** (4), 518–523.

23 Gilbert, P. *et al.* (2001) Assessment of resistance towards biocides following the attachment of micro-organisms to, and growth on, surfaces. *Journal of Applied Microbiology*, **91** (2), 248–254.

24 Gardner, L.R. and Stewart, P.S. (2002) Action of glutaraldehyde and nitrite against sulfate-reducing bacterial biofilms. *Journal of Industrial Microbiology and Biotechnology*, **29** (6), 354–360.

25 Stewart, P.S. (1996) Theoretical aspects of antibiotic diffusion into microbial biofilms. *Antimicrobial Agents and Chemotherapy*, **40** (11), 2517–2522.

26 Lambert, P.A. *et al.* (1993) Chemotherapy of *Pseudomonas aeruginosa* in cystic fibrosis, in *Bacterial Biofilms and their Control in Medicine and Industry* (eds J.T. Wimpenny *et al.*), Bioline, Cardiff, pp. 151–153.

27 Hassett, D.J. *et al.* (1999) *Pseudomonas aeruginosa* biofilm sensitivity to biocides: use of hydrogen peroxide as model antimicrobial agent for examining resistance mechanisms. *Methods in Enzymology*, **310**, 599–608.

28 Elkins, J.G. *et al.* (1999) Protective role of catalase in *Pseudomonas aeruginosa* biofilm resistance to hydrogen peroxide. *Applied and Environmental Microbiology*, **65** (10), 4594–4600.

29 Sondossi, M. *et al.* (1985) Observation of resistance and cross-resistance to formaldehyde and a formaldehyde condensate biocide in *Pseudomonas aeruginosa*. *International Biodeterioration and Biodegradation*, **21**, 105–106.

30 Gilbert, P. *et al.* (1990) Influence of growth rate on susceptibility to antimicrobial agents: biofilms, cell cycle, dormancy, and stringent response. *Antimicrobial Agents and Chemotherapy*, **34** (10), 1865–1868.

31 Brown, M.R. *et al.* (1990) Influence of growth rate on susceptibility to antimicrobial agents: modification of the cell envelope and batch and continuous culture studies. *Antimicrobial Agents and Chemotherapy*, **34** (9), 1623–1628.

32 Gilbert, P. and Brown, M.R. (1980) Cell wall-mediated changes in sensitivity of *Bacillus megaterium* to chlorhexidine and 2-phenoxyethanol, associated with growth rate and nutrient limitation. *Journal of Applied Bacteriology*, **48** (2), 223–230.

33 Giwercman, B. *et al.* (1991) Induction of beta-lactamase production in *Pseudomonas aeruginosa* biofilm. *Antimicrobial Agents and Chemotherapy*, **35** (5), 1008–1010.

34 Govan, J.R. and Fyfe, J.A. (1978) Mucoid *Pseudomonas aeruginosa* and cystic fibrosis: resistance of the mucoid form to carbenicillin, flucloxacillin and tobramycin and the isolation of mucoid variants *in vitro*. *Journal of Antimicrobial Chemotherapy*, **4** (3), 233–240.

35 Huang, C.T. *et al.* (1998) Spatial patterns of alkaline phosphatase expression within bacterial colonies and biofilms in response to phosphate starvation. *Applied and Environmental Microbiology*, **64** (4), 1526–1531.

36 Evans, D.J. *et al.* (1990) Effect of growth-rate on resistance of gram-negative biofilms to cetrimide. *Journal of Antimicrobial Chemotherapy*, **26** (4), 473–478.

37 Evans, D.J. *et al.* (1990) Susceptibility of bacterial biofilms to tobramycin: role of specific growth rate and phase in the division cycle. *Journal of Antimicrobial Chemotherapy*, **25** (4), 585–591.

38 Xu, K.D. *et al.* (1998) Spatial physiological heterogeneity in *Pseudomonas aeruginosa* biofilm is determined by oxygen availability. *Applied and Environmental Microbiology*, **64** (10), 4035–4039.

39 Ashby, M.J. *et al.* (1994) Effect of antibiotics on non-growing planktonic cells and biofilms of *Escherichia coli*. *Journal of Antimicrobial Chemotherapy*, **33** (3), 443–452.

40 Hodgson, A.E. *et al.* (1995) A simple *in vitro* model for growth control of bacterial biofilms. *Journal of Applied Bacteriology*, **79** (1), 87–93.

41 Duguid, I.G. *et al.* (1992) Growth-rate-independent killing by ciprofloxacin of biofilm-derived *Staphylococcus epidermidis*; evidence for cell-cycle dependency. *Journal of Antimicrobial Chemotherapy*, **30** (6), 791–802.

42 Stewart, P.S. (1994) Biofilm accumulation model that predicts antibiotic resistance of *Pseudomonas aeruginosa* biofilms. *Antimicrobial Agents and Chemotherapy*, **38** (5), 1052–1058.

43 Anwar, H. *et al.* (1989) Tobramycin resistance of mucoid *Pseudomonas aeruginosa* biofilm grown under iron limitation. *Journal of Antimicrobial Chemotherapy*, **24** (5), 647–655.

44 Allegrucci, M. and Sauer, K. (2008) Formation of *Streptococcus pneumoniae* non-phase-variable colony variants is due to increased mutation frequency present under biofilm growth conditions. *Journal of Bacteriology*, **190** (19), 6330–6339.

45 Xu, K.D. *et al.* (2000) Biofilm resistance to antimicrobial agents. *Microbiology*, **146** (3), 547–549.

46 McBain, A.J. *et al.* (2000) Emerging strategies for the chemical treatment of microbial biofilms. *Biotechnology and Genetic Engineering Reviews*, **17**, 267–279.

47 Nikaido, H. (1996) Multidrug efflux pumps of gram-negative bacteria. *Journal of Bacteriology*, **178** (20), 5853–5859.

48 George, A.M. and Levy, S.B. (1983) Amplifiable resistance to tetracycline, chloramphenicol, and other antibiotics in *Escherichia coli*: involvement of a non-plasmid-determined efflux of tetracycline. *Journal of Bacteriology*, **155** (2), 531–540.

49 Miller, P.F. and Sulavik, M.C. (1996) Overlaps and parallels in the regulation of intrinsic multiple-antibiotic resistance in *Escherichia coli*. *Molecular Microbiology*, **21** (3), 441–448.

50 Rouch, D.A. *et al.* (1990) Efflux-mediated antiseptic resistance gene qacA from *Staphylococcus aureus*: common ancestry with tetracycline- and sugar-transport proteins. *Molecular Microbiology*, **4** (12), 2051–2062.

51 Chuanchuen, R. *et al.* (2002) The MexJK efflux pump of *Pseudomonas aeruginosa* requires OprM for antibiotic efflux but not for efflux of triclosan. *Journal of Bacteriology*, **184** (18), 5036–5044.

52 Griffith, J.K. *et al.* (1992) Membrane transport proteins: implications of sequence comparisons. *Current Opinion in Cell Biology*, **4** (4), 684–695.

53 Johnson, J.M. and Church, G.M. (1999) Alignment and structure prediction of divergent protein families: periplasmic and outer membrane proteins of bacterial efflux pumps. *Journal of Molecular Biology*, **287** (3), 695–715.

54 Saier, M.H. Jr. and Paulsen, I.T. (2001) Phylogeny of multidrug transporters. *Seminars in Cell and Developmental Biology*, **12** (3), 205–213.

55 Paulsen, I.T. *et al.* (1996) The SMR family: a novel family of multidrug efflux proteins involved with the efflux of lipophilic drugs. *Molecular Microbiology*, **19** (6), 1167–1175.

56 Ma, L. *et al.* (2006) Analysis of *Pseudomonas aeruginosa* conditional psl variants reveals roles for the psl polysaccharide in adhesion and maintaining biofilm structure postattachment. *Journal of Bacteriology*, **188** (23), 8213–8221.

57 Moken, M.C. *et al.* (1997) Selection of multiple-antibiotic-resistant (mar) mutants of *Escherichia coli* by using the disinfectant pine oil: roles of the mar and acrAB loci. *Antimicrobial Agents and Chemotherapy*, **41** (12), 2770–2772.

58 McMurry, L.M. *et al.* (1998) Overexpression of marA, soxS, or acrAB produces resistance to triclosan in laboratory and clinical strains of *Escherichia coli*. *FEMS Microbiology Letters*, **166** (2), 305–309.

59 Maira-Litran, T. *et al.* (2000) Expression of the multiple antibiotic resistance operon (mar) during growth of *Escherichia coli* as a biofilm. *Journal of Applied Microbiology*, **88** (2), 243–247.

60 Maira-Litran, T. *et al.* (2000) An evaluation of the potential of the multiple antibiotic resistance operon (mar) and the multidrug efflux pump acrAB to moderate resistance towards ciprofloxacin in *Escherichia coli* biofilms. *Journal of Antimicrobial Chemotherapy*, **45** (6), 789–795.

61 De Kievit, T.R. *et al.* (2001) Multidrug efflux pumps: expression patterns and contribution to antibiotic resistance in *Pseudomonas aeruginosa* biofilms. *Antimicrobial Agents and Chemotherapy*, **45** (6), 1761–1770.

62 Moyer, C.L. and Morita, R.Y. (1989) Effect of growth rate and starvation-survival on the viability and stability of a psychrophilic marine bacterium. *Applied and Environmental Microbiology*, **55** (5), 1122–1127.

63 Novitsky, J.A. and Morita, R.Y. (1976) Morphological characterization of small cells resulting from nutrient starvation of a psychrophilic marine vibrio. *Applied and Environmental Microbiology*, **32** (4), 617–622.

64 Kjelleberg, S. *et al.* (1982) Effect of interfaces on small, starved marine bacteria. *Applied and Environmental Microbiology*, **43** (5), 1166–1172.

65 Amy, P.S. *et al.* (1983) Starvation-survival processes of a marine vibrio. *Applied and Environmental Microbiology*, **45** (3), 1041–1048.

66 Lleo, M.M. *et al.* (1998) Nonculturable *Enterococcus faecalis* cells are metabolically active and capable of resuming active growth. *Systematic and Applied Microbiology*, **21** (3), 333–339.

67 Matin, A. *et al.* (1989) Genetic basis of starvation survival in nondifferentiating bacteria. *Annual Review of Microbiology*, **43**, 293–316.

68 Piggot, P.J. and Coote, J.G. (1976) Genetic aspects of bacterial endospore formation. *Bacteriological Reviews*, **40** (4), 908–962.

69 Hengge-Aronis, R. (1996) Back to log phase: sigma S as a global regulator in the osmotic control of gene expression in *Escherichia coli*. *Molecular Microbiology*, **21** (5), 887–893.

70 Munro, P.M. *et al.* (1989) Influence of osmoregulation processes on starvation survival of *Escherichia coli* in seawater. *Applied and Environmental Microbiology*, **55** (8), 2017–2024.

71 Trainor, V.C. *et al.* (1999) Survival of *Streptococcus pyogenes* under stress and starvation. *FEMS Microbiology Letters*, **176** (2), 421–428.

72 Roszak, D.B. and Colwell, R.R. (1987) Metabolic activity of bacterial cells enumerated by direct viable count. *Applied and Environmental Microbiology*, **53** (12), 2889–2893.

73 Barer, M.R. and Harwood, C.R. (1999) Bacterial viability and culturability. *Advances in Microbial Physiology*, **41**, 93–137.

74 Roszak, D.B. *et al.* (1984) Viable but nonrecoverable stage of *Salmonella enteritidis* in aquatic systems. *Canadian Journal of Microbiology*, **30** (3), 334–338.

75 Zambrano, M.M. *et al.* (1993) Microbial competition: *Escherichia coli* mutants that take over stationary phase cultures. *Science*, **259** (5102), 1757–1760.

76 Foley, I. *et al.* (1999) General stress response master regulator rpoS is expressed in human infection: a possible role in chronicity. *Journal of Antimicrobial Chemotherapy*, **43** (1), 164–165.

77 Latifi, A. *et al.* (1996) A hierarchical quorum-sensing cascade in *Pseudomonas aeruginosa* links the transcriptional activators LasR and RhIR (VsmR) to expression of the stationary-phase sigma factor RpoS. *Molecular Microbiology*, **21** (6), 1137–1146.

78 Bigger, J.W. (1944) Treatment of staphylococcal infections with penicillin. *Lancet*, **2**, 497–500.

79 Gunnison, J.B. *et al.* (1964) Persistence of *Staphylococcus aureus* in penicillin *in vitro*. *Journal of General Microbiology*, **35**, 335–349.

80 Spoering, A.L. and Lewis, K. (2001) Biofilms and planktonic cells of *Pseudomonas aeruginosa* have similar resistance to killing by antimicrobials. *Journal of Bacteriology*, **183** (23), 6746–6751.

81 Brown, M.R. *et al.* (1969) Step-wise resistance to polymyxin and other agents by *Pseudomonas aeruginosa*. *Journal of General Microbiology*, **55** (3), 17–18.

82 Brozel, V.S. and Cloete, T.E. (1993) Adaptation of *Pseudomonas aeruginosa* to 2,2′-methylenebis (4-chlorophenol). *Journal of Applied Bacteriology*, **74** (1), 94–99.

83 Chuanchuen, R. *et al.* (2001) Cross-resistance between triclosan and antibiotics in *Pseudomonas aeruginosa* is mediated by multidrug efflux pumps: exposure of a susceptible mutant strain to triclosan selects nfxB mutants overexpressing MexCD-OprJ. *Antimicrobial Agents and Chemotherapy*, **45** (2), 428–432.

84 Levy, S.B. (1992) Active efflux mechanisms for antimicrobial resistance. *Antimicrobial Agents and Chemotherapy*, **36** (4), 695–703.

85 Levin, B.R. *et al.* (2000) Compensatory mutations, antibiotic resistance and the population genetics of adaptive evolution in bacteria. *Genetics*, **154** (3), 985–997.

86 Rella, M. and Haas, D. (1982) Resistance of *Pseudomonas aeruginosa* PAO to nalidixic acid and low levels of beta-lactam antibiotics: mapping of chromosomal genes. *Antimicrobial Agents and Chemotherapy*, **22** (2), 242–249.

87 Thanassi, D.G. *et al.* (1995) Role of outer membrane barrier in efflux-mediated tetracycline resistance of *Escherichia coli*. *Journal of Bacteriology*, **177** (4), 998–1007.

5 Mechanisms of Action of Microbicides

Peter A. Lambert

School of Life and Health Sciences, Department of Microbiology, Aston University, Birmingham, UK

Introduction

Understanding the physical and chemical basis of the inter-action(s) between microbicides and microbes is vital for their effective use. Maximum microbicidal performance can be achieved through effective formulation and appropriate usage while emergence of resistance to the microbicides and possible cross-resistance to therapeutic antimicrobials can be minimized [1–3].

The effects of microbicides upon microbial cells are deter-mined by the physical and chemical interactions between the microbicides and microbial components. In some cases it is pos-sible to make a clear association between these properties and the mechanisms of microbicidal action. For example, the detergent and cationic properties of quaternary ammonium compounds (QACs) are responsible for their disruptive action upon micro-bial membranes. This results from interference with hydrophobic and ionic interactions between lipids and proteins in the mem-branes. By contrast, it is the chemical reaction of aldehydes with amino groups on microbial proteins and peptidoglycan that determines their microbicidal action. However, the effects of many microbicides are markedly concentration dependent, with subtle, target-specific effects observed at low concentrations and non-specific cellular disruption at higher concentrations [4]. For example, at very low concentrations the bisphenol, triclosan, exerts specific inhibitory action upon enoyl-acyl carrier protein reductase (FabI), a key microbial enzyme involved in fatty acid biosynthesis [5–8]. At the higher concentrations used for most disinfection purposes, gross membrane disruption and cytoplas-mic precipitation occurs [9]. Another example of multiple, concentration-dependent mechanisms is provided by the bis-biguanide, chlorhexidine. This agent damages the cytoplasmic membrane at low concentrations causing leakage of cytoplasmic components. At higher concentrations it coagulates proteins in the membrane and cytoplasm, resulting in restricted leakage [10, 11]. To ensure that lethal action is obtained, most disinfectants are used at relatively high concentrations, substantially greater than the MIC. At these levels cell death is likely to be caused by non-specific disruptive effects such as membrane damage or protein coagulation rather than by subtle, selective inhibition of individual enzymes [12].

This chapter will consider what is known about the mecha-nisms of lethal action of the major groups of microbicidal agents used as disinfectants, antiseptics or preservatives. Figure 5.1 sum-marizes the different sites of interaction between microbicides

Russell, Hugo & Ayliffe's: Principles and Practice of Disinfection, Preservation and Sterilization, Fifth Edition. Edited by Adam P. Fraise, Jean-Yves Maillard, and Syed A. Sattar.

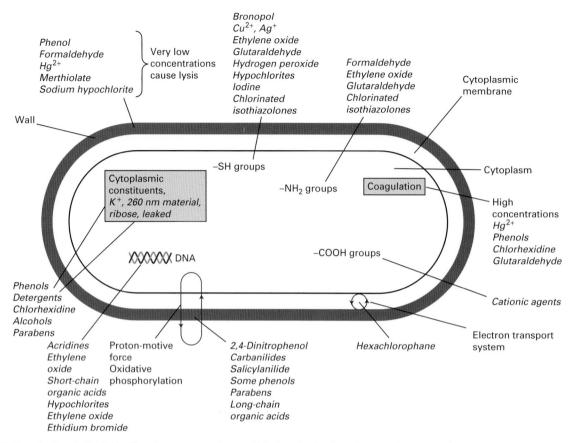

Figure 5.1 Sites of action of microbicides. Note that many agents have multiple sites of action depending upon the concentration.

and microorganisms; note that many agents act upon multiple sites.

Methods for studying the mechanism of action of microbicides

Hugo and colleagues developed the basic experimental approach for investigation of the mechanism of action of microbicides against bacteria [13]. Their classic studies on agents such as chlorhexidine [10, 14, 15] and fentichlor [16–18] illustrate the insight on mechanisms of action that can be gained from such clearly designed experiments. Russell and co-workers extended this approach to study the action of microbicides on a wider range of organisms including mycobacteria [19, 20], spores [21, 22], fungi [23], viruses [24] and protozoa [25–29].

Physical and biochemical approaches to the study of microbicide action

The physical and biochemical methods employed in mechanism of action studies include: (i) analysis of the surface-binding and uptake characteristics; (ii) detection of membrane damage by leakage of cytoplasmic constituents; and (iii) inhibition of key metabolic functions such as respiratory activity. At the molecular

level, microarray-based transcriptome analysis provides information on the global transcriptional response of an organism to microbicide action. Validation and further quantitative analysis of microarray results for selected gene expression can be obtained by quantitative (real-time) polymerase chain reaction (PCR) with reverse transcription to quantify messenger RNA. The appearance of cells under the electron microscope gives an indication of the disruptive action of microbicides upon the outer layers of the cell wall. This is particularly evident in Gram-negative bacteria where blebs or protrusions in the outer membrane caused by agents such as chlorhexidine are readily apparent [30, 31]. Gross loss of cytoplasm and coagulation can also be observed using the electron microscope [32]. An example of the cellular damage caused by chlorhexidine upon *Escherichia coli* is shown in Figure 5.2.

Electron microscopy (EM) has also been used with viruses, whereby the extent and type of damage to virion structure reflects the mechanism of action of the agent. For example, the MADT (morphological alteration and disintegration test) with hepatitis B virus [33, 34] and the use of *Pseudomonas aeruginosa* phage F116 for a more general understanding of structural changes in virions [35].

Alternative approaches for detecting changes in the cell surface include measurement of surface charge (zeta potential) by parti-

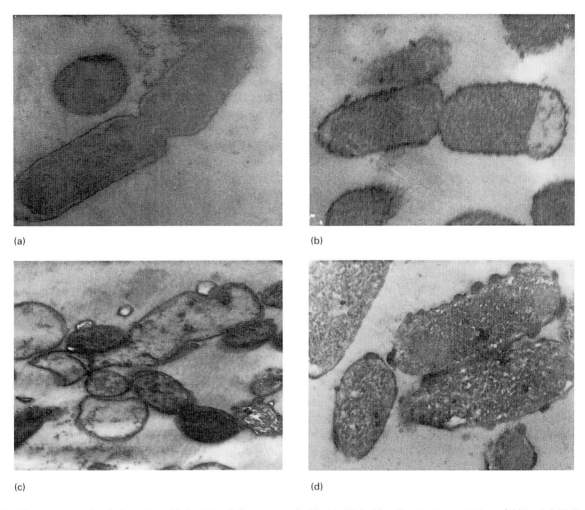

(a)

(b)

(c)

(d)

Figure 5.2 Electron micrographs of thin sections of *Escherichia coli* after treatment for 6 h with chlorhexidine diacetate at concentrations of: (a) 0 μg/ml; (b) 20 μg/ml; (c) 90 μg/ml; and (d) 500 μg/ml (from Hugo and Longworth [15]).

cle microelectrophoresis and surface hydrophobicity by a number of physical methods including contact angle [36, 37]. Energy dispersive analysis of X-ray (EDAX) has also been useful in studying the mechanisms of action of certain chemicals such as chlorhexidine and particularly the action between the biguanides and the protozoan cell [38], viruses [39] and bacteria [32]. Atomic force microscopy may prove to be useful in determining the effects of microbicides upon the cell surface [40–42]. In addition to surface imaging, this technique can be used to probe molecular interaction, physicochemical properties, surface stiffness and macromolecular elasticity [43].

Study of the action of microbicides upon protoplasts and spheroplasts in comparison with whole cells gives an indication of the protective role of the cell wall and can reveal effects upon the cell membrane [44]. The properties and stability of model membranes and membrane fragments [45], including measurements of electrical conductivity [46], and fluorescence [47] can all be useful approaches for the investigation of membrane-active agents. Other biophysical methods such as differential scanning

calorimetry and X-ray diffraction studies of artificial lipid bilayer systems [48] and molecular modeling of interactions [49] can be applied to explore detailed molecular interactions. Electrode-based methods have the advantage of direct measurement of agent action upon cell suspensions. These were first used to detect the earliest signs of membrane damage in terms of potassium leakage from intact cells induced by microbicides [50, 51]. They have been applied to study the action of peptides and natural oils on whole cells [52, 53], model membranes [54] and liposomes [55]. Oxygen electrodes and bioluminescence technology can be used to study the action of microbicides upon cell catabolism and intracellular adenosine triphosphate (ATP) levels [56]. The action of chlorhexidine upon bacteria in dental biofilms has been studied using microelectrodes as real-time biosensors of metabolic activity [57].

Fluorescent staining protocols allow direct analysis of bacterial viability, using confocal fluorescence microscopy, flow cytometry or microplate fluorescence measurements. Dual staining with the LIVE/DEAD BacLight bacterial viability kit involves treating cells with two different DNA-binding dyes (SYTO9 and propidium iodide (PI)). SYTO9 diffuses through the intact cell membrane and binds cellular DNA, producing a green-yellow fluorescence color under UV illumination. PI also binds DNA but is excluded from healthy cells, only entering dead or damaged cells, producing a red color under UV. This dual-staining method allows effective monitoring of viable and dead cells (viability profiling) in real time. Examples of the application of this method are studies of the action of chlorhexidine on dental biofilms [58, 59]. Noyce *et al.* [60], have used the respiratory indicator fluorochrome 5-cyano-2,3-ditolyl tetrazolium (CTC) to study the killing action of copper on *Staphylococcus aureus*. Kim *et al.* [61], have used BacLight and CTC to investigate the action of chlorine and silver ions on *P. aeruginosa* biofilms. An alternative method for measuring bacterial viability using a combination of green fluorescent protein (GFP) and PI has been developed [62]. This allows real-time monitoring of microbicidal activity and distinction between lytic, cidal and static actions [63].

Molecular approaches to the study of microbicide action

Microorganisms respond to environmental stress, including exposure to microbicides, by altering their gene expression [64]. This stress response includes upregulation of genes involved in the repair of cell damage and changing the cells to a less susceptible phenotype [65]. Genome-wide transcriptional analysis and whole-cell proteomics of the effects of microbicides upon microbes give a broad picture of the multiple effects of agents upon gene expression. Transcriptional analysis has been used to investigate the action of a wide range of microbicides including *o*-phenylphenol [66, 67], triclosan [68, 69], chlorhexidine [70], polyhexamethylene biguanide [71], chitosan [72], cetylpyridinium chloride [73] and hydrogen peroxide [74]. However, it is important that interpretation of the data in relation to mechanism of lethal or inhibitory action recognizes the conditions of microbicide concentration and exposure time under which the transcriptional analysis is made. Other regulatory molecules, including the small regulatory RNAs (sRNAs) and small proteins (containing 16–50 amino acids) missed by classic proteomic studies, are involved in the response of bacteria to stress [75, 76]. More than 80 sRNAs and 60 small proteins are encoded in the *E. coli* genome. Although the vast majority of the corresponding genes have no known function, a role in mediating the microbial response to microbicide action seems highly likely.

A systematic molecular approach has been developed to study mechanisms of antibiotic action. This involves transcriptional profiling of conditional mutants of *Bacillus subtilis* and comparison with profiles obtained for a panel of antibiotics of established mechanisms of action [77]. Hutter *et al.* [78] have developed a panel of *B. subtilis* reporter strains that indicate the mechanism of action of antibiotics, and whole-cell biosensors are utilized for the screening of antimicrobials in the pharmaceutical industry [79]. These systems can also be used to investigate the mechanism(s) of action of microbicides, particularly at lower concentrations where gross cellular damage does not occur.

Variable parameters in mechanism of action studies

Many parameters can be varied while studying the mechanisms of action, for example: the effects of microbicide concentration; exposure time; temperature; pH; and the presence of metal ions, metal-chelating agents and microbicide-neutralizing agents. The test organisms chosen and the growth conditions employed can also yield valuable information. Microbicide sensitivity is highly dependent upon the physiological state of the test organism, which in turn can be manipulated by the growth conditions [80–82]. Of particular relevance is the phase of microbial growth. Slowly growing or non-dividing cells are more resistant to antimicrobial agents in general than are rapidly dividing cells. Cells growing as adherent biofilms are far more resistant to microbicides than their freely suspended (planktonic) counterparts [83–87]. Biofilm resistance to microbicides is not due to restricted penetration for all agents. Stewart *et al.* [88] have shown that chlorosulfamate penetrates biofilms well but alkaline hypochlorite does not. The intrinsic microbicide resistance of biofilms is recognized in the design of test systems to evaluate microbicidal activity, where strains, growth conditions and growth phase are increasingly well defined for both suspension and carrier/surface tests [87, 89–94] (refer also to Chapter 4). Where possible, evidence of microbicide efficacy from reliable biofilm models should be considered alongside the more numerous studies on planktonic cells when interpreting mechanism of action studies [95].

The results of a growing body of information on mechanism of action studies have revealed much information on how most of the important groups of microbicidal agents kill microbes. Detailed accounts can be found in a number of excellent reviews [12, 96–101]. The following sections will illustrate different aspects of microbicide action and review the current knowledge of the mechanism(s) of action of the major microbicide groups.

Uptake, binding and penetration

Microbicide uptake can be studied kinetically, where the time course of uptake is investigated, or quantitatively, after a fixed exposure time where an equilibrium between bound and free microbicide is assumed to be established [102, 103]. Figure 5.3 shows the different patterns of adsorption isotherms that can be obtained for equilibrium binding, designated S, L, H, C and Z types [104].

Each type of isotherm can be interpreted in terms of the mechanism of interaction between the microbicide and the microbial surface [103]. Both time course and equilibrium approaches require the availability of sensitive and specific measurement of the microbicide, best achieved where a radiolabeled form is available, plus a means of distinguishing between the bound and unbound agents [105]. Kinetic uptake studies can be directly compared with concurrent assessment of cell viability [16, 106]. Fixed-time equilibrium binding studies can be visualized as adsorption isotherms (plots of bound vs. free microbicide) and

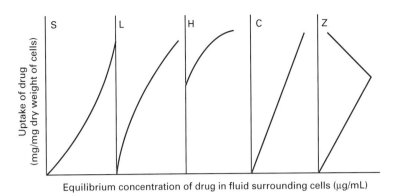

Figure 5.3 Examples of the characteristic patterns of microbicide adsorption isotherms.

interpreted in physicochemical terms [100, 102, 103]. The characteristic shapes of the isotherms (Figure 5.3) give some indication of the mode of binding to the cell surface and have been widely applied [27, 107]. This approach is useful in comparing the binding by different microbicides to a single test organism or the binding of a single agent to different organisms, for example sensitive and resistant strains [108, 109]. Since the interaction of microbicides with microbial cells usually involves penetration of the cell surface and associated surface changes, the interpretation of whole-cell uptake isotherms cannot give detailed information of the effects on intracellular targets. This problem can be overcome by studying binding to isolated cell walls, membranes, cytoplasmic material and to modified cells in which the walls have been partly or completely removed [16, 110]. Measurement of the effects of microbicides upon surface hydrophobicity [111] can be interpreted in terms of binding of the microbicide to the cell surface [112–114].

Action on the cell wall

Some microbicides affect the Gram-negative bacterial cell wall by binding non-covalently to lipid components (e.g. chlorhexidine). The consequences of this physical interaction may be apparent in a change in appearance under EM, especially the formation of surface blebs, protrusions and peeling [32]. Metal ion-chelating agents such as ethylenediamine tetraacetic acid (EDTA) destabilize the outer membrane by removing magnesium ions. The effect is the release of lipopolysaccharide (LPS) containing vesicles, loss of the permeability barrier function of the outer membrane and sensitization of the cells to other agents normally excluded [41, 115]. Similar outer membrane permeabilizing action has been demonstrated for the polyamines naphthylacetylspermine and methoctramine [116]. Other microbicides bind covalently to cell wall components, including peptidoglycan (e.g. aldehydes). The effects are not necessarily apparent in altered appearance (glutaraldehyde is used as a fixative in EM) but the function of the cell wall is affected [12, 117]. Sensitive methods detecting changes in the barrier properties of the cell envelope include increased permeability to substrates for periplasmic

enzymes (e.g. nitrocefin as a substrate for periplasmic β-lactamase) or fluorescent dyes [118–121].

Action on the cell membrane

Leakage of cell constituents

The classic methods for studying the action of membrane-active microbicides involve the measurement of leakage of low molecular weight cell constituents from whole cells [44]. Cytoplasmic components that can be detected by their absorbance of UV light at 260 nm include nucleosides, nucleotides and aromatic amino acids. Their measurement requires the removal of cells and possibly removal of the microbicide itself if it absorbs at this wavelength. Potassium leakage is one of the first indicators of microbicide-induced membrane damage [50]. Leakage is usually rapid following exposure to the microbicide, so measurement of exocellular potassium with an ion-selective electrode without removal of the cells can be an advantage [50, 52, 122–124]. Usually a dose–response relationship can be established where increasing microbicide concentration causes more rapid and extensive leakage of cell constituents. Above a critical concentration of microbicide, coagulation of proteins occurs in the cytoplasm and the membrane, resulting in reduced leakage [125].

It is generally assumed that the sequence of cell-damaging events following exposure of a microbial cell to a microbicide involves progression from sublethal injury to bacteriostasis and bactericidal action. Denyer and Stewart [100] have suggested that the transition from sublethal injury to cell death may result from autocidal mechanisms triggered by the microbicide. Mechanisms suggested include the activation of degradative enzymes and the accumulation of free radicals. Each process may result from the impaired ionic homeostasis generated by the microbicide through potassium leakage or the metabolic imbalance generated by inhibitors of respiration and oxidative phosphorylation. Examples include activation of the latent ribonuclease I by cationic detergents [125] and free radical generation induced by bronopol [126] and isothiazolinones [127]. The porphyrin agent XF-73 causes rapid damage to the cell membrane of *S. aureus*, as demonstrated by leakage of potassium ions and ATP from the cells and response to the BacLight stain for membrane integrity [128]. The ability to cause membrane damage by XF-73 is retained in non-growing, slow-growing and biofilm systems [129].

Inhibition of energy processes

The energized state of bacterial membranes is expressed as the proton-motive force (PMF), composed of an electrical potential and a proton gradient which bacteria maintain across their cytoplasmic membrane to drive vital processes, including active transport of solutes, oxidative phosphorylation and ATP synthesis. The PMF is generated by oxidation–reduction reactions occurring during electron transport. The pH gradient can be measured directly with a glass electrode or by distribution of a weak acid (e.g. benzoic acid) across the membrane. The electrical potential component can be measured by the distribution of membrane potential-sensitive dyes such as rhodamine 123 and bisoxonol [130].

A number of different types of microbicides exert effects upon the PMF across the cytoplasmic membrane. Some lipid-soluble phenols (e.g. 2,4-dinitrophenol) and the protonophore, carbonyl cyanide-3-chlorophenylhydrazone (CCCP), dissipate the PMF by dissolving in the membrane; they uncouple ATP synthesis from electron transport [131]. There is evidence that phenoxyethanol and fentichlor dissipate the PMF at low, bacteriostatic concentrations [132–134] while some organic acids and esters (e.g. sorbic acid and the parabens) collapse the PMF by transporting protons into the cells [135].

Physical methods used to investigate the interaction of microbicides with membranes include differential scanning calorimetry and X-ray diffraction [48] and the monolayer technique for membrane-like systems [136].

Interaction with the cytoplasm

Protein denaturation and coagulation

Aldehydes (formaldehyde, glutaraldehyde, *ortho*-phthalaldehyde) and the sterilizing agents ethylene oxide, propylene oxide and β-propiolactone are all alkylating agents that react readily with amino, carboxyl, sulphydryl and hydroxyl groups on proteins causing irreversible modification of protein structure [101]. Other chemical agents denature proteins by disturbance of the interactions (disulphide bridges, hydrogen bonding, ionic, hydrophobic and hydrophobic interactions) that maintain secondary and tertiary protein structure. Agents that interfere with these interactions can cause irreversible protein coagulation, although the concentrations required to achieve this effect are generally much higher than those needed to cause membrane leakage. Many compounds have been shown to cause cytoplasmic protein coagulation including phenols, QACs, chlorhexidine, halogens, copper and silver ions, and hydrogen peroxide [101]. The effects can be observed in whole cells by light or electron microscopy or by precipitation of cytoplasmic material obtained from

mechanically disrupted cells. Cytoplasmic precipitation may also be apparent in cell-leakage studies of membrane-active agents. The leakage of cytoplasmic material from treated cells generally increases with increasing concentration of membrane-active agent up to a concentration where cytoplasmic precipitation occurs. Further increase in concentration of the agent results in less leakage due to coagulation of the cytoplasm and sealing of the damaged cell membrane. These effects have been reported with QACs and chlorhexidine.

Effects on enzymes

Because of the non-specific nature of protein denaturation by microbicidal agents individual enzymes are not generally thought to be specific targets of action. However, a number of reports showed that triclosan does exert specific effects upon fatty acid biosynthesis at low concentrations. The target enzyme is the enoyl-acyl carrier protein reductase (FabI) in *E. coli* and *Mycobacterium smegmatis*. Various novel classes of agents directed against the FabI target have been developed as promising antibacterials [8, 137, 138]. Concern has been expressed that overuse of triclosan (and other FabI inhibitors) could result in the development of resistance to agents such as isoniazid, which target related enzymes involved in mycolic acid synthesis in mycobacteria. However, triclosan is used at higher concentrations than those that cause selective inhibition of fatty acid synthesis and the antimicrobial action results from non-specific damage to the cytoplasmic membrane [139].

Effects on nucleic acids

Acridine dyes are nucleic acid stains that bind to double-stranded DNA by intercalation between adjacent bases and bind to RNA electrostatically [140]. Polyhexamethylene biguanide binds cooperatively to DNA and RNA [141]. QACs (e.g. cetyltrimethylammonium bromide) bind to nucleic acids and precipitate them; this property is widely exploited in DNA preparations [142]. Formaldehyde and ethylene oxide alkylate amino groups on purines and pyrimidine bases in nucleic acids [143, 144]. Individual base modification results in mutation whereas cell death requires more extensive interference with DNA replication or gene expression. Recovery from alkylation requires oxidative dimethylation [145, 146]. Ozone decomposes in water to yield the hydroxyl and hydrogen peroxy radicals. These reactive species are strong oxidizers and can destroy bacteria through damage of the components in the cell wall, membrane and cytoplasm. Exposure of *Legionella pneumophila* to ozone has been reported to reduce the unsaturated fatty acid content [147]. The activity of ozone towards spores of *Bacillus anthracis* has been reviewed [148]. EM of ozone-treated *B. subtilis* spores suggests the outer spore coat layers are the site of action [148, 149]. Disinfection of *Cryptosporidium* requires high concentrations of ozone, but care must be taken in the treatment of bromide-containing water because ozone forms toxic bromate ions [150]. Ozone is also capable of inducing strand breakage in mammalian DNA [151, 152].

Effects of microbicides on the microbial transcriptome and proteome

The genome-wide transcriptome response of *P. aeruginosa* to sodium hypochlorite-induced oxidative stress has been investigated by the use of DNA microarrays [153]. In addition to a general oxidative stress response to hypochlorite exposure, the organism downregulated virtually all genes related to oxidative phosphorylation and electron transport and upregulated many organic sulfur transport and metabolism genes. Similar methods comparing the toxicogenomic effects with those of other oxidizing agents showed that hypochlorite induced more genome-wide changes than hydrogen peroxide or peracetic acid [154]. Global transcriptome analysis of *Mycobacterium bovis* BCG exposed to hypochlorite has shown significant regulation of oxidative stress response genes such as oxidoreductase, peroxidase and heat-shock proteins as well as lipid transport and metabolism genes [155]. The results also suggested that sodium hypochlorite repressed transcription of genes involved in cell wall mycolic acid synthesis [155]. Transcriptome analysis of the response of *S. aureus* to hydrogen peroxide indicates that the oxidative response includes the induction of genes involved in virulence, DNA repair and anaerobic metabolism [74].

Microarray analysis of the global transcriptomic effects of *ortho*-phenylphenol upon *P. aeruginosa* has shown upregulation of genes involved in swarming motility and anaerobic respiration [66]. Similar studies on the effects of this agent upon *S. aureus* have shown downregulation of the biosynthesis of many amino acids which are required for protein synthesis [67]. Genome-wide transcriptional analysis has given a deeper insight into the multiple effects of triclosan upon the metabolic processes in *S. aureus* [68]. Triclosan downregulated the transcription of genes involved in virulence factor and energy metabolism, while multidrug resistance genes involved in coenzyme transport were upregulated. Furthermore, triclosan downregulated the transcription of genes encoding major lipid metabolism enzymes such as 3-hydroxyacyl-CoA dehydrogenase, acetyl-CoA acetyltransferase, acetyl-CoA synthetase and acetyl-CoA carboxylase, which all play essential roles in *S. aureus* lipid metabolism. Expression of the enoyl-acyl carrier protein (enoyl-ACP) reductase gene *fabI* was not changed suggesting that triclosan may kill *S. aureus* by interfering with its ability to form cell membranes. Microarray studies of *E. coli* and *Salmonella enterica* serovar Typhimurium exposed to triclosan have identified some common responses but also some unexpected species-specific responses [69]. Common responses included increased expression of efflux pump component genes. Species-specific responses included decreased expression of the *fabBAGI* genes in *Salmonella* contrasting with increased expression of the *fabABFH* genes in *E. coli* [69].

Global transcriptomics applied to the effects of 0.008 mM chlorhexidine upon *P. aeruginosa* has shown membrane transport, oxidative phosphorylation and electron transport genes to be downregulated [70]. Various effects were dependent upon the exposure time: after 10 min, DNA repair was downregulated and

the *oprH* gene that blocks the self-promoted uptake of antimicrobials was upregulated. After 60 min, outer membrane protein, the flagellum, pilus, oxidative phosphorylation and electron transport genes were downregulated. The *mexC* and *mexD* genes of the MexCD-OprJ multidrug efflux pump were significantly upregulated after both treatment times.

Target-specific molecular approaches for the study of microbicide action have involved the construction of stress promoter–green fluorescent protein reporter strains. Exposure of *Streptococcus mutans* to hydrogen peroxide and chlorhexidine resulted in upregulation of the serine protease Clp [156]. The protective role of this protease was supported by studies with a *clp* knockout mutant that showed enhanced sensitivity to these agents together with a slower growth rate, hyperaggregation and enhanced biofilm formation.

The global mechanisms of phenol toxicity and tolerance in bacteria have been studied by identification of changes to the whole-cell proteome in *Pseudomonas putida* following exposure to sublethal inhibitory concentrations [157]. Inspection of the two-dimensional gel electrophoresis gels revealed that after 1 h of exposure to phenol the levels of 68 proteins were increased, while the levels of 13 others were reduced. The upregulated proteins included those involved in the oxidative stress response (AhpC, SodB, Tpx, Dsb); general stress response (UspA, HtpG, GrpE, Tig); energetic metabolism (AcnB, AtpH, Fpr, AceA, NuoE, MmsA-1); fatty acid biosynthesis (FabB, AccC-1, FabBx1); inhibition of cell division (MinD); cell envelope biosynthesis (LpxC, VacJ, MurA); transcription regulation (OmpR, Fur); and transport of small molecules (TolC, BraC, AotJ, AapJ, FbpA, OprQ). Among the downregulated proteins were those involved in nucleotide biosynthesis (PurM, PurL, PyrH, Dcd) and cell motility (FliC).

Action of individual classes of microbicidal agents

The actions of the major groups of microbicidal agents used as disinfectants, antiseptics or preservatives are listed in Table 5.1.

Oxidizing agents

Hydrogen peroxide, hypochlorite, peracetic acid and isothiazolones are all oxidizing agents. They owe their microbicidal activity to their oxidizing effects upon proteins, in particular upon the thiol groups of cysteine residues. Thiol groups in cysteine residues are important determinants of protein structure and function. Many vital microbial enzymes, including dehydrogenases, contain reduced cysteine residues at their active sites. Oxidation of the thiol groups results in metabolic inhibition of the cell [158–160]. Structural proteins in the cell wall, membrane and ribosomes may also be affected by disruption of stabilizing disulphide cross-links between cysteine residues [161]. Some bisphenols such as fentichlor and triclosan, as well as bronopol, chlorine, iodine, silver, copper and mercury compounds, also react with thiol groups causing metabolic inhibition [18, 132, 162]. Copper ions cycle

Table 5.1 Interactions between microbicides and microbial cells.

Microbicide	Microbial target	Type of interaction	Effect upon cells
Hydrogen peroxide, peracetic acid, hypochlorite, iodine, organomercurials, silver ions	Thiol groups in proteins	Oxidation of thiol groups to disulfides	Inhibition of key enzymes, modification of structural proteins
Aldehydes, ethylene oxide	Amino groups in proteins and nucleic acids	Alkylation of amino groups in proteins and nucleic acids	Inhibition of enzymes and nucleic acid function
Hypochlorite, chlorine, iodine	Aromatic amino acids in proteins	Halogenation of aromatic amino acids in proteins	Inhibition of key enzymes, modification of structural proteins
EDTA (ethylenediamine tetraacetic acid)	Divalent metal ions (calcium, magnesium) in cell wall and membrane	Specific binding affinity: chelation of metal ions	Wall and membrane damage, inhibition of metalloenzymes
Acridines,	DNA	Intercalation between base pairs	Inhibition of DNA replication
Polyhexamethylene biguanide	DNA and RNA	Cooperative binding	Inhibition of DNA replication
Phenols, alcohols	Cytoplasmic and membrane proteins	Denaturation (and precipitation) of proteins	Enzyme inhibition, membrane damage, cytoplasmic coagulation
Quaternary ammonium compounds, bisbiguanides, chitosan	Lipids in cell membranes	Binding to phosphate head groups and fatty acid chains in phospholipids	Membrane damage, depolarization, leakage of cell constituents, cytoplasmic coagulation at high concentration

between the cuprous and cupric oxidation states under aerobic conditions. This redox cycling generates highly reactive hydroxyl radicals that damage DNA, proteins and lipids [163].

Alkylating and halogenating agents

Chemicals such as formaldehyde and glutaraldehyde react with residues on nucleic acids and proteins by alkylation, an irreversible chemical modification that results in inhibition of metabolism and cell division. Chemical groups on biomolecules that may react with aldehydes include amino, carboxyl, thiol, hydroxyl, imino and amide substituents. Cross-linking of proteins by formaldehyde involves multiple interactions between chemical groups, which leads to aggregation [164, 165].

Metal ion-binding agents

Divalent metal ions play important roles in stabilizing the structure of membrane lipids and ribosomes as well as acting as cofactors to many enzymes. Binding of magnesium to chelating agents such as EDTA results in membrane damage, especially to the outer membrane of Gram-negative bacteria, causing sensitization to other agents, presumably through enhanced uptake [115]. Inclusion of EDTA in microbicide formulations therefore not only aids stability and solubility of the product but may also enhance their microbicidal action. However, concerns over environmental toxicity of EDTA limits its use; the poorly degraded EDTA and increased concentrations of toxic metal ions in wastewaters increase the risk of eutrophication [166].

Nucleic acid-binding agents

The acridine dyes, including the skin antiseptic proflavine and the antimalarial quinacrine, have specific affinity for nucleic acids. They bind to DNA by insertion (intercalation) between base pairs in the double helix, blocking replication and gene expression and protein synthesis [167, 168].

Protein denaturants

Phenols and alcohols denature protein structure by binding to amino acid residues and displacing water molecules [169]. The changes brought about in protein structure depend upon the concentration used. Subtle effects on protein structure result in enzyme inhibition; more marked conformational changes in membrane proteins result in membrane damage and leakage of cell components, whereas total denaturation results in coagulation of proteins in the cytoplasm [170]. Detergents and fatty acids denature proteins by binding to hydrophobic amino acid residues. This results in membrane damage, as shown by lysis of protoplasts [171, 172].

Interaction with lipids

Cationic detergents, QACs and bisbiguanides exert their antimicrobial action through interaction with anionic lipids in the cytoplasmic membrane and the outer membrane of Gram-negative bacteria [173, 174]. Low concentrations cause membrane damage and the leakage of cytoplasmic constituents through disruption of the interactions between lipids and proteins in the membrane structures. At high concentrations these agents cause coagulation of the cytoplasm, presumably through denaturation of proteins. The cationic polysaccharide, chitosan, also damages the cytoplasmic membrane, possibly by binding to the lipoteichoic acid found in many Gram-positive bacteria [72].

Conclusions

In contrast to antibiotics, which exert antimicrobial action through inhibition of a specific target, most microbicides have multiple effects upon microbial cells. However, the demonstration that triclosan inhibits a specific target (FabI) at low concentrations has caused concern that its overuse may select for resistance to the anti-TB agent isoniazid, which also inhibits this target [175–178]. Further concern has arisen from the demonstration that some bacterial drug efflux pumps extrude microbicides as well as antibiotics [179, 180]. Again it is suggested that overuse of microbicides could generate resistance to antibiotics [181–184]. Currently, some studies provide evidence for a link between microbicide and antibiotic resistance [73, 185, 186] but others have shown no convincing evidence for such a link [109, 187–190]. Since the intensity of use of individual microbicides increases the likelihood of resistance development [191], the rotational use of different classes of agents is advisable [192, 193].

References

1 Schweizer, H.P. (2001) Triclosan: a widely used biocide and its link to antibiotics. *FEMS Microbiology Letters*, **202**, 1–7.

2 Russell, A.D. (2003) Biocide use and antibiotic resistance: the relevance of laboratory findings to clinical and environmental situations. *Lancet Infectious Diseases*, **3**, 794–803.

3 Maillard, J.-Y. (2005) Antimicrobial biocides in the healthcare environment: efficacy, usage, policies, and perceived problems. *Therapeutics and Clinical Risk Management*, **1**, 307–320.

4 Russell, A.D. and McDonnell, G. (2000) Concentration: a major factor in studying biocidal action. *Journal of Hospital Infection*, **44**, 1–3.

5 Heath, R.J. *et al.* (1998) Broad spectrum antimicrobial biocides target the FabI component of fatty acid synthesis. *Journal of Biological Chemistry*, **273**, 30316–30320.

6 Heath, R.J. *et al.* (1999) Mechanism of triclosan inhibition of bacterial fatty acid synthesis. *Journal of Biological Chemistry*, **274**, 11110–11114.

7 Slater-Radosti, C. *et al.* (2001) Biochemical and genetic characterization of the action of triclosan on *Staphylococcus aureus*. *Journal of Antimicrobial Chemotherapy*, **48**, 1–6.

8 Payne, D.J. *et al.* (2002) Discovery of a novel and potent class of FabI-directed antibacterial agents. *Antimicrobial Agents and Chemotherapy*, **46**, 3118–3124.

9 Villalain, J. *et al.* (2001) Membranotropic effects of the antibacterial agent triclosan. *Archives of Biochemistry and Biophysics*, **390**, 128–136.

10 Hugo, W.B. and Longworth, A.R. (1966) The effect of chlorhexidine on the electrophoretic mobility, cytoplasmic constituents, dehydrogenase activity and cell walls of *Escherichia coli* and *Staphylococcus aureus*. *Journal of Pharmacy and Pharmacology*, **18**, 569–578.

11 Russell, A.D. and Day, M.J. (1993) Antibacterial activity of chlorhexidine. *Journal of Hospital Infection*, **25**, 229–238.

12 Maillard, J.-Y. (2002) Bacterial target sites for biocide action. *Journal of Applied Microbiology*, **92**, 16S–27S.

13 Hugo, W.B. (1991) A brief history of heat and chemical preservation and disinfection. *Journal of Applied Bacteriology*, **71**, 9–18.

14 Hugo, W.B. and Longworth, A.R. (1964) Effect of chlorhexidine diacetate on "protoplasts" and spheroplasts of *Escherichia coli*, protoplasts of *Bacillus megaterium* and the Gram staining reaction of *Staphylococcus aureus*. *Journal of Pharmacy and Pharmacology*, **16**, 751–758.

15 Hugo, W.B. and Longworth, A.R. (1965) Cytological aspects of the mode of action of chlorhexidine diacetate. *Journal of Pharmacy and Pharmacology*, **17**, 28–32.

16 Hugo, W.B. and Bloomfield, S.F. (1971) Studies on the mode of action of the phenolic antibacterial agent fentichlor against *Staphylococcus aureus* and *Escherichia coli*. I. The adsorption of fentichlor by the bacterial cell and its antibacterial activity. *Journal of Applied Bacteriology*, **34**, 557–567.

17 Hugo, W.B. and Bloomfield, S.F. (1971) Studies on the mode of action of the phenolic antibacterial agent fentichlor against *Staphylococcus aureus* and *Escherichia coli*. II. The effects of fentichlor on the bacterial membrane and the cytoplasmic constituents of the cell. *Journal of Applied Bacteriology*, **34**, 569–578.

18 Hugo, W.B. and Bloomfield, S.F. (1971) Studies on the mode of action of the phenolic antibacterial agent fentichlor against *Staphylococcus aureus* and *Escherichia coli*. III. The effect of fentichlor on the metabolic activities of *Staphylococcus aureus* and *Escherichia coli*. *Journal of Applied Bacteriology*, **34**, 579–591.

19 Fraud, S. *et al.* (2001) Comparison of the mycobactericidal activity of ortho-phthalaldehyde, glutaraldehyde and other dialdehydes by a quantitative suspension test. *Journal of Hospital Infection*, **48**, 214–221.

20 Walsh, S.E. *et al.* (2001) Possible mechanisms for the relative efficacies of ortho-phthalaldehyde and glutaraldehyde against glutaraldehyde-resistant *Mycobacterium chelonae*. *Journal of Applied Microbiology*, **91**, 80–92.

21 Power, E.G. and Russell, A.D. (1990) Sporicidal action of alkaline glutaraldehyde: factors influencing activity and a comparison with other aldehydes. *Journal of Applied Bacteriology*, **69**, 261–268.

22 Williams, N.D. and Russell, A.D. (1993) Revival of *Bacillus subtilis* spores from biocide-induced injury in the germination process. *Journal of Applied Bacteriology*, **75**, 76–81.

23 Russell, A.D. and Furr, J.R. (1996) Biocides: mechanisms of antifungal action and fungal resistance. *Science Progress*, **79**, 27–48.

24 Maillard, J.-Y. and Russell, A.D. (1997) Viricidal activity and mechanisms of action of biocides. *Science Progress*, **80**, 287–315.

25 Khunkitti, W. *et al.* (1996) The lethal effects of biguanides on cysts and trophozoites of *Acanthamoeba castellanii*. *Journal of Applied Bacteriology*, **81**, 73–77.

26 Khunkitti, W. *et al.* (1997) Effects of biocides on *Acanthamoeba castellanii* as measured by flow cytometry and plaque assay. *Journal of Antimicrobial Chemotherapy*, **40**, 227–233.

27 Khunkitti, W. *et al.* (1997) Aspects of the mechanisms of action of biguanides on trophozoites and cysts of *Acanthamoeba castellanii*. *Journal of Applied Microbiology*, **82**, 107–114.

28 Khunkitti, W. *et al.* (1998) *Acanthamoeba castellanii*: growth, encystment, excystment and biocide susceptibility. *Journal of Infection*, **36**, 43–48.

29 Turner, N.A. *et al.* (2000) Emergence of resistance to biocides during differentiation of *Acanthamoeba castellanii*. *Journal of Antimicrobial Chemotherapy*, **46**, 27–34.

30 Richards, R.M. and Cavill, R.H. (1979) Electron-microscope study of the effect of chlorhexidine on *Pseudomonas aeruginosa*. *Microbios*, **26**, 85–93.

31 Richards, R.M. and Cavill, R.H. (1981) Electron microscope study of the effect of benzalkonium, chlorhexidine and polymyxin on *Pseudomonas cepacia*. *Microbios*, **29**, 23–31.

32 Tattawasart, U. *et al.* (2000) Cytological changes in chlorhexidine-resistant isolates of *Pseudomonas stutzeri*. *Journal of Antimicrobial Chemotherapy*, **45**, 145–152.

33 Thraenhart, O. *et al.* (1977) Morphological alteration and desintegration of dane particles after exposure with "Gigasept". A first methological attempt for the evaluation of the virucidal efficacy of a chemical disinfectant against hepatitisvirus B (author's transl.). *Zentralblatt fur Bakteriologie, Mikrobiologie und Hygiene: Originale B*, **164**, 1–21.

34 Thraenhart, O. *et al.* (1978) Influence of different disinfection conditions on the structure of the hepatitis B virus (Dane particle) as evaluated in the morphological alteration and desintegration test (MADT). *Zentralblatt fur Bakteriologie, Mikrobiologie und Hygiene: Originale A*, **242**, 299–314.

35 Maillard, J.-Y. *et al.* (1995) Electronmicroscopic investigation of the effects of biocides on *Pseudomonas aeruginosa* PAO bacteriophage F116. *Journal of Medical Microbiology*, **42**, 415–420.

36 Bruinsma, G.M. *et al.* (2001) Effects of cell surface damage on surface properties and adhesion of *Pseudomonas aeruginosa*. *Journal of Microbiological Methods*, **45**, 95–101.

37 Sharma, P.K. and Rao, K.H. (2002) Analysis of different approaches for evaluation of surface energy of microbial cells by contact angle goniometry. *Advances in Colloid and Interface Sciences*, **98**, 341–463.

38 Khunkitti, W. *et al.* (1999) X-ray microanalysis of chlorine and phosphorus content in biguanide-treated *Acanthamoeba castellanii*. *Journal of Applied Microbiology*, **86**, 453–459.

39 Maillard, J.-Y. *et al.* (1995) Energy dispersive analysis of X-rays study of the distribution of chlorhexidine diacetate and cetylpyridinium chloride on the *Pseudomonas aeruginosa* bacteriophage F116. *Letters in Applied Microbiology*, **20**, 357–360.

40 Amro, N.A. *et al.* (2000) High-resolution atomic force microscopy studies of the *Escherichia coli* 8 outer membrane: structural basis for permeability. *Langmuir*, **16**, 2789–2796.

41 Kotra, L.P. *et al.* (2000) Visualizing bacteria at high resolution. *American Society for Microbiology News*, **66**, 675–681.

42 Li, A. *et al.* (2007) Atomic force microscopy study of the antimicrobial action of Sushi peptides on Gram negative bacteria. *Biochimica et Biophysica Acta*, **1768**, 411–418.

43 Dufrene, Y.F. (2002) Atomic force microscopy, a powerful tool in microbiology. *Journal of Bacteriology*, **184**, 5205–5213.

44 Denyer, S.P. and Hugo, W.B. (1991) Biocide-induced damage to the bacterial cytoplasmic membrane. *Society for Applied Bacteriology Technical Series*, **30**, 171–188.

45 Gilbert, P. *et al.* (1991) Interaction of biocides with model membranes and isolated membrane fragments. *Society for Applied Bacteriology Technical Series*, **27**, 155–170.

46 Gutsmann, T. *et al.* (1999) Molecular mechanisms of interaction of rabbit CAP18 with outer membranes of gram-negative bacteria. *Biochemistry*, **38**, 13643–13653.

47 Giffard, C.J. *et al.* (1996) Interaction of nisin with planar lipid bilayers monitored by fluorescence recovery after photobleaching. *Journal of Membrane Biology*, **151**, 293–300.

48 Lohner, K. and Prenner, E.J. (1999) Differential scanning calorimetry and X-ray diffraction studies of the specificity of the interaction of antimicrobial peptides with membrane-mimetic systems. *Biochimica et Biophysica Acta*, **1462**, 141–156.

49 La Rocca, P. *et al.* (1999) Simulation studies of the interaction of antimicrobial peptides and lipid bilayers. *Biochimica et Biophysica Acta*, **1462**, 185–200.

50 Lambert, P.A. and Hammond, S.M. (1973) Potassium fluxes, first indications of membrane damage in micro-organisms. *Biochemical and Biophysical Research Communications*, **54**, 796–799.

51 Kroll, R.G. and Anagnostopoulos, G.D. (1981) Potassium fluxes on hyperosmotic shock and the effect of phenol and bronopol (2-bromo-2-nitropropan-1,3-diol) on deplasmolysis of *Pseudomonas aeruginosa*. *Journal of Applied Bacteriology*, **51**, 313–323.

52 Cox, S.D. *et al.* (1998) Tea tree oil causes K+ leakage and inhibits respiration in *Escherichia coli*. *Letters in Applied Microbiology*, **26**, 355–358.

53 Orlov, D.S. *et al.* (2002) Potassium release, a useful tool for studying antimicrobial peptides. *Journal of Microbiological Methods*, **49**, 325–328.

54 Breukink, E. *et al.* (1997) The C-terminal region of nisin is responsible for the initial interaction of nisin with the target membrane. *Biochemistry*, **36**, 6968–6976.

55 Silberstein, A. *et al.* (1999) Membrane destabilization assay based on potassium release from liposomes. *Biochimica et Biophysica Acta*, **1461**, 103–112.

56 Dinning, A.J. *et al.* (1998) Pyrithione biocides as inhibitors of bacterial ATP synthesis. *Journal of Applied Microbiology*, **85**, 141–146.

57 Von Ohle, C. *et al.* (2010) Real time microsensor measurement of local metabolic activities in ex vivo dental biofilms exposed to sucrose and treated with chlorhexidine. *Applied and Environmental Microbiology*, **76**, 2326–2334.

58 Hope, C.K. and Wilson, M. (2004) Analysis of the effects of chlorhexidine on oral biofilm vitality and structure based on viability profiling and an indicator of membrane integrity. *Antimicrobial Agents and Chemotherapy*, **48**, 1461–1468.

59 Shen, Y. *et al.* (2009) Evaluation of the effect of two chlorhexidine preparations on biofilm bacteria *in vitro*: a three-dimensional quantitative analysis. *Journal of Endodontics*, **35**, 981–985.

60 Noyce, J.O. *et al.* (2006) Potential use of copper surfaces to reduce survival of epidemic meticillin-resistant *Staphylococcus aureus* in the healthcare environment. *Journal of Hospital Infection*, **63**, 289–297.

61 Kim, J.G. *et al.* (1999) Application of ozone for enhancing the microbiological safety and quality of foods: a review. *Journal of Food Protection*, **62**, 1071–1087.

62 Lehtinen, J. *et al.* (2004) Green fluorescent protein-propidium iodide (GFP-PI) based assay for flow cytometric measurement of bacterial viability. *Cytometry A*, **60**, 165–172.

63 Lehtinen, J. *et al.* (2006) Real-time monitoring of antimicrobial activity with the multiparameter microplate assay. *Journal of Microbiological Methods*, **66**, 381–389.

64 Giuliodori, A.M. *et al.* (2007) Review on bacterial stress topics. *Annals of the New York Academy of Science*, **1113**, 95–104.

65 Russell, A.D. (2003) Similarities and differences in the responses of microorganisms to biocides. *Journal of Antimicrobial Chemotherapy*, **52**, 750–763.

66 Nde, C.W. *et al.* (2008) Toxicogenomic response of *Pseudomonas aeruginosa* to ortho-phenylphenol. *BMC Genomics*, **9**, 473–491.

67 Jang, H.J. *et al.* (2008) Microarray analysis of toxicogenomic effects of ortho-phenylphenol in *Staphylococcus aureus*. *BMC Genomics*, **9**, 411–431.

68 Jang, H.J. *et al.* (2008) Microarray analysis of toxicogenomic effects of triclosan on *Staphylococcus aureus*. *Applied Microbiology and Biotechnology*, **78**, 695–707.

69 Bailey, A.M. *et al.* (2009) Exposure of *Escherichia coli* and *Salmonella enterica* serovar Typhimurium to triclosan induces a species-specific response, including drug detoxification. *Journal of Antimicrobial Chemotherapy*, **64**, 973–985.

70 Nde, C.W. *et al.* (2009) Global transcriptomic response of *Pseudomonas aeruginosa* to chlorhexidine diacetate. *Environmental Science and Technology*, **43**, 8406–8415.

71 Allen, M.J. *et al.* (2006) The response of *Escherichia coli* to exposure to the biocide polyhexamethylene biguanide. *Microbiology*, **152**, 989–1000.

72 Raafat, D. *et al.* (2008) Insights into the mode of action of chitosan as an antibacterial compound. *Applied and Environmental Microbiology*, **74**, 3764–3773.

73 Maseda, H. *et al.* (2009) Mutational upregulation of a resistance-nodulation-cell division-type multidrug efflux pump, SdeAB, upon exposure to a biocide, cetylpyridinium chloride, and antibiotic resistance in *Serratia marcescens*. *Antimicrobial Agents and Chemotherapy*, **53**, 5230–5235.

74 Chang, W. *et al.* (2006) Global transcriptome analysis of *Staphylococcus aureus* response to hydrogen peroxide. *Journal of Bacteriology*, **188**, 1648–1659.

75 Hobbs, E.C. *et al.* (2010) Small RNAs and small proteins involved in resistance to cell envelope stress and acid shock in *Escherichia coli*: analysis of a bar-coded mutant collection. *Journal of Bacteriology*, **192**, 59–67.

76 Hemm, M.R. *et al.* (2010) Small stress response proteins in *Escherichia coli*: proteins missed by classical proteomic studies. *Journal of Bacteriology*, **192**, 46–58.

77 Freiberg, C. *et al.* (2005) Discovering the mechanism of action of novel antibacterial agents through transcriptional profiling of conditional mutants. *Antimicrobial Agents and Chemotherapy*, **49**, 749–759.

78 Hutter, B. *et al.* (2004) Panel of *Bacillus subtilis* reporter strains indicative of various modes of action. *Antimicrobial Agents and Chemotherapy*, **48**, 2588–2594.

79 Urban, A. *et al.* (2007) Novel whole-cell antibiotic biosensors for compound discovery. *Applied and Environmental Microbiology*, **73**, 6436–6443.

80 Gilbert, P. *et al.* (1990) Influence of growth rate on susceptibility to antimicrobial agents: biofilms, cell cycle, dormancy, and stringent response. *Antimicrobial Agents and Chemotherapy*, **34**, 1865–1868.

81 Brown, M.R. *et al.* (1990) Influence of growth rate on susceptibility to antimicrobial agents: modification of the cell envelope and batch and continuous culture studies. *Antimicrobial Agents and Chemotherapy*, **34**, 1623–1628.

82 Evans, D.J. *et al.* (1990) Effect of growth-rate on resistance of gram-negative biofilms to cetrimide. *Journal of Antimicrobial Chemotherapy*, **26**, 473–478.

83 Mah, T.F. and O'Toole, G.A. (2001) Mechanisms of biofilm resistance to antimicrobial agents. *Trends in Microbiology*, **9**, 34–39.

84 Gilbert, P. and McBain, A.J. (2001) Biofilms: their impact on health and their recalcitrance toward biocides. *American Journal of Infection Control*, **29**, 252–255.

85 Gilbert, P. *et al.* (2002) The physiology and collective recalcitrance of microbial biofilm communities. *Advances in Microbial Physiology*, **46**, 202–256.

86 Luppens, S.B. *et al.* (2002) The effect of the growth phase of *Staphylococcus aureus* on resistance to disinfectants in a suspension test. *Journal of Food Protection*, **65**, 124–129.

87 Luppens, S.B. *et al.* (2002) Development of a standard test to assess the resistance of *Staphylococcus aureus* biofilm cells to disinfectants. *Applied and Environmental Microbiology*, **68**, 4194–4200.

88 Stewart, P.S. *et al.* (2001) Biofilm penetration and disinfection efficacy of alkaline hypochlorite and chlorosulfamates. *Journal of Applied Microbiology*, **91**, 525–532.

89 Bloomfield, S.F. *et al.* (1994) An evaluation of the repeatability and reproducibility of a surface test for the activity of disinfectants. *Journal of Applied Bacteriology*, **76**, 86–94.

90 Zelver, N. *et al.* (1999) Measuring antimicrobial effects on biofilm bacteria: from laboratory to field. *Methods in Enzymology*, **310**, 608–628.

91 Gilbert, P. *et al.* (2001) Assessment of resistance towards biocides following the attachment of micro-organisms to, and growth on surfaces. *Journal of Applied Microbiology*, **91**, 248–254.

92 Hamilton, M.A. (2002) Testing antimicrobials against biofilm bacteria. *Journal of AOAC International*, **85**, 479–485.

93 Springthorpe, V.S. and Sattar, S.A. (2005) Carrier tests to assess microbicidal activities of chemical disinfectants for use on medical devices and environmental surfaces. *Journal of AOAC International*, **88**, 182–201.

94 Buckingham-Meyer, K. *et al.* (2007) Comparative evaluation of biofilm disinfectant efficacy tests. *Journal of Microbiological Methods*, **70**, 236–244.

95 Ntsama-Essomba, C. *et al.* (1997) Resistance of *Escherichia coli* growing as biofilms to disinfectants. *Veterinary Research*, **28**, 353–363.

96 Russell, A.D. (1995) Mechanisms of bacterial resistance to biocides. *International Biodeterioration and Biodegradation*, **36**, 247–265.

97 Russell, A.D. (1998) Mechanisms of bacterial resistance to antibiotics and biocides. *Progress in Medicinal Chemistry*, **35**, 133–197.

98 Russell, A.D. (1999) Bacterial resistance to disinfectants: present knowledge and future problems. *Journal of Hospital Infection*, **43**, S57–S68.

99 Russell, A.D. (2002) Mechanisms of antimicrobial action of antiseptics and disinfectants: an increasingly important area of investigation. *Journal of Antimicrobial Chemotherapy*, **49**, 597–599.

100 Denyer, S.P. and Stewart, G.S.A.B. (1998) Mechanisms of action of disinfectants. *International Biodeterioration and Biodegradation*, **41**, 261–268.

101 McDonnell, G. and Russell, A.D. (1999) Antiseptics and disinfectants: activity, action, and resistance. *Clinical Microbiology Reviews*, **12**, 147–179.

102 Denyer, S.P. (1990) Mechanisms of action of biocides. *International Biodeterioration and Biodegradation*, **26**, 89–100.

103 Denyer, S.P. and Maillard, J.-Y. (2002) Cellular impermeability and uptake of biocides and antibiotics in Gram-negative bacteria. *Journal of Applied Microbiology*, **92**, 35S–45S.

104 Giles, C.H. *et al.* (1960) Studies in adsorption. XI. A system of classification of solution adsorption isotherms, and its use in diagnosis of adsorption mechanisms and in measurement of specific areas of solids. *Journal of the Chemical Society*, **111**, 3973–3993.

105 Hiom, S.J. *et al.* (1995) Uptake of 14C-chlorhexidine gluconate by *Saccharomyces cerevisiae*, *Candida albicans* and *Candida glabrata*. *Letters in Applied Microbiology*, **21**, 20–22.

106 Salt, W.G. and Wiseman, D. (1970) The relation between the uptake of cetyltrimethylammonium bromide by *Escherichia coli* and its effects on cell growth and viability. *Journal of Pharmacy and Pharmacology*, **22**, 261–264.

107 Broxton, P. *et al.* (1984) Binding of some polyhexamethylene biguanides to the cell envelope of *Escherichia coli* ATCC 8739. *Microbios*, **163**, 15–22.

108 Sakagami, Y. *et al.* (1989) Mechanism of resistance to benzalkonium chloride by *Pseudomonas aeruginosa*. *Applied and Environmental Microbiology*, **55**, 2036–2040.

109 Loughlin, M.F. *et al.* (2002) *Pseudomonas aeruginosa* cells adapted to benzalkonium chloride show resistance to other membrane-active agents but not to clinically relevant antibiotics. *Journal of Antimicrobial Chemotherapy*, **49**, 631–639.

110 Davies, A. *et al.* (1968) Comparison of the action of vantocil, cetrimide and chlorhexidine on *Escherichia coli* and its spheroplasts and the protoplasts of gram positive bacteria. *Journal of Applied Bacteriology*, **31**, 448–461.

111 Rosenberg, M. (1991) Basic and applied aspects of microbial adhesion at the hydrocarbon : water interface. *Critical Reviews in Microbiology*, **18**, 159–173.

112 Jones, D.S. *et al.* (1991) The effects of three non-antibiotic, antimicrobial agents on the surface hydrophobicity of certain micro-organisms evaluated by different methods. *Journal of Applied Bacteriology*, **71**, 218–227.

113 Majtan, V. and Majtanova, L. (2000) Effect of new quaternary bisammonium compounds on the growth and cell surface hydrophobicity of *Enterobacter cloacae*. *Central European Journal of Public Health*, **8**, 80–82.

114 Anil, S. *et al.* (2001) The impact of chlorhexidine gluconate on the relative cell surface hydrophobicity of oral *Candida albicans*. *Oral Disease*, **7**, 119–122.

115 Vaara, M. (1992) Agents that increase the permeability of the outer membrane. *Microbiological Reviews*, **56**, 395–411.

116 Yasuda, K. *et al.* (2009) Mode of action of novel polyamines increasing the permeability of bacterial outer membrane. *International Journal of Antimicrobial Agents*, **24**, 67–71.

117 Gorman, S.P. *et al.* (1980) Antimicrobial activity, uses and mechanism of action of glutaraldehyde. *Journal of Applied Bacteriology*, **48**, 161–190.

118 Hancock, R.E. and Wong, P.G. (1984) Compounds which increase the permeability of the *Pseudomonas aeruginosa* outer membrane. *Antimicrobial Agents and Chemotherapy*, **26**, 48–52.

119 Lambert, P.A. (1991) Action on cell walls and outer layers. *Society for Applied Bacteriology Technical Series*, **30**, 121–134.

120 Sheppard, F.C. *et al.* (1997) Flow cytometric analysis of chlorhexidine action. *FEMS Microbiology Letters*, **154**, 283–288.

121 Caron, G.N. *et al.* (1998) Assessment of bacterial viability status by flow cytometry and single cell sorting. *Journal of Applied Microbiology*, **84**, 988–998.

122 Lannigan, R. and Bryan, L.E. (1985) Decreased susceptibility of *Serratia marcescens* to chlorhexidine related to the inner membrane. *Journal of Antimicrobial Chemotherapy*, **15**, 559–565.

123 Shapiro, S. and Guggenheim, B. (1995) The action of thymol on oral bacteria. *Oral Microbiology and Immunology*, **10**, 241–246.

124 Cox, S.D. *et al.* (2000) The mode of antimicrobial action of the essential oil of *Melaleuca alternifolia* (tea tree oil). *Journal of Applied Microbiology*, **88**, 170–175.

125 Lambert, P.A. and Smith, A.R. (1976) Antimicrobial action of dodecyldiethanolamine: induced membrane damage in *Escherichia coli*. *Microbios*, **15**, 199–202.

126 Shepherd, J.A. *et al.* (1988) Antibacterial action of 2-bromo-2-nitropropane-1,3-diol (bronopol). *Antimicrobial Agents and Chemotherapy*, **32**, 1693–1698.

127 Chapman, J.S. and Diehl, M.A. (1995) Methylchloroisothiazolone-induced growth inhibition and lethality in *Escherichia coli*. *Journal of Applied Bacteriology*, **78**, 134–141.

128 Ooi, N. *et al.* (2009) XF-73, a novel antistaphylococcal membrane-active agent with rapid bactericidal activity. *Journal of Antimicrobial Chemotherapy*, **64**, 735–740.

129 Ooi, N. *et al.* (2010) XF-70 and XF-73, novel antibacterial agents active against slow-growing and non-dividing cultures of *Staphylococcus aureus* including biofilms. *Journal of Antimicrobial Chemotherapy*, **65**, 72–78.

130 Comas, J. and Vives-Rego, J. (1997) Assessment of the effects of gramicidin, formaldehyde, and surfactants on *Escherichia coli* by flow cytometry using nucleic acid and membrane potential dyes. *Cytometry*, **29**, 58–64.

131 Akiyama, Y. (2002) Proton-motive force stimulates the proteolytic activity of FtsH, a membrane-bound ATP-dependent protease in *Escherichia coli*. *Proceedings of the National Academy of Sciences*, **99**, 8066–8071.

132 Bloomfield, S.F. (1974) The effect of the phenolic antibacterial agent fentichlor on energy coupling in *Staphylococcus aureus*. *Journal of Applied Bacteriology*, **37**, 117–131.

133 Denyer, S.P. and Hugo, W.B. (1977) The mode of action of tetradecyltrimethyl ammonium bromide (CTAB) on *Staphylococcus aureus*. *Journal of Pharmacy and Pharmacology*, **29** (Suppl.), 66 pp.

134 Gilbert, P. *et al.* (1977) The lethal action of 2-phenoxyethanol and its analogues upon *Escherichia coli* NCTC 5933. *Microbios*, **19**, 125–141.

135 Eklund, T. (1985) The effect of sorbic acid and esters of p-hydroxybenzoic acid on the protonmotive force in *Escherichia coli* membrane vesicles. *Journal of General Microbiology*, **131**, 73–76.

136 Maget-Dana, R. (1999) The monolayer technique: a potent tool for studying the interfacial properties of antimicrobial and membrane-lytic peptides and their interactions with lipid membranes. *Biochimica et Biophysica Acta*, **1462**, 109–140.

137 Seefeld, M.A. *et al.* (2001) Inhibitors of bacterial enoyl acyl carrier protein reductase (FabI): 2,9-disubstituted 1,2,3,4-tetrahydropyrido(3,4-b)indoles as potential antibacterial agents. *Bioorganic and Medicinal Chemistry Letters*, **11**, 2241–2224.

138 Miller, W.H. *et al.* (2002) Discovery of aminopyridine-based inhibitors of bacterial enoyl-ACP reductase (FabI). *Journal of Medicinal Chemistry*, **45**, 3246–3256.

139 Suller, M.T. and Russell, A.D. (2000) Triclosan and antibiotic resistance in *Staphylococcus aureus*. *Journal of Antimicrobial Chemotherapy*, **46**, 11–18.

140 Darzynkiewicz, Z. (1990) Differential staining of DNA and RNA in intact cells and isolated cell nuclei with acridine orange. *Methods in Cell Biology*, **33**, 285–298.

141 Allen, M.J. *et al.* (2004) Cooperativity in the binding of the cationic biocide polyhexamethylene biguanide to nucleic acids. *Biochemical and Biophysical Research Communications*, **318**, 397–404.

142 Del Sal, G. *et al.* (1989) The CTAB-DNA precipitation method: a common mini-scale preparation of template DNA from phagemids, phages or plasmids suitable for sequencing. *BioTechniques*, **7**, 514–520.

143 Loshon, C.A. *et al.* (1999) Formaldehyde kills spores of *Bacillus subtilis* by DNA damage and small, acid-soluble spore proteins of the alpha/beta-type protect spores against this DNA damage. *Journal of Applied Microbiology*, **87**, 8–14.

144 van Sittert, N.J. *et al.* (2000) Formation of DNA adducts and induction of mutagenic effects in rats following 4 weeks inhalation exposure to ethylene oxide as a basis for cancer risk assessment. *Mutation Research*, **447**, 27–48.

145 Trewick, S.C. *et al.* (2002) Oxidative demethylation by *Escherichia coli* AlkB directly reverts DNA base damage. *Nature*, **419**, 174–178.

146 Falnes, P.O. *et al.* (2002) AlkB-mediated oxidative demethylation reverses DNA damage in *Escherichia coli*. *Nature*, **419**, 178–182.

147 Domingue, E.L. *et al.* (1988) Effects of three oxidizing biocides on *Legionella pneumophila* serogroup 1. *Applied and Environmental Microbiology*, **54**, 741–747.

148 Rice, R.G. (2002) Ozone and anthrax – knowns and unknowns. *Ozone-Science and Engineering*, **24**, 151–158.

149 Khadre, M.A. and Yousef, A.E. (2001) Sporicidal action of ozone and hydrogen peroxide: a comparative study. *International Journal of Food Microbiology*, **71**, 131–138.

150 von Gunten, U. and Pinkernell, U. (2000) Ozonation of bromide-containing drinking waters: a delicate balance between disinfection and bromate formation. *Water Science and Technology*, **41**, 53–59.

151 Ferng, S.F. (2002) Ozone-induced DNA single strand-breaks in guinea pig tracheobronchial epithelial cells *in vivo*. *Inhalation Toxicology*, **14**, 621–633.

152 Bornholdt, J. *et al.* (2002) Inhalation of ozone induces DNA strand breakage and inflammation in mice. *Mutation Research*, **520**, 63–71.

153 Small, D.A. *et al.* (2007) Toxicogenomic analysis of sodium hypochlorite antimicrobial mechanisms in *Pseudomonas aeruginosa*. *Applied Microbiology and Biotechnology*, **74**, 176–185.

154 Small, D.A. *et al.* (2007) Comparative global transcription analysis of sodium hypochlorite, peracetic acid, and hydrogen peroxide on *Pseudomonas aeruginosa*. *Applied Microbiology and Biotechnology*, **76**, 1093–1105.

155 Jang, H.J. *et al.* (2009) Global transcriptome analysis of the *Mycobacterium bovis* BCG response to sodium hypochlorite. *Applied Microbiology and Biotechnology*, **85**, 127–140.

156 Deng, D.M. *et al.* (2007) The adaptive response of *Streptococcus mutans* towards oral care products: involvement of the ClpP serine protease. *European Journal of Oral Science*, **115**, 363–370.

157 Santos, P.M. *et al.* (2004) Insights into *Pseudomonas putida* KT2440 response to phenol-induced stress by quantitative proteomics. *Proteomics*, **4**, 2640–2652.

158 Thurman, R.B. and Gerba, C.P. (1988) Molecular mechanisms of viral inactivation by water disinfectants. *Advances in Applied Microbiology*, **33**, 75–105.

159 Collier, P.J. *et al.* (1990) Growth inhibitory and biocidal activity of some isothiazolone biocides. *Journal of Applied Bacteriology*, **69**, 569–577.

160 Collier, P.J. *et al.* (1990) Chemical reactivity of some isothiazolone biocides. *Journal of Applied Bacteriology*, **69**, 578–584.

161 Narayan, M. *et al.* (2000) Oxidative folding of proteins. *Accounts of Chemical Research*, **33**, 805–812.

162 Liau, S.Y. *et al.* (1997) Interaction of silver nitrate with readily identifiable groups: relationship to the antibacterial action of silver ions. *Letters in Applied Microbiology*, **25**, 279–283.

163 Espirito Santo, C. *et al.* (2008) Contribution of copper ion resistance to survival of *Escherichia coli* on metallic copper surfaces. *Applied and Environmental Microbiology*, **74**, 977–986.

164 Rossmoore, H.W. and Sondossi, M. (1988) Applications and mode of action of formaldehyde condensate biocides. *Advances in Applied Microbiology*, **33**, 223–277.

165 Jiang, W. and Schwendeman, S.P. (2000) Formaldehyde-mediated aggregation of protein antigens: comparison of untreated and formalinized model antigens. *Biotechnology and Bioengineering*, **70**, 507–517.

166 Eklund, B. *et al.* (2002) Use of ethylenediaminetetraacetic acid in pulp mills and effects on metal mobility and primary production. *Environmental Toxicology and Chemistry*, **21**, 1040–1051.

167 Neidle, S. and Abraham, Z. (1984) Structural and sequence-dependent aspects of drug intercalation into nucleic acids. *CRC Critical Reviews of Biochemistry*, **17**, 73–121.

168 Wilson, W.D. *et al.* (1994) The interaction of intercalators and groove-binding agents with DNA triple-helical structures: the influence of ligand structure, DNA backbone modifications and sequence. *Journal of Molecular Recognition*, **7**, 89–98.

169 Ingram, L.O. and Buttke, T.M. (1984) Effects of alcohols on micro-organisms. *Advances in Microbial Physiology*, **25**, 253–300.

170 Lucchini, J.J. *et al.* (1990) Antibacterial activity of phenolic compounds and aromatic alcohols. *Research in Microbiology*, **141**, 499–510.

171 Gilby, A.R. and Few, A.V. (1960) Lysis of protoplasts of *Micrococcus lysodeikticus* by ionic detergents. *Journal of General Microbiology*, **23**, 19–26.

172 Fay, J.P. and Farias, R.N. (1977) Inhibitory action of a non-metabolizable fatty acid on the growth of *Escherichia coli*: role of metabolism and outer membrane integrity. *Journal of Bacteriology*, **132**, 790–795.

173 Salton, M.R. (1968) Lytic agents, cell permeability, and monolayer penetrability. *Journal of General Physiology*, **52**, 227S–252S.

174 Russell, A.D. (1986) Chlorhexidine: antibacterial action and bacterial resistance. *Infection*, **14**, 212–215.

175 Levy, C.W. *et al.* (1999) Molecular basis of triclosan activity. *Nature*, **398**, 383–384.

176 McMurry, L.M. *et al.* (1999) Genetic evidence that InhA of *Mycobacterium smegmatis* is a target for triclosan. *Antimicrobial Agents and Chemotherapy*, **43**, 711–713.

177 Levy, S.B. (2000) Antibiotic and antiseptic resistance: impact on public health. *Pediatric Infectious Disease Journal*, **19**, S120–S122.

178 Levy, S.B. (2001) Antibacterial household products: cause for concern. *Emerging Infectious Diseases*, **7**, 512–515.

179 Levy, S.B. (2002) Active efflux, a common mechanism for biocide and antibiotic resistance. *Journal of Applied Microbiology*, **92**, 65S–71S.

180 Poole, K. (2002) Mechanisms of bacterial biocide and antibiotic resistance. *Journal of Applied Microbiology*, **92**, 55S–64S.

181 Ng, M.E. *et al.* (2002) Biocides and antibiotics with apparently similar actions on bacteria: is there the potential for cross-resistance? *Journal of Hospital Infection*, **51**, 147–149.

182 Russell, A.D. (2002) Introduction of biocides into clinical practice and the impact on antibiotic-resistant bacteria. *Journal of Applied Microbiology*, **92**, 121S–135S.

183 Maillard, J.-Y. (2007) Bacterial resistance to biocides in the healthcare environment: shall we be concerned? *Journal of Hospital Infection*, **65** (Suppl. 2), 60–72.

184 Maillard, J.-Y. and Denyer, S.P. (2009) Emerging bacterial resistance following biocide exposure: should we be concerned? *Chemica Oggi*, **27**, 26–28.

185 Chuanchuen, R. *et al.* (2008) Susceptibilities to antimicrobials and disinfectants in *Salmonella* isolates obtained from poultry and swine in Thailand. *Journal of Veterinary Medical Science*, **70**, 595–601.

186 McCay, P.H. *et al.* (2010) Effect of subinhibitory concentrations of benzalkonium chloride on the competitiveness of *Pseudomonas aeruginosa* grown in continuous culture. *Microbiology*, **156**, 30–38.

187 Fraise, A.P. (2002) Susceptibility of antibiotic-resistant cocci to biocides. *Journal of Applied Microbiology*, **92**, 158S–162S.

188 Joynson, J.A. *et al.* (2002) Adaptive resistance to benzalkonium chloride, amikacin and tobramycin: the effect on susceptibility to other antimicrobials. *Journal of Applied Microbiology*, **93**, 96–107.

189 Rose, H. *et al.* (2009) Biocide susceptibility of the *Burkholderia cepacia* complex. *Journal of Antimicrobial Chemotherapy*, **63**, 502–510.

190 Cottell, A. *et al.* (2009) Triclosan-tolerant bacteria: changes in susceptibility to antibiotics. *Journal of Hospital Infection*, **72**, 71–76.

191 Block, C. and Furman, M. (2002) Association between intensity of chlorhexidine use and micro-organisms of reduced susceptibility in a hospital environment. *Journal of Hospital Infection*, **51**, 201–206.

192 Murtough, S.M. *et al.* (2001) Biocide rotation in the healthcare setting: is there a case for policy implementation? *Journal of Hospital Infection*, **48**, 1–6.

193 Murtough, S.M. *et al.* (2002) A survey of rotational use of biocides in hospital pharmacy aseptic units. *Journal of Hospital Infection*, **50**, 228–231.

6.1 Mechanisms of Bacterial Resistance to Microbicides

Jean-Yves Maillard

Cardiff School of Pharmacy and Pharmaceutical Sciences, Cardiff University, Cardiff, Wales, UK

Introduction

The use of microbicides in general and the variety of products containing them have increased substantially over the last few years. For example, in Europe the growth in microbicide use has increased steadily in the past 15 years; while the exact tonnage remains unknown for most such chemicals, the market for microbicides as a whole was estimated to be 10–11 billion euros in 2006 [1]. It is also worth noting that the efficacy of a microbicide is rarely evaluated in practice, but is often measured *in vitro* with standard efficacy tests which do not necessarily reflect the final application of a microbicidal product [2]. Taking into consideration the increased usage and the lack of efficacy data in practice, the risk for microbial (bacterial) survival following microbicide exposure in practice is expected to be high.

Bacteria have several mechanisms enabling them to survive the deleterious effects of microbicides and other antimicrobials. When the concentration of the active is high enough, the lethal effect is due to non-specific but irreversible damage to multiple target sites in the bacteria [3–8]. This is in stark contrast to how antibiotics act. Microbicide-resistant bacteria may emerge when the concentration of the active reaches sublethal levels under field conditions either due to dilution, chemical decay or by reaction with other organic and inorganic compounds. In such situations, bacterial mutants with a higher resistance to the active may be selected for; one or more inherent mechanisms may be invoked to reduce the damage by either actively breaking down the active, blocking its entry or by preventing its accumulation inside cells [2, 9–12].

Several mechanisms conferring a decreased susceptibility to chemical microbicides have been identified and are described in more detail below. It is important to note that some of these mechanisms are non-specific and can confer cross-resistance to other antimicrobials, notably antibiotics [13–16]. Bacterial resistance to microbicides has been known for the last 50 years [17–19], often following the improper usage or misuse of such chemicals [18, 20–24]. To date, bacterial resistance has been described for all the microbicides that have been investigated. Unfortunately, and in contrast to antibiotic resistance, thus far the issue of microbicide resistance in healthcare in particular has not received the attention it deserves [25]. As a result, bacterial resistance in environmental and clinical isolates is not routinely investigated even though resistant strains are often isolated following microbicide application. While we have a better understanding of the mechanisms of microbicide resistance *in vitro*, there are still major gaps in our knowledge of their relevance in the field [2, 18, 25].

This section of Chapter 6 aims to review the different mechanisms of resistance to chemical microbicides in bacteria, together with a reflection on the dissemination of resistance and the lack of standard protocols to test for emerging resistance. However, this chapter section will not review bacterial biofilms and bacterial endospores, which are dealt with in Chapters 4 and 6.2, respectively.

Definitions

A major problem associated with the term "resistance" is its definition. The many definitions available are often used interchangeably by academics and professionals, creating much confusion. This conundrum is further compounded due to wide variations in test protocols used to study bacterial resistance to microbicides. In the peer-reviewed literature and other documents, terms referring to "resistance" to microbicides and/or antibiotics include "tolerance", "decreased susceptibility", "reduced susceptibility", "insusceptibility", "multidrug resistance", "intrinsic or innate resistance", "acquired resistance", "acquired reduced susceptibility", "co-resistance" and "cross-resistance". Some of these terms clearly reflect the lack of consensus within the scientific community.

Literally speaking, "resistance" should be defined as the capacity of bacteria to survive the effects of harmful chemical or physical agents. Terms such as "intrinsic", "innate" and "insusceptibility" are appropriate when resistance is due to mechanisms that naturally exist within bacteria. When it is a new property (i.e. not previously encoded within the bacterial genome), resulting from a mutation(s) or the acquisition of mobile genetic elements, the term "acquired" is more suitable.

The following definitions have been proposed by Chapman and colleagues [26, 27], Russell and colleagues [28, 29], Cloete [30] and Maillard [6]. These definitions have also been adopted in Europe [1].

"Reduced susceptibility" and "decreased susceptibility" are terms that reflect the use of minimum inhibitory concentration (MIC) to determine the change in bacterial properties; an increase in MIC denotes an increase in survival of the exposed bacteria. Likewise "tolerance" denotes a reduced susceptibility to an antimicrobial molecule characterized by a raised MIC, or a situation in which a preservative system no longer prevents microbial growth. The term "acquired reduced susceptibility" should not be used.

"Co-resistance", "multidrug resistance" and "cross-resistance" all refer to mechanisms that confer resistance to similar or unrelated chemical antimicrobials. "Co-resistance" indicates the joint transfer of genetic determinants (e.g. integrons, transposons, plasmids) encoding for distinct resistance mechanisms. These genes are then expressed in the recipient bacteria, conferring "cross-resistance" to unrelated antimicrobials. "Multidrug resistance" (MDR) refers to a bacterium that is resistant to different classes of antibiotics, the resistance resulting from different mechanisms. "Cross-resistance" refers to a bacterium that is resistant to unrelated antimicrobials (i.e. microbicides and antibiotics), but with mechanisms of action that are related or overlap.

From a practical point of view, in the laboratory, bacterial resistance has been defined following different observations:
1. Where a strain is not killed or inhibited by a concentration attained *in situ*. In this particular scenario, bacteria survive exposure to a microbicide at the concentration used in practice (i.e. in-use concentration as recommended by the manufacturer). One difficulty with the term "in-use" concentration is the range of concentration of a microbicide found in different products. In addition, the formulation may contain several microbicides or excipients that might potentiate its microbicidal activity.
2. Where a strain is not killed or inhibited by a concentration to which the majority of the strains of that organism are susceptible. This definition is usually used when standard efficacy tests are performed, where the susceptibility of environmental isolates is compared to that of a reference strain.
3. Where bacterial cells are not killed or inhibited by a concentration acting upon the majority of cells in that culture. This definition is widely used where bacterial cells (or just one cell) within a susceptible population are trained to become less susceptible/resistant to a given microbicide. The identification of most of the mechanisms involved in bacterial resistance derives from *in vitro* experiments based on selecting or training a subpopulation.

Occurrence of bacterial resistance to microbicides

Bacterial resistance to microbicides is not a new phenomenon and has been reported since the 1950s, notably with quaternary ammonium compounds (QACs) and biguanides [17–19, 31–34]. Bacterial resistance has also been reported to, among other microbicides, triclosan [35–38], iodophor [39], sodium hypochlorite [40, 41], glutaraldehyde [16, 23, 42–46] and peroxygens [24, 47–49]. Bacterial resistance to all known preservatives has also been described [26, 27, 50, 51].

Most such evidence comes from laboratory investigations, where usually a decrease in susceptibility to a microbicide is observed by measuring an increase in MIC, for example against cationic microbicides [52, 53], isothiazolones [54], phenolics [55–58] hydrogen peroxide or peracetic acid [49]. Studies reporting on the isolation or selection for resistant bacteria to an in-use concentration of a microbicide are scarce and usually concern microbicides that are used in the healthcare environment – such as glutaraldehyde [16, 23, 42], chlorine dioxide [24], chlorhexidine [59–61], triclosan [60, 62], alcohol and iodine [60].

In clinical settings, where bacterial survival following the use of a microbicide has been reported, the failure of the microbicide to kill the bacterial isolates often resulted from the application of a low in-use concentration of the chemical [18, 20–24, 63–67]. A comprehensive review highlighting bacterial outbreaks in the clinical setting from contaminated antiseptics and disinfectants, mainly chlorhexidine and benzalkonium chloride, is available [68].

Bacterial resistance to microbicides has been documented with every microbicide investigated to date. Although the implications of bacteria with a reduced susceptibility is unclear at present, bacterial resistance to a microbicide at "in-use" concentration has led to bacterial infections in patients [16].

Mechanisms of bacterial resistance to microbicides

Principles

It is widely accepted that microbicides have multiple and non-specific target sites against bacteria (see Chapter 5). However, in the case of exposure to sublethal concentrations of a microbicide the bacterial cell may invoke more specific resistance mechanisms [3, 5, 8]. Such a phenomenon is now particularly well documented with triclosan [36, 56, 69–73]. Differences in microbicide interaction with the bacterial cell are important when one considers the development of bacterial resistance. Where multiple interactions occur, it is unlikely that bacterial resistance emerges as the result of mutation or by-pass of metabolic mechanisms. Instead "general" mechanisms aim to decrease the harmful concentration of the microbicide, such as changes in membrane permeability, efflux and degradation [2, 5, 6]. From a bacterial point of view, the objective is to survive microbicide exposure and several mechanisms conferring "resistance" operate synergistically [2, 6, 9–11, 74].

When a low concentration of a microbicide is used, the expression of specific bacterial mechanisms of resistance – such as mutation, by-pass of a metabolic pathway and degradation – can reflect the interaction with a specific target [2, 6]. It should be noted that the concentration of a microbicide is low in certain applications, such as in preservation and the use of microbicides in treated materials, textiles, plastics, etc. The concentration of a microbicide is paramount for its lethal activity [5, 75]. In addition, the effective concentration of a microbicide, and subsequently its bactericidal efficacy, might be severely hampered by a number of external factors, such as level of soiling, type of target surface, air/liquid temperature and contact time [5] (see also Chapter 3). The interaction of a low concentration of a microbicide with the bacterial cell is thus possible following application even when the microbicidal product initially contains a bactericidal concentration of the chemical. Recently, McCay and colleagues [76] highlighted that environmental conditions (e.g. limited nutrients) play an important role in the selection and maintenance of microbicide adaptation.

However, in some instances, phenotypic variation within a bacterial species accounts for the survival of certain isolates.

Cheeseman *et al.* [77] described the variation in the susceptibility of isolates of *Staphylococcus aureus* to alcohol-based hand gels. Some isolates were clearly more resistant, but mechanisms to explain increased survival have not been identified. To some extent, Williams *et al.* [78] came to the same observation when clinical isolates of *S. aureus* were exposed to sodium hypochlorite.

Overview

Mechanisms of bacterial resistance to microbicides have empirically been divided into intrinsic and acquired resistance [79]. Intrinsic resistance is conferred by factors inherent to the bacteria, such as their structure (e.g. presence of an outer membrane in Gram-negative bacteria or lipid-rich outer cell wall in mycobacteria), or encoded by the bacterial genome and (over) expressed following microbicide exposure (e.g. efflux pump) [80, 81]. Bacterial spore resistance to microbicides is also an intrinsic mechanism since the spore structure, with its exosporium and cortex, acts as a barrier to microbicide penetration [82] (see Chapter 6.2).

Acquired bacterial resistance refers to the acquisition of a new resistance mechanism through mutations, often as the result of microbicide exposure, or expression of newly acquired resistance genes from other bacteria [79]. The transfer of new genetic determinants conferring resistance in bacteria has been well described in the literature [19, 83–85], notably the co-transfer of an antibiotic-resistance gene together with a microbicide-resistance gene (i.e. co-resistance) [19, 86, 87]. There is, however, little information on the effect of microbicides on the gene-transfer mechanisms in bacteria. Pearce and colleagues [88] observed that while some microbicides (i.e. chlorhexidine and povidone iodine) at a low "residual" concentration inhibited conjugation and transduction in *S. aureus*, others (i.e. cetrimide) increased genetic transfer efficiency. It is also interesting to note that the concentration of a microbicide that promotes mutation in bacteria might be low. Indeed, a recent investigation showed that active efflux in *Salmonella enterica* serovar Typhimurium induced a higher level of mutations, conferring reduced susceptibility to triclosan [89]. Likewise, Chen and colleagues [90] observed that the emergence of decreased susceptibility to triclosan in *Acinetobacter baumannii* appeared to be dependent on a background of intrinsic triclosan efflux.

The acquisition of new resistance determinants through gene transfer and new properties through mutation, following exposure to microbicides, is of concern since a bacterium with a decreased susceptibility or a resistant phenotype can emerge [1, 91].

Mechanisms

A number of mechanisms conferring bacterial resistance to microbicides have been documented over the last 50 years. New resistance mechanisms, which were originally described for antibiotics, have now been observed following microbicide exposure (e.g. by-pass of metabolic activity). Overall, these mechanisms

Table 6.1.1 Resistance mechanisms in bacteria (based on [1]).

Mechanisms		Nature	Resistance level	Cross-resistance/ co-resistance	References
Change in cell permeability	Decrease in microbicide concentration (that reaches the target sites) • Spores (layers: cortex, spore envelope)	Intrinsic	Highly resistant	Cross-resistance	[3, 4, 30, 92–94]
	Gram-negative bacteria (outer membrane) • Lipopolysaccharides • Proteins (porins) • Fatty acid • Phospholipids	Intrinsic (acquired)	Highly resistant to reduced susceptibility	Cross-resistance	[3–5, 9–11, 54, 75, 95–104]
	Mycobacteria mycoylarabinagalactan				[43, 45, 93, 105–107]
Change in surface properties	Decrease in binding and interaction between microbicide and cell surfaces • Surface charge	Intrinsic	Reduced susceptibility	Cross-resistance to cationic?	[108]
Efflux mechanisms	Decrease in intracellular concentration of a microbicide • Small multidrug resistance (SMR) family (now part of the drug/metabolite transporter (DMT) superfamily) • Major facilitator superfamily (MFS) • ATP-binding cassette (ABC) family • Resistance–nodulation–division (RND) family • Multidrug and toxic compound extrusion (MATE) family	Intrinsic/acquired	Reduced susceptibility	Cross-resistance/ co-resistance	[14, 15, 80, 81, 86, 109–127]
Enzymatic reduction	Decrease in intracellular and exocellular concentration of a microbicide	Intrinsic/acquired	Reduced susceptibility	Co-resistance	[30, 40, 128–130]
Target mutation	Fab1 mutation, e.g. in *Mycobacterium smegmatis*	Acquired	Reduced susceptibility	Neither	[36, 56]
By-pass metabolic activity	Increase in pyruvate synthesis and fatty acid production via an altered metabolic pathway (expression of "triclosan resistance network")	Intrinsic/acquired	Reduced susceptibility	?	[74]

usually contribute to a decrease in concentration of a microbicide to a level that is no longer harmful to the bacterium. These mechanisms are summarized in Table 6.1.1.

Changes in bacterial cell permeability

Changes in bacterial cell permeability to microbicides are associated with decreased susceptibility and resistance and this is a well-established concept for bacterial spores (see Chapter 6.2). It has also been well described in a number of vegetative bacteria [4, 92]. In mycobacteria, the lipid-rich outer cell wall, the presence of a mycoylacylarabinogalactan layer and the composition of the arabinogalactan/arabinomannan within the cell wall account for a reduction of microbicide penetration [4, 43, 45, 93, 95, 105–107]. In Gram-negative bacteria, the role of lipopolysaccharides (LPSs) in decreasing microbicide penetration (e.g. chlorhexidine, QACs, glutaraldehyde) has been well described, notably with studies that have used permeabilizing agents, bacterial protoplasts or transposon mutagenesis [3, 75, 96, 97, 131, 132]. A decrease in bacterial susceptibility to a number of microbicides has also been associated with changes in components of the Gram-negative bacterial outer membrane, including proteins [54, 98, 99], fatty

acids [100–103] and phospholipids [104]; these changes contributing to a change in the membrane ultrastructure [9–11]. Bruinsma *et al.* [108] also described a change in surface charges associated with a decrease in susceptibility of *Pseudomonas aeruginosa* to QACs.

Efflux pump

Efflux pumps are widespread among bacteria and five main classes have been described to date: the drug/metabolite transporter (DMT) superfamily, the major facilitator superfamily (MFS), the adenosine triphospate (ATP)-binding cassette (ABC) family, the resistance–nodulation–division (RND) family and the multidrug and toxic compound extrusion (MATE) family (Figure 6.1.1) [80, 81, 109–113].

The role of efflux pumps is to decrease the amount of harmful substances, including microbicides, from the bacterial cytoplasm to levels that are not damaging for the cell. A number of microbicides have been particularly well documented as exhibiting efflux of microbicides including QACs [76, 114–119, 133] and triclosan [55, 120–124]. A number of bacterial genera have been particularly well studied, including *S. aureus* [83, 114–119],

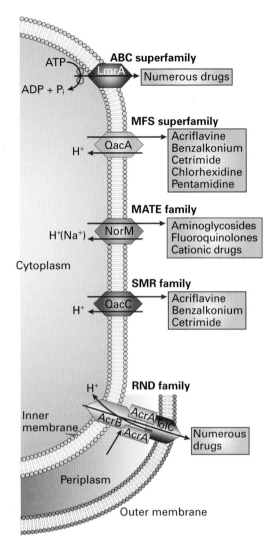

Figure 6.1.1 Efflux pumps (from [80]). Reprinted by permission from Mcmillan Publishers Ltd. Nature Reviews Microbiology; Piddock LJV. Multidrug resistance efflux pumps – not just for resistance. *Nature* **4**, 629–636, copyright 2006.

P. aeruginosa [120, 121, 124–126, 134], *Escherichia coli* [55, 135–138], *S. enterica* serovar Typhimurium [122, 123] and *Acinetobacter baumannii* [139]. The role of efflux in promoting bacterial resistance to microbicides has often been suggested to be limited, since most studies have observed that efflux conferred only a decrease in susceptibility. However, some investigators claim that efflux is responsible for high-level resistance, notably against triclosan [124, 126].

One important consideration is the level of expression of efflux pumps following microbicide exposure. For example, the overexpression of efflux pumps following triclosan exposure has been described in *S. enterica* serovar Typhimurium [13, 122, 123, 140], in *Stenotrophomonas maltophilia* with the overexpression of SmedEF [141] and in *E. coli* with the overexpression of *acrAB* or

marA or *soxS* [13, 55]. In *Campylobacter jejuni*, a clinical strain overexpressing CmeB was shown to have a triclosan MIC of 32 mg/l [142].

Enzymatic degradation
Enzymatic degradation/reduction plays a role in reducing the harmful concentration of a microbicide. Such a mechanism contributes to a decrease in susceptibility to a specific microbicide, although it is unlikely that the expression of such enzymes confers bacterial resistance. Enzymatic inactivation has been described over the years for a number of microbicides, including metallic ions (e.g. silver, copper), which are reduced to the inactive metal [30], aldehydes (e.g. formaldehyde and glutaraldehyde), which are inactivated by aldehyde dehydrogenases [128], peroxygens (e.g. chlorine dioxide, hydrogen peroxide), whose free radicals (e.g. ˙OH) are inactivated by catalases, superoxide dismutase and alkyl hydroperoxidases [48, 129], and the parabens [51, 130].

The co-transfer of resistance genes encoding for metallic reduction enzymes and antibiotic resistance has been observed. The role of metallic ions in maintaining the presence of conjugative plasmid may be questioned but has not been investigated [19, 128].

Change in biosynthetic pathways
There is overall little information on the bacterial resistance associated with a change in (a) metabolic pathway(s). A change in metabolic pathway was previously thought to be a mechanism that only occurs in bacterial resistance to sulfonamides. Codling *et al.* [131] observed with the use of transposon mutagenesis that *Serratia marcescens* insusceptibility to a QAC could be associated with a number of biosynthetic and metabolic pathways, the disruption of which increased bacterial susceptibility. More direct evidence of the change in metabolic pathway associated with a decreased in bacterial susceptibility came from a proteomic study of *S. enterica* interaction with triclosan [74]. Webber and colleagues [74] identified a "triclosan resistance network", which constitutes an alternative pathway to the production of pyruvate and fatty acid. Likewise, Tkachenko *et al.* [143] identified a modification of membrane lipid composition associated with alteration of the expression of various genes involved in the fatty acid metabolism in triclosan-resistant *S. aureus*.

Mutations in a specific target site
The modification of specific bacterial target site in response to microbicide exposure has only been described with triclosan. It is linked to the bisphenol-specific interaction at a low concentration with an enoyl-acyl reductase carrier protein [56, 70–72, 144, 145]. Modification of this enzyme has been associated with decreased susceptibility in a number of bacterial genera [36, 69, 73, 74, 90, 145–148]. It has also been observed that overexpression of *fabI* in *Acinetobacter baumannii* confers reduced susceptibility to triclosan [90].

Induction of gene expression conferring bacterial resistance

The induction of resistance mechanisms following the use of microbicides in practice is of much concern. This is particularly pertinent with regard to the increased usage of products containing a low (inhibitory/subinhibitory) concentration of a microbicide and the presence of low concentrations of microbicides in the environment.

The induction of bacterial resistance has been well documented, although in most occasions a decrease in susceptibility rather than resistance per se was observed. The mechanisms of resistance solicited often result from a bacterial stress-type response to microbicide exposure, including reduced growth rate [149–151], altered gene expression, notably of the efflux pump [13, 76, 122, 123, 140–142, 152], production of guanosine 5′-diphosphate 3′-diphosphate (ppGpp) [153] and DNA repair [41, 154]. Bacterial induction by microbicides can be more complex, involving regulatory genes [13, 49, 55, 74, 138, 155] and changes in metabolic processes [156].

Recently, a number of studies reported a change of gene regulation following microbicide exposure leading to the expression of bacterial virulence determinants [13, 15, 155, 157].

Bacterial biofilms

Bacteria are generally associated with surfaces in a complex community called biofilms. Bacteria in biofilms have been shown to be less susceptible to antibiotics and microbicides than planktonic bacteria [158–160] (see Chapter 4). Decreased susceptibility/resistance to microbicides has been associated with a "biofilm-associated phenotype" [161–163], which is based on several mechanisms: decreased metabolism, quiescence, reduced penetration due to the extracellular polymeric matrix [164, 165], enzymatic inactivation [166, 167];and induction of multidrug-resistant operons and efflux pumps [168] (see Chapter 4). More recently, bacterial swarming motility has been identified as a new factor contributing to bacterial resistance [169].

Change in bacterial populations

Microbicides have also been reported to change the composition of complex biofilms. Although the efficacy of microbicides against bacterial biofilm is dealt with in Chapter 4, it is important to report the selection effects of microbicides within bacterial communities. Moore et al. [170] observed the clonal expansion of pseudomonads to the detriment of Gram-positive species following exposure to polyhexamethylene biguanide, chlorhexidine or Bardac (a QAC) associated with a decrease in microbicide susceptibility. An earlier study from the same group based on a drain microcosm model to study the effect of QACs, reported, however, that the population dynamic and the susceptibility profile of the microcosm to the QACs was not affected [171]. Kümmerer et al. [172] reported a change in bacterial population and a selection of Pseudomonas spp. in activated sludge following exposure to benzalkonium chloride. There is further evidence of bacterial population shift following exposure to triclosan. McBain et al.

[173] investigated the effect of a sublethal concentration (2–4 g/l) of triclosan over a 3-month period against a complex microcosm. A decrease in bacterial diversity and a decrease in susceptibility of the remaining bacterial population were observed. The selectivity of this microbicide has been highlighted in two studies on urinary catheters. While triclosan inhibited growth of Proteus mirabilis, it had little effect on other common bacterial pathogens [174, 175].

Dissemination of resistance

Emerging acquired bacterial resistance to microbicides through the acquisition of new genetic determinants through horizontal and vertical transfers is of great concern. Bacteria can exchange genetic information with three different mechanisms: conjugation, transformation and transduction. Conjugation is particularly efficient among a wide range of bacteria, notably with the exchange of conjugative plasmids and transposons [176–178]. Sidhu et al. [179] demonstrated that staphylococcal resistance to benzalkonium chloride was associated with the presence of plasmids, with some clinical isolates harboring multiresistance plasmids that contain qac, bla and tet resistance genes. It is interesting to note that genetic linkage (co-resistance) between QACs and antibiotic resistance genes (blaZ, aacA-aphD, dfrA, and ble) in clinical and environmental bacterial isolates has been observed [179–181]. The genetic dissemination of resistance genes to QACs encoded on plasmid has been documented in bovine isolates [87] and clinical isolates of S. aureus [182]. The presence of mobile elements conferring resistance to microbicides and other antimicrobials via an efflux mechanism has been found in E. coli [183, 184] and P. aeruginosa [185]. Some mechanisms of bacterial resistance to microbicides, such as efflux and degradation, have been documented to be transferred to other bacteria [79, 177, 186–188]. Microbicides can also contribute to the maintenance of resistance determinants in bacteria [189].

Although, not directly involved with the dissemination of genetic determinants, quorum sensing might have a role to play in the adaption of bacteria to deleterious conditions and decreased susceptibility, with, for example, the formation of biofilms [190–192] and the expression of degradative enzymes. However, the contribution of quorum sensing and emerging planktonic resistance to microbicides might be limited [193].

Measuring bacterial resistance to microbicides

The number of definitions available reflects the differences in test protocols used (Table 6.1.2). Central to these protocols is the concentration of microbicide tested [2, 75, 194]. Concentration is one of the most important factors that affect microbicide activity [6, 8, 12, 194, 195] (see Chapter 3). In terms of development of bacterial resistance, the use of the MIC of a microbicide is often used as a marker [57, 195], although higher concentrations of the active agent are often used in practice. Hence, based on MIC measurement, a decreased in susceptibility to a microbicide or microbicide tolerance can be recorded. The use of MIC measurement has proved useful when a decrease in bacterial susceptibility following repeated exposure to a low concentration of a microbicide or to exposure to incremental concentrations of a microbicide has been investigated [6, 52, 53, 57, 156, 196]. However, using the MIC as a measuring tool, bacterial resistance to a higher in-use concentration (i.e. one that will kill rather than merely inhibit growth) cannot be addressed [2, 6, 194, 195]. Some investigations have clearly highlighted that a bacterial strain showing decreased susceptibility to a microbicide, measured as an increased MIC, remains susceptible to the lethal effect of the same microbicide [59, 197].

In many instances, the determination of the lethal activity of the microbicide or the minimum bactericidal concentration (MBC) is preferable. Indeed, the determination of the lethal activity of a microbicide forms the basis of many standard efficacy test protocols (see Chapter 12). The MBC can provide the basis for comparison between a resistant bacterial strain/isolate and a reference strain and, as such, the nature of resistance (acquired or intrinsic) can be determined. At this point, it is important to note that an effective neutralizer must be used to quench the activity of the microbicide. Failure to do so will provide an overestimation of the lethality of the microbicide (see Chapter 12).

Determination of the inactivation kinetic following exposure to a microbicide, and in particular the shape of the inactivation curve, can provide information as to the nature of resistance of a population of cells and/or the interaction of the microbicide with the cell population (Figure 6.1.2). The presence of a shoulder might indicate the presence of a subpopulation less susceptible to the microbicide, or the presence of aggregates impinging the penetration of a microbicide. The presence of a tail might indicate the presence of a subpopulation resistant to the microbicides, the presence of aggregates impermeable to the microbicide or a depletion of the microbicide. Regrowth in the presence of an excess of microbicide indicates a resistant population (Figure 6.1.2c). Similarly, the use of growth kinetics in the presence of a low (often inhibitory/subinhibitory) concentration of a microbicide provides information on the presence of a resistant subpopulation or changes in bacterial metabolism and phenotypes (Figure 6.1.3). Hence several studies have hypothesized that even a low concentration of a microbicide might have some profound effect on a resistant bacterial cell population, indicating the presence of a susceptible subpopulation or an adaptation/induction process where resistance mechanisms might be expressed to reduce the damaging concentration of a microbicide, enabling exponential growth to resume [6, 59, 198].

Table 6.1.2 Test protocols to determine bacterial resistance to microbicides.

Methodology	Nature of resistance	Mechanisms of "resistance"
Minimum inhibitory concentrations	Decreased susceptibility/ tolerance	Single, mutation (e.g. InhA)
Minimum bactericidal concentrations	Resistance	Multiple
Lethal activity (efficacy test)	Resistance	Multiple
Inactivation kinetic	Resistance	Presence of subpopulation, formation of aggregates
Growth kinetic	Decreased susceptibility/ tolerance	Adaptation, change in metabolic process, expression of mechanisms

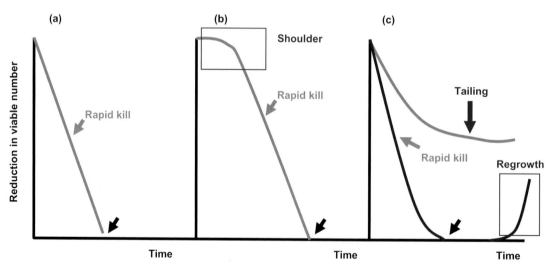

Figure 6.1.2 Inactivation kinetic and mechanisms of resistance. (a) First order of kinetic reaction, rapid kill and no bacterial resistance. (b) Presence of a shoulder indicating less accessible bacteria (e.g. presence of aggregates) or an initially less susceptible subpopulation. Eventually, the subpopulation is killed. (c) Tailing; rapid kill and indication of tailing at the detection limit of the assay followed by regrowth, or tailing indicating the presence of less susceptible isolates or a decrease in microbicide accessibility (e.g. presence of aggregates). Black arrow represents the limit of detection of the assay.

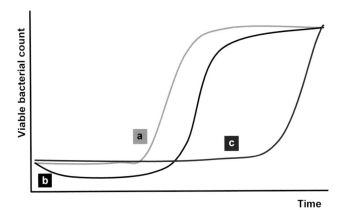

Figure 6.1.3 Growth kinetics and mechanisms of resistance. (a) Bacterial growth curve in the absence of microbicides. (b, c) Bacterial growth curve in the presence of a subinhibitory concentration of a microbicide. (b) Initial decrease in viable number indicating a susceptible subpopulation is being killed. The subsequent lag phase corresponds to the rest of the population to grow and eventually reach the exponential growth phase. (c) The bacterial population needs to respond to the effect of the microbicide before growth can resume, hence the presence of an extended lag phase before the exponential phase. Bacterial response can take the form of overexpression of efflux, degradation, control of porins, etc. – mechanisms that aim to reduce the concentration of a microbicide to a level that is not affecting bacterial growth.

Cross-resistance to unrelated chemicals

The indiscriminate use of microbicides in an increasing number of applications and notably the use of low concentrations has fueled the debate of emerging bacterial cross-resistance to antibiotics used for human and animal medicine [1, 173, 199–208]. Such a concept is not inconceivable since bacteria are adept at responding to external stresses. The adaptation mechanisms in bacterial cells to toxic chemicals might thus confer resistance against structurally non-related molecules [209]. Indeed, there is now solid *in vitro* evidence that bacterial mechanisms conferring a decreased susceptibility or resistance to a microbicide can also lead to resistance to therapeutic concentration of antibiotics [3–7, 210]. Some of the most common mechanisms involved include expression and overexpression of efflux pumps [6, 81] and changes in cell permeability and metabolism. The use of genomic and transcriptomic studies has provided recent advances in our understanding of the effect of microbicides on the induction and expression of specific mechanisms, some of which include the expression of specific mechanisms of antibiotic resistance [13].

Although there is now a body of evidence on mechanisms conferring cross-resistance to microbicides and antibiotics, and on the role of microbicide exposure in expressing such mechanisms, the development of cross-resistance to microbicides is not universal [58] and might depend on the bacterial genera or species and on the microbicides [2, 6]. In addition, emerging cross-resistance following microbicide exposure *in situ* has not been widely studied but has been reported. Carson *et al.* [211]

reported a significant relationship between high QAC MICs and resistance to one or more antibiotics in an environmental study. Duarte *et al.* [16] reported the emergence of *Mycobacterium massilense* resistant to antimycobacterial therapeutic antibiotics and the dissemination of infection caused by this opportunistic pathogen in 38 hospitals. These bacteria, associated with an epidemic of postsurgical infections, were also resistant to 2% glutaraldehyde (used in these institutions for high-level disinfection). Further information on this topic is provided in Chapter 11.

Conclusions

Microbicides are valuable compounds that provide assurance (when used appropriately) that microbial contaminants or infections can be controlled. To this end, microbicides are used effectively in a number of applications in healthcare and the food and water industries. The development of bacterial resistance to microbicides has now been well described, with novel mechanisms such as alteration of a metabolic pathway still emerging. The recent use of genomic and transcriptomic tools in the analysis of bacterial response to microbicides offers a new insight in bacterial adaptation and the expression of mechanisms of resistance and cross-resistance to other antimicrobials.

The impact of bacterial resistance to microbicides in practice has not been well established despite the increase in the indiscriminate use of microbicides. Recent evidence has highlighted a link between microbicide resistance and clinical resistance to antibiotics [16, 211], although not all microbicides might be associated with bacterial resistance and cross-resistance to unrelated antimicrobials *in situ* [212]. It should also be recognized that microbicides are used in complex formulations in practice. The effect of excipients on microbicide activity, let alone on the development of bacterial resistance, is not well established. It is clear, however, that a low concentration (inhibitory/subinhibitory) of a microbicide can lead to the expression of resistance in bacteria. Worryingly, the number of products containing low concentrations of microbicides is increasing. In addition, factors responsible for a decrease in microbicide efficacy (and thus allowing for bacterial survival) are not well understood by manufacturers and end-users [2].

References

1 SCENIHR, Scientific Committee on Emerging and Newly Identified Health Risks (2009) The antibiotic resistance effect of biocides, adopted by the SCENIHR on January 19, 2009.

2 Maillard, J.-Y. and Denyer, S.P. (2009) Emerging bacterial resistance following biocide exposure: should we be concerned? *Chemica Oggi*, **27**, 26–28.

3 Denyer, S.P. and Maillard, J.-Y. (2002) Cellular impermeability and uptake of biocides and antibiotics in Gram-negative bacteria. *Journal of Applied Microbiology*, **92** (Suppl.), 35–45.

4 Lambert, P.A. (2002) Cellular impermeability and uptake of biocides and antibiotics in Gram-positive bacteria and mycobacteria. *Journal of Applied Microbiology*, **92** (Suppl.), 46–55.

5 Maillard, J.-Y. (2002) Bacterial target sites for biocide action. *Journal of Applied Microbiology*, **92** (Suppl.), 16–27.

6 Maillard, J.-Y. (2007) Bacterial resistance to biocides in the healthcare environment: shall we be concerned? *Journal of Hospital Infection*, **65** (Suppl. 2), 60–72.

7 Gilbert, P. and Moore, L.E. (2005) Cationic antiseptics: diversity of action under a common epithet. *Journal of Applied Microbiology*, **99**, 703–715.

8 Maillard, J.-Y. (2005) Biocides: health care application. *Pharmaceutical Journal*, **275**, 639–642.

9 Tattawasart, U. *et al.* (2000) Cytological changes in chlorhexidine-resistant isolates of *Pseudomonas stutzeri*. *Journal of Antimicrobial Chemotherapy*, **45**, 145–152.

10 Tattawasart, U. *et al.* (2000) Membrane changes in *Pseudomonas stutzeri* strains resistant to chlorhexidine diacetate and cetylpyridinium chloride. *International Journal of Antimicrobial Agents*, **16**, 233–238.

11 Braoudaki, M. and Hilton, A.C. (2005) Mechanisms of resistance in *Salmonella enterica* adapted to erythromycin, benzalkonium chloride and triclosan. *International Journal of Antimicrobial Agents*, **25**, 31–37.

12 Maillard, J.-Y. (2005) Usage of antimicrobial biocides and products in the healthcare environment: efficacy, policies, management and perceived problems. *Therapeutics and Clinical Risk Management*, **1**, 340–370.

13 Bailey, A.M. *et al.* (2009) Exposure of *Escherichia coli* and *Salmonella enterica* serovar Typhimurium to triclosan induces a species-specific response, including drug detoxification. *Journal of Antimicrobial Chemotherapy*, **64**, 973–985.

14 Daniel, C. and Ramos, J.L. (2009) Adaptive drug resistance mediated by root-nodulation-cell division efflux pumps. *Clinical Microbiology and Infection*, **15**, 32–36.

15 Maseda, H. *et al.* (2009) Mutational upregulation of a resistance-nodulation-cell division-type multidrug efflux pump, SdeAB, upon exposure to a biocide, cetylpyridinium chloride, and antibiotic resistance in *Serratia marcescens*. *Antimicrobial Agents and Chemotherapy*, **53**, 5230–5235.

16 Duarte, R.S. *et al.* (2009) Epidemic of postsurgical infections caused by *Mycobacterium massiliense*. *Journal of Clinical Microbiology*, **47**, 2149–2155.

17 Adair, F.W. *et al.* (1971) Resistance of *Pseudomonas* to quaternary ammonium compounds. *Applied Microbiology*, **21**, 1058–1063.

18 Russell, A.D. (2002) Introduction of biocides into clinical practice and the impact on antibiotic-resistant bacteria. *Journal of Applied Microbiology*, **92** (Suppl.), 121–135.

19 Chapman, J.S. (2003) Disinfectant resistance mechanisms, cross-resistance, and co-resistance. *International Biodeterioration and Biodegradation*, **51**, 271–276.

20 Sanford, J.P. (1970) Disinfectants that don't. *Annals of Internal Medicine*, **72**, 282–283.

21 Prince, J. and Ayliffe, G.A.J. (1972) In-use testing of disinfectants in hospitals. *Journal of Clinical Pathology*, **25**, 586–589.

22 Centers for Disease Control (1974) *Disinfectant or Infectant: The Label Doesn't Always Say*, National Nosocomial Infections Study, Fourth Quarter, 1973, p. 18.

23 Griffiths, P.A. *et al.* (1997) Glutaraldehyde-resistant *Mycobacterium chelonae* from endoscope washer disinfectors. *Journal of Applied Microbiology*, **82**, 519–526.

24 Martin, D.J.H. *et al.* (2008) Resistance and cross-resistance to oxidising agents of bacterial isolates from endoscope washer disinfectors. *Journal of Hospital Infection*, **69**, 377–383.

25 Cookson, B. (2005) Clinical significance of emergence of bacterial antimicrobial resistance in the hospital environment. *Journal of Applied Microbiology*, **99**, 989–996.

26 Chapman, J.S. (1998) Characterizing bacterial resistance to preservatives and disinfectants. *International Biodeterioration and Biodegradation*, **41**, 241–245.

27 Chapman, J.S. *et al.* (1998) Preservative tolerance and resistance. *International Journal of Cosmetics*, **20**, 31–39.

28 Hammond, S.A. *et al.* (1987) Comparative susceptibility of hospital isolates of gram-negative bacteria to antiseptics and disinfectants. *Journal of Hospital Infection*, **9**, 255–264.

29 Russell, A.D. (2003) Biocide use and antibiotic resistance: the relevance of laboratory findings to clinical environmental situations. *Lancet Infectious Diseases*, **3**, 794–803.

30 Cloete, T.E. (2003) Resistance mechanisms of bacteria to antimicrobial compounds. *International Biodeterioration and Biodegradation*, **51**, 277–282.

31 Stickler, D.J. (1974) Chlorhexidine resistance in *Proteus mirabilis*. *Journal of Clinical Pathology*, **27**, 284–287.

32 Gillespie, M.T. *et al.* (1986) Plasmid-encoded resistance to acriflavine and quaternary ammonium compounds in methicillin-resistant *Staphylococcus aureus*. *FEMS Microbiology Letters*, **34**, 47–51.

33 Randall, L.P. *et al.* (2001) Association between cyclohexane resistance in *Salmonella* of different serovars and increased resistance to multiple antibiotics, disinfectants and dyes. *Journal of Medical Microbiology*, **50**, 919–924.

34 Romao, C.M.C.P.A. *et al.* (2005) Susceptibility of clinical isolates of multiresistant *Pseudomonas aeruginosa* to a hospital disinfectant and molecular typing. *Memorias do Instituto Oswaldo Cruz*, **100**, 541–548.

35 Sasatsu, M. *et al.* (1993) Triclosan-resistant *Staphylococcus aureus*. *Lancet*, **341**, 756.

36 Heath, R.J. *et al.* (1998) Broad spectrum antimicrobial biocides target the FabI component of fatty acid synthesis. *Journal of Biological Chemistry*, **273**, 30316–30320.

37 Bamber, A.I. and Neal, T.J. (1999) An assessment of triclosan susceptibility in methicillin resistant and methicillin sensitive *Staphylococcus aureus*. *Journal of Hospital Infection*, **41**, 107–109.

38 Randall, L.P. *et al.* (2004) Effect of triclosan or a phenolic farm disinfectant on the selection of antibiotic-resistant *Salmonella enterica*. *Journal of Antimicrobial Chemotherapy*, **54**, 621–627.

39 O'Rrourke, E.O. *et al.* (2003) Contaminated iodophor in the operating room. *American Journal of Infection Control*, **31**, 255–256.

40 Motgatla, R.M. *et al.* (1998) Isolation of *Salmonella* resistant to hypochlorous acid from a poultry abattoir. *Letters in Applied Microbiology*, **27**, 379–382.

41 Motgatla, R.M. *et al.* (2002) Mechanisms contributing to hypochlorous acid resistance of a *Salmonella* isolate from a poultry-processing plant. *Journal of Applied Microbiology*, **92**, 566–573.

42 Van Klingeren, B. and Pullen, W. (1993) Glutaraldehyde resistant mycobacteria from endoscope washers. *Journal of Hospital Infection*, **25**, 147–149.

43 Manzoor, S.E. *et al.* (1999) Reduced glutaraldehyde susceptibility in *Mycobacterium chelonae* associated with altered cell wall polysaccharides. *Journal of Antimicrobial Chemotherapy*, **43**, 759–765.

44 Fraud, S. *et al.* (2001) Comparison of the mycobactericidal activity of *ortho*-phthalaldehyde, glutaraldehyde and other dialdehydes by a quantitative suspension test. *Journal of Hospital Infection*, **48**, 214–221.

45 Walsh, S.E. *et al.* (2001) Possible mechanisms for the relative efficacies of ortho-phthalaldehyde and glutaraldehyde against glutaraldehyde-resistant *Mycobacterium chelonae*. *Journal of Applied Microbiology*, **91**, 80–92.

46 Nomura, K. *et al.* (2004) Antibiotic susceptibility of glutaraldehyde tolerant *Mycobacetrium chelonae* from bronchoscope washing machine. *American Journal of Infection Control*, **32**, 185–188.

47 Greenberg, J.T. and Demple, B. (1989) A global response induced in *Escherichia coli* by redox cycling agents overlaps with that induced by peroxide stress. *Journal of Bacteriology*, **171**, 3933–3939.

48 Greenberg, J.T. *et al.* (1990) Positive control of a global antioxidant defence regulon activated by superoxide-generating agents in *Escherichia coli*. *Proceedings of the National Academy of Sciences of the United States of America*, **87**, 6181–6185.

49 Dukan, S. and Touati, D. (1996) Hypochlorous acid stress in *Escherichia coli*: resistance, DNA damage, and comparison with hydrogen peroxide stress. *Journal of Bacteriology*, **178**, 6145–6150.

50 Flores, M. *et al.* (1997) Deterioration of raw materials and cosmetic products by preservative resistant micro-organisms. *International Biodeterioration and Biodegradation*, **40**, 157–160.

51 Hutchinson, J. *et al.* (2004) *Burkholderia cepacia* infections associated with intrinsically contaminated ultrasound gel: the role of microbial degradation of parabens. *Infection Control and Hospital Epidemiology*, **25**, 291–296.

52 Tattawasart, U. *et al.* (1999) Development of resistance to chlorhexidine diacetate and cetylpyridinium chloride in *Pseudomonas stutzeri* and changes in antibiotic susceptibility. *Journal of Hospital Infection*, **42**, 219–229.

53 Thomas, L. *et al.* (2000) Development of resistance to chlorhexidine diacetate in *Pseudomonas aeruginosa* and the effect of "residual" concentration. *Journal of Hospital Infection*, **46**, 297–303.

54 Winder, C.L. *et al.* (2000) Outer membrane protein shifts in biocide-resistant *Pseudomonas aeruginosa* PAO1. *Journal of Applied Microbiology*, **89**, 289–295.

55 McMurry, L.M. *et al.* (1998) Overexpression of *marA*, *soxS*, or *acrAB* produces resistance to triclosan in laboratory and clinical strains of *Escherichia coli*. *FEMS Microbiology Letters*, **166**, 305–309.

56 McMurry, L.M. *et al.* (1999) Genetic evidence that InhA of *Mycobacterium smegmatis* is a target for triclosan. *Antimicrobial Agents and Chemotherapy*, **43**, 711–713.

57 Walsh, S.E. *et al.* (2003) Development of bacterial resistance to several biocides and effects on antibiotic susceptibility. *Journal of Hospital Infection*, **55**, 98–107.

58 Cottell, A. *et al.* (2009) Triclosan-tolerant bacteria: changes in susceptibility to antibiotics. *Journal of Hospital Infection*, **72**, 71–76.

59 Thomas, L. *et al.* (2005) Antimicrobial activity of chlorhexidine diacetate and benzalkonium chloride against *Pseudomonas aeruginosa* and its response to biocide residues. *Journal of Applied Microbiology*, **98**, 533–543.

60 Wisplinghoff, H. *et al.* (2007) Resistance to disinfectants in epidemiologically defined clinical isolates of *Acinetobacter baumannii*. *Journal of Hospital Infection*, **66**, 174–181.

61 Monteros, L.E.E.D.L. *et al.* (2008) Outbreak of infection by extended-spectrum beta-lactamase SHV-5-producing *Serratia marcescens* in a Mexican hospital. *Journal of Chemotherapy*, **20**, 586–592.

62 Lear, J.C. *et al.* (2002) Chloroxylenol- and triclosan- tolerant bacteria from industrial sources. *Journal of Industrial Microbiology and Biotechnology*, **29**, 238–242.

63 Moyer, C.A. *et al.* (1965) Treatment of large burns with 0.5% silver nitrate solution. *Archives of Surgery*, **90**, 812–867.

64 Cason, J.S. *et al.* (1966) Antiseptic and septic prophylaxis for burns: use of silver nitrate and of isolators. *British Medical Journal*, **2**, 1288–1294.

65 Bridges, K. and Lowbury, E.J.L. (1977) Drug-resistance in relation to use of sliver sulfadiazine cream in a burns unit. *Journal of Clinical Pathology*, **30**, 160–164.

66 Klasen, H.J. (2000) A historical review of the use of silver in the treatment of burns. II. Renewed interest for silver. *Burns*, **26**, 131–138.

67 Reiss, I. *et al.* (2000) Disinfectant contaminated with *Klebsiella oxytoca* as a source of sepsis in babies. *Lancet*, **356**, 310.

68 Weber, D.J. *et al.* (2007) Outbreaks associated with contaminated antiseptics and disinfectants. *Antimicrobial Agents and Chemotherapy*, **51**, 4217–4224.

69 McMurry, L.M. *et al.* (1998) Triclosan targets lipid synthesis. *Nature*, **394**, 531–532.

70 Levy, C.W. *et al.* (1999) Molecular basis of triclosan activity. *Nature*, **398**, 384–385.

71 Roujeinikova, A. *et al.* (1999) Crystallographic analysis of triclosan bound to enoyl reductase. *Journal of Molecular Biology*, **294**, 527–535.

72 Stewart, M.J. *et al.* (1999) Structural basis and mechanisms of enoyl reductase inhibition by triclosan. *Journal of Molecular Biology*, **290**, 859–865.

73 Parikh, S.L. *et al.* (2000) Inhibition of InhA, enoyl reductase from *Mycobacterium tuberculosis* by triclosan and isoniazid. *Biochemistry*, **39**, 7645–7650.

74 Webber, M.A. *et al.* (2008) Proteomic analysis of triclosan resistance in *Salmonella enterica* serovar Typhimurium. *Journal of Antimicrobial Chemotherapy*, **62**, 92–97.

75 McDonnell, G. and Russell, A.D. (1999) Antiseptics and disinfectants: activity, action and resistance. *Clinical Microbiology Reviews*, **12**, 147–179.

76 Mc Cay, P.H. *et al.* (2010) Effect of subinhibitory concentrations of benzalkonium chloride on the competitiveness of *Pseudomonas aeruginosa* grown in continuous culture. *Microbiology*, **156**, 30–38.

77 Cheeseman, K.E. *et al.* (2009) Evaluation of the bactericidal efficacy of three different alcohol hand rubs against 57 clinical isolates of *Staphylococcus aureus*. *Journal of Hospital Infection*, **72**, 319–325.

78 Williams, G.J. *et al.* (2009) The use of sodium dichloroisocyanurate, NaDCC, in Welsh ITUs. *Journal of Hospital Infection*, **72**, 279–281.

79 Poole, K. (2002) Mechanisms of bacterial biocide and antibiotic resistance. *Journal of Applied Microbiology*, **92** (Suppl.), 55–64.

80 Piddock, L.J.V. (2006) Multidrug resistance efflux pumps – not just for resistance. *Nature Reviews Microbiology*, **4**, 629–636.

81 Poole, K. (2007) Efflux pumps as antimicrobial resistance mechanisms. *Annals of Medicine*, **39**, 162–176.

82 Maillard, J.-Y. (2010) Incidence of sporicide resistance and risk to the population. *Journal of Hospital Infection*, **77**, 204–209.

83 Lyon, B.R. and Skurray, R.A. (1987) Antimicrobial resistance of *Staphylococcus aureus*: genetic basis. *Microbiology Reviews*, **51**, 88–134.

84 Silver, S. *et al.* (1989) Bacterial ATPases – primary pumps for exploring toxic cations and anions. *Trends in Biochemical Sciences*, **14**, 76–80.

85 White, D.G. and McDermott, P.F. (2001) Biocides, drug resistance and microbial evolution. *Current Opinion in Microbiology*, **4**, 313–317.

86 Kücken, D. *et al.* (2000) Association of *qacE* and *qacEΔ1* with multiple resistance to antibiotics and antiseptics in clinical isolates of Gram-negative bacteria. *FEMS Microbiology Letters*, **183**, 95–98.

87 Bjorland, J. *et al.* (2001) Plasmid-borne *smr* gene causes resistance to quaternary ammonium compounds in bovine *Staphylococcus aureus*. *Journal of Clinical Microbiology*, **39**, 3999–4004.

88 Pearce, H. *et al.* (1999) Effect of biocides commonly used in the hospital environment on the transfer of antibiotic-resistance genes in *Staphylococcus aureus*. *Journal of Hospital Infection*, **43**, 101–108.

89 Karatzas, K.A.G. *et al.* (2008) Phenotypic and proteomic characterisation of multiply antibiotic-resistant variants of *Salmonella enterica* serovar Typhimurium selected following exposure to disinfectants. *Applied and Environmental Microbiology*, **74**, 1508–1516.

90 Chen, Y. *et al.* (2009) Triclosan resistance in clinical isolates of *Acinetobacter baumannii*. *Journal of Medical Microbiology*, **58**, 1086–1091.

91 Russell, A.D. (2002) Antibiotic and biocide resistance in bacteria: comments and conclusion. *Journal of Applied Microbiology*, **92** (Suppl.), 171–173.

92 Champlin, F.R. *et al.* (2005) Effect of outer membrane permeabilisation on intrinsic resistance to low triclosan levels in *Pseudomonas aeruginosa*. *International Journal of Antimicrobial Agents*, **26**, 159–164.

93 Russell, A.D. *et al.* (1997) Microbial susceptibility and resistance to biocides: an understanding. *ASM News*, **63**, 481–487.

94 Russell, A.D. (1990) Bacterial spores and chemical sporicidal agents. *Clinical Microbiology Reviews*, **3**, 99–119.

95 Fraud, S. *et al.* (2003) Effects of ortho-phthalaldehyde, glutaraldehyde and chlorhexidine diacetate on *Mycobacterium chelonae* and *M. abscessus* strains with modified permeability. *Journal of Antimicrobial Chemotherapy*, **51**, 575–584.

96 Munton, T.J. and Russell, A.D. (1970) Effect of glutaraldehyde on protoplasts of *Bacillus megaterium*. *Journal of General Microbiology*, **63**, 367–370.

97 Ayres, H.M. *et al.* (1998) Effect of permeabilizing agents on antibacterial activity against a simple *Pseudomonas aeruginosa* biofilm. *Letters in Applied Microbiology*, **27**, 79–82.

98 Gandhi, P.A. *et al.* (1993) Adaptation and growth of *Serratia marcescens* in contact lens disinfectant solution containing chlorhexidine gluconate. *Applied and Environmental Microbiology*, **59**, 183–188.

99 Brözel, V.S. and Cloete, T.E. (1994) Resistance of *Pseudomonas aeruginosa* to isothiazolone. *Journal of Applied Bacteriology*, **76**, 576–582.

100 Jones, M.W. *et al.* (1989) Resistance of *Pseudomonas aeruginosa* to amphoteric and quaternary ammonium biocides. *Microbios*, **58**, 49–61.

101 Méchin, L. *et al.* (1999) Adaptation of *Pseudomonas aeruginosa* ATCC 15442 to didecyldimethylammonium bromide induces changes in membrane fatty acid composition and in resistance of cells. *Journal of Applied Microbiology*, **86**, 859–866.

102 Guérin-Méchin, L. *et al.* (1999) Specific variations of fatty acid composition of *Pseudomonas aeruginosa* ATCC 15442 induced by quaternary ammonium compounds and relation with resistance to bactericidal activity. *Journal of Applied Microbiology*, **87**, 735–742.

103 Guérin-Méchin, L. *et al.* (2000) Quaternary ammonium compounds stresses induce specific variations in fatty acid composition of *Pseudomonas aeruginosa. International Journal of Food Microbiology*, **55**, 157–159.

104 Boeris, P.S. *et al.* (2007) Modification of phospholipid composition in *Pseudomonas putida* A ATCC 12633 induced by contact with tetradecyltrimethylammonium. *Journal of Applied Microbiology*, **103**, 1048–1054.

105 McNeil, M.R. and Brennan, P.J. (1991) Structure, function and biogenesis of the cell envelope of mycobacteria in relation to bacterial physiology, pathogenesis and drug resistance; some thoughts and possibilities arising from recent structural information. *Research in Microbiology*, **142**, 451–463.

106 Broadley, S.J. *et al.* (1995) Potentiation of the effects of chlorhexidine diacetate and cetylpyridinium chloride on mycobacteria by ethambutol. *Journal of Medical Microbiology*, **43**, 458–460.

107 Russell, A.D. (1996) Activity of biocides against mycobacteria. *Journal of Applied Bacteriology*, **81**, 87–101.

108 Bruinsma, G.M. *et al.* (2006) Resistance to a polyquaternium-1 lens care solution and isoelectric points of *Pseudomonas aeruginosa* strains. *Journal of Antimicrobial Chemotherapy*, **57**, 764–766.

109 Brown, M.H. *et al.* (1999) The multidrug efflux protein NorM is a prototype of a new family of transporters. *Molecular Microbiology*, **31**, 393–395.

110 Borges-Walmsley, M.I. and Walmsley, A.R. (2001) The structure and function of drug pumps. *Trends in Microbiology*, **9**, 71–79.

111 Poole, K. (2001) Multidrug resistance in Gram-negative bacteria. *Current Opinion in Microbiology*, **4**, 500–508.

112 Poole, K. (2002) Outer membranes and efflux: the path to multidrug resistance in Gram-negative bacteria. *Current Pharmaceutical Biotechnology*, **3**, 77–98.

113 McKeegan, K.S. *et al.* (2003) The structure and function of drug pumps: an update. *Trends in Microbiology*, **11**, 21–29.

114 Tennent, J.M. *et al.* (1989) Physical and biochemical characterization of the *qacA* gene encoding antiseptic and disinfectant resistance in *Staphylococcus aureus. Journal of General Microbiology*, **135**, 1–10.

115 Littlejohn, T.G. *et al.* (1992) Substrate specificity and energetics of antiseptic and disinfectant resistance in *Staphylococcus aureus. FEMS Microbiology Letters*, **95**, 259–266.

116 Leelaporn, A. *et al.* (1994) Multidrug resistance to antiseptics and disinfectants in coagulase-negative staphylococci. *Journal of Medical Microbiology*, **40**, 214–220.

117 Heir, E. *et al.* (1998) The *Staphylococcus qacH* gene product: a new member of the SMR family encoding multidrug resistance. *FEMS Microbiology Letters*, **163**, 49–56.

118 Heir, E. *et al.* (1999) The *qacG* gene on plasmid pST94 confers resistance to quaternary ammonium compounds in staphylococci isolated from the food industry. *Journal of Applied Microbiology*, **86**, 378–388.

119 Rouche, D.A. *et al.* (2051) 1990) Efflux-mediated antiseptic gene *qacA* in *Staphylococcus aureus*: common ancestry with tetracycline and sugar transport proteins. *Molecular Microbiology*, **4**, 2062.

120 Chuanchuen, R. *et al.* (2001) Cross-resistance between triclosan and antibiotics in *Pseudomonas aeruginosa* is mediated by multidrug efflux pumps: exposure of a susceptible mutant strain to triclosan selects *nxfB* mutants overexpressing MexCD-OprJ. *Antimicrobial Agents and Chemotherapy*, **45**, 428–432.

121 Chuanchuen, R. *et al.* (2002) The MexJK efflux pump of *Pseudomonas aeruginosa* requires OprM for antibiotic efflux but not for effect of triclosan. *Journal of Bacteriology*, **184**, 5036–5044.

122 Randall, L.P. *et al.* (2007) Commonly used farm disinfectants can select for mutant *Salmonella enterica* serovar Typhimurium with decreased susceptibility to biocides and antibiotics without compromising virulence. *Journal of Antimicrobial Chemotherapy*, **60**, 1273–1280.

123 Webber, M.A. *et al.* (2008) Triclosan resistance in *Salmonella enterica* serovar Typhimurium. *Journal of Antimicrobial Chemotherapy*, **62**, 83–91.

124 Mima, T. *et al.* (2007) Identification and characterization of TriABC-OpmH, a triclosan efflux pump of *Pseudomonas aeruginosa* requiring two membrane fusion proteins. *Journal of Bacteriology*, **189**, 7600–7609.

125 Schweizer, H.P. (1998) Intrinsic resistance to inhibitors of fatty acid biosynthesis in *Pseudomonas aeruginosa* is due to efflux: application of a novel technique for generation of unmarked chromosomal mutations for the study of efflux systems. *Antimicrobial Agents and Chemotherapy*, **42**, 394–398.

126 Chuanchuen, R. *et al.* (2003) High-level triclosan resistance in *Pseudomonas aeruginosa* is solely a result of efflux. *American Journal of Infection Control*, **31**, 124–127.

127 Levy, S.B. (2002) Active efflux, a common mechanism for biocide and antibiotic resistance. *Journal of Applied Microbiology*, **92** (Suppl.), 65–71.

128 Kummerle, N. *et al.* (1996) Plasmid-mediated formaldehyde resistance in *Escherichia coli*: characterization of resistance gene. *Antimicrobial Agents and Chemotherapy*, **40**, 2276–2279.

129 Demple, B. (1996) Redox signaling and gene control in the *Escherichia coli* soxRS oxidative stress regulon – a review. *Gene*, **179**, 53–57.

130 Valkova, N. *et al.* (2001) Hydrolysis of 4-hydroxybenzoic acid esters (parabens) and their aerobic transformation into phenol by the resistant *Enterobacter cloacae* strain EM. *Applied and Environmental Microbiology*, **67**, 2404–2409.

131 Codling, C.E. *et al.* (2004) Identification of genes involved in the resistance *Serratia marcescens* to polyquaternium-1. *Journal of Antimicrobial Chemotherapy*, **54**, 370–375.

132 Stickler, D.J. (2004) Intrinsic resistance of Gram-negative bacteria, in *Principles and Practice of Disinfection, Preservation and Sterilization*, 4th edn (eds A.P. Fraise *et al.*), Blackwell Scientific Publications, Oxford, pp. 154–169.

133 Sundheim, G. *et al.* (1998) Bacterial resistance to disinfectants containing quaternary ammonium compounds. *International Biodeterioration and Biodegradation*, **41**, 235–239.

134 Morita, Y. *et al.* (2003) Induction of mexCD-oprJ operon for a multidrug efflux pump by disinfectants in wild-type *Pseudomonas aeruginosa* PAO1. *Journal of Antimicrobial Chemotherapy*, **51**, 991–994.

135 Moken, M.C. *et al.* (1997) Selection of multiple-antibiotic-resistant (Mar) mutants of *Escherichia coli* by using the disinfectant pine oil: roles of the *mar* and *acrAB* loci. *Antimicrobial Agents and Chemotherapy*, **41**, 2770–2772.

136 Nishino, K. and Yamagushi, A. (2001) Analysis of a complete library of putative drug transporter genes in *Escherichia coli. Journal of Bacteriology*, **183**, 5803–5812.

137 Lomovskaya, O. and Lewis, K. (1992) *emr*, an *Escherichia coli* locus for multidrug resistance. *Proceedings of the National Academy of Sciences of the United States of America*, **89**, 8938–8942.

138 Davin-Regli, A. *et al.* (2008) Membrane permeability and regulation of drug "influx and efflux" in enterobacterial pathogens. *Current Drug Targets*, **9**, 750–759.

139 Rajamohan, G. *et al.* (2010) Novel role of *Acinetobacter baumannii* RND efflux transporters in mediating decreased susceptibility to biocides. *Journal of Antimicrobial Chemotherapy*, **65**, 228–232.

140 Buckley, A. *et al.* (2006) The AcrAB-TolC efflux system of *Salmonella enterica* serovar Typhimurium plays a role in pathogenesis. *Cellular Microbiology*, **8**, 847–856.

141 Sánchez, P. *et al.* (2005) The biocide triclosan selects *Stenotrophomonas maltophilia* mutants that overproduce the SmeDEF multidrug efflux pump. *Antimicrobial Agents and Chemotherapy*, **49**, 781–782.

142 Pumbwe, L. *et al.* (2005) Expression of the efflux pump genes *cmeB, cmeF* and the porin gene *porA* in multiply antibiotic-resistant *Campylobacter* spp. *Journal of Antimicrobial Chemotherapy*, **54**, 341–347.

143 Tkachenko, O. *et al.* (2007) A triclosan-ciprofloxacin cross-resistant mutant strain of *Staphylococcus aureus* displays an alteration in the expression of several cell membrane structural and functional genes. *Research in Microbiology*, **158**, 651–658.

144 Heath, R. *et al.* (1999) Mechanism of triclosan inhibition of bacterial fatty acid biosynthesis. *Journal of Biological Chemistry*, **274**, 11110–11114.

145 Zhu, L. *et al.* (2010) Triclosan resistance of *Pseudomonas aeruginosa* PA01 is due to FabV, a triclosan-resistant enoyl-acyl carrier protein reductase. *Antimicrobial Agents and Chemotherapy*, **54**, 689–698.

146 Heath, R.J. *et al.* (2000) Inhibition of the *Staphylococcus aureus* NADPH-dependent enoyl-acyl carrier protein reductase by triclosan and hexachlorophene. *Journal of Biological Biochemistry*, **275**, 4654–4659.

147 Slater-Radosti, C. *et al.* (2001) Biochemical and genetic characterization of the action of triclosan on *Staphylococcus aureus. Journal of Antimicrobial Chemotherapy*, **48**, 1–6.

148 Massengo-Tiassé, R.P. and Cronan, J.E. (2008) *Vibrio cholerae* FabV defines a new class of enoyl-acyl carrier protein reductase. *Journal of Biological Chemistry*, **283**, 1308–1316.

149 Brown, M.R.W. and William, P. (1985) Influence of substrate limitation and growth-phase on sensitivity to antimicrobial agents. *Journal of Antimicrobial Chemotherapy*, **15**, 7–14.

150 Wright, N.E. and Gilbert, P. (1987) Influence of specific growth rate and nutrient limitation upon the sensitivity of *Escherichia coli* towards chlorhexidine diacetate. *Journal of Applied Bacteriology*, **62**, 309–314.

151 Gomez Escalada, M. *et al.* (2005) Triclosan inhibition of fatty acid synthesis and its effect on growth of *E. coli* and *Ps. aeruginosa. Journal of Antimicrobial Chemotherapy*, **55**, 879–882.

152 Ma, D. *et al.* (1994) Efflux pumps and drug resistance in Gram-negative bacteria. *Trends in Microbiology*, **2**, 489–493.

153 Greenway, D.L.A. and England, R.R. (1999) The intrinsic resistance of *Escherichia coli* to various antimicrobial agents requires ppGpp and σˢ. *Letters in Applied Microbiology*, **29**, 323–326.

154 Allen, M.J. *et al.* (2006) The response of *Escherichia coli* to exposure to the biocide polyhexamethylene biguanide. *Microbiology*, **152**, 989–1000.

155 Jang, H.-J. *et al.* (2008) Microarray analysis of toxicogenomic effects of triclosan on *Staphylococcus aureus. Applied Microbiology and Biotechnology*, **78**, 695–707.

156 Abdel Malek, S.M.A. *et al.* (2002) Antimicrobial susceptibility changes and T-OMP shifts in pythione-passaged planktonic cultures of *Pseudomonas aeruginosa* PAO1. *Journal of Applied Microbiology*, **92**, 729–736.

157 Kastbjerg, V.G. *et al.* (2010) Influence of sublethal concentrations of common disinfectants on expression of virulence genes in *Listeria monocytogenes. Applied and Environmental Microbiology*, **76**, 303–309.

158 Gilbert, P. *et al.* (2003) Formation of microbial biofilm in hygienic situations: a problem of control. *International Biodeterioration and Biodegradation*, **51**, 245–248.

159 Bisset, L. *et al.* (2006) A prospective study of the efficacy of routine decontamination for gastrointestinal endoscopes and the risk factors for failure. *American Journal of Infection Control*, **34**, 274–280.

160 Smith, K. and Hunter, I.S. (2008) Efficacy of common hospital biocides with biofilms of multi-drug resistant clinical isolates. *Journal of Medical Microbiology*, **57**, 966–973.

161 Brown, M.R.W. and Gilbert, P. (1993) Sensitivity of biofilms to antimicrobial agents. *Journal of Applied Bacteriology*, **74** (Suppl.), 87–97.

162 Ashby, M.J. *et al.* (1994) Effect of antibiotics on non-growing planktonic cells and biofilms of *Escherichia coli. Journal of Antimicrobial Chemotherapy*, **33**, 443–452.

163 Das, J.R. *et al.* (1998) Changes in the biocide susceptibility of *Staphylococcus epidermidis* and *Escherichia coli* cells associated with rapid attachment to plastic surfaces. *Journal of Applied Microbiology*, **84**, 852–858.

164 Pan, Y. *et al.* (2006) Resistance of *Listeria monocytogenes* biofilms to sanitizing agents in a simulated food processing environment. *Applied and Environmental Microbiology*, **72**, 7711–7717.

165 Tart, A.H. and Wozniak, D.J. (2008) Shifting paradigms in *Pseudomonas aeruginosa* biofilm research. *Current Topics in Microbiology and Immunology*, **322**, 193–206.

166 Sondossi, M. *et al.* (1985) Observations of resistance and cross-resistance to formaldehyde and a formaldehyde condensate biocide in *Pseudomonas aeruginosa. International Biodeterioration*, **21**, 105–106.

167 Huang, C.T. *et al.* (1995) Nonuniform spatial patterns of respiratory activity within biofilms during disinfection. *Applied and Environmental Microbiology*, **61**, 2252–2256.

168 Maira-Litrán, T. *et al.* (2000) An evaluation of the potential of the multiple antibiotic resistance operon (*mar*) and the multidrug efflux pump *acrAB* to moderate resistance towards ciprofloxacin in *Escherichia coli* biofilms. *Journal of Antimicrobial Chemotherapy*, **45**, 789–795.

169 Lai, S. *et al.* (2009) Swarming motility: a multicellular behaviour conferring antimicrobial resistance. *Environmental Microbiology*, **11**, 126–136.

170 Moore, L.E. *et al.* (2008) *In vitro* study of the effect of cationic biocides on bacterial population dynamics and susceptibility. *Applied and Environmental Microbiology*, **74**, 4825–4834.

171 McBain, A.J. *et al.* (2004) Effects of quaternary-ammonium based formulations on bacterial community dynamics and antimicrobial susceptibility. *Applied and Environmental Microbiology*, **70**, 3449–3456.

172 Kümmerer, K. *et al.* (2002) Use of chemotaxonomy to study the influence of benzalkonium chloride on bacterial populations in biodegradation testing. *Acta Hydrochima et Hydrobiologica*, **30**, 171–178.

173 McBain, A.J. *et al.* (2003) Exposure of sink drain microcosms to triclosan: population dynamics and antimicrobial susceptibility. *Applied and Environmental Microbiology*, **69**, 5433–5442.

174 Jones, G.Ll, *et al.* (2006) Effect of triclosan on the development of bacterial biofilms by urinary tract pathogens on urinary catheters. *Journal of Antimicrobial Chemotherapy*, **57**, 266–272.

175 Stickler, D.J. and Jones, G.L. (2008) Reduced Susceptibility of *Proteus mirabilis* to triclosan. *Antimicrobial Agents and Chemotherapy*, **52**, 991–994.

176 Davison, J. (1999) Genetic exchange between bacteria in the environment. *Plasmid*, **42**, 73–91.

177 Roberts, A.P. and Mullany, P. (2009) A modular master on the move: the Tn916 family of mobile genetic elements. *Trends in Microbiology*, **17**, 251–258.

178 Schlüter, A. *et al.* (2007) Genomics of IncP-1 antibiotic resistance plasmids isolated from wastewater treatment plants provides evidence for a widely accessible drug resistance gene pool. *FEMS Microbiology Reviews*, **31**, 449–477.

179 Sidhu, M.S. *et al.* (2002) Frequency of disinfectant resistance genes and genetic linkage with beta-lactamase transposon Tn552 among clinical staphylococci. *Antimicrobial Agents and Chemotherapy*, **46**, 2797–2803.

180 Paulsen, I.T. *et al.* (1998) Characterization of the earliest known *Staphylococcus aureus* plasmid encoding a multidrug efflux system. *Journal of Bacteriology*, **180**, 3477–3479.

181 Sidhu, M.S. *et al.* (2001) Genetic linkage between resistance to quaternary ammonium compounds and beta-lactam antibiotics in food-related *Staphylococcus* spp. *Microbial Drug Resistance*, **7**, 363–371.

182 Noguchi, N. *et al.* (2005) Susceptibilities to antiseptic agents and distribution of antiseptic-resistance genes *qacA/B* and *smr* of methicillin-resistant *Staphylococcus aureus* isolated in Asia during 1998 and 1999. *Journal of Medical Microbiology*, **54**, 557–565.

183 Hansen, L.H. *et al.* (2005) The prevalence of the OqxAB multidrug efflux pump amongst olaquindox-resistant *Escherichia coli* in pigs. *Microbial Drug Resistance*, **11**, 378–382.

184 Hansen, L.H. *et al.* (2007) Substrate specificity of the OqxAB multidrug resistance pump in *Escherichia coli* and selected enteric bacteria. *Journal of Antimicrobial Chemotherapy*, **60**, 145–147.

185 Laraki, N. *et al.* (1999) Structure of In31, a blaIMP-containing *Pseudomonas aeruginosa* integron phyletically related to In5, which carries an unusual array of gene cassettes. *Antimicrobial Agents and Chemotherapy*, **43**, 890–901.

186 Quinn, T. *et al.* (2006) Multi-drug resistance in *Salmonella enterica*: efflux mechanisms and their relationships with the development of chromosomal resistance gene clusters. *Current Drug Targets*, **7**, 849–860.

187 Hawkey, P.M. and Jones, A.M. (2009) The changing epidemiology of resistance. *Journal of Antimicrobial Chemotherapy*, **64** (Suppl. 1), 3–10.

188 Juhas, M. *et al.* (2009) Genomic islands: tools of bacterial horizontal gene transfer and evolution. *FEMS Microbiology Reviews*, **33**, 376–393.

189 Birošová, L. and Mikulášová, M. (2009) Development of triclosan and antibiotic resistance in *Salmonella enterica* serovar Typhimurium. *Journal of Medical Microbiology*, **58**, 436–441.

190 Davies, D.G. *et al.* (1998) The involvement of cell-to-cell signals in the development of a bacterial biofilm. *Science*, **280**, 295–298.

191 Shih, P.C. and Huang, C.T. (2002) Effects of quorum-sensing deficiency on *Pseudomonas aeruginosa* biofilm formation and antibiotic resistance. *Journal of Antimicrobial Chemotherapy*, **49**, 309–314.

192 MacLehose, H.G. *et al.* (2004) Biofilms, homoserine lactones and biocide susceptibility. *Journal of Antimicrobial. Chemotherapy*, **53**, 180–184.

193 Davies, A.J. and Maillard, J.-Y. (2001) Bacterial adaptation to biocides: the possible role of "alarmones". *Journal of Hospital Infection*, **49**, 300–301.

194 Cerf, O. *et al.* (2010) Tests for determining in-use concentrations of antibiotics and disinfectants are based on entirely different concepts: "resistance" has different meanings. *International Journal of Food Microbiology*, **136**, 247–254.

195 Russell, A.D. and McDonnell, G. (2000) Concentration: a major factor in studying biocidal action. *Journal of Hospital Infection*, **44**, 1–3.

196 Langsrud, S. *et al.* (2003) Bacterial disinfectant resistance – a challenge for the food industry. *International Biodeterioration and Biodegradation*, **51**, 283–290.

197 Lear, J.C. *et al.* (2006) Chloroxylenol- and triclosan-tolerant bacteria from industrial sources – susceptibility to antibiotics and other biocides. *International Biodeterioration and Biodegradation*, **57**, 51–56.

198 Gomez Escalada, M. *et al.* (2005) Triclosan-bacteria interactions: single or multiple target sites? *Letters in Applied Microbiology*, **41**, 476–481.

199 Braoudaki, M. and Hilton, A.C. (2004) Adaptive resistance in *Salmonella enterica* and *Escherichia coli* O157 and cross-resistance to antimicrobial agents. *Journal of Clinical Microbiology*, **42**, 73–78.

200 Braoudaki, M. and Hilton, A.C. (2004) Low level of cross-resistance between triclosan and antibiotics in *Escherichia coli* K-12 and *E. coli* O5 compared to *E. coli* O157. *FEMS Microbiology Letters*, **235**, 305–309.

201 Gilbert, P. and McBain, A.J. (2003) Potential impact of increased use of biocides in consumer products on prevalence of antibiotic resistance. *Clinical Microbiology Review*, **16**, 189–208.

202 Russell, A.D. (2004) Bacterial adaptation and resistance to antiseptics, disinfectants and preservatives is not a new phenomenon. *Journal of Hospital Infection*, **57**, 97–104.

203 Aiello, A.E. *et al.* (2005) Antibacterial cleaning products and drug resistance. *Emerging Infectious Diseases*, **11**, 1565–1570.

204 Aiello, A.E. *et al.* (2007) Consumer antibacterial soaps: effective or just risky? *Clinical Infectious Diseases*, **45** (Suppl. 2), 137–147.

205 Alonso-Hernando, A. *et al.* (2009) Comparison of antibiotic resistance patterns in *Listeria monocytogenes* and *Salmonella enterica* strains pre-exposed and exposed to poultry decontaminants. *Food Control*, **20**, 1108–1111.

206 Weber, D.J. and Rutala, W.A. (2006) Use of germicides in the home and the health care setting: is there a relationship between germicide use and antibiotic resistance? *Infection Control and Hospital Epidemiology*, **27**, 1107–1119.

207 Pumbwe, L. *et al.* (2007) Induction of multiple antibiotic resistance in *Bacteroides fragilis* by benzene and benzene-derived active compounds of commonly used analgesics, antiseptics and cleaning agents. *Journal of Antimicrobial Chemotherapy*, **60**, 1288–1297.

208 Lara, H.H. *et al.* (2010) Bactericidal effect of silver nanoparticles against multidrug-resistant bacteria. *World Journal of Microbiology and Biotechnology*, **26**, 615–621.

209 Walsh, C. and Fanning, S. (2008) Antimicrobial resistance in foodborne pathogens–a cause for concern? *Current Drug Targets*, **9**, 808–815.

210 Fraise, A.P. (2004) Biocide abuse and antimicrobial resistance – a cause for concern. *Journal of Antimicrobial Chemotherapy*, **49**, 11–12.

211 Carson, R.T. *et al.* (2008) Use of antibacterial consumer products containing quaternary ammonium compounds and drug resistance in the community. *Journal of Antimicrobial Chemotherapy*, **62**, 1160–1162.

212 Cole, E.C. *et al.* (2003) Investigation of antibiotic and antibacterial agent cross-resistance in target bacteria from homes of antibacterial product users and non users. *Journal of Applied Microbiology*, **95**, 664–679.

6.2 Resistance of Bacterial Spores to Chemical Agents

Peter Setlow

Department of Molecular, Microbial and Structural Biology, University of Connecticut Health Center, Farmington, CT, USA

Introduction

Dormant spores of the genera *Bacillales* and *Clostridiales* are among the most resistant life forms known. Given that some of these organisms cause food spoilage and/or disease, there has long been interest in mechanisms of spore killing and resistance. A variety of agents will kill spores including UV and γ-radiation, high pressure and wet heat. However, for many applications, in particular for thermosensitive materials, chemicals are the agent of choice for spore killing, with such chemicals commonly termed sporicides. In general, spores are resistant to disinfectants used to kill growing bacteria and are much more resistant to sporicides than are growing cells [1–3]. Resistance to different chemicals is acquired at various times during spore formation, depending on when spore components that are important in resistance are synthesized or assembled. Resistance to sporicides and common disinfectants is lost during spore germination as dormant spores return to active growth. In general, completion of spore germination is required for full loss of resistance to many chemicals, although degradation of DNA-protective proteins early in outgrowth is essential for full loss of resistance to some genotoxic chemicals.

This section will focus on spore resistance to chemical disinfectants and sporicides. Mechanisms of spore resistance to such chemicals will be discussed, as will mechanisms of spore killing by sporicides, focusing primarily on spores of *Bacillus subtilis*. However, there will also be a summary of what is known about mechanisms for chemical killing and resistance of spores of *Clostridium* species. Previous reviews on spore resistance to and killing by chemicals include one in the previous edition of this book, as well as more recent reviews [1–9].

Spore structure

Much work shows that spore chemical resistance is due to novel spore structures and components [1–3]. Consequently, it is useful to review spore structures and components and their key properties. Almost all work on mechanisms of spore resistance and killing has been with spores of *B. subtilis*, and it is reasonable to question whether these results are applicable to spores of other species and genera. Spores of *Bacillales* and *Clostridiales* species share the same general novel structural features (Figure 6.2.1) and components and may therefore be of particular interest.

Russell, Hugo & Ayliffe's: Principles and Practice of Disinfection, Preservation and Sterilization, Fifth Edition. Edited by Adam P. Fraise, Jean-Yves Maillard, and Syed A. Sattar.
© 2013 Blackwell Publishing Ltd. Published 2013 by Blackwell Publishing Ltd.

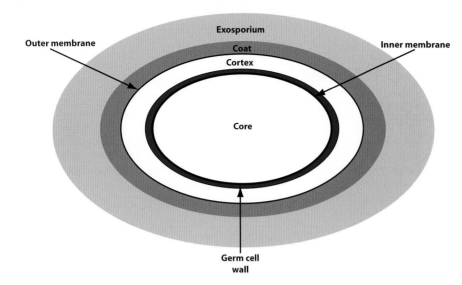

Figure 6.2.1 Schematic structure of a spore of *Bacillus* or *Clostridium* species. Note that spores of some species lack an exosporium, the sizes of the different spore layers are not drawn to scale, and the relative sizes of these layers can vary with the species/ strain as well as the sporulation conditions.

Exosporium

Starting from the outside and working inwards, spores of some species (e.g. pathogens such as *Bacillus cereus* and *Bacillus anthracis*) contain an outermost exosporium composed of proteins and glycoproteins [3, 10, 11], although spores of many species, including *B. subtilis* lack an exosporium. The exosporium proteins are unique to spores and many are unique to the exosporium, although some exosporium proteins are orthologs of proteins in the next spore layer, the coat [10–13]. One role of the exosporium is as a permeability barrier against enzymes and antibodies. In addition, the exosporium of *B. anthracis* spores at least contains enzymes that can detoxify reactive chemicals, and these enzymes can play a role in spore resistance [10, 14].

Coat

The next spore layer is the coat, composed largely of proteins, with ≥70 spore-specific proteins identified in the *B. subtilis* spore coat [10, 11]. In spores of many species, the coat contains several layers and contains large amounts of insoluble protein, some of which is cross-linked. The coat plays a major role in the resistance of spores to enzymes that can degrade the more internal peptidoglycan (PG) layers of spores, and thus protects them against predators [11, 15, 16]. Coat proteins comprise *c.* 50% of spore protein, and may act as reactive armor to detoxify chemicals before they can attack essential spore components further within the spore. Like the exosporium, the coat also contains enzymes that can detoxify reactive chemicals [11].

Outer membrane

Beneath the coat is the spore's outer membrane, derived from the plasma membrane of the mother cell that engulfs the developing spore during sporulation. While this membrane is essential during sporulation, it is probably not important in spore resistance, and may not be a significant permeability barrier in dormant spores [2].

Cortex and germ cell wall

Under the spore's outer membrane there are two layers of PG, the large cortex and the thinner germ cell wall [17]. The germ cell wall PG structure appears identical to that of growing cell wall PG, and while the cortex PG structure is similar to that of germ cell wall PG, it has modifications. One of these modifications, muramic acid-δ-lactam, allows cortex PG to be selectively degraded by endogenous cortex lytic enzymes (CLEs) in the first minutes of spore germination. In contrast, germ cell wall PG lacks muramic acid-δ-lactam and is not degraded by CLEs, eventually becoming the cell wall of the outgrowing spore. Although the spore's PG layers are essential for spore viability, there is no known direct role for PG in spore chemical resistance. It could, however, react with and detoxify chemicals. Cortex PG is involved in some fashion in the maintenance and possibly the establishment of the spore core's low water content, which is important in some spore chemical resistance (discussed further on in this Chapter).

Inner membrane

Beneath the germ cell wall is the spore's inner membrane which acts as a permeability barrier to small molecules, including methylamine and even water [2, 18–20]. This membrane's low permeability plays a major role in spore resistance to chemicals that can kill spores by damaging essential components in the spore's central core. The inner membrane has additional novel properties, for example: (i) fluorescent probes in this membrane are largely immobile; and (ii) the membrane appears to be significantly compressed, since the inner membrane-bounded volume increases 1.5–2-fold early in spore germination without adenosine triphosphate (ATP) synthesis [21]. However, the reasons for the novel properties of the spore's inner membrane are not known; its phospholipid composition is not unique and can be altered without major changes in spore properties [22].

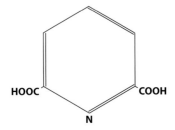

Figure 6.2.2 Structure of dipicolinic acid. Note that at physiological pH the two carboxyl groups will be ionized, and in spores are undoubtedly coordinated to divalent metal ions, predominantly Ca²⁺.

Core

The final spore layer is the central core containing DNA, RNA and most enzymes. There are three novel features of the spore core. First, for spores suspended in water, the percentage of core wet weight as water is only 25–50% (depending on the species), much lower than the water content of a growing cell protoplast (*c.* 80%) [23]. Second, *c.* 25% of the dry weight of the core is a 1:1 complex of pyridine-2,6-dicarboxylic acid (dipicolinic acid or DPA; Figure 6.2.2) with divalent cations, predominantly Ca²⁺ (Ca-DPA) [23]. The developing spore accumulates DPA from the mother cell compartment of the sporulating cell late in sporulation, and DPA accumulation is important in reducing spore core water content [24, 25]. DPA and its associated divalent cations are excreted in the first minutes of spore germination, allowing a significant rise in core water content [3].

The core's low water content is very important in many spore-resistance properties, and is likely essential for spore dormancy as proteins ≥20 kDa in the core are immobile [26]. However, the precise roles that DPA and low core water content play in spore chemical resistance are not clear. To some degree this uncertainty is because the physical states of water and DPA in the spore core are not known. It has been suggested that core water is in a glass-like state [27–29]. However, this idea has not been universally accepted [30], and recent work using nuclear magnetic resonance (NMR) spectroscopy to assess spore core water structure indicates that core water is not in a glass-like state [19]. Presumably the high level of DPA and its associated divalent cations plays a significant role in core water properties, but exactly how is not known. In addition, the great majority, if not all, DPA in the core is generally present as Ca-DPA, and while the concentration of this compound in the core greatly exceeds its solubility, its precise physical state is not known.

Finally, spore DNA is saturated with a spore-specific group of proteins called small acid-soluble spore proteins (SASPs) of the α/β-type, named for the major *B. subtilis* proteins of this type [31]. One or more α/β-type SASPs are found in spores of all *Bacillales* and *Clostridiales* species, and the amino acid sequences of these novel proteins are conserved within and between species but exhibit no significant sequence homology to other proteins. The α/β-type SASPs are synthesized late in sporulation within the developing spore, and the saturation of spore DNA with these

proteins protects the DNA against many, but not all, genotoxic chemicals. In addition to α/β-type SASP, the core of spores of most *Bacillales* species (but not *Clostridiales*) contains high levels of a single other type of SASP, termed a γ-type SASP. This protein is made in parallel with the α/β-type SASPs although its amino acid sequence is very different; it plays no known role in spore resistance. All SASPs are degraded by a SASP-specific protease early in spore outgrowth, and the amino acids ultimately generated are important for spore metabolism and protein synthesis at this time.

Variables affecting spore chemical resistance

A number of variables can affect the chemical resistance of spores, although in many cases the mechanisms behind these effects are unclear. Individual spores in populations of both *Bacillus* and *Clostridium* species also exhibit heterogeneity in their properties, including the timing of spore germination and wet heat resistance [32–36]. It seems reasonable to expect that individual spores in populations will also exhibit heterogeneity in chemical resistance, but this has not been studied.

Species/strain

Many data indicate that spores of different species or different strains of the same species have different chemical resistance [1, 3, 6]. These differences will obviously influence the choice of spores appropriate as surrogates for assessment of the efficacy of chemical treatments, and it is unlikely that spores of one single species will be the ideal surrogate for different chemical treatments.

The reasons for species-specific differences in spore chemical resistance are not known. However, given the importance of the spore coat and the permeability of the spore's inner membrane in *B. subtilis* spore resistance to chemicals, and the general conservation of these structures in spores of different species, it seems likely that differences in these structures are involved in species-specific differences in spore chemical resistance.

Sporulation conditions

Precise sporulation conditions can also affect the chemical resistance of spores; variables such as temperature, the particular sporulation medium, divalent metal ion concentrations in the sporulation medium, and solid versus liquid media all have effects on spore properties [1, 3, 4, 6, 37]. In most cases the mechanisms behind the effects of these variables on spore chemical resistance are not known, although it is known that sporulation temperature affects core water content, while divalent metal ion concentrations in sporulation media can affect the levels of cations associated with DPA [3, 23, 38–40]. Whether these effects on core water content are the reason for the effects of sporulation temperature on spore chemical resistance, and how levels of DPA's associated cations affect spore chemical resistance, are, however, unknown.

Spore purity

Purity of spore preparations can often have marked effects on chemical resistance as measured by standard tests. Presumably impurities can react with and detoxify chemical agents, leading to an apparent increased spore resistance to the chemical agent. Indeed, the addition of blood or serum to spores often increases their apparent chemical resistance, presumably by chemical reactions between impurities and the agent in question [1, 6]. Spore impurities may also include the enzyme catalase, which can reduce hydrogen peroxide concentrations. This is a potentially serious problem as levels of catalase often increase in sporulating cells. Consequently, when sporulating cells lyse, catalase may adsorb to the spore coat/exosporium, and in some cases may even be integral components of the spore's outer layers [10, 11, 14]. In view of the concerns noted above, it is essential that spore preparations used for the assessment of chemical resistance are free of contaminating material.

Spore purity can be assessed in several ways. For example, by microscopic examination to ensure there is minimal contamination with sporulating or growing cells or visible debris. However, microscopic examination will miss material such as nucleic acids and cell wall polymers that are released when sporulating cells lyse and that may adsorb to spores. Also, repeated centrifugation of spore preparations with attention to the appearance of the spore pellet can often indicate that the spore pellet is homogeneous and consists only of single spores, both indications of high spore purity. It should also be kept in mind that in applied uses, spores may be in biological fluids such as blood, fecal matter or soil, and these materials may reduce the sterilization efficacy of chemicals compared with tests with purified spores.

Spore storage and recovery conditions

There are numerous reports that storage of purified spores can alter their chemical resistance [1, 3, 6]. Spores can be stored dry, in water at c. 4°C, in ethanol at low temperatures, or frozen in water. Unfortunately there are no data on the best storage method to ensure stable spore chemical resistance, nor knowledge of what may change during storage that can affect spore chemical resistance.

Another factor that can alter the degree of spore chemical resistance is the conditions used for assessment of spore viability [1, 4, 6]. This is not a major problem for spore resistance to radiation or heat, since simply cooling spores or turning off light sources immediately removes any toxic effect and therefore eliminates further effects on spore recovery. In contrast, toxic chemicals must be inactivated to ensure that residual agents do not affect spore recovery by inactivating the germinated spores and growing cells generated when treated spores are plated on recovery media. A variety of methods can be used to neutralize chemical agents, and it is crucial that the neutralization method allows full recovery of untreated spores. The effects of residual chemical agents can be extremely insidious; for example in one case hydrogen peroxide vapor used for spore treatment in Plexiglas sample chambers was adsorbed by the acrylic glass itself and was then slowly released, affecting subsequent viability studies in the chambers [41].

Problems associated with the recovery of chemically treated spores also go beyond concerns about residual chemical agent, since chemicals often generate spore damage that is only conditionally lethal [2, 6]. Thus the precise pretreatment of spores or recovery media used following chemical exposure can have dramatic effects on spore recovery and thus profound effects on apparent spore chemical resistance. Examples include increased recovery of: (i) glutaraldehyde-treated spores by brief alkali pretreatment [42]; (ii) iodine-treated spores by addition of lactate to the recovery medium [43]; and (iii) alkali-treated spores by pretreatment with lysozyme [44]. A major concern with spore killing by chemicals is thus to ensure that the killed spores are truly dead, and either unable to germinate or only to germinate after long lag times. Use of artificial germinants such as lysozyme can often be helpful in ensuring that, while apparently killed, spores cannot still germinate; in other words, they are indeed dead.

Mechanisms of spore killing by chemicals

Chemicals kill spores by a number of mechanisms including DNA damage, damage to the spore's inner membrane, inactivation of one or more spore germination proteins, and inactivation of key spore core enzymes [2]. It is not surprising that different chemicals kill spores by different mechanisms (Table 6.2.1), and a particular chemical may kill spores by multiple mechanisms. Most work elucidating the mechanisms of spore killing by chemicals has used *B. subtilis* spores, while the use of mutants has facilitated mechanistic studies. It will be important to learn if mechanisms of chemical killing of spores of all *Bacillales* and *Clostridiales* species are the same as for *B. subtilis* spores.

Spore killing by DNA damage

A number of genotoxic chemicals kill *B. subtilis* spores by DNA damage [2] (Table 6.2.1). The evidence for this is that: (i) survivors in spore preparations given a mild treatment by such chemicals have a high percentage of mutations; (ii) loss of DNA repair capacity, often due to the loss of the RecA protein, results in increased sensitivity to the chemical in question; (iii) there is DNA damage in spores killed by such chemicals; and (iv) DNA

Table 6.2.1 Mechanisms of spore killing by various chemicals (from [2]).[a]

Mechanism of spore killing	Examples of chemicals that kill spores by this mechanism
DNA damage	Ethylene oxide, nitrite, formaldehyde
Inner membrane damage	Hypochlorite, ClO_2, ozone, peroxides
Inactivation of core enzymes	Hydrogen peroxide?
Germination apparatus damage	Alkali, dialdehydes
Unknown damage	HCl

[a] Information is for spores of *Bacillus subtilis*.

repair genes are often induced during outgrowth of spores treated with such chemicals. In contrast to the results noted above with chemicals that kill spores by DNA damage, spores treated by many other chemicals, including some that are genotoxic in growing cells such as hydrogen peroxide exhibit: (i) no DNA damage; (ii) no induction of DNA repair genes in spore outgrowth; and (iii) no decrease in resistance when DNA repair capacity is lost.

Spore killing by inactivation of spore core enzymes

Recent work has strongly suggested that it is through inactivation of one or more spore core enzymes that wet heat kills spores of *Bacillus* species [33, 45–47]. There are also data suggesting that some peroxides can inactivate spore core enzymes, with this inactivation accompanying spore killing [48, 49]. However, inactivation of key core enzymes has not been causally connected with spore killing by peroxides or other chemicals.

Spore killing by preventing germination

One obvious way to inactivate spores is to render them incapable of germinating, since germination-defective spores cannot return to life. Many spore germination proteins including CLEs are in the spore's outer layers [3], and such proteins are presumably susceptible to exogenous chemicals. While germination protein inactivation in such a manner does take place, spores that are dead for this reason could come back to life at a later time via very slow germination or could be germinated by an exogenous lytic enzyme.

The evidence that spore killing is due to a spore germination defect is shown by the loss of spores' ability to germinate parallels spore killing and by viable spores that can be recovered from "apparently dead" spores by artificial germination, often with exogenous lysozyme. For several chemicals, including glutaraldehyde, *ortho*-phthalaldehyde and perhaps hydrogen peroxide, inactivation of germination proteins may play some role in spore killing, although recovery of spores treated with these chemicals by artificial germination is never close to 100% [2, 6, 42, 43, 50–52]. However, alkali treatment, at least under relatively mild (for spores!) conditions (1 M NaOH at 24°C for several hours) clearly kills spores by inactivation of CLEs [44]. Apparently alkali-killed *B. subtilis* spores: (i) go through early steps in spore germination; (ii) do not hydrolyze cortex PG during germination; and (iii) can be completely recovered by treatment with low levels of lysozyme.

Spore killing by damage to the inner membrane

The inner membrane is an extremely strong permeability barrier in the spore, preventing loss of core small molecules, and allowing only slow passage of exogenous chemicals into the core [18, 19, 53]. Many chemicals have been suggested to kill spores by damaging this membrane, such that when spores germinate and the core expands, the inner membrane ruptures leading to spore death [2, 53]. Oxidizing agents including hypochlorite, chlorine dioxide, organic hydroperoxides, superoxidized water and ozone probably kill spores by this mechanism [2, 53–56]. The evidence for this mechanism of killing is given by the following:

1. Treated spores do not lose small molecules, in particular DPA, but DPA is released from spores treated by incubation at lower temperatures than from untreated spores.
2. Spores given a mild treatment with such chemicals exhibit lower viability on "stressful" media such as those with high salt or minimal nutrients compared with salt-free or rich media, while untreated spores have similar viability on both high salt and minimal media; this behavior is typical of cells that have suffered some type of membrane damage [57–59].
3. Spores treated with these chemicals exhibit increased permeability to small molecules such as methylamine, and spores' major permeability barrier to methylamine is likely the inner membrane [2, 18, 20, 53].
4. Spores treated with these agents have no DNA damage and often germinate normally, but the killed spores lyse after germination is initiated even if the spores are germinated artificially in a hypertonic medium.

Unfortunately, while available evidence suggests that damage to the inner membrane is the mechanism whereby this group of agents kills spores, the nature of this damage is unknown (although it is not to unsaturated fatty acids) [53]. Interestingly, if this damage is minimal, spores may survive but are sensitized to a subsequent wet heat treatment that is not lethal for untreated spores [53].

Factors important in spore resistance to various chemicals

In addition to the multiple mechanisms of spore killing by chemicals, spore chemical resistance is also due to multiple factors, with the most important factor varying for different chemicals (Table 6.2.2). Factors important in spore chemical resistance include: (i) DNA protection by α/β-type SASPs; (ii) repair of DNA damage during spore outgrowth; (iii) decreased core water content; (iv) the low permeability of the spore's inner membrane; (v) the spore coat; and (vi) enzymes associated with the spore's outer layers. A major factor in resistance of growing bacteria to some chemicals is cytoplasmic detoxifying enzymes such as catalase, superoxide dismutase and alkylhydroperoxide reductase [6, 60, 61]. However, while such enzymes are present in the spore core, they play no role in spore resistance [62], presumably because such enzymes are inactive due to the core's low water content. Mechanisms of spore resistance to specific chemicals are summarized below (conclusions based on work with *B. subtilis* spores unless noted otherwise).

Disinfectants

Disinfectants used to kill growing bacteria on surfaces, hands and instruments, including alcohols, detergents, phenols and chlorhexidine, are almost always inactive against spores, even though the growing cells of spore-formers are sensitive to such agents [1,

Table 6.2.2 Factors important in spore resistance to various chemicals (from [2, 60]).[a]

Type of chemical	Protective factor[b]
Genotoxic chemicals	Low permeability of spore's inner membrane; DNA saturation by α/β-type SASP; DNA repair during spore outgrowth; low core water content
Oxidizing agents	Detoxifying enzymes in spore's outer layers; spore coat protein; low permeability of spore's inner membrane; DNA saturation by α/β-type SASP
Dialdehydes	Spore coats
Disinfectants	Spore coats, perhaps cortex and inner membrane structure
Acids and alkali	Not understood
Supercritical CO_2	Not understood
Plasma	Spore coat; DNA saturation by α/β-type SASP; not yet thoroughly studied

SASP, small acid-soluble spore protein.

[a] Information is for spores of *Bacillus subtilis*.

[b] Not all protective factors are important in protecting against all chemicals of any particular type.

4–7]. Resistance to these disinfectants is acquired at defined times in sporulation, and is lost when spore germination is completed. Precise mechanisms of spore resistance to disinfectants are unknown, but have been inferred from the timing of acquisition of disinfectant resistance during sporulation and seem likely to involve changes in the inner membrane, PG and coat. However, mutants that disrupt spore coat assembly have little to no effect on spore disinfectant resistance.

Genotoxic chemicals

Spores are killed by a variety of genotoxic chemicals, including ethylene oxide (EtO), formaldehyde, hydrogen peroxide and other peroxides, bleach and other halogen-releasing agents [2]. A variety of spore components and structures are important in the protection of spore DNA against potentially genotoxic agents, and the importance of different protective factors varies depending on the chemical.

Ethylene oxide

Spores are killed by EtO via damage to DNA, and DNA repair during outgrowth is an important factor in spore EtO resistance, as *recA* spores are significantly more EtO sensitive than are wild-type spores [63]. Surprisingly, saturation of spore DNA with α/β-type SASP is not involved in DNA protection against EtO. This was concluded from a study of effects of α/β-type SASP on alkylation of DNA either in spores or *in vitro* by ethyl methylsulfonate (EMS), a chemical that alkylates DNA at the same positions as EtO. Spores lacking *c.* 80% of their α/β-type SASP (termed α⁻,β⁻ spores) were as EMS-resistant as were wild-type spores, and saturation of purified DNA with a purified α/β-type SASP did not affect DNA alkylation by EMS. Analysis of a

high-resolution structure of an α/β-type SASP–DNA complex indicates that α/β-type SASP binding does not shield amino groups of purines in DNA's major groove, the predominant sites of DNA alkylation by EMS [64]. Consequently, α/β-type SASPs have no effect on this DNA modification *in vitro* or in spores [63]. However, spores are more resistant to EtO and EMS than are growing cells, and one factor in spore EMS resistance is the low permeability of the spore's inner membrane [20]; presumably this is also true for EtO.

Formaldehyde

Spores are killed by formaldehyde through DNA damage, although the DNA damage has not been identified, and DNA repair is important in spore's formaldehyde resistance [65]. The α/β-type SASPs are important in protecting the spore DNA against formaldehyde, as α⁻,β⁻ spores are more formaldehyde-sensitive than wild-type spores. DPA and/or spore core water content are also important in formaldehyde resistance [17], as is the permeability of the spore's inner membrane, as spores with increased inner membrane permeability have decreased formaldehyde resistance [20]. However, the coat does not play a major role in spore formaldehyde resistance.

Nitrite

Nitrite kills spores by DNA damage, although the precise DNA damage has not been identified [66]. α/β-Type SASP binding to DNA plays a major role in spore DNA protection against nitrite, as does DNA repair in spore outgrowth. Increased permeability of the inner membrane as well as increased core water content are also associated with decreased spore nitrite resistance [19, 38].

Peroxides

Peroxides including hydrogen peroxide and organic hydroperoxides can have genotoxic effects in various cell types [5, 60, 61]. However, these compounds do not kill wild-type spores by DNA damage [67, 68]. The saturation of DNA with α/β-type SASP is the major factor in spore resistance to hydrogen peroxide, as peroxides kill α⁻,β⁻ spores largely by DNA damage. The spore coat plays a minor role in spore resistance to hydrogen peroxide, and an increased core water content and loss of DPA are also associated with decreased hydrogen peroxide resistance [17, 25]. Several studies have also found that UV radiation can act synergistically with hydrogen peroxide in spore killing [69, 70].

Ozone, peracetic acid, bleach and chlorine dioxide

In contrast to results with peroxides, the potentially genotoxic agent peracetic acid does not kill α⁻,β⁻ spores by DNA damage and the mechanism of spore killing by this agent is unclear [67]. Ozone, bleach and chlorine dioxide, which also are potential genotoxic agents, also do not kill α⁻,β⁻ spores by DNA damage, and the coat is important in spore protection against these chemicals [54, 55]. This is also the case for several commercial sporicide formulations including Decon and Oxone™ [71]. These chemicals, with the possible exception of peracetic acid, probably kill spores by damaging the spore's inner membrane (see below).

Hydrogen peroxide

As noted above, hydrogen peroxide does not kill spores by DNA damage despite it being a genotoxic agent. However, it can enter the spore core, as α^-,β^- spores are killed via DNA damage by hydrogen peroxide [68]. This suggests that hydrogen peroxide could kill wild-type spores by damaging one or more proteins in the spore core, and inactivation of core enzymes by peroxides can accompany spore killing [48, 49]. However, it has not been shown that this enzyme inactivation is a cause of spore killing and not simply an event that takes place after spores receive other lethal damage. Hydrogen peroxide treatment also can have effects on both spore germination and outgrowth [52], but again it is not clear if these effects are causes of spore killing. As noted above, catalase in spores' outer layers can assist in protection against hydrogen peroxide. Polycyclic terpenoids, termed sporulenes, associated with *B. subtilis* spores' outer layers (and possibly the outer layers of other spores as well) can also provide protection against hydrogen peroxide [72]. Elevated levels of manganese, most likely in the spore core, also result in higher resistance of spores of *Bacillus megaterium* to hydrogen peroxide, but this is not the case for *B. subtilis* spores [73, 74].

Oxidizing agents other than hydrogen peroxide

A variety of oxidizing agents are or have been proposed to be useful to kill spores in applied settings, including ozone, organic hydroperoxides, superoxidized water, bleach, chlorine dioxide, formulations containing free halogens, dimethyldioxirane, t-butyl hydroperoxide plus a tetra-amido macrocyclic ligand (TAML) activator [75, 76] and a number of commercial formulations [2, 53–56, 66, 77]. Invariably these compounds do not kill spores by DNA damage, but by damaging the spore's inner membrane such that when spores germinate this membrane then ruptures causing spore death [2, 53–56, 66, 76, 77].

The major factor protecting spores against most oxidizing agents is the spore coat, as spores lacking most or their coat protein due to chemical removal or absence of one or more proteins essential for the assembly of major coat layers are generally much more sensitive to oxidizing agents. The spore coats provide less protection against hydrogen peroxide than against other oxidizing agents [78]. As noted above, DNA protection by α/β-type SASPs is a major factor protecting spores against hydrogen peroxide and other peroxides. However, the α/β-type SASPs are generally not important in spore resistance to other oxidizing agents [2, 53–56, 66, 76, 77]. Another factor in spore resistance to some oxidizing agents is the presence of detoxifying enzymes such as catalase and superoxide dismutase in spore outer layers, the latter enzyme in particular in the exosporium of *B. anthracis* spores [10, 11, 14].

While the coat is the major factor in spore resistance to most oxidizing agents, spores lacking the great majority of their coat protein are more resistant to most oxidizing agents than are growing cells. The reason for the residual resistance of "coatless" spores to oxidizing agents is not clear, although it could be the low permeability of the spore's inner membrane [20]. "Coatless" *B. subtilis* spores also retain a significant amount of coat protein that could contribute to the enhanced oxidizing agent resistance of these spores [79].

Dialdehydes

The dialdehydes glutaraldehyde and *ortho*-phthalaldehyde are used in some settings for decontamination of medical instruments [4, 6, 50, 51]. These compounds appear to kill spores by inactivating some germination protein, but which protein and whether there are other mechanisms of spore killing by these agents are not clear [42, 50, 51]. Resistance to these chemicals is highly dependent on the spore coat, as chemically decoated spores or spores that lack much coat protein due to mutation of a major coat assembly protein are much more sensitive to these dialdehydes.

Acid and alkali

Spores are extremely resistant to acids and alkali. The α/β-type SASPs and DNA repair are not important in spore resistance to acid or alkali, and the coat has only a minimal role in spore resistance to these chemicals [44]. However, coat proteins can be extracted by alkali, in particular, so alkali treatment can sensitize spores to agents against which the spore coats are likely major resistance factors [11, 80]. There is also a recent report suggesting that silicate can be taken up by spores of several *Bacillus* species (but not *B. subtilis*), deposited on a spore coat layer, and contribute to spore acid resistance [81].

Alkali can inactivate the CLEs of *B. subtilis* spores and leads to apparent spore death because the treated spores cannot complete germination [44]. In contrast, spore treatment with strong acid causes "acid popping" whereby spores in strong mineral acid actually seem to explode due to rupture of spore's outer layers, with extrusion of spore DNA [44, 82]. However, the mechanism of this "acid popping" is unknown.

Plasma

Low-temperature plasma is gaining popularity for sterilization of heat-sensitive materials, in particular medical devices [83]. A variety of different types of plasma exist, and these can contain many different types of potentially sporicidal components, including UV photons and radical species. Some data indicate that the spore coat, DNA repair and α/β-type SASP can be important in protection against radical species in plasma [83, 84], but precise killing components of plasma other than UV photons have not been identified.

Supercritical carbon dioxide

There has been a moderate amount of work recently on the killing of spores of *Bacillus* species by supercritical CO_2 [85–88]. However, there has been no study of the mechanisms of spore killing by or resistance to this agent, nor on the precise agent actually killing the spores. Supercritical CO_2 alone requires relatively high temperatures to effectively kill spores. However, small amounts of additives such as hydrogen peroxide in supercritical CO_2 allow effective spore killing at moderate temperatures and pressures. In one study [85], the great majority of spores that had their viability reduced by 5-log following exposure to supercritical CO_2 plus hydrogen peroxide exhibited no drastic changes in spore structure or permeability; a killing mechanism was not determined.

Factors important in chemical resistance of spores of clostridium species

While much is known about factors important in the chemical resistance of spores of *Bacillus* species, primarily *B. subtilis* spores, much less is known about factors important in the chemical resistance of *Clostridium* spores. However, the α/β-type SASPs are important in the resistance of *C. perfringens* spores to genotoxic chemicals, including nitrite, hydrogen peroxide and formaldehyde [89–91]. Indeed, a *C. perfringens* α/β-type SASP restores much of the nitrite resistance to *B. subtilis* spores lacking their own major α/β-type SASP [92]. The core's water content is also important in resistance of *C. perfringens* spores to nitrite, and DPA is important in spore resistance to HCl, formaldehyde and hydrogen peroxide [93, 94]. Much of the recent information on the chemical resistance of *C. perfringens* spores was obtained through the use of various molecularly engineered mutant strains. As this technology becomes more widespread, information on the mechanisms of the resistance of spores of other *Clostridium* species should be forthcoming.

Conclusions

Much is now known about mechanisms of bacterial spore killing by, and resistance to, chemicals used for sterilization, but major questions remain unanswered including the following:

1. Are mechanisms of spore killing by and resistance to chemical sporicides similar for spores of different *Bacillus* species as well as for spores of *Clostridium* species? Most work to date has used *B. subtilis* spores with only minimal data for spores of other species.
2. Why is the coat so important in spore resistance to a variety of chemicals? It is hypothesized that spore coat protein acts as reactive armor to detoxify chemicals, but is this hypothesis correct?
3. What is the damage, most likely to the spore's inner membrane, whereby most oxidizing agents kill spores? The spore's inner membrane has a number of novel properties and may have an unusual structure, but the structure of this membrane is not known.
4. How do chemicals such as glutaraldehyde and hydrogen peroxide kill spores? Despite moderate amounts of work on this question and extensive use of such chemicals in sterilization applications, the lethal target(s) of these chemicals remain unknown.
5. How do newer sterilization technologies such as supercritical CO_2 and plasma kill spores? There has been only minimal work

on mechanisms of spore killing by and resistance to these new treatments.
6. What are the mechanisms that prevent spore killing by disinfectants such as alcohols, detergents, phenol and chlorhexidine? There is only minimal knowledge of mechanisms of spore resistance to such agents, despite their widespread use. Since most disinfectants can have severe effects on membranes, it is possible that a spore's likely novel inner membrane structure is important in spore resistance to disinfectants, but this has not been studied.

Overall, while there is certainly more known about mechanisms of spore killing by and spore resistance to chemicals than there was when the previous edition of this book appeared, there is still much to be learned.

Acknowledgments

Work in the author's lab has received generous support over the years in grants from the National Institutes of Health, GM19698, and the Army Research Office.

References

1 Bloomfield, S.F. (1999) Bacterial sensitivity and resistance: resistance of bacterial spores to chemical agents, in *Principles and Practice of Disinfection, Preservation and Sterilization*, 3rd edn (eds A.D. Russell *et al.*), Blackwell Science, London, pp. 303–320.
2 Setlow, P. (2006) Spores of *Bacillus subtilis*: their resistance to radiation, heat and chemicals. *Journal of Applied Microbiology*, **101**, 514–525.
3 Setlow, P. and Johnson, E.A. (2007) Spores and their significance, in *Food Microbiology, Fundamentals and Frontiers*, 3rd edn (eds M.P. Doyle and L.R. Beuchat), ASM Press, Washington, DC, pp. 35–67.
4 Russell, A.D. (2003) Similarities and differences in the responses of microorganisms to biocides. *Journal of Antimicrobial Chemotherapy*, **52**, 750–763.
5 Russell, A.D. (2001) Mechanisms of bacterial insusceptibility to biocides. *American Journal of Infection Control*, **29**, 259–261.
6 McDonnell, G. and Russell, A.D. (1999) Antiseptics and disinfectants: activity, action and resistance. *Clinical Microbiology Reviews*, **12**, 147–179.
7 Brown, K.L. (2000) Control of bacterial spores. *British Medical Bulletin*, **56**, 158–171.
8 Nicholson, W.L. *et al.* (2000) Resistance of *Bacillus* endospores to extreme terrestrial and extraterrestrial environments. *Microbiology and Molecular Biology Reviews*, **64**, 548–572.
9 Maillard, J.-Y. (2011) Innate resistance to sporicides and potential failure to decontaminate. *Journal of Hospital Infection*, **77**, 204–209.
10 Driks, A. (2009) The *Bacillus anthracis* spore. *Molecular Aspects of Medicine*, **30**, 368–373.
11 Henriques, A.O. and Moran, C.P. Jr. (2007) Structure, assembly, and function of the spore surface layers. *Annual Review of Microbiology*, **61**, 555–588.
12 Severson, K.M. *et al.* (2009) Roles of *Bacillus anthracis* spore protein ExsK in exosporium maturation and germination. *Journal of Bacteriology*, **191**, 7587–7596.
13 Chesnokova, O.N. Jr. *et al.* (2009) The spore-specific alanine racemase of *Bacillus anthracis* and its role in suppressing germination during spore development. *Journal of Bacteriology*, **191**, 1303–1310.
14 Cybulski, R.J. *et al.* (2009) Four superoxide dismutases contribute to *Bacillus anthracis* virulence and provide spores with redundant protection from oxidative stress. *Infection and Immunity*, **77**, 274–285.

15 Klobutcher, L.A. *et al.* (2006) The *Bacillus subtilis* spore coat provides "eat resistance" during phagosomal predation by the protozoan *Tetrahymena thermophila*. *Proceedings of the National Academy of Sciences of the United States of America*, **103**, 165–170.

16 Laaberki, M.H. and Dworkin, J. (2008) Role of spore coat proteins in the resistance of *Bacillus subtilis* spores to *Caenorhabditis elegans* predation. *Journal of Bacteriology*, **190**, 6197–6203.

17 Popham, D.L. (2002) Specialized peptidoglycan of the bacterial endospore: the inner wall of the lockbox. *Cellular and Molecular Life Sciences*, **59**, 426–433.

18 Swerdlow, B.M. *et al.* (1981) Levels of H⁺ and other monovalent cations in dormant and germinated spores of *Bacillus megaterium*. *Journal of Bacteriology*, **148**, 20–29.

19 Sunde, E.P. *et al.* (2009) The physical state of water in bacterial spores. *Proceedings of the National Academy Sciences of the United States of America*, **106**, 19334–19339.

20 Cortezzo, D.E. and Setlow, P. (2005) Analysis of factors influencing the sensitivity of spores of *Bacillus subtilis* to DNA damaging chemicals. *Journal of Applied Microbiology*, **98**, 606–617.

21 Cowan, A.E. *et al.* (2004) Lipids in the inner membrane of dormant spores of *Bacillus* species are immobile. *Proceedings of the National Academy of Sciences of the United States of America*, **101**, 7733–7738.

22 Griffiths, K. and Setlow, P. (2009) Effects of modification of membrane lipid composition on *Bacillus subtilis* sporulation and spore properties. *Journal of Applied Microbiology*, **106**, 1600–1607.

23 Gerhardt, P. and Marquis, R.E. (1989) Spore thermoresistance mechanisms, in *Regulation of Prokaryotic Development: Structural and Functional Analysis of Bacterial Sporulation and Germination* (eds I. Smith *et al.*), American Society for Microbiology, Washington, DC, pp. 43–64.

24 Paidhungat, M. *et al.* (2000) Characterization of spores of *Bacillus subtilis* which lack dipicolinic acid. *Journal of Bacteriology*, **182**, 5505–5512.

25 Setlow, B. *et al.* (2006) Role of dipicolinic acid in the resistance and stability of spores of *Bacillus subtilis*. *Journal of Bacteriology*, **188**, 3740–3747.

26 Setlow, P. (2007) I will survive: DNA protection in bacterial spores. *Trends in Microbiology*, **15**, 172–180.

27 Cowan, A.E. *et al.* (2003) A soluble protein is immobile in dormant spores of *Bacillus subtilis* but is mobile in germinated spores: implications for spore dormancy. *Proceedings of the National Academy of Sciences of the United States of America*, **100**, 4209–4214.

28 Sapru, V. and Labuza, T.P. (1993) Glassy state in bacterial spores predicted by polymer glass-transition theory. *Journal of Food Science*, **58**, 445–448.

29 Ablett, S. *et al.* (1999) Glass formation and dormancy in bacterial spores. *International Journal of Food Science and Technology*, **34**, 59–69.

30 Stecchini, M.L. *et al.* (2006) Glassy state in *Bacillus subtilis* spores analyzed by differential scanning calorimetry. *International Journal of Food Microbiology*, **106**, 286–290.

31 Leuschner, R.G.K. and Lillford, P.J. (2003) Thermal properties of bacterial spores and biopolymers. *International Journal of Food Microbiology*, **80**, 131–143.

32 Hornstra, L.M. *et al.* (2009) On the origin of heterogeneity in (preservation) resistance of *Bacillus* spores: input for a "systems" analysis approach of bacterial spore outgrowth. *International Journal of Food Microbiology*, **134**, 9–15.

33 Zhang, P. *et al.* (2010) Characterization of wet heat inactivation of single spores of *Bacillus* species by dual-trap Raman spectroscopy and elastic light scattering. *Applied and Environmental Microbiology*, **76**, 507–514.

34 Ghosh, S. *et al.* (2009) Superdormant spores of *Bacillus* species have elevated wet heat resistance and temperature requirements for heat activation. *Journal of Bacteriology*, **191**, 5584–5591.

35 Ghosh, S. and Setlow, P. (2009) Isolation and characterization of superdormant spores of *Bacillus* species. *Journal of Bacteriology*, **191**, 1787–1797.

36 Ghosh, S. and Setlow, P. (2010) The preparation, germination properties and stability of superdormant spores of *Bacillus cereus*. *Journal of Applied Microbiology*, **108**, 582–590.

37 Rose, R. *et al.* (2007) Comparison of the properties of *Bacillus subtilis* spores made in liquid or on plates. *Journal of Applied Microbiology*, **103**, 691–699.

38 Marquis, R.E. and Shin, S.Y. (1994) Mineralization and responses of bacterial spores to heat and oxidative agents. *FEMS Microbiology Reviews*, **14**, 375–379.

39 Cazemier, A.E. *et al.* (2001) Effect of sporulation and recovery medium on the heat resistance and amount of injury of spores from spoilage bacilli. *Journal of Applied Microbiology*, **90**, 761–770.

40 Melly, E. *et al.* (2002) Analysis of the properties of spores of *Bacillus subtilis* prepared at different temperatures. *Journal of Applied Microbiology*, **92**, 1105–1115.

41 Baron, P.A. *et al.* (2007) Bacterial endospore inactivation caused by outgassing of vapourous hydrogen peroxide from polymethyl methacrylate (Plexiglas). *Letters in Applied Microbiology*, **45**, 485–490.

42 Williams, N.D. and Russell, A.D. (1993) Revival of biocide-treated spores of *Bacillus subtilis*. *Journal of Applied Bacteriology*, **75**, 69–75.

43 Williams, N.D. and Russell, A.D. (1993) Revival of *Bacillus subtilis* spores from biocide-induced injury in the germination process. *Journal of Applied Bacteriology*, **75**, 76–81.

44 Setlow, B. *et al.* (2002) Mechanisms of killing of spores of *Bacillus subtilis* by acid, alkali and ethanol. *Journal of Applied Microbiology*, **92**, 362–375.

45 Coleman, W.H. and Setlow, P. (2009) Analysis of damage due to moist heat treatment of spores of *Bacillus subtilis*. *Journal of Applied Microbiology*, **106**, 1600–1607.

46 Warth, A.D. (1980) Heat stability of *Bacillus cereus* enzymes within spores and in extracts. *Journal of Bacteriology*, **143**, 27–34.

47 Coleman, W.H. *et al.* (2007) How moist heat kills spores of *Bacillus subtilis*. *Journal of Bacteriology*, **189**, 8458–8466.

48 Palop, A. *et al.* (1996) Hydroperoxide inactivation of enzymes within spores of *Bacillus megaterium* ATCC19213. *FEMS Microbiology Letters*, **44**, 283–287.

49 Palop, A. *et al.* (1998) Inactivation of enzymes within spores of *Bacillus megaterium* ATCC19213 by hydroperoxides. *Canadian Journal of Microbiology*, **44**, 465–470.

50 Cabrera-Martinez, R.M. *et al.* (2002) Studies on the mechanisms of the sporicidal action of o-phthalaldehyde. *Journal of Applied Microbiology*, **92**, 675–680.

51 Walsh, S.E. *et al.* (1999) Ortho-phthalaldehyde: a possible alternative to glutaraldehyde for high level disinfection. *Journal of Applied Microbiology*, **86**, 1039–1046.

52 Melly, E. *et al.* (2002) Studies on the mechanism of killing of *Bacillus subtilis* spores by hydrogen peroxide. *Journal of Applied Microbiology*, **93**, 316–325.

53 Cortezzo, D.E. *et al.* (2004) Treatment with oxidizing agents damages the inner membrane of spores of *Bacillus subtilis* and sensitizes the spores to subsequent stress. *Journal of Applied Microbiology*, **97**, 838–852.

54 Young, S.B. and Setlow, P. (2003) Mechanisms of killing of *Bacillus subtilis* spores by hypochlorite and chlorine dioxide. *Journal of Applied Microbiology*, **95**, 54–67.

55 Young, S.B. and Setlow, P. (2004) Mechanisms of *Bacillus subtilis* spore resistance to and killing by aqueous ozone. *Journal of Applied Microbiology*, **96**, 1133–1142.

56 Loshon, C.A. *et al.* (2001) Analysis of killing of spores of *Bacillus subtilis* by a new disinfectant, Sterilox®. *Journal of Applied Microbiology*, **91**, 1051–1058.

57 Hurst, A. (1977) Bacterial injury: a review. *Canadian Journal of Microbiology*, **23**, 935–944.

58 Hurst, A. (1983) Injury, in *The Bacterial Spore*, vol. II, (eds A. Hurst and G.W. Gould), Academic Press, London, pp. 255–274.

59 Shitani, H. (2006) Importance of considering injured microorganisms in sterilization validation. *Biocontrol Science*, **11**, 91–106.

60 Imlay, J.A. (2008) Cellular defenses against superoxide and hydrogen peroxide. *Annual Review of Biochemistry*, **77**, 755–776.

61 Imlay, J.A. (2003) Pathways of oxidative damage. *Annual Review of Microbiology*, **57**, 395–418.

62 Casillas-Martinez, L. and Setlow, P. (1997) Alkyl hydroperoxide reductase, catalase, MrgA, and superoxide dismutase are not involved in resistance of *Bacillus subtilis* spores to heat or oxidizing agents. *Journal of Bacteriology*, **179**, 7420–7425.

63 Setlow, B. *et al.* (1998) Small, acid-soluble spore proteins of the α/β-type do not protect the DNA in *Bacillus subtilis* spores against base alkylation. *Applied and Environmental Microbiology*, **64**, 1958–1962.

64 Lee, K.S. *et al.* (2007) Structure of a protein-DNA complex essential for DNA protection in spores of *Bacillus* species. *Proceedings of the National Academy of Sciences of the United States of America*, **105**, 2806–2811.

65 Loshon, C.A. *et al.* (1999) Formaldehyde kills spores of *Bacillus subtilis* by DNA damage, and small, acid-soluble spore proteins of the α/β -type protect spores against this DNA damage. *Journal of Applied Microbiology*, **87**, 8–14.

66 Tennen, R. *et al.* (2000) Mechanisms of killing of spores of *Bacillus subtilis* by iodine, glutaraldehyde and nitrous acid. *Journal of Applied Microbiology*, **89**, 330–338.

67 Setlow, B. *et al.* (1997) Killing bacterial spores by organic hydroperoxides. *Journal of Industrial Microbiology*, **18**, 384–388.

68 Setlow, B. and Setlow, P. (1993) Binding of small, acid-soluble spore proteins to DNA plays a significant role in the resistance of *Bacillus subtilis* spores to hydrogen peroxide. *Applied and Environmental Microbiology*, **59**, 3418–3423.

69 Bayliss, C.E. and Waites, W.M. (1979) The combined effect of hydrogen peroxide and ultraviolet irradiation on bacterial spores. *Journal of Applied Bacteriology*, **47**, 263–269.

70 Reidmiller, J.S. *et al.* (2003) Characterization of UV-peroxide killing of bacterial spores. *Journal of Food Protection*, **66**, 1233–1240.

71 Young, S.B. and Setlow, P. (2004) Mechanisms of killing of *Bacillus subtilis* spores by Decon and Oxone™, two general decontaminants for biological agents. *Journal of Applied Microbiology*, **96**, 289–301.

72 Bosak, T. *et al.* (2008) A polycyclic terpenoid that alleviates oxidative stress. *Proceedings of the National Academy of Sciences of the United States of America*, **105**, 6725–6729.

73 Ghosh, S. *et al.* (2011) Effects of Mn levels on resistance of *Bacillus megaterium* spores to heat, radiation and hydrogen peroxide. *Journal of Applied Microbiology*, **111**, 663–670.

74 Granger, A.C. *et al.* (2011) Effects of Mn and Fe levels on *Bacillus subtilis* spore resistance and effects of Mn^{2+}, other divalent cations, orthophosphate, and dipicolinic acid on protein resistance to ionizing radiation. *Applied and Environmental Microbiology*, **77**, 32–40.

75 Collins, T.J. and Walter, C. (2006) Little green molecules. *Scientific American*, **294**, 82–90.

76 Paul, M. *et al.* (2007) Killing of spores of *Bacillus subtilis* by tert-butyl hydroperoxide plus a TAML activator. *Journal of Applied Microbiology*, **102**, 954–962.

77 Paul, M. *et al.* (2006) Mechanisms of killing of spores by dimethyldioxirane. *Journal of Applied Microbiology*, **101**, 1161–1168.

78 Riesenman, P.J. and Nicholson, W.L. (2000) Role of the spore coat layers in *Bacillus subtilis* spore resistance to hydrogen peroxide, artificial UV-C, UV-B, and solar UV radiation. *Applied and Environmental Microbiology*, **66**, 620–626.

79 Ghosh, S. *et al.* (2008) Characterization of spores of *Bacillus subtilis* that lack most coat layers. *Journal of Bacteriology*, **190**, 6741–6748.

80 Yardimci, O. and Setlow, P. (2010) Plasma sterilization: opportunities and microbial assessment strategies in medical device manufacturing. *IEEE Transactions in Plasma Science*, **38**, 973–981.

81 Langsrud, S. *et al.* (2000) Potentiation of the lethal effect of peroxygen on *Bacillus cereus* spores by alkali and enzyme wash. *International Journal of Food Microbiology*, **56**, 81–86.

82 Hirota, R. *et al.* (2009) The silicon layer supports acid resistance of *Bacillus cereus* spores. *Journal of Bacteriology*, **192**, 111–116.

83 Robinow, C. (1953) Spore structure as revealed by thin sections. *Journal of Bacteriology*, **66**, 300–311.

84 Roth, S. *et al.* (2010) Characterization of *Bacillus subtilis* spore inactivation in low-pressure, low-temperature gas plasma sterilization processes. *Journal of Applied Microbiology*, **108**, 521–531.

85 Zhang, J. *et al.* (2006) Sterilizing *Bacillus pumilus* spores using supercritical carbon dioxide. *Journal of Microbiological Methods*, **66**, 479–485.

86 Hemmer, J.D. *et al.* (2007) Sterilization of bacterial spores by using supercritical carbon dioxide and hydrogen peroxide. *Journal of Biomedical Materials Research B: Applied Biomaterials*, **80**, 511–518.

87 Zhang, J. *et al.* (2007) Supercritical carbon dioxide and hydrogen peroxide cause mild changes in spore structures associated with high killing rate of *Bacillus anthracis*. *Journal of Microbiological Methods*, **70**, 442–451.

88 Shieh, E. *et al.* (2009) Sterilization of *Bacillus pumilus* spores using supercritical fluid carbon dioxide containing various modifier solutions. *Journal of Microbiological Methods*, **76**, 247–252.

89 Li, J. and McClane, B.A. (2008) A novel small acid soluble protein variant is important for spore resistance of most *Clostridium perfringens* food poisoning isolates. *Public Library of Science Pathology*, **4**, e1000056.

90 Li, J. *et al.* (2009) Further characterization of *Clostridium perfringens* small acid soluble protein-4 (Ssp4) properties and expression. *Public Library of Science One*, **4**, e6249.

91 Paredes-Sabja, D. *et al.* (2008) Role of small, acid-soluble spore proteins in the resistance of *Clostridium perfringens* spores to chemicals. *International Journal of Food Microbiology*, **122**, 333–335.

92 Leyva-Illades, J.F. *et al.* (2007) Effect of a small, acid-soluble spore protein from *Clostridium perfringens* on the resistance properties of *Bacillus subtilis* spores. *Journal of Bacteriology*, **189**, 7927–7931.

93 Parades-Sabja, D. *et al.* (2008) Roles of DacB and Spm proteins in *Clostridium perfringens* spore resistance to moist heat and chemicals. *Applied and Environmental Microbiology*, **74**, 3730–3738.

94 Paredes-Sabja, D. *et al.* (2008) Characterization of *Clostridium perfringens* spores that lack SpoVA proteins and dipicolinic acid. *Journal of Bacteriology*, **190**, 4648–4659.

6.3   Testing of Chemicals as Mycobactericidal Agents

Syed A. Sattar

Centre for Research on Environmental Microbiology (CREM), Faculty of Medicine, University of Ottawa, Ottawa, Ontario, Canada

Introduction

Tuberculosis (TB), already among the most common infectious diseases with 6–9 million new clinical cases globally [1, 2], is an even greater threat now due to the combined influence of the AIDS pandemic [3–6], solid organs transplanted from infected donors [7–9], induced immunosuppression for cancer therapy and organ transplantation [10], malnutrition [11], faster and more frequent international travel [12], higher population density and other on-going societal changes [13–15]. In addition, multidrug-resistant (MDR-TB) and extensively drug-resistant (XDR-TB) strains of *Mycobacterium tuberculosis* are an added challenge to chemotherapy and infection control [16, 17]. Millions more around the world harbor *M. tuberculosis* as latent and asymptomatic cases and contribute further to the pool of potential sources of the pathogen. *Mycobacterium bovis*, primarily a pathogen of bovines, can infect humans as well [18], mainly through the consumption of unpasteurized dairy products [19, 20]. In contrast, leprosy, caused by *Mycobacterium leprae*, has

already been eliminated from many once-endemic regions [21] and it may soon be eradicated.

Apart from those three pathogens, the genus *Mycobacterium* includes many other species variously referred to as "atypical mycobacteria", "mycobacteria other than tuberculosis" (MOTT) and "non-tuberculous mycobacteria" (NTM). This chapter will refer to them as "environmental mycobacteria" to signify their saprophytic and environment-based nature. Such organisms are also called "perikairots" to indicate their environmental origin and opportunistic nature as human pathogens [22]. Environmental mycobacteria are generally slower-growing organisms that achieve prominence in engineered and disinfected systems due to reduced competition from other faster-growing and more readily inactivated bacteria. Thus, ironically, they can benefit from low levels of disinfectant application, for example in potable water. Remarkably, environmental mycobacteria appear to infect humans only upon direct exposure to an environmental source, but are not known to cause secondary cases [23]. Many of the 145 known species of environmental mycobacteria [24] are common in biofilms [25] and there are examples of emerging pathogens being

Russell, Hugo & Ayliffe's: Principles and Practice of Disinfection, Preservation and Sterilization, Fifth Edition. Edited by Adam P. Fraise, Jean-Yves Maillard, and Syed A. Sattar.

found in increasing numbers and in a widening variety of infections in immunosuppressed and also otherwise normal hosts [26]. Lung infections by environmental mycobacteria necessitate additional differential diagnosis to rule out TB [27, 28].

Spread of mycobacteria

Tuberculosis spreads primarily by air [29]. While mycobacteria may survive on environmental surfaces for days to months [30, 31], there are no credible reports of their transmission when such contamination is resuspended and inhaled. Water and soil are the main reservoirs for environmental mycobacteria, with the nose and mouth as well as damaged soft tissue and skin being major portals of entry. Environmental mycobacteria in biofilms in rinse water [32, 33] or inside automated endoscope reprocessors (AERs) themselves can contaminate semicritical medical devices, leading to iatrogenic infections [34, 35], pseudo-outbreaks [36, 37] or misdiagnoses [38]. Improperly reprocessed semicritical devices such as gastroscopes and bronchoscopes can be iatrogenic means of TB spread [34]. Inhalation of environmental mycobacteria in metal-working fluids is a well-recognized cause of hypersensitivity pneumonitis, a debilitating and potentially fatal occupational hazard [39]. An emerging area of concern is that of personal service settings as increasing numbers of cases due to environmental mycobacteria are being reported from improperly processed sharps in tattooing [40], contaminated needles in acupuncture [41] and ill-maintained footbaths for pedicure [42].

Microbicides and mycobacteria

Mycolic acid in mycobacterial cell walls gives them a waxy, hydrophobic and generally less permeable character. This also makes them generally more resistant to penetration by microbicides than other non-sporulating bacteria [43]. In addition, mycobacteria might also be protected from disinfection by their ability to reside and replicate inside eukaryotes such as free-living amoebae [44, 45] (see Chapter 8). A recent report that ascribed the higher resistance to endospores in mycobacteria [46] has been refuted [47], although adequate studies of differences in disinfection sensitivity between actively growing and stressed mycobacteria have not been conducted.

The information summarized above highlights not only the continuing significance of *M. tuberculosis* but also the rapid emergence of environmental mycobacteria as human pathogens. In view of this, the term "tuberculocidal" should be replaced with "mycobactericidal" to more accurately reflect a chemical's microbicidal activity against *Mycobacterium* as a genus.

Testing microbicides against mycobacteria

Chemicals are used to inactivate mycobacteria in water for drinking [48, 49], are added to metal-working fluids to suppress biofilm formation by organisms such as *Mycobacterium immunogenum* [49–51], released into indoor air to decontaminate surfaces and pieces of equipment [52, 53], applied on hard, non-porous environmental surfaces [54], and are used for manual [55] or machine [56] disinfection of medical devices and skin antisepsis. This chapter will discuss only the last three types of uses, with particular focus on information generated in the past decade. The reader is referred to earlier reviews [57, 58] and book chapters [59, 60] for additional details. Any coverage of standard methods and test guidelines for government registration of products with claims of mycobactericidal activity will be limited to those in Europe, Canada and the USA.

Testing chemicals for effectiveness against mycobacteria can be more demanding than similar tests against many other types of organisms. This is primarily due to the hydrophobic nature of mycobacteria that causes them to readily clump together. This clumping phenomenon is more marked with some species of mycobacteria than with others; *M. bovis* is a case in point. Without careful controls, this can result in the overestimation of mycobactericidal activity. Even for other target mycobacteria, it is desirable to include a surface-active agent after disinfectant contact to promote mycobacterial dispersal and proper enumeration of survivors.

Types of tests for mycobactericidal activity

The following types of methods are used to assess the effectiveness of chemicals against mycobacteria.

1. *Suspension tests.* In general, one part of the microbial suspension is mixed with nine parts of the test formulation (for control, saline or a buffer is used instead) and the mixture held at the specified temperature for the required contact time, neutralized to quench any remaining microbicidal activity and then assayed for viable organisms to determine percentage or log_{10} reductions in relation to the control [23, 61]. Although such testing is simpler to perform, it is also a weaker challenge due to an excess of the test formulation, which can more readily inactivate the target cells in suspension even in the presence of an added soil load [61]. Therefore, suspensions tests are more suitable for screening during product development and in establishing the initial promise of formulations for eventual government registration. However, the US Environmental Protection Agency (EPA) accepts data based on suspension tests for registering mycobactericidal claims [62]; Health Canada's recent guidance document on human-use antiseptics lists suspension tests among the protocols for testing the mycobactericidal activity of hand antiseptics [63]. Health Canada's guidance document on disinfectant drugs [64] refers to the somewhat dated standard of the Canadian General Standards Board [65], which includes a suspension test.

2. *In vitro carrier tests.* In these protocols the test organism is first dried on an inanimate carrier for subsequent exposure to the test formulation or a control fluid [54]. The carrier may be placed directly in a recovery broth (with proper neutralizer) or first eluted with an eluent/neutralizer and the eluate assayed for viable organisms. Such protocols represent a stronger challenge to the test formulation as it must first penetrate through the dried inoculum to access the target, a scenario more akin to field conditions [54]. However, carrier test protocols vary widely in the nature and type of carriers, the ratio between the volume of the test formulation and the surface area of a given carrier, the type and level of added soil load, microbial load on carriers, potential for wash-off of viable organisms, and, quite importantly, the level of quantitation feasible for an accurate and reproducible assessment of microbicidal activity in relation to the product performance criterion to be met [54]. In Canada, quantitative *in vitro* carrier testing is now referred for registering environmental surface and medical device disinfectants [64].

3. *Ex vivo tests.* Here, the test organism is first placed on pieces of tissue excised from humans or animals, the inoculum is then dried and exposed to the test formulation to assess its action. Common substrates in *ex vivo* tests are pieces of pig skin [66] or sections of human skin removed during plastic surgery [67, 68]. *Ex vivo* testing is particularly suitable for experimenting with microorganisms and/or chemicals with undocumented or questionable safety for use on human subjects. There are no published reports describing the use of *ex vivo* methods to assess microbicides against mycobacteria.

4. *In vivo tests.* In these methods, the skin of intact animals or human subjects [69] is experimentally contaminated with the test organism, the inoculum is then dried and exposed to the test formulation. Only recently has *in vivo* testing using human subjects been recommended for registration of antiseptics claiming activity against mycobacteria [63, 70].

5. *Simulated use testing.* In this type of protocol external and internal surfaces of semicritical medical devices such as flexible endoscopes are experimentally contaminated with organisms including mycobacteria, and subjected to manual [71] or machine reprocessing [56]. Such testing is required by both Health Canada and the US Food and Drug Administration (FDA) [72] for registration of endoscope disinfectants meant for single use or reuse.

Standard test protocols for mycobactericidal activity

The following bodies in Europe and North America have developed standardized protocols for testing chemicals against mycobacteria to be used on environmental surfaces and medical devices.

AOAC International

Only one method relating to mycobacteria is listed in the 18th edition of the *Official Methods of Analysis* of AOAC International [73]. It is entitled "Tuberculocidal Activity of Disinfectants" (no. 965.12) with First Action status and is awaiting upgrading to Final Action soon. The method, which has not been validated for glutaraldehyde-based products, uses porcelain penicylinders as carriers. Presumptive testing is with *Mycobacterium smegmatis*

(ATCC 19420) and confirmatory tests with *M. bovis* (BCG or equivalent; Organon Teknika Corp., Durham, NC).

ASTM international

ASTM International (formerly known as the American Society for Testing and Materials) has been active for nearly three decades in developing consensus-based standards for testing chemicals as microbicides [70]. It is the only such North America-based organization dealing with antiseptics as well as disinfectants. Several of its standards are now referenced by Health Canada [63, 64], the FDA [72] and the World Health Organization [74]. The Organization for Economic Cooperation and Development (OECD) is now adapting an ASTM method (no. E-2197) for harmonized testing of hard surface disinfectants in its 31 member states [75].

Table 6.3.1 lists ASTM standards for testing the mycobactericidal activity of disinfectants. While it currently does not have any specific standards for testing antiseptics against mycobacteria,

Table 6.3.1 Methods of ASTM International [70] relating to tests against mycobacteria.

Designation (year of last approval)	Title	Scope
E-1837 (2007)	Standard Test Method to Determine Efficacy of Disinfection Processes for Reusable Medical Devices (Simulated Use Test)	Designed for experimental contamination of reusable medical devices with a variety of microorganisms, including mycobacteria, to assess their reductions in manual or machine reprocessing
E-2111 (2005)	Standard Quantitative Carrier Test Method to Evaluate the Bactericidal, Fungicidal, Mycobactericidal, and Sporicidal Potencies of Liquid Chemical Microbicides	Uses the inside bottom surface of glass vials for contamination with the test organism with or without an added soil load. It is designed for use in product development
E-2197 (2011)	Standard Quantitative Disk Carrier Test Method for Determining the Bactericidal, Virucidal, Fungicidal, Mycobactericidal and Sporicidal Activities of Liquid Chemical Germicides	Uses disks of brushed stainless steel as prototypical hard, non-porous surfaces. A soil load is required for testing. Adaptable to other materials with validation
E-2362 (2009)	Standard Practice for Evaluation of Pre-saturated or Impregnated Towelettes for Hard Surface Disinfection	This standard practice is designed to test the combined effect of wiping and disinfection to decontaminate glass slides as representative hard, environmental surfaces. The six test organisms listed include two mycobacteria (*M. bovis* and *M. chelonae*)

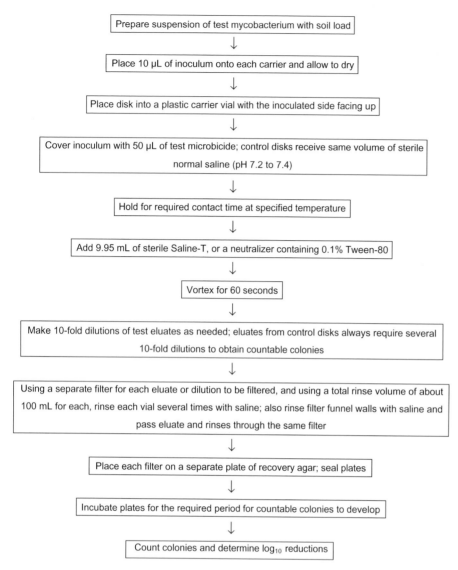

Prepare suspension of test mycobacterium with soil load

↓

Place 10 μL of inoculum onto each carrier and allow to dry

↓

Place disk into a plastic carrier vial with the inoculated side facing up

↓

Cover inoculum with 50 μL of test microbicide; control disks receive same volume of sterile normal saline (pH 7.2 to 7.4)

↓

Hold for required contact time at specified temperature

↓

Add 9.95 mL of sterile Saline-T, or a neutralizer containing 0.1% Tween-80

↓

Vortex for 60 seconds

↓

Make 10-fold dilutions of test eluates as needed; eluates from control disks always require several 10-fold dilutions to obtain countable colonies

↓

Using a separate filter for each eluate or dilution to be filtered, and using a total rinse volume of about 100 mL for each, rinse each vial several times with saline; also rinse filter funnel walls with saline and pass eluate and rinses through the same filter

↓

Place each filter on a separate plate of recovery agar; seal plates

↓

Incubate plates for the required period for countable colonies to develop

↓

Count colonies and determine log₁₀ reductions

Figure 6.3.1 Main steps in the disk-based quantitative carrier test 2 (QCT-2).

Health Canada (see below) recommends the fingerpad method for bactericidal activity (no. E-2276) to test antiseptics against mycobacteria [63] using *Mycobacterium terrae* and *Mycobacterium avium* as surrogates.

Quantitative carrier tests of ASTM international

ASTM International lists two protocols for testing the mycobactericidal activity of environmental surface and medical device disinfectants [70] and they have been described in detail previously [54].

The first of these methods (no. E-2111), referred to as the first tier of the quantitative carrier test (QCT-1), uses the inside bottom surface of flat-bottomed glass vials as the carrier. Ten microliters of the test microbial suspension (with or without an added soil load) is placed in each vial, the inoculum dried and then exposed to 1 ml of the test substance. At the end of the contact time, 9 ml of a diluent/eluent with a neutralizer is added to the vial and a magnet with a knurled surface used to scrape off and recover any inoculum remaining on the glass surface. The

eluent is diluted as needed and the samples are membrane filtered for the recovery and enumeration of colony-forming units. Log₁₀ or percent reductions in the viability of the test organisms are then calculated. Since QCT-1 uses a relatively smooth surface as a carrier and also incorporates a higher volume of test substance in relation to the microbial inoculum, it is recommended for use during product development.

ASTM standard E-2197 [54, 70] is the second tier of the quantitative carrier test (QCT-2). The main steps in the procedure are summarized in Figure 6.3.1. The default carriers in QCT-2 are disks (1 cm in diameter) of magnetized and brushed stainless steel (AISI type 430) to represent the uneven surfaces often encountered in the field to better assess the ability of the test substance to effectively disinfect them. Such disks can be contaminated with a relatively small (10 μl) and precisely measured volume of the challenge organism and also exposed to only 50 μl of the test substance. The magnetized nature of the disks enables one to hold them in place in the carrier vial with the help of a magnet during the washing and rinsing steps of the test procedure. Such disks can be readily sterilized by either autoclaving or dry heat and are recommended for a single use. Similar disks of other types of carrier materials can be used depending on the label claim(s) and the requirements of the target regulatory agency.

Mycobacteria are either discharged in body fluids or embedded in biofilms. Even though medical devices, in particular, are required to be pre-cleaned before disinfection, there are wide variations in the quality of such pre-cleaning. Therefore, QCT-2 also requires a standardized soil load in the challenge microbial suspension to simulate the presence of residues of body fluids or other contaminants on *pre-cleaned* articles to be disinfected [54]. The soil load is a mixture of a large molecular weight protein (bovine albumin), a mucoid substance (bovine mucin) and polypeptides (tryptone or yeast extract) in phosphate buffer with a total protein content roughly equal to that in 5% bovine serum.

Each carrier disk is contaminated with only 10 μl of the microbial suspension in an added soil load and the inoculum dried before exposure to 50 μl of the test substance. The contact time and temperature can be adjusted as needed for testing. The mycobactericidal action of the chemical is arrested immediately at the end of the contact time by the addition of 9.5 ml of an eluent/neutralizer to dilute the test substance 200-fold while chemically neutralizing its activity. Thorough rinsing of the filter holder and the filter membrane itself after the passage of the eluate further reduces the risk from the residues of the test substance.

The member filters are placed separately on the surface of a recovery agar medium and incubated, colonies counted and $\log_{10}$ reductions calculated. QCT-2 can be readily adapted to test formulations to be applied as liquid or foamy sprays on environmental surfaces.

Comité Européean de Normalisation

Comité Européean de Normalisation (CEN), also called the European Committee for Standardization, consists of 31 countries working together to develop voluntary European standards in a variety of areas including methods for testing chemicals as microbicides (Technical Committee no. 216) [76]. The European Medical Devices Directive is the European legal framework that covers regulation of these products and European Norms (ENs) are being developed to assist manufacturers who wish to place their product on the market in Europe. Table 6.3.2 lists CEN methods designed to test antiseptics and disinfectants against mycobacteria.

Guidance on testing and registration of chemicals as mycobactericides

Health Canada
Disinfectants

In August 2007, Health Canada issued an updated guidance document for the testing and registration of hard surface and medical device disinfectants [64]. While it refers to the Canadian General Standards Board's standard CAN/CGSB-2.161-97 [65], it also

Table 6.3.2 CEN [76] standards relating to testing of chemical disinfectants and antiseptics for mycobactericidal activity.

Designation (year of approval)	Title
EN14204 (2004)	Quantitative Suspension Test for the Evaluation of Mycobactericidal Activity of Chemical Disinfectants and Antiseptics used in the Veterinary Area – Test Method and Requirements (phase 2, step 1)
EN14348 (2005)	Quantitative Suspension Test for the Evaluation of Mycobactericidal Activity of Chemical Disinfectants in the Medical Area Including Instrument Disinfectants (phase 2, step 1)
EN14563 (2008)	Quantitative Carrier Test for the Evaluation of Mycobactericidal or Tuberculocidal Activity of Chemical Disinfectants used for Instruments in the Medical Area – Test Method and Requirements (phase 2, step 2)

considers other scientifically valid test protocols in applying this guidance. For instance, it will accept data generated using ASTM's quantitative carrier tests E-2111 and E-2197 (see Table 6.3.1).

Antiseptics

A more recent guidance document from Health Canada concerns the testing of various categories of antiseptics as microbicides [63]. As shown in Table 6.3.3, the organisms listed include two species of mycobacteria and the recommended test protocols are *in vitro* and *in vivo* tests of both CEN and ASTM. Please refer to Chapter 13 for additional details.

United States environmental protection agency

As of January 2009, the EPA's B List of registered products contains 162 claiming activity against *M. tuberculosis*; in List E, 37 of these products are given as claiming activity against *M. tuberculosis*, HIV-1 and hepatitis B virus [62]. The actives listed are caprylic acid, chlorine dioxide, ethanol, glutaraldehyde, hydrochloric acid, hydrogen chloride, hydrogen peroxide, iodine, isopropanol, *para*-chlorometaxylenol, peroxyacetic acid, phenolics, quaternary ammonium compounds (QACs), sodium bromide, sodium chlorite, sodium dichloroisocyanurate, sodium hypochlorite and thymol.

The BEAD (Biological and Economic Analysis Division) Lab of the EPA is currently retesting products with tuberculocidal claims. The methods used for the purpose are summarized in Table 6.3.4.

United States food and drug administration

The FDA has the responsibility for the review and registration of sterilants and high-level disinfectants to be used for the reprocessing of medical devices [72]. High-level disinfectants must show mycobactericidal activity in potency as well as simulated-use tests. Potency testing is based on the AOAC's modified (quantified) Tuberculocidal Activity of Disinfectants Method no. 965.12 or

Table 6.3.3 Health Canada's [63] requirements for testing antiseptics against mycobacteria.[a]

Product category	In vitro (suspension) test		In vivo (fingerpad) test	
	CEN	ASTM	CEN	ASTM
Personal use: self-selected for use by an individual in a domestic setting[b]	EN14476 with a ≥4-log$_{10}$ reduction	ASTM 1052 with a ≥4-log$_{10}$ reduction	EN1499 (for washes) and EN1500 (for rubs) with a ≥2-log$_{10}$ reduction	E-2276 with a ≥2-log$_{10}$ reduction
Commercial use	EN14476 with a ≥4-log$_{10}$ reduction	ASTM 1052 with a ≥4-log$_{10}$ reduction	EN1499 (for handwashes) and EN1500 (for handrubs) with a ≥2-log$_{10}$ reduction	E-2276 with a ≥2-log$_{10}$ reduction
Professional food-handler use	EN14348 with a ≥5-log$_{10}$	Not applicable	EN1499 (for washes) and EN1500 (for rubs) with a ≥3-log$_{10}$ reduction	E-1174 with a ≥3-log$_{10}$ reduction
Professional healthcare use	EN14348 with a 5-log$_{10}$ reduction	Not applicable	EN1499 (for washes) and EN1500 (for rubs) with a ≥3-log$_{10}$ reduction	E-1174 with a ≥3-log$_{10}$ reduction

[a] Testing against both *Mycobacterium avium* and *M. terrae* is required.
[b] Applies only to products beyond the scope of *Antiseptic Skin Cleanser Monograph* by Health Canada.

Table 6.3.4 Test methods used by the Environmental Protection Agency to assess the mycobactericidal activity of microbicides [62].

Title	Particulars	Standard operating procedure (date)
Tuberculocidal Activity of Disinfectants. II Confirmative *in vitro* Test for Determining Tuberculocidal Activity	Based on AOAC International's Method no. 965.12 part II; test organism is *M. bovis* (BCG) dried on porcelain penicylinders	MB-07-05 (March 16, 2010)
Quantitative Suspension Test for Determining Tuberculocidal Efficacy of Disinfectants Against *M. bovis* (BCG)	Based on the method of Ascenzi *et al.* [77]	MB-16-01 (February 6, 2009)
Disinfectant Towelette Test Against *M. bovis* (BCG)	This carrier method, which uses glass slides, is a modification of AOAC method no. 961.02 (2009)	MB-23-01 (February 26, 2010)
Testing of *M. bovis* (BCG) using the Germicidal Spray Products as Disinfectants	This carrier method, which uses glass slides as carriers, is an adaptation of AOAC methods no. 965.12 and 961.02	MB-24-01 (February 26, 2010)

Ascenzi's quantified suspension test [77]. A 6-log$_{10}$ kill of either *M. bovis* or *M. terrae* is required under the test conditions used. The use of other species of mycobacteria is also permitted so long as test data or literature references can be provided to indicate that the resistance of the selected organism to the tested chemical is similar to that of *M. tuberculosis* var. *bovis*. For simulated-use testing [71], the most resistant species of *Mycobacterium* is recommended and a minimum 6-log$_{10}$ reduction in its viability required.

As of March 2009, the FDA lists 30 products registered as high-level disinfectants with general claims for processing reusable medical and dental devices [78]. Such formulations must first show acceptable mycobactericidal activity to qualify as high-level disinfectants. Nearly 57% (17/30) of these products contain 1.12–3.6% glutaraldehyde either alone or in combination with isopropanol or phenol/phenate. The next most common active is *ortho*-phthalaldehyde (0.55–5.75%) as the sole active in 13% (4/30). Ten percent (3/30) contain a mixture of hydrogen peroxide (1.0–8.3%) and peracetic acid (0.08–7.0%). Only one products is based on a mixture of hypochlorite and hypochlorous acid, giving a free chlorine level of 6.75 parts per million.

Table 6.3.5 is a summary of information from selected publications (2001–2010) on the mycobactericidal activities of chemicals [71, 79–89].

Conclusions

TB has re-emerged as a significant threat to global health [13, 90]. Its drug-resistant strains are a particularly serious challenge as chemotherapy is no longer a viable option in dealing with them; progress in developing a safer and more effective vaccine against the disease has also been agonizingly slow [91]. Under the circumstances, interrupting the spread of TB through environmental control presents itself as a viable option. In this regard, proper filtration of indoor air and/or its disinfection using ultraviolet technology show considerable promise in clinics and hospitals, as examples.

Proper chemical disinfection of semicritical medical devices constitutes another crucial aspect of any effective and generic preventive strategy. Even today, many settings either do not reprocess heat-sensitive endoscopes properly or rely upon disinfectants with questionable activity against pathogens such as *M.*

Table 6.3.5 Summary of studies on the mycobactericidal activities of microbicides: 2001–2010.

Reference	Mycobacterial species tested (ATCC number)	Microbicide(s) tested	Test method	Contact time	Summary of results
Bello et al. (2006) [7]	M. smegmatis (19420); M. tuberculosis H37Rv; clinical isolates of M. fortuitum, M. chelonae and M. abscessus	Cidex (2% glutaraldehyde); Cidex-OPA (0.55% o-phthalaldehyde); K-Iler (0.16% dimethyl benzyl lauryl ammonium bromide); Gardex (10% dimethyl benzyl lauryl ammonium bromide); Microplus-Action (5% polymethylene urea); Microplus-Action (5% polymethylene urea)	Quantitative suspension test prEN 14348 in "clean" and "dirty" conditions	5–60 min	Products tested registered as tuberculocides in Venezuela and used in clinical and laboratory settings. Only Cidex and Cidex-OPA produced a >5-$\log_{10}$ reduction in the viability of all species tested in 5 min. All other products failed to do so even after a contact time of 60 min. Authors caution that using ineffective products could result in iatrogenic infections
Garcia de Lomas et al. (2008) [80]	M. terrae (15755)	2-Butanone peroxide (0.5%) as an aqueous solution	Quantitative suspension test EN14476. Soil load was 3 mg/ml bovine serum albumin and 0.03 ml/ml sheep erythrocyte. Product diluent was water with 300 mg/kg $CaCO_3$	60 min	Disinfectant found difficult to neutralize with conventional chemicals; membrane filtration and washing of filters was adopted for the purpose. Mycobactericidal activity was obtained after 60 min at 20°C. Quite likely, the product would require an even longer contact time to meet the generally accepted product performance criterion of ≥6-$\log_{10}$ reduction in viability, thus making it unsuitable for use under most field conditions.
Hernández et al. (2005) [81]	M. tuberculosis H37Rv (25618); M. kansasii (12478); M. chelonae (35752); M. avium-intracellulare (clinical isolate)	2% Korsolex (15.6% dodecyl bispropylene diamine + 5.1% lauryl propylene diamine); prepared and used within 2 h. Concentrations and contact times tested were 1% for 60 min, 2% for 30 min and 3% for 15 min. Acceptable activity was ≥5-$\log_{10}$ reduction	Quantitative suspension as well as carrier tests. Borosilicate disks were used as carriers; a soil load of 7.6 g/l was added to the microbial suspension; distilled water was used instead of the product on control disks. Distilled water and standard hard water (200 ppm $CaCO_3$) were used as the diluent in suspension and carrier tests, respectively	60 min	Minimum of 60 min with a 1% solution was needed in carrier tests against all organisms tested
Hernández et al. (2003) [82]	M. tuberculosis H37Rv (9360); M. avium-intracellulare (clinical isolate)	Perasafe (0.26% peracetic acid); Cidex (2% glutaraldehyde)	Disinfection of flexible fibreoptic bronchoscopes at room temperature after manual cleaning with a neutral detergent. The bacteria were suspended in sputum for experimental contamination of the scopes. Perasafe diluted in tap water to prepare use dilution	10 min	Perasafe proved effective (>4.0-$\log_{10}$ reduction) in 10 min while Cidex required 20 min
Hernández et al. (2008) [83]	M. avium (15769)	Tristel Sporicidal Wipes (200 ppm chlorine dioxide) to disinfect non-lumened semicritical medical devices under clean conditions (0.3 g/l bovine serum albumin)	Modified quantitative carrier test prEN14563 with frosted glass as carriers	30 and 60 s	The wipes were mycobactericidal in 30 s with mechanical action and 60 s without mechanical action; 30 s of wiping needed for a ≥4-$\log_{10}$ reduction
Miner et al. (2010) [84]	M. bovis var. BCG (Organon Teknika); M. terrae (15755); glutaraldehyde-resistant M. chelonae var. abscessus (14472)	≤2.1% glutaraldehyde only, glutaraldehyde in combination with ≤12.0% w/w isopropanol or in combination with ≤5.0% potassium acetate, and glutaraldehyde in combination with both isopropanol and potassium acetate	Suspension test with M. bovis and M. terrae and suture loop test of AOAC International (966.04) for M. chelonae; soil load 5% fetal bovine serum; test temperature 20 and 25°C	2–30 min	Combination of 1.8% w/w glutaraldehyde with 10.6% w/w isopropanol and 4.2% potassium acetate was the most rapidly mycobactericidal, killing 7-$\log_{10}$ of M. terrae within 2 min at 25°C in suspension; the same formulation reduced the viability titer of M. chelonae on polyester suture loops by 6-$\log_{10}$ within 10 min at 20°C

Table 6.3.5 (*Continued*)

Reference	Mycobacterial species tested (ATCC number)	Microbicide(s) tested	Test method	Contact time	Summary of results
Omidbakhsh and Sattar (2006) [85]	*M. bovis* BCG; *M. terrae* (15755)	ACCEL TB (0.5% accelerated hydrogen peroxide)	Tested against *M. bovis* and *M. terrae* using a quantitative suspension test and first tier of the quantitative carrier test (QCT-1; ASTM E-2111), respectively, at 20°C. Soil load was either 5% fetal bovine serum or a mixture of three types of proteins in phosphate buffer	5 min	The formulation reduced the viability titer of *M. bovis* by 6.8-$\log_{10}$ in 5 min in suspension. In QCT-1, *M. terrae* titer was reduced by >6.0-$\log_{10}$ also in 5 min
Rikimaru *et al.* (2002) [86]	Clinical strains of multidrug resistant *M. tuberculosis*; *M. tuberculosis* H37 Rv	Povidone-iodine (PVP-I), cresol, akyldiaminoethyl glycine hydrochloride (AEG) and glutaraldehyde	Suspension test; 0.05 ml of mycobacterial suspension was added to 0.45 ml of disinfectant. Soil load was 2% human serum	1–5 min	PVP-I (0.1–0.2%) required no more than 2 min to reduce the viability titer of all strains tested by ≥3-$\log_{10}$. Cresol (0.5–3%) took 1–5 min to achieve the same level of activity whereas 60 min were needed by AEG (0.1–0.5%). Glutaraldehyde (2%) required 10 min for a 3-$\log_{10}$ kill. There was no quantifiable difference in the disinfectant resistance of sensitive and multidrug resistant strains
Sattar *et al.* (2002) [71]	*M. terrae* (15755)	7% stabilized hydrogen peroxide	A stress test protocol was used in combination with QCT-1 to assess the activity of the disinfectant after 14 days of reuse. Soil load consisted of 2% fetal bovine serum added to the disinfectant bath	25–35 min	The disinfectant collected after 7 days of stress could reduce the viability titer of *M. terrae* by >6.5-$\log_{10}$ after a contact time of 25 min at 20°C. After 14 days of stress, a contact time of 35 min was needed for the same level of mycobactericidal activity
Steinhauer *et al.* (2010) [87]	*M. terrae* (15755) + gfp_m^{2+} gene.	1.5% peracetic acid; a product consisting of a combination of 14% cocospropylenediamine guanidine diacetate, 35% phenoxypropanols and 2.5% benzalkonium chloride	Quantitative carrier test prEN14563. Soil load consisted of 3 mg/ml bovine serum albumin and 0.03 ml/ml sheep erythrocytes	5–60 min	The fluorescence enabled determination of mycobactericidal efficacy within 15 days instead of 21 days
Wang *et al.* (2005) [88]	*M. tuberculosis* H37Ra; CMCC(B) 93020; *M. chelonae* subsp. *abscessus* CMCC(B) 93326	Formulations tested separately contained iodophor (10–40 mg/l), glutaraldehyde (0.25–1%), chlorine (10–80 mg/l), peracetic acid (0.05–2%) and alcohol (30–60%). Distilled water used to prepare in-use dilutions	Suspension test; 0.1 ml of mycobacterial suspension added to 5 ml of disinfectant	1–20 min	*M. chelonae* subsp. *abscessus* proved more resistant to chlorine than *M. tuberculosis* while the two strains showed similar resistance to iodophor, peracetic acid, alcohol and glutaraldehyde. *M. chelonae* subsp. *abscessus* has the potential as a surrogate for *M. tuberculosis* in evaluating mycobactericidal efficacies of disinfectants
Zafer *et al.* (2001) [89]	*M. terrae* (15755) + pBEN(gfp) plasmid	7.5% stabilized hydrogen peroxide; 2.4% alkaline glutaraldehyde; 10% acid glutaraldehyde and 15.5% phenolic	Quantitative suspension test at 22°C	10–20 min	There was good correspondence between the intensity of fluorescence and the numbers of viable organisms in test suspensions, thus allowing for rapid screening of mycobactericidal activity of tested formulations

tuberculosis. This is due to certain deficiencies in the test methods mandated and used to generate data for product registration. Not surprisingly, QACs, with virtually no mycobactericidal activity on their own, still figure prominently as actives in numerous products registered for sale. The rationale for the continued marketing of benzalkonium chloride-based antiseptics has been questioned in the face of numerous cases of iatrogenic infections due to mycobacteria [92].

Environmental mycobacteria are already recognized as significant human pathogens [43, 93, 94] and their impact is likely to increase further with on-going environmental and societal changes [14]. For example, when a community replaces chlorine with monochloramine to disinfect its water for drinking to reduce the levels of regulated disinfection by-products, the types and numbers of environmental mycobacteria in the drinking water distribution system increase [95, 96], likely due to a reduction in the numbers of competing bacterial species.

Unlike the tubercle bacillus, which spreads mainly through air [29] and is not known to replicate outside human or animal hosts, environmental mycobacteria are classic perikairots [22] with a very wide distribution in biofilms in natural and engineered environments [50]. They are inherently more resistant to microbicides and many chemotherapeutic agents as well. Glutaraldehyde-resistant environmental mycobacteria were first isolated from automated endoscope reprocessors by van Klingeren and Pullen [97] and their observations were soon confirmed [98]. More recent reports on the health problems caused by such resistant organisms in Brazil are quite alarming [99, 100] and have much broader implications in view of the continuing use of glutaraldehyde as a high-level disinfectant. It is worth noting here that such microbicide-resistant organisms are showing increased resistance to antibiotics as well [99, 100]. This calls for a critical and immediate assessment of the situation to forestall any further expansion of the already serious problem of microbicide resistance and its potential to generate cross-resistance to antibiotics [101].

The debate on a suitable surrogate for *M. tuberculosis* for testing microbicides is less intense now, possibly because in Europe and in North America there is general consensus on using *M. terrae* and/or *M. avium* for this purpose [54, 102]. It has also been argued that the choice of a surrogate is only one of many factors in the design of a proper microbicide test protocol and that the incorporation of several levels of stringency are essential to abrogate any inherent differences between the actual target pathogen and its surrogate [54]. Since [87] common surrogates for *M. tuberculosis* are relatively slow growing, the fluorescent protein gene has been incorporated into them to reduce the time for disinfectant testing [89].

Mycobacteria as a group present many unique challenges to human health. The re-emergence of drug- and microbicide-resistant strains of the tubercle bacillus is a major setback internationally [103]. Additionally, the true role of environmental mycobacteria in the etiology of many types of diseases is likely underestimated because the routine methods for the processing of clinical samples do not cater to the special needs for laboratory culture. Moreover, infections by environmental mycobacteria are not reportable and so no adequate records are kept. With the well-recognized and growing limitations of chemotherapy, and in the continued absence of effective vaccination, environmental control through the proper use of microbicides is among the limited options available. However, for optimal benefit, better test methods and regulations are needed to select for and use safer and more effective mycobactericides.

Acknowledgments

I thank my colleagues Susan Springthorpe and Jason Tetro for their valuable input and assistance in the preparation of this chapter. I am also most grateful to my family for giving me the time to work on this document.

References

1 Glaziou, P. *et al.* (2009) Global burden and epidemiology of tuberculosis. *Clinics in Chest Medicine*, **30**, 621.

2 Lonnroth, K. *et al.* (2010) Tuberculosis control and elimination 2010–50: cure, care, and social development. *Lancet*, **375**, 1814–1829.

3 Harries, A.D. *et al.* (2010) Tuberculosis 3. The HIV-associated tuberculosis epidemic-when will we act? *Lancet*, **375**, 1906–1919.

4 Lalloo, U.G. and Pillay, S. (2008) Managing tuberculosis and HIV in sub-Sahara Africa. *Current HIV/AIDS Reports*, **5**, 132–139.

5 Laserson, K.F. and Wells, C.D. (2007) Reaching the targets for tuberculosis control: the impact of HIV. *Bulletin of the World Health Organization*, **85**, 377–381.

6 Vitoria, M. *et al.* (2009) The global fight against HIV/AIDS, tuberculosis, and malaria current status and future perspectives. *American Journal of Clinical Pathology*, **131**, 844–848.

7 de Castilla, D.L. and Schluger, N.W. (2010) Tuberculosis following solid organ transplantation. *Transplant Infectious Disease*, **12**, 106–112.

8 Garcia-Goez, J.F. *et al.* (2009) Tuberculosis in solid organ transplant recipients at a tertiary hospital in the last 20 years in Barcelona, Spain. *Transplantation Proceedings*, **41**, 2268–2270.

9 Winthrop, K.L. *et al.* (2004) Transmission of *Mycobacterium tuberculosis* via lung transplantation. *American Journal of Transplantation*, **4**, 1529–1533.

10 Guida, J.P.S. *et al.* (2009) Tuberculosis in renal transplant recipients: a brazilian center registry. *Transplantation Proceedings*, **41**, 883–884.

11 Cegielski, J.P. and McMurray, D.N. (2004) The relationship between malnutrition and tuberculosis: evidence from studies in humans and experimental animals. *International Journal of Tuberculosis and Lung Disease*, **8**, 286–298.

12 Martinez, L. *et al.* (2008) Tuberculosis and air travel: WHO guidance in the era of drug-resistant TB. *Travel Medicine and Infectious Diseases*, **6**, 177–181.

13 Dye, C. *et al.* (2009) Trends in tuberculosis incidence and their determinants in 134 countries. *Bulletin of the World Health Organization*, **87**, 683–691.

14 Falkinham, J.O. (2010) Impact of human activities on the ecology of nontuberculous mycobacteria. *Future Microbiology*, **5**, 951–960.

15 Sattar, S.A. *et al.* (1999) Impact of changing societal trends on the spread of infections in American and Canadian homes. *American Journal of Infection Control*, **27**, S4–S21.

16 Gandhi, N.R. *et al.* (2010) Multidrug-resistant and extensively drug-resistant tuberculosis: a threat to global control of tuberculosis. *Lancet*, **375**, 1830–1843.

17 Centers for Disease Control and Prevention (2009) Plan to combat extensively drug-resistant tuberculosis: recommendations of the Federal Tuberculosis Task Force. *MMWR Recommendations and Reports*, **58**, 1–43.

18 Rua-Domenech, R. (2006) Human *Mycobacterium bovis* infection in the United Kingdom: incidence, risks, control measures and review of the zoonotic aspects of bovine tuberculosis. *Tuberculosis*, **86**, 77–109.

19 Hlavsa, M.C. *et al.* (2008) Human tuberculosis due to *Mycobacterium bovis* in the United States, 1995–2005. *Clinical Infectious Diseases*, **47**, 168–175.

20 Rodwell, T.C. *et al.* (2008) Tuberculosis from *Mycobacterium bovis* in binational communities, United States. *Emerging Infectious Diseases*, **14**, 909–916.

21 Feasey, N. *et al.* (2010) Neglected tropical diseases. *British Medical Bulletin*, **93**, 179–200.

22 Sattar, S.A. and Springthorpe, V.S. (2004) Contribution of the environment to infectious disease transmission, in *Disinfection, Sterilization and Antisepsis: Principles, Practices, Challenges, and New Research* (ed. W.A. Rutala), Association of Practitioners in Infection Control and Epidemiology (APIC), Washington, DC, pp. 148–157.

23 Griffith, D.E. *et al.* (2007) An official ATS/IDSA statement: diagnosis, treatment, and prevention of nontuberculous mycobacterial diseases. *American Journal of Respiratory and Critical Care Medicine*, **175**, 367–416.

24 Euzéby, J.P. (2011) *List of Prokaryotic Names with Standing in Nomenclature – Genus Mycobacterium*, http://www.bacterio.cict.fr/ (accessed October 24, 2011).

25 Feazel, L.M. *et al.* (2009) Opportunistic pathogens enriched in showerhead biofilms. *Proceedings of the National Academy of Sciences of the United States of America*, **106**, 16393–16398.

26 van Duin, D. *et al.* (2010) Nontuberculous mycobacterial blood stream and cardiac infections in patients without HIV infection. *Diagnostic Microbiology and Infectious Disease*, **67**, 286–290.

27 Arend, S.M. *et al.* (2009) Diagnosis and treatment of lung infection with nontuberculous mycobacteria. *Current Opinion in Pulmonary Medicine*, **15**, 201–208.

28 McGrath, E.E. *et al.* (2010) Nontuberculous mycobacteria and the lung: from suspicion to treatment. *Lung*, **188**, 269–282.

29 Escombe, A.R. *et al.* (2009) Upper-room ultraviolet light and negative air ionization to prevent tuberculosis transmission. *PLoS Medicine*, **6**, e43.

30 Archuleta, R.J. *et al.* (2002) The relationship of temperature to desiccation and starvation tolerance of the *Mycobacterium avium* complex. *Archives of Microbiology*, **178**, 311–314.

31 Kramer, A. *et al.* (2006) How long do nosocomial pathogens persist on inanimate surfaces? A systematic review. *BMC Infectious Diseases*, **6**, 130.

32 Vaerewijck, M.J.M. *et al.* (2005) Mycobacteria in drinking water distribution systems: ecology and significance for human health. *FEMS Microbiology Reviews*, **29**, 911–934.

33 Willis, C. (2006) Bacteria-free endoscopy rinse water – a realistic aim? *Epidemiology and Infection*, **134**, 279–284.

34 Vijayaraghavan, R. *et al.* (2006) Hospital outbreak of atypical mycobacterial infection of port sites after laparoscopic surgery. *Journal of Hospital Infection*, **64**, 344–347.

35 Astagneau, P. *et al.* (2001) *Mycobacterium xenopi* spinal infections after discovertebral surgery: investigation and screening of a large outbreak. *Lancet*, **358**, 747–751.

36 Blossom, D.B. *et al.* (2008) Pseudo-outbreak of *Mycobacterium abscessus* infection caused by laboratory contamination. *Infection Control and Hospital Epidemiology*, **29**, 57–62.

37 Chroneou, A. *et al.* (2008) Molecular typing of *Mycobacterium chelonae* isolates from a pseudo-outbreak involving an automated bronchoscope washer. *Infection Control and Hospital Epidemiology*, **29**, 1088–1090.

38 Wang, S.H. *et al.* (2009) Pseudo-outbreak of "Mycobacterium paraffinicum" infection and/or colonization in a tertiary care medical center. *Infection Control and Hospital Epidemiology*, **30**, 848–853.

39 Falkinham, J.O. (2003) Mycobacterial aerosols and respiratory disease. *Emerging Infectious Diseases*, **9**, 763–767.

40 Drage, L.A. *et al.* (2010) An outbreak of *Mycobacterium chelonae* infections in tattoos. *Journal of the American Academy of Dermatology*, **62**, 501–506.

41 Koh, S.J. *et al.* (2010) An outbreak of skin and soft tissue infection caused by *Mycobacterium abscessus* following acupuncture. *Clinical Microbiology and Infection*, **16**, 895–901.

42 Vugia, D.J. *et al.* (2005) Mycobacteria in nail salon whirlpool footbaths, California. *Emerging Infectious Diseases*, **11**, 616–618.

43 Falkinham, J.O. (2009) Surrounded by mycobacteria: nontuberculous mycobacteria in the human environment. *Journal of Applied Microbiology*, **107**, 356–367.

44 Ben Salah, I. and Drancourt, M. (2010) Surviving within the amoebal exocyst: the *Mycobacterium avium* complex paradigm. *BMC Microbiology*, **10**, 99.

45 Lahiri, R. and Krahenbuhl, J.L. (2008) The role of free-living pathogenic amoeba in the transmission of leprosy: a proof of principle. *Leprosy Review*, **79**, 401–409.

46 Ghosh, J. *et al.* (2009) Sporulation in mycobacteria. *Proceedings of the National Academy of Sciences of the United States of America*, **106**, 10781–10786.

47 Traag, B.A. *et al.* (2010) Do mycobacteria produce endospores? *Proceedings of the National Academy of Sciences of the United States of America*, **107**, 878–881.

48 Le Dantec, C. *et al.* (2002) Chlorine disinfection of atypical mycobacteria isolated from a water distribution system. *Applied and Environmental Microbiology*, **68**, 1025–1032.

49 Pryor, M. *et al.* (2004) Investigation of opportunistic pathogens in municipal drinking water under different supply and treatment regimes. *Water Science and Technology*, **50**, 83–90.

50 Falkinham, J.O. (2009) Effects of biocides and other metal removal fluid constituents on *Mycobacterium immunogenum*. *Applied and Environmental Microbiology*, **75**, 2057–2061.

51 Steinhauer, K. and Goroncy-Bermes, P. (2008) Treatment of water-based metalworking fluids to prevent hypersensitivity pneumonitis associated with *Mycobacterium* spp. *Journal of Applied Microbiology*, **104**, 454–464.

52 Hall, L. *et al.* (2007) Use of hydrogen peroxide vapor for deactivation of *Mycobacterium tuberculosis* in a biological safety cabinet and a room. *Journal of Clinical Microbiology*, **45**, 810–815.

53 Kahnert, A. *et al.* (2005) Decontamination with vaporized hydrogen peroxide is effective against *Mycobacterium tuberculosis*. *Letters in Applied Microbiology*, **40**, 448–452.

54 Springthorpe, V.S. and Sattar, S.A. (2007) Application of a quantitative carrier test to evaluate microbicides against mycobacteria. *Journal of AOAC International*, **90**, 817–824.

55 Collins, W.O. (2009) A review of reprocessing techniques of flexible nasopharyngoscopes. *Otolaryngology-Head and Neck Surgery*, **141**, 307–310.

56 Sattar, S.A. *et al.* (2006) Experimental evaluation of an automated endoscope reprocessor with in situ generation of peracetic acid for disinfection of semicritical devices. *Infection Control and Hospital Epidemiology*, **27**, 1193–1199.

57 Russell, A.D. (1996) Activity of biocides against mycobacteria. *Journal of Applied Bacteriology*, **81**, S87–S101.

58 Sattar, S.A. *et al.* (1995) Mycobactericidal testing of disinfectants – an update. *Journal of Hospital Infection*, **30**, 372–382.

59 Hawkey, P.M. (2004) Mycobactericidal agents, in *Principles and Practice of Disinfection, Preservation and Sterilization*, 2nd edn (ed. A.P. Fraise *et al.*), Blackwell Science, Oxford, pp. 191–204.

60 Lauzardo, M. and Rubin, J. (2001) Chapter 26, in *Mycobacterial Disinfection. Disinfection, Sterilization and Preservation*, 5th edn (ed. S.S. Block), Lippincott Williams & Wilkins, Philadelphia, pp. 513–528.

61 Best, M. *et al.* (1988) Comparative mycobactericidal efficacy of chemical disinfectants in suspension and carrier tests. *Applied and Environmental Microbiology*, **54**, 2856–2858.

62 United States Environmental Protection Agency (2009) *EPA's Registered Sterilizers, Tuberculocides, and Antimicrobial Products Against Certain Human Public Health Bacteria and Viruses*, http://www.epa.gov/oppad001/chemregindex.htm.

63 Health Canada (2009) *Guidance Document – Human-Use Antiseptic Drugs*, Health Products and Food Branch, Ottawa.

64 Health Canada (2007) *Guidance Document – Disinfectant Drugs*, Health Products and Food Branch, Ottawa.

65 Canadian General Standards Board (CGSB) (1997) *CAN/CGSB-2.161-M97: Assessment of Efficacy of Antimicrobial Agents for Use on Environmental Surfaces and Medical Devices*, CGSB, Ottawa.

66 Shintre, M.S. *et al.* (2007) Evaluation of an alcohol-based surgical hand disinfectant containing a synergistic combination of farnesol and benzethonium chloride for immediate and persistent activity against resident hand flora of volunteers and with a novel *in vitro* pig skin model. *Infection Control and Hospital Epidemiology*, **28**, 191–197.

67 Graham, M.L. *et al.* (1996) Ex vivo protocol for testing virus survival on human skin: experiments with herpesvirus 2. *Applied and Environmental Microbiology*, **62**, 4252–4255.

68 Messager, S. *et al.* (2004) Use of the "*ex vivo*" test to study long-term bacterial survival on human skin and their sensitivity to antisepsis. *Journal of Applied Microbiology*, **97**, 1149–1160.

69 Sattar, S.A. *et al.* (2000) Activity of an alcohol-based hand gel against human adeno-, rhino-, and rotaviruses using the fingerpad method. *Infection Control and Hospital Epidemiology*, **21**, 516–519.

70 ASTM International (2011) *ASTM Book of Standards Volume 11.05: Pesticides and Alternative Control Agents; Environmental Assessment; Hazardous Substances and Oil Spill Response*, ASTM International, West Conshohocken, PA.

71 Sattar, S.A. *et al.* (2002) Combined application of simulated reuse and quantitative carrier tests to assess high-level disinfection: experiments with an accelerated hydrogen peroxide-based formulation. *American Journal of Infection Control*, **30**, 449–457.

72 United States Food and Drug Administration (2000) *Guidance for Industry and FDA Reviewers. Content and Format of Premarket Notification [510(k)] Submissions for Liquid Chemical Sterilants/High Level Disinfectants.* Center for Devices and Radiological Health, Food and Drug Administration, Washington, DC.

73 AOAC International (2010) *Official Methods of Analysis*, AOAC International, Gaithersburg, MD.

74 World Health Organization (WHO) (2009) *Guidelines on Hand Hygiene in Health Care*, WHO, Geneva.

75 Organization for Economic Co-operation and Development (OECD) (2010) *Biocides: About*, OECD, Paris.

76 Ascenzi J. *et al.* (1987) A more accurate method for measurement of tuberculocidal activity of disinfectants. *Applied and Environmental Microbiology*, **53**, 2189–2192.

77 Comité Européen de Normalisation (2010) *CEN/TC 216 – Published Standards*, http://www.cen.eu/cen/Sectors/TechnicalCommitteesWorkshops/CENTechnicalCommittees/Pages/default.aspx?param=6197&title=CEN/TC%20216.

78 United States Food and Drug Administration (2009) *FDA-cleared Sterilants and High Level Disinfectants with General Claims for Processing Reusable Medical and Dental Devices – March 2009*, http://www.fda.gov/MedicalDevices/DeviceRegulationandGuidance/ReprocessingofSingle-UseDevices/ucm133514.htm.

79 Bello, T. *et al.* (2006) Inactivation of mycobacteria by disinfectants with a tuberculocidal label. *Enfermedades Infecciosas Y Microbiologia Clinica*, **24**, 319–321.

80 Garcia de Lomas, J. *et al.* (2008) Evaluation of the in-vitro cidal activity and toxicity of a novel peroxygen biocide: 2-butanone peroxide. *Journal of Hospital Infection*, **68**, 248–254.

81 Hernández, A. *et al.* (2005) Mycobactericidal and tuberculocidal activity of Korsolex (R) AF, an amine detergent/disinfectant product. *Journal of Hospital Infection*, **59**, 62–66.

82 Hernández, A. *et al.* (2003) In-vitro evaluation of Perasafe (R) compared with 2% alkaline glutaraldehyde against *Mycobacterium* spp. *Journal of Hospital Infection*, **54**, 52–56.

83 Hernández, A. *et al.* (2008) Mycobactericidal activity of chlorine dioxide wipes in a modified prEN 14563 test. *Journal of Hospital Infection*, **69**, 384–388.

84 Miner, N. *et al.* (2010) Aldahol high-level disinfectant. *American Journal of Infection Control*, **38**, 205–211.

85 Omidbakhsh, N. and Sattar, S.A. (2006) Broad-spectrum microbicidal activity, toxicologic assessment, and materials compatibility of a new generation of accelerated hydrogen peroxide-based environmental surface disinfectant. *American Journal of Infection Control*, **34**, 251–257.

86 Rikimaru, T. *et al.* (2002) Efficacy of common antiseptics against multidrug-resistant *Mycobacterium tuberculosis*. *International Journal of Tuberculosis and Lung Disease*, **6**, 763–770.

87 Steinhauer, K. *et al.* (2010) Rapid evaluation of the mycobactericidal efficacy of disinfectants in the quantitative carrier test EN 14563 by using fluorescent *Mycobacterium terrae*. *Applied and Environmental Microbiology*, **76**, 546–554.

88 Wang, G.Q. *et al.* (2005) Comparison of susceptibilities of M-tuberculosis H37Ra and M-chelonei subsp. abscessus to disinfectants. *Biomedical and Environmental Sciences*, **18**, 124–127.

89 Zafer, A.A. *et al.* (2001) Rapid screening method for mycobactericidal activity of chemical germicides that uses *Mycobacterium terrae* expressing a green fluorescent protein gene. *Applied and Environmental Microbiology*, **67**, 1239–1245.

90 Ramon-Pardo, P. *et al.* (2009) Epidemiology of tuberculosis in the Americas: the Stop TB strategy and the Millennium Development Goals. *International Journal of Tuberculosis and Lung Disease*, **13**, 969–975.

91 Russell, D.G. *et al.* (2010) Tuberculosis: what we don't know can, and does, hurt us. *Science*, **328**, 852–856.

92 Tiwari, T.S.P. *et al.* (2003) Forty years of disinfectant failure: outbreak of postinjection *Mycobacterium abscessus* infection caused by contamination of benzalkonium chloride. *Clinical Infectious Diseases*, **36**, 954–962.

93 Jarzembowski, J.A. and Young, M.B. (2008) Nontuberculous mycobacterial infections. *Archives of Pathology and Laboratory Medicine*, **132**, 1333–1341.

94 van Ingen, J. *et al.* (2009) Environmental sources of rapid growing nontuberculous mycobacteria causing disease in humans. *Clinical Microbiology and Infection*, **15**, 888–893.

95 Hermon-Taylor, J. (2009) *Mycobacterium avium* subspecies *paratuberculosis*, Crohn's disease and the Doomsday scenario. *Gut Pathology*, **1**, 15.

96 Pierce, E.S. (2009) Possible transmission of *Mycobacterium avium* subspecies *paratuberculosis* through potable water: lessons from an urban cluster of Crohn's disease. *Gut Pathology*, **1**, 17.

97 Vanklingeren, B. and Pullen, W. (1993) Glutaraldehyde resistant mycobacteria from endoscope washers. *Journal of Hospital Infection*, **25**, 147–149.

98 Griffiths, P.A. *et al.* (1997) Glutaraldehyde-resistant *Mycobacterium chelonae* from endoscope washer disinfectors. *Journal of Applied Microbiology*, **82**, 519–526.

99 Cardoso, A.M. *et al.* (2008) Emergence of nosocomial *Mycobacterium massiliense* infection in Goias, Brazil. *Microbes and Infection*, **10**, 1552–1557.

100 Duarte, R.S. *et al.* (2009) Epidemic of postsurgical infections caused by *Mycobacterium massiliense*. *Journal of Clinical Microbiology*, **47**, 2149–2155.

101 Nomura, K. *et al.* (2004) Antibiotic susceptibility of glutaraldehyde-tolerant *Mycobacterium chelonae* from bronchoscope washing machines. *American Journal of Infection Control*, **32**, 185–188.

102 Griffiths, P.A. *et al.* (1998) *Mycobacterium terrae*: a potential surrogate for *Mycobacterium tuberculosis* in a standard disinfectant test. *Journal of Hospital Infection*, **38**, 183–192.

103 Migliori G.B. *et al.* (2009) Multidrug-resistant and extensively drug-resistant tuberculosis in the West. Europe and United States: epidemiology, surveillance, and control. *Clinical Chest Medicine*, **30**, 637–665.

7 Fungicidal Activity of Microbicides

Sara Fernandes[1], Marta Simões[2], Nicolina Dias[2], Cledir Santos[2] and Nelson Lima[2]

[1] Institute for Molecular and Cell Biology, Porto, Portugal
[2] IBB-Institute for Biotechnology and Bioengineering, Centre of Biological Engineering, Micoteca da Universidade do Minho, Braga, Portugal

Introduction

Fungi are a ubiquitous and diverse group of unique organisms referred as the Eumycota kingdom or, sometimes, as the "fifth kingdom". A highly conservative estimate of fungal species is 1.5×10^6 [1], of which only about 9–10% may have been identified thus far. Fungi range in size from massive underground structures to microscopic, single-celled yeasts.

Several species are routinely used in the manufacture of antibiotics (e.g. penicillin), organic acids (e.g. citric acid), industrial alcohol (e.g. biofuels) and enzymes (e.g. amylases). The organisms are also abundant sources of potential pharmaceuticals such as enzyme inhibitors [2]. They are used as foodstuff directly in the form of mushrooms and "Quorn", the *Fusarium* biomass produced in bioreactors. In addition, fungi are employed in the production of a diverse range of important food products (e.g. cheese, wine, meats, soya sauce). Traditional Chinese medicines, which have huge worldwide markets, include fungi (e.g. *Ganoderma*, *Cordyceps*) and these are being investigated increasingly as novel conventional medicines [3, 4]. One of the most important roles of fungi is in the biodegradation of organic materials in the environment. In this respect, they are found on decaying foodstuff where they may produce toxins (mycotoxins) [5]. Recently, filamentous fungi have received increased attention as drinking water contaminants and the contribution of waterborne fungi to health and water-quality problems are not yet determined completely [6, 7].

Many are also notorious plant pathogens, while others are pathogenic for humans, particularly those who are immunocompromised. Emerging and re-emerging fungal pathogens have been continuously detected and described [8, 9].

General fungal ecology

Fungi display an extraordinary diversity of ecological interactions, but are otherwise alike in being efficient heterotrophs. Along with bacteria, fungi are the primary decomposers, facilitating the flow of energy and the recycling of materials through ecosystems. They occur in many different habitats such as soil, plant surfaces, inside plant tissues and in decaying plant foliage bark and wood. Fungi are also found in marine and aquatic habitats in association with other organisms (e.g. bacteria, algae), and in the digestive tracts and waste of animals [10]. Some fungi can grow under extreme conditions where the majority of organisms would not survive, for example very high or low pH, high salinity and extremely low (−20°C) or high (80°C) temperatures. Xerotolerant species can grow under extremely dry conditions and osmotolerant ones in high solute concentrations. Most fungi are strict aerobes, but species of the chytrid *Neocallimastix*, which inhabit the rumen of herbivorous mammals, are obligate anaerobes [11]. Several aquatic fungi are facultative anaerobes.

Filamentous fungi are able to mechanically penetrate and permeate substrates and the fungal vegetative body then grows rapidly as hyphae. Enzymes excreted by fungal cells can break-down complex polymers such as cellulose and lignin into low molecular weight sources of energy. Fungi have the capacity for indeterminate growth, longevity, resilience and asexual reproduction. The vegetative cells of Eumycota are often multinucleate, containing dissimilar haploid nuclei, and this combination of features gives them an unparalleled capacity for adaptation to varying physiological and ecological circumstances and ensures a high level of genetic diversity.

Fungi often interact with other organisms. As decomposers, they are crucial in the recycling of nutrients. As parasites, pathogens, mutualists or as food sources, they can directly influence the composition and population dynamics of other organisms in a given setting. For example, mycorrhizal fungi function as an interface between the plant and soil, and are essential to the survival of most plants in natural habitats [12].

Fungicidal activity of microbicides

The detrimental role of fungi as contaminations, mycotoxin producers and pathogens requires the use of effective microbicides to prevent and control their spread. Whereas microbicides are those compounds that can kill or control microorganisms in general, "fungistatic" substances are those that specifically inhibit fungal growth and reproduction. "Fungicides", in contrast, can irreversibly inactivate fungi. This section addresses recent developments in the testing of chemicals as fungicides and shows that methods for evaluating microbicides are diverse, indicating a discrepancy in the standardization of testing methods.

Suspension tests, and *in vitro* and *in vivo* carrier tests, have been used in testing chemicals against fungi. While determining minimal inhibitory concentrations (MICs) may be appropriate when evaluating antifungal drugs for therapeutic purposes, such testing is of limited value when testing microbicides, as many such chemicals can react with the constituents of the fungal growth media with an immediate loss of potential fungicidal activity. Suspension tests for fungicidal activity are

predominantly adaptations of bactericidal tests and can be used with a limited number of fungal species [13]. Simmonds in 1951 [14] proposed an *in vitro* method for the evaluation of water-soluble fungicides against *Trichophyton mentagrophytes* as a single test organism. Sisak and Rybnikar [15] reported on the fungicidal effects of several chemicals commonly used against *Trichophyton verrucosum*. Later, Terleckyj and Axler [16] proposed a quantitative neutralization assay for the evaluation of disinfectants against fungi. They considered *T. mentagrophytes* unsuitable for the purpose while suggesting using *Aspergillus fumigatus* instead due to its generally higher resistance to microbicides. Hegna and Clausen [17] modified the Kelsey–Sykes or capacity method (suspension protocol) to assess the fungicidal activity of chemicals.

In 2002, a new suspension method using the Bioscreen optical plate reader was described [18] for screening potential fungicides; the authors claimed the method was rapid, reproducible, quantitative and cost-effective. Recently, Hume *et al.* [19] applied the International Standards Organization's standard ISO 14729:2001 to test five soft contact lens multipurpose disinfectants against 10 ocular isolates of *Fusarium solani* and the ATCC 36031 strain. One of the most widely used fungicidal tests is that of AOAC International [13]. In the United States and Canada, carrier test methods of ASTM International are used to determine the fungicidal and yeasticidal activities of microbicides to be used on environmental surfaces (E-2197) and human skin (E-2613).

Comité Européen de Normalisation (CEN) TC-216 gives details of the European Norm (EN) for a quantitative suspension test (EN1275) to evaluate basic fungicidal or yeasticidal of chemical disinfectants and antiseptics. Table 7.1 lists the standards of CEN/TC-216 for testing fungicidal or yeasticidal activities of chemicals.

Standards

The EN1275 test is intended to determine the activity of commercial formulations or active substances on fungi under the conditions in which they are used. The European fungicidal test uses two test organisms, *Candida albicans* (ATCC 10231) and *Aspergillus niger* (ATCC 16404), and there are two possible techniques for determining the number of surviving organisms, namely the dilution and neutralization technique and the membrane filtration method. However, the critical step in the dilution–neutralization procedure is the preparation of conidial test suspensions, which is particularly cumbersome and time-consuming. Tortorano *et al.* [21] have recently proposed a simplified and reproducible methodology to test microbicides against *A. fumigatus* and compared it to the European guidelines. *Saccharomyces cerevisae* has also been used as a test organism in EN1650 [20] for the purpose of testing fungicidal or yeasticidal activities of chemical disinfectants and antiseptics in food, industrial, domestic and institutional areas. In 2002, EN13697 established the requirements for a quantitative carrier test with a

Table 7.1 Standards for fungicidal or yeasticidal activity published by CEN/TC 216 "Chemical disinfectants and antiseptics".

Area	Application	Standard	Phase/step[a]	Fungal activity
Basic tests		EN1275	Phase 1	Basic fungicidal or yeasticidal activity
Medical	Instrument disinfection	EN13624	Phase2/step1	Fungicidal or yeasticidal activity
	Instrument disinfection	EN14562	Phase2/step 2	Fungicidal or yeasticidal activity
Veterinary	Surface disinfection/immersion of contaminated objects	EN1657	Phase2/step 1	Fungicidal or yeasticidal activity
Food, industrial, domestic and institutional (breweries, beverage and soft drink	Surface disinfection, "cleaning in place"	EN1650	Phase 2/step1	Fungicidal or yeasticidal activity
industry, dairies, cosmetics)	Surface disinfection	EN13697	Phase2/step 2	Bactericidal, yeasticidal or fungicidal activity

[a]The tests carried out in phase 1 are quantitative suspension tests to elucidate the microbicidal efficacy and phase 2 defines the requisite concentration per exposure time [20].

non-porous surface for evaluating bactericidal and/or fungicidal activity of microbicides used in food, industrial, domestic and institutional areas. EN1657 a quantitative suspension test for veterinary applications. EN13624 (directive 93/42/EEC) quantitative suspension test or medical instrument disinfection and EN14562 established test requirements for a quantitative carrier test for the evaluation of fungicidal or yeasticidal activity for instruments used in the medical field.

Scott et al. [22] tested the fungicidal activity of a range of agents used for hard surface and skin disinfection in hospitals in the UK against *T. mentagrophytes* and *A. niger* conidia and *C. albicans* blastospores. The preparations, which contained cetrimide, aqueous solutions of chlorhexidine gluconate (Hibitane) and combinations of these (Savloclens and Savlodil), were only slowly fungicidal, particularly against *T. mentagrophytes* conidia, which were the most resistant of the tested fungi. There are many different fungicidal chemicals as presented below.

Chemicals with fungicidal activity

Acids and alkalis
Acids
Formulations of citric acid ($COOHCH_2COH(CH_2COOH)COOH$) have been used as broad-spectrum disinfectants, with claimed efficacy against fungi, among other microorganisms. Citric acid is also used as a preservative in beverages and as an effective cleaning agent. The acid works in synergy with certain other microbicides, presumably because of its ability to increase permeability across the cell wall.

Acetic acid (CH_3COOH) is a universal metabolic intermediary. It is commonly used by food manufactures as a preservative or acidulent in a variety of products. Fumigation with acetic acid can be extremely effective in killing fungal spores to prevent post-harvest spoilage of produce [23, 24]. For example, such vapors

have been found to inhibit the growth of *Botrytis cinerea* and *Rhizopus stolonifer* (causal agents of soft and gray rots of strawberries, respectively, at 8 and 10 µl/l [23, 24]). According to Morsy et al. [25, 26], acetic acid vapors (8 µl/l) could completely inhibit the growth and conidial germination of *Aspergillus flavus*, *A. niger*, *Aspergillus terreus*, *Fusarium moniliforme*, some *Penicillium* spp. and an *Alternaria* sp. Acetic acid vapors at low concentrations have many qualities that make them an excellent microbicide: first it kills fungal conidia, second it does not damage the fumigated fruit surface, and third it is effective at low temperatures which means that fruit in 1°C cold storage can be effectively treated [23, 24].

Propionic acid (CH_3CH_2COOH) is often used as a preservative in baked goods at concentrations ranging from 0.1% to 0.5%. It is also used as a microbicide. Because of its corrosive nature, it is generally used as a sodium or calcium salt [27].

The acids and acid derivatives demonstrate a range of microbicidal activities, which also depend on their solubility in water or oil/lipid. These effects are important for their use in various emulsions and other formulations. Parabens are fungistatic against yeasts and molds, including *Candida*, *Saccharomyces*, *Trichophyton*, *Penicillium* and *Aspergillus* at concentrations between 100 and 200 µg/ml. In general, short-chain parabens, for example methyl and ethyl derivatives, are less effective than long-chain ones. However, the water solubility of such chemical microbicides decreases as their chain lengths increase [27].

Benzoic acid (C_6H_5COOH) inhibits yeast growth at very low concentrations (0.01–0.02%). Meanwhile, sorbic acid ($CH_3(CH)_4COOH$) inhibits the growth of yeasts and molds to a lesser extent.

Employing acids presents some particular advantages – most of them are non-toxic, non-irritating and are not known to be carcinogenic. Most of the acids, including acetic, propionic, benzoic and sorbic acids, are naturally broken down in the body or the environment and therefore are designated as safe. Some longer-chain acids (e.g. sorbic acid) can irritate mucous membranes at concentrations of ≥0.2% [27]. However, some fungi can use acids, such as lactic and citric acids, as carbon sources for growth, which is a disadvantage.

Alkalis

Alkaline conditions inhibit microbial growth by restricting several metabolic processes. At higher concentrations, alkalis can solubilize microbial walls and membranes causing loss of structure and function and leakage of cytoplasmic materials.

Solutions of NaOH and KOH are routinely used for cleaning and disinfection of various manufacturing surfaces, including purification and separation equipment such as chromatography columns and fractionation vessels [27].

Alkaline cleaning formulations include a variety of bases at low concentrations, such as NaOH, KOH, sodium bicarbonate ($NaHCO_3$) and sodium metasilicate (Na_2SiO_3), which are effective cleaners due to their ability to emulsify and saponify lipids and fats. In addition, they are effective for protein removal from surfaces and can breakdown proteins into peptides.

Despite the facts that alkalis are widely available and inexpensive, they are rarely used directly as microbicides. Depending on their concentration, they can damage skin and mucous membranes, and can even cause severe burns. They are corrosive to several types of surfaces, for example metals and plastics. Reactions with some metals (e.g. tin, aluminum, zinc) can even lead to production of flammable gases and they can cause violent reactions when mixed with certain compounds (e.g. strong acids).

Alcohols

Alcohols have a reactive hydroxyl group (–OH). Ethanol (CH_3CH_2OH), isopropanol ($CH_3CHOHCH_3$) and n-propanol ($CH_3CH_2CH_2OH$) have been extensively used as disinfectants and antiseptics. The microbicidal activity of alcohols increases with the length of the alkyl chain, up to six carbon atoms, and further increases in the chain length reduce activity [28, 29]. The optimal microbicidal efficacy in aqueous solutions is up to 60–90%. Alcohols cause rapid denaturation of proteins and membrane damage, with subsequent interference with metabolism and cell lysis [30].

Salgueiro et al. [31] report on leakage of intracellular material induced by ethanol in S. cerevisae. Susceptibility of yeasts to alcohol was also related to lipid composition and plasma membrane fluidity [32]. An alcohol solution consisting of ethanol and methanol (88%/5%) was used at a final concentration of 28.6% and no survival was found for C. albicans after a 15 min exposure [16]. The authors reported an increase of 53% in the survival of C. albicans when the concentration decreased to 11.6%. Ethanol 70% was shown to be effective against Candida parapsilosis in contaminated hubs of vascular catheters [33]. On the other hand, higher concentrations of alcohols (more than 90%) led to rapid protein coagulation on the outside of the cell wall, preventing further penetration of the microbicidal agent into the cell [27]. Despite their effectiveness on the vegetative form of A. fumigatus [34] and pathogenic yeasts [35] as surface disinfectants, alcohols demonstrate little or no sporicidal activity [27]. Mold ascospores

were resistant to 70% ethanol and such resistance increased with the age of the spores [36].

Biofilms formed by pathogenic fungi can cause serious environmental and health problems and are associated with severe infections. Ethanol concentrations higher than 20% showed complete inhibition of C. albicans biofilm formation [37]. However, some studies have reported on the reduced activity of ethanol on mature yeast biofilms. Recently, Nett et al. [38] noted that a 10-fold higher concentration of ethanol (25–35%) was needed for a 50% reduction in biofilm than the concentration used to kill planktonic cells. Earlier, Théraud et al. [35] reported on the ineffectiveness of ethanol 70% on mixed yeast biofilms. To boost antifungal activity, alcohols can be incorporated into other microbicides, such as chlorine for surface disinfection [39], fluconazol against Candida biofilms [38] and acetic acid for otomycosis therapy [40]. Also, temperature combined with ethanol was shown to exhibit a synergic action against the spores of fungi causing postharvest decay [41].

Aldehydes

Aldehydes remain among the most common microbicides for disinfection of environmental surfaces. Formaldehyde (HCHO) and glutaraldehyde ($OHC(CH_2)_3CHO$) have a virtually complete activity spectrum. The most important use is the disinfection of surfaces, when they are frequently combined with other disinfectants. The activity is by alkylating fungal proteins and DNA.

Formaldehyde

Formaldehyde is a flammable, colorless, reactive and readily polymerized gas at normal temperature and pressure. It is a potent allergen and possibly carcinogenic (International Agency for Research on Cancer (IARC): group 2A) and forms explosive mixtures with air and oxygen at atmospheric pressure. The concentration of formaldehyde used in gaseous sterilization processes is well below the explosive range and it is non-inflammable [42].

The compound is used as a disinfectant and a sterilant in its liquid and gaseous forms. It is used mainly as a water-based solution called formalin, which is 37–40% formaldehyde by weight. This aqueous solution is a fungicide and a bactericide, tuberculocide, virucide and sporicide. Formaldehyde inactivates microorganisms by alkylating the amino and sulfhydril groups of proteins and the nitrogen ring atoms of purine bases. Although formaldehyde-alcohol is a chemical sterilant and formaldehyde is a high-level disinfectant, hospital uses of formaldehyde are limited by its irritating fumes and the pungent odor that is apparent at very low levels (<1 ppm). Notwithstanding this, the fungicide is used in the healthcare setting for preparing viral vaccines (e.g. poliovirus and influenza), as an embalming agent and for preserving anatomic specimens. Historically it was used for sterilizing surgical instruments, especially as a mixture of formaldehyde and ethanol. Other agents used with formaldehyde are chlorine-based disinfectants, glutaraldehyde-based disinfectants, peracetic acid and peracetic acid with hydrogen peroxide [43].

Formaldehyde is supplied as a solution (formalin) or as a polymeric hydrate (paraformaldehyde). In solution, formaldehyde is present as the monohydrate methylene glycol ($CH_2(OH)_2$) and a series of low molecular weight polyoxymethylene glycols. Formalin contains 37–40% formaldehyde and 10–15% methanol to inhibit polymerization [42]. The use of formaldehyde is considered to be cheap, efficient and easy to control.

Paraformaldehyde is a mixture of polyoxymethylene glycols, containing 90–99% formaldehyde. It gradually vaporizes, generating monomeric formaldehyde gas; this depolymerization is accelerated by increasing temperature. Paraformaldehyde, which is a solid polymer of formaldehyde, may be vaporized by heat for the gaseous decontamination of laminar-flow safety cabinets when maintenance work or filter changes require that access is obtained to the sealed portion of the cabinet [43].

Gaseous formaldehyde to be used as a sterilant can be produced by heating formalin or paraformaldehyde. Alternatively, for fumigation of rooms, gaseous formaldehyde can be generated by initiating an exothermic reaction with the addition of a strong oxidizing agent, such as potassium permanganate to formalin [42].

Glutaradehyde

Glutaraldehyde is a saturated dialdehyde that has gained a wide acceptance as a high-level disinfectant and chemical sterilant. Aqueous solutions of glutaraldehyde are acidic and generally in this state are not sporicidal. Only when the 2% aqueous solution is "activated" by alkalizing agents (e.g. sodium bicarbonate) to pH 7.5 to 8.5 does the solution become sporicidal. Once activated, these solutions have a shelf-life of 14–28 days because of the polymerization of the glutaraldehyde molecules at alkaline pH levels. This polymerization blocks the active sites (aldehyde groups) of the glutaraldehyde molecules, which are responsible for its microbicidal activity [43, 44].

Novel glutaraldehyde formulations (e.g. glutaraldehyde-phenate, potentiated acid glutaraldehyde, stabilized alkaline glutaraldehyde) have been produced to overcome the problem of rapid loss of stability, resulting in a usable life of 28–30 days, while generally maintaining excellent microbial activity. It should be realized, however, that antimicrobial activity is also dependent on conditions of use, such as dilution and organic load. Manufacturers' literature for these preparations suggests that neutral or alkaline glutaraldehydes possess microbicidal and anticorrosion properties higher than those of acid glutaraldehydes. The use of glutaraldehyde solutions in hospitals is widespread because of their advantages. These include: (i) excellent microbicidal properties; (ii) being active in the presence of organic matter (e.g. 20% of bovine serum); (iii) non-corrosive action on endoscopic equipment, thermometers and rubber and plastic materials; and (iv) being non-coagulative in proteinaceous material [43]. The microbicidal activity of glutaraldehyde is a consequence of alkylation of the sulfhydryl, hydroxyl, carboxyl and amino groups of cell molecules, which alters RNA, DNA and protein synthesis [43, 44].

Halogens

Halogens such as chlorine, iodine and bromide are important antimicrobial agents widely used as disinfectants and skin antiseptics [27, 30, 45].

Chlorine

Chlorine compounds are the most reactive in water, acting as oxidizing agents of cellular materials and leading to the destruction of vegetative microorganisms including fungi. Sodium hypochlorite (NaOCl), chlorine dioxide and the *N*-chloro compounds such as sodium dichloroisocyanurate (NaDCC), with chloramine-T being used to some extent, are designated as chlorine-releasing agents (CRAs). Antimicrobial efficacy of CRAs increases with temperature and concentration. Optimal microbicidal activity is achieved at a pH range of 4 to 7, in which conditions hypochlorous acid (HOCl) is the dominant chemical species [27]. Inhibition of key enzymatic reactions within the cell and protein denaturation is the proposed mechanism for antimicrobial activity of chlorine active compounds [46].

Bleach (3–6% NaOCl for household; 10–12% for industrial purposes) has been widely used for decades as an inexpensive and safe disinfectant [47]. It has potential in preventing fungal growth in water systems [48], fruits [49] and crops [39]. In surface disinfection of healthcare facilities and medical equipment, bleach remains an important disinfection agent [46]. Bleach disinfection has been used as a sanitation measure taken to further minimize or eliminate airborne fungi producing mycotoxins. One study has focused on the detoxification of aflatoxin molecules produced by an aflatoxigenic strain of *A. flavus*. Complete destruction of aflatoxins was achieved after a 4 h exposure to 156 mg/l NaOCl [50, 51]. As with bacteria, fungal spores are more resistant than hyphae to bleach. In a previous study, conidial resistance of *A. niger*, *A. fumigatus*, *Cladosporium* spp. and *Penicillium oxalicum* to chlorine inactivation was investigated. From these, *A. niger* exhibited the greatest resistance [52]. Viability of spores of *Penicillium brevicompactum* was evaluated using three concentrations of bleach (1%, 5.7% and 10%) at different exposure times. Despite all concentrations being shown to be effective, increasing exposure times (2, 4 and 30 min) were required to achieve death of all spores [53]. In another study, *P. brevicompactum* water biofilms were capable of survival after 15 min in a 2.38 mg/l free chlorine concentration whereas free spores were susceptible to 1.83 mg/l [54].

Sodium hypochlorite (NaOCl) has been used for years in mechanical flushing in dental root canal systems. The efficiency of NaOCl, in concentrations ranging from 1% to 6%, as mouthrinse, root canal irrigation and denture disinfectant against *C. albicans* colonization *in vitro* has been supported by recent studies [55–60]. Strains of *C. albicans* proved to be sensitive to 0.5% NaOCl within 10 s contact time [61]. The decreased efficacy of NaOCl against biofilms of pathogenic yeast was demonstrated by Théraud *et al.* [35]. Only a concentration of 3.8% active chlorine had yeasticidal activity in biofilms of *Cryptococcus* spp., *C. albicans* or *Rhodotorula rubra*.

Other chlorinated derivatives have been explored as alternatives to sodium hypochlorite. In the 1990s, a foam formulation of chlorine dioxide (ClO_2) was found to be effective against common pathogenic postharvest decay fungi occurring in fruit packinghouse surfaces, even on very contaminated surfaces that were not cleaned before sanitization [62]. Wilson *et al.* [63] evaluated the efficacy of fumigation treatment by ClO_2 gas for inactivating "sick building syndrome" related fungi and their mycotoxins. Although ClO_2 was effective for the inactivation of hyphomycete spores of *Penicillium chrysogenum*, *Stachybotrys chartarum*, *Cladosporium cladosporioides* and the majority of ascospores from *Chaetomium* spp., it was found that this sanitizing agent was not able to destroy mycotoxins produced by non-culturable, but still toxic, *S. chartarum*. Chloramine-T used in a concentration of 0.01% did not show microbicidal activity against *A. fumigatus* [21]. Methyl bromide (CH_3Br) has a restricted antimicrobial action as a stable gas for fumigation applications [27]. Investigation on the fungicidal effect of low concentrations of CH_3Br was carried out by Lee and Rieman [64]. Spores of *Aspergillus parasiticus* and *Penicillium rubrum* were killed by a 5-day exposure of CH_3Br 30 at 45 mg/l. However, safety and environmental concerns about CH_3Br toxicity lead researchers to search for more benign alternatives. Methyl iodide (CH_3I) was found to be an ozone-safe alternative for the former soil fumigant (CH_3Br) and was an effective antifungicidal against soilborne plant pathogens [65]. Finally, a combination of methyl iodide with chloropicrin resulted in a synergistic effect against *Fusarium oxysporum* [66].

Iodine

Iodine solutions and iodophors have been widely used as antiseptics as broad-spectrum microbicides, including fungicides, although their exact mechanism of action is unknown [27]. *Sporothrix schenckii* spores were not able to germinate after a treatment with iodine-potassium iodide solution at 5.0 mg/ml. At this concentration the ultrastructure of the cell had changed drastically [67]. More recently, a combination of saturated potassium iodide solution and terbinafine ($C_{21}H_{25}N$) was successfully used in the oral treatment of cutaneous sporotrichosis [68]. The elimination of fungal spores from mangos proved the antifungicidal activity of aqueous iodine solution at 0.5 g/l [43]. Iodophor formulations, for example polyvinylpyrrolidone iodine (1% available iodine) and polyester glycol iodine (0.18% available iodine), resulted in at least 10^4 reductions in the viability of *A. fumigatus* clinical isolates after less than 5 min contact time [21]. However, antimicrobial activity of 10% polyvinylpyrrolidone iodine was significantly less effective in mixed planktonic yeast and yeast biofilms than in pure suspensions of *C. albicans* [35].

Metals

Metals are elements characterized as good conductor of electricity and heat. They form ions and ionic bonds with non-metals. In a metal, atoms readily lose electrons to form cations, which are surrounded by delocalized electrons. This behavior is responsible for the conductivity and for the antimicrobial effects. The anti-infective activity of some heavy metals has been known since antiquity; metal ions, either alone or in complexes, have been used for centuries as microbicides. Copper and silver are the most widely used currently due to the increasing environmental concerns that have limited the applications of the toxic heavy metals.

Copper

Copper (Cu) is essential to plants, animals and human health as it contributes to the function of numerous essential metabolic processes [69, 70]. Also, it demonstrates considerable microbicidal toxicity against microorganisms [71] including fungi. Copper compounds such as copper sulfate, copper carbonate and copper acetate have their most extensive employment in agriculture where they act as fungicides against various fungus diseases of plants. Copper sulfate is one of the most common therapeutics used to treat fungal-infected striped bass and redfish, while two other copper compounds, CuDequest-2041-hydroxide and CuTETA, are applied in biological pollution control of shellfish beds and microbial diseases of shellfish [72]. In hospitals, copper compounds are used to reduce environmental contamination and to eradicate microorganisms responsible for healthcare-associated infections such as *Aspergillus* spp. Copper-8-quinolinolate and some of its derivates have been shown to be fungicidal to *Aspergillus* spp. at concentrations above 0.4 µg/ml [73]. More recently, copper-impregnated clothes proved to be useful in preventing tinea pedis, a dermatophyte infection of the soles of the feet and the interdigital spaces [74].

The mode of action of copper is similar to that of other heavy metals. Toxicity occurs because heavy metal ions bind with greater affinity to negatively charged microbial surfaces than essential metal ions. Therefore the microbicidal action of copper is thought to be related to plasma membrane damage, site-specific mediated damage to nucleic acids, and disruption of essential sulphydryl group-containing proteins. Cell membrane attack can lead to altered permeability manifested as leakage of mobile cellular solutes such as K^+ and disruption of the cell wall resulting in cell death [75]. The capacity of copper to induce DNA damage is due to the fact that the DNA double helix contains binding sites for copper. Consequently, the helical structures are disordered by cross-linking within and between strands by Cu^{2+} that competes with hydrogen bonding present in the DNA molecule [76]. Proteins are also a particular target for Cu^{2+} ions that interact with thiol groups (–SH) disrupting tertiary and secondary structures required for enzymatic activities.

Silver

Silver (Ag) compounds are also broadly used as microbicides. The antimicrobial properties of silver have been know since ancient times and silver antimicrobial activity had many applications prior to the discovery of pharmaceutical antibiotics, when it fell into near disuse. However, as antibiotic-resistant microorganisms have emerged, interest in using the silver ion for antimicrobial purposes has resumed.

Low concentrations of silver are very effective against bacteria but less activity is observed against yeasts and fungi. Widely used microbicidal silver compounds are silver sulfadiazine (AgSD) and silver nitrate ($AgNO_3$). Silver sulfadiazine is historically used as a topical burn cream on second- and third-degree burns. It prevents mixed bacterial infection as well as yeast infections on the damaged skin [77]. Dilute solutions of silver nitrate used to be dropped into newborn babies' eyes at birth to prevent contraction of eye infections [78]. As a consequence of the antimicrobial properties of silver and the development of drug resistance, the preparation of uniform nano-sized silver particles has gained great interest in the formulation of new pharmaceutical products [79]. Many studies have shown their antimicrobial effects [80–85] but the effects of silver nanoparticles against fungal pathogens of the skin are mostly unknown.

Similarly to copper, the microbicidal effect of silver stems from a combination of mechanisms. Positively charged silver ions (Ag^+) have an affinity for electrons and, when introduced into the interior of a microbial cell, they interfere with electron transport in cellular respiration systems. Metal ions bind to the sulfhydryl, amino and carboxyl groups of amino acids, thereby denaturing the proteins they compose. This makes enzymes and other cell proteins ineffective, compromising the biochemical process they control. Cell-surface proteins necessary for the transport of materials across cell membranes are also inactivated as they are denatured.

Oxidizing agents

Many oxidizing agents have potent antimicrobial activity. These include various halogens (like chlorine and iodine) and the peroxygens and other forms of oxygen, which include ozone (O_3), hydrogen peroxide (H_2O_2) and peracetic acid (CH_3COOH). Since their spectrum of activity is very wide, this group of microbicides has become widely used for cleaning, antisepsis, disinfection and sterilization applications.

Ozone

Ozone is a gas and a powerful oxidizing agent that has been used extensively for disinfection of drinking water and municipal wastewater. It was reported as the most effective water-treatment method against fungal spores [86]. Due to its unstable nature and short half-life time, ozone has to be generated "on site". A number of factors determine the amount of ozone required during oxidation; these are pH, temperature, organic load, solvents and accumulated reaction products. Also, high relative humidity is required for microorganisms to be inactivated by ozone gas [87]. Nowadays the maintenance of effective ozone concentrations is possible from the development of ozone generators that also have other applications such as odor control, taste and color remediation, preservation and sanitization of foods, area fumigation, sterilization and disinfection. The toxicity of ozone varies depending on its concentration and the length of exposure. Ozone is a toxic gas that must therefore be monitored in the workplace when it is used to disinfect equipment and installations. Several studies have examined its efficacy by testing different treatments on various

surfaces and microorganisms [88]. Moderate concentrations of ozone in gas form or in ozonated water, respectively 3.0 and 3.5 ppm, are sufficient to eliminate fungi such as *Trichophyton mentagrophytes*, *A. flavus* and *Brettanomyces bruxellensis* [89]. Different studies indicate that ozone is an effective treatment for increasing shelf-life and decreasing fungal deterioration in the postharvest treatment of fresh fruit such as grapes [90], longan fruit [91] and stone fruits [92]. This is due to the resulting lack of residues on the product, unlike the situation with some other fungicides of crops. The effects of ozone on the reduction of sporulation and mycotoxin production by *A. flavus* and *Fusarium moniliforme* [93] have been reported.

Ozone causes oxidation of cell components leading to protein inactivation, cell lysis, perturbation of adenosine triphosphate (ATP) formation and modification of purine and pyrimidine bases in nucleic acids [94].

Hydrogen peroxide

The antimicrobial and/or antiseptic properties of hydrogen peroxide (H_2O_2) have been known for many years because of its efficacy, versatility and safety. Hydrogen peroxide is considered environmentally friendly because it can rapidly degrade into water and oxygen. Although pure solutions are generally stable, most contain stabilizers to prevent decomposition. Hydrogen peroxide is currently used in hospitals to disinfect surfaces and in solution alone or in combination with other chemicals as a highly effective disinfectant. Only low concentrations of hydrogen peroxide are required for it to exhibit broad-spectrum efficacy. Generally, concentrations of hydrogen peroxide below 3% display good fungistatic activity. Higher concentrations of H_2O_2 (10–30%) and longer contact times are required for sporicidal activity [95], although this activity is significantly increased in the gaseous phase. Hydrogen peroxide was shown to have dramatic effects on the viability of quiescent and germinating spores of *A. flavus* [96].

The presence of catalase or other peroxidases – enzymes produced by aerobe microorganisms to protect cells from damage by regulating steady-state levels of metabolically produced hydrogen peroxide – can increase tolerance to lower concentrations of hydrogen peroxide.

Hydrogen peroxide diffuses rapidly through cell membranes and acts as an oxidant by producing hydroxyl free radicals (–OH) that attack essential cell components, including lipids, proteins and DNA, causing cell death. Exposed sulfhydryl groups and double bonds are particularly affected [97]. Hydrogen peroxide was also shown to be responsible for an increase in lactate dehydrogenase leakage and DNA damage in *Aspergillus candidus* [98].

Peracetic acid

Peracetic acid ($C_2H_4O_3$ or PAA) is a mixture of acetic acid (CH_3COOH) and hydrogen peroxide (H_2O_2) in solution. Due to its high oxidizing potential, peracetic acid is broadly effective against microorganisms and is not deactivated by catalase and peroxidase, the enzymes that breakdown hydrogen peroxide. PAA is mainly used in the food industry, where it is applied as a disinfectant. Complete inhibition of germination of *Monilinia laxa* spores in stone fruits was observed with peracetic acid at 0.5 mg/ml after 5 min of contact with spores [99]. Nowadays, PAA is also applied for the disinfection of medical supplies in combination with anticorrosive chemicals to eliminate the corrosivity of peracetic acid, and to prevent biofilm formation in pulp industries [100]. Similarly to hydrogen peroxide, the efficiency of gaseous PAA is greater at lower concentrations than in liquid form even though PAA is considered a more potent microbicide than hydrogen peroxide. Concentrations as low as 0.003% are sufficient for efficient antifungal activity [101].

Although limited work has been done to probe the mode of action of PAA as an antimicrobial agent, it may be speculated that it acts as a microbicide through oxidation and subsequent disruption of microbial cell membranes [97]. It was demonstrated that PAA acts on the bases of the DNA molecule [102]. Furthermore, intracellular PAA may also oxidize essential enzymes; thus vital biochemical pathways, active transport across membranes and intracellular solute levels are impaired [103].

Phenols

Phenols are a class of chemical compounds consisting of a hydroxyl group (–OH) bonded directly to an aromatic hydrocarbon group. Phenolic compounds are classified into different groups based on the structure and functional groups of the phenol. They are fairly insoluble in aqueous solutions, and readily soluble in most organic solvents. Therefore, a combination with soaps, oils and detergents is required for solubilization. The hydroxyl group (–OH) interferes with protein hydrogen bonds inactivating the polymer.

Phenolic-type antimicrobial agents have long been used for their antiseptic, disinfectant or preservative properties. Phenol (C_6H_5OH) is used as an antiseptic in surgical procedures, while salicylic acid is mainly used in skin exfoliants, shampoos and toothpaste. The use of phenols to preserve food additives has also increased [104]. The bisphenols such as hexachlorophene $CH_2(C_6HCl_3OH)_2$ and triclosan $(C_6H_3ClOH)_2O(C_6H_3Cl_2)$ have been widely used; however, because of toxicity concerns, the use of hexachlorophene in consumer products is limited. Triclosan has become the most potent and widely used bisphenol [105]. Triclosan is incorporated into many contemporary consumer and professional healthcare products and also into fabrics, plastics and surgical materials [106].

The spectrum of activity of phenols includes fungi, bacteria and viruses depending on the phenol type. However, it was demonstrated that *A. niger* and *C. albicans* are less susceptible than bacteria [107]. Phenol antifungal action involves damage to the plasma membrane, resulting in leakage of intracellular compounds such as potassium (K^+) leading to cell death [108].

Surfactants

Surfactants or surface-active agents are amphypatic molecules, with two active regions in their molecular structures. One is a hydrocarbon, hydrophobic group and the other is a hydrophilic or polar group. The classification of surfactants is based on the charge or absence of ionization of the hydrophilic group, hence cationic, anionic, non-ionic and amphoteric compounds are respectively categorized. Anionic and non-ionic surfactants have little or no intrinsic antimicrobial activity [27, 109], although some anionic fatty acids had been reported for decades as having fungistatic activity against dermatophytes [110–113]. Indeed, Kull *et al.* [114] reported on the synergistic antifungistatic activity against *Trichophyton mentagrophytes* and *C. albicans* when combining a cationic detergent with an anionic fatty acid chain.

Quatenary ammonium compounds (QACs), also known as cationic surfactants, are well-known active membrane agents and their target site is the fungal cell wall and the plasma membrane of microorganisms, including yeasts [27, 30]. The binding affinity of QACs of different hydrocarbon chains at different concentrations was related to the fungicide effect on *C. albicans*. Differences were related to the critical micelle concentration (CMC) of the compound [115]. Nevertheless, a correlation between microbicidal action of cationic lipids and positive charge on microbial cells suggested different spectra of antimicrobial activity of QACs. A recent study from Codling *et al.* [116] evaluated an antimicrobial potential of two formulations regarding contact lens disinfection. Polyquaternium-1 was found to have predominantly antibacterial activity, although it produced leakage of K^+ ions from *C. albicans* without causing lysis of spheroplasts. Also, myristamidopropyldimethylamine induced possible plasma membrane damage against *A. fumigatus* and *C. albicans*, but the injury was not sufficient to lyse fungal cells. Later, Vieira and Carmona-Ribeiro [117] found that the critical phenomenon determining the antifungal effect of cationic surfactants and lipids was not cell lysis, but rather the change of the cell surface charge from negative to positive. In this study, the presence of anionic sodium dodecyl-sulfate induced cell leakage from *C. albicans*, while cationic hexadecyltrimethylammonium bromide or dioctadecyldimethyl-ammonium decreased significantly and irreversibly cell viability without inducing any lysis or leakage. Recently, the effect of surfactants on aflatoxin production, ergosterol content and sugar consumption by aflatoxigenic *Aspergillus parasiticus* (NRRL 2999) was reported by a study carried out by Tanuja *et al.* [118]. The authors found that spore germination was completely inhibited at 0.01% concentrations of the cationic surfactants, cetyldimethylammonium bromide (CDAB) and dodecyltrimethylammonium bromide. While the later also inhibited the production of ergosterol and toxin, CDAB was found to enhance toxin production at a concentration of 0.001%. Non-ionic surfactants delayed germination at all concentrations tested and inhibited toxin and ergosterol production at 0.001%, although Tween-20 was most effective in inhibiting toxin production on day 7, when toxin production was found to be maximal in the control group.

Biosurfactants are microbial compounds with a wide range of chemical structures that exhibit surface and emulsifying activities. Commercial potentialities in medicine applications from their antimicrobial properties, including to fungi, have been reviewed [119, 120]. A biosurfactant produced by the strains of *Bacillus subtilis* (iturin-A) was found to be an effective antifungal agent against *S. cerevisae* [121–123]. In 1995, Tanaka *et al.* [124] proposed a method of producing iturin-A from *Bacillus amyloliquefaciens* for profound mycoses. Thus, other derivatives of the iturin-like biosurfactant group have the potential to be used as potent antifungal agents. Bacillomicin D and bacillomycin Lc iturin were effective against *A. flavus*, although the different lipid chain length apparently affected the activity of the lipopeptide against other fungi [125].

Microbicide resistance in fungi

The activity of antimicrobial agents is often quantified as a minimum inhibitory concentration (MIC) that is required to inhibit the growth of the target organisms or at a concentration that leaves no detectable survivors after a specified contact time. Resistance to antimicrobial agents is a description of the relative resistance of a microorganism to an agent under a particular set of conditions. Microorganisms differ in their natural sensitivity to chemical agents due to variations in cell structure, physiology and complexity.

A microorganism is intrinsically resistant to a particular microbicide if it lacks critical target sites or the microbicide compounds are unable to accumulate at those targets [126]. On the other hand, resistance can be acquired when microorganisms experience changes in susceptibility that reflect either the conditions under which they were cultivated or exposed. The generation of extrinsic genetic elements that encode such resistance can be responsible for the rapid development of resistance within population groups.

The cell wall composition of fungi confers a high level of intrinsic resistance on these organisms because of the complex structure composed of chitin, glucans and other polymers, with evidence of extensive cross-linking between these components. The wall structure is highly dynamic, changing constantly during cell division, growth and morphogenesis [127]. Reports on drug-resistant clinical isolates of *Aspergillus* spp. have emerged in recent years [128–130]. Ergosterol is also a major and essential component of the cell membrane in most fungi. Changes in sterol pattern observed in *A. fumigatus* were responsible for increased tolerance of azoles as these agents block the ergosterol biosynthesis pathway by inhibiting the enzyme 14α-demethylase, a product of the CYP51 [130]. However, the role of fungal sterols present in the activity of microbicides has not been identified. Low ergosterol content in the cell membrane of *A. terreus* was the postulated mechanism for the poor activity of amphotericin B [131]. The reduced intracellular accumulation of azoles has also been correlated with overexpression of multidrug resistance (MDR) efflux transporter genes of the ATP-binding cassette (ABC) and the major facilitator superfamily (MFS) classes [130]. However, the significance of these transporters remains to be investigated. Even although yeast cell walls present different compositions of glucans in relation to molds, *S. cerevisiae* populations with membranes enriched in ergosterol or stigmasterol and linoleyl residues were shown to be more resistant to ethanol [132]. Changes in glucan

composition, wall thickness and relative porosity also determined the sensitivity of *S. cerevisiae* cells to chlorhexidine [133]. Furthermore, culture age and consequent cell wall thickness and decreased porosity influence the response of *S. cerevisiae* to chlorhexidine; the cells walls are much less sensitive at stationary phase than at logarithmic growth phase [134]. A similar microbicide resistance was achieved by *C. albicans* to the antibiotic amphotericin B as the cells entered the stationary growth phase [135]. Another mechanism of fungal survival and proliferation is the formation of spores in response to low concentrations of fungistatic or fungicidal agents that can be more resistant to microbicides than vegetative fungal cells or hyphae.

Cryptococcus neoformans is an encapsulated yeast resistant to reactive oxygen species produced by H_2O_2 [136]. This capsule enlargement acts as a microbicide barrier, suggesting that other fungal species that were shown to produce capsules such as *Sporothrix*, *Trichosporon* and *Tremella* may present similar mechanisms of resistance.

Copper tolerance in fungi has also been ascribed to diverse mechanisms involving trapping of the metal by cell wall components, altered uptake of copper, extracellular chelation or precipitation by secreted metabolites, and intracellular complexing by metallothioneins and phytochelatins [137]. In *C. albicans* Crd1p is a copper pump that provides the primary source of cellular copper resistance, while the metallothionein copper uptake protein (CUP) binds copper via thiol groups of exposed cysteine groups within the protein [138]. Other fungal enzymes such as formaldehyde dehydrogenases, catalases and peroxidases may be the cause of increased resistance to formaldehyde and hydrogen peroxide [139].

Phenotypic adaptation to intrinsic resistance may be shown by biofilms. In nature, biofilms consist of mixed populations of different types of microorganisms that attach to different surfaces. The mechanisms of resistance of a biofilm include: (i) the reduced access of microbicide molecules to the cells; (ii) modulation of the microenvironment; (iii) production of degradative enzymes that might be effective at lowering microbicide concentrations within the biofilm; (iv) genetic exchange between cells; (v) adaptation and mutation within the biofilm; and (vi) microbicide efflux [140]. *C. albicans* biofilms are commonly seen in biomedical device-associated infections, being highly resistant to microbicides [141]. Apart from *Candida*, other fungi such as *Aspergillus*, *Cladosporium*, *Penicillium*, *Rhodotorula* and *Cryptococcus* are able to form biofilms and eventually become associated with bacterial biofilms in order to establish a cooperation mechanism for survival and proliferation.

Safety, handling and discharge measurements for fungal microbicides

All disinfectants should be used with a high level of safety precautions and only for the intended purpose. Some of them (e.g. alcohols) are flammable and consequently must be stored in a cool, well-ventilated area. Sodium hypochlorite at the concentration used in household bleach (5.25–6.15%) can produce ocular irritation and oropharyngeal, esophageal and gastric burns. Chlorine dioxide is highly irritating to the eyes, nose and throat. Breathing chlorine dioxide vapors can cause coughing, nasal discharge, wheezing, respiratory distress, bronchitis and congestion of the lungs.

The environment is also at risk from some of these chemicals and contamination can occur if proper storage, transportation, disposal management and handling are not undertaken. All chemicals should be disposed as hazardous substances according to the risk assessment details found in the manufacturers' details. Finally, the use of fungal microbicides must follow international and national regulations and guidelines.

References

1 Hawksworth, D.L. (2001) The magnitude of fungal diversity: the 1.5 million species estimate revisited. *Mycological Research*, **105**, 1422–1432.

2 Paterson, R.R.M. (2008) Fungal enzyme inhibitors as pharmaceuticals, toxins, and scourge of PCR. *Current Enzyme Inhibition*, **4**, 46–59.

3 Paterson, R.R.M. (2006) *Ganoderma* – a therapeutic fungal biofactory. *Phytochemistry*, **67**, 1985–2001.

4 Paterson, R.R.M. (2008) *Cordyceps* – a traditional Chinese medicine and another fungal therapeutic biofactory? *Phytochemistry*, **69**, 1469–1495.

5 Paterson, R.R.M. and Lima, N. (2009) Toxicology of mycotoxins, in *Molecular, Clinical and Environmental Toxicology, Vol. 2: Clinical Toxicology* (ed. A. Luch), Birkhauser Verlag Ag, Basel, pp. 31–63.

6 Paterson, R.R.M. *et al.* (2009) Occurrence, problems, analysis and removal of filamentous fungi in drinking water, in *Fungicides* (eds P. de Costa and P. Bezerra), Nova Science Publisher Inc., New York, pp. 379–399.

7 Siqueira, V.M. *et al.* (2011) Filamentous fungi in drinking water, particularly in relation to biofilm formation. *International Journal of Environmental Research and Public Health*, **8**, 456–469.

8 Santos, C. *et al.* (2011) Matrix-assisted laser desorption/ionization time-of-flight intact cell mass spectrometry (MALDI-TOF-ICMS) to detect emerging pathogenic *Candida* species. *Diagnostic Microbiology and Infectious Disease*, **71**, 304–308.

9 Dias, N. *et al.* (2011) Sporotrichosis caused by *Sporothrix mexicana*, Portugal. *Emerging Infectious Diseases*, **17**, 1975–1976.

10 Deacon, J. (2005) *Fungal Biology*, Wiley Blackwell, Edinburgh.

11 Trinci, A.P.J. *et al.* (1994) Anaerobic fungi in herbivorous animals. *Mycological Research*, **98**, 129–152.

12 Gow, N.A.R. and Gadd, G.M. (1995) *The Growing Fungus*, Chapman & Hall, London.

13 Reybrouck, G. (2004) Antifungal activity of disinfectants, in *Principles and Practice of Disinfection, Preservation and Sterilization*, 4th edn (ed. A.P. Fraise *et al.*), Blackwell Publishing, pp. 236–237.

14 Simmonds, W.L. (1951) An *in vitro* method for the evaluation of water soluble fungicides against *Trichophyton*. *Zeitschrift für Hygiene und Infektionskrankheiten*, **132**, S34.

15 Sisak, M. and Rybnikaf, A. (1980) Determination of trichophytocidal efficiency of some disinfection solutions using a simple orientation method. *Acta Veterinaria Brno*, **49**, 245–250.

16 Terleckyj, B. and Axler, D.A. (1987) Quantitative neutralization assay of fungicidal activity of disinfectants. *Antimicrobial Agents and Chemotherapy*, **31**, 794–798.

17 Hegna, I.K. and Clausen, O.G. (1988) An investigation of the bactericidal and fungicidal effects of certain disinfectants by use of a capacity test. *Annales de l'Institut Pasteur/Microbiologie*, **139**, 473–483.

18 Lambert, R.J. *et al.* (2002) Disinfectant testing: use of the Bioscreen Microbiological Growth Analyser for laboratory biocide screening. *Letters in Applied Microbiology*, **26**, 288–292.

19 Hume, E.B.H. *et al.* (2009) Soft contact lens disinfection solution efficacy: clinical *Fusarium* isolates vs. ATCC 36031. *Optometry and Vision Science*, **86**, 415–419.

20 CEN (European Committee for Standardization) (1998) *EN 1650 Chemical Disinfectants and Antiseptics – Quantitative Suspension Test for the Evaluation of Fungicidal Activity of Chemical Disinfectants and Antiseptics used in Food, Industrial, Domestic and Institutional Areas – Test Method and Requirements (phase 2/step 1)*, CEN, Brussels.

21 Tortorano, A.M. *et al.* (2005) *In vitro* testing of fungicidal activity of biocides against *Aspergillus fumigatus*. *Journal of Medical Microbiology*, **54**, 955–957.

22 Scott, E.M. *et al.* (2008) An assessment of the fungicidal activity of antimicrobial agents used for hard-surface and skin disinfection. *Journal of Clinical Pharmacy and Therapeutics*, **11**, 199–205.

23 Sholberg, P.L. *et al.* (1998) Use of acetic acid fumigation to reduce the potential for decay in harvest crops. *Recent Research and Development in Plant Pathology*, **2**, 31–41.

24 Abd-Alla, M.A. (2005) Effect of acetic acid fumigation on common storage fungi of some medicinal and aromatic seeds. *Egyptian Journal of Phytopathology*, **33**, 77–86.

25 Morsy, A.A. *et al.* (1999) Effect of acetic acid on postharvest decay of strawberry fruits. *Egyptian Journal of Phytopathology*, **27**, 117–126.

26 Morsy, A.A. *et al.* (2000) Effect of acetic acid fumigation on common storage fungi of some grains. *Egyptian Journal of Phytopathology*, **28**, 95–106.

27 McDonnell, G. (2007) General considerations, in *Antisepsis, Disinfection, and Sterilization: Types, Action, and Resistance* (ed. G. McDonnell), ASM Press, Washington, DC, pp. 33–43.

28 Ali, Y. *et al.* (2001) Alcohols, in *Disinfection, Sterilization and Preservation*, 5th edn (ed. S.S. Block), Lippincott Williams & Wilkins, Philadelphia, p. 242.

29 Kampf, G. and Kramer, A. (2004) Epidemiologic background of hand hygiene and evaluation of the most important agents for scrubs and rubs. *Clinical Microbiology Reviews*, **17**, 863–893.

30 McDonnell, G. and Russell, D. (1999) Antiseptics and disinfectants: activity, action, and resistance. *Clinical Microbiology Reviews*, **12**, 147–179.

31 Salgueiro, S.P. *et al.* (1988) Ethanol induced leakage in *Saccharomyces cerevisiae*: kinetics and relationship to yeast ethanol tolerance and alcohol fermentation productivity. *Applied and Environmental Microbiology*, **54**, 903–909.

32 Lloyd, D. *et al.* (2004) Effects of growth with ethanol on fermentation and membrane fluidity of *Saccharomyces cerevisiae*. *Yeast*, **9**, 825–833.

33 Salzman, M.B. *et al.* (1993) Use of disinfectants to reduce microbial contamination of Hubs of vascular catheters. *Journal of Clinical Microbiology*, **31**, 475–479.

34 Gangneux, J.-P. *et al.* (2004) Experimental assessment of disinfection procedures for eradication of *Aspergillus fumigatus* in food. *Blood*, **104**, 2000–2002.

35 Théraud, M. *et al.* (2004) Efficacy of antiseptics and disinfectants on clinical and environmental yeast isolates in planktonic and biofilm conditions. *Journal of Medical Microbiology*, **53**, 1013–1018.

36 Bundgaard-Nielsen, K. and Nielsen, P.V. (1996) Fungicidal effect of 15 disinfectants against 25 fungal contaminants commonly found in bread and cheese manufacturing. *Journal of Food Protection*, **59**, 268–275.

37 Mukherjee, P.K. *et al.* (2006) Alcohol dehydrogenase restricts the ability of the pathogen *Candida albicans* to form a biofilm on catheter surfaces through an ethanol-based mechanism. *Infection and Immunity*, **74**, 3804–3816.

38 Nett, J.E. *et al.* (2008) Reduced biocide susceptibility in *Candida albicans* biofilms. *Antimicrobial Agents and Chemotherapy*, **52**, 3411–3413.

39 Andrews, S. *et al.* (1997) Chlorine inactivation of fungal spores on cereal grains. *International Journal of Food Microbiology*, **35**, 153–162.

40 Moghadam, A.Y. *et al.* (2010) Evaluating the effect of a mixture of alcohol and acetic acid for otomycosis therapy. *Jundishapur Journal of Microbiology*, **3**, 66–70.

41 Gabler, F.M. *et al.* (2004) Survival of spores of *Rhizopus stolonifer, Aspergillus niger, Botrytis cinerea* and *Alternaria alternata* after exposure to ethanol solutions at various temperatures. *Journal of Applied Microbiology*, **96**, 1354–1360.

42 Russell, A.D. *et al.* (1999) *Principles and Practice of Disinfection, Preservation and Sterilization*, 3rd edn, Blackwell Science, Oxford.

43 APIC (1996) Guideline for selection and use of disinfectants – guidelines for infection control practice. Reprinted from *American Journal of Infection Control*, **24** (4), 313–342.

44 Rutala, W.A., Weber, D.J. and the Healthcare Infection Control Practices Advisory Committee (HICPAC) (2008) *Guideline for Disinfection and Sterilization in Healthcare Facilities*, CDC, Atlanta, pp. 38–52.

45 Prescott, L.M. *et al.* (1999) Control of microorganisms by physical and chemical agents, in *Microbiology*, 4th edn (eds L.M. Prescott, J.P. Harley and D.A. Klein), WCB McGraw-Hill, Boston, pp. 145–149.

46 Rutala, W.A. and Weber, D.J. (1997) Uses of inorganic hypochlorite (bleach) in health-care facilities. *Clinical Microbiology Reviews*, **10**, 597–610.

47 Racioppi, F. *et al.* (1994) Household bleaches based on sodium hypochlorite: review of acute toxicology and poison control center experience. *Food and Chemical Toxicology*, **32**, 845–861.

48 Niemi, R.M. *et al.* (1982) Actinomycetes and fungi in surface waters and in potable water. *Applied and Environmental Microbiology*, **4**, 378–388.

49 Martinez, C.B. *et al.* (2002) Effects of ozone, iodine and chlorine on spore germination of fungi isolated from mango fruits. *Revista Mexicana de Fitopatologia*, **20**, 60–65.

50 Yang, C.Y. (1972) Comparative studies on the detoxification of aflatoxins by sodium hypochlorite and commercial bleaches. *Applied Microbiology*, **24**, 885–890.

51 Castegnaro, M. *et al.* (1980) *Laboratory Decontamination and Destruction of Aflatoxins B1, B2, G1, G2 in Laboratory Wastes*. International Agency for Research on Cancer, WHO, Lyon.

52 Rosenzweig, W.D. *et al.* (1983) Chlorine demand and inactivation of fungal propagules. *Applied and Environmental Microbiology*, **45**, 182–186.

53 Elbing, P.M. (2008) *Effectiveness of Sodium Hypochlorite Against Spores of Penicillium brevicompactum in an Insect Rearing Facility*. Information Report 0832-7122; GLC-X-8E. Natural Resources Canada, Canadian Reserve Services, Great Lakes Forestry Centre, Sault Ste Marie, Ontario.

54 Siqueira, V.M. and Lima, N. (2011) Efficacy of free chlorine against water biofilms and spores of *Penicillium brevicompactum*, in *Water Contamination Emergencies: Monitoring, Understanding and Acting* (eds U. Borchers and K.C. Thompson), RSC Publishing, Cambridge, pp. 157–168.

55 Valera, M.C. *et al.* (2001) Effect of sodium hypochlorite and five intracanal medications on *Candida albicans* in root canals. *Journal of Endodontics*, **27**, 401–403.

56 Estrela, C. *et al.* (2003) Antimicrobial effect of 2% sodium hypochlorite and 2% chlorhexidine tested by different methods. *Brazilian Dental Journal*, **14**, 58–62.

57 Vianna, M.E. *et al.* (2004) *In vitro* evaluation of the antimicrobial activity of chlorhexidine and sodium hypochlorite. *Oral Surgery, Oral Medicine, Oral Pathology, Oral Radiology and Endodontology*, **97**, 79–84.

58 Ruff, M. *et al.* (2006) *In vitro* antifungal efficacy of four irrigants as a final rinse. *Journal of Endodontics*, **32**, 331–333.

59 Buergers, R. *et al.* (2008) Efficacy of denture disinfection methods in controlling *Candida albicans* colonization *in vitro*. *Acta Odontologica Scandinavica*, **66**, 174–180.

60 Chandra, S.S. *et al.* (2010) Antifungal efficacy of 5.25% sodium hypochlorite, 2% chlorhexidine gluconate, and 17% EDTA with and without an antifungal agent. *Journal of Endodontics*, **36**, 675–678.

61 Radcliffe, C.E. *et al.* (2004) Antimicrobial activity of varying concentrations of sodium hypochlorite on the endodontic microorganisms *Actinomyces israelii, A. naeslundii, Candida albicans* and *Enterococcus faecalis*. *International Endodontic Journal*, **37**, 438–446.

62 Roberts, R.G. and Reymond, S.T. (1994) Chlorine dioxide for reduction of postharvest pathogen inoculum during handling of tree fruits. *Applied and Environmental Microbiology*, **60**, 2864–2868.

63 Wilson, S.C. *et al.* (2005) Effect of chlorine dioxide gas on fungi and mycotoxins associated with sick building syndrome. *Applied and Environmental Microbiology*, **71**, 5399–5403.

64 Lee, W.H. and Rieman, H. (1970) Destruction of toxic fungi with low concentrations of methyl bromide. *Applied Microbiology*, **20**, 845–846.

65 Ohr, H.D. *et al.* (1996) Methyl iodide an ozone-safe alternative to methyl bromide as a soil fumigant. *Plant Disease*, **80**, 731–735.

66 Hutchinson, C.M. *et al.* (2000) Efficacy of methyl iodide and synergy with chloropicrin for control of fungi. *Pest Management Science*, **56**, 413–418.

67 Hiruma, M. and Kagawa, S. (1987) Ultrastructure of *Sporothrix schenckii* treated with iodine-potassium iodide solution. *Mycopathologia*, **97**, 121–127.

68 Coskun, B. *et al.* (2004) Sporotrichosis successfully treated with terbinafine and potassium iodide: case report and review of the literature. *Mycophatologia*, **158**, 53–56.

69 Koch, K.A. *et al.* (1997) Copper-binding motifs in catalysis, transport, detoxification and signaling. *Chemical Biology*, **4**, 549–560.

70 Uauy, R. *et al.* (1998) Essentiality of copper in humans. *American Journal of Clinical Nutrition*, **67**, 952–959.

71 Nicolau, A. *et al.* (1999) Physiological responses of *Tetrahymena pyriformis* to copper, zinc, cycloheximide and Triton X-100. *FEMS Microbiology Ecology*, **30**, 209–216.

72 Borkow, G. and Gabbay, J. (2005) Copper as a biocidal tool. *Current Medicinal Chemistry*, **12**, 2163–2175.

73 Gershon, H. *et al.* (1969) 5-Nitro-8-quinolinols and their copper (II) complexes. Implications of the fungal spore wall as a possible barrier against potential antifungal agents. *Journal of Medical Chemistry*, **6**, 1115–1117.

74 Borkow, G. and Gabbay, J. (2004) Putting copper into action: copper impregnated products with potent biocidal activities. *FASEB Journal*, **18**, 1728–1730.

75 Stohs, S.J. and Bagchi, D. (1995) Oxidative mechanisms in the toxicity of metal ions. *Free Radical Biology and Medicine*, **18**, 321–336.

76 Martin, R.B. and Mariam, Y.H. (1973) *Metal Ions in Biological Systems*, Marcell Decker, New York.

77 Fisher, N.M. *et al.* (2003) Scar-localized argyria secondary to silver sulfadiazine cream. *Journal of American Academy of Dermatology*, **49**, 730–732.

78 Dunn, P. (2000) Dr Carl Credé (1819–1892) and the prevention of ophthalmia neonatorum. *Archives of Diseases in Childhood – Fetal and Neonatal Edition*, **83**, 158–159.

79 Fernandes, S. *et al.* (2010) Fungal nanotechnology, in *Anais do 6° Congresso Brasileiro de Micologia* (eds J.C. Dianese and L.T.P. Santos), Sociedade Brasileira de Micologia, Brasília, pp. 574–578.

80 Chu, C.S. *et al.* (1988) Therapeutic effects of silver nylon dressing with weak direct current on *Pseudomonas aeruginosa* infected burn wounds. *Journal Trauma*, **28**, 1488–1492.

81 Deitch, E.A. *et al.* (1897) Silver nylon cloth: *in vivo* and *in vitro* evaluation of antimicrobial activity. *Journal of Trauma*, **27**, 301–304.

82 Margraff, H.W. and Covey, T.H. (1977) A trial of silver–zinc-allantoine in the treatment of leg ulcers. *Archives of Surgery*, **112**, 699–704.

83 Silver, S. (2003) Bacterial silver resistance: molecular biology and uses and misuses of silver compounds. *FEMS Microbiology Reviews*, **27**, 341–353.

84 Atiyeh, B.S. *et al.* (2007) Effect of silver on burn wound infection control and healing: review of the literature. *Burns*, **33**, 139–148.

85 Law, N. *et al.* (2008) The formation of nano-scale elemental silver particles via enzymatic reduction by *Geobacter sulfurreducens*. *Applied and Environmental Microbiology*, **74**, 7090–7093.

86 Kelley, J. *et al.* (2003) *Identification and Control of Fungi in Distribution Systems*. AWWA Research Foundation and American Water Works Association, Denver, CO.

87 Kuprianoff, J. (1953) The use of ozone for the cold storage of fruit. *Z. Kalentechnik*, **10**, 1–4.

88 Serra, R. *et al.* (2003) Use of ozone to reduce molds in a cheese ripening room. *Journal of Food Protection*, **66**, 2355–2358.

89 Boisrobert, C. (2002) *US Regulatory Review of Ozone Use in the Food Industry. Ozone III: Agricultural and Food Processing Applications of Ozone as an Antimicrobial Agent.*

90 Sarig, P. *et al.* (1996) Ozone for control of postharvest decay of table grape cause by *Rhizopus stolonifer*. *Physiological and Molecular Plant Pathology*, **48**, 403–415.

91 Whangchai, K. *et al.* (2006) Effect of ozone in combination with some organic acids on the control of postharvest decay and pericarp browning of longan fruit. *Crop Protection*, **25**, 821–825.

92 Palou, L. *et al.* (2002) Effect of continuous 0.3 ppm ozone exposure on decay development and physiological responses of peaches and table grapes in cold storage. *Postharvest Biology and Technology*, **24**, 39–48.

93 Mason, L.J. *et al.* (1997) Efficacy of ozone to control insects, molds and mycotoxins, in *Proceeding of the International Conference on Controlled Atmosphere and Fumigation in Stored Products* (eds E.J. Conahaya and A. Navarro), Cyprus Printer Ltd, Nicosia, Cyprus, pp. 665–670.

94 Greene, A.K. *et al.* (1993) A comparison of ozonation and chlorination for the disinfection of stainless steel surfaces. *Journal of Dairy Science*, **76**, 3612–3620.

95 Russell, A.D. (1991) Chemical sporicidal and sporostatic agents, in *Disinfection, Sterilization, and Preservation*, 4th edn (ed. S.S. Block), Lea & Febiger, Philadelphia, pp. 365–376.

96 Jacks, T.J. *et al.* (1999) Effects of chloroperoxidase and hydrogen peroxide on the viabilities of *Aspergillus flavus* conidiospores. *Molecular and Cellular Biochemistry*, **195**, 169–172.

97 Block, S.S. (1991) Peroxygen compounds, in *Disinfection, Sterilization, and Preservation*, 4th edn (ed. S.S. Block), Lea & Febiger, Philadelphia, pp. 167–181.

98 Yen, G.-C. *et al.* (2003) The protective effects of *Aspergillus candidus* metabolites against hydrogen peroxide-induced oxidative damage to Int 407 cells. *Food and Chemical Toxicology*, **41**, 1561–1567.

99 Mari, M. *et al.* (1999) Peracetic acid and chlorine dioxide for postharvest control of *Monilinia laxa* in stone fruits. *Plant Disease*, **83**, 773–776.

100 Malchesky, P.S. (1993) Peracetic acid and its application to medical instrument sterilization. *Artificial Organs*, **17**, 147–152.

101 Kitis, M. (2004) Disinfection of wastewater with peracetic acid: a review. *Environment International*, **30**, 47–55.

102 Tutumi, M. *et al.* (1973) Antimicrobial action of peracetic acid. *Journal of Food Hygienic Society*, **15**, 116–120.

103 Fraser, J.A.L. *et al.* (1984) Use of peracetic acid in operational sewage sludge disposal to pasture. *Water Science and Technology*, **17**, 451–466.

104 Zupko, I. *et al.* (2001) Antioxidant activity of leaves of *Salvia* species in enzyme-dependent and enzyme independent systems of lipid peroxidation and their phenolic constituents. *Planta Medica*, **67**, 366–368.

105 Bhargava, H.N. and Leonard, P.A. (1996) Triclosan: applications and safety. *American Journal of Infection Control*, **24**, 209–218.

106 Jones, R.D. *et al.* (2000) Triclosan: a review of effectiveness and safety in health care settings. *American Journal of Infection Control*, **28**, 184–196.

107 Karabit, M.S. *et al.* (1989) Factorial design in the evaluation of preservative efficacy. *International Journal of Pharmaceutics*, **56**, 169–174.

108 Russell, A.D. and Furr, J.R. (1996) Biocides: mechanisms of antifungal action and fungal resistance. *Science Progress*, **79**, 27–48.

109 Dias, N. *et al.* (2003) Morphological and physiological changes in *Tetrahymena pyriformis* for the *in vitro* cytotoxicity assessment of Triton X-100. *Toxicology in Vitro*, **17**, 357–366.

110 Wyss, O. *et al.* (1945) The fungistatic and fungicidal action of fatty acids and related compounds. *Archives in Biochemistry*, **7**, 415–425.

111 Rothman, S. *et al.* (1946) Mechanism of spontaneous cure in puberty of ringworm of the scalp. *Science*, **104**, 201–203.

112 Peck, S.M. and Russ, W.R. (1947) Propionate-caprylate mixtures in the treatment of dermatomicoses with a review of fatty acid therapy in general. *Archives of Dermatology and Syphilology*, **56**, 601–613.

113 Borick, P.M. *et al.* (1959) Microbiological activity of certain saturated and unsaturated fatty acid salts of tetradecylamine and related compounds. *Applied Microbiology*, **7**, 248–251.

114 Kull, F.C. *et al.* (1961) Mixtures of quaternary ammonium compounds and long-chain fatty acids as antifungal agents. *Applied Microbiology*, **9**, 538–541.

115 Ahlströ, B. *et al.* (1996) Submicellar complexes may initiate the fungicidal effects of cationic amphiphilic compounds on *Candida albicans*. *Antimicrobial Agents and Chemotherapy*, **41**, 544–550.

116 Codling, C.C. *et al.* (2003) Aspects of the antimicrobial mechanisms of action of a polyquaternium and an amidoamine. *Journal of Antimicrobial Chemotherapy*, **51**, 1153–1158.

117 Vieira, D.B. and Carmona-Ribeiro, A.M. (2004) Cationic lipids and surfactants as antifungal agents: mode of action. *Journal of Antimicrobial Chemotherapy*, **58**, 760–767.

118 Tanuja, K. *et al.* (2010) Effect of various surfactants (cationic, anionic and non-ionic) on the growth of *Aspergillus parasiticus* (NRRL 2999) in relation to aflatoxin production. *Mycotoxin Research*, **26**, 155–170.

119 Singh, P. and Cameotra, S.S. (2004) Potential applications of microbial surfactants in biomedical sciences. *Trends in Biotechnology*, **22**, 142–146.

120 Rodrigues, L. *et al.* (2006) Biosurfactants: potential applications in medicine. *Journal of Antimicrobial Chemotherapy*, **57**, 609–618.

121 Besson, F. *et al.* (1976) Characterization of Iturin A in antibiotics from various strains of *Bacillus subtilis*. *Journal of Antibiotics*, **29**, 1043–1049.

122 Besson, F. *et al.* (1979) Antifungal activity upon *Saccharomyces cerevisiae* of Iturin A, Mycosubtilin, Bacillomycin l and of their derivatives; inhibition of this antifungal activity by lipid antagonists. *Journal of Antibiotics*, **32**, 828–833.

123 Latoud, C. *et al.* (1997) Action of Iturin A on membrane vesicles from *Saccharomyces cerevisiae*: activation of phospholipases A and B activities by picomolar amounts of Iturin A. *Journal of Antibiotics*, **41**, 1699–1700.

124 Tanaka, Y. *et al.* (1995) Method of producing Iturin A an antifungal agent for profound mycosis. United State Patent, Patent no. 5470827.

125 Moyne, A.L. *et al.* (2001) Bacillomycin D: an iturin with antifungal activity against *Aspergillus flavus*. *Journal of Applied Microbiology*, **90**, 622–629.

126 Hancock, R.E.W. (1998) Resistance mechanisms in *Pseudomonas aeruginosa* and other nonfermentative gram-negative bacteria. *Clinical Infectious Diseases*, **27**, 93–99.

127 Bernard, M. and Latgé, J.-P. (2001) *Aspergillus fumigatus* cell wall: composition and biosynthesis. *Medical Mycology*, **39**, 9–18.

128 Chamilos, G. and Kontoyiannis, D.P. (2005) Update on antifungal drug resistance mechanisms of *Aspergillus fumigatus*. *Drug Resistance Updates*, **8**, 344–358.

129 Chandrasekar, P.H. (2005) Antifungal resistance in *Aspergillus*. *Medical Mycology*, **43**, 295–298.

130 Ferreira, M.E. *et al.* (2005) The ergosterol biosynthesis pathway, transporter genes and azole resistance in *Aspergillus fumigatus*. *Medical Mycology*, **43**, 313–319.

131 Sutton, D.A. *et al.* (2004) *In vitro* amphotericin B resistance in clinical isolates of *Aspergillus terreus*, a head-to-head comparison of voriconazole. *Clinical Infectious Diseases*, **39**, 743–746.

132 Thomas, D.S. *et al.* (1978) Plasma-membrane lipid composition and ethanol tolerance in *Saccharomyces cerevisiae*. *Archives of Microbiology*, **117**, 239–245.

133 Hiom, S.J. *et al.* (1992) Effects of chlorhexidine diacetate on *Candida albicans*, *C. glabrata* and *Saccharomyces cerevisiae*. *Journal of Applied Bacteriology*, **72**, 335–340.

134 Hiom, S.J. *et al.* (1996) The possible role of yeast cell walls in modifying cellular response to chlorhexidine diacetate. *Cytobios*, **86**, 123–135.

135 Cassone, A. *et al.* (1979) Ultrastructural changes in the cell wall of *Candida albicans* following the cessation of growth and their possible relationship to the development of polyene resistance. *Journal of General Microbiology*, **110**, 339–349.

136 Zaragoza, O. *et al.* (2008) Capsule enlargement in *Cryptococcus neoformans* confers resistance to oxidative stress suggesting a mechanism for intracellular survival. *Cell Microbiology*, **10**, 2043–2057.

137 Cervantes, C. and Gutierrez-Corona, F. (1994) Copper resistance mechanisms in bacteria and fungi. *FEMS Microbiology Reviews*, **14**, 121–137.

138 Riggle, P.J. and Kumamoto, C.A. (2000) Role of a *Candida albicans* P1-type ATPase in resistance to copper and silver ion toxicity. *Journal of Bacteriology*, **182**, 4899–4905.

139 Izawa, S. *et al.* (1996) Importance of catalase in the adaptive response to hydrogen peroxide: analysis of acatalasaemic *Saccharomyces cerevisiae*. *Biochemical Journal*, **320**, 61–67.

140 Russell, A.D. (2003) Similarities and differences in the responses of microorganisms to biocides. *Journal of Antimicrobial Chemotherapy*, **52**, 750–763.

141 Ramage, G. *et al.* (2006) *Candida* biofilms on implanted biomaterials: a clinically significant problem. *FEMS Yeast Research*, **6**, 979–986.

8 Sensitivity and Resistance of Protozoa to Microbicides

Vincent Thomas

STERIS SA, Research and Development, Fontenay-aux-Roses, France

Introduction

The term "protozoa" encompasses a wide variety of unicellular, phylogenetically distant, eukaryotic species that are widespread in nature. Most protozoa are free-living and normal inhabitants of freshwater and soil microbial ecosystems, but some live associated with other organisms in a commensalistic, mutualistic or parasitic lifestyle. Life-threatening infections by protozoa are more likely to develop in the immunocompromised; these include potentially fatal complication of AIDS, but also affect malnourished persons, patients undergoing chemotherapy for malignancy, and those receiving immunosuppressive therapy [1]. In this chapter, the focus is on protozoa that can be directly transmitted to humans through various environmental means (contaminated water, food, environmental surfaces, air, etc.) since in these cases microbicidal treatments can be directly used against protozoa to prevent transmission. Consideration is also given to transmission in animals, as a source of infection to humans via ingestion of undercooked meat. Those protozoa that can only be transmitted by insects or other vectors, through blood transfusion and organ transplantation, or from mother to fetus are not included here.

General descriptions and life cycles

Waterborne parasitic protozoa other than amoebae

Giardia spp. belong to the Diplomonads, and *Cryptosporidium* spp. to the Apicomplexans. In a 2007 study, it was calculated that these obligate parasites accounted for 40.6% and 50.8%, respectively, of waterborne protozoan disease outbreaks reported in the USA and Europe [2]. *Giardia* spp. are common waterborne parasites of humans, with a 2–5% prevalence in industrialized countries and 20–30% in developing countries, and an estimated 200–300 million symptomatic individuals worldwide [3, 4]. Incidence of cryptosporidiosis has ranged from 0.6% to 20%, accounting for up to 20% of all cases of childhood diarrhea in developing countries [5, 6]. Serological studies in the USA have suggested that at least one-third of the population has been exposed to the parasite [7]. Major outbreaks of cryptosporidiosis have occurred in the USA and Europe. For example, the one in 1993 in Milwaukee, Wisconsin, affected >400,000 individuals and an estimated US$96 million in associated costs [8, 9]. *Cryptosporidium* spp. are ubiquitous in the environment; their persistence and resistance to chemical disinfection have made the human pathogenic species *C. parvum* a critical pathogen for the

Russell, Hugo & Ayliffe's: Principles and Practice of Disinfection, Preservation and Sterilization, Fifth Edition. Edited by Adam P. Fraise, Jean-Yves Maillard, and Syed A. Sattar.
© 2013 Blackwell Publishing Ltd. Published 2013 by Blackwell Publishing Ltd.

Table 8.1 Several characteristics of protozoa mentioned in this chapter (adapted from [10, 13, 14]).

Phylogenetic group	Species	Disease/symptoms	Incidence of illness	Dormant forms	Size	Important animal source	Persistence in environment
Alveolates	*Balantidium coli*	Diarrhea, dysentery	Moderate	Cysts	40–60 μm	Yes	Long?
	Cryptosporidium spp.	Diarrhea	Common	Sporulated oocysts	4–6 μm	Yes	Long
	Cyclospora cayetanensis	Protracted diarrhea	Rare	Unsporulated oocyst	8–10 μm	No	Long
	Isospora belli	Diarrhea	Rare	Unsporulated oocysts	14–32 μm	No	Long?
	Sarcocystis spp.	Diarrhea, muscle weakness	Rare	Oocysts, sporocysts (prey), bradyzoites (predators)	7.5–17 μm	Yes	Long
	Toxoplasma gondii	Lymphadenopathy, fever, congenital infections	Common	Unsporulated oocysts	10–12 μm	Yes	Long
Amoebozoa	*Acanthamoeba* spp.	Granulomatous encephalitis (cutaneous and sinus), keratitis	Very rare (encephalitis) to rare (keratitis)	Cysts	13–20 μm	No	Long
	Balamuthia mandrillaris	Granulomatous encephalitis (cutaneous and sinus)	Very rare	Cysts	12–30 μm	No	Long
	Entamoeba histolytica	Dysentery, liver abscess	Common	Cysts	10–15 μm	No	Moderate
	Hartmannella vermiformis	Keratitis (?)	Very rare	Cysts	6–8 μm	No	Long
	Sappinia diploidea	Encephalitis	Very rare	Cysts	13–37 μm	No	Long
Diplomonads	*Giardia lamblia*	Diarrhea, malabsorption	Common	Cysts	12 × 5 μm	Yes	Moderate
Heterolobosea	*Naegleria fowleri*	Primary meningoencephalitis	Very rare	Cysts	7–15 μm	No	Long
	Paravahlkampfia francinae	Primary meningoencephalitis	Very rare	Cysts	15–21 μm	No	Long
Stramenopiles	*Blastocystis hominis*	Diarrhea, abdominal pain, but mostly no symptoms at all	Common	Cysts	4–6 μm	?	Long?
Microsporidia (fungi)	*Encephalitozoon cuniculi* *Encephalitozoon hellem* *Encephalitozoon intestinalis* *Enterocytozoon bieneusi*	Enteritis, hepatitis, peritonitis, keratoconjunctivitis	Rare	Spores	1.8–5 μm	No	Long

drinking water industry, thus being selected as the target for risk-assessment programs [10]. For this reason, and due to the high public health risk linked to *Cryptosporidium* spp. and *Giardia* spp., many studies have investigated the sensitivity of these parasitic protozoa to various disinfection treatments.

Other parasitic protozoa species are generally considered less resistant to microbicides and/or present lower epidemic potential than *Giardia* and *Cryptosporidium* spp. so there are consequently fewer inactivation studies available in the literature. Most of these species also belong to the Apicomplexans but are classified as coccidian parasites, whereas recent studies suggest that *Cryptosporidium* spp. are only distantly related to this group [11]. Coccidians can be transmitted through contaminated water, food and/or soils; they include *Balantidium coli*, *Cyclospora* spp., *Isospora belli*, *Sarcocystis* spp. and *Toxoplasma gondii*. It is estimated that *T. gondii* is as frequently encountered as *Cryptosporidium* spp. in the general population [12] but outbreaks are

rarely described. Altogether, these five species account for c. 3.9% of the outbreaks by water-associated protozoa [2], with the stramenopile species *Blastocystis hominis* being responsible for 0.6% of such outbreaks [2].

These parasitic protozoan all have dormant forms in their life cycle, allowing survival in the environment and permitting spread from one host to another (Table 8.1).

These dormant forms present significant differences that are important to consider for a better understanding of their epidemiology and resistance to microbicides (see the CDC website www.dpd.cdc.gov/dpdx/default.htm for life-cycle illustrations of all protozoa mentioned in this chapter). *B. hominis* and *Giardia* spp. have no sexual multiplication: infective cysts are excreted at the end of the infection cycle and, once ingested by susceptible hosts, they differentiate into actively growing trophozoites that initiate a new infection cycle. Sexual reproduction as conjugation may exist in the case of *B. coli* but it is not well documented and the infective forms are also termed cysts, as for *B. hominis* and *Giardia* spp. [15]. Other Apicomplexans present sexual multiplication, with some differences in the maturity of fertilized forms that are excreted from infected hosts. *Cyclospora* spp., *I. belli* and *T. gondii* form unsporulated non-infective oocysts that are released in the environment and need to differentiate into mature oocysts and sporozoites before infecting new hosts. Differentiation into infective forms takes several days to several weeks and requires specific conditions (e.g. temperature is critical). Conversely, mature oocysts and sporocysts are excreted through stools of hosts infected by *Cryptosporidium* spp. and *Sarcocystis* spp.; as a consequence direct fecal–oral transmission can occur for these two species. Cysts and oocysts can be excreted in very large numbers by infected hosts as demonstrated for *Cryptosporidium* and *T. gondii* with 10^9 to 10^{10} and 10^7 to 10^8 oocysts, respectively [16, 17]. Minimum infective doses are not always known but in those species for which they have been investigated they can be as low as a single oocyst for *T. gondii* in various animal species [18], 10 oocysts for several *Cryptosporidium* isolates experimentally transmitted to immunocompetent volunteers [19], 10 cysts for experimental transmission of *Giardia* to gerbils or to human volunteers [20, 21], 100 cysts for *Isospora suis* in piglets [22], and 100 cysts for *B. hominis* transmitted to rats [23].

Once excreted by infected hosts, dormant forms can survive for weeks to months in the environment, depending on conditions encountered and on the species and strains considered. The most favorable condition for cyst survival is cold freshwater: *Giardia* cysts suspended in either lake or river water remained viable for 2–3 months during winter [24]; *T. gondii* oocysts remained infective up to 54 months in water at 4°C [25]; *Sarcocystis neurona* sporocysts retained viability and ability to infect mice after storage for 7 years at 4°C in buffered saline [26]; and *C. parvum* oocysts remained viable for 7 months when incubated in sterile, deionized water circulating in a 15°C waterbath [27]. Thus, freshwater sources are frequently contaminated with diverse protozoan species: in a recent study conducted in the Paris area, *Cryptosporidium* oocysts and *Giardia* cysts were found in 45.7% and 93.8%, respectively, of a total of 162 river samples, with occasional peaks of high concentration [28]. The dormant forms of several species (mainly *Cryptosporidium*, *Giardia* and *Toxoplasma*) can also survive for extended periods in seawater, potentially contaminating humans through recreational bathing waters or consumption of contaminated oysters [29].

The relatively small size and high microbicide resistance of *Cryptosporidium* oocysts and *Giardia* cysts pose a higher risk for their transmission through drinking and recreational waters, with many outbreaks having been linked to these sources [2]. There is also evidence that *Cyclospora*, *Toxoplasma* and *Blastocystis hominis* can be transmitted by treated drinking water [30–32] but this is not thought to be their main route of spread.

Drying is generally detrimental to the survival of protozoan cysts and oocysts [33, 34]. While the modulation of relative humidity (RH) and air temperature could promote the survival of *Sarcocystis* cysts on environmental surfaces for several months

[35, 36], such surfaces and medical devices are not among the significant vehicles for the spread of protozoan pathogens such as cryptosporidia [37].

Parasitic and free-living amoebae

Other protozoan species that can infect humans are found among the amoebae, a category of monocellular eukaryotic organisms that present many common ecological characters although being phylogenetically distant (see Table 8.1). They have no sexual reproduction and most species also form dormant cysts. Formation of these cysts is necessary for the environmental survival of the parasitic *Entamoeba* spp. and transmission to new hosts; cysts also allow for the environmental persistence of free-living amoebae (FLAs) despite highly variable physical and chemical conditions.

The genus *Entamoeba* belongs to the Amoebozoa supergroup and comprises well-described parasitic species. *Entamoeba histolytica* is responsible for amebic dysentery, a worldwide parasitic infection affecting millions of people and killing 100,000 each year [38]. *Entamoeba*-infected hosts can excrete several million cysts per day [39]; the minimum infective dose is thought to be low (several cysts). These cysts are not as highly resistant to harsh environmental stresses as those of FLAs and transmission is mainly due to poor hygienic conditions, with direct contamination through treated drinking water being only rarely reported [2].

Pathogenic FLAs including *Acanthamoeba* spp., *Balamuthia mandrillaris* and *Sappinia* spp. also belong to the Amoebozoa supergroup [40]. They have been recognized as etiological agents of various diseases. Prevalence of anti-*Acanthamoeba castellanii* antibodies (IgA) in the general population has been observed to be as high as 87.7%, suggesting that we routinely encounter these organisms in our natural environment [41]. *Acanthamoeba* spp. have been associated mainly with keratitis, a rare but sight-threatening corneal infection that can affect immunocompetent individuals. Incidence of the disease has dramatically increased over the last three decades due to the rise in the use of contact lenses, with rates of 0.15 and 1.4 per million in the USA and UK, respectively [42]. In rare instances, FLAs belonging to the genus *Hartmannella* have been isolated from corneal infections, suggesting that other FLA species can induce keratitis [43]. Other infections due to FLA belonging to Amoebozoa occur mainly in the immunocompromised, although several cases of *Balamuthia* encephalitis have been documented in immunocompetent individuals [13, 44]. Granulomatous amebic encephalitis (GAE), disseminated diseases and skin lesions have been reported with *Acanthamoeba* spp. and *B. mandrillaris* [45]. A *Sappinia* species has been reported as the causative agent of severe non-fatal encephalitis in an immunocompetent young male [46]. These infections are very rare, with as few as c. 200 cases reported between the 1960s and 2000 for *Acanthamoeba* GAE and c. 100 cases between the 1990s and 2000 for *Balamuthia* GAE [14].

Naegleria fowleri is another pathogenic FLA species that belongs to the *Heterolobosea* (supergroup Excavata) [47]. It is responsible for primary amebic meningoencephalitis (PAM), a fulminating and frequently fatal infection that can affect immunocompetent individuals [13]. A new FLA species named *Paravahlkampfia francinae* also belongs to *Heteroloboseae* and has been reported as a causative agent of a brain infection in an immunocompetent young male presenting typical symptoms of PAM [48]. These infections are also very rare, with *c.* 200 cases reported between the 1960s and 2000 for *Naegleria* PAM [14]. Brain infections by *Acanthamoeba* spp. and *B. mandrillaris* occur after the entry of amoebae through breaks in the skin or as cysts taken into the respiratory tract [14]. *N. fowleri* infections occur mainly after swimming or diving in contaminated freshwater: amoebae are carried into the nostrils and migrate to the brain along the olfactory nerves [14].

Keratitis is linked mainly to the use of contact lenses that are soaked in solutions with insufficient activity against *Acanthamoeba* spp. [49]. Of note, FLAs have also been recovered from indoor and outdoor air samples [50] and from the nasopharyngeal and oral regions of dental patients [51]. A recent study also demonstrated the presence of amoebae in bronchoaspirate fluid taken from patients after chemotherapy and in samples of bronchoalveolar lavage from patients with respiratory insufficiency [52]. In another study, *Acanthamoeba* spp. were encountered in urine of critically ill patients in intensive care units: 17 of 63 samples collected from urinary catheters were positive for such species [53]. In addition to their intrinsic pathogenicity, *Acanthamoeba* can potentially harbor intracellularly various bacterial, viral and eukaryotic species pathogenic for human and animals [54]. Thus, among 539 bacterial species listed as being pathogenic for humans and/or animals, to date 102 have been described in the literature as being able to resist and potentially proliferate after amoebal ingestion [55]. These include well-known pathogenic species responsible for hospital-acquired infections such as *Acinetobacter* spp., *Enterobacter* spp., *Legionella* spp., various mycobacterial species, *Pseudomonas* spp. and *Serratia* spp. (for a complete review see [55]). Survival of bacteria within amoebal cysts has been demonstrated for several of these species, mainly in mycobacteria [56], and cysts are thus considered as potential reservoirs of pathogenic microorganisms in water networks.

Whereas *Entamoeba histolytica* is an obligate parasite, FLAs are ubiquitous protozoa that proliferate in the environment by grazing on bacterial biofilms. They are normal inhabitants of freshwater sources and soils and can be recovered in high numbers from lakes and rivers [57, 58], and also from ocean sediments [59]. In these environments, the exact composition of the FLA population is dependent on the physicochemical parameters, such as annual temperature fluctuation and pH changes [60, 61]. Compared to cysts of *Entamoeba* spp., FLA cysts are only weakly infective but they present dramatically higher resistance to various stresses and can survive for many years in the environment. This is particularly true for various *Acanthamoeba* species: Mazur *et al.* [62] showed that 14 of 17 encysted acanthamoebal isolates stored at 4°C in water survived for 24 years without apparent loss of virulence in the mouse model; acanthamoebal cysts have also

been reactivated after storage for more than 20 years in a completely dry environment [63]. *Naegleria* spp. are generally considered less resistant to these extreme environmental conditions; in the study published by Chang, drying made pathogenic *Naegleria* trophozoites non-viable instantaneously and cysts non-viable in less than 5 min [64].

It has been demonstrated that although clarification steps used in drinking water production plants dramatically reduce their numbers, FLAs can spread from the water source to the distribution network despite disinfection of water with ozone and chlorine [65–67]. Once in the distribution network, low disinfectant levels have only limited activity on FLAs [68]. They can thus colonize virtually any kind of domestic water system and proliferate by grazing on bacterial biofilms that are also present in these systems [69]. FLAs have been isolated from a number of diverse environments, some containing harsh physical and/or chemical conditions such as elevated temperature (hot tubes, cooling towers) or high concentrations of microbicides. They have been recovered in 13–47% of domestic tapwater samples [70–72], being present in 79–89% of households in the USA [73] and UK [74], respectively, and are mainly isolated from shower heads and kitchen sprayer biofilms. Being ubiquitous, they were also recovered from hospital water networks [75, 76], swimming pools [77], hydrotherapy baths [78], dental unit waterlines [79], eyewash stations [80], cooling towers [81, 82], etc.

Microsporidia

Obligate intracellular parasites termed "microsporidia" were classified as protozoa until recently; however, recent data suggest that they descend from a zygomycete ancestor and have thus been classified as fungi [83]. Despite the recent reclassification of these unusual and ubiquitous microorganisms, we have included them in this chapter due to increasing amounts of data on their inactivation by microbicides.

The group Microsporidia comprises approximately 150 genera and 1200 species, infecting mainly vertebrate and invertebrate hosts. *Enterocytozoon bieneusi* and *Encephalitozoon intestinalis* are the two main species infecting humans (see Table 8.1) but several other opportunistic pathogenic species have been described [1, 84, 85]. Other species infect commercially important animal species including bees, silk worms, salmon and various domesticated mammals [86]. Recent evidence suggests that some Microsporidia have an extant sexual cycle and can also acquire genes from obligate intracellular bacteria when infecting the same eukaryotic cell [87]. Their infective stage is a thick-walled spore-like structure, which is also the only stage that can survive outside their host cell. *E. bieneusi* infections in humans occur mainly through ingestion of the spores, whereas infections by *Encephalitozoon* spp. can also occur through inhalation, sexual transmission, various types of trauma and direct contact via portals such as the eyes [86]. Transplacental transmission has also been reported in animals [85].

Microsporidia can cause symptomatic, potentially severe infections in the immunocompromised, whereas pathogenicity is thought to be limited in immunocompetent persons; increased prevalence has mainly been observed among AIDS patients before the advent of highly active antiretroviral therapy [85]. Seroprevalence in the general population ranges between 1% and 20% [85]. Infection of immunocompromised patients by *E. bieneusi* frequently causes persistent diarrhea, abdominal pain and weight loss; pulmonary infections, cholecystitis and cholangitis are rarely reported [1, 85]. *Encephalitozoon* spp. can cause disseminated microsporidiosis with clinical syndromes including sinusitis, keratoconjunctivitis, encephalitis, tracheobronchitis, interstitial nephritis, hepatitis or myositis [1, 85]. Excretion by symptomatic hosts is thought to be high with, for example, 10^7 spores per single fecal sample in nude rats immunosuppressed with dexamethasone and challenged orally with 10^4 *E. bieneusi* spores [88].

Once excreted, the spores survive well in the environment. Li *et al.* demonstrated that *E. intestinalis* remained infective for at least 12 months when stored at 10°C in distilled water [89]. Infectivity markedly decreased at higher temperatures and viability was not detected after incubation for 3 weeks at 30°C. Interestingly, survival rates of *Encephalitozoon hellem* under the same conditions were similar whereas survival rates of *Encephalitozoon cuniculi* were lower, suggesting differences between different species [89]. This was confirmed in another study demonstrating that *E. intestinalis* and *E. hellem* spores survive better than the spores of *E. cuniculi* in distilled water and in artificial seawater, with a strong effect of temperature and salinity (better survival rates for all species at low temperature and low salinity) [90]. Low temperatures are generally more favorable to spore survival: Kudela *et al.* demonstrated that spores of *E. cuniculi* stored for 2 years at 4°C in sterile distilled water did not show any marked loss of infectivity [91]. Similarly, spores of the fish pathogenic species *Loma salmonae* remained infective after 3 months at 4°C in freshwater and in seawater [92] and the spores of the honeybee pathogenic species *Nosema apis* were still infective after 7 years of storage at 5°C in distilled water [93]. Spores also survive

desiccation for significant periods of time: dried spores of *Nosema ceranae*, another parasite of the honeybee, survived for at least 1 week at room temperature [94]. In some cases, it has been demonstrated that low (but non-freezing) temperatures are detrimental for spore survival to desiccation: dried spores of *E. cuniculi* survived for less than a week at 4°C but at least for 4 weeks at 22°C [95].

Due to the relatively high resistance of their spores, Microsporidia are thought to survive well in the environment and were detected in various surface waters including recreational bathing waters and drinking water sources, but also in groundwater, sewage effluents and in samples taken from various fresh food produces [96–100].

Dormant-form cell wall structures: a key to understanding resistance to microbicides

In most cases, dormant forms of protozoa are the main transmission forms, and these are also the forms with higher resistance to harsh environmental conditions. Transmission electron microscopy of the cyst walls of different protozoa (Figure 8.1) can help us understand the links between the structure and resistance to microbicides. Such studies are difficult with protozoa that cannot be cultivated *in vitro* and for which there are no suitable animal models; *Balantidium coli* and *Blastocystis hominis* are good examples here. *In vitro* induction of encystment can also be difficult and methods are still under investigation for important pathogenic species such as *Entamoeba histolytica* [106]. A brief description of what is known about the various dormant form structures is given below.

Apicomplexans: coccidians

All coccidian oocysts autofluoresce white-blue under UV excitation filters [107]. This suggests that the oocyst wall is essentially consistent in structure across different species of coccidian parasites [108]. Oocysts of coccidian species that belong to the genus

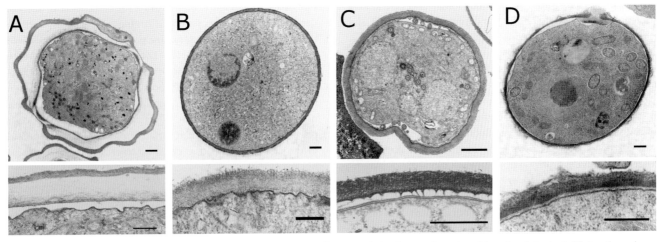

Figure 8.1 Transmission electron microscopy of cysts of various protozoa species (top: general view; bottom: closer view of the cell wall structure). (A) *Acanthamoeba castellanii.* (B) *Entamoeba invadens.* (C) *Giardia intestinalis.* (D) *Naegleria* sp. Bars = 1 μm. (Courtesy of Dr. Chávez-Munguía, Department of Experimental Pathology, Center for Research and Advanced Studies, Mexico City.) (See references [101–105] for further details.)

Eimeria have been extensively studied and are considered as a model for the study of oocyst wall structure of coccidia [109]. Several species that belong to this genus are frequent pathogens of economically important domestic animals (e.g. cattle and chickens) while being non-pathogenic for humans; they can be readily obtained in large numbers for analysis and experimental infections. The mature oocyst wall is bilayered. The electron-dense outer layer is *c.* 200 nm thick in *Eimeria maxima*, whereas the electron-lucent inner layer is around 40 nm thick; an inner zone of *c.* 40 nm separates the outer and inner layers [108, 110]. Biochemical analysis of unsporulated or sporulated *E. maxima* and *Eimeria tenella* oocysts demonstrated 0.6–2.0% carbohydrates, 1.4–7.6% lipids and 90.4–98.3% proteins [109]. In both species the carbohydrate content of sporulated oocysts was made up of 4.3–5% mannose, 33.7–37.4% galactose and 58.3–61.3% glucose, whereas the carbohydrate profile of unsporulated oocyst walls was dominated by galactose (62.3–67.6%), followed by glucose (26–27.9%) and mannose (6.4–9.8%) [109]. Sporulated oocysts of both species contained a number of fatty acids including palmitic, stearic, oleic, linoleic, behenic and lignoceric acids; non-saponifiable lipids such as cholestadiene, cholestane and cholesterol were also detected [109]. These compounds were found at similar percentages in sporulated oocysts of both species, with the exception of oleic and palmitic acids which more abundant in *E. tenella*, whereas cholestane and cholesterol were more abundant in *E. maxima* [109]. Unsporulated oocysts of both species had similar lipid levels but completely lacked linoleic acid. Protein content of *Eimeria* spp. oocyst walls has also been investigated. It has been demonstrated that two tyrosine-rich precursor glycoproteins, GAM56 and GAM82, that are present in various *Eimeria* species, are proteolytically processed into smaller glycoproteins which are incorporated into the oocyst wall [111, 112]. High concentrations of dityrosine and 3,4-dihydroxyphenylalanine (DOPA) have been detected in oocyst extracts suggesting, together with the detection of a UV autofluorescence in intact oocysts, dityrosine– and possibly DOPA–protein cross-links in the oocyst wall [111]. A 22 kDa protein has also been described; it is dominated by histidine and proline residues, its gene is present in high copy number and it might be involved in stabilizing extracellular structures via cross-links between histidine and catechols, as described for insect cuticles [113].

Although *gam56* and *gam82* homologs have not been identified in the genomes of other coccidians, the observation that the oocyst walls of these coccidia autofluoresce blue under UV light suggests that they share a common mechanism of oocyst wall assembly involving protein–tyrosine cross-links [108]. Additionally, the presence of seven cysteine-rich extracellular proteins related to COWP-1 (see below) in the *T. gondii* oocyst wall suggests that this species might have a cell wall with similarities to that of *Cryptosporidium* [114, 115]. The oocyst wall of *T. gondii* is comprised of three distinct layers: a 20–50 nm thick electron-dense outer layer, a 8–10 nm thick electron-lucent middle layer, and a 50–90 nm thick moderately electron-dense inner layer [116].

Apicomplexans: Cryptosporidium

The oocyst cell wall provides a protective barrier for infective *Cryptosporidium*. Recent investigations proposed the oocyst wall to be composed of an outer glycocalyx layer (*c.* 8 nm), a lipid hydrocarbon layer (*c.* 4 nm), a protein layer (*c.* 13 nm) and a structural polysaccharide inner layer (*c.* 25–40 nm) [117]. The expanded glycocalyx layer external to the outer bilayer is easily removed and not present in all oocysts; it is suspected that immunogenicity and the surface chemistry of oocysts vary depending on the presence or absence of this outer glycocalyx matrix [117]. In the same study proteins represented 7.5% of total oocyst wall and yielded five major bands, while wall residues obtained after lipid extraction yielded 12 major bands, likely resulting from the release of lipoproteins during the lipid extraction process [117]. Nine *Cryptosporidium* oocyst wall proteins (COWPs) have been identified, and it has been demonstrated that COWP1 and COWP8 are selectively localized in the inner layer of the oocyst wall [114, 118]. These proteins are characterized by tandem arrays of cysteine-rich domains, with intermolecular disulfide bonds being a potential source of oocyst wall rigidity [118]. Oocyst walls also contain 2% hexose: glucose, galactose, mannose, talose, glucofuranose, D-glucopyranose and D-mannopyranose were detected [117]. Hexadecanoic, octadecanoic, 9-octadecenoic and 11,14-eicosandienoic acids are the most abundant fatty acids in the oocyst wall [117] and are also present in whole oocysts [119]. Importantly, four fatty alcohols were also detected in oocyst walls [117]. Based on these analyses, the authors proposed a model for the *C. parvum* oocyst wall and suggested that similarities in lipid composition and acid-fast staining between *C. parvum* and mycobacteria may indicate that the two organisms share structural mechanisms conferring resistance to microbicides [117].

Diplomonads: Giardia

In *Giardia*, the cyst wall thickness varies from 300 to 500 nm. It is formed by an outer filamentous layer and an inner membranous layer including three membranes that enclose the periplasmic space (see Figure 8.1) [101, 120]. Biochemical analysis demonstrated that the cyst wall is composed of carbohydrates in the form of *N*-acetyl galactosamine polymers [121], and cyst wall proteins 1, 2 and 3 (CWPs) [122–124]. These proteins have 14–16 Cys residues and similar leucine-rich repeats, they form disulfide-bonded oligomers, with CWP2 possibly acting as an aggregation factor for CWP1 and CWP3. Another protein, the high cysteine non-variable surface protein (VSP) cyst protein (HCNCp) that resembles trophozoite variant surface proteins, has been localized in the cyst wall of mature cysts; however its function remains unclear [125].

Amoebae

The cyst wall of *Entamoeba invadens*, a model for the human pathogen *Entamoeba histolytica*, is a single 120–150 nm thick and continuous fibrillar layer closely associated to the plasma membrane (see Figure 8.1) [102, 103]. It is composed of fibrils of chitin and three cystein-rich, chitin-binding lectins (CBDs) called Jacob,

Jessie3 and chitinase [126]. The recent study published by Chatteriee *et al.* proposed a "wattle and daub" model to explain *Entamoeba* cyst wall formation. In the first "foundation" phase, Jacob lectins are bound to the surface of encysting amoebae. In the second "wattle" phase, Jacob lectins cross-link chitin fibrils that are deposited on the surface of encysting amoebae. In the third "daub" phase, the cyst wall is solidified and made impermeable to small molecules by the addition of the Jessie3 lectin, which has an N-terminal CBD that binds chitin and a unique C-terminal domain that appears to cause self-aggregation [126].

In *Acanthamoeba* spp. the cyst wall consists of a double-layered structure (see Figure 8.1). The ectocyst is 250–300 nm thick and also presents a 30–40 nm thick superficial layer with compact fibrous structure [104]. The endocyst is 200–300 nm thick; it is composed of fine (6–10 nm diameter) fibrils forming a granular matrix and contains cellulose [104]. The *Acanthamoeba* cyst wall contains approximately 33% protein, 4–6% lipid, 35% carbohydrates, 8% ash and 20% unidentified material [127]. These amounts vary depending on the species and strains considered [128]. Detailed analysis of the carbohydrate content of *Acanthamoeba castellanii* cyst walls revealed a high percentage of galactose and glucose, in addition to small amounts of mannose and xylose [129]. Linkage analysis revealed several types of glycosidic linkages including the 1,4-linked glucosyl conformation, indicative of cellulose [129]. *Balamuthia mandrillaris* mature cysts have a tripartite wall consisting of an outer loose ectocyst, a thick inner endocyst and a fibrillar middle mesocyst [130]. It has been demonstrated to contain a much lower percentage of carbohydrates than those of *Acanthamoeba* species: 0.3% dry weight carbohydrates consisting of glucose, mannose and traces of galactose [131]. Linkage analysis also demonstrated the presence of cellulose and possibly other unidentified branched oligo- or polysaccharides [131]. Interestingly, *Balamuthia* cysts present resistance to treatments that compares to resistance of *Acanthamoeba* cysts (see below), supporting the hypothesis that cellulose plays an important role in high resistance to microbicides.

Of note, a selective immunocytochemical marker failed to detect cellulose in cyst walls of representative species of *Naegleria* and *Hartmannella*, which are generally considered less resistant than *Acanthamoeba* spp. [132]. It has been reported that the cyst walls of most *Naegleria* spp. consist of a double layer: the ectocyst is irregular and approximately 25 nm thick, and the endocyst is 200–450 nm thick and appears layered [133, 134] (see Figure 8.1). However, it has been reported that the outer layer of the cyst wall present in the cysts of *Naegleria gruberi* is absent in the cysts of *Naegleria fowleri* and *Naegleria jadini* [135], and recent analysis suggest that the *Naegleria* cyst wall is formed only as a single, thick, fibrillar layer with detached irregular thin loops that might have been confounded with a real ectocyst [105]. Although detailed analysis of *Naegleria* spp. cyst walls remains unknown, they are thought to contain chitin since, despite the absence of cellulose, they are stained by calcofluor white M2R, indicating the presence of another kind of β-1-4-linked polysaccharide [105].

Microsporidia

At the end of intracellular multiplication, microsporidia differentiate into resistant spore forms that are protected by a thick spore wall composed of a glycoprotein-rich outer layer (exospore, 25–30 nm thick) and a chitin-rich inner layer (endospore, 30–35 nm thick) [136]. These mature spores are very small (2–7 μm by 1.5–5 μm). They possess an extrusion apparatus – a unique feature of microsporidia allowing injection of infective sporoplasm into the host cell cytoplasm [137]. This rigid spore wall, in addition to providing mechanical resistance, is thus involved in host cell recognition and initiation of the infection process [136, 138]. Two proteins have been identified in the exospore of *Encephalitozoon* spp.: spore wall protein 1 (SWP1) and SWP2 present 10 conserved cysteines in the N-terminal domain, suggesting similar secondary structures [136, 139]. Furthermore the C-terminal domain of SWP2 has a unique region containing 50 repeating 12- or 15-amino-acid units that lacks homology to known protein motifs [139]. One of the endospore proteins (SWP3, also termed EnP2) is predicted to be *O*-glycosylated and glycosylphosphatidylinositol-anchored to the plasma membrane; it contains only two cysteine residues [140, 141]. Another endospore protein (EnP1) is cysteine-rich and is postulated to be involved in spore wall assembly by disulfide bridging [141]. It has been demonstrated that this protein contains multiple heparin-binding motifs and that it binds host cell surfaces via glycosaminoglycans [142]. The third protein identified in endospores is associated with the plasma membrane of developing spores; it is a putative chitin deacetylase (EcCDA) supposed to deacetylate chitin into chitosan that interacts with other cell wall components [143]. This enzymatic activity has been described in other fungi and could account for the extreme rigidity and resistance of the parasite wall to various stresses such as freezing, heating and extreme pH [143].

Sensitivity and resistance of protozoa to microbicides

One of the main problems to address when comparing the efficacy of microbicides against microorganisms is the evaluation of differences between methods used by researchers and the impact on their results. This is particularly true when considering protozoa (including microsporidia) as there are no well-standardized test methods described for this purpose. For example, various methods aiming at quantifying the residual infectivity of Apicomplexans after disinfection have been described, including animal infectivity assay, excystation, staining with fluorogenic vital dyes, reverse transcription polymerase chain reaction (PCR), combination of cell culture and quantitative real-time PCR (cc-qPCR) and others [27, 144, 145]. Accuracy of these methods can vary from one organism to another but also depends on the microbicidal treatment evaluated [146]. Methods used to evaluate efficacy of disinfectants against *Acanthamoeba* cysts have also been demonstrated to be highly variable, leading to inconsistency in efficacy results from one study to another. Critical parameters include tested amoebal strains, composition of media used to grow the amoebae and prepare cysts, age of th ecysts, and methods used to evaluate cyst viability after treatments [147–150]. In addition to these limitations, it should always been kept in mind that the killing effect of microbicide formulations and exposure conditions can differ substantially even if these formulations have similar concentrations of microbicide. This is especially true and has been largely demonstrated for products used for contact lens disinfection, thus highlighting the critical importance of "non-active" ingredients, notably surfactants, for the microbicidal activity of formulations (see for example [151]). Another important point to consider is that most common antiseptics and disinfectants have not been tested against various protozoa, unlike bacteria and other classes of pathogens. Possible exceptions here are several studies on contact lens disinfectants against *Acanthamoeba* spp.

Chemical microbicides
Cationic microbicides
These positively charged molecules bind strongly to the negatively charged cell walls and particularly membranes of microorganisms, resulting in disruption of the target cell by perturbation of these sites [152]. They are widely used in a range of applications, including antimicrobial soaps, microbicidal wound dressings, mouthwashes, hair-care products, environmental surface disinfectants and preservatives [153]. Notably, biguanides (mainly chlorhexidine and polyhexamethylene biguanides) are used at low concentrations as preservatives in contact lens solutions but also at higher concentrations as curing treatments for patients suffering from amoebal keratitis. In contrast, quaternary ammonium compounds (QACs) have been less well studied despite their widespread use as surface disinfectants and preservatives.

Trophozoites of *Acanthamoeba* spp., *A. castellanii*, *A. polyphaga* and *A. culbertsoni*, have been found to be susceptible to relatively low concentrations (0.005–0.006%) of chlorhexidine (CHG) [154–157]. A QAC-based formulation has been demonstrated to be effective against trophozoites of various *Acanthamoeba* and *Naegleria* species but was not tested against their cysts [158]. Whereas cationic microbicides generally present good activity against *Acanthamoeba* trophozoites, resistance to these compounds develops when trophozoites encyst, corresponding to increasing cellulose levels in cyst walls [159]. Efficacy data of cationic microbicides against amoebal cysts vary from one study to another: Penley *et al.* reported that *A. polyphaga* cysts persisted in disinfecting solutions preserved with chlorhexidine for at least 2 days [155] whereas Silvany *et al.* reported a good efficacy of solutions containing chlorhexidine even after short exposure [156]. These differences may be due to the effect of formulation. CHG 0.005% in formulation with thimerosal 0.001% (an organomercury compound) and/or ethylenediamine tetraacetic acid (EDTA) 0.1% has been reported to be effective against acanthamoebal cysts [160, 161]. Polyhexamethylene biguanide (PHMB) was described as trophocidal and cysticidal against the cysts of various

Acanthamoeba spp. including *A. castellanii*, *A. polyphaga* and clinical isolates of *Acanthamoeba* spp. associated with keratitis [162–168]. However, low concentrations of PHMB (0.00005%) and the quaternary ammonium polyquaternium-1 (0.055–0.001%) were also reported to be inactive against *A. castellanii*, *A. polyphaga* and *A. culbertsoni* [154–156, 160, 169, 170]. These low concentrations are used in multipurpose solutions for contact lenses and several investigations demonstrated that some of these solutions were not cysticidal within the manufacturer's recommended contact time [171–173]. Of note, a national outbreak of *Acanthamoeba* keratitis was detected in the USA in 2007 and has been linked to the use of a 0.0001% PHMB-based multipurpose contact lens solution presenting limited efficacy against *Acanthamoeba* cysts [49]. A study comparing the relative efficacy of this and other products based on polymeric biguanides and CHG demonstrated that none of them was effective against the cysts of *A. castellanii*, *A. polyphaga* and *Acanthamoeba hatchetti* even after 24 h of exposure [151]. The QAC benzalkonium chloride was shown to be effective at a concentration of 0.04% against the trophozoites and cysts of *A. castellanii* [160, 167, 168] and *A. polyphaga* [168]. Lower concentrations (0.003–0.004%) were found to be non-cysticidal [154, 155, 157], although Turner *et al.* showed the minimum cysticidal concentration for *A. castellanii* was 0.004% [159].

A QAC-based formulation has been demonstrated to be effective against *Cryptosporidium* oocysts after a 1 h contact at 37°C (excystation index was used as a measure of efficacy) [174]. Conversely, another QAC-based formulation did not show any activity against *Cryptosporidium* oocysts after a 10 min contact at 20°C (infectivity was used as a measure of efficacy) [175]. Treatments with formulations containing 2% CHG or 6% benzyl ammonium chloride were not effective against the sporocysts of *Sarcocystis neurona* [176]. Treatment with 0.1% cetyltrimethyl ammonium for 24 h did not completely kill *T. gondii* oocysts [17]. Conversely, benzyldimethyltetradecyl ammonium at 0.001% demonstrated complete inactivation of *Giardia* cysts after 10 min of contact at 24°C (excystation index was used as a measure of efficacy) [146]. Several commercial formulations containing various kinds of QACs were also demonstrated to be effective against the spores of *Encephalitozoon intestinalis* within 5–15 min [177, 178].[000]

Halogen compounds: chlorine, bromine and iodine
Chlorine, bromine and iodine are halogens that are widely used for their microbicidal action. When dissolved in water these actives generate reactive species presenting strong micobicidal activity. The exact mode of action of these agents has not been elucidated but oxidation is a major effect [153]. The initial levels of organic and inorganic molecules present in water can strongly influence the microbicidal efficacy of halogens since they will react with these molecules. pH is also a critical parameter since it will change the proportions of halogen species that do not have the same microbicidal efficacy. For example, at pH 4 to 7 the predominant form for chlorine will be HOCl, which is also the most potent microbicidal species; the microbicidal activity of

chlorine will thus be better between these pH values. Temperature is also important, with lower efficacy at lower temperatures.

Differences in the microbicidal activity of chlorine against FLAs have been reported, with trophozoites and cysts of *Acanthamoeba* spp. being less susceptible than those of *Naegleria* spp. [158, 179]. Mogoa *et al.* demonstrated that the size of *Acanthamoeba* trophozoites exposed to 5 mg/ml chlorine decreased, that more than 90% of the cells were permeabilized and that intracellular thiol levels were increased [180]. Moreover, they found that more than 99.9% of the cells were no longer cultivable after exposure, suggesting that approximately 10% of these treated cells were in a viable (since not permeabilized) but non-cultivable state. Electron microscopy showed cell condensation, loss of pseudopodia and organelle (mitochondria, nucleus) modification [180].

Various studies on the effects of chlorine at concentrations commonly found in water distribution networks (1–5 ppm) clearly demonstrated its inefficiency against acanthamoebal cysts at those low residual doses [68, 71, 72, 179]. However those concentrations are more active against acanthamoebal trophozoites [181] and cysts of other FLA species: Chang *et al.* reported that exposure to 1–7 mg/l free chlorine for 5–30 min was cysticidal against *Naegleria* spp. [64]. Monochloramine at 0.8 mg Cl_2/l has been reported to be active (>3-log reduction) against trophozoites of two *Acanthamoeba* spp., but one of three strains displayed higher resistance with only a 1- to 2-log reduction [181]. Monochloramine at 3.9 mg/l also killed *Naegleria lovanensis* cysts within 1 h [182]. Importantly, this microbicide has also been demonstrated to induce a viable-but-non-cultivable (VBNC) state in *Legionella pneumophila* that could then be resuscitated by co-culture with *A. castellanii* [183]. High doses of chlorine used for hyperchlorination of water were demonstrated to be effective against the cysts of several FLA species: chlorine at 10 mg/l (free and combined) was reported to be effective against *Hartmannella vermiformis* cysts after 30 min of exposure [184]. Cysts of *Acanthamoeba* spp. have repeatedly been reported to resist very high doses of chlorine, with exposures to 100 mg/l for 10 min [185] or 50 mg/l for 18 h [186] being ineffective. Importantly, it has also been demonstrated that *Acanthamoeba* cysts can protect various mycobacterial species from high concentrations of chlorine [56]. Interestingly, limited activity of chlorine was also reported against the cysts and trophozoites of *Balamuthia mandrillaris*, a species phylogenetically close to *Acanthamoeba* spp. but presenting a different cell wall composition [131, 187].

Recent comparative studies have demonstrated that 25,000 ppm sodium hypochlorite was fully effective against the cysts of all *Acanthamoeba* strains after 10 min of exposure, whereas exposure at 2500 ppm for 30 min did not yield complete cyst inactivation for the most resistant strains studied [188].

Low concentrations of bromine and iodine have limited activity against cysts of *Acanthamoeba* spp. whereas they have partial cysticidal activity against *Naegleria* spp. [179, 189, 190]. A recent study demonstrated that povidone-iodine alone or in formulation inhibits the growth of *Acanthamoeba* spp. trophozoites; 50%

inhibitory concentrations varied according to the strains tested, ranging between 90 and 370 ppm for povidone-iodine alone, and between 60 and 195 ppm for the formulation [191]. In contrast, the study published by Gatti *et al.* in 1998 demonstrated that povidone-iodine has very variable activity against the trophozoites and cysts of *Acanthamoeba* spp. depending on the strains and species tested [192]. When diluted in water, a 0.031–0.062% concentration was required to inactivate the trophozoites of the most sensitive strain, whereas 2.5–5% was required for the most resistant ones. Concerning cysts, active concentrations ranged between <0.25% and >10% [192].

Stringer *et al.* compared the activities of bromine, iodine and chlorine against cysts of *Entamoeba* spp. using an excystation index [39]. They concluded that in the absence of interfering substances bromine is a superior cysticide and its action is less influenced by pH compared with iodine and chlorine. A 15 min contact time with 2 mg/l of bromine resulted in a 3-log inactivation of cysts at both pH 6 and 8. The inactivation rate was identical for the same concentration of chlorine at pH 6, but a >60 min contact time was required to achieve a 2-log reduction at pH 8. Iodine at pH 8 was ineffective, and at pH 6 more than 40 min of contact was required to achieve a 3-log reduction with 2 mg/l. Efficacy was dramatically different in the presence of sewage effluent: under those conditions only iodine at 13.7 mg/l and pH 6 was efficient whereas it was not cysticidal at pH 8; bromine and chlorine were not cysticidal at pH 6 or 8, suggesting that these actives quickly react with organic compounds, leaving only traces of reactive species insufficient to inactivate cysts [39].

Cysts of *Cryptosporidium* have been largely demonstrated to be resistant to free chlorine and monochloramine, with CT values of 800–900 [193], 7200 [194] and 9380 mg/min/l [195] for 1-, 2- and 3-log inactivation, respectively [196]. Likewise hypochlorites are non-cysticidal against *Cryptosporidium* spp. even after long exposures (>1 h) to high concentrations (>5%) [197, 198]. A recent study reported that the heat-shock protein Hsp70 is overexpressed in *Cryptosporidium* oocysts exposed to chlorine [199]. Cysts of *Giardia* spp. are less resistant to chlorine, as similarly described for other microbicides. The mouse pathogenic species *Giardia muris* has been used as a surrogate to the human pathogenic species *Giardia lamblia*. CT values of 50–71, 25–45 and 177–223 mg/min/l were required to achieve 2-log reductions of *G. muris* cysts with chlorine at pH 5, 7 or 9, respectively [200]. Cysticidal activity is decreased at lower temperatures, with 447–1014 mg/min/l required to achieve the same reduction at 5°C and pH 7 [200]. CT values of 139–182, 149–291 and 117–1495 mg/min/l were required to achieve 2-log reductions of *G. lamblia* (harvested from gerbils) with chlorine at pH 5, 7 or 9, respectively [201]. Using electron microscopy, it has been demonstrated that exposure of *G. lamblia* cysts to chlorine rapidly induced cyst wall damage, plasmalemma breakage, lysis of peripheral vacuoles, and nuclear degradation [202].

Giardia cysts and *Cryptosporidium* oocysts were exposed to 13–18 mg/l iodine for 20 min, resulting in a 3-log inactivation of *Giardia* in "clean" water at 23–25°C and pH 9 [203]. In worst-case water containing organic compounds, only 35% of the cysts were inactivated at 4°C and pH 5, with 50 min being required to achieve a 3-log reduction in these conditions. Only 10% of *Cryptosporidium* oocysts were inactivated after a 20-min exposure and 66–81% after 240 min [203]. Another study showed less than 1-log inactivation of *C. parvum* oocysts exposed at 16 mg iodine/l for 35 min; a dose of 29 mg/l for the same contact time was required to achieve a 2-log inactivation [204]. Finally, a 10% povidone-iodine-based product could not completely inactivate *Cryptosporidium* oocysts even after 10 h exposure [205]. Methyl bromide, a highly toxic fumigant could inactivate 10^6 *Cryptosporidium* oocysts after a 24 h exposure [206].

Recent studies suggest that *T. gondii* oocysts are the most resistant coccidian parasites to chlorine, with exposure of 10^4 oocysts to 100 mg/l chlorine for 24 h at 22°C and pH 7.2 failing to abolish infectivity [207]. Tincture of iodine at 2% for 10 min also failed to kill *Toxoplasma* oocysts, whereas 2% for 3 h or 7% for 10 min succeeded [17]. *Blastocystis hominis* cysts have been demonstrated to survive exposure to 2.2 ppm chlorine in sterile distilled water for 3 h [208], and *Sarcocystis neurona* oocysts treated with 5.25% sodium hypochlorite or betadine (1% iodine) for 1–6 h were still infectious [176]. Although *Balantidium coli* cysts are supposed to be resistant to chlorine [15], data to support this resistance could not be confirmed.

Concerning microsporidia, human pathogenic species have been demonstrated to be efficiently inactivated by chlorine, with CT values required for 2-log inactivation ranging from 12.8 mg/min/l at pH 6 to 68.8 mg/min/l at pH 8 [209–211]. Conversely, other species can be more resistant, with minimal concentrations of ≥100 and ≥1500 mg/l required to inactivate most spores of the fish pathogenic species *Pseudoloma neurophilia* and *Glugea anomala*, respectively [212]. It has also been reported that another fish pathogenic species *Loma salmonae* survives exposure to 150 mg iodine/l for 25 min [213].

Oxidizing agents

Widely used microbicides to be considered in this category will include chlorine dioxide, ozone, hydrogen peroxide and peracetic acid. They all release very active molecules that react with cell surfaces and potentially penetrate within cells, causing irreversible damage to and inactivation of microorganisms. Oxidizing agents are used in nearly all areas requiring microbial control, including treatment of water for drinking, antisepsis and decontamination of environmental surfaces and medical devices [153].

Chlorine dioxide is used mainly to treat drinking water and as a gas for room fumigation. It should not be taken for granted that its activity is the same as a liquid and as a gas [149]. Concentrations of about 2–3 mg/l of water were effective against the trophozoites of *Acanthamoeba* and *Naegleria* with a contact time of 30 min [158]. Lower concentrations (0.4 mg/l) demonstrated decreased efficacy against the trophozoites of *Acanthamoeba* spp., with only 0.5 to 1.5-log reductions achieved for two of three strains and a >3-log reduction observed for the third strain only

[181]. Good activity has also been reported against *Naegleria gruberi* cysts, with a 5.5 mg/min/l CT required to obtain a 99% inactivation [214]. The same active had only limited effect on *Acanthamoeba polyphaga* cysts exposed to 5 mg/l for 60 min [215], and continuous injection in water pipes at 0.5 mg/l did not completely inactivate FLAs [68]. Chlorine dioxide is generally considered more active than chlorine against the oocysts of *Cryptosporidium* [196]; however, exposure of *Cryptosporidium* oocysts to 0.4 mg/l chlorine dioxide for 30 min failed to abolish infectivity [216]. Similarly, exposure at 1.3 mg/l chlorine dioxide for 1 h yielded only a 1-log inactivation [194]. Chauret *et al.* reported that CT values of 75, 550 and 1000 mg min/l (i.e. theoretical exposures at concentrations of 1.5, 9.1 and 16.7 mg/l for 1 h) were required to achieve approximately a 2-log of inactivation with *Cryptosporidium* oocysts from different sources [217]. These values vary depending on temperature, with decreased efficacy at low temperatures [218]. Interestingly, inactivation of *Cryptosporidium* oocysts was not improved when using sequential treatments with chlorine dioxide followed by free chlorine or monochloramine, suggesting that these actives target similar chemical groups in the oocyst wall [219]. Chlorine dioxide at high concentration has been demonstrated to be active against the spores of *Nosema bombycis*, a microsporidian infecting silkworms [220]. Exposure at 15 mg/l resulted in complete inactivation of their spores within 30 min; exposed spores displayed loss of lipids from the outer shell and a decrease in adenosine triphospatase (ATPase) levels, followed by the spores losing large amounts of proteins, DNA, polysaccharide and ions [220]. The viability (measured by cell infectivity assay) of *Cryptosporidium* and *Encephalitozoon intestinalis* exposed to 4.1 mg/l of chlorine dioxide gas for 20 min was reduced by 2.6–3.3-log and 3.6–4.6-log, respectively. Intriguingly, the same treatment had no effect on the excystation rate of *Cyclospora* [221].

Ozone, another potent oxidizer, is used primarily in the treatment of a limited volume of circulating water; ozone decay rates are strongly influenced by organic matter in water [222] and it has only very low (if any) residual activity. Furthermore, its activity is dramatically reduced at low temperatures. It has been demonstrated that continuous exposure to 0.4–0.5 mg/l ozone in such applications rapidly inactivated cysts of all *Naegleria* and most *Acanthamoeba* (with the exception of *A. polyphaga* CCAP 1501/3a) strains tested [223, 224]. Activity of ozone against the cysts of *A. polyphaga* has been confirmed by others; however, such a treatment did not completely kill the cysts after a 2 h exposure [215]. Field investigations demonstrated that ozone considerably decreases numbers of FLA cysts entering a drinking water plant [66], but lack of residual activity allows regrowth of amoebae in treated water [68, 225]. In a comparative study by Wickramanayake *et al.*, *N. gruberi* cysts proved more resistant than those of *Giardia muris*, with, respectively, 7.5 and 1.05 min required for a 99% reduction in viability with 0.2 mg/l of ozone at 25°C and pH 7; excystation rate was used to measure *G. muris* cyst inactivation [223]. Another study evaluated residual infectivity of cysts after ozonation and demonstrated that *Giardia lamblia* and its surrogate *G. muris* presented similar susceptibilities to ozone, with a 1.25 mg/l ozone concentration recommended to inactivate more than 3-log of cysts for both the species [226]. Scanning electron microscopy demonstrated that exposure of *Giardia* cysts to an initial dose of 1.5 mg/l ozone in water rapidly leads to degradation of essential proteins and also structural modifications of the cyst wall, resulting in complete abolition of infectivity within 1 min [202, 227]. *C. parvum* oocysts were demonstrated to be 30 times more resistant to ozone than *Giardia* cysts, with more than 90% inactivation (as measured by infectivity) achieved by treating oocysts with 1 mg/l of ozone for 5 min [194, 196].

A synergistic effect was observed when using ozone followed by monochloramine or chlorine, suggesting that these actives have separate targets on the cyst wall [228, 229]. Interestingly, *Toxoplasma* oocysts seem very resistant to ozone since exposure of 10^4 oocysts to 6 mg/l ozone for 12 min failed to abolish infectivity [207]. This was confirmed in further studies [230] and raises interesting questions about relations between cell wall structures and observed differences between the levels of resistance to such treatments. Treatment of *Eimeria colchici* oocysts with ozone was observed to partially inhibit the growth and infectivity of the oocysts [231], and a good efficacy was observed against spores of *E. intestinalis* [209]. In a study comparing the activity of ozone against field isolates representing various protozoa species, Khalifa *et al.* demonstrated that infectivity of *Giardia*, *Cryptosporidia* and *Microsporidium* was completely abolished after overnight exposure to water previously treated with 1 mg/l ozone for 9 min, while the infectivity of *Cyclospora* and *Blastocystis* was markedly (but not completely) reduced [232]. This study has important limitations (different initial numbers of spores, cysts and oocysts exposed to treatments), but to our knowledge this is the only study in which an attempt was made to compare the microbicidal effects of ozone against a number of different protozoan species. Humidified ozone is also used as an area fumigant and in sterilization processes, but investigations of such processes against protozoa in vegetative or dormant forms have not been published to date.

Hydrogen peroxide formulations are commonly used for the disinfection of contact lenses. As a consequence, the trophocidal and cysticidal activity of liquid hydrogen peroxide against *Acanthamoeba* spp. has been well studied [156, 161, 168, 169, 172, 233, 234]. Activity has been reported to depend upon the type of formulation and contact time [233], with two studies reporting commercial products containing 3% hydrogen peroxide to be ineffective against *Acanthamoeba* spp. within the 30 min contact time recommended by manufacturers [160, 235]. Longer contact times are generally required and other 3% hydrogen peroxide-based formulations were effective after a 6–24 h contact (depending on solution and *Acanthamoeba* species tested) [151]. Peroxide is also used as an environmental surface disinfectant, in direct liquid dilution and in formulation, which can also vary in activity. One report recently demonstrated that short exposures to 7.5% hydrogen peroxide had only limited activity against cysts of various *Acanthamoeba* isolates, with the most resistant strains

presenting a less than 1-log reduction after a 30 min exposure [188]. Conversely, a 2% hydrogen peroxide-based formulation (RESERT XL) had very good activity after only a 10 min exposure at room temperature, again demonstrating the critical impact of formulation on microbicidal activity [188]. It has been reported that the cysticidal activity of 3% hydrogen peroxide is enhanced by the addition of potassium iodide and various peroxidases [236]. Similarly, a recent study reported that treatment of *A. polyphaga* cysts with hydrogen peroxide 0.4% or acidified nitrite 2 mg/ml for 6 h is poorly cysticidal (≤1-log reduction) whereas a combination of both actives yielded a 4-log reduction after 1 h [237].

Hydrogen peroxide as a gas has been demonstrated to be effective against *A. polyphaga* and *A. castellanii* cysts [238]. Hydrogen peroxide has also been reported to efficiently inactivate *Cryptosporidium* oocysts after exposures at 3–7.5% for relatively short times of 10–30 min [175, 198], or at lower concentrations (0.025–0.03% in various fruit juices) for longer times (2–6 h at 4°C) [239, 240]. Hydrogen peroxide combined with plasma has been demonstrated to be efficient against *Cryptosporidium* cysts [175, 241]. Spores of *Encephalitozoon intestinalis* were demonstrated to be completely inactivated (>5-log reduction) after exposure to 0.5% hydrogen peroxide for 1 min [177]; spores of *Encephalitozoon cuniculi* were also completely inactivated after exposure to 1% hydrogen peroxide for 30 min (shorter times were not tested), suggesting that microsporidia are efficiently inactivated by this active [95]. Conversely, cysts of *Sarcocystis gigantea* were apparently unaffected after exposure to 3% hydrogen peroxide for 48 h [35].

Peracetic acid (PAA) is very active and presents rapid microbicidal activity against various microorganisms at low concentrations [153]. Unformulated PAA was demonstrated to be effective against *Acanthamoeba* and *Naegleria* trophozoites after exposure to 15 mg/l for 2 h, but activity against *Acanthamoeba* cysts required longer incubation (18 h) and higher concentration (150 mg/l). A commercial PAA-based product used at room temperature killed all the trophozoites of *A. polyphaga* within 30 min, but failed to completely inactivate the cysts within 24 h [242]. Other FLA species seem more susceptible to inactivation by PAA, and cysticidal activity against *Naegleria lovanensis* was observed after exposure to 5.3 mg/l for 1 h [182]. PAA alone at 0.2% has relatively good activity against the cysts of most *Acanthamoeba* after a 10 min exposure, with the exception of several strains presenting high resistance [188]. However, even these strains were successfully inactivated using a 0.2% PAA formulation for a 10 min exposure at 55°C (whereas exposure at 55°C without any active yielded <1-log reduction) [188]. PAA also presents good activity against the cysts of *Giardia* [243]. Activity of PAA-based formulations against *Cryptosporidium* oocysts has been reported as moderate (0.2% PAA, cell infectivity assay) to high (0.35% PAA, excystation assay) and depends upon the temperature used for exposures [175, 244]. A formulation containing 25% hydrogen peroxide plus 5% PAA used at 10% in distilled water led to complete loss of infectivity of *Cryptosporidium* oocysts exposed for 10 min

[245]. *T. gondii* oocysts were not killed after exposure to 5% PAA for 24 h; however, they were fully inactivated after a 48 h exposure [246], as were the spores of *E. intestinalis* after 5–15 min exposure to a PAA-based formulation [177].

Aldehydes

Three aldehydes are commonly used as disinfectants and/or sterilants: glutaraldehyde, *ortho*-phthalaldehyde (OPA) and formaldehyde (or formalin, containing formaldehyde in solution) [153]. From bacterial studies, these microbicides act by cross-linking with proteins and inhibiting synthesis of DNA, RNA and other macromolecules. Due to differences in its structure, OPA is thought to have better bacterial penetration than glutaraldehyde and consequently better mycobactericidal activity, but lower activity against bacterial endospores [153].

Only a few studies have tested aldehydes against FLAs. A commercial formulation of 2% glutaraldehyde showed poor activity against the trophozoites of *A. polyphaga* after an exposure of 30 min to 3 h [242]. Similarly, 2% glutaraldehyde alone or in formulation was not effective against the cysts of most *Acanthamoeba* tested after 10–30 min exposures [188]. A more intriguing result was that trophozoites of most tested isolates also resisted this concentration for 30 min, this concentration being even less effective than against the cysts [188]. A possible explanation for this difference is that glutaraldehyde acts on cysts by cross-linking cyst wall structures and impairing excystation, without necessarily killing encysted amoebae. The corresponding trophozoites are less affected, possibly due to a different cell wall structure or an active glutaraldehyde detoxification pathway. Tiewchaloren *et al.* demonstrated that trophozoites of *Naegleria fowleri* survived exposure to formaldehyde at 0.05% for 60 min at 37°C, whereas they were completely inactivated after exposure to formaldehyde at 0.1% under the same test conditions [247]. In the work by Aksozek and colleagues, 10% formalin (as a preservative liquid) was reported to be cysticidal within 30 min against *A. castellanii* [234].

A commercial formulation containing 2.5% activated glutaraldehyde could completely inactivate 10^4 *Cryptosporidium* oocysts with a 10 h exposure, whereas survivors were still observed when 0^5 or 10^6 oocysts were tested under the same conditions [205]. A commercial product containing a mixture of formaldehyde and glutaraldehyde did not succeed in inactivating *Cryptosporidium* oocysts after a 2 h exposure [248]. Formaldehyde as a gas also demonstrated limited activity [206]. Importantly, activity of aldehydes is lower in the presence of added organic matter [249]; this could be due to the cross-linking of such organics potentially creating a protective matrix around the microbial target.

Sporocysts of *Sarcocystis neurona* were not inactivated by 10% formalin [176], nor were sporocysts of *Sarcocystis gigantea* [35]. This same active was not active against *Toxoplasma* oocysts when used at the same concentration for 48 h; however, it became fully active after a 48 h exposure [246]. Formalin at 10% was fully active against the spores of *Encephalitozoon cuniculi* within 10 min [250], as was 1% or 0.3% formaldehyde within 30 min [95].

Alcohols

Alcohols are compounds with a hydroxyl group attached to a saturated carbon atom. Ethanol, isopropanol and *n*-propanol are common antiseptics and disinfectants. A major part of their activity is achieved by forming hydrogen bonds with proteins, leading to loss of structure and function and coagulation [153]. As shown in studies with bacteria, the microbicidal activity of alcohols is generally better at levels of 60–70%; higher concentrations may be less efficient due to the coagulation of proteins on the outside of the cell wall, thus preventing further penetration of the microbicide into the cell [153].

Products with 20% isopropyl alcohol showed good activity against the cysts of *Acanthamoeba castellanii* and *Acanthamoeba culbertsoni* after an exposure of hours [154, 234]. Another study noted good activity of 70% ethanol used for only 10 min against the cysts of various *Acanthamoeba* spp. [188]. Whether encysted amoebae are truly killed or if ethanol impairs excystation by fixing ectocyst structures remains to be determined. The same exposure conditions with the same active were ineffective against *Cryptosporidium* oocysts [175], as were exposures to 37% methanol and 70% isopropanol for 33 min [198]. Exposure to 70% ethanol for 48 h was not effective in inactivating *Toxoplasma* oocysts, nor was exposure to 99% ethanol for 12 h, methanol for 6 h, or *n*-butyl or isoamyl alcohols for 48 h [246]. Exposures to 99% ethanol or 95% ethanol + 5% PAA for 24 h, or to methanol for 12 h, completely inactivated *Toxoplasma* oocysts, whereas exposure to *n*-propyl alcohol for 48 h resulted in partial loss of infectivity [246]. Ethanol and methanol at 10% in water were not effective against the sporocysts of *Sarcocystis gigantea* after a 48 h exposure, whereas they presented good activity at 90% concentration [35]. Isopropyl alcohol at 90% in water presented limited activity even after 48 h of exposure [35]. Exposure of *Encephalitozoon cuniculi* spores to 70% ethanol for 30 s rendered them non-infectious [251]. Full activity was also observed for *Encephalitozoon intestinalis* spores exposed to 70% ethanol for 5 min [178].

Various microbicides

Other categories of chemicals have been tested against a variety of protozoa. Ammonia is relatively efficient against cysts and oocysts but might require long exposures and/or high concentrations. For example, an exposure of longer than 8 days at 24°C to a 0.1% solution of ammonia wasneeded to achieve a >5-log reduction in the viability of *Cryptosporidium* oocysts [252], a 48 h exposure to a 10% solution to inactivate *S. gigantea* sporocysts [35], a 1 h exposure to a 29.5% solution to kill *S. neurona* sporocysts [176], and a 30 min exposure to a 5% solution to inactivate *T. gondii* oocysts [246].

Isothiazolones consist of a range of microbicides extensively used in the water industry. As a consequence, their cysticidal activity, as well as their activity against intracellular bacterial pathogens, has been investigated. Cysts of environmental isolates of *Acanthamoeba hatchetti* and *Cochliopodium bilimbosum* were shown to be resistant to an isothiazolin derivative (5-chloro-2-

methyl-4-isothiazolin-3-one) used according to the manufacturer's recommendations for the disinfection of cooling tower waters [253, 254] and were shown to reproduce faster at a low concentration of the microbicide [254]. Diamidines have been shown to be trophocidal against FLAs but they are not cysticidal [165, 255–258]. Although propamidine is poorly cysticidal, other homologous microbicides, such as hexamidine and octamidine, appeared to have greater activity [257]. Ethylene oxide gas applied with a concentration of 450–500 mg/l at 55–60°C was fully active against *Cryptosporidium* oocysts [175], as was a mixture of 88% Freon and 12% ethylene oxide gas applied for 5 h at 54.4°C and 30% humidity against cysts of *A. polyphaga* and *A. castellanii* [259].

Physical microbicides

High temperatures

Protozoa are readily killed at the temperatures (>100°C) and contact times (>15 min) routinely used in heat-based disinfection and sterilization procedures to decontaminate medical devices, for example [259]. Lower temperatures have variable effects depending on the species tested.

Raising the temperature from 9 to 55°C over 15–20 min abolished the infectivity of *Cryptosporidium* oocysts in calf feces, cecal contents and ileal scrapings; inocula held at 45°C for 5–20 min also lost their infectivity [260]. *Giardia* cysts were rapidly inactivated when held at 56°C [146], as were *T. gondii* oocysts exposed to 55°C for 2 min or 60°C for 1 min [25]. Turner *et al.* [159] observed that trophozoites of *A. castellanii* were inactivated following a 30 min exposure at 46°C, while a temperature of 56°C was necessary to inactivate the same number of the cysts. Aksozek *et al.* [234] reported that a temperature of 65°C for more than 5 min was cysticidal for *A. castellanii*, while Ludwig *et al.* [235] reported that cysts of *A. castellanii* and *A. polyphaga* were inactivated only after exposure to moist heat for 10 min at 80°C. The same exposure conditions did not completely inactivate thermotolerant *Acanthamoeba* spp. cysts in other studies [185]. *Balamuthia mandrillaris* trophozoites may be more resistant to heat since a temperature of 60°C was not trophocidal within 60 min; however, a temperature of 80°C maintained for at least 60 min did inactivate the cysts [187]. *Naegleria* spp. are generally considered more sensitive to heat [64, 76]. *Entamoeba histolytica* cysts were found to have thermal death times at 65 and 100°C of 5 min and 10 s in water, respectively [261]. *Sarcocystis neurona* oocysts were still infective to mice when heated at 50°C for 60 min or 55°C for 5 min; heating at 55°C for 15 min and 60°C for 1 min rendered them non-infective [176]. Other studies reported that pork meat containing sarcocysts of *Sarcocystis miescheriana*, and possibly of *Sarcocystis suihominis*, require cooking at a minimum of 70°C for 15 min for complete inactivation [262].

Ultraviolet radiation

As for other organisms, UV radiation induces thymine dimers potentially inhibiting normal replication and transcription in the DNA of *Cryptosporidium* [263]. At given doses, these lesions

cannot be completely repaired by the parasite despite the presence of UV repair genes in its genome [264], and UV has consequently been described to be very efficient at inactivating *Cryptosporidium* oocysts. When exposed to medium-pressure doses of 60 mJ/cm^2 or higher, *C. parvum* did not exhibit resistance to and/or reactivation following treatment [265]. Interestingly, it was also confirmed that *C. parvum* did not repair UV damage [266] and Craik *et al.* measured oocyst inactivation ranging from 3.4-log to >4.9-log depending on different preparations of protozoal cultures [267]. They reported that the water type and temperature, the concentration of oocysts in the suspension, and the UV radiation level did not have a significant impact on oocyst inactivation.

Similar results on the activity of UV were observed with cysts of *Giardia muris* and *Giardia lamblia* [265, 268, 269]. However, it has also been reported that different strains of the same *Giardia* species can present different levels of susceptibility to UV [270], and *Giardia* spp. may have the ability to repair DNA damage induced by low- or medium-pressure UV rays [265, 271]. These findings could have a significant impact, with UV doses demonstrated to be effective in the literature being less efficient in complex processes such as treatment of wastewater effluents [272].

The solar disinfection ("SODIS") technique consists of storing contaminated drinking water in transparent plastic containers that are placed in direct sunlight for up to 8 h before consumption. It has been demonstrated to be efficient against the oocysts of *C. parvum* and the cysts of *G. muris* [273]. The non-toxic photocatalyst TiO$_2$ can be coated on plastic containers to enhance and accelerate the inactivation rate [274]. The technique is also efficient against the cysts of *Entamoeba histolytica* and *Entamoeba dispar* [275], even if these parasites possess genes encoding DNA-repair proteins that are upregulated after short exposures to UV [276].

While UV radiation is frequently used for water disinfection, its activity against FLAs has not been as widely reported as that for other protozoa such as *C. parvum*. Hijnen *et al.* have provided a comprehensive overview of the ability of UV radiation to inactivate cysts and reported that *Acanthamoeba* spp. are highly UV resistant [277]. UV exposure has good activity against trophozoites [278], but cysts are much more resistant. For example, *Acanthamoeba* spp. cysts were demonstrated to be resistant to exposure to UVC at 253.7 nm, 1.1 mJ/s/cm^2 [279]; *A. castellanii* cysts were shown to be resistant to UVB irradiation (800 mJ/cm^2) and *Balamuthia mandrillaris* cysts to exposure at 200 mJ/cm^2 UV irradiation [187]. Other studies reported a 4-log$_{10}$ reduction in the viability of *A. polyphaga* cysts after exposure to 40 mJ/cm^2 [280], suggesting there might be some differences between the sensitivity of different strains and species.

SODIS and solar photocatalytic (TiO$_2$) disinfection methods were demonstrated to be effective against the trophozoites of *A. polyphaga* but the cysts were unaffected [281]. A further study confirmed that exposure of *A. polyphaga* cysts to simulated solar irradiation in water (85 mJ/s^1/cm^2) does not achieve cyst inactivation when the temperature is kept below 40°C but gives better results at 45°C (1.2-log reduction after 6 h), 50°C (>3.6-log reduction after 6 h) and 55°C (>3.3-log reduction after 4 h) [282]. Sixty-one percent of *Naegleria gruberi* cysts were still alive after UV irradiation with 21.6 mJ/cm^2, and treating amoebae with inhibitors of DNA repair mechanisms improved UV irradiation efficacy [283]. Photosensitized inactivation of *Acanthamoeba palestinensis* in the cystic stage has also been demonstrated by incubating cysts with tetracationic Zn(II) phthalocyanine before exposure to 600–700 nm wavelength light sources [284].

Inactivation of *T. gondii* oocysts occurred with exposure to pulsed and continuous UV radiation, as evidenced by mouse bioassay; however, some oocysts retained their viability even at doses of >500 mJ/cm^2 [18]. Other authors reported a 4-log reduction of infectivity both by mouse bioassay and cell culture assay at 40 mJ/cm^2 [230]. When exposed to 254 nm UV, spores of *Encephalitozoon intestinalis*, *Encephalitozoon cuniculi* and *Encephalitozoon hellem* exhibited 3.2-log reductions in viability at UV fluences of 60, 140 and 190 mJ/cm^2 [285]. Good activity of UV against the spores of *E. intestinalis* has also been reported in other studies [286, 287]. Sporocysts of *Sarcocystis gigantea* were inactivated after an exposure to 240 mJ/cm^2 [35].

Gamma radiation

Gamma radiation can be used for a variety of disinfection and sterilization processes in a wide range of applications (food and beverages, pharmaceuticals, medical devices, etc.). They are high-energy sources, being highly penetrating and rapidly biocidal [153].

The effect of γ-radiation on *Cryptosporidium* and others coccidian species has been described in several studies. Interestingly, it was reported in some cases that irradiated oocysts could still infect cells or animals but sporozoites lose their capacity to reproduce, thus resulting in the absence of propagation in infected organisms. This was the case in the study by Kato *et al.*, with oocysts that received 2 kGy irradiation excysting at the same rates as non-irradiated oocysts, infecting cells but unable to replicate [288]. Another study reported that higher doses of radiation are required for oocyst inactivation, with oocysts irradiated with less than 10 kGy inducing infections in mice [289]. Recent studies suggest that higher infectivity of irradiated oocysts in the mouse model could be due to DNA repair [290]. *Giardia lamblia* cysts might be less resistant than *Cryptosporidium* oocysts to γ-radiation, with cysts that received doses of radiation ranging from 0.25 to 2 kGy with a recovery period of 6 h or less being unable to infect gerbils. DNA repair was evidenced with cysts that were irradiated at 0.25 kGy and allowed to recover at room temperature for 24 h or longer, being infective [291]. *Eimeria acervulina* is used as a surrogate for *Cyclospora cayetanensis* decontamination studies; γ-irradiation of *E. acervulina* sporulated oocysts at a dose of 0.5 kGy was partially effective in abolishing infectivity, but was completely effective at 1.0 kGy and higher [292]. Oocysts of various *T. gondii* strains were rendered non-viable at 0.4 kGy, with no effect of temperature during irradiation [293]. As described

for *Cryptosporidium*, a further study by the same authors demonstrated that unsporulated oocysts irradiated at 0.4–0.8 kGy sporulated but were not infective to mice. Sporulated oocysts irradiated at 0.4 kGy were able to excyst, and sporozoites were infective but not capable of inducing a viable infection in mice [294]. As for *Eimeria* spp., it has been suggested that irradiated *Toxoplasma* oocysts can be used as a vaccination tool to elicit cellular immunity against the parasite [295, 296]. *A. castellanii* cysts were resistant to 2.5 kGy of γ-irradiation [234], and *Naegleria gruberi* cysts have been demonstrated to resist X-ray irradiation with a dose of 17.4 kGy [283], suggesting that some if not all FLAs have very efficient DNA repair mechanisms. Li *et al.* observed inactivation of the spores of microsporidia by g-irradiation: they reported complete inactivation of *Encephalitozoon cuniculi* and *E. intestinalis* after exposure to 1.5 and 2.0 kGy, respectively; *E. hellem* was significantly inactivated after exposure to 3.0 kGy but complete inhibition was not obtained [297].

High pressures

High hydrostatic pressure (HHP) is used mainly in the food industry for the processing of fresh food products potentially contaminated with various microorganisms. HHP has been demonstrated to be effective against *C. parvum* oocysts, with more than a 4-log reduction in oocysts exposed to 5.5×10^8 Pa for 60 s [298]. Exposure of oyster tissue contaminated with 2.10^7 oocysts to 5.5×10^8 Pa for 180 s produced a 93.3% decrease in the numbers of mouse pups developing *C. parvum* infection after feeding the processed samples [299]. Exposure at 5.5×10^8 Pa for 120 s at 40°C abolished the infectivity of 10^6 *Eimeria acervulina* oocysts when tested in chickens [300], whereas exposure at 5.5×10^8 Pa for 120 s at a lower temperature dramatically reduced the infectivity [301]. Several studies by Lindsay *et al.* reported the effects of HHP against *T. gondii* oocysts: they observed that a minimum pressure of 3 to 4×10^8 Pa during 30–90 s was generally required to inactivate oocysts contaminating various matrices (ground pork, raspberries, etc.) [302–304]. The spores of *E. cuniculi* were inactivated after an exposure to 3.45×10^8 Pa for 1 min [305].

Other treatments

A number of other physical treatments have been reported in the literature, some of which are further described. Microwaves have been used against *C. parvum* and *Cyclospora cayetanensis* oocysts, displaying various levels of activity depending on temperature reached during the treatment [306]; the major activity appears to be due directly to the effects of heat. Trophozoites as well as cysts of several *Acanthamoeba* strains were effectively killed by only 3 min of microwave irradiation [307]. Pulsed electric fields have been used against *Naegleria lovaniensis* trophozoites [308]; however, this is not a particularly challenging organism when compared with other protozoa. Cryotherapy (repeated quick freezing to around −100°C) has been used to treat the cysts of *Acanthamoeba* spp. *in vitro* and in clinical settings but was not fully effective [309, 310]. Repeated freeze–thawing cycles were also demonstrated to have limited cysticidal activity against

Table 8.2 Relative sensitivity of protozoa to microbicides.v[a]

Species	Cationic microbicides	Halogen compounds			Oxidizing agents				Aldehydes			Alcohols			Ammonia	Physical treatments			
		Cl₂	Br₂	I₂	ClO₂	O₃	H₂O₂	PAA	Formal.	Gluta.	OPA	Ethanol	Isoprop.	Methanol		Heat	UV	Gamma	Pressure
Cryptosporidium spp.	M	H		H	H	M	L	M	M	H	M	H	H	H	M	L	L	M	L
Cyclospora cayetanensis						M^b												L to M^b	L^b
Sarcocystis spp.	H	H			H		H	H	H			M	H	M	H	L to M	M		
Toxoplasma gondii		H		M	H	H	H	H	H			H				L	M to H	L	
Acanthamoeba spp.	M	H		H	H	M	M	M	M	H	M	L	L		M	M	M to H	M	L
Balamuthia mandrillaris		H														M	H		
Entamoeba histolytica		M	L	M												L to M	L		
Giardia lamblia	L	M		M		L		L								L	L to M		
Naegleria spp	M	M				L		L								L	M		
Blastocystis hominis	M	M				M													
Microsporidia	L	L to H			L to M	L	L	L	L			L				L	L	L to M	L

Resistance: H, high resistance; M, moderate resistance; L, low resistance. Treatments: Cl₂, chlorine; Br₂, bromine; I₂, iodine; ClO₂, chlorine dioxide; O₃, ozone; H₂O₂, hydrogen peroxide; PAA, peracetic acid; Formal., formaldehyde; Gluta., glutaraldehyde; OPA, *ortho*-phtalaldehyde; Isoprop., isopropanol; UV, ultraviolet irradiation; Gamma, γ-irradiation. Heat treatments evaluated mostly consisted of moist heat.

[a] These estimations are mainly based on research papers cited in this chapter and are given as an illustration of results described in these reports. It should be kept in mind that sensitivity to microbicides can vary according to species/strains tested, the test methods and the microbicide application method (formulation, pH, temperature etc); these estimations should consequently not be taken for universally granted.

[b] The surrogate species *Eimeria acervulina* was used in these tests.

Balamuthia mandrillaris (five cycles from −80° to 37°C) [187] and against *A. castellanii* (five cycles from −160 to 45°C) [234].

Conclusions

As highlighted in this chapter, dormant forms of protozoa (including microsporidia) are a particularly difficult challenge for chemical and physical microbicidal processes. These microorganisms present unique cell wall structures that contribute to the observed resistance to treatments, not unlike bacterial and fungal spores in many cases. These structures are still not completely elucidated; they vary from one organism to another (and likely from one strain to another) and might explain the dramatic differences observed in the activity of the treatments (e.g. high resistance of *T. gondii* oocysts to ozone) (Table 8.2). Furthermore, little is known about any intracellular mechanisms allowing protection or repair of any damage induced by microbicides. In some cases, the vegetative (trophozoites) forms of these organisms have also been described as having surprising resistance profiles to widely used microbicides such as glutaraldehyde. The lack of approved standards to test the activity of microbicides against these organisms, and particularly those that can be difficult to grow in the laboratory, is a problem that needs to be addressed. An important point to consider is the transposition of the results of lab-based evaluations to real-life situations where the conditions encountered, and also the variations in the applications of the products and processes, could readily compromise the microbicidal action.

Protozoa have been described to interact with other individual microbial species or even microbial consortia that could limit the action of microbicides. For example, it has been demonstrated that protozoan oocysts (*C. parvum*) and cysts (*Giardia lamblia*) can be captured within single-species (*Pseudomonas aeruginosa*) and multispecies biofilms [311, 312] and that seasonal variations in the composition of the complex biofilms in particular can influence the attachment and detachment dynamics of *C. parvum* oocysts [313]. It is well known that biofilms can protect microorganisms from the action of microbicides and this phenomena may need to be taken into account when testing certain applications [314]. It has also been reported that oocysts of *C. parvum* are predated by other protozoa (*Acanthamoeba* spp.) and rotifers, and that these organisms could thus act as protective carriers of *Cryptosporidium* oocysts [315, 316]. Predation by *Acanthamoeba* spp. has also been reported for *T. gondii* oocysts [317], and microorganisms resembling microsporidia were detected in amoebae that belong to the *Vannella* genus [318, 319]. The fate of amoebae within bacterial biofilms has not been investigated in detail and it is consequently not known if they can embed deep into the biofilms or if they only graze upon bacteria exposed at the surface of biofilms. Recent reports suggest that in addition to drinking water networks, amoebae can also colonize medical devices such as urinary catheters [53], thus possibly bringing potential pathogenic species closer to vulnerable individuals. The demonstrated association of amoebae with non-tuberculous mycobacteria is also a major concern, especially knowing that these often naturally occurring microbicide-resistant bacteria survive within microbicide-resistant cysts [320].

Protozoa are generally not considered during the development of disinfection and sterilization processes, despite their ubiquitous nature and the pathogenic potential of many species. Thus much work is still needed to increase our understanding of these microorganisms for developing better and safer means of preventing and controlling their environmental spread. The ecology of protozoa in water systems and the impact of microbicides have to be approached from a global perspective. This is suggested to include studies investigating the interaction of physical and chemical microbicides with dormant and active forms of protozoa and the mechanisms of resistance to disinfection, as well as the survival of protozoa in complex microbial biofilms. Finally, the standardization of cyst and oocyst production and the methods for testing the activity of microbicides against protozoa are required to generate meaningful and reproducible data.

References

1 Stark, D. *et al.* (2009) Clinical significance of enteric protozoa in the immuno-suppressed human population. *Clinical Microbiology Reviews*, **22**, 634–650.

2 Karanis, P. *et al.* (2007) Waterborne transmission of protozoan parasites: a worldwide review of outbreaks and lessons learnt. *Journal of Water and Health*, **5**, 1–38.

3 Bouzid, M. *et al.* (2008) Detection and surveillance of waterborne protozoan parasites. *Current Opinion in Biotechnology*, **19**, 302–306.

4 Lane, S. and Lloyd, D. (2002) Current trends in research into the waterborne parasite *Giardia*. *Critical Reviews in Microbiology*, **28**, 123–147.

5 Rose, J.B. *et al.* (2002) Risk and control of waterborne cryptosporidiosis. *FEMS Microbiology Reviews*, **26**, 113–123.

6 Mosier, D.A. and Oberst, R.D. (2000) Cryptosporidiosis. A global challenge. *Annals of the New York Academy of Sciences*, **916**, 102–111.

7 Rose, J.B. (1997) Environmental ecology of *Cryptosporidium* and public health implications. *Annual Review of Public Health*, **18**, 135–161.

8 Corso, P.S. *et al.* (2003) Cost of illness in the 1993 waterborne *Cryptosporidium* outbreak, Milwaukee, Wisconsin. *Emerging Infectious Diseases*, **9**, 426–431.

9 Mac Kenzie, W.R. *et al.* (1994) A massive outbreak in Milwaukee of Cryptosporidium infection transmitted through the public water supply. *New England Journal of Medicine*, **331**, 161–167.

10 Medema, G. *et al.* (2009) *Risk Assessment of Cryptosporidium in Drinking Water*, vol. WHO/HSE/WSH/09.04, World Health Organization, Geneva.

11 Leander, B.S. (2008) Marine gregarines: evolutionary prelude to the apicomplexan radiation? *Trends in Parasitology*, **24**, 60–67.

12 Karanis, P. (2006) A review of an emerging waterborne medical important parasitic protozoan. *Japanese Journal Protozoology*, **39**, 5–19.

13 Schuster, F.L. and Visvesvara, G.S. (2004) Free-living amoebae as opportunistic and non-opportunistic pathogens of humans and animals. *International Journal for Parasitology*, **34**, 1001–1027.

14 Schuster, F.L. and Visvesvara, G.S. (2004) Amebae and ciliated protozoa as causal agents of waterborne zoonotic disease. *Veterinary Parasitology*, **126**, 91–120.

15 Schuster, F.L. and Ramirez-Avila, L. (2008) Current world status of *Balantidium coli*. *Clinical Microbiology Reviews*, **21**, 626–638.

16 Smith, H.V. and Rose, J.B. (1998) Waterborne cryptosporidiosis: current status. *Parasitology Today*, **14**, 14–22.

17 Jones, J.L. and Dubey, J.P. (2010) Waterborne toxoplasmosis – recent developments. *Experimental Parasitology*, **124**, 10–25.

18 Wainwright, K.E. *et al.* (2007) Physical inactivation of *Toxoplasma gondii* oocysts in water. *Applied and Environmental Microbiology*, **73**, 5663–5666.

19 Okhuysen, P.C. *et al.* (1999) Virulence of three distinct *Cryptosporidium parvum* isolates for healthy adults. *Journal of Infectious Diseases*, **180**, 1275–1281.

20 Hoff, J.C. 3rd. *et al.* (1985) Comparison of animal infectivity and excystation as measures of *Giardia muris* cyst inactivation by chlorine. *Applied and Environmental Microbiology*, **50**, 1115–1117.

21 Schaefer, F.W. *et al.* (1991) Determination of *Giardia lamblia* cyst infective dose for the Mongolian gerbil (*Meriones unguiculatus*). *Applied and Environmental Microbiology*, **57**, 2408–2409.

22 Worliczek, H.L. *et al.* (2009) Age, not infection dose, determines the outcome of *Isospora suis* infections in suckling piglets. *Parasitology Research*, **105** (Suppl. 1), S157–S162.

23 Yoshikawa, H. *et al.* (2004) Fecal–oral transmission of the cyst form of *Blastocystis hominis* in rats. *Parasitology Research*, **94**, 391–396.

24 deRegnier, D.P. *et al.* (1989) Viability of *Giardia* cysts suspended in lake, river, and tap water. *Applied and Environmental Microbiology*, **55**, 1223–1229.

25 Dubey, J.P. (1998) *Toxoplasma gondii* oocyst survival under defined temperatures. *Journal of Parasitology*, **84**, 862–865.

26 Elsheikha, H.M. *et al.* (2004) Viability of *Sarcocystis neurona* sporocysts after long-term storage. *Veterinary Parasitology*, **123**, 257–264.

27 Jenkins, M. *et al.* (2003) Comparison of tests for viable and infectious *Cryptosporidium parvum* oocysts. *Parasitology Research*, **89**, 1–5.

28 Mons, C. *et al.* (2009) Monitoring of *Cryptosporidium* and *Giardia* river contamination in Paris area. *Water Research*, **43**, 211–217.

29 Fayer, R. *et al.* (2004) Zoonotic protozoa: from land to sea. *Trends in Parasitology*, **20**, 531–536.

30 Huang, P. *et al.* (1995) The first reported outbreak of diarrheal illness associated with *Cyclospora* in the United States. *Annals of Internal Medicine*, **123**, 409–414.

31 Bowie, W.R. *et al.* (1997) Outbreak of toxoplasmosis associated with municipal drinking water. The BC Toxoplasma Investigation Team. *Lancet*, **350**, 173–177.

32 Leelayoova, S. *et al.* (2004) Evidence of waterborne transmission of *Blastocystis hominis*. *American Journal of Tropical Medicine and Hygiene*, **70**, 658–662.

33 Robertson, L.J. *et al.* (1992) Survival of *Cryptosporidium parvum* oocysts under various environmental pressures. *Applied and Environmental Microbiology*, **58**, 3494–3500.

34 Martinaud, G. *et al.* (2009) Circadian variation in shedding of the oocysts of *Isospora turdi* (Apicomplexa) in blackbirds (*Turdus merula*): an adaptive trait against desiccation and ultraviolet radiation. *International Journal for Parasitology*, **39**, 735–739.

35 McKenna, P.B. and Charleston, W.A. (1992) The survival of *Sarcocystis gigantea* sporocysts following exposure to various chemical and physical agents. *Veterinary Parasitology*, **45**, 1–16.

36 Savini, G. *et al.* (1996) Viability of the sporocysts of *Sarcocystis cruzi* after exposure to different temperatures and relative humidities. *Veterinary Parasitology*, **67**, 153–160.

37 Weber, D.J. and Rutala, W.A. (2001) The emerging nosocomial pathogens *Cryptosporidium*, *Escherichia coli* O157:H7, *Helicobacter pylori*, and hepatitis C: epidemiology, environmental survival, efficacy of disinfection, and control measures. *Infection Control and Hospital Epidemiology*, **22**, 306–315.

38 WHO/PAHO/UNESCO (1997) WHO/PAHO/UNESCO report. A consultation with experts on amoebiasis. Mexico City, Mexico, 28–29 January, 1997. *Epidemiological Bulletin*, **18**, 13–14.

39 Stringer, R.P. *et al.* (1975) Comparison of bromine, chlorine, and iodine as disinfectants for amoebic cysts, in *Disinfection: Water and Wastewater* (ed. J.D. Johnson), Ann Arbor Science Publishers Inc., Ann Arbor, MI, pp. 193–209.

40 Pawlowski, J. and Burki, F. (2009) Untangling the phylogeny of amoeboid protists. *Journal of Eukaryotic Microbiology*, **56**, 16–25.

41 Brindley, N. *et al.* (2009) *Acanthamoeba castellanii*: high antibody prevalence in racially and ethnically diverse populations. *Experimental Parasitology*, **121**, 254–256.

42 Dart, J.K. *et al.* (2009) *Acanthamoeba* keratitis: diagnosis and treatment update 2009. *American Journal of Ophthalmology*, **148**, 487–99 e2.

43 Aitken, D. *et al.* (1996) Amebic keratitis in a wearer of disposable contact lenses due to a mixed *Vahlkampfia* and *Hartmannella* infection. *Ophthalmology*, **103**, 485–494.

44 Marciano-Cabral, F. and Cabral, G. (2003) *Acanthamoeba* spp. as agents of disease in humans. *Clinical Microbiology Reviews*, **16**, 273–307.

45 Visvesvara, G.S. *et al.* (2007) Pathogenic and opportunistic free-living amoebae: *Acanthamoeba* spp., *Balamuthia mandrillaris*, *Naegleria fowleri*, and *Sappinia diploidea*. *FEMS Immunology and Medical Microbiology*, **50**, 1–26.

46 Gelman, B.B. *et al.* (2003) Neuropathological and ultrastructural features of amebic encephalitis caused by *Sappinia diploidea*. *Journal of Neuropathology and Experimental Neurology*, **62**, 990–998.

47 Hampl, V. *et al.* (2009) Phylogenomic analyses support the monophyly of Excavata and resolve relationships among eukaryotic "supergroups". *Proceedings of the National Academy of Sciences of the United States of America*, **106**, 3859–3864.

48 Visvesvara, G.S. *et al.* (2009) *Paravahlkampfia francinae* n. sp. masquerading as an agent of primary amoebic meningoencephalitis. *Journal of Eukaryotic Microbiology*, **56**, 357–366.

49 Verani, J.R. *et al.* (2009) National outbreak of *Acanthamoeba* keratitis associated with use of a contact lens solution, United States. *Emerging Infectious Diseases*, **15**, 1236–1242.

50 Kingston, D. and Warhurst, D.C. (1969) Isolation of amoebae from the air. *Journal of Medical Microbiology*, **2**, 27–36.

51 Rivera, F. *et al.* (1984) Pathogenic and free-living protozoa cultured from the nasopharyngeal and oral regions of dental patients. *Environmental Research*, **33**, 428–440.

52 Lanocha, N. *et al.* (2009) The occurrence *Acanthamoeba* (free living amoeba) in environmental and respiratory samples in Poland. *Acta Protozoologica*, **48**, 271–279.

53 Santos, L.C. *et al.* (2009) *Acanthamoeba* spp. in urine of critically ill patients. *Emerging Infectious Diseases*, **15**, 1144–1146.

54 Greub, G. and Raoult, D. (2004) Microorganisms resistant to free-living amoebae. *Clinical Microbiology Reviews*, **17**, 413–433.

55 Thomas, V. *et al.* (2010) Free-living amoebae and their intracellular pathogenic microorganisms: risks for water quality. *FEMS Microbiology Reviews*, **34**, 231–259.

56 Adekambi, T. *et al.* (2006) Survival of environmental mycobacteria in *Acanthamoeba polyphaga*. *Applied and Environmental Microbiology*, **72**, 5974–5981.

57 Rodriguez-Zaragoza, S. (1994) Ecology of free-living amoebae. *Critical Reviews in Microbiology*, **20**, 225–241.

58 Ettinger, M.R. *et al.* (2003) Distribution of free-living amoebae in James River, Virginia, USA. *Parasitology Research*, **89**, 6–15.

59 Liu, H. *et al.* (2006) Genetic diversity of *Acanthamoeba* isolated from ocean sediments. *Korean Journal of Parasitology*, **44**, 117–125.

60 Kyle, D.E. and Noblet, G.P. (1986) Seasonal distribution of thermotolerant free-living amoebae. I. Willard's Pond. *Journal of Protozoology*, **33**, 422–434.

61 Kyle, D.E. and Noblet, G.P. (1987) Seasonal distribution of thermotolerant free-living amoebae. II. Lake Issaqueena. *Journal of Protozoology*, **34**, 10–15.

62 Mazur, T. *et al.* (1995) The duration of the cyst stage and the viability and virulence of *Acanthamoeba* isolates. *Tropical Medicine and Parasitology*, **46**, 106–108.

63 Sriram, R. *et al.* (2008) Survival of *Acanthamoeba* cysts after desiccation for more than 20 years. *Journal of Clinical Microbiology*, **46**, 4045–4048.

64 Chang, S.L. (1978) Resistance of pathogenic *Naegleria* to some common physical and chemical agents. *Applied and Environmental Microbiology*, **35**, 368–375.

65 Hoffmann, R. and Michel, R. (2001) Distribution of free-living amoebae (FLA) during preparation and supply of drinking water. *International Journal of Hygiene and Environmental Health*, **203**, 215–219.

66 Thomas, V. *et al.* (2008) Biodiversity of amoebae and amoebae-resisting bacteria in a drinking water treatment plant. *Environmental Microbiology*, **10**, 2728–2745.

67 Corsaro, D. *et al.* (2009) Novel *Chlamydiales* strains isolated from a water treatment plant. *Environmental Microbiology*, **11**, 188–200.

68 Thomas, V. *et al.* (2004) Amoebae in domestic water systems: resistance to disinfection treatments and implication in *Legionella* persistence. *Journal of Applied Microbiology*, **97**, 950–963.

69 Barbeau, J. and Buhler, T. (2001) Biofilms augment the number of free-living amoebae in dental unit waterlines. *Research in Microbiology*, **152**, 753–760.

70 Jeong, H.J. and Yu, H.S. (2005) The role of domestic tap water in *Acanthamoeba* contamination in contact lens storage cases in Korea. *Korean Journal of Parasitology*, **43**, 47–50.

71 Shoff, M.E. *et al.* (2008) Prevalence of *Acanthamoeba* and other naked amoebae in South Florida domestic water. *Journal of Water and Health*, **6**, 99–104.

72 Trzyna, W.C. *et al.* (2010) *Acanthamoeba* in the domestic water supply of Huntington, West Virginia, U.S.A. *Acta Protozoologica*, **49**, 9–15.

73 Stockman, L.J. *et al.* (2010) Prevalence of *Acanthamoeba* spp. and other free-living amoebae in household water, Ohio, USA-1990–1992. *Parasitology Research*, **170**, 197–200.

74 Kilvington, S. *et al.* (2004) *Acanthamoeba* keratitis: the role of domestic tap water contamination in the United Kingdom. *Investigative Ophthalmology and Visual Science*, **45**, 165–169.

75 Thomas, V. *et al.* (2006) Biodiversity of amoebae and amoebae-resisting bacteria in a hospital water network. *Applied and Environmental Microbiology*, **72**, 2428–2438.

76 Rohr, U. *et al.* (1998) Comparison of free-living amoebae in hot water systems of hospitals with isolates from moist sanitary areas by identifying genera and determining temperature tolerance. *Applied and Environmental Microbiology*, **64**, 1822–1824.

77 Vesaluoma, M. *et al.* (1995) Microbiological quality in Finnish public swimming pools and whirlpools with special reference to free living amoebae: a risk factor for contact lens wearers? *British Journal of Ophthalmology*, **79**, 178–181.

78 Scaglia, M. *et al.* (1983) Isolation and identification of pathogenic *Naegleria australiensis* (*Amoebida, Vahlkampfiidae*) from a spa in northern Italy. *Applied and Environmental Microbiology*, **46**, 1282–1285.

79 Singh, T. and Coogan, M.M. (2005) Isolation of pathogenic *Legionella* species and legionella-laden amoebae in dental unit waterlines. *Journal of Hospital Infection*, **61**, 257–262.

80 Paszko-Kolva, C. *et al.* (1991) Isolation of amoebae and *Pseudomonas* and *Legionella* spp. from eyewash stations. *Applied and Environmental Microbiology*, **57**, 163–167.

81 Barbaree, J.M. *et al.* (1986) Isolation of protozoa from water associated with a legionellosis outbreak and demonstration of intracellular multiplication of *Legionella pneumophila*. *Applied and Environmental Microbiology*, **51**, 422–424.

82 Berk, S.G. *et al.* (2006) Occurrence of infected amoebae in cooling towers compared with natural aquatic environments: implications for emerging pathogens. *Environmental Science and Technology*, **40**, 7440–7444.

83 Lee, S.C. *et al.* (2008) Microsporidia evolved from ancestral sexual fungi. *Current Biology*, **18**, 1675–1679.

84 Mathis, A. *et al.* (2005) Zoonotic potential of the microsporidia. *Clinical Microbiology Reviews*, **18**, 423–445.

85 Didier, E.S. (2005) Microsporidiosis: an emerging and opportunistic infection in humans and animals. *Acta Tropica*, **94**, 61–76.

86 Didier, E.S. *et al.* (2004) Epidemiology of microsporidiosis: sources and modes of transmission. *Veterinary Parasitology*, **126**, 145–166.

87 Lee, S.C. *et al.* (2009) Generation of genetic diversity in microsporidia via sexual reproduction and horizontal gene transfer. *Communicative and Integrative Biology*, **2**, 414–417.

88 Feng, X. *et al.* (2006) Serial propagation of the microsporidian *Enterocytozoon bieneusi* of human origin in immunocompromised rodents. *Infection and Immunity*, **74**, 4424–4429.

89 Li, X. *et al.* (2003) Infectivity of microsporidia spores stored in water at environmental temperatures. *Journal of Parasitology*, **89**, 185–188.

90 Fayer, R. (2004) Infectivity of microsporidia spores stored in seawater at environmental temperatures. *Journal of Parasitology*, **90**, 654–657.

91 Koudela, B. *et al.* (1999) Effect of low and high temperatures on infectivity of *Encephalitozoon cuniculi* spores suspended in water. *Folia Parasitologica*, **46**, 171–174.

92 Shaw, R.W. *et al.* (2000) Viability of *Loma salmonae* (Microsporidia) under laboratory conditions. *Parasitology Research*, **86**, 978–981.

93 Revell, I.L. (1960) Longevity of refrigerated *Nosema* spores – *Nosema apis*, a parasite of honey bees. *Journal of Economic Entomology*, **53**, 1132–1133.

94 Fenoy, S. *et al.* (2009) High-level resistance of *Nosema ceranae*, a parasite of the honeybee, to temperature and desiccation. *Applied and Environmental Microbiology*, **75**, 6886–6889.

95 Waller, T. (1979) Sensitivity of *Encephalitozoon cuniculi* to various temperatures, disinfectants and drugs. *Lab Animal*, **13**, 227–230.

96 Jedrzejewski, S. *et al.* (2007) Quantitative assessment of contamination of fresh food produce of various retail types by human-virulent microsporidian spores. *Applied and Environmental Microbiology*, **73**, 4071–4073.

97 Graczyk, T.K. *et al.* (2007) Quantitative evaluation of the impact of bather density on levels of human-virulent microsporidian spores in recreational water. *Applied and Environmental Microbiology*, **73**, 4095–4099.

98 Fournier, S. *et al.* (2000) Detection of microsporidia in surface water: a one-year follow-up study. *FEMS Immunology and Medical Microbiology*, **29**, 95–100.

99 Dowd, S.E. *et al.* (1998) Confirmation of the human-pathogenic microsporidia *Enterocytozoon bieneusi*, *Encephalitozoon intestinalis*, and *Vittaforma corneae* in water. *Applied and Environmental Microbiology*, **64**, 3332–3335.

100 Dowd, S.E. *et al.* (2003) Confirmed detection of *Cyclospora cayetanesis*, *Encephalitozoon intestinalis* and *Cryptosporidium parvum* in water used for drinking. *Journal of Water and Health*, **1**, 117–123.

101 Chavez-Munguia, B. *et al.* (2004) The ultrastructure of the cyst wall of *Giardia lamblia*. *Journal of Eukaryotic Microbiology*, **51**, 220–226.

102 Chavez-Munguia, B. *et al.* (2007) Ultrastructure of cyst differentiation in parasitic protozoa. *Parasitology Research*, **100**, 1169–1175.

103 Chavez-Munguia, B. *et al.* (2003) Ultrastructural study of *Entamoeba invadens* encystation and excystation. *Journal of Submicroscopic Cytology and Pathology*, **35**, 235–243.

104 Chavez-Munguia, B. *et al.* (2005) Ultrastructural study of encystation and excystation in *Acanthamoeba castellanii*. *Journal of Eukaryotic Microbiology*, **52**, 153–158.

105 Chavez-Munguia, B. *et al.* (2009) Ultrastructural study of the encystation and excystation processes in *Naegleria* sp. *Journal of Eukaryotic Microbiology*, **56**, 66–72.

106 Aguilar-Diaz, H. *et al.* (2010) *In vitro* induction of *Entamoeba histolytica* cyst-like structures from trophozoites. *PLoS Neglected Tropical Diseases*, **4**, e607.

107 Ortega, Y.R. and Sanchez, R. (2010) Update on *Cyclospora cayetanensis*, a foodborne and waterborne parasite. *Clinical Microbiology Reviews*, **23**, 218–234.

108 Belli, S.I. *et al.* (2006) The coccidian oocyst: a tough nut to crack! *Trends in Parasitology*, **22**, 416–423.

109 Mai, K. *et al.* (2009) Oocyst wall formation and composition in coccidian parasites. *Memorias do Instituto Oswaldo Cruz*, **104**, 281–289.

110 Ferguson, D.J. *et al.* (2003) The development of the macrogamete and oocyst wall in *Eimeria maxima*: immuno-light and electron microscopy. *International Journal for Parasitology*, **33**, 1329–1340.

111 Belli, S.I. *et al.* (2003) Roles of tyrosine-rich precursor glycoproteins and dityrosine- and 3,4-dihydroxyphenylalanine-mediated protein cross-linking in development of the oocyst wall in the coccidian parasite *Eimeria maxima*. *Eukaryotic Cell*, **2**, 456–464.

112 Belli, S.I. *et al.* (2009) Conservation of proteins involved in oocyst wall formation in *Eimeria maxima*, *Eimeria tenella* and *Eimeria acervulina*. *International Journal for Parasitology*, **39**, 1063–1070.

113 Krucken, J. *et al.* (2008) Excystation of *Eimeria tenella* sporozoites impaired by antibody recognizing gametocyte/oocyst antigens GAM22 and GAM56. *Eukaryotic Cell*, **7**, 202–211.

114 Templeton, T.J. *et al.* (2004) The *Cryptosporidium* oocyst wall protein is a member of a multigene family and has a homolog in *Toxoplasma*. *Infection and Immunity*, **72**, 980–987.

115 Spano, F. (2009) Development of new diagnostic tools for the diagnosis of *Toxoplasma gondii* infections, in *Fourth Workshop of National Reference Laboratories for Parasites*, May 28–29, 2009, Istituto Superiore di Sanità, Rome.

116 Speer, C.A. *et al.* (1998) Ultrastructure of the oocysts, sporocysts, and sporozoites of *Toxoplasma gondii*. *Journal of Parasitology*, **84**, 505–512.

117 Jenkins, M.B. *et al.* (2010) Significance of wall structure, macromolecular composition, and surface polymers to the survival and transport of *Cryptosporidium parvum* oocysts. *Applied and Environmental Microbiology*, **76**, 1926–1934.

118 Spano, F. *et al.* (1997) Cloning of the entire COWP gene of *Cryptosporidium parvum* and ultrastructural localization of the protein during sexual parasite development. *Parasitology*, **114** (5), 427–437.

119 Mitschler, R.R. *et al.* (1994) A comparative study of lipid compositions of *Cryptosporidium parvum* (Apicomplexa) and Madin-Darby bovine kidney cells. *Journal of Eukaryotic Microbiology*, **41**, 8–12.

120 Adam, R.D. (2001) Biology of *Giardia lamblia*. *Clinical Microbiology Reviews*, **14**, 447–475.

121 Jarroll, E.L. *et al.* (1989) *Giardia* cyst wall-specific carbohydrate: evidence for the presence of galactosamine. *Molecular and Biochemical Parasitology*, **32**, 121–131.

122 Sun, C.H. *et al.* (2003) Mining the *Giardia lamblia* genome for new cyst wall proteins. *Journal of Biological Chemistry*, **278**, 21701–21708.

123 Lujan, H.D. *et al.* (1995) Identification of a novel *Giardia lamblia* cyst wall protein with leucine-rich repeats. Implications for secretory granule formation and protein assembly into the cyst wall. *Journal of Biological Chemistry*, **270**, 29307–29313.

124 Mowatt, M.R. *et al.* (1995) Developmentally regulated expression of a *Giardia lamblia* cyst wall protein gene. *Molecular Microbiology*, **15**, 955–963.

125 Davids, B.J. *et al.* (2006) A new family of giardial cysteine-rich non-VSP protein genes and a novel cyst protein. *PLoS One*, **1**, e44.

126 Chatterjee, A. *et al.* (2009) Evidence for a "wattle and daub" model of the cyst wall of *Entamoeba*. *PLoS Pathogens*, **5**, e1000498.

127 Neff, R.J. and Neff, R.H. (1969) The biochemistry of amoebic encystation. *Symposia of the Society for Experimental Biology*, **23**, 51–81.

128 Barrett, R.A. and Alexander, M. (1977) Resistance of cysts of amoebae to microbial decomposition. *Applied and Environmental Microbiology*, **33**, 670–674.

129 Dudley, R. *et al.* (2009) Carbohydrate analysis of *Acanthamoeba castellanii*. *Experimental Parasitology*, **122**, 338–343.

130 Visvesvara, G.S. *et al.* (1993) *Balamuthia mandrillaris*, N. G., N. Sp., agent of amebic meningoencephalitis in humans and other animals. *Journal of Eukaryotic Microbiology*, **40**, 504–514.

131 Siddiqui, R. *et al.* (2009) The cyst wall carbohydrate composition of *Balamuthia mandrillaris*. *Parasitology Research*, **104**, 1439–1443.

132 Linder, M. *et al.* (2002) Use of recombinant cellulose-binding domains of *Trichoderma reesei* cellulase as a selective immunocytochemical marker for cellulose in protozoa. *Applied and Environmental Microbiology*, **68**, 2503–2508.

133 Schuster, F. (1963) An electron microscope study of the amoebo-flagellate, *Naegleria gruberi* (Schardinger). II. The cyst stage. *Journal of Protozoology*, **10**, 313–320.

134 Visvesvara, G.S. *et al.* (2005) Morphologic and molecular identification of *Naegleria dunnebackei* n. sp. isolated from a water sample. *Journal of Eukaryotic Microbiology*, **52**, 523–531.

135 Marciano-Cabral, F. (1988) Biology of *Naegleria* spp. *Microbiological Reviews*, **52**, 114–133.

136 Bohne, W. *et al.* (2000) Developmental expression of a tandemly repeated, glycine- and serine-rich spore wall protein in the microsporidian pathogen *Encephalitozoon cuniculi*. *Infection and Immunity*, **68**, 2268–2275.

137 Bigliardi, E. and Sacchi, L. (2001) Cell biology and invasion of the microsporidia. *Microbes and Infection*, **3**, 373–379.

138 Hayman, J.R. *et al.* (2005) Role of sulfated glycans in adherence of the microsporidian *Encephalitozoon intestinalis* to host cells *in vitro*. *Infection and Immunity*, **73**, 841–848.

139 Hayman, J.R. *et al.* (2001) Developmental expression of two spore wall proteins during maturation of the microsporidian *Encephalitozoon intestinalis*. *Infection and Immunity*, **69**, 7057–7066.

140 Xu, Y. *et al.* (2006) Identification of a new spore wall protein from *Encephalitozoon cuniculi*. *Infection and Immunity*, **74**, 239–247.

141 Peuvel-Fanget, I. *et al.* (2006) EnP1 and EnP2, two proteins associated with the *Encephalitozoon cuniculi* endospore, the chitin-rich inner layer of the microsporidian spore wall. *International Journal for Parasitology*, **36**, 309–318.

142 Southern, T.R. *et al.* (2007) EnP1, a microsporidian spore wall protein that enables spores to adhere to and infect host cells *in vitro*. *Eukaryotic Cell*, **6**, 1354–1362.

143 Brosson, D. *et al.* (2005) The putative chitin deacetylase of *Encephalitozoon cuniculi*: a surface protein implicated in microsporidian spore-wall formation. *FEMS Microbiology Letters*, **247**, 81–90.

144 Shahiduzzaman, M. *et al.* (2010) Combination of cell culture and quantitative PCR (cc-qPCR) to assess disinfectants efficacy on *Cryptosporidium* oocysts under standardized conditions. *Veterinary Parasitology*, **167**, 43–49.

145 Labatiuk, C.W. *et al.* (1991) Comparison of animal infectivity, excystation, and fluorogenic dye as measures of *Giardia muris* cyst inactivation by ozone. *Applied and Environmental Microbiology*, **57**, 3187–3192.

146 Sauch, J.F. *et al.* (1991) Propidium iodide as an indicator of *Giardia* cyst viability. *Applied and Environmental Microbiology*, **57**, 3243–3247.

147 Anger, C. and Lally, J.M. (2008) *Acanthamoeba*: a review of its potential to cause keratitis, current lens care solution disinfection standards and methodologies, and strategies to reduce patient risk. *Eye and Contact Lens*, **34**, 247–253.

148 Hughes, R. *et al.* (2003) *Acanthamoeba polyphaga* strain age and method of cyst production influence the observed efficacy of therapeutic agents and contact lens disinfectants. *Antimicrobial Agents and Chemotherapy*, **47**, 3080–3084.

149 Buck, S.L. *et al.* (2000) Methods used to evaluate the effectiveness of contact lens care solutions and other compounds against *Acanthamoeba*: a review of the literature. *CLAO Journal*, **26**, 72–84.

150 Pumidonming, W. *et al.* (2010) *Acanthamoeba* strains show reduced temperature tolerance after long-term axenic culture. *Parasitology Research*, **106**, 553–559.

151 Johnston, S.P. *et al.* (2009) Resistance of *Acanthamoeba* cysts to disinfection in multiple contact lens solutions. *Journal of Clinical Microbiology*, **47**, 2040–2045.

152 Gilbert, P. and Moore, L.E. (2005) Cationic antiseptics: diversity of action under a common epithet. *Journal of Applied Microbiology*, **99**, 703–715.

153 McDonnell, G. (2007) *Antisepsis, Disinfection and Sterilization: Types, Action and Resistance*, ASM Press, Washington, DC.

154 Connor, C.G. *et al.* (1991) Effectivity of contact lens disinfection systems against *Acanthamoeba culbertsoni*. *Optometry and Vision Science*, **68**, 138–141.

155 Penley, C.A. *et al.* (1989) Comparative antimicrobial efficacy of soft and rigid gas permeable contact lens solutions against *Acanthamoeba*. *CLAO Journal*, **15**, 257–260.

156 Silvany, R.E. *et al.* (1990) The effect of currently available contact lens disinfection systems on *Acanthamoeba castellanii* and *Acanthamoeba polyphaga*. *Ophthalmology*, **97**, 286–290.

157 Hugo, E.R. *et al.* (1991) Quantitative enumeration of acanthamoeba for evaluation of cyst inactivation in contact lens care solutions. *Investigative Ophthalmology and Visual Science*, **32**, 655–657.

158 Cursons, R.T. *et al.* (1980) Effect of disinfectants on pathogenic free-living amoebae: in axenic conditions. *Applied and Environmental Microbiology*, **40**, 62–66.

159 Turner, N.A. *et al.* (2000) Emergence of resistance to biocides during differentiation of *Acanthamoeba castellanii*. *Journal of Antimicrobial Chemotherapy*, **46**, 27–34.

160 Zanetti, S. *et al.* (1995) Susceptibility of *Acanthamoeba castellanii* to contact lens disinfecting solutions. *Antimicrobial Agents and Chemotherapy*, **39**, 1596–1598.

161 Brandt, F.H. *et al.* (1989) Viability of *Acanthamoeba* cysts in ophthalmic solutions. *Applied and Environmental Microbiology*, **55**, 1144–1146.

162 Elder, M.J. *et al.* (1994) A clinicopathologic study of *in vitro* sensitivity testing and *Acanthamoeba* keratitis. *Investigative Ophthalmology and Visual Science*, **35**, 1059–1064.

163 Hay, J. *et al.* (1994) Drug resistance and *Acanthamoeba* keratitis: the quest for alternative antiprotozoal chemotherapy. *Eye*, **8** (5), 555–563.

164 Seal, D. *et al.* (1996) Successful medical therapy of *Acanthamoeba* keratitis with topical chlorhexidine and propamidine. *Eye*, **10** (4), 413–421.

165 Kim, S.Y. and Hahn, T.W. (1999) *In vitro* amoebicidal efficacy of hexamidine, polyhexamethylene biguanide and chlorhexidine on 10 ocular isolates of *Acanthamoeba*. *Investigative Ophthalmology and Visual Science*, **40**, 1392–1300.

166 Burger, R.M. *et al.* (1994) Killing acanthamoebae with polyaminopropyl biguanide: quantitation and kinetics. *Antimicrobial Agents and Chemotherapy*, **38**, 886–888.

167 Khunkitti, W. *et al.* (1996) The lethal effects of biguanides on cysts and trophozoites of *Acanthamoeba castellanii*. *Journal of Applied Bacteriology*, **81**, 73–77.

168 Silvany, R.E. *et al.* (1991) Effect of contact lens preservatives on *Acanthamoeba*. *Ophthalmology*, **98**, 854–857.

169 Davies, J.G. *et al.* (1990) Evaluation of the anti-Acanthamoebal activity of five contact lens disinfectants. *International Contact Lens Clinic*, **17**, 14–20.

170 Cengiz, A.M. *et al.* (2000) Co-incubation of *Acanthamoeba castellanii* with strains of *Pseudomonas aeruginosa* alters the survival of amoeba. *Clinical and Experimental Ophthalmology*, **28**, 191–193.

171 Kilvington, S. (1998) Reducing the risk of microbial keratitis in soft contact lens wearers. *Optician*, **217**, 28–31.

172 Niszl, I.A. and Markus, M.B. (1998) Anti-*Acanthamoeba* activity of contact lens solutions. *British Journal of Ophthalmology*, **82**, 1033–1038.

173 Buck, S.L. *et al.* (1998) Amoebicidal activity of a preserved contact lens multipurpose disinfecting solution compared to a disinfection/neutralisation peroxide system. *Contact Lens and Anterior Eye*, **21**, 81–84.

174 Holton, J. *et al.* (1994) Efficacy of selected disinfectants against mycobacteria and cryptosporidia. *Journal of Hospital Infection*, **27**, 105–115.

175 Barbee, S.L. *et al.* (1999) Inactivation of *Cryptosporidium parvum* oocyst infectivity by disinfection and sterilization processes. *Gastrointestinal Endoscopy*, **49**, 605–611.

176 Dubey, J.P. *et al.* (2002) Effects of high temperature and disinfectants on the viability of *Sarcocystis neurona* sporocysts. *Journal of Parasitology*, **88**, 1252–1254.

177 Ortega, Y.R. *et al.* (2007) Efficacy of a sanitizer and disinfectants to inactivate *Encephalitozoon intestinalis* spores. *Journal of Food Protection*, **70**, 681–684.

178 Santillana-Hayat, M. *et al.* (2002) Effects of chemical and physical agents on viability and infectivity of *Encephalitozoon intestinalis* determined by cell culture and flow cytometry. *Antimicrobial Agents and Chemotherapy*, **46**, 2049–2051.

179 De Jonckheere, J. and van de Voorde, H. (1976) Differences in destruction of cysts of pathogenic and nonpathogenic *Naegleria* and *Acanthamoeba* by chlorine. *Applied and Environmental Microbiology*, **31**, 294–297.

180 Mogoa, E. *et al.* (2010) *Acanthamoeba castellanii*: cellular changes induced by chlorination. *Experimental Parasitology*, **126**, 97–102.

181 Dupuy, M. *et al.* (2011) Efficiency of water disinfectants against *Legionella pneumophila* and *Acanthamoeba*. *Water Research*, **45**, 1087–1094.

182 Ercken, D. *et al.* (2003) Effects of peracetic acid and monochloramine on the inactivation of *Naegleria lovaniensis*. *Water Science and Technology*, **47**, 167–171.

183 Alleron, L. *et al.* (2008) Long-term survival of *Legionella pneumophila* in the viable but nonculturable state after monochloramine treatment. *Current Microbiology*, **57**, 497–502.

184 Kuchta, J.M. *et al.* (1993) Impact of chlorine and heat on the survival of Hartmannella vermiformis and subsequent growth of *Legionella pneumophila*. *Applied and Environmental Microbiology*, **59**, 4096–4100.

185 Storey, M.V. *et al.* (2004) The efficacy of heat and chlorine treatment against thermotolerant *Acanthamoebae* and *Legionellae*. *Scandinavian Journal of Infectious Diseases*, **36**, 656–662.

186 Kilvington, S. and Price, J. (1990) Survival of *Legionella pneumophila* within cysts of *Acanthamoeba polyphaga* following chlorine exposure. *Journal of Applied Bacteriology*, **68**, 519–525.

187 Siddiqui, R. *et al.* (2008) *Balamuthia mandrillaris* resistance to hostile conditions. *Journal of Medical Microbiology*, **57**, 428–431.

188 Coulon, C. *et al.* (2010) Resistance of *Acanthamoeba* cysts to disinfection treatments used in health care settings. *Journal of Clinical Microbiology*, **48**, 2689–2697.

189 Perrine, D. *et al.* (1980) [Comparative *in vitro* activity of chlorine and bromine on the cysts of free-living amoebae.] *Comptes Rendus des Seances de la Societe de Biologie et de Ses Filiales*, **174**, 297–303.

190 Lim, L. *et al.* (2000) Antimicrobial susceptibility of 19 Australian corneal isolates of *Acanthamoeba*.*Clinical and Experimental Ophthalmology*, **28**, 119–124.

191 Martín-Navarro, C.M. *et al.* (2010) *Acanthamoeba* spp.: efficacy of Bioclen FR One Step®, a povidone-iodine based system for the disinfection of contact lenses. *Experimental Parasitology*, **126**, 109–112.

192 Gatti, S. *et al.* (1998) *In vitro* effectiveness of povidone-iodine on *Acanthamoeba* isolates from human cornea. *Antimicrobial Agents and Chemotherapy*, **42**, 2232–2234.

193 Hirata, T. *et al.* (2000) Effects of ozonation and chlorination on viability and infectivity of *Cryptosporidium parvum* oocysts. *Water Science and Technology*, **41**, 39–46.

194 Korich, D.G. *et al.* (1990) Effects of ozone, chlorine dioxide, chlorine, and monochloramine on *Cryptosporidium parvum* oocyst viability. *Applied and Environmental Microbiology*, **56**, 1423–1428.

195 Gyürék, L.L. *et al.* (1997) Modeling chlorine inactivation requirements of *Cryptosporidium parvum* oocysts. *Journal of Environmental Engineering*, **123**, 865–875.

196 Erickson, M.C. and Ortega, Y.R. (2006) Inactivation of protozoan parasites in food, water, and environmental systems. *Journal of Food Protection*, **69**, 2786–2808.

197 Fayer, R. (1995) Effect of sodium hypochlorite exposure on infectivity of *Cryptosporidium parvum* oocysts for neonatal BALB/c mice. *Applied and Environmental Microbiology*, **61**, 844–846.

198 Weir, S.C. *et al.* (2002) Efficacy of common laboratory disinfectants on the infectivity of *Cryptosporidium parvum* oocysts in cell culture. *Applied and Environmental Microbiology*, **68**, 2576–2579.

199 Bajszar, G. and Dekonenko, A. (2010) Stress-induced Hsp70 gene expression and inactivation of *Cryptosporidium parvum* oocysts by chlorine-based oxidants. *Applied and Environmental Microbiology*, **76**, 1732–1739.

200 Leahy, J.G. *et al.* (1987) Inactivation of *Giardia muris* cysts by free chlorine. *Applied and Environmental Microbiology*, **53**, 1448–1453.

201 Rubin, A.J. *et al.* (1989) Inactivation of gerbil-cultured *Giardia lamblia* cysts by free chlorine. *Applied and Environmental Microbiology*, **55**, 2592–2594.

202 Li, Y. *et al.* (2004) Morphological changes of *Giardia lamblia* cysts after treatment with ozone and chlorine. *Journal of Environmental Engineering and Science*, **3**, 495–506.

203 Gerba, C.P. *et al.* (1997) Efficacy of iodine water purification tablets against *Cryptosporidium* oocysts and *Giardia* cysts. *Wilderness and Environmental Medicine*, **8**, 96–100.

204 Butkus, M.A. *et al.* (2005) Do iodine water purification tablets provide an effective barrier against *Cryptosporidium parvum*? *Military Medicine*, **170**, 83–86.

205 Wilson, J.A. and Margolin, A.B. (1999) The efficacy of three common hospital liquid germicides to inactivate *Cryptosporidium parvum* oocysts. *Journal of Hospital Infection*, **42**, 231–237.

206 Fayer, R. *et al.* (1996) Gaseous disinfection of *Cryptosporidium parvum* oocysts. *Applied and Environmental Microbiology*, **62**, 3908–3909.

207 Wainwright, K.E. *et al.* (2007) Chemical inactivation of *Toxoplasma gondii* oocysts in water. *Journal of Parasitology*, **93**, 925–931.

208 Zaki, M. *et al.* (1996) Resistance of *Blastocystis hominis* cysts to chlorine. *Journal of the Pakistan Medical Association*, **46**, 178–179.

209 John, D.E. *et al.* (2005) Chlorine and ozone disinfection of *Encephalitozoon intestinalis* spores. *Water Research*, **39**, 2369–2375.

210 Johnson, C.H. *et al.* (2003) Chlorine inactivation of spores of *Encephalitozoon* spp. *Applied and Environmental Microbiology*, **69**, 1325–1326.

211 Wolk, D.M. *et al.* (2000) A spore counting method and cell culture model for chlorine disinfection studies of *Encephalitozoon* syn. *Septata intestinalis. Applied and Environmental Microbiology*, **66**, 1266–1273.

212 Ferguson, J.A. *et al.* (2007) Spores of two fish microsporidia (*Pseudoloma neurophilia* and *Glugea anomala*) are highly resistant to chlorine. *Diseases of Aquatic Organisms*, **76**, 205–214.

213 Shaw, R.W. *et al.* (1999) Iodophor treatment is not completely efficacious in preventing *Loma salmonae* (Microsporidia) transmission in experimentally challenged chinook salmon, *Oncorhynchus tshawytscha* (Walbaum). *Journal of Fish Diseases*, **22**, 311–313.

214 Chen, Y.S.R. *et al.* (1985) Inactivation of *Naegleria gruberi* cysts by chlorine dioxide. *Water Research*, **19**, 783–789.

215 Loret, J.F. *et al.* (2008) Elimination of free-living amoebae by drinking water treatment processes. *European Journal of Water Quality*, **39**, 37–50.

216 Peeters, J.E. *et al.* (1989) Effect of disinfection of drinking water with ozone or chlorine dioxide on survival of *Cryptosporidium parvum* oocysts. *Applied and Environmental Microbiology*, **55**, 1519–1522.

217 Chauret, C.P. *et al.* (2001) Chlorine dioxide inactivation of *Cryptosporidium parvum* oocysts and bacterial spore indicators. *Applied and Environmental Microbiology*, **67**, 2993–3001.

218 Ruffell, K.M. *et al.* (2000) Inactivation of *Cryptosporidium parvum* oocysts with chlorine dioxide. *Water Research*, **34**, 868–876.

219 Corona-Vasquez, B. *et al.* (2002) Sequential inactivation of *Cryptosporidium parvum* oocysts with chlorine dioxide followed by free chlorine or monochloramine. *Water Research*, **36**, 178–188.

220 Wang, Z. *et al.* (2010) Inactivation and mechanisms of chlorine dioxide on *Nosema bombycis. Journal of Invertebrate Pathology*, **104**, 134–139.

221 Ortega, Y.R. *et al.* (2008) Efficacy of gaseous chlorine dioxide as a sanitizer against *Cryptosporidium parvum, Cyclospora cayetanensis*, and *Encephalitozoon intestinalis* on produce. *Journal of Food Protection*, **71**, 2410–2414.

222 von Gunten, U. (2003) Ozonation of drinking water: part I. Oxidation kinetics and product formation. *Water Research*, **37**, 1443–1467.

223 Wickramanayake, G.B. *et al.* (1984) Inactivation of *Naegleria* and *Giardia* cysts in water by ozonation. *Journal – Water Pollution Control Federation*, **56**, 983–988.

224 Langlais, B. and Perrine, D. (1986) Action of ozone on trophozoites and free amoeba cysts, whether pathogenic or not. *Ozone: Science and Engineering*, **8**, 187–198.

225 Grillot, R. and Ambroise-Thomas, P. (1980) [Free-living amoebae in the Grenoble area swimming pool water. Influence of the "winter–summer" use and of the sterilising procedure (author's translation).] *Revue d'Epidemiologie et de Sante Publique*, **28**, 185–207.

226 Finch, G.R. *et al.* (1993) Comparison of *Giardia lamblia* and *Giardia muris* cyst inactivation by ozone. *Applied and Environmental Microbiology*, **59**, 3674–3680.

227 Widmer, G. *et al.* (2002) Structural and biochemical alterations in *Giardia lamblia* cysts exposed to ozone. *Journal of Parasitology*, **88**, 1100–1106.

228 Driedger, A.M. *et al.* (2001) Inactivation of *Cryptosporidium parvum* oocysts with ozone and monochloramine at low temperature. *Water Research*, **35**, 41–48.

229 Li, H. *et al.* (2001) Sequential inactivation of *Cryptosporidium parvum* using ozone and chlorine. *Water Research*, **35**, 4339–4348.

230 Dumetre, A. *et al.* (2008) Effects of ozone and ultraviolet radiation treatments on the infectivity of *Toxoplasma gondii* oocysts. *Veterinary Parasitology*, **153**, 209–213.

231 Liou, C.T. *et al.* (2002) Effect of ozone treatment on *Eimeria colchici* oocysts. *Journal of Parasitology*, **88**, 159–162.

232 Khalifa, A.M. *et al.* (2001) Effect of ozone on the viability of some protozoa in drinking water. *Journal of the Egyptian Society of Parasitology*, **31**, 603–616.

233 Hughes, R. and Kilvington, S. (2001) Comparison of hydrogen peroxide contact lens disinfection systems and solutions against *Acanthamoeba polyphaga. Antimicrobial Agents and Chemotherapy*, **45**, 2038–2043.

234 Aksozek, A. *et al.* (2002) Resistance of *Acanthamoeba castellanii* cysts to physical, chemical, and radiological conditions. *Journal of Parasitology*, **88**, 621–623.

235 Ludwig, I.H. *et al.* (1986) Susceptibility of *Acanthamoeba* to soft contact lens disinfection systems. *Investigative Ophthalmology and Visual Science*, **27**, 626–628.

236 Hughes, R. *et al.* (2003) Enhanced killing of *Acanthamoeba* cysts with a plant peroxidase-hydrogen peroxide-halide antimicrobial system. *Applied and Environmental Microbiology*, **69**, 2563–2567.

237 Heaselgrave, W. *et al.* (2010) Acidified nitrite enhances hydrogen peroxide disinfection of *Acanthamoeba*, bacteria and fungi. *Journal of Antimicrobial Chemotherapy*, **65**, 1207–1214.

238 Thomas, V. and McDonnell, G. (2008) Efficacy of hydrogen peroxide gas against amoebal cysts and amoebae-associated mycobacteria. Poster presented at 108th ASM General Meeting, Boston, USA, 1–5 June.

239 Kniel, K.E. *et al.* (2004) Effect of hydrogen peroxide and other protease inhibitors on *Cryptosporidium parvum* excystation and *in vitro* development. *Journal of Parasitology*, **90**, 885–888.

240 Kniel, K.E. *et al.* (2003) Effect of organic acids and hydrogen peroxide on *Cryptosporidium parvum* viability in fruit juices. *Journal of Food Protection*, **66**, 1650–1657.

241 Vassal, S. *et al.* (1998) Hydrogen peroxide gas plasma sterilization is effective against *Cryptosporidium parvum* oocysts. *American Journal of Infection Control*, **26**, 136–138.

242 Greub, G. and Raoult, D. (2003) Biocides currently used for bronchoscope decontamination are poorly effective against free-living amoebae. *Infection Control and Hospital Epidemiology*, **24**, 784–786.

243 Briancesco, R. *et al.* (2005) Peracetic acid and sodium hypochlorite effectiveness in reducing resistant stages of microorganisms. *Central European Journal of Public Health*, **13**, 159–162.

244 Holton, J. *et al.* (1995) Efficacy of "Nu-Cidex" (0.35% peracetic acid) against mycobacteria and cryptosporidia. *Journal of Hospital Infection*, **31**, 235–237.

245 Quilez, J. *et al.* (2005) Efficacy of two peroxygen-based disinfectants for inactivation of *Cryptosporidium parvum* oocysts. *Applied and Environmental Microbiology*, **71**, 2479–2483.

246 Ito, S. *et al.* (1975) Disinfectant effects of several chemicals against *Toxoplasma* oocysts. *Japanese Journal of Veterinary. Science*, **37**, 229–234.

247 Tiewcharoen, S. and Junnu, V. (1999) Factors affecting the viability of pathogenic *Naegleria* species isolated from Thai patients. *Journal of Tropical Medicine and Parasitology*, **22**, 15–21.

248 Castro-Hermida, J.A. *et al.* (2006) Evaluation of two commercial disinfectants on the viability and infectivity of *Cryptosporidium parvum* oocysts. *Veterinary Journal*, **171**, 340–345.

249 Wilson, J. and Margolin, A.B. (2003) Efficacy of glutaraldehyde disinfectant against *Cryptosporidium parvum* in the presence of various organic soils. *Journal of AOAC International*, **86**, 96–100.

250 Shadduck, J.A. and Polley, M.B. (1978) Some factors influencing the *in vitro* infectivity and replication of *Encephalitozoon cuniculi. Journal of Protozoology*, **25**, 491–496.

251 Jordan, C.N. *et al.* (2006) Activity of bleach, ethanol and two commercial disinfectants against spores of *Encephalitozoon cuniculi. Veterinary Parasitology*, **136**, 343–346.

252 Jenkins, M.B. *et al.* (1998) Inactivation of *Cryptosporidium parvum* oocysts by ammonia. *Applied and Environmental Microbiology*, **64**, 784–788.

253 Sutherland, E.E. and Berk, S.G. (1996) Survival of protozoa in cooling tower biocides. *Journal of Industrial Microbiology*, **16**, 73–78.

254 Srikanth, S. and Berk, S.G. (1993) Stimulatory effect of cooling tower biocides on amoebae. *Applied and Environmental Microbiology*, **59**, 3245–3249.

255 Gray, T.B. *et al.* (1996) Amoebicidal efficacy of hexamidine, compared with PHMB, chlorhexidine, propamidine and paromycin. *Investigative Ophthalmology and Visual Science*, **37**, 875.

256 Osato, M.S. *et al.* (1991) *In vitro* evaluation of antimicrobial compounds for cysticidal activity against *Acanthamoeba. Reviews of Infectious Diseases*, **13** (Suppl. 5), S431–S435.

257 Perrine, D. *et al.* (1995) Amoebicidal efficiencies of various diamidines against two strains of *Acanthamoeba polyphaga. Antimicrobial Agents and Chemotherapy*, **39**, 339–342.

258 Wysenbeek, Y.S. *et al.* (2000) The reculture technique: individualizing the treatment of *Acanthamoeba* keratitis. *Cornea*, **19**, 464–467.

259 Meisler, D.M. *et al.* (1985) Susceptibility of *Acanthamoeba* to surgical instrument sterilization techniques. *American Journal of Ophthalmology*, **99**, 724–725.

260 Anderson, B.C. (1985) Moist heat inactivation of *Cryptosporidium* sp. *American Journal of Public Health*, **75**, 1433–1434.

261 Jones, M.F. and Newton, W.L. (1950) The survival of cysts of *Endamoeba histolytica* in water at temperatures between 45 degrees C. and 55 degrees C. *American Journal of Tropical Medicine and Hygiene*, **30**, 53–58.

262 Saleque, A. *et al.* (1990) Effect of temperature on the infectivity of *Sarcocystis miescheriana* cysts in pork. *Veterinary Parasitology*, **36**, 343–346.

263 Al-Adhami, B.H. *et al.* (2007) Detection of UV-induced thymine dimers in individual *Cryptosporidium parvum* and *Cryptosporidium hominis* oocysts by immunofluorescence microscopy. *Applied and Environmental Microbiology*, **73**, 947–955.

264 Rochelle, P.A. *et al.* (2004) Irreversible UV inactivation of *Cryptosporidium* spp. despite the presence of UV repair genes. *Journal of Eukaryotic Microbiology*, **51**, 553–562.

265 Belosevic, M. *et al.* (2001) Studies on the resistance/reactivation of *Giardia muris* and *Cryptosporidium parvum* oocysts exposed to medium-pressure ultraviolet radiation. *FEMS Microbiology Letters*, **204**, 197–203.

266 Shin, G.A. *et al.* (2001) Low-pressure UV inactivation and DNA repair potential of *Cryptosporidium parvum* oocysts. *Applied and Environmental Microbiology*, **67**, 3029–3032.

267 Craik, S.A. *et al.* (2001) Inactivation of *Cryptosporidium parvum* oocysts using medium- and low-pressure ultraviolet radiation. *Water Research*, **35**, 1387–1398.

268 Linden, K.G. *et al.* (2002) UV disinfection of *Giardia lamblia* cysts in water. *Environmental Science and Technology*, **36**, 2519–2522.

269 Mofidi, A.A. *et al.* (2002) The effect of UV light on the inactivation of *Giardia lamblia* and *Giardia muris* cysts as determined by animal infectivity assay (P-2951-01). *Water Research*, **36**, 2098–2108.

270 Li, D. *et al.* (2007) Comparison of levels of inactivation of two isolates of *Giardia lamblia* cysts by UV light. *Applied and Environmental Microbiology*, **73**, 2218–2223.

271 Li, D. *et al.* (2008) Survival of *Giardia lamblia* trophozoites after exposure to UV light. *FEMS Microbiology Letters*, **278**, 56–61.

272 Li, D. *et al.* (2009) Infectivity of *Giardia lamblia* cysts obtained from wastewater treated with ultraviolet light. *Water Research*, **43**, 3037–3046.

273 McGuigan, K.G. *et al.* (2006) Batch solar disinfection inactivates oocysts of *Cryptosporidium parvum* and cysts of *Giardia muris* in drinking water. *Journal of Applied Microbiology*, **101**, 453–463.

274 Mendez-Hermida, F. *et al.* (2007) Disinfection of drinking water contaminated with *Cryptosporidium parvum* oocysts under natural sunlight and using the photocatalyst TiO2. *Journal of Photochemistry and Photobiology. B, Biology*, **88**, 105–111.

275 Mtapuri-Zinyowera, S. *et al.* (2009) Impact of solar radiation in disinfecting drinking water contaminated with *Giardia duodenalis* and *Entamoeba histolytica/dispar* at a point-of-use water treatment. *Journal of Applied Microbiology*, **106**, 847–852.

276 Weber, C. *et al.* (2009) Effects of DNA damage induced by UV irradiation on gene expression in the protozoan parasite *Entamoeba histolytica*. *Molecular and Biochemical Parasitology*, **164**, 165–169.

277 Hijnen, W.A. *et al.* (2006) Inactivation credit of UV radiation for viruses, bacteria and protozoan (oo)cysts in water: a review. *Water Research*, **40**, 3–22.

278 Maya, C. *et al.* (2003) Evaluation of the UV disinfection process in bacteria and amphizoic amoebae inactivation. *Water Science and Technology: Water Supply*, **3**, 285–291.

279 Hwang, T.S. *et al.* (2004) Disinfection capacity of PuriLens contact lens cleaning unit against *Acanthamoeba*. *Eye and Contact Lens*, **30**, 42–43.

280 Loret, J.F. *et al.* (2008) Amoebae-resisting bacteria in drinking water: risk assessment and management. *Water Science and Technology*, **58**, 571–577.

281 Lonnen, J. *et al.* (2005) Solar and photocatalytic disinfection of protozoan, fungal and bacterial microbes in drinking water. *Water Research*, **39**, 877–883.

282 Heaselgrave, W. *et al.* (2006) Solar disinfection of poliovirus and *Acanthamoeba polyphaga* cysts in water – a laboratory study using simulated sunlight. *Letters in Applied Microbiology*, **43**, 125–130.

283 Hillebrandt, S. and Muller, I. (1991) Repair of damage caused by UV- and X-irradiation in the amoeboflagellate *Naegleria gruberi*. *Radiation and Environmental Biophysics*, **30**, 123–130.

284 Ferro, S. *et al.* (2006) Photosensitized inactivation of *Acanthamoeba palestinensis* in the cystic stage. *Journal of Applied Microbiology*, **101**, 206–212.

285 Marshall, M.M. *et al.* (2003) Comparison of UV inactivation of spores of three *Encephalitozoon* species with that of spores of two DNA repair-deficient *Bacillus subtilis* biodosimetry strains. *Applied and Environmental Microbiology*, **69**, 683–685.

286 Huffman, D.E. *et al.* (2002) Low- and medium-pressure UV inactivation of microsporidia *Encephalitozoon intestinalis*. *Water Research*, **36**, 3161–3164.

287 John, D.E. *et al.* (2003) Development and optimization of a quantitative cell culture infectivity assay for the microsporidium *Encephalitozoon intestinalis* and application to ultraviolet light inactivation. *Journal of Microbiological Methods*, **52**, 183–196.

288 Kato, S. *et al.* (2001) Chemical and physical factors affecting the excystation of *Cryptosporidium parvum* oocysts. *Journal of Parasitology*, **87**, 575–581.

289 Yu, J.R. and Park, W.Y. (2003) The effect of gamma-irradiation on the viability of *Cryptosporidium parvum*. *Journal of Parasitology*, **89**, 639–642.

290 Lee, S.U. *et al.* (2010) Rejoining of gamma-ray-induced DNA damage in *Cryptosporidium parvum* measured by the comet assay. *Experimental Parasitology*, **125**, 230–235.

291 Sundermann, C.A. and Estridge, B.H. (2009) Inactivation of *Giardia lamblia* cysts by cobalt-60 irraditaion. *Journal of Parasitology*, **96**, 425–428.

292 Lee, M.B. and Lee, E.H. (2001) Coccidial contamination of raspberries: mock contamination with *Eimeria acervulina* as a model for decontamination treatment studies. *Journal of Food Protection*, **64**, 1854–1857.

293 Dubey, J.P. and Thayer, D.W. (1994) Killing of different strains of *Toxoplasma gondii* tissue cysts by irradiation under defined conditions. *Journal of Parasitology*, **80**, 764–767.

294 Dubey, J.P. *et al.* (1998) Effect of gamma irradiation on unsporulated and sporulated *Toxoplasma gondii* oocysts. *International Journal for Parasitology*, **28**, 369–375.

295 Gilbert, J.M. *et al.* (1998) Biological effects of gamma-irradiation on laboratory and field isolates of *Eimeria tenella* (Protozoa; Coccidia). *Parasitology Research*, **84**, 437–441.

296 Hiramoto, R.M. Jr. *et al.* (2002) 200 Gy sterilised *Toxoplasma gondii* tachyzoites maintain metabolic functions and mammalian cell invasion, eliciting cellular immunity and cytokine response similar to natural infection in mice. *Vaccine*, **20**, 2072–2081.

297 Li, X. *et al.* (2002) Effects of gamma radiation on viability of *Encephalitozoon* spores. *Journal of Parasitology*, **88**, 812–813.

298 Slifko, T.R. *et al.* (2000) Effect of high hydrostatic pressure on *Cryptosporidium parvum* infectivity. *Journal of Food Protection*, **63**, 1262–1267.

299 Collins, M.V. *et al.* (2005) The effect of high-pressure processing on infectivity of *Cryptosporidium parvum* oocysts recovered from experimentally exposed Eastern oysters (*Crassostrea virginica*). *Journal of Eukaryotic Microbiology*, **52**, 500–504.

300 Kniel, K.E. *et al.* (2007) High hydrostatic pressure and UV light treatment of produce contaminated with *Eimeria acervulina* as a *Cyclospora cayetanensis* surrogate. *Journal of Food Protection*, **70**, 2837–2842.

301 Shearer, A.E.H. *et al.* (2007) Effects of high hydrostatic pressure on *Eimeria acervulina* pathogenicity, immunogenicity and structural integrity. *Innovative Food Science and Emerging Technologies*, **8**, 259–268.

302 Lindsay, D.S. *et al.* (2008) Effects of high pressure processing on *Toxoplasma gondii* oocysts on raspberries. *Journal of Parasitology*, **94**, 757–758.

303 Lindsay, D.S. *et al.* (2006) Effects of high-pressure processing on *Toxoplasma gondii* tissue cysts in ground pork. *Journal of Parasitology*, **92**, 195–196.

304 Lindsay, D.S. *et al.* (2005) Effects of high pressure processing on infectivity of *Toxoplasma gondii* oocysts for mice. *Journal of Parasitology*, **91**, 699–701.

305 Jordan, C.N. *et al.* (2005) Effects of high-pressure processing on *in vitro* infectivity of *Encephalitozoon cuniculi*. *Journal of Parasitology*, **91**, 1487–1488.

306 Ortega, Y.R. and Liao, J. (2006) Microwave inactivation of *Cyclospora cayetanensis* sporulation and viability of *Cryptosporidium parvum* oocysts. *Journal of Food Protection*, **69**, 1957–1960.

307 Hiti, K. *et al.* (2001) Microwave treatment of contact lens cases contaminated with acanthamoeba. *Cornea*, **20**, 467–470.

308 Vernhes, M.C. *et al.* (2002) Elimination of free-living amoebae in fresh water with pulsed electric fields. *Water Research*, **36**, 3429–3438.

309 Meisler, D.M. *et al.* (1986) Susceptibility of *Acanthamoeba* to cryotherapeutic method. *Archives of Ophthalmology*, **104**, 130–131.

310 Matoba, A.Y. *et al.* (1989) The effects of freezing and antibiotics on the viability of *Acanthamoeba* cysts. *Archives of Ophthalmology*, **107**, 439–440.

311 Searcy, K.E. *et al.* (2006) Capture and retention of *Cryptosporidium parvum* oocysts by *Pseudomonas aeruginosa* biofilms. *Applied and Environmental Microbiology*, **72**, 6242–6247.

312 Helmi, K. *et al.* (2008) Interactions of *Cryptosporidium parvum*, *Giardia lamblia*, vaccinal poliovirus type 1, and bacteriophages phiX174 and MS2 with a drinking water biofilm and a wastewater biofilm. *Applied and Environmental Microbiology*, **74**, 2079–2088.

313 Wolyniak, E.A. *et al.* (2010) Seasonal retention and release of *Cryptosporidium parvum* oocysts by environmental biofilms in the laboratory. *Applied and Environmental Microbiology*, **76**, 1021–1027.

314 Russell, A.D. (2003) Similarities and differences in the responses of microorganisms to biocides. *Journal of Antimicrobial Chemotherapy*, **52**, 750–763.

315 Gomez-Couso, H. *et al.* (2007) *Acanthamoeba* as a temporal vehicle of *Cryptosporidium*. *Parasitology Research*, **100**, 1151–1154.

316 Stott, R. *et al.* (2003) Predation of *Cryptosporidium* oocysts by protozoa and rotifers: implications for water quality and public health. *Water Science and Technology*, **47**, 77–83.

317 Winiecka-Krusnell, J. *et al.* (2009) *Toxoplasma gondii*: uptake and survival of oocysts in free-living amoebae. *Experimental Parasitology*, **121**, 124–131.

318 Hoffmann, R. *et al.* (1998) Natural infection with microsporidian organisms (KW19) in *Vannella* spp. (Gymnamoebia) isolated from a domestic tap-water supply. *Parasitology Research*, **84**, 164–166.

319 Michel, R. *et al.* (2000) *Vannella* sp. harboring *Microsporidia*-like organisms isolated from the contact lens and inflamed eye of a female keratitis patient. *Parasitology Research*, **86**, 514–520.

320 Thomas, V. and McDonnell, G. (2007) Relationship between mycobacteria and amoebae: ecological and epidemiological concerns. *Letters in Applied Microbiology*, **45**, 349–357.

9 Virucidal Activity of Microbicides

Jean-Yves Maillard[1], Syed A. Sattar[2] and Federica Pinto[1]

[1] Cardiff School of Pharmacy and Pharmaceutical Sciences, Cardiff University, Cardiff, Wales, UK

[2] Centre for Research on Environmental Microbiology, Faculty of Medicine, University of Ottawa, Ottawa, Ontario, Canada

Introduction

Viruses are significant among pathogens of humans. In addition to causing substantial morbidity and mortality, they regularly lead to much economic damage [1, 2]. "New" viruses continue to be discovered as etiological agents of serious diseases [3], while the emergence of natural recombinants of influenza viruses, for example, poses a constant threat of pandemics [4]. "Old" viruses are now being incriminated as the primary or cofactors in the causation of certain human ailments such as cancers [5] and neurological disorders [6].

Most cases of viral infections are subclinical or asymptomatic while excreting infectious viral particles in the surroundings, and this makes it virtually impossible to identify and treat/isolate such cases. Chronic carriers of bloodborne pathogens such as hepatitis B and C and the human immunodeficiency virus (HIV) also represent important sources of such viruses [7, 8]. Unhygienic conditions and overcrowding greatly favor the spread of viral infections, as exemplified by improperly maintained institutional settings such as children's daycare centers, hospitals and nursing homes [9].

Viruses generally have a low minimal infective dose [10]. While vaccination against several viral diseases has been remarkably successful [11], safe and effective vaccines remain unavailable against many such infections. The limited success with antiviral chemotherapy achieved thus far is seriously threatened by the rapid emergence of drug resistance [12, 13]. These factors together re-emphasize the need for microbicides for controlling and preventing the spread of viral diseases. However, our understanding of the activity and the mechanisms of action of microbicidal chemicals against viruses of human origin remain quite fragmentary. Also, information on the virucidal activity of microbicides is often extrapolated from data based on testing against other microorganisms, bacteria in particular [14]. Such an approach is often difficult to justify in view of many fundamental differences in the size, structure and chemistry of bacteria and viruses.

Microbicides (disinfectants and antiseptics) active against viruses are termed "virucides". This chapter will focus on the potency and potential of microbicides to interrupt the transmission of human pathogenic viruses as well as on the mechanisms of action of virucidal chemicals.

Interrupting the spread of viruses with microbicides

Viruses vary widely in their ability to survive outside the host [15–20]. Generally speaking, the longer they can remain viable in the environment the greater is the risk of their spread from environmental sources [9]. This is where proper decontamination of environmental surface and medical devices (e.g. endoscopes) with microbicides can play a role in environmental control [21]. Viruses that spread directly via air, food, injections or direct venereal/non-venereal person-to-person contact are less amenable to such control. Disinfection of potable water is crucial in preventing the spread of enteric viral infections [22–24].

Microbicides are also essential in the inactivation of viruses in an increasing variety of pharmaceutical products derived from animal and human origin, in tissue for transplantation and in gene transfer medicinal products (GTMPs). For example, the possible presence of HIV and hepatitis B and C viruses (HBV and HCV) must be eliminated from blood-derived products (e.g. human antithrombin III, human coagulation factor VII, VIII, IX and XI, dried prothrombin complex, dried fibrinogen, normal immunoglobulin, human α_1-proteinase inhibitor, human von Willebrand factor) and urine-derived urofollitropin [25]. For such products, the use of microbicides may be only one of many strategies employed during production to eliminate viruses [26–30]. The validation of virus removal/inactivation is a crucial part of the product quality assurance [25, 31].

Viruses contaminate surfaces by: (i) direct contact deposition from the contaminated secretion or excretion of an infected host; (ii) transfer via other animate or inanimate surfaces; (iii) deposition from contaminated fluids in contact with the surface; or (iv) deposition from large- or small-particle aerosols. When contaminated surfaces are treated, the nature and properties of the surface also become factors in the disinfection process (see Chapter 3). Likewise, viruses are always discharged in body secretions and/or excretions of infected hosts and such organic matrices may enhance their survival in the environment while also providing them greater protection against microbicides [17, 32–35]. Relative humidity (RH) is also an important factor to consider for the virucidal action of gaseous microbicides. Morino *et al.* [36] observed that low RH (45–55%) prevented the inactivation of feline calicivirus dried on hard surfaces in soiling by gaseous chlorine dioxide (ClO_2; 8 ppm for 24 h). However, an RH of 75–85% was sufficient to kill the virus with a ClO_2 concentration of 0.08 ppm under the same test conditions.

In the healthcare environment, surfaces are generally considered important only if they are in areas where there are highly susceptible individuals, for example neonatal intensive care units, burn units, operating suites, etc. [37]. Environmental surfaces are generally considered to be less important as vehicles of virus transmission, and only low-level disinfection is practiced [38]. However, patients with a persistent viral infection have been shown to contribute to the continuous contamination of their environment, and as such the efficacy of an appropriate disinfection regime is paramount [39]. The role of contaminated hands in the transmission of viruses has long been well established [40–50] and emphasizes the role of hand hygiene to interrupt the transmission of healthcare-associated infections [38, 51–56]). Little attention is, however, paid to the possible (re)contamination of hands by contact with other contaminated surfaces, although it has been demonstrated to occur readily [47, 49, 57].

In addition, it is well recognized that handwashing technique is usually poor [58, 59] and that healthcare personnel do not wash their hands frequently enough [58], although compliance has increased [60] (see Chapter 19.1). The antimicrobial efficacy of antiseptics on skin and in particular their virucidal activity is not well documented, partly because of the lack of, and the difficulty in, testing antiseptic products.

Likewise, the failure of disinfection of surgical instruments and medical devices that allow viral transmission to patients has been well documented [61–70].

The use of microbicides to interrupt the transmission of viral infections in the healthcare environment is thus paramount and it is unfortunate that, by comparison to the activity of microbicides against bacteria, the virucidal efficacy of commonly used microbicides has been little studied.

Evaluation of virucidal activity

Microbicides are used extensively to prevent the spread of infections. The bactericidal, fungicidal or virucidal activity of particular chemical compounds cannot be reliably predicted from their chemical composition alone and standardized testing procedures are required to evaluate their efficacy. Since many non-enveloped viruses can be more resistant to microbicides than vegetative bacteria, recommendations based solely on bactericidal tests might not be appropriate. There are few internationally accepted tests for the evaluation of virucides, reflecting the complexity of testing procedures and the difficulty of standardizing the many variables involved. However, there are many national recommendations for the testing of virucidal activity, such as AFNOR (Association Française de Normalisation) in France, DVV (Deutshe Veringung zür Bekämpfung der Viruskrankheiten) in Germany and DEFRA (Department of Environment, Food and Rural Affairs) in the UK. In North America, such recommendations come from Health Canada, the US Environmental Protection Agency (EPA) and the US Food and Drug Administration (FDA).

While suspension test protocols are available to assess the virucidal activity of microbicides, they should be used only in the preliminary screening of formulations. Ideally, any tests for virucidal activity should simulate as closely as possible the conditions that prevail in the field. Therefore, formulations meant for use on environmental surfaces should be examined using carriers prototypical of common hard surfaces [71]. Likewise, skin antiseptics should be tested using *ex vivo* [72] or *in vivo* [73, 74] systems. In reality, even when laboratory-based studies indicate the virucidal potential of microbicides, tests often fail to examine the disinfectant under simulated use conditions, and clinical trials necessary to establish effectiveness [75] are invariably lacking. This lack of in-use tests is not surprising since protocols, scale and significance of a study might be difficult to appreciate even when the control of vegetative bacteria is investigated (see Chapter 11).

Viral propagation, detection and enumeration

Propagation of viruses

Being obligate parasites, viruses require living, susceptible cells for replication. The need for mammalian cell cultures when working with viruses of human and animal origin demands additional skills, facilities and expense. While cell cultures are often used these days for routine work with most viruses, some viruses require the use of embryonated eggs and laboratory animals; influenza viruses and the rabies virus are good examples here. Some viruses, for example the human norovirus, cannot yet be grown either in cell cultures or animal models, and human subjects are used to culture it [76].

Detection of viruses

Many viruses produce degenerative changes when replicating in cell cultures; these changes, which are readily visible under a light microscope, are referred to as the cytopathic effects (CPEs). The CPE, therefore, is a reliable and readily visible indicator of the presence and replication of an infectious virus. Viruses of different groups produce distinct types of CPE and this can help in the presumptive identification of viruses. It should, however, be noted that certain types of viruses can infect and replicate in cell cultrures without producing any readily visible CPEs. While a variety of indirect means can be used to detect the presence of such non-cytopathogenic viruses, such approaches are rarely used in testing microbicides against viruses. Molecular approaches such as the polymerase chain reaction (PCR) are used in testing virucides such as human norovirus, for example, but such means cannot differentiate between inactivated and still infectious viruses [77], a crucial factor in assessing microbicides.

Enumeration of viruses

Proper quantitation of the level of infectious viruses is crucial in assessing the virucidal activity of a microbicide. This is often accomplished using either the most probable number (MPN) method or plaque assays. The MPN-based assays are easier to perform as they require inoculation of test samples and controls into several individual cell cultures in tubes or cluster plates and examining them for CPEs after an appropriate period of incubation. The plaque assay, based on counting foci of infection produced by individual infectious viral particles, generates more precise results but requires greater skill and added materials and manipulations to perform it properly. The infectivity titer is expressed as plaque-forming units (pfu) per unit volume.

Use of mammalian cell culture systems

The use of mammalian cell cultures to propagate viruses imposes some additional challenges when the virucidal activity of an agent is investigated. Mammalian cells are often very sensitive to chemical disinfectants and therefore microbicides must be removed, diluted to non-toxic levels or neutralized before testing for infectious virus (Figure 9.1). Dilution is an appropriate method for overcoming cytotoxicity but requires a high titer of test virus. Neutralization of the disinfectant is an alternative to dilution, but neutralizing compounds must themselves be free of cytotoxic effects. Virucidal testing employing neutralizing compounds requires the following protocol: (i) virus alone; (ii) virus and disinfectant; (iii) disinfectant alone; (iv) virus, disinfectant and neutralizer; (v) neutralizer alone; and (vi) virus and neutralizer. Samples from each of these preparations should be tested. The significance of any cytopathic effects should be interpreted with reference to the changes induced by disinfectant or neutralizer alone or in combination with virus.

Dialysis has been proposed as a method for removing or reducing the concentration of disinfectant in virucidal tests to a level that would not interfere with the growth of cell cultures. Gel filtration, using a cross-linked dextran gel, has been employed for the separation of virus and disinfectant [78–80]. Ultrafiltration has been used as a method of overcoming the limitations of dilution of the disinfectant [81]. In this procedure, the virus suspension and disinfectant are mixed, and the mixture is sampled after specified incubation intervals. The sample aliquot is diluted in phosphate-buffered saline to stop the reaction, concentrated at 4°C by ultrafiltration, and titrated for virus survival. Other possible methods of separating virus from disinfectant include density-gradient ultracentrifugation, preparative isoelectric focusing and a range of electrophoretic procedures, using support media of appropriate pore size.

Use of virus surrogates

Surrogates have been used to study viruses that are particularly difficult to propagate *in vitro*, especially those that can only replicate in an animal. For example, the duck hepatitis B virus has been used as a model to test the efficacy of microbicides against hepadnaviruses [82–84]. The feline calicivirus has been used as a surrogate for the human norovirus [85]. Parallels have also been drawn between mammalian viruses and bacteriophages (see Chapter 4). The use of viral surrogates as an alternative to highly pathogenic viruses or difficult to propagate viruses, if not entirely satisfactory, nevertheless provides useful and much needed information.

In Canada (http://www.hc-sc.gc.ca/dhp-mps/prodpharma/applic-demande/guide-ld/disinfect-desinfect/disinf_desinf-eng.php) surrogate viruses can be used to make general claims of virucidal activity. However, the US EPA requires that every virus to be listed on a product label must be individually tested, with the exception of surrogates for HBV (http://www.epa.gov/oppad001/pdf_files/hbvprotocol.pdf), HCV (http://www.epa.gov/oppad001/pdf_files/hepcbvdvpcol.pdf) and the human norovirus (http://www.epa.gov/oppad001/pdf_files/initial_virucidal_test.pdf).

Virucidal tests and their significance

As mentioned earlier, ideally, a virucidal testing protocol should represent *in situ* conditions, although in reality this is rarely the case and useful information has to be extrapolated from laboratory testing conditions. There are several reasons for such a practice, some inherent to testing methodologies and their significance

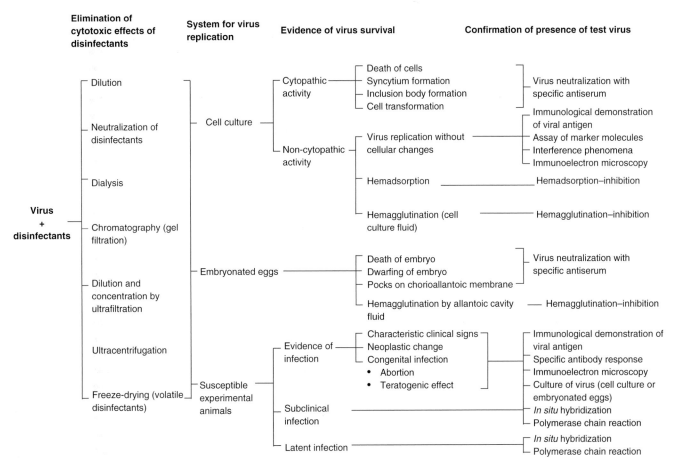

Figure 9.1 Major steps in testing microbicides against viruses

and some related to viruses. Furthermore, one of the fundamental questions is what virus strain to test as some are more difficult to propagate or more resistant to chemical inactivation than others. Another question is what virus concentration and detection/ enumeration technique should be used? One has to bear in mind that not all virus particle might be infectious; that is the number of infectious particles might be different. The sensitivity of the test method for assessing virus survival or inactivation may determine the reliability of the results obtained. Choice of the right protocol has also a financial consequence, and some techniques might bring additional costs; for example, cell tissue culture for slow-growing viruses, use of fluorescent markers, etc.

Several tests can be distinguished depending upon the purpose of the study: protocols that evaluate solely the virucidal activity of an agent; tests that mimic in-use conditions for which factors such as temperature, exposure time, pH, concentration and presence of soil load can be controlled. In addition, when dealing with viruses, it is important to remember that the toxic effect of the chemical agent needs to be eliminated when cell cultures are used for recovering the surviving viruses (see Figure 9.1). A particularly important factor, which may influence the interpretation of test results, is the degree of aggregation of virus particles in the

test system [86]. Neutralization/removal of the active immediately at the end of the contact time must also be validated.

Finally, the criterion set for virucidal efficacy is somewhat arbitrary. A number of investigators have proposed a 3-$\log_{10}$ reduction in titer as being adequate [82, 87–89], although other protocols recommend a reduction of infectivity by a factor of 4-$\log_{10}$ [90, 91].

Virucidal testing methods

There are no standardized procedures agreed internationally for assessing the virucidal activity of chemical disinfectants. Methods used include suspension tests and carrier methods [87, 88, 92–94]. Plaque-suppression tests and bacteriophage test systems have also been used to a lesser extent.

Suspension tests

In suspension tests, a virus suspension of specified concentration is usually mixed with dilutions of the active agents for a set contact time. Parameters such as pH, concentration of viruses and virucides, exposure time, temperature and soil load are easily controlled and may vary to simulate practical conditions of use. Suspension tests are particularly recommended for those viruses that are inactivated by drying. Neutralization or removal of the active agent is necessary to control the time of exposure accurately but mainly to avoid any toxicity if a cell culture, embryonated eggs or animals are used to recover the surviving viruses.

It is recommended that the virus concentration used in suspension experiments be at least 10^4 and that the protocol should allow for replicate sampling. Test results should be reported as the reduction in virus titer, expressed as $\log_{10}$, attributed to the activity of disinfectant and should be calculated by an accepted statistical method. The formation of virus aggregates, sometimes caused by the disinfectant used, especially if it precipitates proteins, needs to be considered and may play an important survival role in suspension tests (as discussed in Chapter 6.1). Suspension tests generally only furnish the minimum requirements for virus inactivation, and for practical recommendations carrier methods should be employed. Furthermore, it has been pointed out that in suspension test methods significant differences in inactivation occur both within and between laboratories [95].

Carrier tests

Viruses are often found contaminating environmental surfaces. In this respect, virucides, and especially those intended for use on dry environmental surfaces, should be tested using carrier methods, which might reflect better simulated use conditions [96, 97]. One limitation of carrier tests relates to loss in viability of viruses during the drying of the inoculated carriers. This makes it essential to start with a sufficiently high titer of infectious virus in the inoculum to ensure that enough infectious virus is left to meet the product performance criterion required.

There are several carrier protocols that have been described, but in general these methods can be divided according to whether an animate or an inanimate surface is used [94]. Among inanimate surfaces, carrier rings, cylinders and disks of stainless steel, glass and plastic have been used [94, 98–104]. The virucidal activity of antiseptics has also been tested on the hands [73, 105–107] and fingers [74, 105, 108, 109] of human subjects and an *ex vivo* test has been used to study herpesvirus survival on human skin [72].

In an inanimate surface carrier test, a known concentration of a viral suspension is placed on a hard, non-porous surface, allowed to dry and then treated with the virucide. Alternatively, the carriers may be immersed in a virus suspension and then dried. As for the suspension test, parameters such as the addition of soil load, concentration and contact time can be controlled. In addition, a wide range of surfaces can be used representing *in situ* conditions. It is generally recommended that a recoverable virus titer of at least 10^4 be used on the test surface and at least a 3-$\log_{10}$ reduction in viral titer, without cytotoxicity, be obtained [103].

Obvious ethical reasons require that there be much care in selecting and using human subjects in *in vivo* testing of virucidal chemicals. Further, these tests tend to be expensive to run and the use of *ex vivo* technologies might offer numerous advantages [72, 97, 110, 111].

Plaque-suppression tests

The principle of this method is that a layer of host cells on a suitable agar medium is infected with virus. Small disks of filter paper treated with disinfectant are applied. After a designated incubation period, the disks are removed and the agar is stained with a suitable dye in order to observe plaque suppression and also possible toxicity to host cells [112]. This method can be applied to a range of viruses, including vaccinia, herpes and Newcastle disease viruses [113, 114].

Approved tests for virucidal activity

A limited number of tests are recognized by professional groups or governments for approval of virucides: in the UK, the Ministry of Agriculture, Fisheries and Food (1970) recommendations, in France, AFNOR [115] and in Germany, the DVV [116]. In the USA, the FDA does not mention viruses in its final monograph on topical antimicrobials [117]; the official testing methodology is given by the EPA. Other recognized protocols are now available, such as the prEN14476 for the testing of virucides in a suspension test [91], on hands or on fingertips [74]. However, the range of methods available, and especially the diversity of viruses used, make it particularly difficult to compare the virucidal efficacy between chemical disinfectants [118, 119].

In the USA, the testing of virucidal activity makes use of a great variety of viruses, not all of which may spread through contaminated environmental surfaces. A 10^3 reduction in viral concentration is then required to demonstrate virucidal activity in a carrier test. In Europe, model viruses are used in suspension tests. In Germany, the DVV guidelines make use of adenovirus type 2, vaccinia virus and papovavirus SV40. A 10^4 reduction in viral concentration is required in a suspension test. However, previous recommendations from the German Society of Veterinary Medicine guidelines [120] use a virus suspension of 10^6 ID$_{50}$ in 20% bovine serum; two non-enveloped viruses are used (enteric cytopathogenic bovine orphan virus and infectious canine hepatitis virus) and two enveloped viruses (Newcastle disease virus and vaccinia virus). In France, the virucidal testing of chemical disinfectants (AFNOR T72-180) requires the use of poliovirus type 1 (vaccine strain), adenovirus type 5 and vaccinia virus [115].

The development of an ideal testing procedure for virucidal disinfectants presents many technical problems. A suitable test virus, easily grown to high titers and representative of a given family, with appropriate attributes of stability and safety, is not easily identifiable. Because of the diversity of viruses encountered in human and veterinary medicine, test viruses representing the more important families should be included in a standardized protocol. Virus concentration, contact time, temperature, bioburden and the method of exposing virus to disinfectant should be clearly specified.

The Organization for Economic Cooperation and Development (OECD) is currently considering a carrier test method for harmonization of microbicide testing in all its member states (http://www.oecd.org/LongAbstract/0,3425,en_2649_34377_44162962_1_1_1_1,00.html).

Assessment of virucidal activity with bacteriophages

Bacterial viruses (bacteriophages) have often been used alongside or instead of mammalian viruses to test the virucidal activity of disinfectants [121]. Some bacteriophages such as the MS2 coliphages [122–125] or the *Bacteroides fragilis* phage B40-8 [126–131] have also been used as indicators for enteroviruses in wastewater and polluted water. Others have been used as surrogates because of their structure. For example, the coliphage MS2 has been used as an alternative for poliovirus in virucidal testing procedures since it is structurally similar to the poliovirus [132]. The coliphage PRD-1 was used to assess microbial transmission from surface to hand and from hand to lip [133]. Furthermore, the complex structure of some phages (e.g. tailed phage), their ease of culture and other characteristics make these viruses prime candidates to study the virucidal mechanisms of action of chemical disinfectants [121](see also below).

There are multiple examples of microbicide efficacy studies using bacteriophages as surrogates either alone or together with mammalian viruses. The coliphages T2, MS2 and ØX174 were used by Lepage and Romond [134] to test the virucidal activity of iodophor, aldehyde, hypochlorite, quaternary ammonium and amphoteric compounds. The coliphage ØX174 has been used in both suspension and carrier tests to determine the virucidal activity of disinfectants [135]. The MS2 coliphage has also been used as a test virus for evaluating the virucidal activity of disinfectants in handwashing procedures [136].

Virucidal efficacy of microbicides

Not all microbicides show virucidal activity. The activity of a virucide depends upon a number of factors, some inherent to the chemical nature of the microbicides (e.g. concentration, pH, contact time, relative humidity), some inherent to the conditions on application (e.g. type of surfaces, temperature, soiling) (see Chapter 3) and some inherent to the structure and genome content of the viral particle.

The virucidal efficacy of microbicidal products might be difficult to predict. The specific viral contaminants are usually unknown, although in particular cases specific viruses are associated with specific settings, for example rotavirus and hepatitis A virus in daycare, and HBV, HCV and HIV in blood products [29, 68, 137–139]. In addition, the level of viral inactivation to achieve depends very much upon the infectivity of the virus. There is a high variation in the infectious dose depending upon the pathogenicity of the viral particle and the immune status of the host [140].

Viral inactivation implies that there is a permanent loss of infectivity following exposure to a microbicide. However, it does not necessarily imply the complete destruction of viral structure (see below). To understand the interaction between viruses and microbicides, inactivation kinetics have proved useful [86, 141] but generally have not been widely investigated. This is unfortu-nate since the information provided by such studies has contributed greatly to our knowledge of the virucidal activity of microbicidal products, and the conclusions from such studies are still valid today. With the exception of certain slow-acting microbicides, virus inactivation generally occurs rapidly or not at all. Hence a first-order kinetic can sometimes be observed, but generally multiple-hit or multicomponent patterns are described [86]. Such a non-linear kinetic often reflects the presence of viral aggregates, and on occasion an alteration in disinfectant stability, viral conformational alteration or change in the experimental methodology. The study of viral kinetics of inactivation by microbicide is particularly important for those applications where either a rapid kill is required before the complete neutralization or/and removal of the microbicides (e.g. blood products, medical devices), or a long-term efficacy is required using a low concentration of a microbicide (e.g. preservation of multidose vaccine). It can be noted that physical methods to eliminate viruses (e.g. heat sterilization) offer a better sterility assurance than the use of chemical microbicides (see Chapter 15). For surface disinfection, practical considerations limit the use of optimal conditions (e.g. high concentration, long contact time) for microbicides. For example, it is unlikely that surfaces can be soaked for hours or that the use of wipes will limit contact time to a few seconds [142, 143].

An early study by Klein and Deforest [144] provided general observations about the virucidal activity of microbicides. Viruses were divided into three classes depending upon their susceptibility to microbicides: (i) the enveloped viruses, which are the most susceptible; (ii) large non-enveloped viruses; and (iii) small non-enveloped viruses, which are the least susceptible. Although the number of viruses and microbicides investigated was small, their conclusions are still valid today. Since then, a number of efficacy studies have been performed and have confirmed the general susceptibility trend of viruses towards microbicides. It is usually accepted that enveloped viruses are inactivated more easily than non-enveloped viruses [14]. This simplistic classification of virucidal activity does not provide fine distinctions between the susceptibility of similar viruses to microbicidal products, notably at a low concentration. For example, enveloped viruses might often be more resilient to microbicide inactivation depending upon the type of environmental conditions – natural or simulated [103]. Some small non-enveloped viruses, for example the hepatitis A virus [103, 145–148], are more resistant to microbicides than other picornaviruses [14]. Further information on viral susceptibility to microbicides is given by Springthorpe and Sattar [87], Bellamy [149] and Maillard [14]. Highly reactive microbicides (e.g. oxidizers) are generally considered to have a much higher antimicrobial activity (see Chapter 2). Table 9.1 gives a summary of the classes of microbicides, indicating their potential for controlling viral contamination. The selection and use of microbicides to control virus contaminants requires a clear understanding of the potency and limitations of the active ingredients and an understanding of the effect of individual components of a given formulation. Furthermore, they also require

Table 9.1 Disinfectants used for the control of human pathogenic viruses.

Disinfectant class	Uses	Properties	Activity	References
Halogens				
Chlorine	• Water disinfection • General purpose disinfection • General sanitation in food service and manufacture • Often recommended as the standard disinfectant for inactivation of viral pathogens	• Used as chlorine gas or sodium hypochlorite solution • Relatively low residual toxicity • Stability of hypochlorite solutions affected by chlorine concentration and pH • Hypochlorous acid, favoured at low pH, is most active germicidal species • Oxidizing agent	• Wide-spectrum virucide at sufficient concentration • Activity affected by presence of reducing agents and temperature • Readily neutralized by exposure to organic material or UV radiation • Many studies on chlorine inactivation of viruses have ignored the organic material which is naturally present in the field • Increased levels needed in the presence of hard water and organic matter	[80, 101, 150–172]
Monochloramine	• Water disinfection	• Formed by the addition of ammonia after the chlorine gas	• Reacts only slowly with organic material; generally poor virucide • May have some advantages in areas where residual needs to be maintained	[125, 168, 173–177]
Chlorine dioxide	• Water disinfection • General purpose disinfectant and sporicide	• Suggested to have advantages over chlorine for some applications • Prepared on site	• May be similar in activity to sodium hypochlorite for many viruses	[36, 80, 178, 179]
Organochlorines	• General purpose disinfection • Disinfection of swimming pools (sodium dichlorodiisocyanurate) • Sanitizers in food and dairy industry (chloramine T)	• Act as demand-type disinfectants	• Reacts more slowly with biological material and therefore is less efficient as disinfectant • May have some advantages in areas where considerable organic soil exists	[80, 103]
Bromine and mixed halides	• Limited use	• Addition to chlorine-based products improves efficiency		[180, 181]
Iodine/iodophores	• Regarded as essential "drug" by World Health Organization for its disinfection properties as a topical antiseptic • In acidic solution as a sanitizer • Viral inactivation in blood products	• Analogous to chlorine but reactions are more complex • Inorganic iodine mostly replaced by iodophores, in which iodine is a loose complex with a carrier molecule (usually a neutral organic polymer). This permits greater solubility and sustained release of the active germicidal species • Surface active properties of carrier may improve wetting and soil-penetrating properties • Oxidizes –SH groups; unsaturated carbon bonds • Tends to stain skin	• Although affected, iodine compounds are less inhibited by organic matter than other halogens • In dilute solution, may act like free iodine, whereas in a more concentrated solution it behaves as a demand-type disinfectant • Neutralized by reducing agents • Addition of alcohol can improve virucidal properties	[80, 101, 169, 180, 182–194]
Phenolics	• General purpose germicides	• Complex group of chemicals • Not systematically studied as virucides	• Activity very formulation dependent • Also depends on temperature, concentration, pH, level of organic matter, etc. • Cationic and non-ionic surfactants neutralize activity • Enveloped viruses more susceptible • Need to test against specific viruses because it is difficult to generalize	[80, 169, 185, 195–198]

Table 9.1 (*Continued*)

Disinfectant class	Uses	Properties	Activity	References
Alcohols	• Used alone or in formulations to potentiate the activity of other active ingredients • General purpose disinfectant • Antiseptic in topical preparations and waterless handwashes	• As length of aliphatic chain increases, there is increased activity on lipophilic viruses, but the reverse is generally true for non-enveloped hydrophilic viruses • Ethanol is most commonly used alcohol	• Acts on envelope and denatures proteins • Not markedly affected by contaminating organic matter • Affected by dilution • Ethanol at a concentration of at least 70% is a wide-spectrum virucide • Surface active agents may improve penetration on dried material	[73, 80, 101, 109, 161, 169, 170, 198–212]
Aldehydes	• Production of inactivated viral vaccines • Fumigation (formaldehyde, paraformaldehyde) • Sterilization of tissues and medical devices (glutaraldehyde) • Topicals that release formaldehyde • Disinfection of medical instruments, notably endoscopes, before reuse (glutaraldehyde)	• Glutaraldehyde is a dialdehyde that acts more rapidly than formaldehyde and is capable of cross-linking molecules • Stable in acid solution but more active at alkaline pH • Binds to proteins through amide and amino groups • Most glutaraldehyde used at *c.* 2% for high-level disinfection	• Activity increases with temperature • React readily with proteins • Wide spectrum of activity against viruses when used at appropriate concentration • Activity decreases rapidly as product diluted on reuse • Prolonged contact needed at lower concentrations • Activity improved by addition of surface active agents or inorganic cations	[80, 101, 103, 154, 174, 205, 212–226]
Acids	• Mainly used for pH modulation in formulations • Toiletbowl cleaners • Constituents of anionic surfactant or iodophore preparations • Organic acids in food and pharmaceuticals	• Use limited by corrosion • Phosphoric acid often used because deposits resist corrosion • Organic acids are potentially more important than generally recognized	• Many viruses are susceptible to low pH; small variations can affect results • Nature of acid affects activity • Nature of diluent can affect activity • Can be affected by residuals from prior cleaning by alkaline cleaners	[80, 160, 161, 198, 227–231]
Alkalis	• Used mainly to modulate pH of formulations • Domestic and industrial sanitizers and cleaners	• Use limited by corrosion • pH levels up to 13 or higher are used	• Many viruses are susceptible to high pH	[80, 101, 103, 231, 232]
Anionic surfactants	• Used in phenolic disinfectants and acidic anionic surfactant sanitizers • Potential use as topical microbicide	• Primary effects on lipid envelope • Also affect proteins (capsid) • Often used in conjunction with phosphoric acid	• Active against enveloped but not non-enveloped viruses • Nature of acids in formulation can affect activity	[80, 103, 160, 233–236]
Cationic surfactants	• Constituents of many consumer products • Dilute aqueous solutions used as topicals for skin and mucous membranes • Hard surface disinfectants • Can be used in alcoholic solution	• Quaternary ammonium group, with hydrogen groups replaced by alkyl or aryl substituents • Most active are those with single long hydrocarbon chain (C8–C16) • Surface active properties • Concentrations of up to 20,000 parts/10^6 are used, but concentrations of 400–800 parts/10^6 are more common because of costs	• Efficiency reduced by soap • Readily neutralized by proteins • Should be applied to chemically clean surfaces unless formulated as disinfectant cleaners • Mainly useful against enveloped viruses; non-enveloped viruses are refractory • Activity of alcoholic solutions are similar to alcohols	[73, 80, 101, 103, 161, 169, 182, 201, 233, 237–246]
Amphoteric compounds	• More widely used in Europe than in North America	• Amphoteric surfactants with amino acids substituted with long-chain alkyl amine groups	• Activity mainly against enveloped viruses • Activity poor against most non-enveloped viruses	[80]

(*Continued*)

Table 9.1 (*Continued*)

Disinfectant class	Uses	Properties	Activity	References
Peroxides and peracids				
Hydrogen peroxide	• Long known as disinfectant/ antiseptic; formerly unstable; new preparations are highly stabilized • Many potential uses • Disinfection of plastics, implants and contact lenses • Used in food industry lines • Some experimental use in water disinfection • Used in low-temperature gas plasma sterilizers	• Potent oxidant which is usually considered to act through the formation of hydroxyl radicals • Very formulation dependent, acts slowly as pure chemical; 3–6% used for disinfection and 6–25% used for sterilization; care needed in handling higher concentrations	• Not widely studied as virucide • Synergism with ultrasound reported for bacteria, not studied for viruses	[22, 84, 101, 185, 217, 247–252]
Peracids	• Similar to peroxides • Many uses, from sewage disinfection to sterilization in healthcare; used in dialysis machines and on food contact surfaces	• Contain varying amounts of hydrogen peroxide; peracetic acid is the most common oxidizer; pungent odor; hazardous to handle • Tumor promoter and possible co-carcinogen	• Generally considered as potent virucide in appropriate concentrations • Powdered preparations are less potent than liquids • Not as affected by organic material as some other disinfectants	[101, 217, 247, 253–256]
Ozone	• Water disinfection • Used in food industry • Potential use as an antiseptic	• Powerful and fast-acting oxidizing agent • Unstable, therefore, must be generated on site	• Strong and broad-spectrum virucidal activity	[257–264]
Chlorhexidine and polymeric biguanides	• Widely used in aqueous solution as topical in hygienic handwash preparations • In alcoholic solution used as waterless handwash or for preoperative skin preparation • Alcoholic solution useful in critical care • Sometimes used for general purpose disinfection	• Available as dihydrochloride, diacetate or gluconate • Gluconate most soluble and most common • Low oral and percutaneous toxicity	• Activity reduced in presence of anions; often contains cationic surfactants to avoid a decrease in activity • Acts at level of envelope; virucidal activity poor in aqueous solution, and confined to enveloped viruses • Alcoholic solutions inactivate similar viruses to alcohols • PHMB binds to protein capsid • Viral aggregates are formed	[73, 80, 182, 184, 265–272]
β-Propiolactone	• Has been used for production of inactivated viral vaccines; possible value when hazardous agents are known to be present • Potential use for disinfection of blood products	• As lactone, it alkylates nucleic acids • In aqueous solution, lactone bydrolyzed to inactive products • Possible carcinogen • Purity and storage history important	• Rate and extent of activity dependent on concentration and temperature • Higher concentrations needed when proteins are present	[272–277]
Ethylene oxide	• Used for gas sterilization process • Sterilization of bone and tissue allograft	• Alkylation of –SH groups		[30, 278]

PHMB, polyhexamethylene biguanide.

knowledge of the type of material to be decontaminated and assurance that the selected treatment will not affect its property, safety and integrity. It should be re-emphasized that viruses are usually embedded in organic materials that might affect the overall virucidal efficacy of a formulation [195, 213]. Finally, it must be remembered that the efficacy of virucides *in situ* is often extrapolated from *in vitro* studies using semipurified virus preparations.

Mechanisms of virucidal action

Generally, there is a paucity of information on the mechanisms of action of virucides. Most of the information available has usually derived from the mechanisms of action of microbicides against unrelated microorganisms such as bacteria and yeast. Viruses are considered to have a simple structure and are divided into families

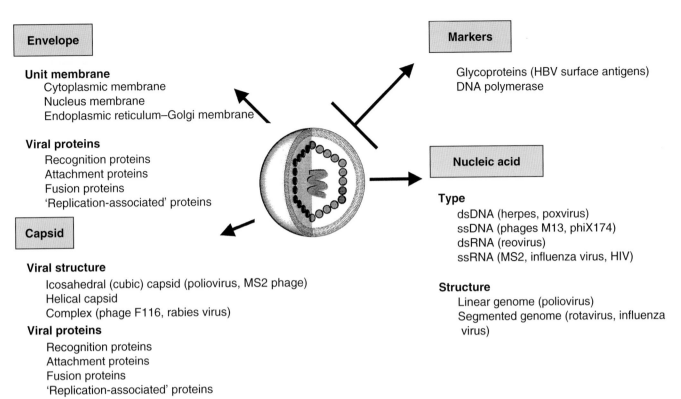

Figure 9.2 Potential viral target sites for virucidal activity. dsDNA/RNA, double-stranded DNA/RNA; HBV, hepatitis B virus; HIV, human immunodeficiency virus; ssDNA/RNA, single-stranded DNA/RNA.

on the basis of size, capsid symmetry, type and form of nucleic acid and mode of replication [279]. As mentioned above, enveloped viruses are more sensitive than non-enveloped viruses to microbicides. Such generalization is more difficult to apply to non-enveloped viruses, although larger viruses are generally considered more susceptible than small ones [14]. One of the major structural factors affecting virucidal efficacy is the presence of several "coats" and their nature, which make, for example, certain rotaviruses particularly resilient to disinfection [80, 150–153, 257]. In addition, it has been observed that viruses belonging to the same group sometimes show different sensitivities to a particular virucide under the same disinfection conditions [199, 280].

Differences in virus preparation might also account for the variability in virucide susceptibility. For example, different results were obtained when HIV was tested cell-free or cell-associated. HIV association with T-lymphocyte cell line influenced the IC_{50} of polyhexamethylene biguanide (PHMB), which decreased from 0.18% to 0.01% against cell-free and cell-associated, respectively [265].

Viral structures and targets

It is generally accepted that viruses present fewer target sites to microbicides than larger and more complex microorganisms. Furthermore, viruses do not have any metabolic activity, which further reduces the number of target sites available to microbicides, notably those that affect the proton-motive force (e.g. 2,4-dinitrophenol, carbanilides, salicylanilides) and the electron-

transport system (e.g. hexachlorophene) of other microorganisms. Nevertheless, viruses still offer multiple target sites to the action of microbicides. The number and nature of target site damage following exposure to a microbicide are likely to be concentration dependent. The segregation of viruses according to their susceptibility to microbicides [88, 144] indicates that specific target structures are important for viral survival or infectivity (Figure 9.2). Generally, the structures that offer target sites for virucides can be separated into: (i) the envelope (when present); (ii) (glyco)protein receptors; (iii) the capsid or virus coats; and (iv) the viral genome.

The susceptibility of enveloped viruses to microbicides is due to the lipidic nature of the envelope, which is derived from the host cell. There is little information on the specific interaction(s) of microbicides with the viral envelope. It is, however, accepted that many microbicides will cause disruption/lysis of the viral envelope, effectively inactivating the virus (Figure 9.3). Such a statement is based on observations that lipophilic viruses are more readily inactivated by most microbicidal agents [14, 103, 182, 200, 214] and knowledge of the interactions of microbicides with the bacterial cytoplasmic membrane [281].

The inactivation of non-enveloped viruses by microbicides most probably results from damage to either their structural or functional proteins, which are necessary for infection and replication (Figure 9.4). Capsid proteins account for 60–90% of the total virus mass. The virucidal activity of microbicides appears to be relatively similar against non-enveloped viruses [103, 199,

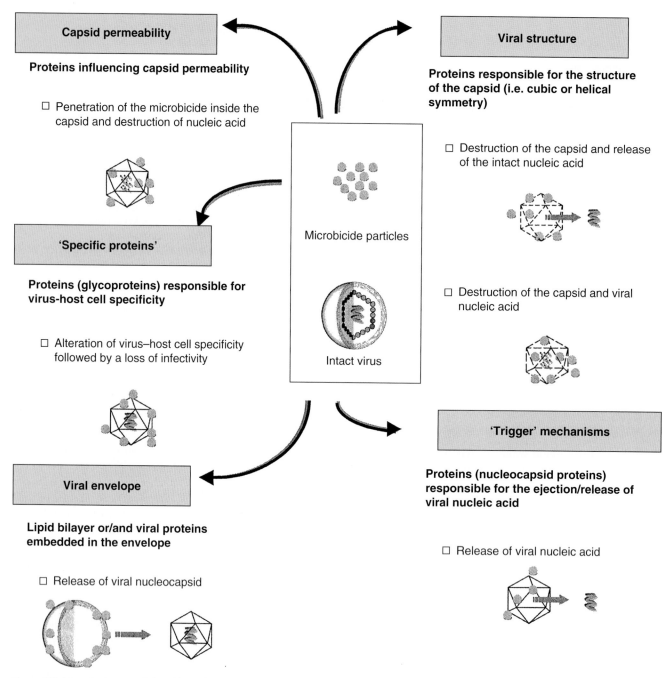

Figure 9.3 Interaction between viral particles and microbicides. HBcAg, HBV core antigen; HBsAg, HBV surface antigen; HBV, hepatitis B virus.

282], with larger non-enveloped viruses often being more readily killed than smaller ones [14, 283, 284]. Differences in susceptibility within similar non-enveloped viruses may be related to structural differences of the capsid core, different inactivation energy (see Chapter 4), availability and number of targets exposed to virucides, and the accessibility and sensitivity of the nucleic acid core to the agent. Ultimately, the viral genome should be damaged to ensure the complete inactivation of the virus (Figure 9.4). The type of nucleic acid might also affect viral susceptibility to microbicides. Viral RNA is usually closely associated with the viral capsid. Damage to the capsid will affect the RNA genome integrity through a shearing process.

Bacterial viruses (bacteriophages) have been used as surrogates for human viruses for the study of microbicide interactions with viral particles because of their ease of culture and rapid propagation to high concentrations [121]. Their complex structures have been useful in understanding the mechanisms of action of virucides [121, 266, 267, 285–289] and most of our understanding of virus-microbicide interactions is derived from the study of bacteriophages.

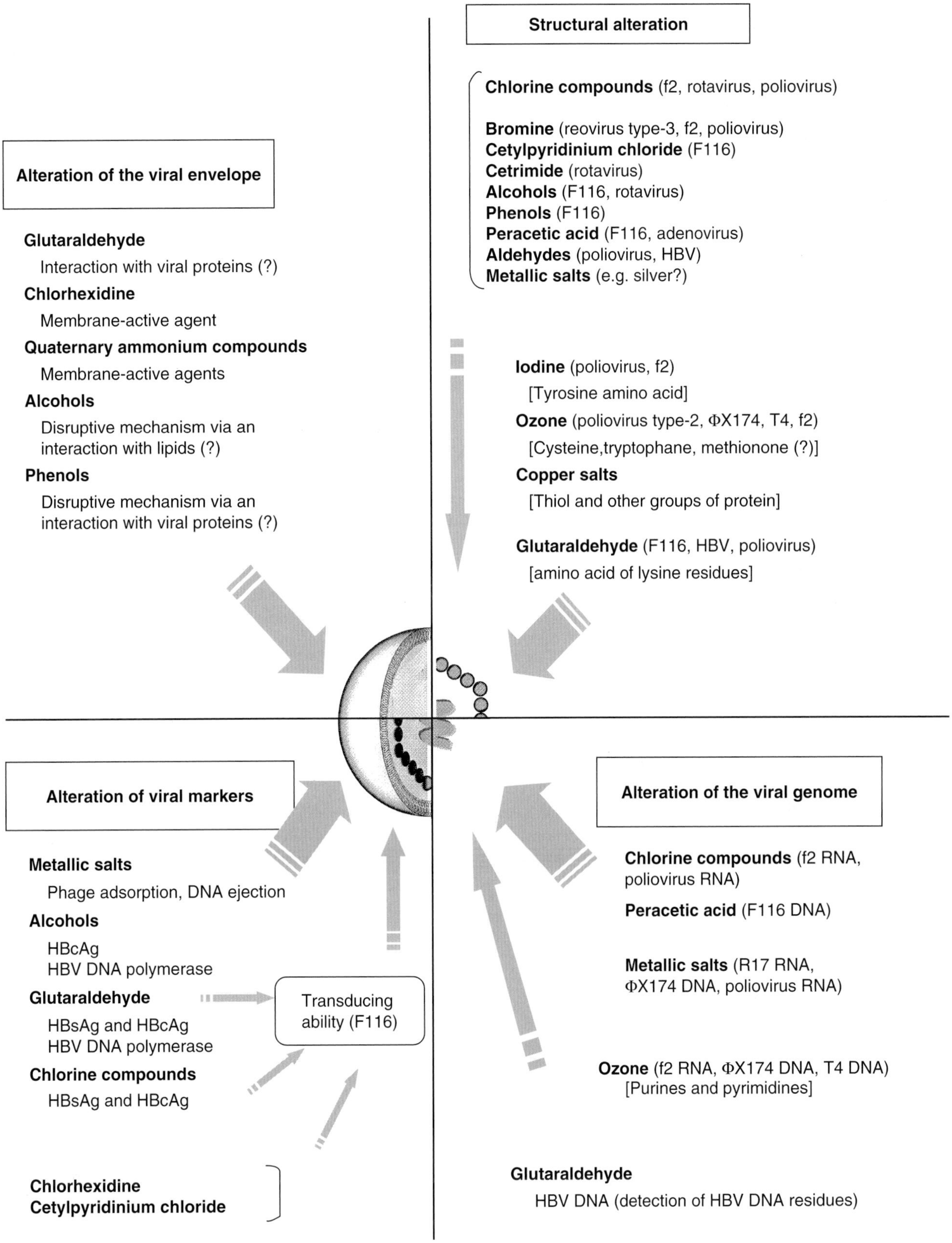

	Structural alteration

Chlorine compounds (f2, rotavirus, poliovirus)

Bromine (reovirus type-3, f2, poliovirus)
Cetylpyridinium chloride (F116)
Cetrimide (rotavirus)
Alcohols (F116, rotavirus)
Phenols (F116)
Peracetic acid (F116, adenovirus)
Aldehydes (poliovirus, HBV)
Metallic salts (e.g. silver?)

Alteration of the viral envelope

Glutaraldehyde
  Interaction with viral proteins (?)
Chlorhexidine
  Membrane-active agent
Quaternary ammonium compounds
  Membrane-active agents
Alcohols
  Disruptive mechanism via an
  interaction with lipids (?)
Phenols
  Disruptive mechanism via an
  interaction with viral proteins (?)

Iodine (poliovirus, f2)
  [Tyrosine amino acid]
Ozone (poliovirus type-2, ΦX174, T4, f2)
  [Cysteine,tryptophane, methionone (?)]
Copper salts
  [Thiol and other groups of protein]

Glutaraldehyde (F116, HBV, poliovirus)
  [amino acid of lysine residues]

Alteration of viral markers

Metallic salts
  Phage adsorption, DNA ejection
Alcohols
  HBcAg
  HBV DNA polymerase
Glutaraldehyde
  HBsAg and HBcAg
  HBV DNA polymerase
Chlorine compounds
  HBsAg and HBcAg

Transducing
ability (F116)

Chlorhexidine
Cetylpyridinium chloride

Alteration of the viral genome

Chlorine compounds (f2 RNA,
poliovirus RNA)

Peracetic acid (F116 DNA)

Metallic salts (R17 RNA,
ΦX174 DNA, poliovirus RNA)

Ozone (f2 RNA, ΦX174 DNA, T4 DNA)
  [Purines and pyrimidines]

Glutaraldehyde
  HBV DNA (detection of HBV DNA residues)

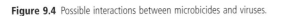

Figure 9.4 Possible interactions between microbicides and viruses.

Mechanisms of action of microbicides against viruses

The understanding of the interaction of microbicides with the viral particles has often relied on studies performed on other microorganisms. There has been very little novel information since the early studies performed in the 1960s and 1970s. The mechanisms of action of microbicides against viruses are summarized in Figure 9.4. Overall, most microbicides will interact with the viral envelope (when present), the viral capsid and nucleocapsid, but not necessarily against the viral genome. This might be an issue, since some viral genomes are known to remain infectious when released from the capsid.

The virucidal effects of microbicides vary greatly, not only between virus families but also sometimes within a family. The use of bacteriophages, however, offers many advantages and they constitute excellent tools for studying the efficacy and mechanisms of action of virucides [121, 266, 267].

Aldehydes

Glutaraldehyde (GTA) has been used extensively for high-level disinfection because of its broad spectrum of microbicidal activity; consequently, its mechanisms of action, mainly against bacteria, but also against viruses, has been well studied (see Chapter 5). GTA has been shown to react with the α-amino groups of amino acids, the N-terminal amino groups of some peptides and the sulfhydryl group of cysteine. Such interactions result in heavily cross-linked proteins on the cell surface, thus disrupting the normal function of the cells, including metabolic and respiratory processes.

GTA has a broad range of virucidal activity against enveloped viruses [14, 79, 214, 215], large non-enveloped viruses [80, 87, 213, 216, 290–292] and small non-enveloped viruses [14, 79, 114, 145, 214, 217, 293–295]. The mechanism(s) of action of GTA against viruses leading to viral inactivation can be highlighted with the study of the interaction of the GTA molecule with specific viral markers (see Figure 9.3), although the relationship between viral inactivation and alteration of a particular target site remains unclear.

Gross damage to the viral structures

The use of 4% GTA has been shown to change both the appearance and the physical properties of the foot-and-mouth disease virus, although the reason for the appearance of larger particles remained unclear [296]. Likewise, the buoyant density of the poliovirus was affected by prolonged exposure to 4% GTA [297] but not shorter exposure [298]. Such a change in appearance was linked to differential permeability to phosphotungstic acid [297]. Thraenhart and colleagues [299] showed that the morphology of hepatitis B virus "Dane particles" was severely altered by succinaldehyde. Long exposure to the aldehyde resulted in a loss of the characteristic substructure following the disintegration of the outer membrane, and asymmetrical enlargement of the space between the outer membrane and the HBV core. The effect of microbicides against the structure of HBV Dane particles has been divided into three groups according to the severity of

damage: (i) alteration of the outer shell; (ii) alteration of all sub-structures; and (iii) loss of all substructures. However, there was little correlation between the extent of damage caused to the viral particle following exposure to GTA and loss of virus infectivity [297]. The use of electron microscopy (EM) has been useful in investigating microbicide–virus interactions. Similar to the use of EM described above, Maillard *et al.* [285] studied the effects of GTA against the *Pseudomonas aeruginosa* PAO F116 bacteriophage. A concentration of 1% produced a higher number of empty heads (i.e. intact structures with no material packaged inside) (Figure 9.5b). It was suggested that GTA triggered the mechanism, causing the genome to be ejected from the phage particles [285]. GTA was shown to affect specifically two F116 proteins (molecular weight 59,100 and 10,900) which are possibly associated with the release of F116 nucleic acid [288].

Interaction with viral antigens

Two percent alkaline GTA (Cidex), 2% alkaline GTA with surface active ingredients (Cidex Formula 7) and formaldehyde (2.02%) have been shown to alter the hepatitis B virus surface (HBsAg) and core antigens (HBcAg) [300]. A decrease in HBV antigens following treatment with formaldehyde was also described by Frösner *et al.* [301]. Although the exact physical and chemical mechanism of action of GTA was not explained, it was suggested that GTA probably reacted chemically with HbsAg and HBcAg sites containing lysine residues. GTA is known for its ability to cross-link proteins [302], the reaction involving lysine and hydroxylysine residues and GTA in the relative amounts of 4 M GTA to 1 mol lysine [303]. Similarly, GTA was shown to affect the antigenicity of HAV [304]. However, it was noted that reduction in viral antigenicity and reduction in infectivity were difficult to correlate. Indeed, the detection range (i.e. only virus contamination of $>10^7$ to 10^8 virus/ml) of the HbsAg radioimmunoassay, which is often used for the testing of virucides, is far above the minimum infective dose for HBV (i.e. 10–100 virus particles).

Interactions with capsid proteins

Chambon *et al.* [305] showed that low concentrations of GTA (0.005–0.10%) caused the formation of high molecular weight complexes between capsid proteins of poliovirus type 1 and echovirus type 25. It was suggested that cross-linkages between capsid polypeptides of the poliovirus were caused by accessibility to GTA of lysine residues of VP1 and VP3. Furthermore, the three-dimensional structure of the poliovirus shows that two exposed loops, one in VP1 and the other in VP3, contain lysine residues immediately accessible to GTA [306], and that such a disposition might account for the intermolecular cross-linkage of the two polypeptides [305]. Capsid proteins of the poliovirus VP1, VP2 and VP3 contained, respectively, 15, 5 and 10 lysine residues [307], and GTA cross-links essentially with the ε-amino groups of lysine residues of proteins [303]. Similarly the amino acid sequence of the hepatitis A virus structural protein VP1 was shown to contain lysine [308] and as such is also likely to react with GTA. In echovirus type 25, variations of the location of

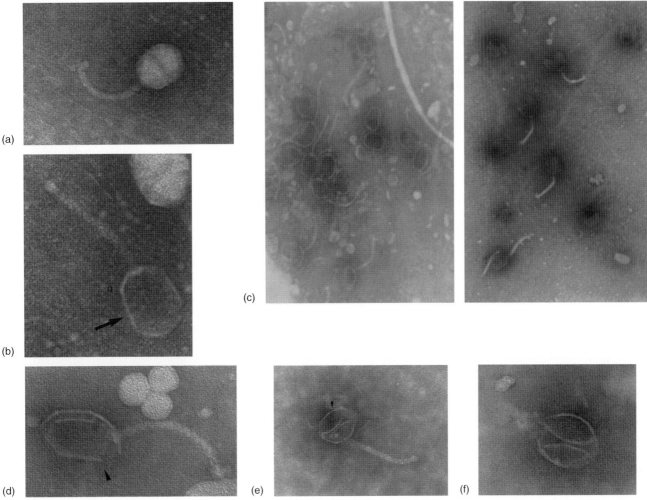

Figure 9.5 Electron microscopical evidence of viral damage by microbicides [285]. (a) Intact F116 bacteriophage with distinct and well-defined head and tail structures. (b) Intact F116 structure with empty head (arrow), typically observed after treatment with glutaraldehyde. (c) F116 with fractured head, typically observed after treatment with a quaternary ammonium compound or alcohol. (d) Close-up details of F116 with fractured head (arrowhead). (e) F116 with folded head structure (arrowhead), typically observed after treatement with alcohol or phenol. (f) F116 with folder head and damaged tail, typically observed after treatment with phenol or peracetic acide. Magnifications: (a,b,d–f) ×400,000; (c) ×80,000.

lysine residues on the VP1 capsid proteins [309] might account for small conformational changes explaining the intratypic differences in GTA susceptibility [310].

Interactions with viral markers

Howard and colleagues [311] showed that a GTA-based disinfectant (Kohrsolin) reduced the activity of HBV DNA polymerase and possibly denatured HBcAg. The aldehyde-based compound was also shown to affect the structure of HBV particles. It was suggested that chemical changes of markers (e.g. DNA polymerase, HBcAg) might precede gross morphological changes.

Interactions with viral nucleic acid

Bailly *et al.* [293] showed that 1% GTA was ineffective against the poliovirus type 1 RNA. Similarly, Maillard *et al.* [289] showed that the nucleic acid extracted from the capsid of the *P. aeruginosa* F116 bacteriophage remained undamaged after a challenge with 1% GTA. However, another study demonstrated that low concentrations of GTA (0.05–1%) were sufficient to inhibit the transduction ability of the phage F116 [287]. It was emphasized that the inhibition of transduction might be caused by the alteration of a protein target responsible for the process, rather than an alteration of the phage genome. Charrel and colleagues [154] showed that a 2% GTA formulation produced an extensive genomolysis of the HCV genome. Differences in protocol used and a formulation effect might account for such a discrepancy in results since the crosslinking ability of GTA, which is used extensively as a fixative, notably for EM preparation, cannot explain extensive lysis to the DNA structure.

Mechanisms of action of ortho-*phthalaldehyde*

Ortho-phthalaldehyde (OPA) is a broad-spectrum dialdehyde, although its virucidal activity has not been particularly studied [312]. OPA produces a 3-log$_{10}$ reduction in adenovirus type 8 viability after 1 min of exposure [213] and is virucidal against the duck hepatitis B virus and bovine viral diarrhea virus after 5 min contact time [313]. OPA is also a cross-linking agent, although to a lesser extent than GTA. OPA is thought to penetrate bacterial cells more effectively than GTA, accounting for a better and more rapid bactericidal efficacy [314]. The virucidal mechanism(s) of action of OPA has not been studied, although it is possible that the dialdehyde cross-links the capsid surface and/or penetrates the nucleocapsid, thus damaging structural and functional proteins.

Halogen-releasing agents

Chlorine compounds

In the healthcare setting, sodium hypochlorite is often the microbicide of choice in conditions where hazardous agents are known to be, or suspected of being, present [315]. High sodium hypochlorite concentrations are used with 10,000 ppm available chlorine for blood spillages and 1000 ppm for surface disinfection for surfaces contaminated with viruses other than hepatitis viruses and HIV [316, 317]. Where viruses such as Lassa or Ebola are suspected to be present, a concentration of 5000 ppm for emergency use has been recommended. In the USA, the Occupational Safety and Health Administration states that blood spills must be disinfected using an EPA-registered tuberculocidal disinfectant, a disinfectant with HBV/HIV inhibition claim, or a solution of 5.25% sodium hypochlorite diluted between 1:10 and 1:100 with water [318].

In a number of studies, chlorine was shown to inactivate the viral genome. Olivieri and colleagues [319] showed that chlorine inactivated naked f2 RNA at the same rate as it did in the intact phage. Similarly, it was observed that poliovirus type 1 RNA was degraded into fragments within the capsid after exposure to chlorine (1 mg/l). Taylor and Butler [180] suggested that chlorine dioxide and bromine chloride affected poliovirus viral nucleic acid since the structure of the virus remained unaltered. Indeed poliovirus inactivation preceded any severe morphological changes following exposure to a high concentration of chlorine [180]. Degradation of poliovirus RNA as well a viral inactivation was shown to be concentration dependent when challenged with chlorine dioxide [178]. It was found that the untranslated regions 5'- and 3'-UTR of the poliovirus genome, their spatial organization (native vs. denatured), size and location, affected the amount and severity of the damage caused by chlorine dioxide [178]. Likewise, chlorine has also been shown to inactivate the HAV genome, which resulted in the loss of the 5″ non-translated regions [155]. Charrel *et al.* [154] demonstrated severe damage to the HCV genome following hypochlorite treatment.

Other investigations highlighted, however, the lack of activity of chlorine against the viral genome. O'Brien and Newman [320] showed that chlorine had no effect on RNA extracted from poliovirus. Floyd *et al.* [321] showed that the capsid of the poliovirus type 1 was broken following challenge with similar concentrations of chlorine. Tenno *et al.* [322] suggested that the mechanism of action of chlorine against the poliovirus was via slight structural alteration of the capsid, since viral RNA remained infectious after virus inactivation by the microbicide. Alvarez and O'Brien [323] showed that poliovirus RNA was released from the capsid as a result, and not as a cause, of virus inactivation by chlorine. They suggested that the apparent discrepancy in chlorine virucidal effect resulted from variations in chlorine concentrations used in the different studies. Chlorine has been shown to cause gross morphological alterations in HBV structure [299] and other viruses [324]. Rodgers *et al.* [325] found that sodium hypochlorite rapidly removed the outer coat of rotavirus. Sodium hypochlorite (0.525% v/v) has been shown to severely alter HBV markers such as HbsAg and HBcAg [300]. Page *et al.* [156] investigated the inactivation kinetic of adenovirus type 2 exposed to chlorine. A complex three-phase inactivation was observed. It was hypothesized that the first phase, characterized by a rapid inactivation rate, corresponds to damage to coat proteins containing amine, thiol and other functional groups by hypochlorous acid. The second and third phase, characterized by a slower rate of inactivation, might be associated with conformational change of proteins and genome damage caused by reaction with secondary oxidizing species, such as organic chloramines.

The mechanism of action of hypochlorite might also be dependent on the type of viruses. Nuanualsuwan and Cliver [326] observed that hypochlorite significantly damaged the genome of the poliovirus type 1 and feline calcivirus, and significantly reduced the infectivity of both viruses. However, hepatitis A virus treatment with hypochlorite resulted in no measurable damage to the viral genome, although viral infectivity was reduced [326]. Similar results were observed with poliovirus type 1 and the Norwalk virus treated with monochloramine [125].

Whether chlorine and sodium hypochlorite damage viral RNA before virus structural alterations or not, these microbicides were shown to be rapidly virucidal at low concentrations against a number of viruses such as HIV [327, 328], pseudorabies, parvoviridae [79], rotavirus [80, 150, 329] and picornaviridae [114, 145, 157, 294, 329].

Iodine compounds

Taylor and Butler [180] showed that iodine caused severe morphological changes to the poliovirus structure. Gross morphological damage after virus treatment with iodine was also observed by Shirai and colleagues [324]. The conformational change of MS2 virus treated by iodine might be reversible and might result in an increase in virion infectivity when iodine is removed [330]. The larger atomic radius of iodine might account for the structural alterations, although it might prevent its diffusion through the capsid to possible target sites inside the virion. The mechanism of action of iodine appeared largely to affect the viral capsid rather than viral nucleic acid. Indeed, Alvarez and O'Brien [331] proposed that iodine might inactivate poliovirus by disrupting the protein coat rather than the nucleic acid. Olivieri *et al.* [319] showed that the target site of iodine on the f2 coliphage was the amino acid tyrosine of the capsid moiety, with almost no effect on f2 viral RNA. The amino acids tyrosine and histidine of the viral coat have been proposed as the specific targets for iodine [332, 333]. Sriwilaijaroen *et al.* [183] showed that povidone-iodine inactivated the human and avian influenza A viruses by altering viral hemagglutinin and viral neuraminidase catalytic hydrolysis, preventing viral entry into the host.

Bromine compounds

Sharp and colleagues [334] suggested that bromine (0.2–0.4 mg/l) damaged the capsid proteins of reovirus type 3 and possibly induced a loss of RNA. Olivieri *et al.* [319] proposed that the primary site of bromine inactivation was more likely to be the protein moiety of the f2 coliphage. Similarly, Keswick *et al.* [181] showed that high concentrations of bromine chloride (10–20 mg/l) produced a structural degradation of the poliovirus. It was also found that poliovirus RNA remained infectious after treatment with bromine chloride (0.3 mg/l). However, it was suggested that structural degradation and loss of infectivity were not necessarily correlated, since lower concentrations of bromine chloride (0.3–5 mg/l) inactivated the poliovirus without causing structural alterations.

Biguanides

Chlorhexidine

Chlorhexidine is a membrane active agent, which has been shown to affect the cytoplasmic membrane of bacteria, inducing the leakage of intracellular components (see Chapter 5). Chlorhexidine is likely to interact with the viral envelope, inducing envelope lysis and the release of the viral capsid (see Figures 9.3 and 9.4). This explains why chlorhexidine is virucidal against enveloped viruses [182, 184, 268, 269, 335] but not necessarily against non-enveloped viruses [80, 93, 145, 294, 336]. The lack of activity of chlorhexidine against non-enveloped viruses might be caused by a reversible adsorption of the molecule to the viral capsid. A structural study with the phage F116 showed that chlorhexidine diacetate (1%) caused little structural damage to the phage [285]. Similarly, phage proteins [288] and nucleic acid [289] were not affected when phage particles were challenged with the bisbiguanide. An energy-dispersive analysis of X-rays (EDAX) study showed that the chlorhexidine molecules did not bind strongly and did not penetrate inside the phage particles [286]. However, low concentrations of chlorhexidine probably interacted with some component of the viral capsid or tail, resulting in an inhibition of the transduction ability of F116 [287].

Polyhexamethylene biguanides and other biguanides

Polyhexamethylene biguanides (PHMBs) and substituted biguanides have been shown to be virucidal against enveloped viruses [337, 338]. Their efficacy might depend on the test conditions and viral strains. Valluri *et al.* [270] observed that PHMB (200 ppm)

was active against the herpes simplex virus (HSV) *in vitro* but not when tested *in vivo*. Such results might be explained by the partial inactivation of PHMB by soiling (fluid) rather than a lack of virucidal activity. Krebs *et al.* [265] observed difference in PHMB inactivation of HIV depending on whether the virus was associated with cells or not. In addition, it was shown that different strains of HIV required different concentrations of PHMB to be inactivated [265]. The length of the alkyl chain in substituted biguanides affects virucidal efficacy [338], although the reason for such a difference in activity is not clear.

Biguanides including PHMB have been described to have limited virucidal efficacy against non-enveloped viruses [266, 267, 270, 339]. Interestingly the activity of PHMB against the MS2 bacteriophage was found to be temperature dependent. Microbicide activity can increase with temperature and can be measured by the temperature coefficient Q_{10} (see Chapter 3). However, in the study by Pinto *et al.* [266], the increase in PHMB activity with rising temperature was linked to a decrease in the presence of viral aggregates. It is, however, possible that a high temperature produced some conformational changes of the viral capsid, increasing the sensitivity of MS2 to the microbicide, although this was not observed using EM on bacteriophages exposed to PHMB [267].

The mechanisms of action of PHMB against viruses have not been described. It is likely that PHMB will cause lysis of the viral envelope in a mechanism similar to that of chlorhexidine [14], although Thakkar *et al.* [340] described a specific interaction between PHMB and HIV-1, whereby the biguanide inhibited virus infection by interacting with the HIV-1 co-receptor CXCR4 on the host cell. PHMB (800 ppm) was shown to affect F116 bacteriophage structural protein and to cause structural alteration to the capsid, resulting notably in a broken head [339] (see Figure 9.5c,d). Capsid damage in the MS2 bacteriophage was also observed, although no alterations were detected to the primary structure of capsid proteins even though PHMB was shown to bind capsid proteins [267]. In adenovirus type 5 PHMB (800 ppm) was shown to disrupt specifically the minor coat protein VI, which mediates the rupture of the endosomal membrane to allow the entry of the virus into the cytoplasm [339].

A mechanism of action has been proposed for PHMB interaction with non-enveloped viruses [339]. Most viruses are negatively charged at the pH at which PHMB is used (i.e. pH 7 to 8) according to their isoelectric point (pI). Initially electrostatic and then hydrophobic forces seemed to be involved in the attachment of PHMB to the viral capsid. Such an interaction leads to an increase in viral hydrophobicity and to the formation of viral aggregates [267]. This has been demonstrated with a strong interaction of PHMB with the viral capsid and a concurrent increase in viral aggregates [267, 339]. With small non-enveloped virus such as the MS2 bacteriophage, PHMB inactivation was shown to be temperature dependent [266]. After the formation of viral aggregates following PHMB exposure, small conformational changes to the quaternary and tertiary structures occur and result in a small decrease in virus viability. As temperature

Table 9.2 Viral inactivation energy and susceptibility to microbicides (from [136, 195, 280, 336, 339, 341–352].

Virus	MW (Da)	Size (nm)	Envelope	Structural proteins	Inactivation energy (KJ/ mol)	Log$_{10}$ reduction in viability (exposure time in minutes)		
						Biguanide	QAC	Iodine
MS2	3.6×10^6	25	No	2	50.5	1.5 (30)	0.23 (0.6)	2.74 (0.5)
Adenovirus type 5	150×10^6	100	No	11	88	1 (30)	2.74 (30)	2.2 (15)
Poliovirus type 1	6.8×10^6	30	No	4	145	<3	0.83 (10)	5 (10)
Coronavirus	400×10^6	120–160	Yes	5	30	2.1 (15)	0.5 (30)	>4 (2)

QAC, quaternary ammonium compound.

increases, the higher thermal energy (i.e. high kinetic energy) causes bacteriophages to disperse uniformly and increases PHMB interaction with more viral particles, increasing virucidal activity. With larger viruses, such as the adenovirus type 5, another mechanism of inactivation occurs [339]. Following the formation of viral aggregates, PHMB interacts with the minor coat protein VI, causing a precise breakage in the capsid of a limited number of viral particles. An increase in temperature was shown to have only a small effect on virucidal activity [339]. Such a variation in PHMB virucidal activity between MS2 and adenovirus might be explained by a difference in their inactivation energy, 50.5 kJ/mol and 88 kJ/mol, respectively. Thus a higher kinetic energy needs to be produced to breakup the viral structure of adenovirus type 5 [339].

Table 9.2 shows the inactivation energy of four different viruses and their susceptibility to biguanides and an iodine-based microbicide. A high energy level is required to inactivate poliovirus and adenovirus, which are usually considered to be less susceptible to virucides. Such a theory might be useful in predicting virus susceptibility to microbicides and which mechanism of action is involved in breaking up the capsid, although more examples are needed.

Quaternary ammonium compounds

Quaternary ammonium compounds (QACs) are surface active agents and, like the biguanides, they are more active against lipophilic viruses [80, 201, 237, 324, 327]. QAC activity against non-enveloped viruses might be limited [238]. The mechanisms of virucidal action of QACs have been poorly studied. Cetylpyridinium chloride (CPC) produced a severe alteration of the capsid of the F116 bacteriophage [285](see Figure 9.5c,d), as well as alteration of the phage–protein band pattern [288] and the transduction ability of the phage [287]. However, CPC had no effect on the phage genome [289]. Similarly, another QAC, cetrimide, was shown to alter the structure of rotavirus [325].

Alcohols

There is little information on the virucidal mechanisms of action of alcohols, despite the recent increase in the number of products available for hand antisepsis. Their activity against

principally enveloped viruses [202] suggests that the viral envelope might be a major target site. Indeed, several alcohols have been shown to react with the bacterial cytoplasmic membrane (see Chapter 5).

Their activity against non-enveloped viruses might be partially due to an alteration of viral substructure. Ethanol was shown to remove rapidly the outer coat of the rotavirus [325]. Ethanol and isopropanol altered structurally the capsid of the phage F116 in a similar manner, producing a high number of folded and fractured capsids [285](see Figure 9.5e). However, alcohol did not affect the substructures of HBV [353]. An alcohol-based disinfectant (Sterillium) was also found to reduce the activity of HBV DNA polymerase and, to a lesser extent, possibly to denature HBcAg [311]. Ethanol and isopropanol were shown to be ineffective against the F116 nucleic acid [289]. Ito et al. [354] observed that HBV DNA was still isolated after treatment with ethanol. They postulated that the decrease of HBV infectivity by ethanol was caused by the inhibition of virus binding to hepatocytes.

Phenolics

The virucidal activity of phenolic compounds has not been widely investigated, and some reports are sometimes controversial [87]. Phenols including some essential oils have been shown to be virucidal against lipid-enveloped viruses [80, 185, 268, 355]. Phenols have not been described to have a high efficacy against non-enveloped viruses, although complete inactivation of norovirus was achieved only at a concentration of only 0.17% in one study [196].

Phenolic compounds might interact with the envelope of viruses in a similar way to their interaction with the prokaryotic membrane (see Chapter 5). Investigations on the efficacy and mechanisms of action of essential oil-based products against several enveloped and non-enveloped viruses highlighted that the observed virucidal activity was probably related to damage caused to the viral envelope [356–358]. Maillard et al. showed that phenol did not alter the nucleic acid or the transduction process [287, 289] of the P. aeruginosa F116 bacteriophage, although it might have a wide range of effects on capsid proteins, as demonstrated in an EM investigation [285] (see Figure 9.5c,f).

Oxidizing agents

Oxidizing agents (peracetic acid, hydrogen peroxide, ozone) are highly reactive microbicides, which are likely to react with, and damage, proteins of the viral nucleocapsid and viral envelope by oxidizing sulfur and amino groups (see Chapter 5).

Peracetic acid has a wide spectrum of virucidal action including non-enveloped viruses [87, 151, 213, 217, 247, 253, 359]. However, some viruses have been shown to be more resilient to peracetic acid [145]. Peracetic acid severely damages the structure of vaccinia virus and adenovirus [253] and produces distinct alterations of the F116 phage structure [285](see Figure 9.5f). Peracetic acid was shown to damage specific F116 phage proteins [288] and its nucleic acid [289]. It completely denatures adenovirus hexon proteins at a high concentration (0.5%) following 60 min of exposure. Lower concentrations resulted in partial degradation of the adenovirus proteins [360]. However, it failed to inactive adenovirus genome even after 1 h of exposure at a concentration of 0.5% [280].

The virucidal activity and mechanisms of action of hydrogen peroxide have not been widely studied. In addition, there might be some important differences in activity and mechanisms of action between the liquid and gaseous forms of hydrogen peroxide (see Chapter 2). Poliovirus was found to be resistant to liquid hydrogen peroxide [294]. Vapor hydrogen peroxide at a low concentration was virucidal (6-$\log_{10}$ reduction in viability) against MS2 bacteriophage dried onto a stainless disk within 60 min [361]. Hydrogen peroxide vapor (10 ppm) was shown to be virucidal against H1N1 influenza viruses [248]. However, liquid hydrogen peroxide failed to reduce the infectivity of H5N1 avian influenza virus [185].

Ozone is a powerful oxidant that has been used for disinfection (see Chapter 2). Lipid peroxidation, caused by primary and secondary ozone-mediated reactive oxygen species, appeared to be involved in the deterioration of enveloped viruses, such as herpes simplex virus and vaccinia virus [258]. Ozone was also found to react strongly with proteins, damaging the nucleocapsid of enveloped and non enveloped viruses through oxidative changes [258]. Riesser et al. [362] reported that the capsid protein of the poliovirus type 2 was damaged following ozonation, subsequently inhibiting virus host cell specificity and virus uptake. DeMik and DeGroot [363] also demonstrated damage to the coliphage ØX174 protein coat following treatment with ozone. Deleterious alterations of the bacteriophage DNA were also reported. It has been suggested that ozone had damaging effects on purine and pyrimidine bases and reacted more strongly with DNA than with RNA [364]. Similarly, studies investigating the effect of ozone against the bacteriophage T4 showed that the oxidizing agent damaged its capsid protein, releasing the viral nucleic acid, which was subsequently inactivated [365]. Kim et al. [366] showed that treatment of the f2 coliphage with an ozone concentration of 0.8 mg/l for 30 s resulted in broken capsids and damaged RNA. The extent of capsid damage was concentration and contact time dependent. Mudd et al. [367] reported that alteration of proteins challenged with ozone was caused by a reaction with cysteine, tryptophane and methionine. Damage to the f2 capsid was proposed as a consequence of the alteration of these amino acids, contained in the coat proteins [366]. Interestingly, it was demonstrated that RNA extracted from the phage prior to ozone treatment was less susceptible than RNA within ozonated bacteriophages. Such a damaging effect might be explained by the interaction between capsid protein and viral RNA, and the generation of shearing forces contributing to RNA damage during the breaking up of the capsid. Similar findings were observed with poliovirus exposed to ozone. Roy et al. [368] showed that two polypeptide chains of the poliovirus capsid, VP1 and VP2, were damaged by ozonation, although the RNA breakage into short chains appeared to be the major cause of poliovirus inactivation. Looking at the kinetics of inactivation of enteroviruses by ozone, it is thought that ozone penetrates the capsid and reaches the nucleic acid core where damage occurs [369].

Metallic salts

Silver salts

The virucidal activity of silver has been demonstrated not only against several enveloped viruses, such as the herpesvirus, vaccinia virus, influenza A virus and pseudorabies virus, but also against bovine enteroviruses [370]. The virucidal properties of silver might be explained by the oxidation and denaturation of sulphydryl groups. It has been postulated that viral inactivation might result from metal ions binding electron donor groups on proteins and nucleic acids [370]. Silver has also been shown to bind phage DNA [371, 372], and phage inactivation by silver nitrate might be explained by its cross-linking ability with the DNA helix [373]. Since DNA and RNA viruses are affected by silver, its virucidal mechanism of action might be more complex than just an effect on viral nucleic acid. An alteration of capsid proteins is likely, especially since the metallic salt has to penetrate within the capsid to alter the viral genome.

Silver-based nanotechnology

There is a growing interest in using silver-based nanotechnology for water disinfection and other disinfection processes. The microbicidal activity of silver nanoparticles seemed to be related to degradation of bacterial lipopolysaccharides, resulting in an increase in membrane permeability, better penetration and subsequent DNA damage [374]. Silver nanoparticles have also been shown to be virucidal [375, 376] although their size and spatial arrangement appeared to affect efficacy [377]. In HIV-1, silver nanoparticles inhibited the virus from binding to the host cells by interacting with the sulfur-bearing residues of the gp120 glycoprotein knob, indicating reaction with thiol groups [375].

Copper salts

The virucidal action of copper ions might involve the binding of copper to thiol or other groups in proteins, leading to an alteration of the protein complex [370] and inhibition of protein/enzymatic function [378]. Copper ion was shown to be virucidal against avian influenza virus (H9N2) reducing viability by 3 to 4-log$_{10}$ within 3 and 6h, respectively, and caused morphological changes to the viral structure [378]. Copper ions have also been reported to have a strong affinity with DNA and to denature DNA reversibly in low-ionic-strength solutions. There are several reports showing that the combination of copper (II) with other compounds produces cleavage of viral nucleic acid in R17 (i.e. via RNA degradation), ØX174 (i.e. via ssDNA scission), λ DNA bacteriophages (i.e. via cleavage) and poliovirus RNA (i.e. via scission) [370]. Samuni et al. [379] also reported that the action of copper (II) resulted in impaired phage adsorption and DNA injection. In addition, it was suggested that copper ions might affect viral capsid proteins by site-specific Fenton mechanisms producing hydroxyl radicals [380]. It should be noted that the ability of heavy metal ions to react with viral nucleic acid depends strongly upon the accessibility of viral nucleic acid to these ions.

Other compounds
Acids
Viruses are usually sensitive to low pH. Citric and phosphoric acids have been shown to inactivate foot-and-mouth disease virus [381] and hydrochloric acid inactivates human rotavirus and vesicular stomatitis virus [87]. Organic acids, such as salicylic acid, pyroglutamic acid and glutaric acid, have virucidal activity against rhinovirus for up to 3–6h after its application on hands [227]. Because the viral capsid is composed mainly of proteins, it is not surprising that a variation of pH will produce a conformational change of the viral capsid. However, such a conformational change might sometimes be associated with a decrease in viral susceptibility (see above). A drastic change in the conformational state might ultimately alter capsid integrity. Giranda et al. [228] showed that the mechanism of action of acids is based on the interaction with capsid proteins in rhinovirus, specifically with VP4 protein, inducing conformational changes and a loss of infectivity.

Ethylene oxide
Ethylene oxide (EtO) gas is used for the gaseous sterilization of heat labile products. EtO gas was shown to inactivate the bacteriophage ØX174 [278] and several viruses (HIV-1, bovine viral diarrhea, reovirus type 3, duck hepatitis B virus, poliomyelitis, canine parvovirus) [30]. EtO gas is an alkylating microbicide thath interacts with the amino, carboxyl, sulfhydryl and hydroxyl groups in bacterial proteins and with nucleic acids (see Chapter 5). It is likely that its virucidal efficacy is based on the same mechanisms.

Other virucidal processes

Physical agents such as heat and irradiation can inactivate viruses. Thermal processes are used for eliminating viruses such as HIV from bloodborne and other pharmaceutical and medicinal products. Most viruses are sensitive to heat and are readily inactivated following exposure at 60°C for 30 min or less [382], although some such as the hepatitis B virus, hepatitis A virus [383] and adenovirus type 2 and 5 [384], can survive long exposure to higher temperature, probably because of the number of viral particles present at one time. UV and ionizing radiations (e.g. γ-rays, accelerated electrons) can also be used to eliminate viruses, following alteration/damage to the viral genome (see Chapter 15).

Viral resistance to microbicides

The extent to which viruses can escape a disinfection process has not been widely studied. Most of the studies available concern virus survival following disinfection in practice, where an unsatisfactory cleaning or disinfection regime has been used, leading to the presence of soiling which ultimately affects the activity of microbicides [195, 385]. However, there are a few factors associated with the virus that might lead to a slight or large increase in viral resistance to disinfection (Figure 9.6), the most important of which is viral aggregation.

Viral aggregation
Viruses are often found aggregated within, or when released from, their host cells [86, 386, 387]. Viruses in body fluids and on naturally contaminated surfaces are often found as clumps or aggregates [86]. The shape of viral inactivation kinetics might indicate the presence of viral aggregates [151, 388]. A number of factors affect the formation of viral aggregates: (i) virus species and serotype; (ii) viral surface charge; (iii) virus concentration; (iv) type of microbicide; and (v) chemical properties of the surrounding medium, such pH, ionic strength and the nature of ions [389]. The isoelectric point (pI) of the virus is an important contributing factor, which correlates well with clumping [339, 390]. Viruses located at the center of an aggregate are more likely to withstand the deleterious effect of microbicides as they are less accessible to the microbicide [14]. It has been postulated that, for spherical viruses, clumps containing more than 16 virions might show some resistance to microbicides as only 16 spheres identical in diameter to the virion can confer protection to a central virion [86]. The size of the viral aggregates is certainly important in the development of resistance to disinfection, as observed by Sharp et al. [334] with reovirus challenged with bromine, and by Jensen et al. [391] with coxsackie virus following chlorination. The microbicide itself might induce the formation of viral aggregates. Pinto et al. [267, 339] showed that the size of viral aggregates increases with increasing concentrations of PHMB, reaching micrometer size with 800 ppm of the biguanide. Keswick et al. [329] showed that the presence of viral aggregates was likely to be responsible for the resistance of Norwalk virus to chlorination (Figure 9.6). Persistence of poliovirus infectivity after formaldehyde treatment has been associated with clumping [392]. Copper and silver ions might also promote viral aggregation [393]. It has been reported

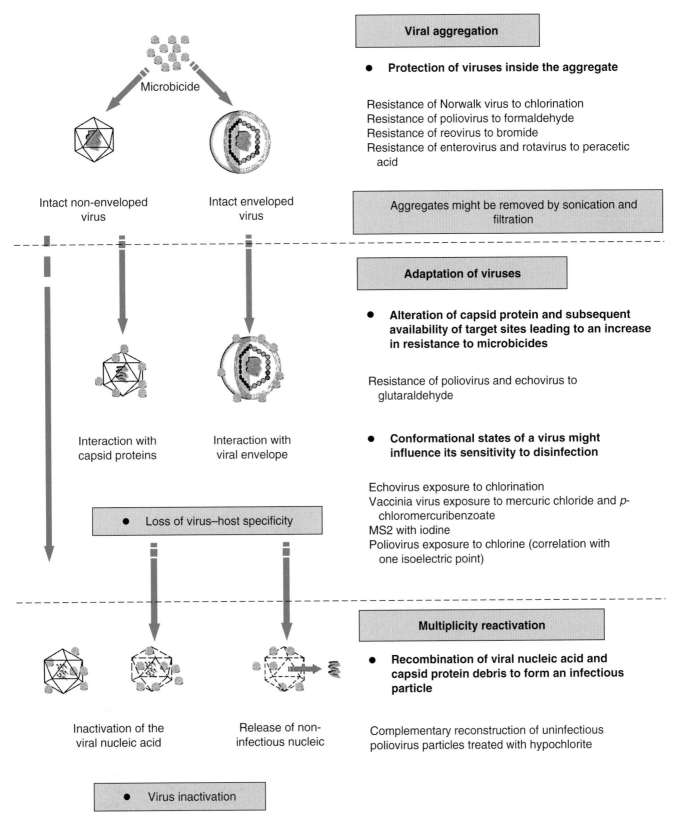

Figure 9.6 Possible mechanisms of viral resistance to microbicides.

that divalent and trivalent cations can induce the formation of aggregates [394, 395]. The presence of viral aggregates has a practical implication for the results of efficacy tests, as clumping might overestimate the activity of a virucide; that is one viral clump might be identified as one infective particle [267, 396].

Other mechanisms

Adaptation of viruses to microbicides

Viruses might adapt to some extent to new environmental conditions and become genetically stable. However, a genetic rather than an environmental basis for virus resistance to disinfectants has not yet been established. Change in virus susceptibility could occur via a morphological change of the viral structure, via an altered interaction with the host cell or an increase in virus protection as discussed above (Figure 9.6). The presence of a residual concentration of a microbicide is of particular interest. Repeated exposures to inadequate levels of a disinfectant have been shown to produce poliovirus isolates with a decreased susceptibility to chlorine [158]. Maillard *et al.* [397] reported the adaptation of F116 bacteriophages to increasing concentrations of sodium hypochlorite solution. Chambon *et al.* [398] suggested that the resistance to GTA (0.1%) of two echovirus 25 isolates was due to the difference in cross-linking formation of the capsid polypeptides.

Viruses also exist in different forms, depending on the pH. A change of the isoelectric point is likely to affect the availability of target sites, thus affecting microbicide activity [86] as well as promoting clumping. Vrisjen *et al.* [399] suggested that some viruses have several isoelectric points and there is evidence of correlation between one of the isoelectric points and the sensitivity to disinfection [400]. Young and Sharp [401] reported that echovirus had three conformational states. The virucidal efficiency of chlorine disinfection depended on the viral structural state. Poliovirus type 1 possesses two isoelectric points associated with two conformational states, A and B, the latter being related to virus inactivation [402].

Removal of the selective pressure might also result in an increase of virus infectivity. This phenomenon of apparent rebound might relate to a mechanism of action involving a reversible conformational change (see Figure 9.4) and was observed with vaccinia virus treated with mercuric chloride and *p*-chloromercuribenzoate [403] and with MS2 virus treated with iodine [330].

Even if the selection of viruses which are genetically more resistant to disinfectants is subsequently shown to be a common phenomenon, it is unlikely to be more important for virus protection against disinfectants than the nature and protection of the surrounding organic and particulate matter.

Multiplicity reactivation

Young and Sharp [401] noticed that clumping of an echovirus after partial viral inactivation by hypochlorite significantly increased the viral concentration. The clumping of non-infectious virions, producing random damage to their capsid proteins or their nucleic acid, can result in complementary reconstruction of an infectious particle by hybridization of the gene pool of the

inactivated virions. This phenomenon, first described by Luria in 1947, is the basis of multiplicity reactivation [370] (see Figure 9.6) and underlines the necessity of rendering the viral nucleic acid non-infectious [86].

Conclusions

The selection and use of microbicides for the control of microorganisms, including viruses, require a clear understanding of the potency and limitations of individual chemical formulations [38]. They also require knowledge of the material that has to be decontaminated and assurance that its treatment with the selected chemical will not compromise its subsequent safety and integrity [404]. It must also be re-emphasized that contamination of surfaces with organic or inorganic soils or the presence of organic materials in solution will tend to interfere with and limit the virucidal potential of many microbicides, as well as shielding contaminating viruses from microbicide contact. This is particularly important since some viruses, such as HBV, have a very low minimum infective dose. Finally, the reader is cautioned about extrapolating potential for microbicide effectiveness in the field from *in vitro* studies conducted on relatively pure virus preparations. Similarly, the effectiveness of topical agents should be assessed under clinically relevant conditions, using *in vivo* or *ex vivo* systems whenever possible.

The development of an ideal testing procedure for virucidal disinfectants presents many technical problems. A suitable test virus, easily grown to high titers and representative of a given family, with appropriate attributes of stability and safety, is not easily identifiable. Because of the diversity of viruses encountered in human and veterinary medicine, test viruses representing the more important families should be included in a standardized protocol. Virus concentration, contact time, temperature, bioburden and the method of exposing virus to disinfectant should be clearly specified.

A better understanding of virucide interaction with the virus particle is needed. At present, several tests rely on the detection of viral markers such as antigens, nucleic acid or viral enzymes, although viral infectivity might not relate to the inactivation to viral markers. Likewise, structural damage to the capsid might not reflect a loss in infectivity. Too few studies on the mechanisms of action of virucides have highlighted that chemical disinfectants might not necessarily inactivate viral nucleic acid, although damage to the viral capsid might be extensive. This is particularly pertinent as the nucleic acid of some viruses is known to be infectious. Furthermore, studies of the mechanisms of action of microbicides against viruses have highlighted the difficulty in selecting an adequate viral model. The use of bacteriophages, however, offers many advantages and they constitute excellent tools for studying the efficacy and mechanisms of action of virucides.

Despite the complexity of the task, study of the mechanisms of action of microbicides against viruses remains important if the overall virucidal activity of such agents and our understanding of viral resistance to disinfection are to improve.

References

1 Fendrick, A.M. *et al.* (2003) The economic burden of non-influenza-related viral respiratory tract infection in the United States. *Archives of Internal Medicine*, **163**, 487–494.

2 Nwachuku, N. and Gerba, C.P. (2006) Health risks of enteric viral infections in children. *Review in Environmental Contamination and Toxicology*, **186**, 1–56.

3 Sattar, S.A. (2007) Hierarchy of susceptibility of viruses to environmental surface disinfectants: a predictor of activity against new and emerging viral pathogens. *Journal of AOAC International*, **90**, 1655–1658.

4 Tumpey, T.M. and Belser, J.A. (2009) Resurrected pandemic influenza viruses. *Annual Reviews of Microbiology*, **63**, 79–98.

5 Bergonzini, V. *et al.* (2010) View and review on viral oncology research. *Infectious Agents and Cancer*, **24**, 5–11.

6 Johnson, R.T. and Power, C. (2008) Emerging issues in neurovirology: new viruses, diagnostic tools, and therapeutics. *Neurologic Clinics*, **26**, 855–864.

7 Chen, D.S. (2010) Toward elimination and eradication of hepatitis B. *Journal of Gastroenterology and Hepatology*, **25**, 19–25.

8 Ferri, C. *et al.* (2010) The A, B, Cs of viral hepatitis in the biologic era. *Current Opinion in Rheumatology*, **22**, 443–450.

9 Sattar, S.A. (2005) Viruses as nosocomial pathogens: the environmental connection. *Hygiene and Medizin*, **30**, 189–194.

10 Graham, D.Y. *et al.* (1987) Minimal infective dose of rotavirus. *Archives of Virology*, **92**, 261–271.

11 Lauring, A.S. *et al.* (2010) Rationalizing the development of live attenuated virus vaccines. *Nature Biotechnology*, **28**, 573–579.

12 Das, K. *et al.* (2010) Structures of influenza A proteins and insights into antiviral drug targets. *Nature Structural and Molecular Biology*, **17**, 530–538.

13 Shafer, R.W. and Schapiro, J.M. (2008) HIV-1 drug resistance mutations: an updated framework for the second decade of HAART. *AIDS Review*, **10**, 67–84.

14 Maillard, J.-Y. (2001) Virus susceptibility to biocides: an understanding. *Reviews in Medical Microbiology*, **12**, 63–74.

15 Kramer, A. *et al.* (2006) How long do nosocomial pathogens persist on inanimate surfaces? A systematic review. *BMC Infectious Diseases*, **6**, 130.

16 Boone, S.A. and Gerba, C.P. (2007) Significance of fomites in the spread of respiratory and enteric viral disease. *Applied and Environmental Microbiology*, **73**, 1687–1696.

17 Tiwari, A. *et al.* (2006) Survival of two avian respiratory viruses on porous and nonporous surfaces. *Avian Diseases*, **50**, 284–287.

18 Mocé-Llivina, L. *et al.* (2006) A membrane-based quantitative carrier test to assess the virucidal activity of disinfectants and persistence of viruses on porous fomites. *Journal of Virological Methods*, **135**, 49–55.

19 Clay, S. *et al.* (2006) Survival on uncommon fomites of feline calicivirus, a surrogate of noroviruses. *American Journal of Infection Control*, **34**, 41–43.

20 Müller, A. *et al.* (2008) Stability of human metapneumovirus and human coronavirus NL63 on medical instruments and in the patient environment. *Journal of Hospital Infection*, **69**, 406–408.

21 Sattar, S.A. (2004) Microbicides and the environmental control of nosocomial viral infections. *Journal of Hospital Infection*, **56** (Suppl.), 64–69.

22 Koivunen, J. and Heinonen-Tanski, H. (2005) Inactivation of enteric microorganisms with chemical disinfectants, UV irradiation and combined chemical/UV treatments. *Water Research*, **39**, 1519–1526.

23 Thurston-Enriquez, J.A. *et al.* (2005) Inactivation of enteric adenovirus and feline calicivirus by ozone. *Water Research*, **39**, 3650–3656.

24 Springthorpe, V.S. and Sattar, S.A. (2007) Virus removal during drinking water treatment, in *Human Viruses in Water* (ed. A. Bosch), Elsevier, New York, pp. 109–126.

25 British Pharmacopoeia Commission (2010) *British Pharmacopoeia*, The Stationery Office, London.

26 Burstyn, D.G. and Hageman, T.C. (1996) Strategies for viral removal and inactivation. *Developments in Biological Standardization*, **88**, 73–79.

27 Horowitz, B. and Ben-Hur, E. (1996) Viral inactivation of blood components: recent advances. *Transfusion Clinique et Biologique*, **3**, 75–77.

28 Manabe, S. (1996) Removal of virus through novel membrane filtration method. *Developments in Biological Standardization*, **88**, 81–90.

29 Edens, A.L. (2000) Occupational safety and health administration: regulations affecting healthcare facilities, in *Disinfection, Sterilization and Antisepsis: Principles and Practice in Healthcare Facilities* (ed. W.A. Rutala), APIC, Minneapolis, pp. 49–58.

30 Moore, T.M. *et al.* (2004) Viruses adsorbed on musculoskeletal allografts are inactivated by terminal ethylene oxide disinfection. *Journal of Orthopaedic Research*, **22**, 1358–1361.

31 Walter, J.K. *et al.* (1996) Process scale considerations in evaluation studies and scale up. *Developments in Biological Standardization*, **88**, 99–108.

32 Bond, W.W. *et al.* (1981) Survival of hepatitis B virus after drying and storage for one week. *Lancet*, **1**, 550–551.

33 Ansari, S.A. *et al.* (1991) Survival and vehicular spread of human rotavirus: possible relation to seasonality of outbreaks. *Reviews in Infectious Diseases*, **13**, 448–461.

34 Abad, F.X. *et al.* (1994) Survival of enteric viruses on environmental fomites. *Applied and Environmental Microbiology*, **60**, 3704–3710.

35 Abad, F.X. *et al.* (2001) Potential role of fomites in the vehicular transmission of human astroviruses. *Applied and Environmental Microbiology*, **67**, 3904–3907.

36 Morino, H. *et al.* (2009) Inactivation of feline calicivirus, a norovirus surrogate, by chlorine dioxide gas. *Biocontrol Science*, **14**, 147–153.

37 Maillard, J.-Y. (2005) Usage of antimicrobial biocides and products in the healthcare environment: efficacy, policies, management and perceived problems. *Therapeutics and Clinical Risk Management*, **1**, 340–370.

38 Rutala, W.A. and Weber, D.J. (2000) Overview of the use of chemical germicides in healthcare, in *Disinfection, Sterilization and Antisepsis: Principles and Practice in Healthcare Facilities* (ed. W.A. Rutala), APIC, Minneapolis, pp. 1–15.

39 Cheng, F.W.T. *et al.* (2008) Prolonged shedding of respiratory syncytial virus in immunocompromised children: implication for hospital infection control. *Journal of Hospital Infection*, **70**, 383–385.

40 Naikoba, S. and Hayward, A. (2001) The effectiveness of interventions aimed at increasing handwashing in healthcare workers – a systematic review. *Journal of Hospital Infection*, **47**, 173–180.

41 Hendley, J.O. *et al.* (1973) Transmission of rhinovirus colds by self-inoculation. *New England Journal of Medicine*, **288**, 1361–1364.

42 Gwaltney, J.M. *et al.* (1978) Hand-to-hand transmission of rhinovirus colds. *Annals of Internal Medicine*, **88**, 463–467.

43 Gwaltney, J.M. and Hendel, J.O. (1982) Transmission of experimental rhinovirus infection by contaminated surfaces. *American Journal of Epidemiology*, **116**, 828–833.

44 Samadi, A.R. *et al.* (1983) Detection of rotavirus in the handwashings of attendants of children with diarrhea. *British Medical Journal*, **286**, 188.

45 Hutto, C. *et al.* (1986) Isolation of cytomegalovirus from toys and hands in a day care center. *Journal of Infectious Diseases*, **154**, 527–530.

46 Sattar, S.A. and Springthorpe, V.S. (1996) Transmission of viral infection through animate and inanimate surfaces and infection control through chemical disinfection, in *Modelling Disease Transmission and its Prevention by Disinfection* (ed. J.C. Hurst), Cambridge University Press, New York, pp. 224–257.

47 Mbithi, J.N. *et al.* (1992) Survival of hepatitis A virus on human hands and its transfer on contact with animate and inanimate surfaces. *Journal of Clinical Microbiology*, **30**, 757–763.

48 Hall, C.B. *et al.* (1980) Possible transmission by fomites of respiratory syncytial virus. *Journal of Infectious Diseases*, **141**, 98–102.

49 Ansari, S.A. *et al.* (1988) Rotavirus survival on human hands and transfer of infectious virus to animate and non-porous inanimate surfaces. *Journal of Clinical Microbiology*, **26**, 1513–1518.

50 Pancic, F. *et al.* (1980) Role of infectious secretions in the transmission of rhinovirus. *Journal of Clinical Microbiology*, **12**, 467–471.

51 Cliver, D.O. and Kostenbader, K.D. (1984) Disinfection of virus on hands for the prevention of foodborne disease. *International Journal of Food Microbiology*, **1**, 75–87.

52 Zagora, M. *et al.* (1999) Handwashing with soap or alcoholic solutions? A randomised clinical trial of its effectiveness. *American Journal of Infection Control*, **27**, 258–261.

53 Simmons, B. *et al.* (1990) The role of handwashing in prevention of endemic intensive-care unit infections. *Infection Control and Hospital Epidemiology*, **11**, 589–594.

54 Anon. (2002) Guideline for hand hygiene in health-care settings. Recommendations of the Health-care Infection Control Practices Advisory Committee and the HICPAC/SHIA/APIC/IDSA Hand Hygiene Task Force. *Morbidity and Mortality Weekly Report*, **51** (No. RR16), Centers for Disease Control and Prevention, Atlanta, GA.

55 Kampf, G. *et al.* (2009) Hand hygiene for the prevention of nosocomial infections. *Deutsches Ärzteblatt International*, **106**, 649–655.

56 Boyce, J.M. (2000) Scientific basis for handwashing with alcohol and other waterless antiseptic agents, in *Disinfection, Sterilization and Antisepsis: Principles and Practice in Healthcare Facilities* (ed. W.A. Rutala), APIC, Minneapolis, pp. 140–150.

57 Nicas, M. and Best, D. (2008) A study quantifying the hand-to-face contact rate and its potential application to predicting respiratory tract infection. *Journal of Occupational and Environmental Hygiene*, **5**, 347–352.

58 Pittet, D. (2001) Compliance with hand disinfection and its impact on hospital-acquired infections. *Journal of Hospital Infection*, **48** (Suppl. A), 40–46.

59 Cheeseman, K.E. *et al.* (2009) Evaluation of the bactericidal efficacy of three different alcohol hand rubs against 57 clinical isolates of *Staphylococcus aureus*. *Journal of Hospital Infection*, **72**, 319–325.

60 Karabay, O. *et al.* (2005) Compliance and efficacy of hand rubbing during in-hospital practice. *Medical Principles and Practice*, **14**, 313–317.

61 Schabrun, S. and Chipchase, L. (2006) Healthcare equipment as a source of nosocomial infection: a systematic review. *Journal of Hospital Infection*, **63**, 239–245.

62 Roll, M. *et al.* (1995) Nosocomial spread of hepatitis B virus (HBV) in a haemodialysis unit confirmed by HBV DNA sequencing. *Journal of Hospital Infection*, **30**, 57–63.

63 De Lamballerie, X. *et al.* (1996) Nosocomial transmission of hepatitis C virus in haemodialysis patients. *Journal of Medical Virology*, **49**, 296–302.

64 Bronowicki, J.P. *et al.* (1997) Patient-to-patient transmission of hepatitis C virus during colonoscopy. *New England Journal of Medicine*, **337**, 237–240.

65 Blanchard, A. *et al.* (1998) Molecular evidence for nosocomial transmission of human immunodeficiency virus from a surgeon to one of his patients. *Journal of Virology*, **72**, 4537–4540.

66 Rabkin, C.S. *et al.* (1988) Outbreak of echovirus 11 infection in hospitalized neonates. *Pediatric Infectious Diseases*, **7**, 186–190.

67 Rey, J.F. (1999) Endoscopic disinfection – a worldwide problem. *Journal of Clinical Gastroenterology*, **28**, 291–297.

68 Arenas, M.D. *et al.* (2001) Nosocomial transmission of hepatitis C virus: dialysis, machines, staff or both? *Nefrologia*, **21**, 476–484.

69 Muscarella, L.F. (2001) Recommendations for preventing hepatitis C virus infection: analysis of a Brooklyn endoscopy clinic's outbreak. *Infection Control and Hospital Epidemiology*, **22**, 669–669.

70 Delarocque-Astagneau, E. *et al.* (2002) Outbreak of hepatitis C virus infection in a hemodialysis unit: potential transmission by the hemodialysis machine? *Infection Control and Hospital Epidemiology*, **23**, 328–334.

71 Springthorpe, V.S. and Sattar, S.A. (2005) Carrier tests to assess microbicidal activities of chemical disinfectants for use on medical devices and environmental surfaces. *Journal of AOAC International*, **88**, 182–201.

72 Graham, M.L. *et al.* (1996) *Ex vivo* protocol for testing virus survival on human skin: experiments on herpes virus 2. *Applied and Environmental Microbiology*, **62**, 4252–4255.

73 Ansari, S.A. *et al.* (1989) *In vivo* protocol for testing efficacy of handwashing agents against viruses and bacteria: experiments with rotavirus and *Escherichia coli*. *Applied and Environmental Microbiology*, **55**, 3113–3118.

74 Sattar, S.A. and Ansari, S.A. (2002) The fingerpad protocol to assess hygienic hand antiseptics against viruses. *Journal of Virological Methods*, **103**, 171–181.

75 Haley, R.W. *et al.* (1985) The efficacy of infection surveillance and control programs in preventing nosocomial infections in US hospitals. *American Journal of Infection Control*, **121**, 182–205.

76 Lopman, B.A. *et al.* (2002) Human caliciviruses in Europe. *Journal of Clinical Virology*, **24**, 137–160.

77 Richards, G.P. (1999) Limitations of molecular biological techniques for assessing the virological safety of foods. *Journal of Food Protection*, **62**, 691–697.

78 Blackwell, J.H. and Chen, J.H.S. (1970) Effects of various germicidal chemicals on H.Ep.2 cell cultures and herpes simplex virus. *Journal of the Association of Official Analytical Chemists*, **53**, 1229–1236.

79 Brown, T.T. (1981) Laboratory evaluation of selected disinfectants as virucidal agents against porcine parvovirus, pseudorabiesvirus, and transmissible gastroenteritis virus. *American Journal of Veterinary Research*, **42**, 1033–1036.

80 Springthorpe, V.S. *et al.* (1986) Chemical disinfection of human rotaviruses: efficacy of commercially-available products in suspension tests. *Journal of Hygiene*, **97**, 139–161.

81 Boudouma, M. *et al.* (1984) A simple method for the evaluation of antiseptic and disinfectant virucidal activity. *Journal of Virological Methods*, **9**, 271–276.

82 Murray, S.M. *et al.* (1991) Duck hepatitis B virus: a model to assess efficacy of disinfectants against hepadnavirus activity. *Epidemiology and Infection*, **106**, 435–443.

83 Chaufour, X. *et al.* (1999) Evaluation of disinfection and sterilization of reusable engioscopes with the duck hepatitis B model. *Journal of Vascular Surgery*, **30**, 277–282.

84 Vickery, K. *et al.* (1999) Inactivation of duck hepatitis B virus by hydrogen peroxide gas plasma sterilization system: a laboratory and "in use" testing. *Journal of Hospital Infection*, **41**, 317–322.

85 Doultree, J.C. *et al.* (1999) Inactivation of feline calicivirus, a Norwalk virus surrogate. *Journal of Hospital Infection*, **41**, 51–57.

86 Thurman, R.B. and Gerba, C.P. (1988) Molecular mechanisms of viral inactivation by water disinfectants. *Advances in Applied Microbiology*, **33**, 75–105.

87 Springthorpe, V.S. and Sattar, S.A. (1990) Chemical disinfection of virus-contaminated surfaces. *Critical Reviews in Environmental Control*, **20**, 169–229.

88 Prince, H.N. *et al.* (1991) Principles of viral control and transmission, in *Disinfection, Sterilization and Preservation*, 4th edn (ed. S.S. Block), Lea & Febiger, Philadelphia, pp. 411–444.

89 Pugh, J.C. *et al.* (1999) Use of surrogate models for testing efficacy of disinfectants against HBV. *American Journal of Infection Control*, **27**, 375–376.

90 Anon. (1982) Richtlinie des Bundesgesundheitsamts und der Deutschen Vereinigung zur Bekämpfung der Viruskrankheiten e.V. zur Prüfung von chemischen Desinfektionsmitteln auf Wirksamkeit gegen Viren. *Bundesgesundheitsblatt*, **25**, 397–398.

91 Anon. (2002) *Chemical Disinfectants and Antiseptics. Virucidal Quantitative Suspension Test for Chemical Disinfectants and Antiseptics used in Human Medicine*. Test Method and Requirements (phase 2, step 1). *prEN 14476*, CEN, Brussels.

92 Grossgebauer, K. (1970) Virus disinfection, in *Disinfection* (ed. M.A. Bernarde), Marcel Dekker, New York, pp. 103–148.

93 Papageorgiou, G.T. *et al.* (2001) New method for evaluation of virucidal activity of antiseptics and disinfectants. *Applied and Environmental Microbiology*, **67**, 5844–5848.

94 Sattar, S.A. *et al.* (2003) A disc-based quantitative carrier test method to assess the virucidal activity of chemical germicides. *Journal of Virological Methods*, **112**, 3–12.

95 Bloomfield, S.F. and Looney, E. (1992) Evaluation of the repeatability and reproducibility of European suspension test methods for antimicrobial activity of disinfectants and antiseptics. *Journal of Applied Bacteriology*, **73**, 87–93.

96 van Klingeren, B. *et al.* (1998) Assessment of the efficacy of disinfectants on surfaces. *International Biodeterioration and Biodegradation*, **41**, 289–293.

97 Sattar, S.A. and Springthorpe, V.S. (2000) New methods for efficacy testing of disinfectants and antiseptics, in *Disinfection, Sterilization and Antisepsis: Principles and Practice in Healthcare Facilities* (ed. W.A. Rutala), APIC, Minneapolis, pp. 173–186.

98 Lorenz, D.E. and Jann, G.J. (1964) Use-dilution test and Newcastle disease virus. *Applied Microbiology*, **12**, 24–26.

99 Slavin, G. (1973) A reproducible surface contamination method for disinfectant tests. *British Veterinary Journal*, **129**, 13–18.

100 Chen, J.H.S. and Koski, T.A. (1983) Methods of testing virucides, in *Disinfection, Sterilization and Preservation*, 3rd edn (ed. S.S. Block), Lea & Febiger, Philadelphia, pp. 981–997.

101 Lloyd-Evans, N. *et al.* (1986) Chemical disinfection of human rotavirus-contaminated surfaces. *Journal of Hygiene*, **97**, 163–173.

102 Allen, L.B. *et al.* (1988) A simple method of drying virus on inanimate objects for virucidal testing. *Journal of Virological Methods*, **19**, 239–248.

103 Sattar, S.A. *et al.* (1989) Chemical disinfection of non-porous inanimate surfaces experimentally contaminated with four human pathogenic viruses. *Epidemiology and Infection*, **102**, 493–505.

104 Anon. (1995) Richtlinie des Robert-Koch-Institutes zur Prüfung der Viruzidie von chemischen Flächendesinfektionsmitteln und Instrumentendesinfktionsmitteln, die in die Liste gemäß §10c des Bundesseuchengesetzes aufgenommen werden sollen. *Bundesgesundheitsblatt*, **6**, 242.

105 Schürmann, W. and Eggers, H.J. (1983) Antiviral activity of an alcoholic hand disinfectant. Comparison of the *in vitro* suspension test with the *in vivo* experiments on hands, and on individual fingertips. *Antiviral Research*, **3**, 25–41.

106 Schürmann, W. and Eggers, H.J. (1985) An experimental study of the epidemiology of enteroviruses: water and soap washing of poliovirus type 1-contaminated hand, its effectiveness and kinetics. *Medical Microbiology and Immunology*, **174**, 221–236.

107 Steinmann, J. *et al.* (1995) Two *in vivo* protocols for testing virucidal efficacy of handwashing and hand disinfection. *Zentralblatt für Hygiene und Umweltmeizin*, **196**, 425–436.

108 ASTM (American Society for Testing and Materials) (1996) *Standard Test Method to Determine the Virus-Eliminating Effectiveness of Liquid Hygienic Handwash Agents using the Fingerpads of Adult Panelists*, Designation E-1838-95, ASTM, West Conshohocken, PA.

109 Sattar, S.A. *et al.* (2000) Activity of an alcohol based hand gel against human adeno-, rhino-, and rotaviruses using the fingerpad method. *Infection Control and Hospital Epidemiology*, **21**, 516–519.

110 Maillard, J.-Y. *et al.* (1998) Antimicrobial efficacy of biocides tested on skin using an *ex-vivo* test. *Journal of Hospital Infection*, **40**, 313–323.

111 Messager, S. *et al.* (2001) Determination of the antibacterial efficacy of several antiseptics tested on skin using the "ex-vivo" test. *Journal of Medical Microbiology*, **50**, 284–292.

112 Sykes, G. (1965) *Disinfection and Sterilization*, Chapman & Hall, London, pp. 291–308.

113 Tyler, R. and Ayliffe, G.A.J. (1987) A surface test for virucidal activity: preliminary study with herpesvirus. *Journal of Hospital Infection*, **9**, 22–29.

114 Tyler, R. *et al.* (1990) Virucidal activity of disinfectants. *Journal of Hospital Infection*, **15**, 339–345.

115 AFNOR (Association Française de Normalisation) (1989) *Antiseptiques et désinfectants utilisés à l'état liquide, miscibles à l'eau. Détermination de l'activité virucide vis-à-vis des virus de vertebras*, NFT72-180, AFNOR, Paris La Défence, Paris.

116 Anon. (1990) Guidelines of bundesgesundheitsamt (BGA; German federal health office) and Deutche Vereinigung zur Bekämpfung der Viruskrankheiten e.V. (DVV; German Association for the Control of Virus Diseases) for testing the effectiveness of chemical disinfectants against viruses. *Zentralblatt für Hygiene und Umweltmedizin*, **189**, 554–562.

117 US Food and Drug Administration (FDA) (1994) *Tentative Final Monograph for Health-care Antiseptic Products, June 1994*, US FDA, Washington, DC.

118 Soule, H. *et al.* (1998) Virus survival in hospital environment: an overview of the virucide activity of disinfectants used in liquid form. *Annales de Biologie Clinique*, **56**, 693–703.

119 Steinmann, J. (2001) Some principles of virucidal testing. *Journal of Hospital Infection*, **48** (Suppl. A), 15–17.

120 Schliesser, T. (1979) Testing of chemical disinfectants for veterinary medicine. *Hygiene and Medizin*, **4**, 51–56.

121 Maillard, J.-Y. (1996) Bacteriophages: a model system for human viruses. *Letters in Applied Bacteriology*, **23**, 1.

122 Kott, Y. (1981) Viruses and bacteriophages. *Science of the Total Environment*, **18**, 13–23.

123 Lazarova, V. *et al.* (1998) Advanced wastewater disinfection technologies: short and long term efficiency. *Water Science and Technology*, **38**, 109–117.

124 Tree, J.A. *et al.* (1997) Virus inactivation during disinfection of wastewater by chlorination and UV irradiation and the efficacy of F+ bacteriophage as a viral indicator. *Water Science and Technology*, **35**, 227–232.

125 Shin, G.A. and Sobsey, M.D. (1998) Reduction of norwalk virus, poliovirus 1 and coliphage MS2 by monochloramine disinfection of water. *Water Science and Technology*, **38**, 151–154.

126 Pintó, R.M. *et al.* (1991) The use of bacteriophages of *Bacteroides fragilis* as indicators of the efficiency of virucidal products. *FEMS Microbiology Letters*, **66**, 61–65.

127 Finch, G.R. and Fairbairn, N. (1991) Comparative inactivation of poliovirus type 3 and MS2 coliphage in demand-free phosphate buffer by using ozone. *Applied and Environmental Microbiology*, **57**, 3121–3126.

128 Jofre, J. *et al.* (1995) Potential usefulness of bacteriophages that infect *Bacteroides fragilis* as model organisms for monitoring virus removal in drinking treatment plants. *Applied and Environmental Microbiology*, **61**, 3227–3231.

129 Abad, F.X. *et al.* (1997) Disinfection of human enteric viruses on fomites. *FEMS Microbiology Letters*, **156**, 107–111.

130 Grabow, W.O.K. (2001) Bacteriophages: update on application as models for viruses in water. *Water SA*, **22**, 251–268.

131 Storey, M.V. and Ashbolt, N.J. (2001) Persistence of two model enteric viruses (B40-8 and MS-2 bacteriophages) in water distribution pipe biofilms. *Water Science and Technology*, **43**, 133–138.

132 Jones, M.V. *et al.* (1991) The use of bacteriophage MS2 as a model system to evaluate virucidal hand disinfectants. *Journal of Hospital Infection*, **17**, 279–285.

133 Rusin, P. *et al.* (2002) Comparative surface-to-hand and fingertip-to-mouth transfer efficiency of gram-positive bacteria, gram-negative bacteria, and phage. *Journal of Applied Microbiology*, **93**, 585–592.

134 Lepage, C. and Romond, C. (1984) Détermination de l'activité virucide: intérêt du bactériophage comme modèle viral. *Pathologie Biologie*, **32**, 631–635.

135 Bydžovská, O. and Kneiflová, J. (1983) Assessment of viral disinfection by means of bacteriophage ØX 174. *Journal of Hygiene, Epidemiology, Microbiology and Immunology*, **27**, 60–68.

136 Davies, J.G. *et al.* (1993) Preliminary study of test methods to assess the virucidal activity of skin disinfectants using poliovirus and bacteriophages. *Journal of Hospital Infection*, **25**, 125–131.

137 Cardo, D.M. and Bell, D.M. (1997) Bloodborne pathogens transmission in healthcare workers. *Infectious Disease Clinics of North America*, **11**, 331–346.

138 Sanchez-Tapias, F.M. (1999) Nosocomial transmission of hepatitis C virus. *Journal of Hepatology*, **31** (Suppl. 1), 107–112.

139 Rosen, H.R. (2000) Primer on hepatitis C for hospital epidemiology. *Infection Control and Hospital Epidemiology*, **21**, 229–234.

140 Barker, J. *et al.* (2001) Spread and prevention of some common viral infections in community facilities and domestic homes. *Journal of Applied Microbiology*, **91**, 7–21.

141 Gyurek, L.L. and Finch, G.R. (1998) Modeling water treatment chemical disinfection kinetics. *Journal of Environmental Engineering-Asce*, **124**, 783–793.

142 Williams, G.J. *et al.* (2009) The use of sodium dichloroisocyanurate, NaDCC, in Welsh ITUs. *Journal of Hospital Infection*, **72**, 279–281.

143 Williams, G.J. *et al.* (2009) Limitations of the efficacy of surface disinfection in the healthcare settings. *Infection Control and Hospital Epidemiology*, **30**, 570–573.

144 Klein, M. and Deforest, A. (1963) The inactivation of viruses by germicides, in *Proceedings of the 49th Midyear Meeting of the Chemical Specialties Manufacturers Association*, Chicago, pp. 116–118.

145 Mbithi, J.N. *et al.* (1990) Chemical disinfection of hepatitis A virus on environmental surfaces. *Applied and Environmental Microbiology*, **56**, 3601–3604.

146 Mbithi, J.N. *et al.* (1993) Bactericidal, virucidal and mycobactericidal activity of alkaline glutaraldehyde under reuse in an endoscopy unit. *Journal of Clinical Microbiology*, **31**, 2988–2995.

147 Mbithi, J.N. *et al.* (1993) Comparative *in vivo* efficiency of hand-washing agents against hepatitis A virus (HM-175) and poliovirus type 1 (Sabin). *Applied and Environmental Microbiology*, **59**, 3463–3469.

148 Bigliardi, L. and Sansebastiano, G. (2006) Study on inactivation kinetics of hepatitis A virus and enteroviruses with peracetic acid and chlorine. New ICC/PCR method to assess disinfection effectiveness. *Journal of Preventive Medicine and Hygiene*, **47**, 56–63.

149 Bellamy, K. (1995) A review of the test methods used to establish virucidal activity. *Journal of Hospital Infection*, **30** (Suppl.), 389–396.

150 Berman, D. and Hoff, J.C. (1984) Inactivation of simian rotavirus SA-11 by chlorine, chlorine dioxide and monochloramine. *Applied and Environmental Microbiology*, **48**, 317–323.

151 Harakeh, M.S. (1984) Inactivation of enteroviruses, rotaviruses and bacteriophages by peracetic acid in a municipal sewage effluent. *FEMS Microbiology Letters*, **23**, 27–30.

152 Harakeh, M. and Butler, M. (1984) Inactivation of human rotavirus, SA-11 and other enteric viruses in effluent by disinfectants. *Journal of Hygiene*, **93**, 157–163.

153 Raphael, R.A. *et al.* (1987) Lack of human rotavirus inactivation by residual chlorine in municipal drinking water systems. *Revue Internationale de Science de l'Eau*, **3**, 67–69.

154 Charrel, R.N. *et al.* (2001) Evaluation of disinfectant efficacy against hepatitis C virus using a RT-PCR-based method. *Journal of Hospital Infection*, **49**, 129–134.

155 Li, J.W. *et al.* (2002) Mechanisms of inactivation of hepatitis A virus by chlorine. *Applied and Environmental Microbiology*, **68**, 4951–4955.

156 Page, M.A. *et al.* (2009) Kinetics of adenovirus type 2 inactivation with free chlorine. *Water Research*, **43**, 2916–2926.

157 Peterson, D.A. *et al.* (1983) Effect of chlorine treatment on infectivity of hepatitis A virus. *Applied and Environmental Microbiology*, **45**, 223–227.

158 Bates, R.C. *et al.* (1977) Development of poliovirus having increased resistance to chlorine inactivation. *Applied and Environmental Microbiology*, **34**, 849–853.

159 Clarke, N.A. *et al.* (1956) The inactivity of purified type 3 adenovirus in water by chlorine. *American Journal of Hygiene*, **64**, 314–319.

160 Herniman, K.A.J. *et al.* (1973) The action of heat, chemicals and disinfectants on swine vesicular disease virus. *Veterinary Record*, **93**, 620–624.

161 Wright, H. (1970) Inactivation of vesicular stomatitis virus by disinfectants. *Applied Microbiology*, **19**, 96–98.

162 Evans, D.H. *et al.* (1977) Disinfection of animal viruses. *British Veterinary Journal*, **133**, 356–359.

163 Engelbrecht, R.S. *et al.* (1980) Comparative inactivation of viruses by chlorine. *Applied and Environmental Microbiology*, **40**, 249–256.

164 Gowda, N.M.M. *et al.* (1981) Inactivation of poliovirus by chloramine-T. *Applied and Environmental Microbiology*, **42**, 469–476.

165 Fauris, C. *et al.* (1982) Parameters influencing poliovirus inactivation by chlorine. *Comptes Rendu de l'Académie des Sciences (Paris)*, **295**, 73–76.

166 Churn, C.C. *et al.* (1984) The inactivation kinetics of H-1 parvovirus by chlorine. *Water Research*, **18**, 195–203.

167 Grabow, W.O.K. *et al.* (1984) Inactivation of hepatitis A virus, other enteric viruses and indicator organisms in water by chlorination. *Water Science and Technology*, **17**, 657–664.

168 Sobsey, M.D. *et al.* (1991) Inactivation of cell-associated and dispersed hepatitis A virus in water. *Journal of the American Water Works Association*, **83**, 64–67.

169 Krilov, L.R. and Harkness, S.H. (1993) Inactivation of respiratory syncytial virus by detergents and disinfectants. *Pediatric Infectious Diseases Journal*, **12**, 582–584.

170 Ceisel, R.J. *et al.* (1995) Evaluating chemical inactivation of viral agents in handpiece splatter. *Journal of the American Dental Association*, **126**, 197–202.

171 Rutala, W.A. (1996) APIC guideline for the selection and use of disinfectants. *American Journal of Infection Control*, **24** (Suppl.), 313–342.

172 Selkon, J.B. *et al.* (1999) Evaluation of the antimicrobial activity of a new super-oxidized water, Sterilox®, for the disinfection of endoscope. *Journal of Hospital Infection*, **41**, 59–70.

173 Sobsey, M.D. *et al.* (1988) Inactivation of hepatitis-A virus and model viruses in water by free chlorine and monochloramine. *Water Science and Technology*, **20**, 385–391.

174 Chepurnov, A.A. *et al.* (1995) Effects of some physical and chemical factors on inactivation of ebola virus. *Russian Progress in Virology*, **2**, 40–43.

175 Springthorpe, S. *et al.* (2001) Comparison of static and dynamic disinfection models for bacteria and viruses in water of varying quality. *Water Science and Technology*, **43**, 147–154.

176 Sirikanchana, K. *et al.* (2008) Effect of exposure to UV-C irradiation and monochloramine on adenovirus serotype 2 early protein expression and DNA replication. *Applied and Environmental Microbiology*, **74**, 3774–3782.

177 Sirikanchana, K. *et al.* (2008) Inactivation kinetics of adenovirus serotype 2 with monochloramine. *Water Research*, **42**, 1467–1474.

178 Simonet, J. and Gantzer, C. (2006) Degradation of the poliovirus 1 genome by chlorine dioxide. *Journal of Applied Microbiology*, **4**, 862–870.

179 Huang, J.L. *et al.* (1997) Disinfection effect of chlorine dioxide on viruses, algae and animal planktons in water. *Water Research*, **31**, 455–460.

180 Taylor, G.R. and Butler, M. (1982) A comparison of the virucidal properties of chlorine, chlorine dioxide, bromine chloride and iodine. *Journal of Hygiene, Cambridge*, **89**, 321–328.

181 Keswick, B.H. *et al.* (1981) Mechanism of poliovirus inactivation by bromine chloride. *Applied and Environmental Microbiology*, **42**, 824–829.

182 Wood, A. and Payne, D. (1998) The action of three antiseptics/disinfectants against enveloped and non-enveloped viruses. *Journal of Hospital Infection*, **38**, 283–295.

183 Sriwilaijaroen, N. *et al.* (2009) Mechanisms of the action of povidone-iodine against human and avian influenza a viruses: its effects on hemagglutination and sialidase activities. *Virology Journal*, **6**, 124–134.

184 Kawana, R. *et al.* (1997) Inactivation of human viruses by povidone-iodine in comparison with other antiseptics. *Dermatology*, **195**, 29–35.

185 Wanaratana, S. *et al.* (2010) The inactivation of avian influenza virus subtype H5N1 isolated from chickens in Thailand by chemical and physical treatments. *Veterinary Microbiology*, **140**, 43–48.

186 Hsu, Y.-C. *et al.* (1966) Some bactericidal and virucidal properties of iodine not affecting infectious RNA and DNA. *American Journal of Epidemiology*, **82**, 317–328.

187 Jordan, F.T.W. and Nassar, T.J. (1973) The survival of infectious bronchitis (IB) virus in an iodophor disinfectant and the influence of certain components. *Journal of Applied Bacteriology*, **36**, 335–341.

188 Wallbank, A.M. *et al.* (1978) Wescodyne: lack of activity against poliovirus in the presence of organic matter. *Health Laboratory Science*, **15**, 133–137.

189 Sobsey, M.D. *et al.* (1991) Comparative inactivation of hepatitis A virus and other enteroviruses in water by iodine. *Water Science and Technology*, **24**, 331–337.

190 Highsmith, F.A. *et al.* (1994) Inactivation of lipid-enveloped and non-lipid-enveloped model viruses in normal human plasma by cross-linked starch-iodine. *Transfusion*, **34**, 322–327.

191 Highsmith, F. *et al.* (1995) Iodine-mediated inactivation of lipid-enveloped and nonlipid-enveloped viruses in human antithrombin-III concentrate. *Blood*, **86**, 791–796.

192 Wutzler, P. *et al.* (2000) Virucidal and chlamydicidal activities of eye drops with povidone-iodine liposome complex. *Ophthalmic Research*, **32**, 118–125.

193 Lombardi, M.E. *et al.* (2008) Inactivation of avian influenza virus using common detergents and chemicals. *Avian Diseases*, **52**, 118–123.

194 Belliot, G. *et al.* (2008) Use of murine norovirus as a surrogate to evaluate resistance of human norovirus to disinfectants. *Applied Environmental Microbiology*, **74**, 3315–3318.

195 Weber, D.J. *et al.* (1999) The effect of blood on the antiviral activity of sodium hypochlorite, a phenolic, and a quaternary ammonium compound. *Infection Control and Hospital Epidemiology*, **20**, 821–827.

196 Whitehead, K. and McCue, K.A. (2010) Virucidal efficacy of disinfectant actives against feline calicivirus, a surrogate for norovirus, in a short contact time. *American Journal of Infection Control*, **38**, 26–30.

197 Drulak, M.W. *et al.* (1984) The effectiveness of six disinfectants in the inactivation of reovirus 3. *Microbios*, **41**, 31–38.

198 Hendley, J.O. *et al.* (1978) Evaluation of virucidal compounds for inactivation of rhinovirus on hands. *Antimicrobial Agents and Chemotherapy*, **14**, 690–694.

199 Wolff, H.H. *et al.* (2001) Hepatitis A virus: a test method for virucidal activity. *Journal of Hospital Infection*, **48** (Suppl. A), 18–22.

200 Klein, M. and Deforest, A. (1983) Principles of viral inactivation, in *Disinfection, Sterilization and Preservation* (ed. S.S. Block), Lea & Febiger, Philadelphia, pp. 422–434.

201 Dellanno, C. *et al.* (2009) The antiviral action of common household disinfectants and antiseptics against murine hepatitis virus, a potential surrogate for SARS coronavirus. *American Journal of Infection Control*, **37**, 649–652.

202 Steinmann, J. *et al.* (2010) Virucidal activity of 2 alcohol-based formulations proposed as hand rubs by the World Health Organization. *American Journal of Infection Control*, **38**, 66–68.

203 Kurtz, J.B. (1979) Virucidal effects of alcohols against echovirus 11. *Lancet*, **i**, 496–497.

204 Kurtz, J.B. *et al.* (1980) The action of alcohols on rotavirus, astrovirus and enterovirus. *Journal of Hospital Infection*, **1**, 321–325.

205 Brade, L. *et al.* (1981) Zur relativen Wirksam keit von Desinfektion-mitteln gegenuber Rotaviren. *Zentralblatt für Bakteriologie, Mikrobiologie und Hygiene (Orig. B)*, **174**, 151–159.

206 Sattar, S.A. *et al.* (1986) Institutional outbreaks of rotavirus diarrhea: possible role of fomites and environmental surfaces as vehicles for virus transmission. *Journal of Hygiene*, **96**, 277–289.

207 Bellamy, K. *et al.* (1993) A test for the assessment of "hygienic" hand disinfection using rotavirus. *Journal of Hospital Infection*, **24**, 201–210.

208 van Bueren, J. *et al.* (1994) Inactivation of human immunodeficiency virus type 1 by alcohols. *Journal of Hospital Infection*, **28**, 137–148.

209 Kampf, G. *et al.* (2002) Spectrum of antimicrobial activity and user acceptability of the hand disinfectant agent Sterillium® Gel. *Journal of Hospital Infection*, **52**, 141–147.

210 Van Engelenburg, F.A.C. *et al.* (2002) The virucidal spectrum of a high concentration alcohol mixture. *Journal of Hospital Infection*, **51**, 121–125.

211 Liu, P. *et al.* (2010) Effectiveness of liquid soap and hand sanitizer against Norwalk virus on contaminated hands. *Applied Environmental Microbiology*, **76**, 394–399.

212 Sidwell, R.W. *et al.* (1970) Potentially infectious agents associated with shearling bedpads. I. Effect of laundering with detergent-disinfectant combinations on polio and vaccinia viruses. *Applied Microbiology*, **19**, 53–59.

213 Rutala, W.A. *et al.* (2006) Efficacy of hospital germicides against adenovirus 8, a common cause of epidemic keratoconjunctivitis in health care facilities. *Antimicrobial Agents and Chemotherapy*, **50**, 1419–1424.

214 Howie, R. *et al.* (2008) Survival of enveloped and non-enveloped viruses on surfaces compared with other micro-organisms and impact of suboptimal disinfectant exposure. *Journal of Hospital Infection*, **69**, 368–376.

215 Payan, C. *et al.* (2001) Inactivation of hepatitis B virus in plasma by hospital in-use chemical disinfectants assessed by a modified HepG2 cell culture. *Journal of Hospital Infection*, **47**, 282–287.

216 Gorman, S.P. *et al.* (1980) Antimicrobial activity, uses and mechanism of action of glutaraldehyde. *Journal of Applied Bacteriology*, **48**, 161–190.

217 Magulski, T. *et al.* (2009) Inactivation of murine norovirus by chemical biocides on stainless steel. *BMC Infectious Diseases*, **9**, 107–114.

218 Saitanu, K. and Lund, E. (1975) Inactivation of enterovirus by glutaraldehyde. *Applied Microbiology*, **29**, 571–574.

219 Thraenhart, O. and Kuwert, E. (1975) Virucidal activity of the disinfectant "Gigasept" against different enveloped and non-enveloped RNA- and DNA-viruses pathogenic for man. I. Investigation in the suspension test. *Zentralblatt für Bakteriologie und Hygiene, I. Abteilung (Originale B)*, **161**, 209–232.

220 Mahnel, H. and Kunz, W. (1976) Suitability of carriers for the examination of disinfectants against viruses. *Berliner und Münchener Tierärztliche Wochenschrift*, **89**, 138–142.

221 Mahnel, H. and Kunz, W. (1976) Suitability of carriers for the examination of disinfectants against viruses. *Berliner und Münchener Tierärztliche Wochenschrift*, **89**, 149–152.

222 Drulak, M. *et al.* (1978) The relative effectiveness of commonly used disinfectants in inactivation of echovirus 11. *Journal of Hygiene*, **81**, 77–87.

223 Drulak, M. *et al.* (1978) The relative effectiveness of commonly used disinfectants in inactivation of coxsackievirus B5. *Journal of Hygiene*, **81**, 389–397.

224 Hanson, P.J.V. *et al.* (1994) Enteroviruses, endoscopy and infection control: an applied study. *Journal of Hospital Infection*, **27**, 61–67.

225 Deva, A.K. *et al.* (1996) Establishment of an in-use testing method for evaluating disinfection of surgical instruments using the duck hepatitis B model. *Journal of Hospital Infection*, **33**, 119–130.

226 Jülich, W.-D. and von Woedtke, T. (2001) Reprocessing of thermosensitive materials – efficacy against bacterial spores and viruses. *Journal of Hospital Infection*, **48** (Suppl. A), 69–79.

227 Turner, R.B. *et al.* (2004) Efficacy of organic acids in hand cleansers for prevention of rhinovirus infections. *Antimicrobial Agents and Chemotheraphy*, **48**, 2595–2598.

228 Giranda, V.L. *et al.* (1992) Acid-induced structural changes in human rhinovirus 14: possible role in uncoating. *Proceedings of the National Academy of Sciences of the United States of America*, **89**, 10213–10217.

229 Hayden, G.F. *et al.* (1985) Rhinovirus inactivation by nasal tissues treated with virucide. *Antiviral Research*, **5**, 103–109.

230 Dick, E.C. *et al.* (1986) Interruption of transmission of rhinovirus colds among human volunteers using virucidal paper handkerchiefs. *Journal of Infectious Diseases*, **153**, 352–356.

231 Jannat, R. *et al.* (2005) Inactivation of adenovirus type 5 by caustics. *Biotechnology Progress*, **21**, 446–450.

232 Alphin, R.L. *et al.* (2009) Inactivation of avian influenza virus using four common chemicals and one detergent. *Poultry Science*, **88**, 1181–1185.

233 Fellowes, O.N. (1965) Some surface-active agents and their virucidal effect on foot-and-mouth disease virus. *Applied Microbiology*, **13**, 694–697.

234 Piret, J. *et al.* (2000) *In vitro* and *in vivo* evaluations of sodium lauryl sulfate and dextran sulfate as microbicides against herpes simplex and human immunodeficiency viruses. *Journal of Clinical Microbiology*, **38**, 110–119.

235 Piret, J. *et al.* (2002) Sodium lauryl sulfate, a microbicide effective against enveloped and non-enveloped viruses. *Current Drug Targets*, **3**, 17–30.

236 Butcher, W. and Ulaeto, D. (2005) Contact inactivation of orthopoxviruses by household disinfectants. *Journal of Applied Microbiology*, **99**, 279–284.

237 Rabenau, H.F. *et al.* (2005) Efficacy of various disinfectants against SARS coronavirus. *Journal of Hospital Infection*, **61**, 107–111.

238 Girard, M. *et al.* (2010) Attachment of noroviruses to stainless steel and their inactivation, using household disinfectants. *Journal of Food Protection*, **73**, 400–404.

239 Kirchhoff, H. (1968) The effect of quaternary ammonium compounds on Newcastle disease virus and parainfluenza virus. *Deutsche Tierärztliche Wochenschrift*, **75**, 160–165.

240 Oxford, J.S. *et al.* (1971) Inactivation of influenza and other viruses by a mixture of virucidal compounds. *Applied Microbiology*, **21**, 606–610.

241 Poli, G. *et al.* (1978) Virucidal activity of some quaternary ammonium compounds. *Drug Research*, **28**, 1672–1675.

242 Anderson, L.J. and Winkler, W.G. (1979) Aqueous quaternary ammonium compounds and rabies treatment. *Journal of Infectious Diseases*, **139**, 494–495.

243 Kennedy, M.A. *et al.* (1995) Virucidal efficacy of the newer quaternary ammonium compounds. *Journal of the American Animal Hospital Association*, **31**, 254–258.

244 Jimenez, L. and Chiang, M. (2006) Virucidal activity of a quaternary ammonium compound disinfectant against feline calicivirus: a surrogate for norovirus. *American Journal of Infection Control*, **34**, 269–273.

245 Malik, Y.S. *et al.* (2006) Disinfection of fabrics and carpets artificially contaminated with calicivirus: relevance in institutional and healthcare centres. *Journal of Hospital Infection*, **63**, 205–210.

246 Pratelli, A. (2007) Action of disinfectants on canine coronavirus replication *in vitro*. *Zoonoses Public Health*, **54**, 383–386.

247 Sauerbrei, A. *et al.* (2006) Validation of biocides against duck hepatitis B virus as a surrogate virus for human hepatitis B virus. *Journal of Hospital Infection*, **64**, 358–365.

248 Rudnick, S.N. *et al.* (2009) Inactivating influenza viruses on surfaces using hydrogen peroxide or triethylene glycol at low vapor concentrations. *American Journal of Infection Control*, **37**, 813–819.

249 Mentel, R. and Schmidt, J. (1973) Investigations on rhinovirus inactivation by hydrogen peroxide. *Acta Virologica*, **17**, 351–354.

250 Hall, R.M. and Sobsey, M.D. (1993) Inactivation of hepatitis A virus and MS2 by ozone and ozone-hydrogen peroxide in buffered water. *Water Science and Technology*, **27**, 371–378.

251 Heckert, R.A. *et al.* (1997) Efficacy of vaporized hydrogen peroxide against exotic animal viruses. *Applied and Environmental Microbiology*, **63**, 3916–3918.

252 Smith, C.A. and Pepose, J.S. (1999) Disinfection of tonometers and contact lenses in the office setting: are current techniques adequate? *American Journal of Ophthalmology*, **127**, 77–84.

253 Wutzler, P. and Sauerbrei, A. (2000) Virucidal efficacy of a combination of 0.2% peracetic acid and 80% (v/v) ethanol (PAA-ethanol) as a potential hand disinfectant. *Journal of Hospital Infection*, **46**, 304–308.

254 Kline, L.B. and Hull, R.N. (1960) The virucidal properties of peracetic acid. *American Journal of Clinical Pathology*, **33**, 30–33.

255 Sporkenbach, J. *et al.* (1981) The virus inactivating efficacy of peracids and peracidous disinfectants. *Zentralblatt für Bakteriologie, Mikrobiologie und Hygiene (Orig. B)*, **173**, 425–439.

256 Zanetti, F. *et al.* (2007) Disinfection efficiency of peracetic acid (PAA): inactivation of coliphages and bacterial indicators in a municipal wastewater plant. *Environmental Technology*, **28**, 1265–1271.

257 Khadre, M.A. and Yousef, A.E. (2002) Susceptibility of human rotavirus to ozone, high pressure, and pulsed electric field. *Journal of Food Protection*, **65**, 1441–1446.

258 Murray, B.K. *et al.* (2008) Virion disruption by ozone-mediated reactive oxygen species. *Journal of Virological Methods*, **153**, 74–77.

259 Helmer, R.D. and Finch, G.R. (1993) Use of MS2 coliphage as a surrogate for enteric viruses in surface waters disinfected with ozone. *Ozone Science and Engineering*, **15**, 279–293.

260 Kim, J.G. *et al.* (1999) Application of ozone for enhancing the microbiological safety and quality of foods: a review. *Journal of Food Protection*, **62**, 1071–1087.

261 Kashiwagi, K. *et al.* (2001) Safety of ozonated solution as an antiseptic of the ocular surface prior to ophthalmic surgery. *Ophthalmologica*, **215**, 351–356.

262 James, L. *et al.* (2002) Ozone: a potent disinfectant for application in food industry – an overview. *Journal of Scientific and Industrial Research*, **61**, 504–509.

263 Lénès, D. *et al.* (2010) Assessment of the removal and inactivation of influenza viruses H5N1 and H1N1 by drinking water treatment. *Water Research*, **44**, 2473–2486.

264 Lim, M.Y. *et al.* (2010) Characterization of ozone disinfection of murine norovirus. *Applied Environmental Microbiology*, **76**, 1120–1124.

265 Krebs, F.C. *et al.* (2005) Polybiguanides, particularly polyethylene hexamethylene biguanide, have activity against human immunodeficiency virus type 1. *Biomedecine and Pharmacotherapy*, **59**, 438–445.

266 Pinto, F. *et al.* (2010) Effect of surfactants, temperature and sonication on the virucidal activity of polyhexamethylene biguanide against the bacteriophage MS2. *American Journal of Infection Control*, **38**, 393–398.

267 Pinto, F. *et al.* (2010) PHMB microbicide exposure leads to viral aggregation. *Journal of Applied Microbiology*, **108**, 1080–1088.

268 Baqui, A.A.M.A. *et al.* (2001) *In vitro* effect of oral antiseptics on human immunodeficiency virus-1 and herpes simplex virus type 1. *Journal of Clinical Periodontology*, **28**, 610–616.

269 Grayson, M.L. *et al.* (2009) Efficacy of soap and water and alcohol-based hand-rub preparations against live H1N1 influenza virus on the hands of human volunteers. *Clinical Infectious Diseases*, **48**, 285–291.

270 Valluri, S. *et al.* (1997) *In vitro* and *in vivo* effects of polyhexamethylene biguanide against herpes simplex virus infection. *Cornea*, **16**, 556–559.

271 Bailey, A. and Longson, M. (1972) Virucidal activity of chlorhexidine on strains of herpes virus hominis, poliovirus and adenovirus. *Journal of Clinical Pathology*, **25**, 76–78.

272 Dawson, F.W. *et al.* (1959) Virucidal activity of beta-propiolactone vapour. I. Effect of beta-propiolactone on Venezuelan equine encephalitis virus. *Applied Microbiology*, **7**, 199–201.

273 Dawson, F.W. *et al.* (1960) Virucidal activity of beta-propiolactone vapor. II. Effect on the biological agents of smallpox, yellow fever, psittacosis and Q fever. *Applied Microbiology*, **8**, 39–41.

274 Lloyd, G. *et al.* (1982) Physical and chemical methods of inactivating Lassa virus. *Lancet*, **i**, 1046–1048.

275 Scheidler, A. *et al.* (1998) Inactivation of viruses by beta-propiolactone in human cryo poor plasma and IgG concentrates. *Biologicals*, **26**, 135–144.

276 Lawrence, S.A. (1999) Beta-propiolactone and aziridine: their applications in organic synthesis and viral inactivation. *Chimica Oggi*, **17**, 51–54.

277 Quinn , P.J. and Carter, M.E. (1999) Evaluation of viricidal activity, in *Principles and Practice of Disinfection, Preservation and Sterilization*, 3rd edn (ed. A.D. Russell *et al.*), Blackwell Science, Oxford, pp. 197–206.

278 Bienek, C. *et al.* (2007) Development of a bacteriophage model system to investigate virus inactivation methods used in the treatment of bone allografts. *Cell and Tissue Banking*, **8**, 15–24.

279 Murphy, F.A. *et al.* (1995) Virus taxonomy: classification and nomenclature of viruses. *Archives of Virology*, **140** (Suppl. 10), 1.

280 Sauerbrei, A. *et al.* (2004) Sensitivity of human adenoviruses to different groups of chemical biocides. *Journal of Hospital Infection*, **57**, 59–66.

281 Maillard, J.-Y. (2002) Bacterial target sites for biocide action. *Journal of Applied Microbiology*, **92** (Suppl.), 16–27.

282 Mahnel, H. (1979) Variations in resistance of viruses from different groups to chemico-physical decontamination methods. *Infection*, **7**, 240–246.

283 Thurston-Enriquez, J.A. *et al.* (2003) Chlorine inactivation of adenovirus type 40 and feline calicivirus. *Applied and Environmental Microbiology*, **69**, 3979–3985.

284 Eterpi, M. *et al.* (2009) Disinfection efficacy against parvoviruses compared with reference viruses. *Journal of Hospital Infection*, **73**, 64–70.

285 Maillard, J.-Y. *et al.* (1995) Electron-microscopic investigation of the effect of biocides on *Pseudomonas aeruginosa* PAO bacteriophage F116. *Journal of Medical Microbiology*, **42**, 415–420.

286 Maillard, J.-Y. *et al.* (1995) Analysis of X-rays: study of the distribution of chlorhexidine and cetylpyridinium chloride on the *Pseudomonas aeruginosa* bacteriophage F116. *Letters in Applied Microbiology*, **20**, 357–360.

287 Maillard, J.-Y. *et al.* (1995) The effects of biocides on the transduction of *Pseudomonas aeruginosa* PAO by F116 bacteriophage. *Letters in Applied Microbiology*, **21**, 215–218.

288 Maillard, J.-Y. *et al.* (1996) The effects of biocides on proteins of *Pseudomonas aeruginosa* PAO bacteriophage F116. *Journal of Applied Bacteriology*, **80**, 291–295.

289 Maillard, J.-Y. *et al.* (1996) Damage to *Pseudomonas aeruginosa* PAO1 bacteriophage F116 DNA by biocides. *Journal of Applied Bacteriology*, **80**, 540–544.

290 Bond, W.W. *et al.* (1983) Inactivation of hepatitis B virus by intermediate-to-high level disinfectant chemicals. *Journal of Clinical Microbiology*, **18**, 535–538.

291 Kobayashi, H. and Tsuzuki, M. (1984) The effects of disinfectants and heat on hepatitis B virus. *Journal of Hospital Infection*, **5**, 93–94.

292 Kobayashi, H. *et al.* (1984) Susceptibility of hepatitis B virus to disinfectants or heat. *Journal of Clinical Microbiology*, **20**, 214–216.

293 Bailly, J.-L. *et al.* (1991) Activity of glutaraldehyde at low concentrations (<2%) against poliovirus and its relevance to gastrointestinal endoscope disinfection procedures. *Applied and Environmental Microbiology*, **57**, 1156–1160.

294 Best, M. *et al.* (1994) Feasibility of a combined carrier test for disinfectants: studies with a mixture of five types of microorganisms. *American Journal of Infection Control*, **22**, 152–162.

295 Maillard, J.-Y. *et al.* (1994) Effect of biocides on MS2 and K coliphages. *Applied and Environmental Microbiology*, **60**, 2205–2206.

296 Sangar, D.V. *et al.* (1973) Reaction of glutaraldehyde with foot and mouth disease virus. *Journal of Genetic Virology*, **21**, 399–406.

297 Wouters, M. *et al.* (1973) Distortion of poliovirus particles by fixation with formaldehyde. *Journal of General Virology*, **18**, 211–214.

298 Baltimore, D. and Huang, A.S. (1968) Isopycnic separation of subcellular components from poliovirus-infected and normal HeLa cells. *Science*, **162**, 572–574.

299 Thraenhart, O. *et al.* (1977) Morphological alteration and disintegration of Dane particles after exposure with "Gigasept": a first methodological attempt for the evaluation of the virucidal efficacy of a chemical disinfectant against hepatitis virus B. *Zentralblatt für Bakteriologie, Parasitenkunde, Infektionskrankheinten und Hygiene. I. Abteilung Originale, Reike*, **164**, 1–21.

300 Adler-Storthz, K. *et al.* (1983) Effect of alkaline glutaraldehyde on hepatitis B virus antigens. *European Journal of Clinical Microbiology*, **2**, 316–320.

301 Frösner, G. *et al.* (1982) Destroying of antigenicity and influencing the immunochemical reactivity of hepatitis B virus antigens (HBsAg, HBcAg, HBeAg) through disinfectants – a proposed method for testing. *Zentralblatt für Bakteriologie, Parasitenkunde, Infektionskrankheinten und Hygiene. I. Abteilung Originale, Reike*, **176**, 1–14.

302 Richards, F.M. and Knowles, J.R. (1968) Glutaraldehyde as a protein cross-linking reagent. *Journal of Molecular Biology*, **37**, 231–233.

303 Korn, A.H. *et al.* (1972) Glutaraldehyde: nature of the reagent. *Journal of Molecular Biology*, **65**, 525–529.

304 Passagot, J. *et al.* (1987) Effect of glutaraldehyde on the antigenicity and infectivity of hepatitis A virus. *Journal of Virological Methods*, **16**, 21–28.

305 Chambon, M. *et al.* (1992) Activity of glutaraldehyde at low concentrations against capsid proteins of poliovirus type 1 and echovirus type 25. *Applied and Environmental Microbiology*, **58**, 3517–3521.

306 Hogle, J.M. *et al.* (1985) Three-dimensional structure of poliovirus at 2.9 resolution. *Science*, **229**, 1358–1365.

307 Racaniello, V.R. and Baltimore, D. (1981) Molecular cloning of poliovirus cDNA and determination of the complete nucleotide sequence of the viral genome. *Biochemistry*, **78**, 4887–4891.

308 Linemeyer, D.L. *et al.* (1985) Molecular cloning and partial sequencing of hepatitis A viral cDNA. *Journal of Virology*, **54**, 247–255.

309 Chambon, M. *et al.* (2004) Virucidal efficacy of glutaraldehyde against enteroviruses is related to the location of lysine residues in exposed structures of the VP1 capsid protein. *Applied and Environmental Microbiology*, **70**, 1717–1722.

310 Chambon, M. *et al.* (1997) Comparative sensitivities of sabin and mahoney poliovirus type 1 prototype strains and two recent isolates to low concentrations of glutaraldehyde. *Applied and Environmental Microbiology*, **63**, 3199–3204.

311 Howard, C.R. *et al.* (1983) Chemical inactivation of hepatitis B virus: the effect of disinfectants on virus-associated DNA polymerase activity, morphology and infectivity. *Journal of Virological Methods*, **7**, 135–148.

312 Walsh, S.E. *et al.* (1999) *ortho*-Phthalaldehyde: a possible alternative to glutaraldehyde for high-level disinfection. *Journal of Applied Microbiology*, **86**, 1039–1046.

313 Roberts, C.G. *et al.* (2008) Virucidal activity of ortho-phthalaldehyde solutions against hepatitis B and C viruses. *American Journal of Infection Control*, **36**, 223–226.

314 Fraud, S. *et al.* (2003) Effects of *ortho*-phthalaldehyde, glutaraldehyde and chlorhexidine diacetate on *Mycobacterium chelonae* and *M. abscessus* strains

with modified permeability. *Journal of Antimicrobial Chemotherapy*, **51**, 575–584.

315 World Health Organization (WHO) (1993) *Laboratory Biosafety Manual*, 2nd edn, WHO, Geneva, Chapter 9.

316 Breuer, J. and Jeffries, D.J. (1990) Control of viral infections in hospital. *Journal of Hospital Infection*, **16**, 191–221.

317 Philpott-Howard, J. and Casewell, M. (1995) *Hospital Infection Control*, W.B. Saunders, London, pp. 86–87.

318 Anon. (1997) *Occupational Safety and Health Administration Memorandum. EPA-registered Disinfectants for HIV/HBV*, February 28, http://www.osha.gov/index.html

319 Olivieri, V.P. *et al.* (1975) The comparative mode of action of chlorine, bromine, and iodine on f2 bacterial virus, in *Disinfection – Water and Wastewater* (ed. J.D. Johnson), Ann Arbor Science Publisher, Ann Arbor, MI, pp. 145–162.

320 O'Brien, R.T. and Newman, J. (1979) Structural and compositional changes associated with chlorine inactivation of polioviruses. *Applied and Environmental Microbiology*, **38**, 1034–1039.

321 Floyd, R.D. *et al.* (1979) Inactivation by chlorine of single poliovirus particles in water. *Environmental Sciences and Technology*, **13**, 438–442.

322 Tenno, K.M. *et al.* (1979) The mechanisms of poliovirus inactivation by hypochlorous acid, in *Proceedings of the 3rd Conference on Water Chlorination: Environmental Impact and Health Effects* (eds R. Jolley *et al.*), Ann Arbor Science Publisher, Ann Arbor, MI, pp. 665–675.

323 Alvarez, M.E. and O'Brien, R.T. (1982) Effects of chlorine concentration on the structure of poliovirus. *Applied and Environmental Microbiology*, **43**, 237–239.

324 Shirai, J. *et al.* (2000) Effects of chlorine, iodine, and quaternary ammonium compound disinfectants on several exotic disease viruses. *Journal of Veterinary Medical Science*, **62**, 85–92.

325 Rodgers, F.G. *et al.* (1985) Morphological response of human rotavirus to ultra-violet radiation, heat and disinfectants. *Journal of Medical Microbiology*, **20**, 123–130.

326 Nuanualsuwan, S. and Cliver, D.O. (2002) Pretreatment to avoid positive RT-PCR results with inactivated viruses. *Journal of Virological Methods*, **104**, 217–225.

327 Resnick, L. *et al.* (1986) Stability and inactivation of HTLV-III/LAV under clinical and laboratory environments. *Journal of the American Medical Association*, **255**, 1887–1891.

328 Bloomfield, S.F. *et al.* (1990) Evaluation of hypochlorite-releasing disinfectants against the human immunodeficiency virus (HIV). *Journal of Hospital Infection*, **15**, 273–278.

329 Keswick, B.H. *et al.* (1985) Inactivation of Norwalk virus in drinking water by chlorine. *Applied and Environmental Microbiology*, **50**, 261–264.

330 Brion, G.M. and Silverstein, J. (1999) Iodine disinfection of a model bacteriophage, MS2, demonstrating apparent rebound. *Water Research*, **33**, 169–179.

331 Alvarez, M.E. and O'Brien, R.T. (1982) Mechanisms of inactivation of poliovirus by chlorine dioxide and iodine. *Applied and Environmental Microbiology*, **44**, 1064–1071.

332 Hsu, Y. (1964) Resistance of infectious RNA and transforming DNA to iodine which inactivates f2 phage and cells. *Nature*, **203**, 152–153.

333 Cramer, W.N. *et al.* (1976) Chlorination and iodination of poliovirus and f2. *Journal of Water Pollution Control Federation*, **48**, 61–76.

334 Sharp, D.G. *et al.* (1975) Nature of the surviving plaque-forming unit of reovirus in water containing bromine. *Applied Microbiology*, **29**, 94–101.

335 Park, J.B. and Park, N.-H. (1989) Effect of chlorhexidine on the *in vitro* and *in vivo* herpes simplex virus infection. *Oral Surgery*, **67**, 149–153.

336 Sickbert-Bennett, E.E. *et al.* (2005) Comparative efficacy of hand hygiene agents in the reduction of bacteria and viruses. *American Journal of Infection Control*, **33**, 67–77.

337 Pilcher, K.S. *et al.* (1961) Studies of chemical inhibitors of influenza virus moltiplication: I. Biguanides and related compounds. *Antimicrobial Agents and Chemotherapy*, **11**, 381–389.

338 Fara, G.M. *et al.* (1974) Antiviral activity of selected biguanide derivatives. *Pharmacological Research Communications*, **6**, 117–126.

339 Pinto, F. (2010) *Mechanisms of action of polyhexamethylene biguanide-based biocide against non-enveloped virus*. PhD thesis, Welsh School of Pharmacy, Cardiff University.

340 Thakkar, N. *et al.* (2009) Specific interactions between the viral coreceptor CXCR4 and the biguanide-based compound NB325 mediate inhibition of human immunodeficiency virus type 1 infection. *Antimicrobial Agents and Chemotherapy*, **53**, 631–638.

341 van den Worm, S.H.E. *et al.* (2006) Cryo electron microscopy reconstructions of the Leviviridae unveil the densest icosahedral RNA packing possible. *Journal of Molecular Biology*, **363**, 558–565.

342 Cusack, S. (2005) Adenovirus complex structures. *Current Opinion in Structural Biology*, **15**, 237–243.

343 Ansardi, D.C. and Morrow, C.D. (1993) Poliovirus capsid proteins derived from P1 precursors with glutamine-valine cleavage sites have defects in assembly and RNA encapsidation. *Journal of Virology*, **67**, 7284–7297.

344 Laude, H. *et al.* (1990) Molecular biology of transmissible gastroenteritis virus. *Veterinary Microbiology*, **23**, 147–154.

345 Anders, R. and Chrysikopoulos, C.V. (2006) Evaluation of the factors controlling the time-dependent inactivation rate coefficients of bacteriophage MS2 and PRD1. *Environmental Science and Technology*, **40**, 3237–3242.

346 Svensson, U. and Persson, R. (1984) Entry of adenovirus 2 into Hela cells. *Journal of Virology*, **51**, 687–694.

347 Tsang, S.K. *et al.* (2001) Kinetic analysis of the effect of poliovirus receptor on viral uncoating: the receptor as a catalyst. *Journal of Virology*, **75**, 4984–4989.

348 Laude, H. (1981) Thermal inactivation studies of a coronavirus, transmissible gastroenteritis virus. *Journal of General Virology*, **56**, 235–240.

349 Narang, H.K. and Codd, A.A. (1983) Action of commonly used disinfectants against enteroviruses. *Journal of Hospital Infection*, **4**, 209–212.

350 Geller, C. *et al.* (2009) A new Sephadex-based method for removing microbicidal and cytotoxic residues when testing antiseptics against viruses: experiments with a human coronavirus as a model. *Journal of Virological Methods*, **159**, 217–226.

351 Valot, S. *et al.* (2000) A simple method for the *in vitro* study of the virucidal activity of disinfectants. *Journal of Virological Methods*, **86**, 21–24.

352 Kariwa, H. *et al.* (2004) Inactivation of SARS coronavirus by means of povidone-iodine, physical conditions, and chemical reagents. *Japanese Journal of Veterinary Research*, **52**, 105–112.

353 Thraenhart, O. *et al.* (1978) Influence of different disinfection conditions on the structure of the hepatitis B virus (Dane particle) as evaluated in the morphological alteration and disintegration test (MADT). *Zentralblatt für Bakteriologie, Parasitenkunde, Infektionskrankheinten und Hygiene. I. Abteilung Originale, Reike*, **242**, 299–314.

354 Ito, K. *et al.* (2002) Effect of ethanol on antigenicity of hepatitis B virus envelope proteins. *Japanese Journal of Infectious Diseases*, **55**, 117–121.

355 Schnitzler, P. *et al.* (2001) Antiviral activity of Australian tea tree oil and eucalyptus oil against herpes simplex virus in cell culture. *Die Pharmazie*, **56**, 343–347.

356 Hayashi, K. *et al.* (1995) Virucidal effects of the steam distillate from *Houttuynia cordata* and its components on HSV-1, influenza virus and HIV. *Planta Medica*, **61**, 237–241.

357 Dennison, D.K. *et al.* (1995) The antiviral spectrum of listerine antiseptic. *Oral Surgery Oral Medicine Oral Pathology Oral Radiology and Endodontics*, **79**, 442–448.

358 Siddiqui, Y.M. *et al.* (1996) Effect of essential oils on the enveloped viruses: antiviral activity of oregano and clove oils on herpes simplex virus type 1 and Newcastle disease virus. *Medical Science Research*, **24**, 185–186.

359 Baldry, M.G.C. *et al.* (1991) The activity of peracetic acid on sewage indicator bacteria and viruses. *Water Science Technology*, **24**, 353–357.

360 Sauerbrei, A. *et al.* (2007) Hexon denaturation of human adenoviruses by different groups of biocides. *Journal of Hospital Infection*, **65**, 264–270.

361 Pottage, T. *et al.* (2010) Evaluation of hydrogen peroxide gaseous disinfection systems to decontaminate viruses. *Journal of Hospital Infection*, **74**, 55–61.

362 Riesser , V.W. *et al.* (1976) Possible mechanism of poliovirus inactivation by ozone, in *Forum on Ozone Disinfection* (eds E.G. Fochtman *et al.*), International Ozone Institute, New York, pp. 186–192.

363 DeMik, G. and DeGroot, I. (1977) Mechanism of inactivation of bacteriophage ØX174 and its DNA in aerosols by ozone and ozomised cyclohexene. *Journal of Hygiene, Cambridge*, **78**, 191–211.

364 Christensen, E. and Giese, A. (1954) Changes in adsorption spectra of nucleic acids and their derivatives following exposure to ozone and ultraviolet radiations. *Archives of Biochemistry and Biophysics*, **51**, 208–216.

365 Sproul, O.J. *et al.* (1982) The mechanism of ozone inactivation of water borne viruses. *Water Science Technology*, **14**, 303–314.

366 Kim, C.H. *et al.* (1980) Mechanism of ozone inactivation of bacteriophage f2. *Journal of Environmental Microbiology*, **39**, 210–218.

367 Mudd, J.B. *et al.* (1969) Reaction of ozone with amino acids and proteins. *Atmospheric Environment*, **3**, 669–681.

368 Roy, D. *et al.* (1981) Mechanism of enteroviral inactivation by ozone. *Applied Environmental Microbiology*, **41**, 718–723.

369 Roy, D. *et al.* (1981) Kinetics of enteroviral inactivation by ozone. *Journal of the Environmental Engineering Division*, **107**, 887–901.

370 Thurman, R.B. and Gerba, C.P. (1989) The molecular mechanisms of copper and silver ion disinfection of bacteria and viruses. *Critical Reviews of Environmental Control*, **18**, 295–315.

371 Rahn, R.O. and Landry, L.C. (1973) Ultraviolet irradiation of nucleic acid complexed with heavy atoms. 11. Phosphorescence and photodimerization of DNA complexed with Ag. *Photochemistry and Photobiology*, **18**, 29–38.

372 Rahn, R.O. *et al.* (1973) Ultraviolet irradiation of nucleic acid complexed with heavy atoms. III. Influence of Ag^+ and Hg^{2+} on the sensitivity of phage and of transforming DNA to ultraviolet radiation. *Photochemistry and Photobiology*, **18**, 39–41.

373 Fox, C.L. and Modak, S.M. (1974) Mechanisms of silver sulphadiazine action on burn wound infections. *Antimicrobial Agents and Chemotherapy*, **5**, 582–588.

374 Li, Q. *et al.* (2008) Antimicrobial nanomaterials for water disinfection and microbial control: potential applications and implications. *Water Research*, **42**, 4591–4602.

375 Elechiguerra, J.L. *et al.* (2005) Interaction of silver nanoparticles with HIV-1. *Journal of Nanobiotechnology*, **29**, 3–6.

376 Rogers, J.V. *et al.* (2008) A preliminary assessment of silver nanoparticle inhibition of monkeypox virus plaque formation. *Nanoscale Research Letters*, **3**, 129–133.

377 De Gusseme, B. *et al.* (2010) Biogenic silver for disinfection of water contaminated with viruses. *Applied and Environmental Microbiology*, **76**, 1082–1087.

378 Horie, M. *et al.* (2008) Inactivation and morphological changes of avian influenza virus by copper ions. *Archives of Virology*, **153**, 1467–1472.

379 Samuni, A. *et al.* (1983) On the cytotoxicity of vitamin C and metal ions. *European Journal of Biochemistry*, **137**, 119–124.

380 Samuni, A. *et al.* (1984) Roles of copper and superoxide anion radicals in the radiation-induced inactivation of T7 bacteriophage. *Radiation Research*, **99**, 562–572.

381 Russell, A.D. (1998) Microbial sensitivity and resistance to chemical and physical agents, in *Topley and Wilson's Microbiology and Microbial Infections*, vol. 2, 9th edn (eds A. Balows and B.I. Duerden), Edward Arnold, London, pp. 149–184.

382 Song, H. *et al.* (2010) Thermal stability and inactivation of hepatitis C virus grown in cell culture. *Virology Journal*, 7, 40–52.

383 Shimasaki, N. *et al.* (2009) Inactivation of hepatitis A virus by heat and high hydrostatic pressure: variation among laboratory strains. *Vox Sanguinis*, **96**, 14–19.

384 Sauerbrei, A. and Wutzler, P. (2008) Testing thermal resistance of viruses. *Archives of Virology*, **154**, 115–119.

385 Roberts, C.G. (2000) Studies on the bioburden on medical devices and the importance of cleaning, in *Disinfection, Sterilization and Antisepsis: Principles and Practice in Healthcare Facilities* (ed. W.A. Rutala), APIC, Minneapolis, pp. 63–69.

386 Williams, F.P. (1985) Membrane-associated viral complexes observed in stools and cell cultures. *Applied and Environmental Microbiology*, **50**, 523–526.

387 Hoff, J.C. and Akin, E.W. (1986) Microbial mechanisms of resistance to disinfectants: mechanisms and significance. *Environmental Health Perspectives*, **69**, 7–13.

388 Sharp, D.G. (1968) Multiplicity reaction of animal viruses. *Progress in Medical Virology*, **10**, 64–109.

389 Gassilloud, B. and Gantzer, C. (2005) Adhesion–aggregation and inactivation of poliovirus 1 in groundwater stored in a hydrophobic container. *Applied and Environmental Microbiology*, **71**, 912–920.

390 Floyd, R. and Sharp, D.G. (1979) Viral aggregation: buffer effects in the aggregation of poliovirus and reovirus at low and high pH. *Applied and Environmental Microbiology*, **38**, 395–401.

391 Jensen, H. *et al.* (1980) Inactivation of coxsackie viruses B3 and B5 in water by chlorine. *Applied and Environmental Microbiology*, **40**, 633–640.

392 Salk, J.E. and Gori, J.B. (1960) A review of theoretical, experimental and practical considerations in the use of formaldehyde for inactivation of poliovirus. *Annals of New York Academy of Sciences*, **83**, 609–637.

393 Abad, F.X. *et al.* (1994) Disinfection of human enteric viruses in water by copper and silver combination with low levels of chlorine. *Applied and Environmental Microbiology*, **60**, 2377–2383.

394 Floyd, R. and Sharp, D.C. (1977) Aggregation of poliovirus and reovirus by dilution in water. *Applied and Environmental Microbiology*, **33**, 159–167.

395 Tang, J.X. *et al.* (2002) Metal ion-induced lateral aggregation of filamentous viruses fd and M13. *Biophysical Journal*, **83**, 566–581.

396 Moldenhauer, D. (1984) Quantitative evaluation of the effects of disinfectants against viruses in suspension experiments. *Zentralblatt für Bakteriologie und Hygiene, I. Abteilung Originale*, **B179**, 544–554.

397 Maillard, J.-Y. *et al.* (1998) Resistance of *Pseudomonas aeruginosa* PAO1 phage F116 to sodium hypochlorite. *Journal of Applied Microbiology*, **85**, 799–806.

398 Chambon, M. *et al.* (1994) Comparative sensitivity of the echovirus type 25 JV-4 prototype strain and two recent isolates to glutaraldehyde at low concentrations. *Applied and Environmental Microbiology*, **60**, 387–392.

399 Vrisjen, R. *et al.* (1983) pH dependent aggregation and electrofocusing of poliovirus. *Journal of Genetic Virology*, **64**, 2339–2342.

400 Butler, M. *et al.* (1985) Electrofocusing of viruses and sensitivity to disinfection. *Water Science Technology*, **17**, 201–210.

401 Young, D.C. and Sharp, D.G. (1985) Virion conformational forms and the complex inactivation kinetics of echovirus by chlorine in water. *Applied and Environmental Microbiology*, **49**, 359–364.

402 Mandel, B. (1971) Characterization of type 1 poliovirus by electrophoretic analysis. *Virology*, **44**, 554–568.

403 Allison, A.C. (1962) Observations of viruses by sulfhydryl reagents. *Virology*, **17**, 176–183.

404 Fraise, A.P. (1999) Choosing disinfectants. *Journal of Hospital Infection*, **43**, 255–264.

10 Transmissible Spongiform Encephalopathies and Decontamination

Gerald McDonnell

Research and Technical Affairs, STERIS Ltd, Basingstoke, UK

Introduction

Prion diseases

Transmissible spongiform encephalopathies (TSEs), also referred to as transmissible degenerative encephalopathies (TDEs) or prion diseases, are a distinct group of fatal neurological diseases of mammals that share many unusual features (Table 10.1) [1]. They are transmissible, although the mechanisms and extent of transmission seem to vary from disease to disease.

"Encephalopathy" is a disease or disorder of the brain and "spongiform" the presentation of diseased neural tissue from histological analysis in such cases. Although the presentation and progression of these diseases can vary from disease to disease and also individual to individual, they are all characterized by similar signs of neurological degeneration. In humans, these include dementia, personality changes and memory loss, followed by various physical impairments such as loss of balance/coordination (ataxia) and jerking-movements (myoclonus). Similar manifestations are seen in animals. Once these initial clinical signs begin, the progress in the severity of the disease may take a few weeks to several years. To date, these diseases are always fatal. Their diagnosis is difficult and histology of brain tissue is necessary to confirm cases, as demonstrated by the loss of brain structure (spongiform appearance due to neutron cell loss), astrocytosis (as a response to neuron cell loss) and amyloid/protein plaque deposition.

Human diseases include sporadic Creutzfeldt–Jakob disease (sCJD), variant Creutzfeldt–Jakob disease (vCJD), familial Creutzfeldt–Jakob disease (fCJD), Gerstmann–Sträussler–Scheinker syndrome (GSS), fatal familial insomnia (FFI) and kuru. Epidemiologically, they are described as affecting humans worldwide at a collective frequency of 1–3 in a million people/year. In many countries the published rates for these diseases may be less, although this is more likely due to the difficulty in disease diagnosis than actual lower incidence in those populations. CJD is the most common form of TSE in humans, being initially described in the 1920s. It is generally sporadic in occurrence and though it is more common in those of 60 years or older, cases have been recorded in younger (<30 years) persons as well. Iatrogenic cases have been described, demonstrating the transmissible nature of these diseases, linked to reusable medical devices and transplanted tissues/biological materials (e.g. dura mater grafts and growth hormones [2]). Further, approximately 10% of cases are known to have a genetic link, which can be identified in higher risk groups. During the 1990s a distinct form of CJD (now known as variant CJD or vCJD) was described [3] and has been the focus of much research. This disease was observed in younger people and had subtle differences in clinical presentation and on

Russell, Hugo & Ayliffe's: Principles and Practice of Disinfection, Preservation and Sterilization, Fifth Edition. Edited by Adam P. Fraise, Jean-Yves Maillard, and Syed A. Sattar.

Table 10.1 Examples of the most common transmissible spongiform encephalopathies (TSEs).

Disease	Hosts	Notes
Scrapie	Sheep, goats	One of the most widely studied diseases, both its transmission and progression in sheep as well as a laboratory model for prion investigations. The disease name derives from the scratching of infected animals during disease progression
Transmissible mink encephalopathy (TME)	Mink	A rare disease described in mink
Chronic wasting disease (CWD)	Deer, elk, moose	TSE disease particularly in cervids (deer). Reports of the incidence of CWD have been increasing from the first description in the 1960s from Colorado, USA, spreading into neighboring states
Bovine spongiform encephalopathy (BSE)	Cattle	Commonly known as "mad cow disease" and probably the most famous TSE. Responsible for a large outbreak of disease in cattle during the 1980s, particularly in the UK. Is widely accepted to have been transmitted to humans by contaminated meat products, leading to a similar disease (vCJD) outbreak
Kuru	Humans	A unique disease linked to a Papua New Guinea tribe, commonly related to cannibalism of individuals with another TSE (CJD)
Creutzfeldt–Jakob disease (CJD)	Humans	The most common TSE in humans, which occurs spontaneously in most cases but also genetically and iatrogenically
Variant (or new variant) Creutzfeldt–Jakob disease (vCJD or nvCJD)	Humans	Human disease similar yet distinct to CJD and widely accepted to have been transmitted to humans via meat products contaminated with BSE
Gerstmann–Straussler–Scheinker (GSS)	Humans	Rare human disease, distinct from CJD, with known genetic transmission
Fatal familial insomnia	Humans	Rare human disease, distinct from CJD, with known genetic transmission

histological examination of brain tissue in comparison with "classic" CJD. vCJD is now widely accepted to be associated with the transmission of an animal TSE (bovine spongiform encephalopathy or BSE in cattle) into humans by contaminated meat products (see below).

Kuru is another disease of note in humans, being confined to the Fore tribe of Papua New Guinea [4]. Kuru predominantly affected women and children of both sexes, with only 2% of cases in adult males. Kuru was always fatal and, in affected villages, was the commonest cause of death among women who had more frequent contact with brain tissue during ritualistic cannibalism. The disease is now considered eradicated due the banning of such a practice. It remains unclear as to whether the brain tissue was actually consumed in a cannibalistic fashion or was simply smeared on the bodies of the mourners [5]. More recent studies show that the age of onset of disease in kuru can range from 5 to over 60 years, suggesting that genetic and other susceptibility factors may play a role during the transmission/onset of disease, similar to other TSEs [6].

In animals, the most widely studied TSE is scrapie in sheep, which can result in losses of up to 30% of infected flocks [7]. Scrapie was first described in 1732 and its name comes from the sheep scraping itself to relieve the intense itching associated with the disease. It has been identified in sheep flocks worldwide, with the notable exception (to date) of Australia and New Zealand. It is believed to spread directly between animals through contact or indirectly by ingestion of contaminated materials. The scrapie protein is speculated to persist in the environment for decades [8]. More is known about scrapie as a natural disease in sheep and as an experimental disease in rodents, with the latter being widely used for laboratory investigations of TSEs.

Transmissible mink encephalopathy (TME) originally occurred sporadically among ranch-bred mink in North America and Europe, and resulted in very high mortality rates [9]. A link between the disease and a previously unrecognized scrapie-like infection in cattle in the United States has been suggested [10]. Chronic wasting disease (CWD) was first found in captive deer in Colorado in 1967 [11] and was later identified in several US states and Canadian provinces. Epidemiological evidence suggests that CWD is continuing to spread among cervid populations in North America. Diseased animals first show weight loss and then other clinical signs typical of TSEs. The mechanisms of transmission are not fully understood, but ingestion of grass contaminated with prion-containing feces of infected animals is the most likely means [11]. Blood and urine from contaminated animals are also infectious. Humans may contract CWD through consuming infected venison and develop an ailment similar to CJD [12, 13]; however, others believe that CWD prions are unable to cross the species barrier between cervids and humans [14].

Of particular notoriety is BSE, a TSE of cattle. The first cases of BSE were identified in England in the early 1980s, and the disease was later found to spread through the use of bovine-derived meat and bone-meal in cattle feed [15]. A ban on the use of such material for feeding ruminants in the UK was introduced in 1988, and was extended to all farmed species in 1996. Nevertheless, about 185,000 cases had occurred in British cattle by 2009. Although BSE clearly originated in England, the disease had also been detected by June 2002 to varying degrees in the indigenous cattle populations of all European Union (EU) states. BSE had also been previously detected at a significant level in Switzerland. By October 2009, the disease had also been detected at lower levels not only in other non-EU European countries but also in Israel (one case), Japan (35 cases), Canada (18 cases) and the USA (two cases). These findings suggest that those EU member states (and Switzerland) that first experienced BSE in the early 1990s are likely to have imported BSE-prion-contaminated cattle feed from the UK during the late 1980s. The much later identification of the disease in other EU states, other European countries, Israel and Japan suggests that this was propagated by a "second wave" of exportation of animal feed products from EU states; these were considered (until recently) to be BSE-free because the exportation of such products from the UK had been prohibited in the early 1990s. BSE also appears to have been transmitted in the past to domestic cats and to captive exotic felids and ruminants born in Britain.

The origins of BSE remain unknown. It has been suggested that the UK BSE outbreak may have originated from a unique scrapie strain, through the rendering of sheep and cattle carcasses into cattle feed [16]. Other suggestions include the natural selection of an atypical strain of BSE in cattle [17]. Recently, a new atypical BSE disease in cattle has been described, known as BASE [17, 18]. Interestingly, these forms of BSE remain mostly asymptomatic in aging cattle and have been identified in Europe and North America. In animal experiments to date, BASE demonstrates a shorter survival, and a different clinical evolution, histopathology and PrP^{res} pattern than that observed with classic BSE or vCJD strains [19].

The possibility that BSE might be zoonotically transmissible to humans was suggested by the occurrence of a few cases of a new form of CJD (vCJD) that was originally confined to the UK [3]. Not only had the new form of the disease affected an unusually younger age group but the clinical and neuro-histopathological features are quite distinct from the traditional form of sporadic CJD. The probable association between BSE and vCJD was suggested [20]. These studies showed that the BSE and vCJD agents had identical phenotypic properties when injected into mice, and that these were different from any of the previously mouse-passaged TSE strains [21]. By 2009, 170 cases of vCJD had been recorded in Great Britain, 25 cases had occurred in France, and 1–5 cases had been reported in Ireland, Italy, the USA, Canada, Saudi Arabia, Japan, the Netherlands, Portugal and Spain. Epidemiologically, the incidence of vCJD in the UK peaked in 2000 (28 cases) and has subsequently declined, with one case in 2008 and two in 2009; however, there remains much speculation regarding a potential second wave of the epidemic in a larger subgroup of the population.

A feature of all TSEs is that a normal animal glycoprotein (PrP^c), which is particularly expressed at a high level in neurons, converts to a protease-resistant form (often referred to as PrP^{res} when associated with scrapie) as a consequence of infection [22] and accumulates progressively in brain and a variety of other tissues. The level of accumulation is highest within the central nervous system (CNS) and is associated topographically with neuronal vacuolation [23]. This is the principal lesion that is detectable by histological examination and is thought to cause the fatal neurological dysfunction which is a clinical hallmark for the

TSEs. This leads to the remarkable proposal that these diseases were caused by small proteinaceous infectious particles known as "prions" [24]. The term prion refers to the unit of infection and is coined from the words "proteinaceous" and "infectious".

Agent characteristics
What is the disease-causing agent?
The unconventional nature of scrapie and its associated agent has long been recognized [25]. Scrapie and other TSEs were originally described as "slow" viruses, being associated with diseases having long incubation periods, slow but progressive development of disease and leading to severe illness or death. Interestingly, experiments failed to identify any typical microbial cause for these diseases, despite their infectious nature, and the immune system did not appear to play a role in protection. To date, the precise molecular nature of the agents that cause TSEs has not been determined, but a conventional viral etiology has been largely excluded because no agent-specific nucleic acids have been detected for any of the TSE agents. Nor have agent-specific antibodies been detected in naturally infected hosts.

An abnormal protease-resistant form of a normal host protein is strongly implicated in the pathological process. PrP^c is a normal glycoprotein that is associated with cell membranes and is expressed in a various types of cells. The highest level of expression is in neurons, but its exact normal function is unknown. Experiments in mice had suggested that the protein was non-essential, but many subtle and important functions have been subsequently suggested [26]. These include cellular trafficking of copper, oxidative stress control, roles in the immune system (e.g. T-cell functions), hematopoietic stem cell renewal, CNS structure and functions (e.g. neuron morphology, adhesion, circadian rhythms, synaptic transmissions) and long-term memory. PrP^c is predominantly found attached to the cell plasma membrane as an extracellular glycoprotein, with a smaller fraction of the protein located intracellularly. During TSE infection, PrP^c is converted to an abnormal protease-resistant form (PrP^{res}) that accumulates progressively, particularly within the CNS because it resists catabolic degradation. This conversion is a change in secondary/tertiary structure and the levels of intracellular PrP significantly increases, which is subsequently linked with neurotoxicity.

Because PrP^{res} usually (but interestingly, not always) co-purifies with infectivity, it is now widely accepted that the transmissible agent is solely comprised of PrP^{res}, and is devoid of any additional specific nucleic acids. This is the essential basis of the "prion" hypothesis [24]. The hypothesis argues that PrP^{res} per se is the infectious agent, and that its introduction into, or spontaneous generation within, a previously uninfected host causes a post-translational conformational modification of PrP^c to PrP^{res} by some unknown mechanism; the amino acid sequences of PrP^c and PrP^{res} are the same. The importance of PrP protein in the development of disease was demonstrated by the inability of scrapie infectivity to replicate in mice in which the PrP gene had been ablated [27]. PrP clearly plays an important role in these diseases, but there remains much evidence to suggest that other cellular (or indeed non-cellular) components may be involved in the process. First, investigators have shown that PrPres is capable of generating the infectious form of PrP *in vitro*, but it appears to differ significantly in infectivity and structure. Indeed, the structure of PrPres (or PrP in its converted form) has been difficult to study, but recent evidence has shown important structural differences between naturally occurring and synthetic (recombinant) prions [28]. Various other factors could be involved in the conversion process itself and/or associated with the infectious structure of PrPres. The known hydrophobic nature of PrPres could encourage the association of other molecules that may be associated with or even determine the phenomenon of strain specificity that is described later in this chapter. The association of important informational molecules with PrPres is certainly a model that was preferred in the past [29–31]. More recently, evidence for the presence and role of associated molecules has come to light and is more widely accepted [32, 33]. These include various polysaccharides, lipids (cholesterol, sphingolipids), nucleic acids (DNA and RNA) and even other proteins ("protein X"). As a recent example, a transmission study was conducted with the 263K scrapie hamster model to search for a putative prion-associated factor indispensable for infectivity [33]. Recombinant prion protein was reproducibly shown to transmit disease when converted *in vitro* in a solution containing PrPres-derived RNA material. The RNA molecules consisted of two fractions with an average length of about *c.* 27 and *c.* 55 nucleotides. The authors concluded that the "prion" could indeed be a nucleoprotein, but it may not be specific in nature.

It has long been suggested that prion diseases were associated with an infectious agent, either indirectly or directly. The "virino" theory proposes that, although PrPres is probably a required component of the infectious agent, there is the likely requirement for additional informational molecule(s) such as nucleic acids to convey strain-specific information; these may also trigger the change from PrPc to PrPres [34]. The virino model invokes the need for only very small informational molecules, which would be difficult to detect, and argues that informational molecules such as nucleic acids are essential in explaining the diversity of strains and the mutations that are known to occur with scrapie agent in mice of the same PrP genotype [35]. Other reports have suggested co-infection with microorganisms as being important for disease progression, such as *Helicobacter pylori* [36], *Spiroplasma* [37] and other pathogens [38].

Prion strain variation
Multiple strains of prions have been identified to date and remain to be isolated as research continues into these diseases [39]. However, it should be noted that the present number of recognized strains has arisen coincidentally as a result of general research into TSEs rather than through a rigorous "strain-hunting" exercise. Thus, it is likely that there are many other strains yet to be identified. Strains are not just differentiated based on their origin (e.g. from a scrapie, CJD or vCJD case). In fact,

many strains that have been passaged and investigated within rodents of the same PrP genotype can be distinguished by many factors, including their incubation periods, the distribution and severity of lesions in the brain, clinical manifestations, ease of transmission to new species and even susceptibility to thermal and chemical inactivation [39, 40]. An interesting example is the fact that vCJD prion isolates from humans readily transmit disease when introduced into wild-type mice, while similar isolates from sCJD cases do not. There appear to be many factors that require further investigation to understand the nature of these strains and their implications from a species barrier (or not) point of view.

With regard to the strain-specific properties of TSE agents relating to their relative degrees of thermostability, it is significant that these properties (as well as other strain characteristics) remained the same regardless of whether they were passaged in mice strains that were congenic and differed genetically only with regard to the chemical nature of the PrP protein that they produced [41]. In one study, five different strains were compared for moist- and dry-heat sterilization resistance; this suggested particular differences in moist-heat inactivation rates [42]. Chemical and enzymatic differences in the susceptibility of different prion strains to degradation have also been shown [43, 44]. It is important to note that the test methods used in these and other cases all utilized prion-contaminated brain homogenates. The presence of different sources of brain tissue may have an important role in the "resistance" observed in combination with or distinct from the prion agent itself. Despite this, these results not only are scientifically intriguing but are an important practical consideration in the development of test methods that may be used for testing the effectiveness of decontamination methods against prions.

Given that prions are considered to be simple proteins void of any genetic elements, the concept of specific strains occurring may be initially challenging to accept. Proponents of the virino hypothesis argue that strain-specific characteristics must be conveyed by informational molecules that are independent of the host, but none have been identified. Indeed, the presence of such a wide range of strains was often in contrast to the protein-only hypothesis. In support of the protein-only hypothesis, there is evidence to suggest that prions are subject to mutational and selective amplification [45]. This is not limited to slight differences in the primary structures (as determined genetically) of the PrP protein itself. Studies with TME have shown that two strains of the agent can convert hamster PrPc to PrPres in a cell-free system and pass on strain-specific information in the form of differing enzyme cleavage sites for the PrPres molecules [46]. The authors suggest that this confirms that a messenger molecule, such as a nucleic acid, is not required for conveying strain-specific information. Another theory that has been proposed to explain strain variation within the framework of the prion hypothesis is that PrPres glycosylation patterns confer strain specificity [47]. This theory is based on the suggestion that different strains of scrapie agent target different areas of the brain, and that there are diversely glycosylated forms of PrP^res in scrapie-infected brain [48]. The hypothesis is that different subsets of neurons express differently glycosylated forms of PrP^c, and that when the host is challenged with PrP^res this will interact preferentially with PrP^c molecules that have a matching glycosylation pattern, thus perpetuating strain characteristics. However, some strains target the same areas of the brain. Also, strain specificity is preserved in infectivity that is recovered from lymphoreticular tissues such as spleen. Although the TSEs are essentially neurological diseases in terms of their clinical manifestations, the disease process customarily involves infection of the lymphoreticular system before neuro-invasion occurs. Current evidence indicates that infection of the spleen is associated with agent replication (or accumulation) within the follicular dendritic cells [49, 50], and one would not expect this single cell type to have the capacity to donate diverse glycosylation patterns to PrP^res. There is clearly a need to determine unequivocally how the "inherited" information that defines the strain-specific properties of TSE agents is processed.

General considerations
Survival in the environment
As will be described later in the chapter, many of the TSE agents are remarkably resistant to conventional disinfection and sterilization procedures that are normally considered effective for all other types of microorganisms. Infectivity has been reported from prion-contaminated brain macerates incinerated at 600°C for 15 min [51]. It is, therefore, not surprising that drying and even desiccation of prion-contaminated materials have little effect on their infectivity [52, 53] and can even increase their resistance to heat and chemical inactivation methods [54]. This may explain the genesis of outbreaks of scrapie in sheep grazed on pastures that had been fallow for years [7], and the spread of CWD in the cervid population of North America [55, 56]. In the case of CWD, levels of prions can be detected in grass samples in the vicinity of affected herds [11]. Scrapie agent has also been shown to maintain a significant degree of viability after burial for 3 years [57] and the sCJD agent remains highly infectious after being held at room temperature for 28 months [58]. Scrapie agent survives in a desiccated state for at least 30 months [59]. Resistance and infectivity of prions may also be affected by interaction with other types of structures and minerals [60]. For example, a 10-fold increase in the survival of prions in soil samples was reported in the presence of manganese [61]. Given their persistent nature, it may also be suggested that such survival could contribute to the rare but ubiquitous sporadic cases of CJD of unknown etiology.

Investigations into transmission
As discussed above, the environment may be considered a significant reservoir for prions and as a source of infectious material to animal and human populations. Given the incubation time of TSEs, which is often as long as a few decades, it is difficult to link an outbreak to any particular source. It is clear from studies with scrapie and CWD, including laboratory, field and epidemiological studies, that prions are more than likely to be transmitted by close contact between animals (in particular through open wounds) and/or via contaminated surfaces such as soil and grass. The impact of these studies on the risks associated with drinking water or wastewater contamination is unknown. This may be important, as cleaning with water is a general recommendation in animal and human situations where prion contamination is known. Water contamination has been shown from environmental samples in CWD epidemic areas, as well as samples from an associated water treatment facility [62]. In contrast, a simulated, indirect study in wastewaters (sludge) suggested that detectable amyloid fibrils were reduced over time [63]. However, this study was not conducted with actual prion fibrils. Overall, there is little known of the risks associated with water contamination with prions and the potential for transmission to occur.

It is now widely accepted that meat or meat-containing food products are a risk for prion transmission. Although initially considered controversial, the BSE epidemic in cattle in the UK, and subsequent outbreak of vCJD in humans, has been strongly linked with prion-contaminated meat products [64]. BSE transmission to cattle is believed to have been through the consumption of meat and bone-meal prepared from the rendering of animal tissue (presumably brain and spinal cord material in particular). It is widely believed that this was due to a difference in the heating temperature/time used during the rendering process, where lower temperatures and shorter times may have been used. However, changes also included moving from a batch to a continuous process and the removal of a solvent extraction method for some materials [65]. Overall, we may never know the exact reason for the outbreak or indeed the original source of the prion contamination. What is known, epidemiologically and from subsequent laboratory studies, is that the disease spread through contaminated foodstuffs and then was subsequently transmitted to humans by contaminated meat and/or meat products. This is also a likely source of transmission of the same strain to cats and other animals. The mechanisms of uptake in the intestine, including proliferation in Peyer's patches, have been reasonably well described in the literature [66]. Similar risks have been proposed from the consumption of deer meat and the potential transmission of CWD to humans, although this remains to be confirmed [12].

Transmission of prion diseases has been shown with various body tissues, experimentally in the laboratory and in clinical practice. In human diseases such as CJD these have been particularly associated with tissues of the CNS [67, 68]. Such tissues include brain material, particularly when associated with devices used during neurosurgical/investigational procedures, eye surgery (corneal transplantation), dura mater grafts and pituitary hormone therapy. These reports should not be surprising, considering that the highest titers of prion protein precipitates are observed in the CNS of diseased subjects. Other tissues, even those with known or at high risk of TSEs, have traditionally been considered to have low or even no risk of contamination or infectivity [69]. This is the basis for current clinical decisions regarding the reuse, decontamination and/or disposal of contaminated instruments/surfaces. This perspective may need to be reconsidered for at least three reasons. First, most cases of CJD and other TSEs are sporadic in nature, which means that during the incubation and initial development of disease these cases remain asymptomatic while still cross-contaminating devices. Some suggest this a likely explanation in reports of iatrogenic cases with an unidentifiable source [70]. Second, detection technologies have improved over the last 10 years and further investigations have suggested that higher titers of prion may be present in various peripheral tissues/organs (including blood) during earlier, non-symptomatic stages of disease. The significantly higher levels of prion precipitation appear to build up in the CNS during the later stages of disease [71, 72]. With improved detection, even body fluids (e.g. urine) and tissues previously considered to be non-infectious in CJD patients have now been shown to have detectable levels of prions [73]. Third, the tissue distribution of vCJD has been known for some time to be different to that of classic CJD cases [74]. Higher levels of PrP^{res} could be detected, although at significantly lower levels than in the brain, in a wider range of tissues such as tonsils, spleen, lymph nodes, retina and optic nerve. In addition, possible cases of vCJD transmission by blood transfusion have been reported [75], building on previous experimental studies with animals demonstrating clinical and preclinical signs of disease in a sheep model [76]. The impact of blood and blood-fractionation products on the transmission of TSEs is an important area for further studies and risk mitigation [77]. Furthermore, tissue distribution in animal diseases such as scrapie and CWD is significantly different, including environmental persistence as described above, and could provide further risks. In all, the arguments in favor of standard precautions against the risks of prion contamination in various clinical and industrial applications are mounting and may become more practical with the development of practical prion-effective decontamination methods [78].

Iatrogenic transmission of TSEs by the surgical use of cross-contaminated, reusable instruments has been reported both experimentally [52, 53] and clinically [79]. Most of these investigation and cases to date have been directly related to instruments contaminated with brain material from CJD patients or TSE-infected animals. Considering the rare nature of CJD, of notable example is a report from the 1970s of disease transmission over a number of years from the same set of intracerebral electrodes [80]. It was established during this investigation that contamination of the electrodes occurred in an older patient, although the reprocessing methods used at that time following this procedure may not have been optimal given our current knowledge of the nature of these diseases. In this case the device was cleaned by and then reprocessed using chemicals such as alcohol and formaldehyde, both known to have a cross-linking mechanism of action, particularly on proteins. However, these practices should not be considered as being unusual even today where various types of aldehydes and alcohols are widely used for disinfection and

sterilization [78]. What was striking was that CJD transmission was confirmed, or at least highly expected, in two younger patients on whom these devices had been used in the subsequent 3 months (both dying within approximately 18 months following surgery). Moreover, the same devices were identified and removed from use some 3 years following the initial contamination and were shown to transmit the disease to an experimental chimpanzee following implantations. Further studies have suggested that transmission may have occurred in at least four other cases from use of neurosurgical instruments despite the multiple cycles of normal cleaning and sterilization methods used in hospitals [81]. Given the sporadic and rare nature of these diseases, it is remarkable to consider that such cases have been documented in the literature. Some epidemiological investigations have suggest that many surgical procedures present a significant risks of TSE transmission and that cases of sCJD may indeed be related to accidental transmission [82].

Practical considerations in decontamination studies

General

TSE agents are remarkably resistant to inactivation as shown in the studies reported to date. However, as these agents are rarely tested in their purified state, it is difficult to know to what degree their resistance is intrinsic and how much it is influenced by the protective effect of the host tissue to which they are intimately bound. It is well known, for example, that when microorganisms are in the presence of various types of organic or inorganic soils they present unusual resistance to disinfection and sterilization, including steam sterilization (particularly with inorganic soils). Host tissues themselves can contain a variety of proteins, lipids, carbohydrates, etc. With particular significance in prion decontamination studies, brain material is known to have a high lipid/hydrophobic nature that itself can create a barrier to removal and inactivation methods. In addition, particularly with prions, the hydrophobic nature of the cell membrane domains with which infectivity is associated will also encourage the formation of aggregates in homogenized tissue preparations [83]. The protective effect of such aggregates has been recognized for conventional viruses [84] and may at least partly explain the resistance of TSE agents. Decontamination experiments have involved various tissue preparation methods, such as crude brain macerates, 20% homogenates, 10% tissue supernatants, and biochemically processed or ultracentrifuged material including microsomal fractions. Autoclaving studies have confirmed that the presence of tissue has an impeding effect on inactivation of scrapie agent. Gravity-displacement autoclaving of scrapie-infected mouse brain macerate (22A strain) at 126°C for 30 min resulted in a loss of 10^2 infective dose for 50% (ID$_{50}$)/g [85]. When autoclaved at 100 or 105°C as 10% homogenate (i.e. 10-fold less tissue and infectivity per unit volume), the titer losses were 2.5 and 3.5 log$_{10}$, respectively (D.M. Taylor and A.G. Dickinson, unpublished data).

Further, exposure times and conditions have been varied, and the temperature for chemical treatment has been generally either 4°C or room temperature, occasionally with mechanical stirring. Temperature and the presence of other chemicals are known to play both a negative and positive role in affecting prion decontamination [86, 87]. It should be expected that the results using these materials as well as the variability from one preparation to another will be significant.

No standard methods exist for carrying out decontamination studies. This is not unusual in microbiology, as there are no universal methods that are accepted as confirming bactericidal, virucidal and sporicidal activities. There are locally recognized test methods such as the AOAC International's microbiological methods [88] and the European antiseptic and disinfectant test methods. Similarly, some countries have recognized different test methods, such as in Germany where recommendations regarding suspension and surface test methods have been published [89]. Other countries have highlighted the need to test multiple strains of prions, due to concerns over the higher resistance of different strains to decontamination. The most widely used methods to date are suspension studies (using a prion-contaminated suspension directly exposed to a liquid or physical process) or surface studies (using wire or other surfaces contaminated with a prion suspension, usually brain homogenate). Prion preparations have been shown to have a high affinity for surfaces and can be difficult to remove [53]. Surface decontamination has therefore been particularly well studied, for example using a contaminated wire model [43, 52, 53]. These studies have yielded some interesting conclusions, such as the difficulty in cleaning prion contamination from a surface and that some types of cleaning chemistries can increase the resistance of prion infectivity to subsequent disinfection/sterilization methods [53, 90].

It is often assumed that procedures shown to be effective with partially purified infectivity are equally applicable for dealing with crude tissue contamination, but this is unwarranted [91]. Decontamination experiments should mimic the most adverse conditions, thus enhancing the prospect of detecting residual infectivity after exposure to partially inactivating procedures. Such conditions usually employ the use of brain tissue macerates or homogenates. Reticuloendothelial tissues can also be contaminated, although at a lower level and depending on the stage of disease. It is unknown whether there are differences in the degree of protection afforded to the TSE agents by different tissues. An example is seen with validation studies relating to the presence of TDE infectivity in blood or blood products; it is clearly inappropriate to use crude infected brain-tissue as the "spike" material. The effect of the presence of various types of tissues such as in blood is not known. Infectivity has been associated with blood and blood components and has been associated with iatrogenic transmission [75, 76]. For validation studies relating to blood, it would seem appropriate to use partially purified infectivity rather than crude tissue preparations, although the purification method may not reflect the true distribution of PrP^{res} in a natural blood sample.

It is important that recommended test methods used to test prion decontamination should reflect the proposed application. Decontamination methods can be used for a wide range of applications, from device reprocessing (such as used for reusable medical and dental instruments), general surface decontamination (e.g. mortuary, abattoir or laboratory facilities), biopharmaceutical production, tissue preparation (e.g. blood fractionation) and even whole animal/body digestion. Independent of the application, the methods used should provide the required balance of efficacy, safety and compatibility. For example, a method using high concentrations of alkali at high temperatures may be practical for whole carcass treatment but will be very damaging for surgical devices. Likewise, the risks of iatrogenic transmission may be considered low when incineration is used in comparison to the reuse of neurosurgical instruments that have been previously used on a patient with a known TSE disease.

Test methods

Various methods have been used to detect and quantify prions in decontamination studies, which can be considered as being *in vitro* or *in vivo*. *In vitro* tests include a variety of basic biochemical methods to detect PrP, such as western blots, using antibodies raised against the protein. There are a wide variety of antibodies that have been mapped to various locations along the PrP protein which can be used for detection (Figure 10.1). However, to date, antibody-based methods do not differentiate between the non-infectious and the infectious form of PrP as the primary structure is identical. The protease-resistant nature of PrP^{res} is therefore used to differentiate its presence from PrP^c, in particular using proteinase K as a powerful protease. It is important to note that PrP^{res} demonstrates a greater resistance to proteinase K, but will degrade over time depending on the test conditions used. Therefore this method can often present some misleading results. For example, only a portion of PrP^{res} (the hydrophobic core) has been shown to be protease resistant and therefore the choice of antibody can be important (as shown in Figure 10.1). This method can, however, be used to study or optimize any physical effects on PrP^{res} itself but in general is not always predictive of a priocidal effect [53]. In some cases, western blot analysis has shown what appears to be degrading effects on PrP^{res} but these test fractions remained infectious on animal infectivity assays. In contrast, some inactivation methods (particularly using phenolics) had no obvious effects on PrP^{res} in western blot analysis but were non-infectious *in vivo*. A further limitation of western blotting procedures is that these methods are much less sensitive than described *in vivo* assays by a factor of at least 1000, if not greater; estimates of the detection range using western blots would be >10^4 infectious doses.

In vivo (bioassay) models are more reliable and consistent for the detection of TSE infectivity. These procedures produce reliably reproducible results in different laboratories provided that standard methodologies are applied [43, 92]. A typical outline of decontamination bioassays are shown in Figure 10.2.

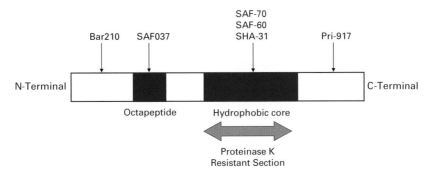

Figure 10.1 Representation of the PrP protein and associated antibodies used for western blot detection. Note the hydrophobic core is the only section in PrP^{res} with high resistance to proteinase K digestion.

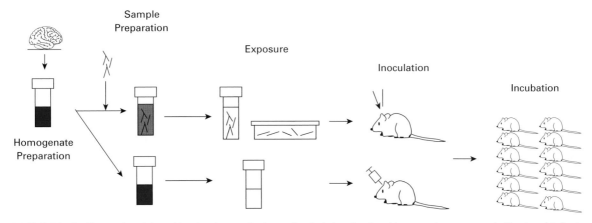

Figure 10.2 Typical *in vivo* (bioassays) models used in prion decontamination studies. Brain (or other tissue) homogenates are prepared, either inoculated onto surfaces or used directly as a suspension for exposure to chemical/physical decontamination methods, inoculated into animals and monitored over time for progression of disease in comparison with controls.

In these tests, exposed prion homogenates (in suspension or dried into a support, such as stainless steel wires) are injected into sensitive animals (usually intracerebrally, although various other sites of injection can be used). A variety of TSE strains have been used for this purpose. In contrast to the situation with many other TSEs, distinct strains of mouse-passaged scrapie agents have been cloned in rodents, and have reproducible biological characteristics [93]. Because high titers of infectivity in brain tissue combined with a short incubation period are a feature of the 263K strain of scrapie agent in hamsters, it has been regarded as an optimal and representative model for decontamination studies [43, 53, 94]. However, this is complicated by the fact that incubation periods can be extremely prolonged when only small amounts of infectivity survive after the agent is exposed to partially inactivating procedures [90]. There is evidence to suggest that some TSE agent isolates or strains differ significantly in their susceptibility to inactivation by chemical and thermal methods [43, 44, 95]. For example, the 22A strain of scrapie agent in mice is known to be relatively thermostable [85, 95] and was previously considered to be the most appropriate model for studying thermal destruction of the TDE agents, even though infectivity titers in brain are lower than for 263K [96]. However, more recent data

suggest that the 301V strain of mouse-passaged BSE agent may be an alternative because it achieves high infectivity titers, has a relatively short incubation period when inoculated at high titer and is extremely resistant to heat inactivation [41]. In contrast, some chemical and even enzymatic inactivation methods may demonstrate greater resistance to scrapie than BSE/vCJD strains ([43, 86]; G. McDonnell *et al.*, unpublished data).

Under well-defined experimental conditions, specific strains of rodent-passaged scrapie agents display consistently reproducible inverse relationships between the dose of infectivity administered and the subsequent incubation period before the onset of clinical disease [97]. This consistency is reproducible within different laboratories, provided that the methodologies used are exactly the same [43, 92]. For any given model, the amount of infectivity present in an inoculum can usually be calculated by comparing the incubation period of the recipients with an "incubation period assay" graph, without the need for titration. Unfortunately, this procedure may not always be applied to infectivity exposed to chemical or physical treatments, because these can radically extend the dose–response curves for treated, compared with untreated, agents [98]. The same conclusions have been arrived at as a result of other studies involving chemical or physical treatments of scrapie agent [99–105]. This means that a meaningful assessment of the amount of infectivity remaining after exposure to partially inactivating procedures can only be obtained by full titration and observing the assay animals for extended periods. Such a method has been developed based on the hamster-adapted scrapie strain 263K and can be easily standardized. In this case, residual infectivity adsorbed on stainless steel wires has been measured by inoculating individual wires intracerebrally into rodents. The time to terminal disease was studied in comparison to controls contaminated with serial dilutions of the original inoculum to determine levels of infectivity reduction [43, 52, 53]. This test method was used to confirm the efficacy of certain World Health Organization (WHO) reference decontamination procedures, and to investigate novel cleaning and disinfection procedures. Despite this, the disadvantages of these types of tests are primarily the costs associated and the extended incubation times (1–2 years in hamster and mice studies, and even longer in studies with other animals such as experimental chimpanzees).

In recent years, two other test methods have been described that may bridge the gaps between western blot and *in vivo* assays: cell culture assays and PMCA (protein misfolding cyclic amplification assay). The assaying of prions in cell culture, particularly known as standard scrapie cell assay (SSCA) although the test is not limited to scrapie strains, is based on the use of various cell lines that are susceptible to prion strains [106, 107]. Prions can thus be "grown" by a series of passages through these cell lines to reach detectable levels by traditional biochemical (western blot) methods. It is estimated that these assays are faster and cheaper than bioassays, with at least equivalent sensitivity. PMCA is a further *in vitro* method, based on the fact that PrPres acts as an initiator (or chaperone) of the change in PrPc structure to the protease-resistant form [108, 109]. In this assay, low doses of PrPres are detected by a series of amplification steps, not dissimilar to polymerase chain reaction (PCR) methods using for the detection of DNA signatures. Samples containing PrPres are mixed with a solution of PrPc, allowed to incubate (to allow for the change in structure of PrPc) and therefore aggregate, and then disaggregated (by sonication/chemical means) and re-incubated in repeated cycles. This allows for a build-up of PrPres that can be detected by traditional western blotting. These assays are not only important in the fundamental understanding and detection of prion diseases but are also under development for use in decontamination studies (investigating the presence of PrPres following decontamination in suspension and surface tests). Further investigations are required – in particular correlation studies with *in vivo* assays and results to date of effective/ineffective decontamination methods – for their acceptance as reliable alternatives to bioassays.

Inactivation methods

Inactivation studies on TSE agents are conducted to obtain information regarding their molecular nature or to establish meaningful decontamination protocols. In the past, the former generally used partially purified materials, whereas the latter involved preparations of relatively crude infected brain tissue. Prion inactivation studies are considered in further detail in this section.

Physical inactivation methods
Gamma and ultraviolet irradiation
The proposed lack of a nucleic acid is often support by the statement that prions are resistant to the effects of various forms of radiation, in particular UV (200–400 nm wavelength) and γ (<10 pm) radiation. It is often assumed that radiation methods specifically target nucleic acids as their principle mechanism of action, but this is certainly not their only effect as other macromolecules such as proteins are also affected [87]. Despite this, when CJD, kuru and scrapie agents were exposed to γ (150 kGy) or UV irradiation (254 nm wavelength, 100 kJ/m^2) infectivity was recoverable [110]; the TME agent was equally resistant [111]. Such exposures represent what would be a gross degree of overkill for conventional microorganisms, although in all cases a significant reduction in prion infectivity was observed. For example, isolated samples of kuru, scrapie and CJD prions were reported to be highly resistant to radiation, although a quantitative decrease in prion tiers was observed on increasing the dose of γ-radiation from 50 to 200 kGy [112]. In these reports it is clear that the test methodology (presence of soil, brain material, aggregates, etc.) can have a significant impact. UV light in particular is known to be poorly penetrating in comparison to γ-radiation due to their respective energy levels. The resistance of TSE agents may be attributable at least partially to protective mechanisms afforded by the intimate association of these agents with cell membranes [113] and the tendency of infected tissue fragments to form aggregates; these would need to receive as many radiation "single hits" as there are infectious units within such aggregates to achieve inactivation [114].

Many earlier reports on the effects of γ-radiation on prions should be read in some detail, as they actually looked at the effects in whole animals on the progression of the disease rather than direct decontamination effects. There has been some recent interest in studying the effects of UV radiation on prion protein structure due to the potential link of prion disease development and oxidative stress. Some investigators have reported unfolding and aggregation effects [115] due to the protein structure effects of UV light. Other earlier reports suggested that the effects of UV radiation observed in their studies may be linked to the presence of a highly protected nucleic acid associated with infectivity [116]. Finally, it should be remembered that UV radiation, as an example, can lead to the localized generation of ozone and other reactive species that may have indirect effects on infectivity. For example, a UV–ozone study in soil samples suggested a dramatic decrease in prion infectivity, although persistence was also observed [117]. Overall, the interpretation of irradiation data has caused considerable debate [118].

Although further investigations and optimization of the effects of γ and UV radiation may lead to the optimization of these methods (e.g. the effects of surface pre-cleaning followed by irradiation), it is unclear if these methods can have any practical application for the routine inactivation of TSE agents.

Microwave irradiation

Although the inactivating effect of microwave irradiation on conventional microorganisms is generally considered to be attributable to the heat generated, a number of investigators have concluded some effects from non-thermal mechanisms [119–122]. Despite these reports, the major action of microwaves appears to be the local generation of moist heat (steam) and not direct heating of a surface itself. Of particular interest are the effects observed in a microwave-treated water sample, observed as an extremely rapid rise in temperature to the temperature required (up to boiling). These effects are different to the direct effects of steam under various temperatures and times of contact, as the effects on protein will vary in heated and direct steam-exposed samples. To date, only one study has investigated the effects of microwave irradiation on one scrapie strain (22A). However, no significant degree of inactivation was observed after the exposure of undiluted, infected brain tissue or 10% saline homogenates [123]. These results seem to match investigations of simply heating and boiling similar samples of scrapie and vCJD brain homogenates both *in vitro* and *in vivo* (G. McDonnell, unpublished data).

Dry heat

Thermal studies involving the transfer of heat from water to samples in glass containers have shown that, at temperatures up to 100°C, there is only a small effect on sCJD [124] and scrapie agents [25]. However, in more sophisticated studies, significant degrees of inactivation were observed at temperatures ranging between 84 and 97°C, depending upon the strain of scrapie agent used [125]. Overall, the effects of dry heat over extended periods of time or direct incineration appear to be effective methods of prion decontamination, despite the presence of soil. Only a small amount of infectivity was recoverable after a homogenate of hamster brain infected with the 263K strain of scrapie agent was exposed to dry heat at a temperature of 360°C for 1 h [126]. It should be noted that the brain homogenate had been lyophilized before heating, which may have further increased thermostability [127]. In contrast, when 7 mg samples of (non-lyophilized) macerated mouse brain infected with the ME7 strain of scrapie agent were exposed to dry heat, there was no detectable infectivity after an exposure to 200°C for 1 h, even though some infectivity had survived exposure to 160°C for 24 h or 200°C for 20 min [128]. Subsequent studies with the 263K and 301V strains showed a significant amount of infectivity survived exposure to hot air at a temperature of 200°C for 1 h [129]. The survival of lyophilized infectivity after exposure to 36°C [126] led to speculation that the effectiveness of incineration for inactivating scrapie-like agents might need to be questioned. In

more recent studies [130] it was reported that traces of scrapie infectivity could be detected after 263K-infected brain tissue had been exposed to 600°C for 15 min in a muffle-furnace. Because such a process would be expected to reliably destroy all forms of organic material, it was hypothesized that an inorganic "fossilized" form of PrP^{res} might retain sufficient structural integrity to trigger the conversion of normal PrP into the disease-specific form. In conclusion, although incineration can be an effective method, it is clear that infectivity at low levels can remain despite such aggressive methods.

Moist-heat (steam) sterilization

Steam is one of the most widely used sterilization technologies, but how it is used can vary. It is therefore important in understanding experiments with steam sterilization that such variables are considered and not just the steam temperature and cycle exposure time. In all steam processes, important variables include the preconditioning of a load to be sterilized (such as the effective removal of air and other gases that can interfere with the penetration of steam and the adequate attainment of the required temperature throughout the load) and even the quality of the water used to generate the steam [87]. Of further interest are the various treatments that can occur with contaminated samples and surfaces prior to exposure with steam, such as pre-drying, pre-cleaning and the use of TSE-contaminated brain homogenates versus isolated precipitates of prion infectivity. In reviewing the literature, these variables are generally not considered when conducting prion decontamination studies, particularly in earlier studies, and they may therefore contribute to the inconsistency of reported results (examples are shown in Table 10.2). In prion decontamination studies, steam sterilization testing has been traditionally referred to as gravity-displacement autoclaving (describing a method of using steam to remove air by gravity, where an autoclave is a chamber in which the steam process is conducted) and porous-load autoclaving (where air removal is assisted using a vacuum pump). What is not provided are details of the exact process used – such as times, levels of pressure during the conditioning cycle, exact temperatures attained in the samples tested, etc. – which can have a significant effect on the success of the cycle tested. Therefore, reports in the literature should be considered critically.

For example, gravity-displacement autoclaving at 126°C for 2 h inactivates the 139A strain of scrapie agent but not the more "thermostable" 22A strain [85], which is inactivated only after 4 h exposure [133]. Guinea-pig-passaged CJD agent and the hamster-passaged 263K strain of scrapie agent were reported to be inactivated at 132°C for 1 h [103]. Consequently, this procedure was adopted as a standard for CJD agent decontamination in the USA [94], and has been used as a general decontamination procedure for TSE agents. However, subsequent studies with the 263K strain of scrapie agent have shown that, although high levels of inactivation are achieved, the use of this procedure does not guarantee complete inactivation [90, 134]. In studies designed to determine the relative thermostability patterns of four different

Table 10.2 A comparison of prion inactivation studies using steam sterilization.

Test conditions	Test method	Published result	Reference
Gravity-displacement autoclave at 121°C, 15 min	CJD brain homogenate (guinea-pig model)	<4-log$_{10}$ infectivity removed; ineffective	[103]
Gravity-displacement autoclave at 121°C, 30 min	CJD brain homogenate (mouse model)	>3.1-log$_{10}$ infectivity removed; effective	[131]
Gravity displacement at 126°C, 15 min	Scrapie (two strains) brain mascerate (hamster model)	1.8- and 5.9-log$_{10}$ infectivity removed; ineffective	[85]
Gravity-displacement autoclave at 126°C, 30 min	Scrapie (two strains) brain mascerate (hamster model)	2.1 and 5.9 infectivity removed; ineffective	[85]
Porous-load autoclave at 136°C, 4 min	Scrapie (two strains) brain mascerate (hamster model)	No transmission (>7-log$_{10}$ infectivity removed); effective	[85]
Porous-load autoclave at 136°C, 8 min	Scrapie (two strains) brain mascerate (hamster model)	No transmission (>7 log$_{10}$ infectivity removed); effective	[85]
Porous-load autoclave at 134°C, 18 min	Scrapie (263K) brain mascerate (hamster model)	Transmission (<7-log$_{10}$ infectivity removed); ineffective	[132]
Porous load autoclave at 138°C, 1 h	BSE (301V) brain mascerate (mouse model)	Transmission, ineffective	[41]

mouse-passaged strains of scrapie agent and the 301V strain of mouse-passaged BSE agent, these strains were subjected to gravity-displacement autoclaving at 126°C for 30 min. The ME7 strain did not survive, but the others showed varying degrees of survival. Thus, 22C was found to be less stable than 139A which, in turn, was less stable than 22A. 301V was by far the most stable strain [41].

Data indicating that porous-load autoclaving at 136°C for *c.* 4 min inactivates both the 139A and 22A strains of scrapie agent [85] were used to formulate the UK standard for inactivation of CJD agent by porous-load autoclaving (i.e. 134–138°C for 18 min), which has been widely adopted internationally. Further studies involving hamster and mouse brain infected with scrapie agents and bovine brain infected with BSE agent, have indicated that this standard may also be unreliable [135]. Infectivity was detectable in samples exposed to 134–138°C for up to 1 h. It is clear that the test method, not just the exposure conditions, can be important in understanding these results. The major difference between these studies was that the average weight of the brain macerates used in the former was 50 mg [85, 135]. In the more recent studies, this was increased to 340 mg because this was considered to be more representative of a worst-case veterinary situation in practice. Also, previous experience with porous-load autoclaving had indicated that inactivation of samples of intact brain in this weight range would be effective [132]. Following the completion of even more recent porous-load autoclaving studies it was recognized that, because the samples were 340 mg brain macerates, there had been the potential for a significant amount of smearing and drying of infected tissue on glass surfaces prior to autoclaving, and that this would have been greater than in the earlier study in which 50 mg samples were used. As stated earlier, it is known that the drying of scrapie infectivity onto glass surfaces enhances thermostability [127]. Since the drying of infectivity onto surfaces is exactly what would occur in practice, it is considered that the more recent data are relevant. Surprisingly,

the 22A strain of scrapie agent and the 301V strain of BSE agent became enhanced when autoclaved at 138°C, compared with 134°C [136]. This was presumably due to the drying of portions of the brain macerates onto glass surfaces before autoclaving The fixation by steam of the proteins in these areas of the samples would have been extremely efficient and rapid, arguably more so at the higher temperature. It is proposed that, paradoxically, the fixation effect actually protects infectivity from further inactivation by the steam process. Similarly, prior fixation in ethanol [91] or formalin [132] has been shown to enhance considerably the resistance of scrapie agents to inactivation by autoclaving. Depending on the application, these data indicate that the practice of porous-load autoclaving at 134–138°C for 18 min on its own may not always be reliable.

Overall, it can be concluded that steam can be an effective process against prions, despite showing unusual resistance when compared with microorganisms such as bacterial endospores. The effect of temperature is inconclusive, but it would appear from the data discussed above that higher temperatures (up to 134°C) and longer exposure times are effective. However, lower temperatures have not been widely tested. Some experiments with boiling (at 100°C for up to 1 h, where contaminated surfaces where initially cleaned, heated to 100°C and then boiled for 30 and/or 60 min) showed no reduction in scrapie *in vivo* wire studies when compared with surfaces only cleaned (G. McDonnell, unpublished data). In contrast, higher temperatures may be less effective, as suggested in detailed studies on the thermostability of prion-infected brain homogenates exposed to various steam temperature conditions over time (Figure 10.3).

Finally, over the last few years a number of *in vivo* studies have investigated the effects of steam sterilization against prion infectivity when contaminated onto wires, to simulate a reusable device surface. These studies have confirmed that 134°C for 18 min can be an effective method, but residual infectivity is often detected [53, 90]. However, two further unexpected conclusions have been made from these and other recent studies. The first is the effect of hydration. When wires where exposed "dry" to the sterilization cycle (simulating the typical presentation of a device to steam) at 134°C for 18 min, infectivity was significantly reduced but not fully. In contrast, complete reduction in infectivity was observed when wires where placed into water and exposed as such to the same sterilization cycle. This effect has been shown to be reproducible (E. Comoy *et al.*, personal communication). It is suggested that these results are due to the slower heating effects under water immersion conditions, which may prevent the clumping effects observed in dry exposed wires [53]. The second conclusion is the significant effects of pre-cleaning on the success or failure of the steam sterilization cycle (Table 10.3). From these

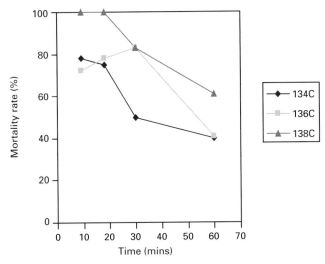

Figure 10.3 The transmission of prion disease (% mortality rate) on exposure to steam at various temperatures and sterilization exposure times. In these studies 375 mg of infected brain homogenate material was dried onto a glass surface, exposed, recovered and inoculated. (Based on [42].)

Table 10.3 The impact of cleaning on the steam sterilization resistance of surface-contaminated prion infectivity. All tests were conducted as previously described [53, 90] at use dilution/exposure times as recommended by the manufacturer and include data from these reports and unpublished data (G. McDonnell, unpublished data).

Treatment	Infectivity reduction (log$_{10}$)
Water washing	<1
Water washing + 134°C × 4 min	*c.* 3
Water washing + 134°C × 18 min	*c.* 5.5
Enzyme cleaner 1	*c.* 4.5
Enzyme cleaner 2	*c.* 1
Enzyme cleaner 1 + 134°C × 18 min	>6
Enzyme cleaner 2 + 134°C × 18 min	*c.* 3
Alkaline cleaning 1	*c.* 3
Alkaline cleaning 2	*c.* 4
Alkaline cleaning 1 + 134°C × 4 min	*c.* 6
Alkaline cleaning 2 + 134°C × 4 min	>6

results it can be concluded that water washing had little impact in reducing infectivity, but subsequent steam sterilization at longer exposure times were partially effective. The effects of cleaning with enzymatic-based detergents ranged in activity, but the effects of one cleaner appeared to increase the resistance of remaining infectivity to steam sterilization. The alkaline cleaners appeared to also reduce infectivity and were effective even at routine steam sterilization cycle conditions (134°C for 3–4 min). The specific effects of cleaning chemistries are described further below.

Overall, from these results, it can be seen that steam sterilization on its own can be effective in significantly reducing the levels of prion infectivity on surfaces, even under worst case test conditions. Despite this, close attention needs to be paid to any prior treatment that is recommended to be done or routinely used prior to steam sterilization. Prior treatment may include a variety of chemicals, such as cleaning chemistries, as recommended in WHO and indeed all international recommendations regarding the handling of TSE-contaminated devices, in particular when used in human surgical, high-risk procedures [69]. Cleaning chemistries that have been shown to reduce the risks associated with TSE infectivity can be safely used, in particular when combined with subsequent steam sterilization and even at routinely used autoclave cycles (e.g. 134°C for 3–4 min). Conversely, some cleaning formulations may have the opposite effects, by increasing the resistance of the prion material to steam inactivation.

Chemical inactivation methods

Similar to physical inactivation methods, prions are considered highly resistant to various types of chemicals (also known as microbicides) that are widely used for decontamination processes. It is important to note that in most cases (and in particular when considering liquids) these chemicals are not used on their own, but are used in formulations and/or under controlled process conditions. A formulation may be defined as a combination of ingredients, including active and inert ingredients, into a product for an intended use (e.g. cleaning chemistries and disinfectants). Process conditions can include temperature, humidity, pH, concentration, exposure time, etc. For traditional cleaning and antimicrobial activity, these variables play an important role depending on the various types of chemicals or defined products [87]. It should be expected that such variables can also play a significant role in the activity of chemicals against prion infectivity. In older studies, the effects of various types of chemicals were generally tested on their own, while more recent studies have begun to demonstrate that significant optimization or indeed negative effects can be observed when various chemicals are tested in different formulations or defined process conditions.

Acids and bases

It is widely accepted that prions can resist strong acids. Little inactivation of the hamster-passaged 263K scrapie agent was detected when exposed to 1 M hydrochloric acid at room temperature for periods ranging from 1 h [103] to 153 h [137]. This situation was not significantly changed when the agent was exposed to 8 M hydrochloric acid for 1 h [137]. These reports matched earlier studies that showed the infectivity titer of a mouse-passaged scrapie agent was little affected by exposure at room temperature over the pH range 2 to 10 [138]. Interestingly, a significant degree of inactivation of the hamster-passaged agent was achieved by 1 M hydrochloric acid in an hour when the exposure temperature was increased to 65°C [137]. These results suggest that further investigations of the effects of acids (various types under different formulation and exposure conditions) may be worth investigating to optimize the activity of acids against prions. For example, a recent study reported significant infectivity reduction of acidic sodium dodecyl sulfate (SDS) solutions for cleaning followed by autoclaving for 15 min against human sCJD prions bound to stainless steel wires [44].

More efficient and consistent effects have been shown using various types of alkali and alkaline formulations. In general, various types of alkali are considered effective against prions and are widely used for this purpose in laboratory, industrial and clinical applications [53, 69, 90]. The effects of alkalis are not surprising, considering their mechanism of action through the potent degradation of proteins and other biological molecules. The most widely cited method is 1 M NaOH for 1 h, although lower concentrations and contact times have also been validated for other purposes. Despite this, variability in infectivity reduction has also been reported. For example, a 1 h exposure to 1 M NaOH (pH 14) inactivated a guinea-pig-passaged CJD agent and the hamster-passaged 263K strain of scrapie agent [103]. However, the sensitivity of these bioassays was substantially reduced because it proved necessary to dilute the samples to render them non-toxic for the recipient animals. Other reports have shown residual infectivity following treatment of 263K scrapie agent with 1 M NaOH [134, 139], even after periods of up to 24 h [140]. Similarly, rodent-passaged CJD infectivity has been reported to survive exposure to 1 M [141] or 2 M NaOH [142]. Work with NaOH, involving the mouse-passaged (ME7) and hamster-passaged (263K) strains of scrapie agent and BSE-infected bovine brain [135], has demonstrated that, if the pH of the samples is carefully neutralized, they can be injected without further dilution. Under these circumstances, infectivity was shown to survive exposure to 2 M NaOH for up to 2 h. With the 263K strain of scrapie agent, although more than 5-$\log_{10}$ of infectivity was lost following such treatments, around 4-$\log_{10}$ survived. Others have suggested more aggressive treatments by combining sodium hydroxide with auto-claving to give complete inactivation of large tissue samples (including whole animals). The successful inactivation of a CJD agent by a sequential process involving exposure to 1 M NaOH, followed by gravity-displacement autoclaving at 121°C for 30 min has been described [131]. Not surprisingly, when a scrapie strain was autoclaved at 121°C for 30 min in the presence of 2 M NaOH (without a prior holding period in NaOH), inactivation was achieved (D.M. Taylor, personal communication). There are practical problems relating to this procedure, such as the potential exposure of operators to splashing with NaOH, the eventual

Table 10.4 Reduction in surface prion contamination with various alkaline cleaning formulations.

Test conditions	Alkaline pH	Infectivity reduction ($\log_{10}$)
Deconex 28 ALKA ONE (1%; 65°C; 10 min)	c. 12	3
Deconex 28 ALKA ONE (1%; 70°C; 10 min)	c. 12	6.5
HAMO 100 (0.8%; 43°C; 7.5 min)	c. 10.5	>7
HAMO 100 (0.4%; 4°C; 5 min)	c. 10.5	5
Prolystica Alkaline 10 × (0.08%; 65°C; 5 min)	c. 10	5
Prolystica Alkaline 10 × (0.08%; 65°C; 5 min) and steam sterilization (134°C × 4 min)	c. 10	>7

deleterious effect on the autoclave chamber and, in particular, that this method should not be used on medical devices due to damage to metals/plastics. This method can be used for large tissue samples and may be further optimized for surface applications by combining lower alkali concentrations with higher temperatures.

The impact of formulation has been demonstrated with various types of alkaline cleaning chemistries. These formulations can contain a variety of alkalis (such as KOH and NaOH), as well as various types of buffers, chelating agents and surfactants. These formulations have been particularly tested for medical device applications, in the routine cleaning of surgical instruments [43, 86, 143]. It has been suggested that formulations with pH >10 can be effective in reducing the risk of surface prion contamination on medical devices, although this may be an oversimplification. As an example, a summary of *in vivo* infectivity reductions (all using the same test method) observed with various alkaline cleaners and their respective pH levels is shown in Table 10.4. From these results it can be seen that the product pH does not correlate to the observed reduction in activity and also that the product can vary depending on the concentration and temperature tested. In these cases, formulation effects play an important role in prion removal and inactivation from surfaces. It is therefore important to verify that such products can be effective, irrespective of their pH. Further, as the routine reprocessing cycle for reusable medical devices includes cleaning followed by steam sterilization, it would appear that using such cleaners can allow for further additional reduction in infectivity by a regular steam cycle.

Alkylating agents

Alkylating agents are not theoretically considered to be effective due to their mechanism of action as cross-linking or fixing agents. Indeed, the viability of scrapie agent after exposure to 0.35% formalin (used for tissue fixation) has been described, but it can even survive more rigorous treatments, for example immersion of infected brain tissue for 974 days in 20% formol-saline (D.M. Taylor and A.G. Dickinson, personal communication). The agents of CJD and TME are equally resilient, the former surviving at least

1 year in 10% formol-saline [58]; the latter survived formol fixation for at least 6 years [144]. BSE is also known to be relatively resistant, having survived an exposure to 10% formol-saline for 2 years [145]. Although the titer of surviving infectivity was not measured in any of these studies, it could be concluded generally from the number of affected animals and their incubation periods that little inactivation had occurred. In the one study where titer reduction was measured, only 1.5-$\log_{10}$ of infectivity was lost when scrapie-infected hamster brain was exposed to 10% formol-saline for 48 h [126]. Of particular note, published reports of the iatrogenic transmission of CJD on medical devices that had been reprocessed using formaldehyde (and alcohol), suggest that the formaldehyde may have been responsible for its persistent nature on these devices over a number of years [80]. It would seem likely that infectious material, even at low levels, had been fixed onto the device surface and remained infectious during the repeated use of these devices over time.

Scrapie infectivity survived an exposure to 12.5% unbuffered glutaraldehyde (pH 4.5) for 16 h [95], nor was CJD agent inactivated by a 14-day exposure to 5% buffered histological glutaraldehyde at pH 7.3 [146]. 2% glutaraldehyde buffered to pH 8 is a widely used disinfectant, but tests to date have not shown any effects in reducing the risks of surface prion contamination (G. McDonnell, unpublished data). The impact of these tests being conducted in the presence of high levels of soil should not be underestimated, as it is unlikely that the microbicide penetrated into the material sufficiently to have any significant effect in reducing infectivity. Other alkylating agents such as acetylethyleneimine [25] and β-propiolactone [147] have had little effect on scrapie agent when tested. Further, despite its widespread use as a sterilization agent, ethylene oxide exposure caused very little loss of CJD [148] or scrapie infectivity [133]. In the case of ethylene oxide gas, the control of temperature, gas concentration and humidity levels (in excess of 70%) are known to be particularly important in effective antimicrobial activity and have yet to be tested against prions.

Detergents

Various types of detergents have been tested for their direct effects on prions. Mild detergents had little effect on TSE agents [113], but SDS had some effect on CJD [149] and scrapie [113] infectivity; this was enhanced by heat [85] and also under acidic pH conditions [44]. Boiling infected tissue homogenates for 3 min in 3% SDS was completely effective [150]. However, survival of infectivity was detected after 50 mg samples of macerated scrapie-infected brain tissue were boiled (or autoclaved at 121°C) in 5% SDS [151]. Although there was a substantial loss of infectivity after the autoclaving process, this was not complete.

"Detergents" can refer to a wide variety of surface-active (surfactant) agents such as SDS, but also to cleaning formulations. The impact of these detergents on prion infectivity can have theoretical positive and negative effects. Indeed, the impact of alkaline cleaning formulations has already been discussed above, with significant results [53, 90, 143]. The true effects of the various surfactants used in these formulations is not known, but it can be proposed to be associated with dispersion (allowing for access of the alkali activity), assisting removal of prion-contaminated material from surfaces, and even partial effects on disrupting the structure of the prion protein. These effects have not only been shown with alkali, but also with other potential actives such as proteolytic enzymes. As an example, a specific enzymatic formulation (Klenzyme®) was shown to be very effective at removing prion contamination from surfaces but had little to no effect on degrading the prion protein [53]. In contrast, some recently described formulations containing mixtures of surfactants, chelating agents and enzymes have shown removal and prion protein degradation activity under some test conditions (G. McDonnell and N. Kaiser, unpublished data).

Halogens

In addition to NaOH, sodium hypochlorite (chlorine) solutions are widely used as anti-prion chemicals. Solutions containing up to 25,000 ppm of available (active) chlorine have been reported to inactivate guinea-pig-passaged CJD agent and the hamster-passaged 263K strain of scrapie agent [103]. In an extensive study with two strains of mouse-passaged scrapie agent, it was demonstrated that a solution containing 14,000 ppm available chlorine was effective in 30 min, leading to the recommendation that 20,000 ppm for 1 h should be used in practice [85]. Such strong solutions are corrosive to metals, but the less corrosive chlorine-releasing compound, sodium dichloroisocyanurate (NaDCC), has been reported to be equally effective for bacterial inactivation at equivalent levels of available chlorine [152]. Consequently, a study was conducted using two sources of BSE-infected brain tissue, which were exposed for 30–120 min to solutions of sodium hypochlorite or NaDCC containing comparable levels of available chlorine (ranging from 8250 to 16,500 ppm.). No infectivity was detectable in any of the hypochlorite-treated samples, but infectivity was recoverable from samples that had been treated for up to 120 min with NaDCC solutions containing up to 16,500 ppm available chlorine [153]. It was shown that, at the end of the various exposure periods, the NaDCC solutions had released 3.5 times less chlorine than the hypochlorite solutions on average. Greater effects have been shown using lower hypochlorite concentrations in formulation with surfactants and other components (as described with CIP150, a hypochlorite-containing cleaning formulation [43]).

Unlike chlorine, only a modest reduction in scrapie infectivity was obtained using 2% iodine in sodium iodide for 4 h [154]. Similar results were observed with scrapie and CJD agents, using an iodophor containing 0.8% iodine [127]. To date, other halogens (in particular bromide) have not been reported to have been tested but may be of interest for investigation given the parallels in mechanisms of action to chlorine.

Organic solvents

Numerous studies, particularly with scrapie agent, have shown that organic solvents generally have little effect on TSE infectivity. Experimental exposures have included 1h with acetone [155], 2 weeks with 5% chloroform [133], 16h with ether [156], 2 weeks with 4% phenol [133] and 2 weeks with ethanol [95]. In studies relating to the historical use of organic solvents by the rendering industry, to enhance the yield of tallow from the raw materials, it was found that even hot organic solvents provided a very limited degree of inactivation of mouse-passaged BSE and scrapie agents. This was not significantly enhanced by the subsequent exposure of the raw materials to dry heat and steam [157]. The solvents tested were hexane, heptane, perchloroethylene and petroleum.

Of notable exception is a specific phenolic-containing disinfectant (known as Environ® LpH), which has been shown to be particularly effective against prions both in brain homogenate suspension [134] and surface-contaminated [53] infectivity studies. It is interesting to note that in mechanism of action studies that the formulation was shown to have no obvious effects on the structure or size of the prion protein [53]. The anti-prion effect appears to be due to a unique mixture of phenolic compounds in one formulation, whereas a similar yet distinct formulation was shown to not be effective [158].

Oxidizing agents

Initial studies with various types of oxidizing agents did not show remarkable effects against prions. Exposure of scrapie agents to chlorine dioxide (50ppm for 24h) had only a partial reduction in infectivity [154]. Treatment of scrapie with 3% hydrogen peroxide for 24h caused little inactivation [148]. Scrapie-infected brain homogenates were not inactivated by concentrations of up to 18% peracetic acid, but 2% inactivated intact brain tissue [159]. These apparently anomalous results may demonstrate the protective effect of aggregation under some of the conditions tested. Despite these initial results, subsequent studies have shown significant activity. Initially, this was partially shown with a peracetic acid formulation when tested *in vitro* (western blot) at 50°C [160]; this was subsequently verified in infectivity assays [53]. Mechanisms of action studies suggested that these effects may be due to the fragmentation of proteins by this formulation, but only at temperature greater than 40°C and less than 60°C [161]. However, some caution is required in interpreting these results in that peracetic acid under some conditions/formulations can lead to protein cross-linking while under others it can aid in surface protein removal and degradation.

Similar effects have been reported for hydrogen peroxide in liquid and gas form [53, 162]. Liquid hydrogen peroxide up to 50–60% had little to no effect in activity, although formulations with much lower concentrations of peroxide in combination with copper were particularly effective both *in vitro* and *in vivo* [163]. It is likely that further formulation effects with hydrogen peroxide will also be shown to have efficacy, both in cleaning and disinfection efficacy. In contrast, hydrogen peroxide in gas form has been shown to be an effective microbicide against prions, both under atmospheric [53] and vacuum conditions [162]. This difference between liquid and gas peroxide also

appears to be due to differences in their mode of action; specifically, liquid peroxide (under the conditions tested) appears to cause oxidation of amino acid side-chains in proteins, while gas peroxide causes peptide bond breakdown [162]. Despite this, hydrogen peroxide gas sterilization processes have not all been shown to be effective, which may be due to distinct differences in exposure conditions during each process. For example, the AMSCO V-Pro1 process (at full and half cycle conditions [162]; G. McDonnell, unpublished data) and the STERRAD NX process are effective, but a similar STERRAD 100S is not [90, 164]. They all use hydrogen peroxide gas for sterilization, but in different ways: the V-Pro1 claims to provide unsaturated gas conditions; the STERRAD 100S uses saturated gas but also uses plasma following gas exposure; and the STERRAD NX process uses a concentrated peroxide gas for sterilization followed by plasma [87] (see Chapter 15.3). These subtle differences appear to be important and may be due to the presence of saturated conditions (liquid and gas peroxide) leading to limitations in prion neutralization. Overall, these results confirm that hydrogen peroxide gas can be an effective method against prions, but exposure or process conditions can dramatically affect efficacy.

Other oxidizing agents have been the focus of some initial research on their effects against prions, but remain to be published in the peer-reviewed literature. These include ozone, chlorine dioxide gas, nitrous oxide and true plasmas. Ozone, for example, has shown some preliminary effects under western blot analysis for prion protein degradation, although these initial reports remain to be verified; combinations of ozone and UV light over extended exposure periods has also had some success [117]. Plasmas are energized gases that can have potent antimicrobial activity, in particular those based on oxygen, nitrogen, other inert gases (such as helium and argon) and mixtures thereof (see Chapter 15.4). Plasmas have been recommended due to their ability to degrade biological molecules such as proteins, although this will depend on the choice of gas used to generate the plasma, as well as the method of application, exposure time, etc. [165]. Some studies have focused on the potential application of plasmas for cleaning applications, in particular argon–oxygen mixtures [166]. Argon/oxygen plasma-treated surfaces contaminated with brain homogenates showed excellent cleaning effects with or without pre-cleaning with water (although water immersion alone was previously shown to have little benefit in prion reduction [53]). *In vitro* studies in Japan have suggested that nitrogen gas plasma exposure could partially remove/inactivate surfaces inoculated with high levels of scrapie (H. Shintani, personal communication). Various mixtures of gas plasma (including argon, oxygen, nitrogen or hydrogen) have also shown particular effects against prions *in vitro* while argon/oxygen mixtures were efficient in eliminating any detectable PrPres [165]. Interestingly, plasmas based on gas mixtures of argon with nitrogen or hydrogen were not efficient. It is useful to note that the mechanisms of action of these gas plasmas are proposed to be more related to UV radiation than the generation of various active (oxidizing/reducing) chemical species (see Chapter 15.3). Further, plasmas based on oxygen were the most effective both *in vitro* and *in vivo*, presumably through physical etching (removal) phenomena, having a rather higher effect than the oxidizing agent species effects. It is clear that such processes require further investigations and practical implementation for high-risk applications.

A final microbicide in this group that may have some potential benefits is based on a photo-Fenton reagent based on titanium dioxide, itself a powerful antimicrobial agent [166]. Initial studies *in vitro* have suggested that the oxidizing agent activity could significantly reduce the detection of PrP^res. A similar type of Fenton reaction has been described in formulations containing hydrogen peroxide and copper [163].

Oxidizing salts

Oxidizing salts have been tested for their effect on TSE agents, with conflicting results. For example, the report that sodium metaperiodate has a considerable effect on scrapie infectivity [167] is contradicted by several other studies [148, 168]. Similarly, a claim that potassium permanganate inactivates all CJD and scrapie infectivity in homogenates of brain tissue [127] is challenged by data from other experiments [85, 148]. Overall, these and other similar microbicides require further investigation.

Chaotropes

The claim that urea is an effective chemical in reducing scrapie infectivity [113] is not supported by other studies that have been reviewed [103]. High concentrations (>4 mol/l) of guanidine thiocyanate (GdnSCN) are known to be relatively effective with infected brain homogenates. Lower concentrations or the use of less chaotropic salts such as guanidine hydrochloride (GdnHCl) are less effective. PrP^res was denatured in 2–4 M GdnHCl, depending on the degree of purification, final pH, etc., and this correlated with some loss of infectivity. It has been reported that 0.4 M GdSCN may be employed as a disinfectant for some types of surgical instruments [169], but this is not practically used. The study on which this claim was based did not involve the use of contaminated instruments, but used 10% homogenates of CJD-infected hamster brain [170]. Also, the sensitivity of the bioassays was reduced 200-fold by the need to dilute the treated brain homogenates to avoid toxicity in the assay animals, and the experiment was incomplete at the time of publication. More recent studies have shown an advantage in the use of urea (8 M) in the treatment of biological fluids, as part of a process including sedimentation, denaturation and ultracentrifugation [170].

Proteolytic enzymes

One of the hallmarks of prion infectivity and the prion protein is resistance to the effects of proteolytic enzymes (or proteases). This is used as a method to distinguish the normal PrP^c from its misfolded, protease-resistant form in western blot studies. Resistance is not ultimate, in that longer exposure times at higher protease concentrations can show prion degradation, which has encouraged further investigations of various protease and

protease formulations for their activity against prions. Proteases such as trypsin on their own have little effect on TSE agents [113, 171], producing titer losses of <1-log₁₀, which are insignificant. Broad-spectrum proteases such as pronase [113] and proteinase K [172] can significantly reduce infectivity titers after prolonged digestion times. A combination of proteinase K and pronase, in conjunction with SDS, has been shown to degrade PrP^res material from highly concentrated vCJD-infected brain preparations to below detection levels [173]. Others have shown the impact of formulation effects such as the combination of chelating agents and certain proteases (G. McDonnell and N. Kaiser, unpublished data). A number of researchers have investigated the potential use of alkaline proteases such as keratinases [174, 175] and other serine proteases [93, 176, 177], with some success. For example, some subtilisins (at 55°C, 14h at a pH of 7.9) had some limited activity, with greater results suggested at higher pH levels (>9.0 [176]). Similarly, a thermostable protease at pH 10 and 12 had greater activity in comparison to proteinase K [93]. These results suggest that the type of enzyme as well as the process conditions used for exposure can have a significant effect on reducing prion infectivity. Overall, many of these reports need to be verified by testing for prion inactivation in animal models or investigated to optimize the activity observed by process and/or formulation effects.

Future perspectives in prion decontamination

Prions may not be considered to be what are currently defined as microorganisms, but at the same time they are transmissible and unusually resistant to physical and chemical decontamination methods. There is much to learn regarding the true nature and detection of these agents and their associated diseases. On the decontamination side, what has been shown in recent years is that these agents may not be as resistant as previously reported, although they may require separate consideration to classic microorganisms. For example, optimal inactivation methods for prions (or protein denaturation/degradation) may not be the same as those applied to bacteria, viruses and bacterial endospores [78, 87]. Examples include efficient inactivation and removal of prion infectivity by simple cleaning formulations that are considered to have poor efficacy against more resistant microorganisms. Similarly, some methods such as hydrogen peroxide gas and steam sterilization can be very efficient against these organisms, as well as prions when optimized. Overall, there is much scope for investigations into further cleaning, disinfection and sterilization processes effective against prions, in particular balancing the priocidal effects with safety, compatibility, regulatory and cost requirements for various applications.

Despite this, some caution is required. It has been shown that combined effects, typically applied in decontamination practices such as cleaning followed by an antimicrobial process, can have both positive and negative effects [143]. Further slight changes in the formulation of liquid chemicals, exposure conditions and applications of a given method or product can be significant (in a positive or negative sense). Test methodology is an important factor, as in any antimicrobial investigation, as false positive or negative results can be misleading. For this particular reason, standardized test methodology and particularly alternatives to *in vivo* bioassay methods are important to develop.

Prion decontamination techniques will also depend on the applications that are being considered, ranging from laboratory, device, environmental surfaces, industrial and tissue situations. In the decontamination of reusable instruments (such as surgical and dental devices), it is already important that standard precautions are applied to reduce the potential risk of prion infectivity being transmitted on device surfaces. These methods include validated cleaning and sterilization processes [78]. Practical prion decontamination strategies are already commonplace in various industrial and manufacturing environments that may be considered at risk (including blood fractionation and any processes that may use materials from a human or animal source). Veterinary, laboratory and environmental applications may require further consideration, due to unique challenges in these areas. These include the handling of high concentrations of research prion samples in laboratories or whole animal treatment systems in treating known infected herds. However, even in these areas there are practical methods identified to significantly reduce any risks.

Parallels with other protein-precipitating diseases

Prions have been considered to be unique examples of unusual forms of "infectious" or transmissible agents that are characterized by misfolded proteins. Such proteins subsequently precipitate, causing cell death and tissue damage, with particular consequences to neural tissues. TSEs such as CJD in humans and scrapie in sheep are considered rare diseases, but there are other similar diseases that show similar effects but have not (or not yet) been shown to be transmissible. This conjecture has been a subject of some recent debate [177–180]. There are actually a number of human disorders/diseases where protein precipitation does play an important role in their development, but these have not been considered to be transmissible in nature (Table 10.5). Of particular note are the neurodegenerative diseases Alzheimer's and Parkinson's. Although a true transmissible nature of these diseases remains to be definitively accepted, there is some evidence to suggest that the presence of associated misfolded proteins in Alzheimer's disease can lead to a seeding mechanism not unlike that proposed with prions [181, 182]. Further evidence suggests that such a mechanism could also be transferred by contaminated surfaces [183]. In Alzheimer's disease this is proposed to be due to the proteolytic digestion of amyloid precursor protein (APP) to produce peptides known as β-amyloid. Two peptides, β-amyloid 40 and 42, are produced and the latter has been shown to be neurotoxic. A similar mechanism has been described with amyloidosis [180]. Further research is required in

Table 10.5 Example of other diseases associated with protein-precipitation.

Disease	Protein precipitation	Notes
Alzheimer's disease	Amyloid β-peptide	Some experimental evidence suggests a potential transmissible nature
Parkinson's disease	α-Synuclein	No evidence of transmissibility
Cataracts	Crystallins	No evidence of transmissibility
Systemic amyloidosis	Amyloid-A (AA) and apolipoprotein AII (apoAII) amyloid	Some experimental evidence suggests a potential transmissible/acceleration nature
Tauopathies	Tau	Some experimental evidence suggests a potential transmissible/acceleration nature

this area to verify these reports and the associated mechanisms in the initiation and development of these diseases. Verification of these results would also require investigations of the effects of the various disinfection and sterilization methods on such agents.

References

1 Aguzzi, A. and Calella, A.M. (2009) Prions: protein aggregation and infectious diseases. *Physiology Reviews*, **89**, 1105–1152.

2 Panà, A. and Jung, M. (2005) Prion diseases and iatrogenic infections I. A review. *Igiene e sanità pubblica*, **61**, 325–377.

3 Will, R.G. *et al.* (1996) A new variant of Creutzfeldt–Jakob disease in the UK. *Lancet*, **347**, 921–925.

4 Alpers, M. (1987) Epidemiology and clinical aspects of kuru, in *Prions: Novel Infectious Pathogens Causing Scrapie and Creutzfeldt–Jakob Disease* (eds S.B. Prusiner and M.P. McKinlay), Academic Press, London, pp. 451–465.

5 Taylor, D.M. (1989) Phenolized formalin may not inactivate Creutzfeldt–Jakob disease infectivity. *Neuropathology and Applied Neurology*, **15**, 585–586.

6 Collinge, J. *et al.* (2006) Kuru in the 21st century – an acquired human prion disease with very long incubation periods. *Lancet*, **367**, 2068–2074.

7 Palsson, P.A. (1979) Rida (scrapie) in Iceland and its epidemiology, in *Slow Transmissible Disease of the Nervous System*, vol. 1 (eds S.B. Prusiner and W.J. Hadlow), Academic Press, London, pp. 357–366.

8 Detwiler, L.A. and Baylis, M. (2003) The epidemiology of scrapie. *Revue Scientifique et Technique (International Office of Epizootics)*, **22**, 121–143.

9 Eckroade, R.J. *et al.* (1979) Experimental transmissible mink encephalopathy: brain lesions and their sequential development in mink, in *Slow Transmissible Diseases of the Nervous System*, vol. 1, (eds S.B. Prusiner and W.J. Hadlow), Academic Press, London, pp. 409–449.

10 Marsh, R.F. *et al.* (1991) Epidemiological and experimental studies on a new incident of transmissible mink encephalopathy. *Journal of General Virology*, **72**, 589–594.

11 Williams, E.S. and Young, S. (1980) Chronic wasting disease of captive mule deer: a spongiform encephalopathy. *Journal of Wildlife Diseases*, **16**, 89–98.

12 Belay, E.D. *et al.* (2004) Chronic wasting disease and potential transmission to humans. *Emerging Infectious Diseases*, **10**, 977–984.

13 Belay, E.D. *et al.* (2001) Creutzfeldt–Jakob disease in unusually young patients who consumed venison. *Archives of Neurology*, **58**, 1673–1678.

14 Race, B. *et al.* (2009) Susceptibilities of nonhuman primates to chronic wasting disease. *Emerging Infectious Diseases*, **15**, 1366–1376.

15 Wilesmith, J.W. *et al.* (1988) Bovine spongiform encephalopathy: epidemiological studies. *Veterinary Record*, **123**, 638–644.

16 ACDP (1994) *Precautions for Work with Human and Animal Transmissible Spongiform Encephalopathies*, London: HMSO.

17 Capobianco, R. *et al.* (2007) Conversion of the BASE prion strain into the BSE strain: the origin of BSE? *PLoS Pathogens*, **3**, 31.

18 Lombardi, G. *et al.* (2008) Intraspecies transmission of BASE induces clinical dullness and amyotrophic changes. *PLoS Pathogens*, **4**, e1000075.

19 Comoy, E.E. *et al.* (2008) Atypical BSE (BASE) transmitted from asymptomatic aging cattle to a primate. *PLoS ONE*, **3**, e3017.

20 Bruce, M.E. *et al.* (1997) Transmissions in mice indicate that "new variant" CJD is caused by the BSE agent. *Nature*, **389**, 498–501.

21 Asante, E.A. *et al.* (2006) Dissociation of pathological and molecular phenotype of variant Creutzfeldt–Jakob disease in transgenic human prion protein 129 heterozygous mice. *Proceedings of the National Academy of Sciences of the United States of America*, **103**, 10759–10764.

22 Carp, R.I. *et al.* (1985) Nature of the scrapie agent: current status of facts and hypotheses. *Journal of General Virology*, **66**, 1357–1368.

23 Bruce, M.E. *et al.* (1989) Precise targeting of the pathology of the sialoglycoprotein, PrP, and vacuolar degeneration in mouse scrapie. *Neuroscience Letters*, **102**, 1–6.

24 Prusiner, S.B. (1982) Novel proteinaceous infectious particles cause scrapie. *Science*, **216**, 136–144.

25 Stamp, J.T. *et al.* (1959) Further studies on scrapie. *Journal of Comparative Pathology*, **69**, 268–280.

26 Zomosa-Signoret, V. *et al.* (2008) Physiological role of the cellular prion protein. *Veterinary Research*, **39**, 9.

27 Bueler, H. *et al.* (1993) Mice devoid of PrP are resistant to scrapie. *Cell*, **73**, 1339–1347.

28 Wille, H. *et al.* (2009) Natural and synthetic prion structure from X-ray fiber diffraction. *Proceedings of the National Academy of Sciences of the United States of America*, **106**, 16990–16995.

29 Bruce, M.E. *et al.* (1994) Transmission of bovine spongiform encephalopathy and scrapie to mice; strain variation and the species barrier. *Philosophical Transactions of the Royal Society B*, **343**, 405–411.

30 Chesebro, B. (1998) BSE and prions; uncertainties about the agent. *Science*, **279**, 42–43.

31 Farquhar, C.F. *et al.* (1998) Straining the prion hypothesis. *Nature*, **391**, 345–346.

32 Geoghegan, J.C. *et al.* (2007) Selective incorporation of polyanionic molecules into hamster prions. *Journal of Biological Chemistry*, **282**, 36341–36353.

33 Simoneau, S. *et al.* (2009) Small critical RNAs in the scrapie agent. *Nature Proceedings*, posted June 16, http://precedings.nature.com/documents/3344/version/1 (accessed June 12, 2012).

34 Dickinson, A.G. and Outram, G.W. (1979) The scrapie replication-site hypothesis and its implications for pathogenesis, in *Slow Transmissible Diseases of the Nervous System*, vol. 2 (eds S.B. Prusiner and W.J. Hadlow), Academic Press, London, pp. 13–21.

35 Dickinson , A.G. *et al.* (1989) Further evidence that scrapie agent has an independent genome, in *Unconventional Virus Diseases of the Central Nervous System* (eds L.A. Court *et al.*), Abbaye de Melleray, Moisdon la Rivière, France, pp. 446–460.

36 Konturek, P.C. *et al.* (2005) *Helicobacter pylori* upregulates prion protein expression in gastric mucosa: a possible link to prion disease. *World Journal of Gastroenterology*, **11**, 7651–7656.

37 Bastian, F.O. *et al.* (2007) *Spiroplasma* spp. from transmissible spongiform encephalopathy brains or ticks induce spongiform encephalopathy in ruminants. *Journal of Medical Microbiology*, **56**, 1235–1242.

38 Manuelidis, L. *et al.* (2009) The kuru infectious agent is a unique geographic isolate distinct from Creutzfeldt–Jakob disease and scrapie agents. *Proceedings of the National Academy of Sciences of the United States of America*, **106**, 13529–13534.

39 Aguzzi, A. (2008) Prion diseases of humans and farm animals: epidemiology, genetics, and pathogenesis. *Journal of Neurochemistry*, **97**, 1726–1739.

40 Bruce, M.E. (1993) Scrapie strain variation and mutation. *British Medical Bulletin*, **49**, 822–838.

41 Taylor, D.M. *et al.* (1999) The thermostability of scrapie-like agents is dependent upon the strain and not on the PrP genotype, in *Abstracts of a European Commission Symposium on the Characterisation and Diagnosis of Prion Diseases in Animals and Man, 23–25 September, Tubingen*, p. 169.

42 Fernie, K. *et al.* (2007) Comparative studies on the thermostability of five strains of transmissible-spongiform-encephalopathy agent. *Biotechnology and Applied Biochemistry*, **47**, 175–183.

43 McDonnell, G. *et al.* (2005) Cleaning investigations to reduce the risk of prion contamination on manufacturing surfaces and materials. *European Journal of Parenteral and Pharmaceutical Sciences*, **10**, 67–72.

44 Peretz, D. *et al.* (2006) Inactivation of prions by acidic sodium dodecyl sulfate. *Journal of Virology*, **80**, 322–331.

45 Li, J. *et al.* (2009) Darwinian evolution of prions in cell culture. *Science*, **327**, 869–872.

46 Bessen, R.A. *et al.* (1995) Non-genetic propagation of strain-specific properties of scrapie prion protein. *Nature*, **375**, 698–700.

47 Hecker, R. *et al.* (1992) Replication of distinct scrapie prion isolates is region-specific in brains of transgenic mice and hamsters. *Genes and Development*, **6**, 1213–1228.

48 Endo, T. *et al.* (1989) Diversity of oligosaccharide structures linked to asparagines of the scrapie prion protein. *Biochemistry*, **28**, 8380–8388.

49 Fraser, H. *et al.* (1989) Transmission of bovine spongiform encephalopathy to mice. *Veterinary Record*, **123**, 472.

50 McBride, P.A. *et al.* (1992) PrP protein is associated with follicular dendritic cells of spleens and lymph nodes in uninfected and scrapie-infected mice. *Journal of Pathology*, **168**, 413–418.

51 Brown, P. *et al.* (2004) Infectivity studies of both ash and air emissions from simulated incineration of scrapie-contaminated tissues. *Environmental Sciences and Technology*, **38**, 6155–6160.

52 Zobeley, E. *et al.* (1999) Infectivity of scrapie prions bound to a stainless steel surface. *Molecular Medicine*, **5**, 240–243.

53 Fichet, G. *et al.* (2004) Novel methods for disinfection of prion-contaminated medical devices. *Lancet*, **364**, 521–526.

54 Asher D.M. *et al.* (1987) Attempts to disinfect surfaces contaminated with etiological agents of the spongiform encephalopathies, in *Abstracts of the VIIth International Congress of Virology*, Edmonton, p. 147.

55 Miller, M.W. *et al.* (2004) Environmental sources of prion transmission in mule deer. *Emerging Infectious Diseases*, **10**, 1003–1006.

56 Saunders, S.E. *et al.* (2008) Prions in the environment: occurrence, fate and mitigation. *Prion*, **2**, 162–169.

57 Brown, P. and Gajdusek, D.C. (1991) Survival of scrapie virus after 3 years' interment. *Lancet*, **337**, 269–270.

58 Tateishi, J. *et al.* (1980) Properties of the transmissible agent derived from chronic spongiform encephalopathy. *Annals of Neurology*, **7**, 390–391.

59 Wilson, D.R. *et al.* (1950) Studies in scrapie. *Journal of Comparative Pathology*, **60**, 267–282.

60 Wiggins, R.C. (2009) Prion stability and infectivity in the environment. *Neurochemical Research*, **34**, 158–168.

61 Davies, P. and Brown, D.R. (2009) Manganese enhances prion protein survival in model soils and increases prion infectivity to cells. *PLoS ONE*, **4**, e7518.

62 Nichols, T.A. *et al.* (2009) Detection of protease-resistant cervid prion protein in water from a CWD-endemic area. *Prion*, **3**, 171–183.

63 Morales-Belpaire, I. and Gerin, P.A. (2008) Fate of amyloid fibrils introduced in wastewater sludge. *Water Research*, **42**, 4449–4456.

64 Ricketts, M.N. (2004) Public health and the BSE epidemic. *Current Topics in Microbiology and Immunology*, **284**, 99–119.

65 Department for Environment, Food and Rural Affairs (DEFRA) (2001) *Review of the Origin of BSE*, http://archive.defra.gov.uk/foodfarm/farmanimal/diseases/atoz/bse/controls-eradication/causes.htm (accessed May, 2012).

66 Ano, Y. *et al.* (2009) Uptake and dynamics of infectious prion protein in the intestine. *Protein and Peptide Letters*, **16**, 247–255.

67 Baron, H. *et al.* (2000) Prions, in *Disinfection, Sterilization and Preservation*, 5th edn (ed. S.S. Block), Lippincott Williams & Wilkins, Philadelphia, pp. 659–674.

68 Sutton, J.M. *et al.* (2006) Methods to minimize the risks of Creutzfeldt–Jakob disease transmission by surgical precedures: where to set the standard? *Clinical Infectious Diseases*, **43**, 737–764.

69 World Health Organization (WHO) (1999) WHO Infection Control Guidelines for Transmissible Spongiform Encephalopathies 2000, Report of a WHO Consultation, Geneva, March 23–26, 1999, WHO/CDS/CSR/APH/2000/3, http://www.who.int/csr/resources/publications/bse/WHO_CDS_CSR_APH_2000_3/en/ (accessed May 25, 2012).

70 Hamaguchi, T. *et al.* (2009) The risk of iatrogenic Creutzfeldt–Jakob disease through medical and surgical procedures. *Neuropathology*, **29**, 625–631.

71 González, L. *et al.* (2009) High prevalence of scrapie in a dairy goat herd: tissue distribution of disease-associated PrP and effect of PRNP genotype and age. *Veterinary Research*, **40**, 65.

72 Caplazi, P. *et al.* (2004) Biology of PrPsc accumulation in two natural scrapie-infected sheep flocks. *Journal of Veterinary Diagnostic Investigation*, **16**, 489–496.

73 Dabaghian, R. *et al.* (2008) Detection of proteinase K resistant proteins in the urine of patients with Creutzfeldt–Jakob and other neurodegenerative diseases. *Prion*, **2**, 170–178.

74 Wadsworth, J.D. *et al.* (2001) Tissue distribution of protease resistant prion protein in variant Creutzfeldt–Jakob disease using a highly sensitive immuno-blotting assay. *Lancet*, **358**, 171–180.

75 Hewitt, P.E. *et al.* (2006) Creutzfeldt–Jakob disease and blood transfusion: results of the UK Transfusion Medicine Epidemiological Review study. *Vox Sanguinis*, **91**, 221–230.

76 Houston, F. *et al.* (2000) Transmission of BSE by blood transfusion in sheep. *Lancet*, **356**, 999–1000.

77 Coste, J. *et al.* (2009) Subgroup on TSE. A report on transmissible spongiform encephalopathies and transfusion safety. *Vox Sanguinis*, **96**, 284–291.

78 McDonnell, G. (2008) Prion disease transmission: can we apply standard precautions to prevent or reduce risks? *Journal of Perioperative Practice*, **18**, 298–304.

79 Will, R.G. (2003) Acquired prion disease: iatrogenic CJD, variant CJD, kuru. *British Medical Bulletin*, **66**, 255–265.

80 Bernoulli, C. *et al.* (1977) Danger of accidental person-to-person transmission of Creutzfeldt–Jakob disease by surgery. *Lancet*, **1**, 478–479.

81 Weissmann, C. *et al.* (2002) Transmission of prions. *Proceedings of the National Academy of Sciences of the United States of America*, **99**, 16378–16383.

82 Mahillo-Fernandez, I. *et al.* (2008) Surgery and risk of sporadic Creutzfeldt–Jakob disease in Denmark and Sweden: registry-based case–control studies. *Neuroepidemiology*, **31**, 229–240.

83 Rohwer, R.G. and Gajdusek, D.C. (1980) Scrapie, virus or viroid: the case for a virus, in *In Search of the Cause of Multiple Sclerosis and other Chronic Diseases of the CNS*, Proceedings of the 1st International Symposium of the Hertie Foundation, Frankfurt, September 1979, Verlag Chemie, Weinheim, pp.335–355.

84 Salk, J.E. and Gori, J.B. (1960) A review of theoretical, experimental, and practical considerations in the use of formaldehyde for the inactivation of poliovirus. *Annals of the New York Academy of Sciences*, **83**, 609–637.

85 Kimberlin, R.H. *et al.* (1983) Disinfection studies with two strains of mouse-passaged scrapie agent. *Journal of the Neurological Sciences*, **59**, 355–369.

86 Fichet, G. *et al.* (2007) Investigations of a prion infectivity assay to evaluate methods of decontamination. *Journal of Microbiological Methods*, **7**, 511–518.

87 McDonnell, G. (2007) *Antisepsis, Disinfection, and Sterilization: Types, Action, and Resistance*, ASM Press, Washington, DC.

88 AOAC International (2007) *Official Methods of Analysis of AOAC International*, 18th edn, Revision 2, AOAC International, Gaithersburg, MD.

89 Bertram, J.M. *et al.* (2004) Inactivation and removal of prions when processing medical devices: proposal for testing and declaration of suitable procedures under discussion. *Bundesgesundhedbl Gesundheitforch Gesundheitsschutz*, **47**, 36–40.

90 Yan, Z.X. *et al.* (2004) Infectivity of prion protein bound to stainless steel wires: a model for testing decontamination procedures for transmissible spongiform encephalopathies. *Infection Control and Hospital Epidemiology*, **25**, 280–283.

91 Taylor, D.M. (1996) Transmissible subacute spongiform encephalopathies: practical aspects of agent inactivation, in *Transmissible Subacute Spongiform Encephalopathies: Prion Disease. Third International Symposium on Subacute Spongiform Encephalopathies* (eds L. Court and D. Dodet), Prion Diseases, Paris, pp. 479–482.

92 Taylor, D.M. *et al.* (2000) Closely similar values obtained when the ME7 strain of scrapie agent was titrated in parallel by two different individuals in separate laboratories using two sublines of C57BL mice. *Journal of Virological Methods*, **86**, 35–40.

93 Dickinson, J. *et al.* (2009) Decontamination of prion protein (BSE301V) using a genetically engineered protease. *Journal of Hospital Infection*, **72**, 65–70.

94 Rosenberg, R.N. *et al.* (1986) Precautions in handling tissues, fluids, and other contaminated materials from patients with documented or suspected Creutzfeldt–Jakob disease. *Annals of Neurology*, **19**, 75–77.

95 Taylor, D.M. *et al.* (2002) Thermostability of mouse-passaged BSE and scrapie is independent of host PrP genotype: implications for the nature of the causal agents. *Journal of General Virology*, **83**, 3199–3204.

96 Taylor, D.M. (1986) Decontamination of Creutzfeldt–Jakob disease agent. *Annals of Neurology*, **20**, 749.

97 Outram, G.W. (1976) The pathogenesis of scrapie in mice, in *Slow Virus Diseases of Animals and Man* (ed. R.H. Kimberlin), North Holland, Amsterdam, pp. 325–357.

98 Taylor, D.M. and Fernie, K. (1996) Exposure to autoclaving or sodium hydroxide extends the dose–response curve of the 263K strain of scrapie agent in hamsters. *Journal of General Virology*, **77**, 811–813.

99 Dickinson, A.G. and Fraser, H. (1969) Modification of the pathogenesis of scrapie in mice by treatment of the agent. *Nature*, **222**, 892–893.

100 Kimberlin, R.H. (1977) Biochemical approaches to scrapie research. *Trends in Biochemical Sciences*, **2**, 220–223.

101 Lax, A.J. *et al.* (1983) Can scrapie titers be calculated accurately from incubation periods? *Journal of General Virology*, **64**, 971–973.

102 Somerville, R.A. and Carp, R.I. (1983) Altered scrapie infectivity estimates by titration and incubation period in the presence of detergents. *Journal of General Virology*, **64**, 2045–2050.

103 Brown, P. *et al.* (1986) Newer data on the inactivation of scrapie virus or Creutzfeldt–Jakob disease virus in brain tissue. *Journal of Infectious Diseases*, **153**, 1145–1148.

104 Pocchiari, M. *et al.* (1991) Combination filtration and 6M urea treatment of human growth hormone effectively minimizes risk from potential Creutzfeldt–Jakob disease virus. *Hormone Research*, **35**, 161–166.

105 Taylor, D.M. (1993) Inactivation of SE agents. *British Medical Bulletin*, **49**, 810–821.

106 Mahal, S.P. *et al.* (2008) Assaying prions in cell culture: the standard scrapie cell assay (SSCA) and the scrapie cell assay in end point format (SCEPA). *Methods in Molecular Biology*, **459**, 49–68.

107 Edgeworth, J.A. *et al.* (2008) Highly sensitive, quantitative cell-based assay for prions adsorbed to solid surfaces. *Proceedings of the National Academy of Sciences of the United States of America*, **106**, 3479–3483.

108 Aguzzi, A. (2007) Prion biology: the quest for the test. *Nature Methods*, **4**, 614–616.

109 Barria, M.A. *et al.* (2009) De novo generation of infectious prions *in vitro* produces a new disease phenotype. *PLoS Pathogens*, **5**, e1000421.

110 Latarjet, R. (1979) Inactivation of the agents of scrapie, Creutzfeldt–Jakob disease, and kuru by radiations, in *Slow Transmissible Disease of the Nervous System*, vol. 2 (eds S.B. Prusiner and W.J. Hadlow), Academic Press, London, pp. 387–407.

111 Marsh, R.F. and Hanson, R.P. (1969) Physical and chemical properties of the transmissible mink encephalopathy agent. *Journal of Virology*, **3**, 176–180.

112 Gibbs, C.J. *et al.* (1978) Unusual resistance to ionizing radiation of the viruses of kuru, Creutzfeldt–Jakob disease, and scrapie. *Proceedings of the National Academy of Sciences of the United States of America*, **75**, 6268–6270.

113 Millson, G.C. *et al.* (1976) The physico-chemical nature of the scrapie agent, in *Slow Virus Diseases of Animals and Man* (ed. R.H. Kimberlin), North-Holland, Amsterdam, pp. 243–266.

114 Rohwer, R.G. (1983) Scrapie inactivation kinetics – an explanation of scrapie's apparent resistance to inactivation – a re-evaluation of estimates of its small size, in *Virus Non Conventionnels et Affections du Système Nerveux Central* (eds L.A. Court and E. Cathala), Masson, Paris, pp. 84–113.

115 Redecke, L. *et al.* (2009) UV-light-induced conversion and aggregation of prion proteins. *Free Radical Biology and Medicine*, **46**, 1353–1361.

116 Bellinger-Kawahara, C. *et al.* (1987) Purified scrapie prions resist inactivation by UV irradiation. *Journal of Virology*, **61**, 159–166.

117 Johnson, C.J. *et al.* (2009) Ultraviolet-ozone treatment reduces levels of disease-associated prion protein and prion infectivity. *BMC Research Notes*, **6**, 121.

118 Alper, T. (1987) Radio- and photobiological techniques in the investigation of prions, in *Prions: Novel Infectious Pathogens Causing Scrapie and Creutzfeldt–Jakob Disease* (eds S.B. Prusiner and M.P. McKinlay), Academic Press, London, pp. 113–146.

119 Culkin, F. and Fung, D.Y.C. (1975) Destruction of *Escherichia coli* and *Salmonella typhimurium* in microwave cooked soups. *Journal of Milk and Food Technology*, **38**, 8–15.

120 Diprose, M.F. and Benson, F.A. (1984) The effect of externally applied electrostatic fields, microwave radiation and electric currents on plants, with special reference to weed control. *Botanical Reviews*, **50**, 171–223.

121 Latimer, J.M. and Matsen, J.M. (1977) Microwave oven irradiation as a method for bacterial decontamination in a clinical microbiology laboratory. *Journal of Clinical Microbiology*, **6**, 340–342.

122 Rosaspina, S. *et al.* (1994) The bactericidal effect of microwaves on *Mycobacterium bovis* dried on scalpel blades. *Journal of Hospital Infection*, **26**, 45–50.

123 Taylor, D.M. and Diprose, M.F. (1996) The response of the 22A strain of scrapie agent to microwave irradiation compared with boiling. *Neuropathology and Applied Neurobiology*, **22**, 256–258.

124 Tateishi, J. *et al.* (1987) Experimental Creutzfeldt–Jakob disease: inducation of amyloid plaques in rodents, in *Prions: Novel Infectious Pathogens Causing Scrapie and Creutzfeldt–Jakob Disease* (eds S.B. Prusiner and M.P. McKinlay), Academic Press, New York, pp. 415–426.

125 Somerville, R.A. *et al.* (2002) Characterization of thermodynamic diversity between transmissible spongiform encephalopathy agent strains and its theoretical implications. *Journal of Biological Chemistry*, **277**, 11084–11089.

126 Brown, P. *et al.* (1990) Resistance of scrapie agent to steam autoclaving after formaldehyde fixation and limited survival after ashing at 360°C: practical and theoretical implications. *Journal of Infectious Diseases*, **161**, 467–472.

127 Asher, D.M. *et al.* (1981) Effects of several disinfectants and gas sterilisation on the infectivity of scrapie and Creutzfeldt–Jakob disease, in *Abstracts of the Twelfth World Congress of Neurology*, Kyoto, p. 225.

128 Taylor, D.M. *et al.* (1966) The effect of dry heat on the ME7 strain of scrapie agent. *Journal of General Virology*, **77**, 3161–3164.

129 Steele, P.J. *et al.* (1999) Survival of BSE and scrapie agents at 200°C, in *Abstracts of a Meeting of the Association of Veterinary Teachers and Research Workers.* Scarborough, p.21.

130 Brown, P. *et al.* (2000) New studies on the heat resistance of hamster-adapted scrapie agent; threshold survival after ashing at 600°C suggests an inorganic template of replication. *Proceedings of the National Academy of Sciences of the United States of America*, **97**, 3418–3421.

131 Taguchi, E. *et al.* (1991) Proposal for a procedure for complete inactivation of the Creutzfeldt–Jakob disease agent. *Archives of Virology*, **119**, 297–301.

132 Taylor, D.M. and McConnell, I. (1988) Autoclaving does not decontaminate formol-fixed scrapie tissues. *Lancet*, **i**, 1463–1464.

133 Dickinson, A.G. (1976) Scrapie in sheep and goats, in *Slow Virus Diseases of Animals and Man* (ed. R.H. Kimberlin), North Holland, Amsterdam, pp. 209–241.

134 Ernst, D.R. and Race, R.E. (1993) Comparative analysis of scrapie agent inactivation. *Journal of Virological Methods*, **41**, 193–202.

135 Taylor, D.M. (1994) Survival of mouse-passaged bovine spongiform encephalopathy agent after exposure to paraformaldehyde-lysine-periodate and formic acid. *Veterinary Microbiology*, **44**, 111–112.

136 Taylor, D.M. (2000) Inactivation of transmissible degenerative encephalopathy agents; A review. *Veterinary Journal*, **159**, 10–17.

137 Appel, T.R. *et al.* (1999) Acid inactivation of hamster scrapie prion rods, in *Abstracts of a Symposium on Characterization and Diagnosis of Prion Diseases in Animals and Man*, Tubingen, p.169.

138 Mould, D.L. and Dawson AMcL, S.W. (1965) Scrapie in mice: the stability of the agent to various suspending media, pH and solvent extraction. *Research in Veterinary Science*, **6**, 151–154.

139 Diringer, H. and Braig, H. (1989) Infectivity of unconventional viruses in dura mater. *Lancet*, **i**, 439–440.

140 Prusiner, S.B. *et al.* (1984) Prions: methods for assay, purification, and characterisation, in *Methods in Virology*, vol. VIII, (eds K. Maramorosch and H. Koprowski), Academic Press, New York, pp. 293–345.

141 Tamai, Y. *et al.* (1988) Inactivation of the Creutzfeldt–Jakob disease agent. *Annals of Neurology*, **24**, 466.

142 Tateishi, J. *et al.* (1988) Inactivation of the Creutzfeldt–Jakob disease agent. *Annals of Neurology*, **24**, 466.

143 Fichet, G. *et al.* (2007) Wirksame Reinigungsverfahren zur verringerung des risikos ener prionen-übertragung durch chirurgische instrumente. *Zentral Sterilisation*, **15** (6), 418–437.

144 Burger, D. and Gorham, J.R. (1977) Observation on the remarkable stability of transmissible mink encephalopathy virus. *Research in Veterinary Science*, **22**, 131–132.

145 Fraser, H. *et al.* (1992) Transmission of bovine spongiform encephalopathy and scrapie to mice. *Journal of General Virology*, **173**, 1891–1897.

146 Amyx, H.L. *et al.* (1981) Some physical and chemical characteristics of a strain of Creutzfeldt–Jakob disease in mice, in *Abstracts of the Twelfth World Congress of Neurology*, Kyoto, p. 255.

147 Haig, D.A. and Clarke, M.C. (1968) The effect of β-propiolactone on the scrapie agent. *Journal of General Virology*, **3**, 281–283.

148 Brown, P. *et al.* (1982) Chemical disinfection of Creutzfeldt–Jakob disease virus. *New England Journal of Medicine*, **306**, 1279–1282.

149 Walker, A.S. *et al.* (1983) Conditions for the chemical and physical inactivation of the K.Fu. strain of the agent of Creutzfeldt–Jakob disease. *American Journal of Public Health*, **73**, 661–665.

150 Tateishi, J. *et al.* (1991) Practical methods for chemical inactivation of Creudtzfeldt–Jakob disease pathogen. *Microbiology and Immunology*, **35**, 163–166.

151 Taylor, D.M. *et al.* (1999) Survival of scrapie agent after exposure to sodium dodecyl sulphate and heat. *Veterinary Microbiology*, **67**, 13–16.

152 Coates, D. (1985) A comparison of sodium hypochlorite and sodium dichloroisocyanurate products. *Journal of Hospital Infection*, **6**, 31–40.

153 Taylor, D.M. *et al.* (1994) Decontamination studies with the agents of bovine spongiform encephalopathy and scrapie. *Archives of Virology*, **139**, 313–326.

154 Brown, P. *et al.* (1982) Effects of chemicals, heat and histopathological processing on high-infectivity hamster-adapted scrapie virus. *Journal of Infectious Diseases*, **145**, 683–687.

155 Hunter, G.D. and Millson, G.C. (1964) Further experiments on the comparative potency of tissue extracts from mice infected with scrapie. *Research in Veterinary Science*, **5**, 149–153.

156 Gajdusek, D.C. and Gibbs, C.J. (1968) Slow, latent and temperature virus infections of the central nervous system, in *Infections of the Nervous System* (ed. H.M. Zimmerman), Williams & Wilkins, Baltimore, pp. 254–280.

157 Taylor, D.M. *et al.* (1998) Solvent extraction as an adjunct to rendering: the effect on BSE and scrapie agents of hot solvents, followed by dry heat and steam. *Veterinary Record*, **143**, 6–9.

158 Race, R.E. and Raymond, G.J. (2004) Inactivation of transmissible spongiform encephalopathy (prion) agents by environ LpH. *Journal of Virology*, **78**, 2164–2165.

159 Taylor, D.M. (1991) Resistance of the ME7 scrapie agent to peracetic acid. *Veterinary Microbiology*, **27**, 19–24.

160 Antloga, K. *et al.* (2000) Prion disease and medical devices. *ASAIO Journal*, **46**, S69–S72.

161 McDonnell, G. (2006) Peroxygens and other forms of oxygen: their use for effective cleaning, disinfection and sterilization, in *New Microbicides Development: the Combined Approach of Chemistry and Microbiology*, ACS Symposium Series (ed. P.C. Zhu), Oxford University Press, New York, pp. 292–308.

162 Fichet, G. *et al.* (2007) Prion inactivation using a new gaseous hydrogen peroxide sterilisation process. *Journal of Hospital Infection*, **67**, 278–386.

163 Lehmann, S. *et al.* (2009) New hospital disinfection processes for both conventional and prion infectious agents compatible with thermosensitive medical equipment. *Journal of Hospital Infection*, **72**, 342–350.

164 Rogez-Kreuz, C. *et al.* (2009) Inactivation of animal and human prions by hydrogen peroxide gas plasma sterilization. *Infection Control and Hospital Epidemiology*, **30**, 769–777.

165 McDonnell, G. and Comoy, E. (2010) Inactivation of prions, in *Sterilization and Disinfection by Plasma: Sterilization Mechanisms, Biological and Medical Application* (eds H. Shintani and A. Sakudo), Nova Science, Hauppauge, NY, pp. 61–73.

166 Baxter, H.C. *et al.* (2005) Elimination of transmissible spongiform encephalopathy infectivity and decontamination of surgical instruments by using radio-frequency gas-plasma treatment. *Journal of General Virology*, **86**, 2393–2399.

167 Hunter, G.D. *et al.* (1969) Further studies of the infectivity and stability of extracts and homogenates derived from scrapie affected mouse brains. *Journal of Comparative Pathology*, **79**, 101–108.

168 Adams, D.H. *et al.* (1972) Periodate – an inhibitor of the scrapie agent? *Research in Veterinary Science*, **13**, 195–198.

169 Manuelidis, L. (1998) Cleaning CJD-contaminated instruments. *Science*, **281**, 1961.

170 Seeger, H. *et al.* (2008) Prion depletion and preservation of biological activity by preparative chaotrope ultracentrifugation. *Biologicals*, **36**, 403–411.

171 Hunter, G.D. and Millson, G.C. (1967) Attempts to release the scrapie agent from tissue debris. *Journal of Comparative Pathology*, **77**, 301–307.

172 Prusiner, S.B. *et al.* (1981) Scrapie agent contains a hydrophobic protein. *Proceedings of the National Academy of Sciences of the United States of America*, **78**, 6675–6679.

173 Jackson, G.S. *et al.* (2005) An enzyme-detergent method for effective prion decontamination of surgical steel. *Journal of General Virology*, **86**, 869–878.

174 Yoshioka, M. *et al.* (2007) Characterization of a proteolytic enzyme derived from a *Bacillus* strain that effectively degrades prion protein. *Journal of Applied Microbiology*, **102**, 509–515.

175 Langeveld, J.P. *et al.* (2003) Enzymatic degradation of prion protein in brain stem from infected cattle and sheep. *Journal of Infectious Diseases*, **188**, 1782–1789.

176 Pilon, J.L. *et al.* (2009) Feasibility of infectious prion digestion using mild conditions and commercial subtilisin. *Journal of Virological Methods*, **161**, 168–172.

177 McLeod, A.H. *et al.* (2004) Proteolytic inactivation of the bovine spongiform encephalopathy agent. *Biochemical and Biophysical Research Communications*, **317**, 1165–1170.

178 Aguzzi, A. (2009) Cell biology: beyond the prion principle. *Nature*, **459** (7249), 924–925.

179 Scheibel, T. and Buchner, J. (2006) Protein aggregation as a cause for disease. *Handbook of Experimental Pharmacology*, **172**, 199–219.

180 Soto, C. *et al.* (2006) Amyloids, prions and the inherent infectious nature of misfolded protein aggregates. *Trends in Biochemical Sciences*, **31**, 150–155.

181 Walker, L.C. (2002) Modeling Alzheimer's disease and other proteopathies *in vivo*: is seeding the key? *Amino Acids*, **23**, 87–93.

182 Meyer-Luehmann, J. *et al.* (2008) Exogenous induction of cerebral β-amyloidogenesis is governed by agent and host. *Science*, **313**, 1781–1784.

183 Eisele, Y.S. *et al.* (2009) Induction of cerebral beta-amyloidosis: intracerebral versus systemic Abeta inoculation. *Proceedings of the National Academy of Sciences of the United States of America*, **106**, 12926–12931.

11 Microbicides – the Double-edged Sword: Environmental Toxicity and Emerging Resistance

Jean-Marie Pagès[1], Jean-Yves Maillard[2], Anne Davin-Regli[1] and Susan Springthorpe[3]

[1]UMR-MD1, Aix-Marseille Université Transporteurs Membranaires, Chimiorésistance et Drug-Design, Facultés de Médecine et de Pharmacie, Marseille, France
[2]Cardiff School of Pharmacy and Pharmaceutical Sciences, Cardiff University, Cardiff, Wales, UK
[3]Centre for Research on Environmental Microbiology, University of Ottawa, Ottawa, Ontario, Canada

Introduction

The worldwide dissemination of multidrug-resistant (MDR) pathogens has severely reduced the efficacy of our antibiotic arsenal and increased the frequency of therapeutic failure. Today, antibiotic resistance is a major concern in the anti-infective treatment of both humans and animals. Misuse and overuse of antibiotics is widely blamed as the sole reason for this widespread resistance, although microbicide usage has recently been implicated as a possible contributing factor [1].

The development and use of microbicidal products are of immense benefit to human and animal health, and to associated economic activities [1]. However, the widespread use of microbicidal products also entails a number of negative aspects such as the potential for toxicity to humans and the environment and their sublethal environmental residues leading to the emergence of microbial resistance [1].

In a global context, microorganisms are regularly exposed to natural or anthropogenic physical and chemical elements detrimental to their growth and survival. Antimicrobials (e.g. antibiotics, peptides, hydrogen peroxide) from natural sources usually exert their inhibitory effects within their immediate vicinity. In contrast, humans have been much less discriminating in how they use both natural and synthetic antibiotics and microbicides in increasing ways. This mounting and widening use is fueled primarily by a better understanding of microbe-led degradation of our surroundings and continuing discoveries of microbial pathogens and their potential for serious harm. Of course, the widespread press coverage of these issues and their negative impacts on human health have provided microbicide manufacturers in particular unprecedented marketing opportunities [2]. The widening varieties and increasing quantities of such chemicals that we use in domestic and professional settings will ultimately enter the waste stream.

All types of microorganisms, with their relatively small but pliable genomes and short generation times, have evolved a number of strategies to deal with damaging chemicals. While some possess intrinsic resistance to such chemicals, others deal with them by acquiring mobile resistance-conferring genetic elements through horizontal gene transfer, modifying membrane permeability, overexpressing efflux pumps, detoxification outside the cell, or by altering or multiplying cellular targets [2]. Chapter 6.1 provides more information on this topic and also discusses terms such as "resistance", "cross-resistance", "co-resistance", "tolerance" and "reduced susceptibility".

One of the most important factors in the development and spread of microbial resistance (or enhancing survival) in the environment is whether or not a toxic chemical is maintained for any significant period at sublethal concentrations to allow the selection for and persistence of resistance, through gene expression, mutation, etc. Since mutation itself is a random event, it is the selection that is important in driving entrenchment and spread of resistance. This is widely recognized for antibiotics as antibiotic resistance emerges and disseminates almost immediately following their field applications [3–5]. Serious concerns about antibiotic resistance and its impact on nosocomial, community-acquired and foodborne pathogens are now well recognized and have been raised at both national and international levels as well as in the popular press.

Bacteria in particular can also increase their mutation rate significantly during the starvation phase due to failures in mismatch repair; the resulting "mutator" phenotype that arises is then already primed for secondary mutations [6]. Mismatch repair mutants often undergo more conjugation and recombination events [7]. This might readily contribute to the development of antimicrobial resistance; conversely, cells primed to further mutations are also more vulnerable to extinction. Direct linkage between mismatch repair mutants and antimicrobial resistance was suggested previously but only recently has any potential link been demonstrated [8]; in this case, overexpression of an efflux pump resulted simultaneously in antibiotic resistance, protection against reactive oxygen species and a decrease in mutation rate. It is worth noting that "mutator" phenotypes might be selected within a host to whom antibiotics may also be administered [9].

This chapter aims to put into context the use of microbicides and subsequent effects on bacteria in particular and the consequences for the environment. It should be noted that while the main focus has been and continues to be on human pathogens, pathogens of economically important animals and crops, as well as those of wildlife, are likely to be significantly affected as well. Aquatic species might be especially vulnerable. While it is not the main target of this chapter to discuss hazards to persons from occupational or other microbicide exposure, it is pertinent that this be mentioned as a part of the downside of microbicide use. Microbicidal products are often used in high concentrations and direct toxic exposures, especially of young children, are not uncommon. These chemicals can also give rise to numerous side effects in those who use them regularly [10], and even low-level exposures through food and water by ingestion of the microbicides or their toxic and mutagenic by-products are recognized risks [11], although reports remain scarce. There are some regulations on the presence of by-products in the environment, notably in drinking water where the presence of trihalomethanes as by-products of water disinfection is regulated. However, the only hazards regulated are those that are recognized and many more disinfectant by-products remain to be investigated.

Applications of biocidal products and fate in the environment

Microbicides are a very diverse group of chemicals [1]. Such chemicals are rarely used on their own and are often a part of a formulation to optimize or increase their delivery, activity or to negate side effects such as smell, toxicity or corrosiveness. Yet, most studies on the development of microbial resistance to microbicides are based on the chemical alone and rarely on formulations containing it [12].

Microbicides have a wide variety of applications – including infection control, water and wastewater treatment, food production and preparation for market, microbial control in manufacturing and other industries, and disinfection or preservation of degradable substances – everything from household cleaners, personal care products and consumer plastics to transportation vehicles, building substrates and oil and gas exploration. Increases in microbicide use are forecast to continue. Consequently, the risks of microbicide use leading to the selection of resistant organisms followed by their selection and dissemination are of increasing concern [1, 2, 12].

In the healthcare setting, microbicidal products are used for the disinfection of medical devices, environmental surfaces, disinfection of skin and mucosa (antisepsis) as well decontamination of hospital wards. The Spaulding classification [13], which takes into account the degree of infection risk from a particular item (divided into critical, semi-critical and non-critical) and the level of disinfection required, holds true today, with some recent concerns on its relevance to current products and practices [14–19].

While the significance of environmental surfaces as vehicles for pathogens is still questioned by some, there is increasing evidence that such surfaces can be potential means of spread of a variety of pathogens in healthcare settings, in particular [20, 21]. This increasing appreciation of environmental surfaces in the spread of pathogens has spawned the development and aggressive marketing of a wide range of microbicide-containing surfaces (see Chapter 20). Then there is the burgeoning marketing of microbicidal wipes for use on skin and environmental surfaces [22, 23].

Microbicides are used in numerous consumer products such as cosmetics, personal care products, household products and textiles. In the European Union (EU) the use of microbicides as preservatives in cosmetics is regulated by the Cosmetics Directive (see Chapter 18). The use of microbicides in household products such as dishwashing liquids and powders, liquid soaps, shampoos and many others has seen recent and substantial increases in use with claims against innumerable pathogens. Antimicrobial surfaces are also being sold for use in domestic settings, such as cutting boards, plastic containers for food storage, toilet seats, shower curtains and various textiles as examples.

Microbicide use is, of course, common in food preservation and for environmental hygiene in settings where food is produced, manufactured and served. In the EU, microbicides used during food production are regulated under the Biocidal Products Directive (see Chapter 14.1). Microbicides are applied in the decontamination of carcasses; in 2008, the European Food Safety Authority BIOHAZ panel noted the lack of information on the ability of such microbicides to generate microbial resistance and cross-resistance [24, 25]. Disinfection of water in recreational areas regularly relies on the use of chemical disinfectants (see Chapter 19.5). The use of disinfectants for potable water is regulated by the Drinking Water Directive (98/83/EC) in the EU.

In animal husbandry, farm buildings, barns, equipment and vehicles are all chemically disinfected to reduce the risk of spread of animal pathogens. It is often difficult to assess the effectiveness and real benefits of such applications and to get accurate measures on the types and amounts of chemicals used for these purposes in order to properly determine any potential impacts on humans and the environment. On farms, the use of microbicide-containing teat-dips is common and so is the use of preservatives for eggs and semen.

A large range of microbicide use includes the disinfection/decontamination of environmental surfaces, their use as anti-biofouling agents during industrial processes, the preservation of building materials (including antimicrobial coating or impregnated surfaces), water disinfection and wastewater treatment. In the EU, the amounts of microbicides used for these different applications cannot be estimated because of the absence of reporting requirements. The European Commission has produced an assessment of human and environmental risks linked to the use of microbicides (report available at http://ec.europa.eu/environment/biocides/pdf/report_use.pdf; accessed July 2011). This overview is based on the minimum annual production/import volumes of microbicides in the EU.

High concentrations of microbicides have been reported in river water and wastewater effluents [26–28]. The bisphenol triclosan in these environmental locations has been particularly well investigated, and concentrations have been found ranging from 1.4 to 40,000 ng/l in surface water, up to 85,000 ng/l in wastewater and 133,000 μg/kg in biosolids from wastewater treatment plants [29]. These concentrations are high enough to produce a selective pressure on the microbial microcosm. Long-term exposures to low concentrations of microbicides have been found to change the bacterial composition of complex microcosms [30, 31].

Differences and similarities in antimicrobial actions

While microbicides are a very diverse group of chemicals [1], the focus here is on commercially-produced bactericidal/bacteriostatic agents. In contrast to how antibiotics exert their antimicrobial action, microbicides as a class are often much less discriminating in the targets they attack [32, 33] (see also Chapter 4). Electrophilic microbicides react with critical enzymes and inhibit growth and metabolism, with cell death occurring immediately or after several hours of contact. For example, the modification of functional groups from proteins and nucleic acids by oxidation or precipitation are characteristic of heavy metals (copper, silver, mercury), halogens (chlorine, bromine), oxidizers (ozone, peroxides), aldehydes, carbamates and isothiazolones [32]. Membrane-active microbicides directly affect cell membranes by a lytic effect (e.g. surfactants, phenols, biguanides, alcohols, quaternary ammonium compounds (QACs)) or a protonophoric interaction (e.g. weak acids, parabens, pyrithiones). This quite simple classification of the mechanisms of action does not consider that some microbicides have multiple effects. For example, QACs also bind to, and denature (solubilization and depolymerization), proteins and enzymes [32, 34–37]. Microbicides, especially those used as sporicides, are highly reactive and are thought to disrupt many functions and structures simultaneously (see Chapter 4).

The key mechanisms of bacterial resistance to antibiotics are well understood, but the same cannot be said about how bacteria become resistant to microbicides [12]. However, it turns out that the strategies used by bacteria to survive the deleterious effects of sublethal levels of antibiotics and microbicides have much in common [2, 12, 33, 38, 39]. This alone suggests that, in general terms and in theory, resistance developed originally against an antibiotic may manifest itself as resistance to a microbicidal chemical as well and vice versa. However, the available evidence shows that while bacteria with reduced susceptibility to microbicides also show an increased resistance to antibiotics, antibiotic-resistant bacteria have not been shown to develop increased insusceptibility to microbicides. This may well be because microbicides are often used in higher concentrations and they also have the ability to attack multiple targets on bacterial cells simultaneously.

It is important to understand the molecular and genetic bases for the selection of antibiotic-resistant bacteria by microbicides and to have a clear picture of the corresponding health risks. It is equally important to decipher the genetic, biochemical and physiological bases of mechanisms conferring microbicide resistance to pathogens in order to combat the emergence and dissemination of resistant pathogens that limit the efficiency of our antibacterial weapons [1].

Microbicide concentration and bacterial susceptibility

Effects of Low Concentrations of a Microbicide
Although microbicide concentration is key to its effective use [12, 40], it is crucial to remember that the microbicide concentration applied may not necessarily be the level the target pathogen encounters. Therefore, it is very important to consider how the microbicide is delivered.

The reduced availability of a microbicide through bacterial biofilms [2, 41, 42] has already been mentioned (see Chapter 5). What is often less apparent are the other factors that affect the bioavailability of a microbicide, such as formulation and the presence of organic matter and diluent (e.g. ionic content of water/hard water). Microbicides are used in formulations (i.e. microbicidal products) usually, but not always, at a high concentration for application on surfaces or the disinfection of liquids (i.e. application of microbicides in suspension). With advances in formulations and delivery methods, one might consider that a microbicide delivered should be thought of as a dose (concentration × volume) rather than simply as concentration. For example, some microbicides are recommended by manufacturers to be applied on a surface via the use of a wipe. Test data are rarely, if ever, obtained using a wipe test, and when results are available using a wipe efficacy test, microbicidal efficacy has been shown to be limited [22, 23, 43]. The nature and cleanliness of the microbicide applicator and how it is used are key to the dose of microbicide that will be delivered to the surface. The microbicide volume delivered on a surface is also important to consider as well as the time for application. The exposure time recommended in standard tests (see Chapter 12) is often not representative of microbicide application on surfaces in reality [22, 23, 44, 45]. In practice, failure to deliver sufficient microbicide to kill the target organisms will result in microorganisms surviving on the surface [46] and their possible selection [2, 47, 48], and, depending on the delivery method, it might result in distributing microorganisms over a wider area [22]. It is thus paramount that label instructions include accurate information on product dilution, usage (including detailed procedure and minimum contact time required) and storage.

Numerous reports on bacterial resistance to microbicides have been based on measuring the minimum inhibitory concentration (MIC). MICs are largely used for determining antibiotic susceptibility; for microbicides MICs provide evidence of the alteration of bacterial susceptibility to a microbicide (see Chapter 6.1). However, there can be considerable variations in the MIC values for a microbicide exposure within a single species or even among laboratories working with the same strain. Where the MIC of a microbicide differs widely from its minimum bactericidal concentration (MBC), the use of a concentration close to the MIC might result in selection for microorganisms with reduced susceptibility; this is particularly pertinent when the type of microorganism present is unknown [12]. In many studies the level of microbial resistance could be increased following repeated exposure to low concentrations of a microbicide or to its increasing (gradient) concentrations [2, 49–53].

Concentrations of Microbicides in the Environment

Virtually all antimicrobials or their by-products are eventually discharged into the environment, either directly to water or through sewage treatment plant effluents. In many instances the volume of water or sewage is large enough that the concentration(s) of microbicides might be below stressful levels for bacteria, but this is not always the case. Examples where bacteria are likely exposed to microbicide levels that might be stressful include wastes from cooling towers, farms, pulp and paper mills, and various industries including gas and oil drilling. The injection of largely undisclosed mixtures of microbicides (including aldehydes) and other toxic chemicals during the fracking (hydraulic fracturing) process for gas extraction has recently drawn public concern for the safety of groundwater.

As mentioned above, triclosan has been found at low concentrations in a number of settings [27, 29]. Often those concentrations are at the stressful level for bacteria. To date, there have been no antimicrobial susceptibility studies investigating microbial microcosms in these environments.

The acquisition of resistance determinants in the environment is of concern. Environmental bacterial isolates from a reed bed exposed to QACs from a wool-finishing mill have been shown to have high levels of resistance to QACs, and class 1 integron incidence was significantly higher for bacteria pre-exposed to QACs [54]. Gaze *et al.* [55] reported a high prevalence of class 1 integrons and demonstrated the potential importance of detergents. These authors estimated that more than 1×10^{19} bacteria carrying class 1 integrons enter the UK environment from sewage sludge each year. The presence of conjugative plasmids has also been associated with co-resistance between a number of microbicides such as cationic compounds, metallic salts (e.g. organomercurials) and antibiotics [50, 56, 57].

However, to date, there have not been any comprehensive studies linking microbicides in the environment and antibiotic resistance.

Microbicides and antimicrobial resistance in bacteria

General Considerations

Microbicide resistance in bacteria has been described since the 1950s and a number of mechanisms for such resistance have been described (see Chapter 6.1). Most of the evidence regarding bacterial resistance to microbicides comes from laboratory-based studies, which report a change of susceptibility in a wide range of bacterial pathogens such as *Staphylococcus aureus*, *Pseudomonas aeruginosa*, *Escherichia coli*, *Salmonella enterica*, etc. against a wide range of microbicides (see Chapter 6.1). The role of bacterial biofilms in bacterial survival and persistence has been particularly well addressed (see Chapter 6.2). Evidence for the effects of microbicides on altering antibiotic susceptibility profiles *in situ* is scarce. In a study performed in the community, a significant relationship was highlighted between high MICs to QACs, high MICs to triclosan and resistance to one or more antibiotics [58]. More recently, an outbreak of *Mycobacterium massiliense* in a number of hospitals in Brazil linked antibiotic resistance with glutaraldehyde resistance [59].

Some resistance mechanisms expressed in bacteria constitutively or as a result of environmental stresses, notably exposure to microbicides, have a broad spectrum of action and contribute not only to resistance to microbicides but also to resistance to unrelated compounds such as antibiotics [12, 60]. For example, to reduce the intracellular concentration of antibacterial molecules under an inhibitory concentration threshold, Gram-negative bacteria can regulate the permeability of their membranes by decreasing the expression of porins (membrane pore-forming proteins involved in antibiotic uptake) and altering the lipopolysaccharide structure or overexpressing efflux pumps [12, 60–63]. These modifications contribute to the resistance against antibiotics and microbicides [2, 64, 65].

Expression and Overexpression of Efflux Pumps and Other Systems

Efflux pumps, because of their broad-spectrum substrates, are increasingly associated with resistance [66–68]. In *Salmonella*, triclosan-selected strains have been shown to be less susceptible to antibiotics than the wild-type [69, 70]. Changes in antibiotic susceptibility profiles have also been observed following exposure to a low concentration of other microbicides [67, 68]. In triclosan-selected *Stenotrophomonas* clones, the overexpression of an efflux pump (SmeDEF) involved in antibiotic resistance has been described [71]. Other investigations described *P. aeruginosa* overexpressing multidrug efflux systems during exposure to chlorhexidine [72]. Expression and overexpression of other multigenic systems such as *soxRS* and *oxyR* [73] have also been implicated in bacterial resistance. In *S. aureus*, Huet *et al.* [74] described that transcription of efflux pump genes is stimulated during exposure of clinical isolates to low concentrations of a variety of microbicides and dyes. In a recent study, Bailey *et al.* [75] demonstrated that the exposure of *E. coli* and *S. enterica* cells to triclosan induces a species-specific response corresponding to an increase of the expression of efflux pump genes. A recent report showed that the triclosan resistance could involve distinct mechanisms including the overexpression and mutagenesis of *fab1* and the production of the active efflux pump AcrAB/TolC in *Salmonella* [76]. In bacterial biofilms, triclosan could also upregulate the transcription of *acrAB*, of *marA* (the major regulator of the genetic cascade controlling multidrug resistance) and of the cellulose synthesis coding genes *bcsA* and *bcsE*. In *E. coli* exposure to polyhexamethylene biguanide induced the alteration of transcriptional activity in a number of genes, notably in the *rhs* gene involved in repair/binding of nucleic acid [77]. Some of the mechanisms that play a major role in microbicide and antibiotic resistance are controlled by diverse genetic cascades that share common key gene regulators (*soxS*, *marA*) [60, 78, 79]. A transcriptional analysis has demonstrated that paraquat is able to induce the expression of several genes that are directly involved in antibiotic resistance [80]. In addition, activation of the *soxRS* regulon with paraquat treatment increased resistance to ampicillin, nalidixic acid, chloramphenicol and tetracycline in laboratory strains of *E. coli* and *S. enterica*. The *soxRS* regulon was also connected to antibiotic resistance in clinical strains [81]. In a recent study, the exposure of *E. coli* and

S. enterica cells to triclosan was able to modify expression of regulator genes (*soxS*) involved in the genetic control of antibiotic resistance [75].

Physiological and Metabolic Changes

A change in bacterial physiology, including small colonies, alteration of growth rates and altered gene expression, have been described during bacterial exposure to microbicides [82]. Exposure to isothiazolones changed metabolic processes in *P. aeruginosa* [49]. *Serratia marcescens* insusceptibility to a QAC was proposed to be dependent in part on a number of biosynthetic pathways [83]. In *S. enterica*, a "triclosan resistance network", which constitutes an alternative pathway to the production of pyruvate and fatty acid, has been described [76]. Likewise, in *S. aureus*, a modification of the membrane lipid composition associated with the alteration of expression of various genes involved in fatty acid metabolism has been associated with triclosan resistance [84]. A change in metabolic pathways in bacteria exposed to triclosan is, overall, not surprising when one considers the specific mechanism of action of triclosan at a low concentration [85, 86].

Conclusions

The emergence of microbicide resistance and the persistence of mobile genetic elements containing resistance genes have important implications for human and animal health in terms of surviving pathogens and the potential dissemination of antimicrobial resistance. The selective pressure exerted by exposure to microbicides has been associated with the selection of less susceptible or resistant bacteria. This has been exacerbated with increasing use and sometimes misuse of microbicides worldwide. A large number of studies have reported the resistance to microbicides in specific applications including healthcare, consumer products, food production and animal husbandry [1].

Microbicides used in a very large number of applications will eventually be released in the environment together with their by-products, despite existing regulations (e.g. BPD and REACH, see Chapter 14.1). In the environment, sewage and biosolid residuals combine with microbial pathogens and various chemicals, including microbicides and antibiotics. It is disappointing that, to date, there have been no investigations on the antimicrobial phenotypes of bacteria isolated from these environments.

There are now genetic and bacteriological data to demonstrate the involvement of microbicides in the selection of resistant bacterial strains. Such information strongly indicates that prudence in the use of microbicides is needed in order to preserve their efficacy and to limit the emergence and dissemination of resistant bacteria.

This chapter dealt with bacteria and did not address the development of resistance to other classes of microorganisms such as fungi, protozoa and viruses (see Chapters 8 and 9). For those microorganisms, investigations in the development of resistance following microbicide exposure are scarce.

References

1 SCENIHR (Scientific Committee on Emerging and Newly Identified Health Risks) (2009) The antibiotic resistance effect of biocides, adopted by the SCENIHR on January 19, 2009. http://ec.europa.eu/health/ph_risk/committees/04_scenihr/docs/scenihr_o_021.pdf

2 Maillard, J.-Y. (2007) Bacterial resistance to biocides in the health care environment: should it be of genuine concern? *Journal of Hospital Infection*, **65** (Suppl. 2), 60–72.

3 Falagas, M.E. and Bliziotis, I.A. (2007) Pandrug-resistant Gram-negative bacteria: the dawn of the post-antibiotic era? *International Journal of Antimicrobial Agents*, **29**, 630–636.

4 Jansen, W.T. *et al.* (2006) Bacterial resistance: a sensitive issue complexity of the challenge and containment strategy in Europe. *Drug Resistance Update*, **9**, 123–133.

5 Chopra, I. *et al.* (2008) Treatment of health-care-associated infections caused by Gram-negative bacteria: a consensus statement. *Lancet Infectious Diseases*, **8**, 133–139.

6 Llorens, J.M.N. *et al.* (2010) Stationary phase in Gram negative bacteria. *FEMS Microbiology Reviews*, **34**, 476–495.

7 Feinstein, S.I. and Brooks, K.B. (1986) Hyper-recombining recipient strains in bacterial conjugation. *Genetics*, **113**, 13–33.

8 Guelfo, J.R. *et al.* (2010) A MATE-family efflux pump rescues the *Escherichia coli* 8-oxoguanine-repair-deficient mutator phenotype and protects against H$_2$O$_2$ killing. *PLoS Genetics*, **6** (5), e1000931.

9 Jolivet-Gougeon, A. *et al.* (2011) Bacterial hypermutation: clinical implications. *Journal of Medical Microbiology*, **60**, 563–573.

10 Preller, L. *et al.* (1996) Disinfectant use as a risk factor for atopic sensitization and symptoms consistent with asthma: an epidemiological study. *European Respiratory Journal*, **9**, 1407–1413.

11 Bove, G.E. *et al.* (2007) Case control study of the geographic variability of exposure to disinfectant byproducts and risk for rectal cancer. *International Journal of Health Geographics*, **6**, 6–18.

12 Maillard, J.-Y. and Denyer, S.P. (2009) Emerging bacterial resistance following biocide exposure: should we be concerned? *Chemica Oggi*, **27**, 26–28.

13 Spaulding, E.H. (1968) Chemical disinfection of medical and surgical materials, in *Disinfection, Sterilization and Preservation* (eds C.A. Laurence and S.S. Block), Lea & Febiger, Philadelphia, pp. 517–531.

14 Allerberger, F. *et al.* (2002) Routine surface disinfection in health care facilities: should we do it? *American Journal of Infection Control*, **30**, 318–319.

15 Dettenkoffer, M. *et al.* (2004) Does disinfection of environmental surfaces influence nosocomial infection rates? A systematic review. *American Journal of Infection Control*, **32**, 84–89.

16 Dharan, S. *et al.* (1999) Routine disinfection of patients' environmental surfaces. Myth or reality? *Journal of Hospital Infection*, **42**, 113–117.

17 Rutala, W.A. and Weber, D.J. (2001) Surface disinfection: should we do it? *Journal of Hospital Infection*, **48** (Suppl. A), 64–68.

18 Rutala, W.A. and Weber, D.J. (2004) The benefits of surface disinfection. *American Journal of Infection Control*, **32**, 226–231.

19 Boyce, J.M. (2007) Environmental contamination makes an important contribution to hospital infection. *Journal of Hospital Infection*, **65** (Suppl. 2), 50–54.

20 Talon, D. (1999) The role of the hospital environment in the epidemiology of multi-resistant bacteria. *Journal of Hospital Infection*, **43**, 13–17.

21 Hota, B. (2004) Contamination, disinfection and cross-colonization: are hospital surfaces reservoirs for nosocomial infection? *Clinical Infectious Diseases*, **39**, 1182–1189.

22 Williams, G.J. *et al.* (2009) Limitations of the efficacy of surface disinfection in the healthcare settings. *Infection Control and Hospital Epidemiology*, **30**, 570–573.

23 Siani, H. *et al.* (2011) Efficacy of "sporicidal" wipes against *Clostridium difficile*. *American Journal of Infection Control*, **39**, 212–218.

24 EFSA (European Food Safety Authority) (2008) *Assessment of the Possible Effect of the Four Antimicrobial Treatment Substances on the Emergence of Antimicrobial Resistance*, Scientific Opinion of the Panel on Biological Hazards, published 2 April 2008; adopted 6 March 2008.

25 EFSA (European Food Safety Authority) (2008) Scientific opinion of the panel on biological hazards on a request from the European Food Safety Authority on foodborne antimicrobial resistance as a biological hazard. *EFSA Journal*, **765**, 1–87.

26 Pedrouzo, M. *et al.* (2009) Ultra-high-performance liquid chromatography and mass spectrometry for determining the presence of eleven personal care products in surface and wastewaters. *Journal of Chromatography A*, **1216**, 6994–7000.

27 Kumar, K.S. *et al.* (2010) Mass loadings of triclosan and triclocarbon from four wastewater treatment plants to three rivers and landfill in Savannah, Georgia, USA. *Archives of Environmental Contamination and Toxicology*, **58**, 275–285.

28 Wilson, B. *et al.* (2009) The partitioning of triclosan between aqueous and particulate bound phases in the Hudson River Estuary. *Marine Pollution Bulletin*, **59**, 207–212.

29 SCCS (Scientific Committee on Consumer Safety) (2010) *Preliminary Opinion on Triclosan (Antimicrobial Resistance)*, March 23, http://ec.europa.eu/health/scientific_committees/consumer_safety/docs/sccs_o_023.pdf.

30 McBain, A.J. *et al.* (2004) Effects of quaternary-ammonium based formulations on bacterial community dynamics and antimicrobial susceptibility. *Applied and Environmental Microbiology*, **70**, 3449–3456.

31 McBain, A.J. *et al.* (2003) Exposure of sink drain microcosms to triclosan: population dynamics and antimicrobial susceptibility. *Applied and Environmental Microbiology*, **69**, 5433–5442.

32 Maillard, J.-Y. (2002) Bacterial target sites for biocidal action. *Journal of Applied Microbiology*, **92** (Suppl.), 16–27.

33 Russell, A.D. (2003) Biocide use and antibiotic resistance: the relevance of laboratory findings to clinical environmental situations. *Lancet Infectious Diseases*, **3**, 794–803.

34 Aiello, A.E. and Larson, E. (2003) Antibacterial cleaning and hygiene products as an emerging risk factor for antibiotic resistance in the community. *Lancet Infectious Diseases*, **3**, 501–506.

35 Aiello, A.E. *et al.* (2005) Antibacterial cleaning products and drug resistance. *Emerging Infectious Diseases*, **11**, 1565–1570.

36 Aiello, A.E. *et al.* (2007) Consumer antibacterial soaps: effective or just risky? *Clinical Infectious Diseases*, **45** (Suppl. 2), 137–147.

37 Levy, S.B. (2000) Antibiotic and antiseptic resistance: impact on public health. *Pediatric Infectious Disease Journal*, **19** (Suppl.), 120–122.

38 Russell, A.D. (2002) Antibiotic and biocide resistance in bacteria: comments and conclusion. *Journal of Applied Microbiology*, **92** (Suppl.), 171–173.

39 Sheldon, A.T., Jr. (2005) Antiseptic "resistance": real or perceived threat? *Clinical Infectious Diseases*, **40**, 1650–1656.

40 Russell, A.D. and McDonnell, G. (2000) Concentration: a major factor in studying biocidal action. *Journal of Hospital Infection*, **44**, 1–3.

41 Anderson, G.G. and O'Toole, G.A. (2008) Innate and induced resistance mechanisms of bacterial biofilms. *Current Topics in Microbiology and Immunology*, **322**, 85–105.

42 Tart, A.H. and Wozniak, D.J. (2008) Shifting paradigms in *Pseudomonas aeruginosa* biofilm research. *Current Topics in Microbiology and Immunology*, **322**, 193–206.

43 Panousi, M.N. *et al.* (2009) Use of alcoholic wipes during aseptic manufacturing. *Letters in Applied Microbiology*, **48**, 648–651.

44 Williams, G.J. *et al.* (2009) The use of sodium dichloroisocyanurate, NaDCC, in Welsh ITUs. *Journal of Hospital Infection*, **72** (3), 279–281.

45 Cheeseman, K.E. *et al.* (2009) Evaluation of the bactericidal efficacy of three different alcohol hand rubs against 57 clinical isolates of *Staphylococcus aureus*. *Journal of Hospital Infection*, **72**, 319–325.

46 Maillard, J.-Y. (2011) Innate resistance to sporicides and potential failure to decontaminate. *Journal of Hospital Infection*, **77**, 204–209.

47 Chapman, J.S. (2003) Disinfectant resistance mechanisms, cross-resistance, and co-resistance. *International Biodeterioration and Biodegradation*, **51**, 271–276.

48 Maillard, J.-Y. (2005) Antimicrobial biocides in the health care environment: efficacy, policies, management and perceived problems. *Therapeutics and Clinical Risk Management*, **1**, 307–320.

49 Abdel Malek, S.M. *et al.* (2002) Antimicrobial susceptibility changes and T-OMP shifts in pythione-passaged planktonic cultures of *Pseudomonas aeruginosa* PAO1. *Journal of Applied Microbiology*, **92**, 729–736.

50 Langsrud, S. *et al.* (2003) Bacterial disinfectant resistance – a challenge for the food industry. *International Biodeterioration and Biodegradation*, **51**, 283–290.

51 Tattawasart, U. *et al.* (1999) Development of resistance to chlorhexidine diacetate and cetylpyridinium chloride in *Pseudomonas stutzeri* and changes in antibiotic susceptibility. *Journal of Hospital Infection*, **42**, 219–229.

52 Thomas, L. *et al.* (2000) Development of resistance to chlorhexidine diacetate in *Pseudomonas aeruginosa* and the effect of "residual" concentration. *Journal of Hospital Infection*, **46**, 297–303.

53 Walsh, S.E. *et al.* (2003) Development of bacterial resistance to several biocides and effects on antibiotic susceptibility. *Journal of Hospital Infection*, **55**, 98–107.

54 Gaze, W.H. *et al.* (2005) Incidence of class-1 integrons in a quaternary ammonium compound-polluted environment. *Antimicrobial Agents and Chemotherapy*, **49**, 1802–1807.

55 Gaze, W.H. *et al.* (2011) Impacts of anthropogenic activity on the ecology of class 1 integrons and integron-associated genes in the environment. *ISME Journal*, **5**, 1253–1261.

56 Beveridge, T.J. *et al.* (1997) Metal–microbe interactions: contemporary approaches. *Advances in Microbial Physiology*, **38**, 177–243.

57 Misra, T.K. (1992) Bacterial resistances to inorganic mercury salts and organomercurials. *Plasmid*, **27**, 4–16.

58 Carson, R.T. *et al.* (2008) Use of antibacterial consumer products containing quaternary ammonium compounds and drug resistance in the community. *Journal of Antimicrobial Chemotherapy*, **62**, 1160–1162.

59 Duarte, R.S. *et al.* (2009) Epidemic of postsurgical infections caused by *Mycobacterium massiliense*. *Journal of Clinical Microbiology*, **47**, 2149–2155.

60 Poole, K. (2007) Efflux pumps as antimicrobial resistance mechanisms. *Annals of Medicine*, **39**, 162–176.

61 Pagès, J.M. *et al.* (2008) The porin and the permeating antibiotic: a selective diffusion barrier in Gram-negative bacteria. *Nature Reviews. Microbiology*, **6**, 893–903.

62 Nikaido, H. (2003) Molecular basis of bacterial outer membrane permeability revisited. *Microbiology and Molecular Biology Reviews*, **67**, 593–656.

63 Piddock, L.J. (2006) Clinically relevant chromosomally encoded multidrug resistance efflux pump in bacteria. *Clinical Microbiology Reviews*, **19**, 382–402.

64 Thorrold, C.A. *et al.* (2007) Efflux pump activity in fluoroquinolone and tetracycline resistant *Salmonella* and *E. coli* implicated in reduced susceptibility to household antimicrobial cleaning agents. *International Journal of Food Microbiology*, **113**, 315–320.

65 Tumah, H.N. (2009) Bacterial biocide resistance. *Journal of Chemotherapy*, **21**, 5–15.

66 Maira-Litrán, T. *et al.* (2000) An evaluation of the potential of the multiple antibiotic resistance operon (mar) and the multidrug efflux pump acrAB to moderate resistance towards ciprofloxacin in *Escherichia coli* biofilms. *Journal of Antimicrobial Chemotherapy*, **45**, 789–795.

67 Randall, L.P. *et al.* (2007) Commonly used farm disinfectants can select for mutant *Salmonella enterica* serovar Typhimurium with decreased susceptibility to biocides and antibiotics without compromising virulence. *Journal of Antimicrobial Chemotherapy*, **60**, 1273–1280.

68 Randall, L.P. *et al.* (2004) Effect of triclosan or a phenolic farm disinfectant on the selection of antibiotic-resistant *Salmonella enterica*. *Journal of Antimicrobial Chemotherapy*, **54**, 621–627.

69 Karatzas, K.A. *et al.* (2008) Phenotypic and proteomic characterization of multiply antibiotic-resistant variants of *Salmonella enterica* serovar Typhimurium selected following exposure to disinfectants. *Applied and Environmental Microbiology*, **74**, 1508–1516.

70 Karatzas, K.A. *et al.* (2007) Prolonged treatment of *Salmonella enterica* serovar Typhimurium with commercial disinfectants selects for multiple antibiotic resistance, increased efflux and reduced invasiveness. *Journal of Antimicrobial Chemotherapy*, **60**, 947–955.

71 Sánchez, P. *et al.* (2005) The biocide triclosan selects *Stenotrophomonas maltophilia* mutants that overproduce the SmeDEF multidrug efflux pump. *Antimicrobial Agents and Chemotherapy*, **49**, 781–782.

72 Fraud, S. *et al.* (2008) MexCD-OprJ multidrug efflux system of *Pseudomonas aeruginosa*: involvement in chlorhexidine resistance and induction by membrane-damaging agents dependent upon the AlgU stress response sigma factor. *Antimicrobial Agents and Chemotherapy*, **52**, 4478–4482.

73 Dukan, S. and Touati, D. (1996) Hypochlorous acid stress in *Escherichia coli*: resistance, DNA damage, and comparison with hydrogen peroxide stress. *Journal of Bacteriology*, **178**, 6145–6150.

74 Huet, A.A. *et al.* (2008) Multidrug efflux pump overexpression in *Staphylococcus aureus* after single and multiple *in vitro* exposures to biocides and dyes. *Microbiology*, **154**, 3144–3153.

75 Bailey, A.M. *et al.* (2009) Exposure of *Escherichia coli* and *Salmonella enterica* serovar Typhimurium to triclosan induces a species-specific response, including drug detoxification. *Journal of Antimicrobial Chemotherapy*, **64**, 973–985.

76 Webber, M.A. *et al.* (2008) Triclosan resistance in *Salmonella enterica* serovar Typhimurium. *Journal of Antimicrobial Chemotherapy*, **62**, 83–91.

77 Allen, M.J. *et al.* (2006) The response of *Escherichia coli* to exposure to the biocide polyhexamethylene biguanide. *Microbiology*, **152**, 989–1000.

78 Li, X.Z. and Nikaido, H. (2009) Efflux-mediated drug resistance in bacteria: an update. *Drugs*, **69**, 1555–1623.

79 Oethinger, M. *et al.* (1998) Association of organic solvent tolerance and fluoroquinolone resistance in clinical isolates of *Escherichia coli*. *Molecular Microbiology*, **16**, 45–55.

80 Pomposiello, P.J. *et al.* (2001) Genome-wide transcriptional profiling of the *Escherichia coli* responses to superoxide stress and sodium salicylate. *Journal of Bacteriology*, **183**, 3890–3902.

81 Koutsolioutsou, A. *et al.* (2005) Constitutive *soxR* mutations contribute to multiple-antibiotic resistance in clinical *Escherichia coli* isolates. *Antimicrobial Agents and Chemotherapy*, **49**, 2746–2752.

82 Seaman, P. *et al.* (2007) Small-colony variants: a novel mechanism for triclosan resistance in methicillin-resistant *Staphylococcus aureus*. *Journal of Antimicrobial Chemotherapy*, **59**, 43–50.

83 Codling, C.E. *et al.* (2004) Identification of genes involved in the susceptibility of *Serratia marcescens* to polyquaternium-1. *Journal of Antimicrobial Chemotherapy*, **54**, 370–375.

84 Tkachenko, O. *et al.* (2007) A triclosan-ciprofloxacin cross-resistant mutant strain of *Staphylococcus aureus* displays an alteration in the expression of several cell membrane structural and functional genes. *Research in Microbiology*, **158**, 651–658.

85 Gomez Escalada, M. *et al.* (2005) Triclosan inhibition of fatty acid synthesis and its effect on growth of *E. coli* and *P. aeruginosa*. *Journal of Antimicrobial Chemotherapy*, **55**, 879–882.

86 Gomez Escalada, M. *et al.* (2005) Triclosan-bacteria interactions: single or multiple target sites? *Letters in Applied Microbiology*, **41**, 476–481.

12   Evaluation of Antimicrobial Efficacy

Lawrence Staniforth

Campden BRI, Chipping Campden, UK

Introduction

Disinfection is commonly defined as "a process by which micro-organisms are killed, so that their numbers are reduced to a level which is neither harmful to health nor to the quality of perishable goods". However, this definition is vague, more qualitative than quantitative, and thus there is no general agreement on what disinfection really means – and that is part of the problem. Perhaps due to terminology and language rather than the lack of scientific discourse, the above definition may perhaps be better described as "the common purpose of disinfection".

Disinfectants are tested to ensure that they are capable of delivering the degree of protection required by the user or promised by their manufacturers or suppliers. Although many identical disinfectants are used in many different countries, a general internationally accepted test scheme does not exist [1]. Many countries have their own government testing laboratories with their own national standards for testing disinfectants. A disinfectant that is passed for use in one country may not necessarily pass in another.

In 2000 the Organization for Economic Cooperation and Development (OECD) performed a survey of available disinfection methods and found more than 70 methods in use or in development for testing bactericidal disinfectants alone (this excludes sporicidal, fungicidal, mycobactericidal or virucidal test methods).

Within Europe there has been a drive to standardize terminology and thus testing, starting with the Council of Europe's so-called European suspension test (1987) [2]. This test differed little from the preceding tests, except for attempting to add more rigors to the testing systems. Prescriptions for the organic load in clean and dirty conditions were stipulated to more accurately reflect possible in-use scenarios. With the introduction of the Biocidal Products Directive (now known as the BPD/BPR) the European Committee for Standardization (CEN) formed Technical Committee (TC) 216 concerned with the testing of chemical disinfectants and antiseptics.

According to resolution BT 192/1990, the aim of CEN TC 216 is "standardization of the terminology, requirements, test methods including potential efficacy under in-use conditions, recommendations for use and labeling in the whole field of chemical disinfection and antiseptics. Areas of activity include agriculture (but not crop protection chemicals), domestic service, food hygiene and other industrial fields, institutional, medical and veterinary applications" [3]. CEN TC 216 has three working groups:
- CEN TC 216/WG 1 – Medical.
- CEN TC 216/WG 2 – Veterinary.
- CEN TC 216/WG 3 – Food hygiene, industrial, domestic and institutional.

Russell, Hugo & Ayliffe's: Principles and Practice of Disinfection, Preservation and Sterilization, Fifth Edition. Edited by Adam P. Fraise, Jean-Yves Maillard, and Syed A. Sattar.
© 2013 Blackwell Publishing Ltd. Published 2013 by Blackwell Publishing Ltd.

The methods used by the different working groups are similar, differing in the scope of organisms tested, the temperature, the contact times and the interfering substances. All try to simulate the particular application area as closely as possible. Adopted testing schemes are supposed to supplant all previous suspension testing schemes within EU countries.

In the USA, the Environmental Protection Agency (EPA) classifies disinfectants (often referred to as "germicides") as either high, intermediate or low level. High-level disinfectants (HLDs) kill all classes of microorganisms, except large numbers of bacterial spores; HLDs are now mainly under the jurisdiction of the US Food and Drug Administration (FDA). Intermediate-level disinfectants kill mycobacteria, other types of vegetative bacteria and most viruses. Low-level disinfectants kill some types of viruses and vegetative bacteria only [4].. Test methods used in the USA include those from ASTM International (formerly known as the American Society for Testing and Materials) and AOAC International (formerly known as the Association of Official Analytical Chemists).

Testing of disinfectants for their microbicidal activity is, in principle, easy, but in reality quite complex. There are a myriad of factors to deal with to ensure the repeatability and reliability of the test. Although rarely mentioned, the fundamental basis of the disinfection test is that disinfectants obey rate laws. That is to say, the rate of disinfection is dependent on the concentration of the active chemical, the time the disinfectant is in contact with the microbe, the ambient temperature, etc. The basic rate law used to examine disinfectants is the Chick–Watson law [5–7]. This law suggests that as disinfection proceeds, the number of survivors will fall exponentially at a rate governed by the rate constant and the disinfectant concentration. A plot of the log survivors against time gives the classic semi-log plot of inactivation kinetics.

$$N_s = N_0 \exp(-kB^n - t)$$

where N_s are the surviving number of microbes, N_0 is the initial inoculum number used, k is the disinfectant rate constant, B is the disinfectant concentration, n is the dilution coefficient and t is the contact time.

Phelps [5] argued that disinfectant testing should take account of the effect of temperature, concentration and time of contact; however, experimental prudence suggested otherwise. In essence, disinfectant tests have been standardized so that the effects of variables such as temperature have been reduced to the extent that their effect is assumed to be minimum or negligible. Only through such strict standards can a reliable test be obtained, it was argued.

Yet, after a hundred years of testing, disinfection tests are still notorious for their poor degree of reproducibility. On writing about the Rideal–Walker test, Croshaw [8] stated "its reproducibility is well established; although this is of the order of 30% it is no worse than that of most other disinfectant tests". Standards that have been published include contributions from ASTM International [9], AOAC International [10], the German Society for

Hygiene and Microbiology (DGHM) [11], the French Association of Normalization (AFNOR) [12], the German Veterinary Society [13] and the British Standards Institution (BSI) [14–18].

The outcome of a test of disinfectant efficacy is, essentially, a pass–fail criterion. It is not the intention to conduct intensive scientific studies; the test is done merely to confirm or deny the ability of, or the claims made for, the prowess of a commercial or prototype disinfectant. It is the construction of the testing procedures that ensures that disinfectants are tested by the most appropriate method. There are a multitude of methods to choose from; however, the actual choice may be decided by the prevailing national or international standard. Although these are the test methods used to decide whether a particular disinfectant can be used for a specific purpose, many industries and academic institutes, which research and develop new disinfectants or formulations, use the same methods. A thorough examination of disinfectant tests and all the literature that has accumulated to validate or refute them would fill a good size book in its own right. A chapter must therefore necessarily skim the essence of the literature, without, hopefully, reducing the chapter to mere musings. Within this survey, an examination of the testing structures and their reliabilities is attempted. Some detailed reviews can be found by the authorships of Ayliffe [19], Reuter [20], Cremieux and Fleurette [21], Mulberry [22] and Springthorpe and Sattar [23].

Classification of disinfectant tests

There are three principal stages in disinfectant testing.
1. Primary testing or screening begins with suspension tests to determine activity against indicator organisms (e.g. *Staphylococcus aureus* and *Pseudomonas aeruginosa*).
2. Laboratory tests simulating possible in-use scenarios determines whether the disinfectant can be active for a given application, that is the conditions of a particular use are recreated by selecting appropriate challenge organisms, interfering substances, temperature and contact time.
3. Field tests (*in loco* tests). These tests can be costly and it is difficult to ensure any degree of standardization/repeatability (and therefore reliability). While there are a number of examples of field trials, no one method would be suitable for all application areas, thus guidelines upon how to plan and run a field trial may be more applicable than a standard method.

CEN TC216 disinfection tests follow these stages or phases. Phase 1 tests EN1040 (bactericidal) and EN1275 (fungicidal) are common to all application areas and are basic suspension tests. Phase 2 tests are split into two parts – in phase 2, step 1, a more involved suspension test is carried out, introducing four challenge organisms (with scope to add additional organisms). Factors such as water hardness and interfering substances are also considered (dependent upon the area of use). In phase 2, step 2, practical tests such as "surface disinfection with no mechanical action" are performed using a carrier test principle. As yet there is no standard method for a surface test with mechanical action. In this phase there are also tests for disinfectant handsoaps such as EN1499 and handrubs such as EN1500.

Primary and secondary testing methods: suspension

Preliminary tests are the most simple of the tests and often involve nothing more than ascertaining whether a given concentration of disinfectant/microbicidal active has killed all microbes in a given time. The types of tests normally carried out can be divided into two groups: suspension and surface (carrier) tests. In a suspension test (e.g. BS EN1040 [24]) one part of a bacterial suspension is added to four to nine parts of a test concentration of disinfectant; after a predetermined exposure time an aliquot of the mixture is removed, the disinfectant in the aliquot is neutralized and the mixture examined to determine the extent of microbial inactivation.

Capacity tests (e.g. Kelsey–Sykes) are a form of suspension test where the test dilution of the disinfectant is loaded, stepwise, with several additions of a bacterial suspension. After each addition the reaction mixture is subcultured for survivors. Successive additions of bacteria allow the determination of when the disinfecting ability (capacity) of the microbicidal agent has been exhausted.

Suspension tests

The basic idea behind the suspension test is to mix an inoculum with a disinfectant for a period of time, and then check for survivors. If the survivors are enumerated then a quantitative suspension test is achieved, otherwise the test, at its most basic, is used to give an indication of survival (e.g. visual growth of survivors in a tube of broth). Rigor is added through a standardized inoculum (preparation and size), specified disinfectant concentration(s), time(s) of contact, temperature(s), water hardness and "soil". Not withstanding these standardizations, the lack of reliability of these tests often results in even the type of glassware used being specified.

The qualitative suspension test is a useful first indicator of activity and can be used as a quick screening tool to gauge the range of the active concentration for a given scenario (inclusive of contact time). However, since enumeration is not carried out, a population that is injured and exhibits a long lag before commencement of growth, may be indistinguishable from a lone survivor multiplying, hence these tests are really indicative rather than qualitative. Subculturing of tubes can show whether this has occurred [25], but the test is no longer a quick indicative measurement. A variety of qualitative suspension test methods have been published, principally from the German institutions [10, 12].

By simple enumeration, a basic test becomes quantitative and given that many suspension tests can be automated there should be no real reason to perform qualitative testing. Many quantitative suspension tests have been described in the last four decades [26]. After the exposure of test organism to the disinfectant, survivors can be counted by two techniques, either by direct culture

or by membrane filtration. The microbicidal effect (ME) is the decimal log reduction in the number of viable microorganisms relative to an untreated control in a given contact time:

$$ME = \log NC - \log ND$$

where log NC is the decimal log of the number of colony-forming units in the untreated control(s) and log ND the decimal log number of colony-forming units counted after exposure to the disinfectant.

Most of the microbicidal tests used for routine and research purposes are quantitative suspension tests, in which the number of survivors is determined by direct culture. In Europe, several tests were widely used, often with regional variation and even laboratory variation depending on the desired outcome of the test. The Dutch standard suspension test became quite widely used throughout Europe and beyond [27]. The test was known as the 5-5-5 because of the requirements for the use of five organisms and the achievement of 5-log reductions in 5 min of contact time. The organisms tested tended to reflect the particular arena in which the disinfectant was to be used, for example food industry or healthcare.

Other widely used quantitative suspension tests were those of AFNOR and DGHM [26]. The criterion of the French AFNOR test NF T 72-150 [12] is, like the Dutch test, a reduction of 5-log after a reaction time of 5 min. Under the auspices of the Committee of the International Colloquium on the Evaluation of Disinfectants in Europe, a new *in vitro* test was developed in 1975 [28, 29], which served as a basis for the quantitative suspension test of the DGHM guidelines [30]. Meanwhile, in the UK, the Kelsey–Sykes capacity test [2] was prevalent, the Chick–Martin test scheme was updated and phenol coefficients were still looked for (the Rideal–Walker test).

CEN TC216 suspension testing of disinfectants has been established and supplants all previous member state methods. In phases 1 and 2 (step 1), the methodology for suspension testing is given. All the tests within the CEN TC216 framework set out obligatory conditions of challenge organisms, type of water (water of standard hardness or sterile distilled water), level and type of interfering substance, contact temperature and contact times. However, they also have scope for the addition of extra organisms, interfering substances, etc.

In phase 1 testing, there are only two test organisms, *P. aeruginosa* (ATCC 15442) and *S. aureus* (ATCC 6538). The contact time is 5 min but can be supplemented with other times. Also, the pour-plate technique is followed, but, if no suitable neutralizer is found, the membrane filtration technique is applied for determining the number of survivors after disinfection (a technique developed by AFNOR in test NF T 72-171 [12]). In this case, the reaction mixture is filtered through a membrane filter, which retains the bacteria on its surface, and is then rinsed with sterile, physiological saline to physically separate the surviving organisms and the disinfectant. The main advantage of this procedure is that neutralization by inactivators becomes unnecessary. However, there is the assumption that the disinfectants can be washed off quickly. With surfactants, or with compounds with a large water–oil partition coefficient, this may not be the case, so care is required. The membrane filtration step is also an integral part of certain types of carrier tests of ASTM International [31].

As an example of the BS EN1276 test method (phase 2, step 1) used in a research environment, Taylor *et al.* [32] used the method to study the in-use concentrations of 18 commercial disinfectants routinely used in food-processing arenas. The researchers augmented the test by studying the efficacy at 10°C as well as the stipulated 20°C. Only 13 disinfectants passed the test in both clean and dirty conditions at 20°C when tested against *P. aeruginosa*. At 10°C, in addition there were a further two failures. This study is notable because it first evaluates the efficacies under standard conditions, produces the basal results (clean conditions), then evaluates the effect of soil and then compares these results to those reflecting usage conditions.

The European standardization of disinfectant testing through the adoption of EN testing by the various European members, for example BS EN 1276 [17], allows all countries to finally agree on laboratory results. The importance of this standard can be seen with the withdrawal of previous British standards, for example BSI 541 [33], BS 808 [34], BS 6471 [35] and DD 177 [14] which were methods for the determination of Rideal–Walker coefficients, use of the Chick–Martin test, determination of the microbicidal effect of quaternary ammonium compounds (QACs) and a disinfectant test method for the food industry, respectively, all withdrawn and replaced by EN1276. The removal of BS 541 [32] means that, finally, the phenol coefficient method has been consigned to the history books, at least in the UK and USA.

Reproducibility of suspension testing

The reproducibility problems of suspension tests still exist and large discrepancies between test results regularly occur. Often such irreproducibility, and perhaps the frustration this brings, results in calls for yet another type of testing regime. The repeatability of the testing regimes has been investigated by many workers (e.g. [1, 36–45]). For example, in the study of Taylor *et al.* [32] several commercial disinfectant products failed the basic suspension test. A study by Jacquet and Reynaud [46] using AFNOR 72-170 [47] found similar failures. Given that the manufacturers or suppliers of disinfectants have had to test their products, why do some simply fail at the stipulated in-use concentration? Part of the problem may be the various test methods available: some may be easier to pass than others – which is yet another reason to harmonize testing methods. However, the lack of reproducibility appears endemic within testing regimes. Most studies examining the statistics of pass–fail have sought answers through the examination of the inoculum preparation, the counting method and the methods of neutralization. However, many such studies have failed to provide unequivocal evidence of any particular cause.

If, after a more rigorous standardization of the disinfectant, reproducibility still remains problematic then the source of the errors may be within the basic assumptions of the testing regimes and these are explored below.

The basic equations of disinfection relate log reduction to concentration, time and temperature of the experiment. The temperature dependence of a disinfection experiment follows an Arrhenius-type dependency.

$$K_T = K_{20}Q^{(t-20)}$$

where K_T is the disinfection rate constant at temperature T, K_{20} is the disinfection rate constant at 20°C and Q is the temperature coefficient per degree. The temperature coefficient is also often referred to as Q_{10}, the change in rate for a 10-degree change. For phenolics Q_{10} is approximately 5; for alcohols it can be as high as 50 [48, 49].

The concentration–dependence of the disinfection is often non-linear, for example phenolics have a dilution coefficient of between 5 and 8 [50]. The dilution coefficient is rarely, if ever, quoted in disinfection testing. The standard size of the inoculum used in many suspension tests is quoted as being between 1×10^8 and 5×10^8/ml, which is then diluted 1:10 in the actual contact vessel. What is the effect on the repeatability of this range? When "interfering" substances are added to simulate "dirty" conditions, disinfection is curtailed. Yet, there are few studies that examine the magnitude of the interaction between soil/microbes and disinfectant. If each of these "fixed" parameters – temperature, concentration, inoculum size and amount of soil – were to vary by a small amount it can be shown that sizeable effects on the outcome of the suspension test can be expected.

Figure 12.1 shows the effect that small changes in temperature and concentration (e.g. weighing errors) can have on the outcome of a disinfection test. Hypothetical disinfectants A and B have rate constants of 1, dilution coefficients of 1 and 6, and temperature coefficients of 2 and 5, respectively. The calculated difference between 18 and 22°C is 1.4-log reductions for A and 3.3-log reductions for B. The difference between 0.98% and 1.02% are 0.2-log and 1.1-log reductions for A and B, respectively.

Inoculum size can have a dramatic effect on the outcome of the disinfection test. Johnston *et al.* [51] studied the effect of the size of the initial inoculum (1.0×10^7/ml to 5.0×10^7/mL) on the disinfection efficacy of sodium dodecyl sulfate (SDS). After 18 min of contact >5-log reductions were recorded with the test containing 1.0×10^7/ml, whereas less than 2-log reductions were seen with the test containing 5.0×10^7/ml. Interestingly, extrapolation of the data suggests that if the inoculum level was approximately 6.0×10^7/mL, then no disinfection (i.e. no log reductions) would be observed.

Blooomfield *et al.* [41], in an effort to understand some of the reasons for the inherent errors of the test, studied, at length, the effect of inoculum preparation. The results of an examination of the disinfection of *P. aeruginosa* with alcohol by a single operator, done in triplicate on five different days were given. They suggested that day-to-day variability arose through variations in the phenotype generated from the laboratory stock culture, but also from

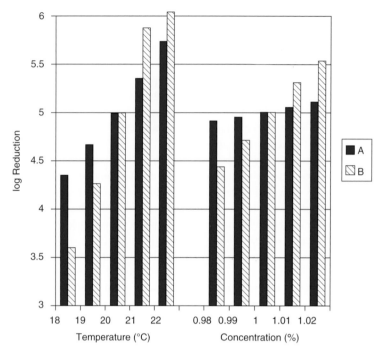

Figure 12.1 Effect of small changes in temperature and disinfectant concentration on the efficacy of two hypothetical microbicides, A and B.

lack of standardization of conditions used to harvest and prepare test inocula. They further hypothesized that alterations in the genotype caused by storage conditions may also contribute to the lack of reproducibility.

Although statistical analysis was performed on many of the data, the effect of the initial inoculum size was not included. Although the test required a range between 1.0×10^7 and 5.0×10^7 organisms/ml, the reported range was 7.4×10^6 to 9.5×10^6 organisms/ml. Using a simple linear regression model, which includes the initial inoculum size as well as the concentration of the alcohol as variables, this small inoculum range was found to be statistically significant.

$$ME = -9.024 + 0.334C$$

$$r^2 = 0.691 \,(\text{microbicide only})$$

$$ME = 22.39 + 0.334C - 4.52 \log I_0$$

$$r^2 = 0.778 \,(\text{microbicide and inocula})$$

where ME is microbicidal effect, C is alcohol concentration (%) and $\log I_0$ is the decimal log of the initial inoculum size. This simple model shows that as the initial inoculum increases, the ME decreases. The difference between the highest and lowest inoculum size for a given concentration of microbicide was calculated to be 0.5-log reductions. Although extrapolation of any interpolating model is not recommended, in this case extrapolation to include the recommended test range of 1×10^7 to 5×10^7 is illuminating. For any concentration of alcohol, according to this model, there is a 3-log reduction difference between the

lowest inoculum level (1.0×10^7 organisms/ml) and the highest (5.0×10^7 organisms/ml).

Small changes in the "fixed" values of disinfectant tests can significantly change the outcome of the test. Payne *et al.* [52] used the phase 2, step 1 CEN TC216 test (using *P. aeruginosa* and *S. aureus*) to compare the efficacy of several disinfectants against clinical isolates. The size of the starting inocula used ranged between 1.0×10^8 and 2.0×10^8/ml and the results obtained appeared to be reproducible.

Capacity tests

Capacity tests attempt to simulate the practical situations of housekeeping and instrument disinfection. A predetermined volume of bacterial suspension is added to the use-dilution of the agent, and after a given exposure time the mixture is sampled for survivors, mostly in a semiquantitative way, by inoculating several culture broths. After a certain period, a second addition of the bacterial suspension is made and a new subculture is made after the same reaction time; several additions with subcultures are carried out. Although capacity tests are *in vitro* tests, they closely resemble real-life situations, and in most instances are used as tests confirming the use-dilution.

The Kelsey–Sykes [53, 54] is the most widely used capacity test, not only in the UK (e.g. BS 6905 [2]), but also elsewhere in Europe. The original method was modified in 1969 [55] and improved in 1974 [56]. The bacteria in these tests are suspended in standard hard water for the test under clean conditions, and in a yeast suspension for the test under dirty conditions (BS 6905 [2]).

A theoretical point on capacity tests

The Kelsey–Sykes test [2, 53, 56], used to estimate the concentration of disinfectants, which may be recommended for use under dirty conditions in hospitals, is a fairly typical capacity test, as is the AOAC test [10]. In the BSI test the bacteria are suspended in a yeast suspension and the disinfectant is diluted in hard water, the initial volume being 3 ml. The reaction time is 8 min and a new addition of 1 ml of bacterial suspension is carried out 2 min after the subculture of the preceding addition; subcultures are done by transferring a 0.02 ml aliquot portion to each of five subculture tubes. The general idea is to gauge at which point the organic load becomes too much for the capacity of the disinfectant. The dilution coefficient is not considered in these tests.

Consider two further hypothetical disinfectants, C and D, each with a disinfectant constant of 0.5 and dilution coefficients of 1 and 6. In 10 min, at a concentration of 1% each will give 5-log reductions. If after 10 min 1 ml of a new bacterial culture is added, disinfectants C and D now contain 0.67%. The maximum log reductions achievable in 10 min with the disinfectants are now 3.35 and 0.45 for C and D, respectively. The power of the disinfectant has been lost whether or not the organic load (i.e. the inoculum) is added.

Surface (carrier) testing

The formation and elaboration of surface tests is not difficult, but most of them have a limited application since they are found to be poorly reproducible. Factors influencing the resistance of the test microorganism to a disinfectant are more easily recognized in *in vitro* tests, but in the practical tests it can be difficult, if not impossible, to standardize them. Drying of organisms on the surface often results in a decrease in their viability. The changes will be influenced by many factors, such as the drying time, the air temperature and relative humidity, the intrinsic humidity of the carrier itself, the suspending medium of the cells and the growth phase of the organisms. Although repeatability in one laboratory may be reasonable, collaborative trials in different laboratories show that reproducibility is not easily attained [57, 58].

Carrier test

In a carrier test, (e.g. the AOAC use-dilution test) an object (a penicylinder) is artificially contaminated with the test organism and the inoculum dried. The carrier is then immersed in the disinfectant at the test dilution for a period of time followed by a check for survivors.

In Germany, DGHM guidelines [59] are based on the technique of the Hygiene Institute of Mainz [11] and use standard operating-theater tiles or PVC floor covering contaminated with a standardized inoculum. Another practical test for surface disinfection is the AFNOR (1989) test NF T 72-190 (determining bactericidal, fungicidal and sporicidal action) [12]. Other tests are the Dutch quantitative carrier test [60], the Leuven test [61] and the quantitative surface disinfectant test (QSDT) [62].

The CEN TC216 Working Group 3, which gave rise to EN1276, included a new surface disinfectant test, EN13697, the carriers being small, circular, stainless steel surfaces. Although a collaborative study gave satisfying results [63, 64], further refining of the technique was suggested. The use-dilution method of the AOAC [10] is a much used carrier test. However, extreme variability of the results obtained by this test (as with all other surface tests) among different laboratories, especially in the case of *P. aeruginosa* is problematic. Increased standardization did not result in dramatic improvements [39]. The original test was modified slightly [22] and the AOAC hard surface carrier test (HSCT) can now be used in place of the use-dilution method under certain circumstances [65]. An increased standardization of the inoculum used has improved matters [66–68].

After reviewing a number of carrier test methods, a group set up by the OECD is now considering a quantitative carrier test for harmonization of hard surface disinfectant testing in its member states (minutes of 6th meeting of the OECD Microbicide Task Force 6-7/9/2010, Paris).

A full listing of the many surface tests available would be unimaginative and perhaps lead to confusion: many variations of standard surface tests are used to examine, essentially, the same phenomenon. However, the article or microbe under test may, by necessity, require more stringent regimes, for example mycobacteria and bacterial spores on invasive medical equipment. The results of the carrier test on "standardized" objects are used as an indication of the potential outcome on a more sophisticated surface, for example an endoscope.

Non-standard methods for investigating microbicidal activity

Disinfectant tests look for the reduction in "viability" of the test microorganism: qualitatively through simple turbidity and quantitatively through enumeration on agar-based media. In the former technique, one cell (theoretically) or many cells will be ultimately responsible for growth and development of turbidity, whereas in the latter it is assumed that each surviving cell is eventually responsible for the development of a colony in the case of bacteria and fungi or a focus of infection in a host cell monolayer in the case of viruses.

In general, traditional methods for culturing microorganisms can be laborious, time-consuming and quite costly, with incubation at an appropriate temperature for 24 h (or longer) adding to the length of time needed to determine whether, and to what extent (or if), a microbicidal effect has been achieved. Further, bacterial spores have to germinate and grow into vegetative cells before cell division takes place [69], and many mycobacterial species are notoriously slow growers [70]. It is, therefore, an attractive idea to consider whether viability can be detected far more rapidly than by conventional procedures [71]. While many "non-standard methods" lack regulatory recognition and the ability to make label claims, they are extremely useful as screening tools when developing new formulations or looking at new chemistries.

Biochemical methods

Microbes metabolize nutrients in the culture media and excrete waste products. An alternative to enumeration is to directly measure, biochemically, the alterations in the microbial environment or microbial metabolism following an inimical process. Quastel and Whetham [72] studied the action of microbicides on the dehydrogenases of *E. coli*, which led to further studies in this field [73]. The principle of triphenyltetrazolium chloride (TTC) reduction by bacteria was utilized by Hurwitz and McCarthy [74] in developing a rapid test for evaluating biocidal activity against *E. coli*. In essence, cells exposed to a microbicide are removed by filtrate, excess microbicide is quenched and the filter transferred to a growth medium containing TTC. During subsequent incubation at 37°C, formazan is extracted and color development measured spectrophotometrically. The method permits a 2–3-$\log_{10}$ reduction cycle to be followed and inactivation kinetics to be calculated. The incubation period takes about 4–5 h to provide a minimum detection level of *c*. 10^5 cfu/ml.

Methods that detect the activity of the enzymes β-galactosidase and β-δ-glucuronidase to indicate the presence of total coliforms and *E. coli*, respectively, are used in public health microbiology [75], allowing a modest saving of time over the normal culture methods. By using more sensitive equipment, the detection of enzyme activity and, hence, bacteria can be done using specific markers, for example methylumbelliferone labels [76–78]. Fiksdal *et al.* [79] and Davies and Apte [80] describe fluorimetric methods able to detect low numbers of coliforms in less than 60 min; Farnleitner *et al.* [81] discuss a method for the detection of *E. coli* in 25 min using β-δ-glucuronidase.

Although such methods allow the rapid estimation of microbial numbers, the analysis of inactivation kinetics may be difficult – the discrimination between viable and non-viable cells, based on a single enzymatic assay, may not be achievable. Lisle *et al.* [82] used a variety of techniques to probe the viability of *E. coli* O157:H7. They stress that using a single method to study physiological activity and relating that to a specific viability is tenuous, since the term "viability" can describe a wide range of states.

Physical methods

When bacteria grow, they produce metabolites, which alter the conductivity of the medium, a property first observed in 1898. With the use of modern electrical measuring equipment, this 19th century observation has been put to use as a rapid impedance microbiology technique [83]. However, use of charged antimicrobials, such as silver ions or cationic surfactant microbicides, can lead to interpretive problems.

Microcalorimetry, as a rapid analytical method for microbicide testing, is based upon the principle that bacteria and other microorganisms produce heat when they metabolize [84]. Microcalorimeters can detect the small amount of heat produced [85]. Any surviving cells, following an inimical treatment, will, during subsequent incubation, metabolize and generate heat. Morgan *et al.* [86] used microcalorimetry to examine the effect of microbicides on *Streptococcus mutans* and suggested that the data obtained by this technique gave a "better indication of antimicrobial efficacy than merely determining concentrations at which an antimicrobial agent is bacteriostatic or bactericidal".

Discriminatory counting techniques

The principle of the direct epifluorescent filtration technique (DEFT) is that viable microorganisms fluoresce (orange-red) when stained with acridine orange, whereas non-viable cells do not [87–89]. Thus, examination and counting of cells under a fluorescence microscope can provide a quantitative assessment of the number of viable cells present. In practice, the liquid to be tested is filtered through a membrane filter, which is then stained with acridine orange and examined microscopically [90].

The method has been used in microbiological quality control, for the rapid estimation of microbial counts in foods, beverages, meat and poultry and for detecting organisms in urine and in intravenous fluids. Couto and Hogg [91], due to problems with acridine orange, used two fluorescers (a commercially available system SYTO 9 and propidium iodide) as a rapid detection method for bacteria in wine. Using both the traditional plating methods and the DEFT technique, inactivation kinetics were shown to be similar – that is not method dependent. Decker [92] who compared several dye systems also used SYTO 9 and propidium iodide to examine the state of viability of *Streptococcus sanguinis* and *S. mutans*. Thiriat *et al.* [93] used 4′,6-diamidino-2-phenylindole in conjunction with propidium iodide to study the viability of *Giardia* cysts, having quantified the numbers using an immunofluorescence technique.

Flow cytometry

Several reviews have appeared that discuss the principles of flow cytometry [94–96]. The method has been used to evaluate antibacterial and antiprotozoal activity. In a typical flow cytometry system, individual particles pass through an illumination zone at the rate of several thousand cells per second; appropriate detectors measure the magnitude of a pulse representing the extent of light scattered. By "labeling" the cells with fluorescent molecules, for example an appropriate dye, that have high specificity to one particular cellular constituent, it is possible to measure the content of that constituent [97].

Flow cytometry can be used to detect viable and dead microbial cells, and has been employed to assess the lethal effects of biguanides and other microbicides on spores and trophozoites of *Acanthamoeba castellanii* [98] and the damaging effects of antibiotics on bacteria [99].

Bioluminescence

Some marine bacteria can emit light. A segment of DNA was isolated from *Photobacterium* (*Vibrio*) *fischeri* and cloned into *E. coli*, which was thereby provided with a bioluminescent phenotype [100]. Bioluminescence provides a direct measure of viability and a rapid means of measuring bacterial response to inimical treatments [101–103]. The procedure has been used to measure the effects of phenol [102] and other microbicides [104] on bioluminescent *E. coli* and to compare the results with those obtained by conventional plating experiments. Decimal reduction times (*D*-values) obtained by the two methods were identical, and both procedures could be used for determining concentration exponents (dilution coefficients, h-values) with equal confidence. Bioluminescence thus provides a rapid method for evaluating biocidal activity and can detect a 5-$\log_{10}$ reduction in viability from a starting inoculum of around 10^7 cfu/ml.

The system has now been expanded to bacterial spores and sporicidal activity [105]. Dark spores of *Bacillus* spp. are produced from phenotypically bioluminescent vegetative cells, since spores do not possess the energy to drive the light reaction [106]. During germination of *lux*-containing spores, however, bioluminescence is produced. Highly luminescent *Bacillus subtilis* cells have been constructed that can express a *luxAB* fusion gene from vegetative or sporulation-specific promoters. These *B. subtilis* spores have been used to monitor ethylene oxide sterilization and the use of a germination-specific promoter element, rather than a vegetative cell-specific promoter element, is claimed to enable sublethally injured spores to be detected [105].

Quantitative optical density

Optical density (OD) has traditionally been used as an indicative measure of biocidal effectiveness, essentially giving a growth/no growth criterion. Most microbiological laboratories have access to instruments that measure OD, whereas access to other, more elaborate (and usually more expensive) equipment capable of monitoring growth may be limited. Lambert *et al.* [107] used an OD reader to examine disinfection kinetics by relating the log reduction of a standard test inoculum to a serially diluted control. Essentially the OD reader was able to replace the need for plating. Furthermore, results comparable to those obtained by traditional methods could be obtained with a 10 h incubation. This method is an example of a rapid, reliable and reproducible suspension test, based on standard methods (e.g. BS EN1276), but capable of giving fast screening and an increase in the quality of the data [108, 109]. As with the standard test methods, the influence of soil can be accommodated [110]. The effect of inoculum size can also be quantified [51]. The development of a set of mathematical models with which to interpret the data increases the utility of the method [111].

Conclusions

The number of tests described and their diversity show that there is still a lack of agreement among workers on the standardization of all the components of a testing method. The EU has taken some important steps in introducing standard testing procedures for its member countries and now the OECD Task Force on Microbicides has started to consider and develop methods. However, as

long as there is an absence of a general agreement on method, different tests will be used and varying results will be obtained.

It must be highlighted that test methods are designed to evaluate the appropriateness of a disinfectant for its purpose. This has been complicated by the introduction of on-site actives generation (e.g. hypochlorous acid, chlorine dioxide, ozonated water) and the development of whole-room disinfection systems, which in our opinion have come a long way since fogging with QACs. Be it misting or vaporization of gases, these methods of disinfection do not comply with our traditional ideas of disinfectants. Where actives and methods of application have been shown to make a positive contribution to cleanliness, control of contaminants and disinfection in a given application, appropriate methods of determining their efficacy and limitations should be developed for the laboratory.

The development of rapid methods for evaluating biocidal activity and the evolution of physical analytical techniques in microbiology provide a future platform for the advancement of microbicide science. It should also be borne in mind that a rapid method without an increase in the quality of the data obtained or without concomitant advances in data analyses is simply speeding up the status quo.

Acknowledgments

The author thanks R. J. W. Lambert who wrote the original chapter in the last edition, on which this one is based.

References

1 Reybrouck, G. (1991) International standardization of disinfectant testing: is it possible? *Journal of Hospital Infection*, **18** (Suppl. A), 280–288.
2 BSI (British Standards Institution) (1987) *Estimation of Concentration of Disinfectants Used in "Dirty" Conditions in Hospitals by the Modified Kelsey–Sykes Test*, BS 6905, BSI, London.
3 European Committee for Standardization (CEN) (2010) *Antiseptique et Desinfectants*, AFNOR/172/T72Q CF/CEN TC 216, CEN, Brussels.
4 Rutala, W.A. and Weber, D.J. (2008) *Guideline for Disinfection and Sterilization in Healthcare Facilities, 2008*, Centers for Disease Control and Prevention, Atlanta, GA.
5 Phelps, E.B. (1911) The application of certain laws of physical chemistry in the standardization of disinfectants. *Journal of Infectious Diseases*, **8**, 27–38.
6 Chick, H. (1908) An investigation of the laws of disinfection. *Journal of Hygiene (Cambridge)*, **8**, 92–158.
7 Watson, H.E. (1908) A note on the variation of the rate of disinfection with change in the concentration of the disinfectant. *Journal of Hygiene (London)*, **8**, 536–342.
8 Croshaw, B. (1981) Disinfectant testing with particular reference to the Rideal–Walker and Kelsey–Sykes tests, in *Disinfectants: their Use and Evaluation of Effectiveness* (eds C.H. Collins et al.), Academic Press, London, pp. 1–15.
9 ASTM International (2011) *Annual Book of Standards*, vol. 11.05, ASTM International, Conshohocken, PA.
10 AOAC International (2011) *Official Methods of Analysis*, 18th edn, AOAC, Gaithersburg, MD.
11 Borneff, J. and Werner, H.-P. (1977) Entwicklung einer neuen Pr methode für Flächendesinfektionsverfahren. VII. Mitteilung: Vorschlag der Methodik.

Zentralblatt für Bakteriologie, Parasitenkunde, Infektionskrankheiten und Hygiene, I. Abteilung Originale, Reihe B, **165**, 97–101.

12 AFNOR (Association Française de Normalisation) (1989) *Recueil de normes françaises. Antiseptiques et désinfectants*, 2nd edn, AFNOR, Paris.

13 DVG (Deutsche Veterinärmedizinische Gesellschaft) (1988) *Richtlinien für die Prüfung chemischer Desinfektionsmittel*, 2nd edn, DVG, Giessen, Germany.

14 Anon. (1988) *Method of Test for the Antimicrobial Activity of Disinfectants in Food Hygiene*, DD 177, British Standards Institute, London.

15 Anon. (1994) *Chemical Antiseptics and Disinfectants – Basic Fungicidal Activity – Test Method and Requirement*. Provisional European Norm, EN1275, British Standards Institute, London.

16 Anon. (1994) *Chemical Antiseptic and Disinfectants – Quantitative Suspension Test for the Evaluation of Bactericidal Activity of Chemical Disinfectants and Antiseptics for Use in the Veterinary Field – Test Method and Requirements Provisional European Norm*, EN1656, British Standards Institute, London.

17 Anon. (1996) *Chemical Disinfectants and Antiseptics – Quantitative Suspension Test for the Evaluation of Bactericidal Activity of Chemical Disinfectants and Antiseptics Used in Food, Industrial, Domestic and Institutional Areas – Test Method and Requirements*. European Committee for Standardization, EN1276, British Standards Institute, London.

18 Anon. (1997) *Quantitative Suspension Test for the Evaluation of Bactericidal Activity of Chemical Disinfectants and Antiseptics Used in Food, Industrial, Domestic and Institutional Areas – Test Method and Requirements (Phase 2, Step 1)*, BS EN1276, British Standards Institute, London.

19 Ayliffe, G.A.J. (1989) Standardization of disinfectant testing. *Journal of Hospital Infection*, **13**, 211–216.

20 Reuter, G. (1989) Anforderungen an die Wirksamkeit von Desinfektionsmitteln für den lebensmittelverar-beitenden Bereich. *Zentralblatt für Bakteriologie, Parasitenkunde, Infektionskrankheiten und Hygiene, I. Abteilung Originale, Reibe B*, **187**, 564–577.

21 Cremieux, A. and Fleurette, J. (1991) Methods of testing disinfectants, in *Disinfection, Sterilization and Preservation*, 4th edn (ed. S.S. Block), Lea & Febiger, Philadelphia, pp. 1009–1027.

22 Mulberry, G.K. (1995) Current methods of testing disinfectants, in *Chemical Germicides in Health Care* (ed. W.A. Rutala), Association for Professionals in Infection Control, Washington, DC, pp. 224–235.

23 Springthorpe, V.S. and Sattar, S.A. (2005) Carrier tests to assess microbicidal activities of chemical disinfectants for use on medical devices and environmental surfaces. *Journal of AOAC International*, **88**, 182–201.

24 Anon. (2005) *Chemical Antiseptics and Disinfectants – Basic Bactericidal Activity Test Method and Requirement*. Provisional European Norm, EN1040, British Standards Institute, London.

25 Reybrouck, G. (1975) A theoretical approach of disinfectant testing. *Zentralblatt für Bakteriologie, Parasitenkunde, Infektionskrankheiten und Hygiene, I. Abteilung Originale, Reihe B*, **160**, 342–367.

26 Reybrouck, G. (1980) A comparison of the quantitative suspension tests for the assessment of disinfectants. *Zentralblatt für Bakteriologie, Parasitenkunde, Infektionskrankheiten und Hygiene, I. Abteilung Originale, Reihe B*, **170**, 449–456.

27 van Klingeren, B. *et al.* (1977) A collaborative study on the repeatability and the reproducibility of the Dutch standard-suspension-test for the evaluation of disinfectants. *Zentralblatt fur Bakteriologie Origale B*, **164**, 521–548.

28 Reybrouck, G. and Werner, H.-P. (1977) Ausarbeitung eines neuen quantitativen in-vitro-Tests für die bakteriologische Prüfung chemischer Desinfektionsmittel. *Zentralblatt für Bakteriologie, Parasitenkunde, Infektionskrankheiten und Hygiene, I. Abteilung Originale, Reihe B*, **165**, 126–137.

29 Reybrouck, G. *et al.* (1979) A collaborative study on a new quantitative suspension test, the *in vitro* test, for the evaluation of the bactericidal activity of chemical disinfectants. *Zentralblatt für Bakteriologie, Parasitenkunde, Infektionskrankheiten und Hygiene, I. Abteilung Originale, Reihe B*, **168**, 463–479.

30 Borneff, J. *et al.* (1981) Directives for the testing and evaluation of chemical disinfection methods – 1st part (1.1.1981). I. *In vitro* tests. II. Tests under medical practice conditions. 1. Hygienic hand disinfection. 2. Surgical hand disinfection. *Zentralblatt fur Bakteriologie, Mikrobiologie und Hygiene B*, **172**, 534–562.

31 Springthorpe, V.S. and Sattar, S.A. (2005) Carrier tests to assess microbicidal activities of chemical disinfectants for use on medical devices and environmental surfaces. *Journal of AOAC International*, **88**, 182–201.

32 Taylor, J.H. *et al.* (1999) A comparison of the bactericidal efficacy of 18 disinfectants used in the food industry against *Escherichia coli* O157:H7 and *Pseudomonas aeruginosa* at 10 and 20°C. *Journal of Applied Microbiology*, **87**, 718–725.

33 BSI (British Standards Institution) (1985) *Determination of the Rideal–Walker Coefficient of Disinfectants*, BS 541, BSI, London.

34 BSI (British Standards Institution) (1986) *Assessing the Efficacy of Disinfectants by the Modified Chick–Martin Test*, BS 808, BSI, London.

35 BSI (British Standards Institution) (1984) *Method for Laboratory Evaluation of Disinfectant Activity of Quaternary Ammonium Compounds*, BS 6471, BSI, London.

36 Groschel, D.H.M. (1983) Caveat emptor: do your disinfectants work? *Infection Control*, **4**, 144.

37 Rutala, W.A. and Cole, E.C. (1984) Antiseptics and disinfectants – safe and effective? *Infection Control*, **5**, 215–218.

38 Rutala, W.A. and Cole, E.C. (1987) Ineffectiveness of hospital disinfectants against bacteria: a collaborative study. *Infection Control*, **8**, 501–506.

39 Cole, E.C. *et al.* (1988) Disinfectant testing using a modified use-dilution method: collaborative study. *Journal of the Association of Official Analytical Chemists*, **71**, 1187–1194.

40 Bloomfield, S.F. (1995) Reproducibility and predictivity of disinfection and biocide tests, in *Microbiological Quality Assurance Screening and Bioassay: a Guide Towards Relevance and Reproducibility of Inocula* (eds M.R.W. Brown and P. Gilbert), CRC Press, Boca Raton, FL, pp. 189–215.

41 Bloomfield, S.F. *et al.* (1995) Development of reproducible test inocula for disinfectant testing. *International Biodeterioration and Biodegradation*, **36**, 311–331.

42 Bloomfield, S.F. and Looney, E. (1992) Evaluation of the repeatability and reproducibility of European suspension test for antimicrobial activity of disinfectants and antiseptics. *Journal of Applied Bacteriology*, **73**, 87–93.

43 Holah, J.T. (1995) Progress report on CEN/TC 216/Working Group 3: disinfectant test methods for food hygiene, institutional, industrial and domestic applications. *International Biodeterioration and Biodegradation*, **35**, 355–365.

44 Jeffrey, D.J. (1995) European disinfectant testing- collaborative trials. *International Biodeterioration and Biodegradation*, **36**, 367–374.

45 Langsrud, S. and Sundheim, G. (1998) Factors influencing a suspension test method for antimicrobial activity of disinfectants. *Journal of Applied Microbiology*, **85**, 1006–1012.

46 Jacquet, C. and Reynaud, A. (1994) Difference in the sensitivity to eight disinfectants of *Listeria monocytogenes* strains as related to their origin. *International Journal of Food Microbiology*, **22**, 79–83.

47 Cremieux, A. *et al.* (1987) Value of a standard exudate in the *in vitro* study of antiseptics. *Pathologie et Biologie (Paris)*, **35** (5 Pt 2), 887–890.

48 Bean, H.S. (1967) Type and characteristics of disinfectants. *Journal of Applied Bacteriology*, **30**, 6–16.

49 Russell, A.D. (1999) Factors influencing the efficacy of antimicrobial agents, in *Principles and Practice of Disinfection, Preservation and Sterilization* (eds A.D. Russell *et al.*), Blackwell Science, Oxford, pp. 95–123.

50 Hugo, W.B. and Denyer, S.P. (1987) Concentration exponent of disinfectants and preservatives (biocides), in *Preservatives in the Food, Pharmaceutical and Environmental Industries* (eds R.G. Board *et al.*), Blackwell Scientific Publications, Oxford, pp. 281–291.

51 Johnston, M.D. *et al.* (2000) One explanation for the variability of the bacterial suspension test. *Journal of Applied Microbiology*, **88**, 237–242.

52 Payne, D.N. *et al.* (1999) An evaluation of the suitability of the European suspension test to reflect *in vitro* activity of antiseptics against clinically significant organisms. *Journal of Applied Microbiology*, **28**, 7–12.

53 Kelsey, J.C. *et al.* (1965) A capacity use-dilution test for disinfectants. *Monthly Bulletin of the Ministry of Health and the Public Health Laboratory Service*, **24**, 152–160.

54 Kelsey, J.C. and Maurer, I.M. (1966) An in-use test for hospital disinfectants. *Monthly Bulletin of the Ministry of Health and the Public Health Laboratory Service*, **25**, 180–184.

55 Kelsey, J.C. and Sykes, G. (1969) A new test for the assessment of disinfectants with particular reference to their use in hospitals. *Pharmaceutical Journal*, **202**, 607–609.

56 Kelsey, J.C. and Maurer, I.M. (1974) An improved (1974) Kelsey–Sykes test for disinfectants. *Pharmaceutical Journal*, **207**, 528–530.

57 Reybrouck, G. (1986) Uniformierung der Prüfung von Desinfektionsmitteln in Europa. *Zentralblatt für Bakteriologie, Parasitenkunde, Infektionskrankheiten und Hygiene, I. Abteilung Originale Reihe B*, **182**, 485–498.

58 Reybrouck, G. (1990) The assessment of the bactericidal activity of surface disinfectants. III. Practical tests for surface disinfection. *Zentralblatt für Hygiene und Umweltmedizin*, **190**, 500–510.

59 DGNM (Deutshe Gesellschaft fur Hygiene und Mikrobiologie) (1991) *Prufung und Bewertung chemischer Desinfektionsverfahren*, Stand: 12.7.1991, MHP-Verlag, Wiesbaden.

60 van Klingeren, B. (1978) Experience with a quantitative carrier test for the evaluation of disinfectants. *Zentralblatt fur Bakteriologie B*, **167**, 514–527.

61 Reybrouck, G. (1990) The assessment of the bactericidal activity of surface disinfectants. I. A comparison of three practical tests. *Zentralblatt für Hygiene und Umweltmedizin*, **190**, 479–491.

62 Reybrouck, G. (1990) The assessment of the bactericidal activity of surface disinfectants. II. Two other practical tests. *Zentralblatt für Hygiene und Umweltmedizin*, **190**, 492–499.

63 Bloomfield, S.E. *et al.* (1993) Comparative testing of disinfectants using proposed European surface test methods. *Letters in Applied Microbiology*, **17**, 119–125.

64 Bloomfield, S.F. *et al.* (1994) An evaluation of the repeatability and reproducibility of a surface test for the activity of disinfectants. *Journal of Applied Bacteriology*, **76**, 86–94.

65 Beloian, A. (1993) General referee reports. Disinfectants. *Journal of AOAC International*, **76**, 97–98.

66 Beloian, A. (1995) General referee reports. Disinfectants. *Journal of AOAC International*, **78**, 179.

67 Rubino, J.R. *et al.* (1992) Hard surface carrier test for efficiency testing of disinfectants: collaborative study. *Journal of AOAC International*, **75**, 635–645.

68 Hamilton, M.A. *et al.* (1995) Hard surface carrier test as a quantitative test of disinfection: a collaborative study. *Journal of AOAC International*, **78**, 1102–1109.

69 Russell, A.D. (1990) Bacterial spores and chemical sporicidal agents. *Clinical Microbiology Reviews*, **3**, 99–119.

70 Grange, J.M. (1996) The biology of the genus *Mycobacterium*. *Journal of Applied Bacteriology Symposium Supplement*, **81**, 1S–9S.

71 Lloyd, D. and Hayes, A.J. (1995) Vigour, vitality and viability of micro-organisms. *FEMS Microbiology Letters*, **133**, 1–7.

72 Quastel, J.H. and Whetham, M.D. (1925) Dehydrogenases produced by resting bacteria. *Biochemical Journal*, **19**, 520–531.

73 Sykes, G. (1939) The influence of germicides on the dehydrogenases of *Bact. coli*. *Journal of Hygiene (Cambridge)*, **39**, 463–469.

74 Hurwitz, S.J. and McCarthy, T.J. (1986) 2,3,5-Triphenyltetrazolium chloride as a novel tool in germicide dynamics. *Journal of Pharmaceutical Sciences*, **75**, 912–916.

75 Edberg, S.C. and Edberg, M.M. (1988) A defined substrate technology for the enumeration of microbial indicators of environmental pollution. *Yale Journal of Biology and Medicine*, **61**, 389–399.

76 Apte, S.C. and Batley, G.E. (1994) Rapid detection of sewage contamination in marine waters using a fluorimetric assay of β-δ-galactosidase activity. *Science of the Total Environment*, **141**, 175–180.

77 Apte, S.C. *et al.* (1995) Rapid detection of faecal coliforms in sewage using a colorimetric assay of β-δ-galactosidase. *Water Research*, **29**, 1803–1806.

78 Davies, C.M. and Apte, S.C. (1999) Field evaluation of a rapid portable test for monitoring fecal coliforms in coastal waters. *Environmental Toxicology*, **14**, 355–359.

79 Fiksdal, L. *et al.* (1997) Rapid detection of coliform bacteria and influence of non-target bacteria. *Water Science and Technology*, **35**, 415–418.

80 Davies, C.M. and Apte, S.C. (2000) An evaluation of potential interferences in a fluorometric assay for the rapid detection of thermotolerant coliforms in sewage. *Letters in Applied Microbiology*, **30**, 99–104.

81 Farnleitner, A.H. *et al.* (2001) Rapid enzymatic detection of *Escherichia coli* contamination in polluted river. *Letters in Applied Microbiology*, **33**, 246–250.

82 Lisle, J.T. *et al.* (1999) The use of multiple indices of physiological activity to access viability in chlorine disinfected *Escherichia coli* O157:H7. *Letters in Applied Microbiology*, **29**, 42–47.

83 Silley, P. and Forsythe, S. (1996) Impedance microbiology – a rapid change for microbiologists. *Journal of Applied Bacteriology*, **80**, 233–243.

84 Beezer, A.E. (1980) *Biological Microcalorimetry*, Academic Press, London.

85 Perry, B.F. *et al.* (1980) Bioassay of phenol disinfectants by flow microcalorimetry. *Microbios*, **29**, 81–87.

86 Morgan, T.D.A.E. *et al.* (2001) A microcalorimetric comparison of the anti-*Streptococcus mutans* efficacy of plant extracts and antimicrobial agents in oral hygiene formulations. *Journal of Applied Microbiology*, **90**, 53–58.

87 Pettipher, G.L. *et al.* (1980) Rapid membrane filtration-epifluorescent microscopy technique for direct enumeration of bacteria in raw milk. *Applied and Environmental Microbiology*, **39**, 423–429.

88 Pettipher, G.L. *et al.* (1989) DEFT: recent developments for foods and beverages, in *Rapid Microbiological Methods for Foods, Beverages and Pharmaceuticals* (eds C.J. Stannard *et al.*), Society for Applied Bacteriology, Technical Series No. 25, Blackwell Scientific Publications, Oxford, pp. 33–45.

89 Denyer, S.P. *et al.* (1989) Medical and pharmaceutical applications of the direct epifluorescent filter technique (DEFT), in *Rapid Microbiological Methods for Foods, Beverages and Pharmaceuticals* (eds C.J. Stannard *et al.*), Society for Applied Bacteriology, Technical Series No. 25, Blackwell Scientific Publications, Oxford, pp. 59–71.

90 Pettipher, G.L. (1986) Review: the direct epifluorescent filter technique. *Journal of Food Technology*, **21**, 535–546.

91 Couto, J.A. and Hogg, T. (1999) Evaluation of a commercial fluorochromic system for the rapid detection and estimation of wine lactic acid bacteria by DEFT. *Letters in Applied Microbiology*, **28**, 23–26.

92 Decker, E.M. (2001) The ability of direct fluorescence-based, two colour assays to detect different physiological states of oral streptococci. *Letters in Applied Microbiology*, **33**, 88–192.

93 Thiriat, L. *et al.* (1998) Determination of *Giardia* cyst viability in environmental and faecal samples by immunofluorescence, fluorogenic dyes staining. *Letters in Applied Microbiology*, **26**, 237–242.

94 Lloyd, D. (1993) *Flow Cytometry in Microbiology*, Springer Verlag, London.

95 McSherry, J.J. (1994) Uses of flow cytometry in microbiology. *Clinical Microbiology Reviews*, **7**, 576–604.

96 Davey, H.M. and Kell, D.B. (1996) Flow cytometry and cell sorting of heterogeneous microbial populations: the importance of single-cell analyses. *Microbiology Reviews*, **60**, 641–696.

97 Shapiro, H.M. (1990) Flow cytometry in laboratory technology: new directions. *ASM News*, **56**, 584–586.

98 Khunkitti, W. *et al.* (1997) Effects of biocides on *Acanthamoeba castellanii* as measured by flow cytometry and plaque assay. *Journal of Antimicrobial Chemotherapy*, **40**, 227–233.

99 Suller, M.T.E. *et al.* (1997) A flow cytometric study of antibiotic-induced damage and the development of a rapid antibiotic susceptibility test. *Journal of Antimicrobial Chemotherapy*, **40**, 77–83.

100 Engebrecht, J. *et al.* (1983) Bacterial bioluminescence-isolation and generic analysis of functions from *Vibrio fischeri*. *Cell*, **32**, 773–781.

101 Stewart, G.S.A.B. (1990) *In vivo* bioluminescence: new potentials for microbiology. *Letters in Applied Microbiology*, **10**, 1–8.

102 Stewart, G.S.A.B. *et al.* (1991) Mechanisms of action and rapid biocide testing, in *Mechanisms of Action of Chemical Biocides* (eds S.P. Denyer and W.B. Hugo), Society for Applied Bacteriology, Technical Series No. 27, Wiley-Blackwell, Oxford, pp. 319–329.

103 Stewart, G.S.A.B. *et al.* (1996) The bacterial *lux* gene bioluminescent biosensor. *ASM News*, **62**, 297–301.

104 Walker, A.J. *et al.* (1992) Bioluminescent *Listeria monocytogenes* provide a rapid assay for measuring biocide efficacy. *FEMS Microbiology Letters*, **70**, 251–255.

105 Hill, P.J. *et al.* (1994) Bioluminescence and spores as biological indicators of inimical processes. *Journal of Applied Bacteriology Symposium Supplement*, **76**, 1295–1345.

106 Carmi, O.A. *et al.* (1987) Use of bacterial luciferase to establish a promoter probe vehicle capable of nondestructive realtime analysis of gene expression in *Bacillus* spp. *Journal of Bacteriology*, **169**, 2165–2170.

107 Lambert, R.J.W. *et al.* (1998) Disinfectant testing: use of the bioscreen microbiological growth analyser for laboratory biocide screening. *Letters in Applied Microbiology*, **26**, 288–292.

108 Lambert, R.J.W. *et al.* (1999) A kinetic study of the effect of hydrogen peroxide and peracetic acid against *Staphylococcus aureus* and *Pseudomonas aeruginosa* using the Bioscreen disinfection method. *Journal of Applied Microbiology*, **87**, 782–786.

109 Lambert, R.J.W. and Johnston, M.D. (2000) Disinfection kinetics: a new hypothesis and model for the tailing of log-survivor/time curves. *Journal of Applied Microbiology*, **88**, 907–913.

110 Lambert, R.J.W. and Johnston, M.D. (2001) The effect of interfering substances on the disinfection process: a mathematical model. *Journal of Applied Microbiology*, **91**, 548–555.

111 Lambert, R.J.W. (2001) Advances in disinfection testing and modelling. *Journal of Applied Microbiology*, **91**, 351–363.

13 Assessing the Efficacy of Professional Healthcare Antiseptics: a Regulatory Perspective

Albert T. Sheldon

Antibiotic and Antiseptic Consultants, Inc., Cypress, TX, USA

Introduction

The 19th century witnessed Ignaz Semmelweis (1818–1865) propose the infectious etiology of puerperal sepsis, and by suggesting a simple antiseptic procedure whereby physicians delivering babies washed their hands with chlorinated lime, he achieved marked reductions in morbidity and mortality in obstetrics wards [1]. Several subsequent studies provided the needed scientific evidence to justify the adoption of topical antimicrobial drug products in the general practice of medicine [2–4]. These studies demonstrated that proper use of such products reduced the spread of many types of infections.

The development of standardized *in vitro* and *in vivo* test methods to better understand and properly assess the microbicidal activities of antiseptics followed. Using *in vitro* tests, Kroing and Paul evaluated the influence of temperature, drug product concentration and contact time on microbial kill [5]. They proposed the need to achieve optimized growth of the surviving test microorganism and proper neutralization of the antiseptic's microbicidal action to ensure accuracy and reducibility in results. These principles were among the guideposts for developing standardized test protocols. Good early examples of the application of these principles are the works of Rideal and Walker, and of Chick and Martin [6, 7].

Subsequent work by ASTM International (formerly known as the American Society for Testing and Materials) and the European Committee for Standardization (CEN) culminated in the formulation and validation of standardized methods for assessing various types of antiseptics [8, 9]. Several of these methods are now recommended by regulatory agencies for use in generating data for product registration purposes. In this chapter, the term "antiseptic" refers to any antimicrobial-containing product that is safe and effective when applied to the human skin and is capable of preventing transmission of organisms that cause infections in specific use environments. This chapter focuses on antiseptic drug products used in healthcare.

North American regulatory process

Canada

The authority of Health Canada (HC) to regulate the safety, efficacy and quality of therapeutic products is described in the Foods and Drug Act and Regulations [10]. Review of antiseptics is the responsibility of Health Canada's Health Products and Foods Branch (HPFB), which evaluates the evidence and determines whether the potential benefits of the therapeutic agent outweigh risks associated with product use. The stages of a therapeutic drug development program range from pre-clinical trials to

Russell, Hugo & Ayliffe's: Principles and Practice of Disinfection, Preservation and Sterilization, Fifth Edition. Edited by Adam P. Fraise, Jean-Yves Maillard, and Syed A. Sattar.

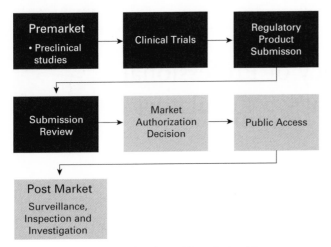

Figure 13.1 The Health Canada and United States Food and Drug Administration therapeutic drug product regulatory path.

post-authorization surveillance, inspection and investigation, as described in Figure 13.1.

The regulatory path available to an antiseptic depends on whether the active ingredient is defined as a new drug. A new drug is a brandname or proprietary product created by a company and patented, rather than reproduced by competitors. Such products are regulated under New Drug Submission (NDS) regulations. Antiseptic drug products not meeting the definition of a "new drug" and containing an active ingredient with an established safety and efficacy profile for a recognized use are regulated under the Drug Identification Number (DIN) regulations. If the antiseptic drug product contains a natural product and is the subject of a monograph, it is regulated by the National Health Products Directorate of Health Canada.

United States of America

The regulatory path followed for antiseptic product development is not unlike that in Canada and is dependent on the status of the active ingredients under evaluation and the indication sought. Several paths are available in the USA, as regulated by the Food and Drug Administration (FDA). The first is the over-the-counter (OTC) drug review process, which is an ongoing review of OTC drug products marketed prior to May 11, 1972 [11]. If an antiseptic product was sold OTC prior to this date, and the product label made drug claims of safety and effectiveness for specific uses, the agency must develop a monograph describing conditions that allow assessment of these claims. Upon publication of a final monograph (Final Rule), all products not conforming to the safety and efficacy requirements either are removed from the market or evidence is provided to prove the product meets requirements for safety and efficacy specified in the monograph. In 1994, the FDA published a tentative final monograph (TFM) for healthcare antiseptic drug products describing conditions, specifications and claims under which are listed antiseptic active

ingredients considered safe and effective [12]. The monograph limits the development of antiseptic claims to those for surgical handscrubs, healthcare personnel handwashes, patient preoperative skin prepping, and skin prepping prior to injection.

If an antiseptic ingredient is not addressed in the Final Rule, then two regulatory options exist: (i) the manufacturer may petition to amend the Final Rule to include the active; or (ii) the antiseptic may be developed under Section 505 of the Federal Food, Drug, and Cosmetic Act as a new drug [11]. As with the monograph regulatory process, the development of claims is limited to surgical handscrubs, healthcare personnel handwashes, patient preoperative skin preps, and skin preps for injection. Irrespective of the regulatory path taken, the antiseptic product is labeled in compliance with OTC drug-labeling regulations.

European Union regulatory process

Companies wishing to market antiseptics in Europe prior to the establishment of the European Union (EU) were required to meet individual safety and efficacy requirements established by each country. This was an expensive and repetitive task as the regulatory requirements of each country could vary considerably. On February 7, 1992, the Treaty of the European Union (92/c 191/01) was established among 12 member countries [13]. Title II of the treaty provided, in Article G, amendment of the European Economic Community Treaty by establishing five institutions, including the European Parliament and the Council of the European Union. The European Parliament and Council issued Directive 98/8/EC concerning the placing of biocidal products on the market (Biocidal Products Directive, BPD) in 1998 [14]. The directive provides provisions for submission of a dossier by an applicant to a competent authority of a member state and an authorization or registration process to market low-risk microbicides in the member territories, provided the active substance is listed in Annex I, IA or IB of the Directive. Also provided in Annex V of the Directive is a list of 23 product types with an indicative set of descriptions within each type; biocidal products intended for human hygienic purposes are listed as product type 1 (PT1), and these are the subject of this chapter. Paragraph 51 of Annex VI of the BPD provides a requirement for the assessment of the efficacy of microbicides using methods accepted by Member States or standard methods developed by the International Standards Organization (ISO), CEN or other international standards-setting organizations. However, the BPD does not provide clear directions on the scientific and administrative requirements for authorization or registration. Thus, the European Commission issued technical notes for guidance (TNsG) addressing the implementation of authorization, entry of active substances in the appropriate annexes, development of annexes relating to data requirements and description of common principles for the evaluation of biocidal products. *TNsG on Data Requirements* describes the minimum common core dataset required for all substances and product types, and data requirements for low-risk biocidal products relative to the proposed labeling claims, and most importantly, the methods to support these claims [15]. Clarification was provided in *TNsG on Data Requirements* recommending CEN standard test methods for the evaluation of PT1 biocidal claims. Finally, *TNsG on Product Evaluation*, a guidance to aid Competent Authorities in Member States to carry out their obligations when considering applications for the authorization and registration of biocidal products, was issued [16]. Because international agreement as to what constitutes a valid labeling claim or methods used to assess efficacy of label claims did not exist, this TNsG provided detailed guidance to the assessment of efficacy for authorization and registration of PT1 microbicides.

Annex IIA and IIB of the Directive also requires assessment for possible emergence of resistance to microbicides. Hence, studies that assess the possibility for emergence of resistance among target pathogens are required, as well as the development of strategies, to address possible emergence and limitations that resistance may impose on microbicide product efficacy [14, 17]. As PT1 biocidal products used to control microorganisms may be prone to the emergence of resistance, the nature and level of resistance is explored using *in vitro* standard reference bacteriostatic and bactericidal methods, and genetic methods for characterizing the phenotypic and genotypic mechanisms of resistance [17].

Antiseptics in healthcare settings: why are they needed?

The spread of infections in healthcare settings results from cross-contamination and transmission of microorganisms via the hands of healthcare workers [18–20]. Multiple epidemics have been traced to contaminated hands of healthcare personnel, including surgeons [21–23]. Further, the relationship of hand-washing and concomitant reductions of the microbiota of hands to reductions in incidence of nosocomial infection is suggested [18, 24, 25]. Thus, one of the most fundamental infection control practices for preventing cross-infection in the medical and scientific communities is handwashing to kill and/or remove transient organisms acquired from patients or the environment [26]. In addition, surgical site infections (SSIs) can be traced back to the operation itself, and may be exogenous in origin and associated with the surgical process, or endogenous from the patient's own skin or intestinal flora [13, 27, 28]. The immediate objective of antiseptic preoperative skin preparation prior to surgery is to reduce the incidence of SSIs by reducing a patient's endogenous skin flora.

Thus, antiseptic products are designed for use in healthcare environments with specific objectives in mind. These objectives define the use of the product, which may include: (i) use by healthcare personnel to prevent transmission of transient contaminative microorganisms acquired during the conduct of daily activities; (ii) use by surgeons and surgical suite personnel to prevent transmission of transient and resident microorganisms to the patient; and (iii) use for preoperative skin prepara-

tion to reduce the transient and resident microbial flora of the patient's own skin, thereby reducing the probability of SSI [29–31]. Keeping these objectives in mind, regulatory agencies adopt *in vitro* and *in vivo* test methods designed to determine antiseptic characteristics versus nosocomial pathogens and other transient and resident microbiota encountered in specific-use environments.

Scientific methods used by regulatory agencies to assess antiseptic effectiveness
North American Perspective

The regulatory testing requirements of Health Canada and the FDA for healthcare personnel, surgical scrub and preoperative skin preparation antiseptic products are dependent on claims made by the manufacture on product labels. The testing and labeling requirements for such claims are described in the Health Canada *Guidance Document: Human-Use Antiseptic Drugs* and the FDA TFM published in the Federal Register [11, 32]. The claims allowed on the label for professional-use healthcare products, the testing methods used to justify these claims, and the minimum efficacy requirements that must be met are presented in Tables 13.1 and 13.2 for Health Canada, and in Tables 13.3–13.5 for the FDA.

Prior to exposure of subjects to investigational antiseptics in clinical trials, both regulatory agencies require assessment of the performance characteristic of the investigational antiseptic using *in vitro* methods specified in Tables 13.1, 13.3 and 13.4. As presented in Table 13.1, Health Canada requires *in vitro* testing versus all organisms listed for the specified category of use. If, for example, the "healthcare personal use" category is desired then EN13727 (bacteria), EN14348 (mycobacteria), EN13624 (fungi) and EN14476 (viruses) are the methods used to evaluate a product's effectiveness against challenges from the battery of surrogate organisms listed, which, in many cases, are those associated with nosocomial infection. At a minimum, the investigational antiseptic must achieve the $\log_{10}$ reduction specified for each pathogen group. The laboratory test methods recommended by Health Canada are standardized, quantitative, suspension tests specifically designed to evaluate the -cidal activity of the test antiseptic.

Conversely, the regulatory strategy for assessing *in vitro* effectiveness adopted by the FDA is the minimal inhibitory concentration (MIC) and time-kill kinetic tests (Tables 13.3 and 13.4). In the MIC evaluation, the test antiseptic is serially diluted and evaluated against a select battery of organisms associated with nosocomial infections, and the lowest concentration that inhibits growth (MIC) is determined (Table 13.3). Included in the MIC study design is the requirement to evaluate the test antiseptic product vehicle and a marketed product as a positive control. The FDA also requires assessment of the rate of kill using time-kill kinetic studies, but an acceptable end-point is not specified, nor is a preferred test method (Table 13.4). Data derived from these studies are used by the FDA only to characterize the intrinsic activity of the antiseptic. The results of these studies cannot be

Table 13.1 Health Canada *in vitro* testing recommendations to obtain specified claims on professional healthcare use product labels (adapted from [32]).

In vitro claim for healthcare use products		Accepted *in vitro* test method		Acceptable ≥$\log_{10}$ reduction requirement	Surrogate test microorganism
		ASTM	CEN		
General healthcare personnel use or Surgical scrub used with or without water or Patient preoperative skin preparation used with or without water	Bacteria	Not applicable	EN13727	5	*Acinetobacter* spp. *Bacteroides fragilis* *Enterococcus faecium* ATCC 6057 *Enterococcus hirae* ATCC 10541 *Escherichia coli* K-12 NCTC 10538 *Haemophilus influenzae* *Klebsiella pneumoniae* and other species *Micrococcus luteus* ATCC 7468 *Proteus mirabilis* ATCC 14153 *Pseudomonas aeruginosa* ATCC 15442/27583 *Serratia marcescens* ATCC 14756 *Staphylococcus aureus* ATCC 6538/29213 *Staphylococcus epidermidis* ATCC 12228 *Staphylococcus haemolyticus* *Staphylococcus hominis* *Staphylococcus saprophyticus* *Streptococcus pneumoniae* *Streptococcus pyogenes*
	Fungi	Not applicable	EN13624	4	*Candida albicans* ATCC 10231 *Aspergillus niger* ATCC 16404
General healthcare personnel use	Mycobacteria	Not applicable	EN14348	5	*Mycobacterium avium* ATCC 15769 *Mycobacterium terrae* ATCC15755
	Viruses	E1052	EN14476	4	Bovine viral diarrhea virus Duck hepatitis B virus Hepatitis A VR-2903 Herpes simplex viruses type 1 VR-733 Herpes simplex viruses type 2 Influenzae A virus VR-544 Influenzae B virus Human adenovirus type 2 VR-2 Murine norovirus Papovavirus SV40 Polio virus type 1 Respiratory syncytial virus VR-26 Rhinovirus VR-1147 Rotavirus VR-2018 Sabine Mahoney–Pette strain VR-1562
$\log_{10}$ or percent reduction	Bacteria Mycobacteria Fungi/viruses	This labeling claim is allowed if testing for the specific healthcare category desired is performed, the product meets the efficacy requirement for acceptable $\log_{10}$ reduction stated for each claim, and if multiple indications are sought, efficacy outcomes must meet the most stringent criteria for each category			
Organism-specific	Bacteria Mycobacteria Fungi Viruses	This labeling claim is allowed if testing for the specific healthcare category desired is performed, the product meets the efficacy requirement for acceptable $\log_{10}$ reduction stated for each claim, and if multiple indications are sought, efficacy outcomes must meet the most stringent criteria for each category			Organisms highlighted on the product label
Persistence	Bacteria Fungi	This labeling claim is allowed if testing for the specific healthcare category desired is performed, the product meets the efficacy requirement for acceptable $\log_{10}$ reduction stated for each claim, and if multiple indications are sought, efficacy outcomes must meet the most stringent criteria for each category			This labeling claim is allowed if testing for the specific healthcare category desired is performed and if multiple indications are sought, efficacy outcomes must meet the most stringent criteria for each category

Table 13.2 Health Canada *in vivo* testing recommendation to obtain specified claims on professional healthcare use product labels (adapted from [32]).

In vivo claim for professional healthcare use product		Accepted *in vivo* test method		Acceptable ≥$\log_{10}$ reduction requirement	Surrogate test microorganism
		ASTM	CEN		
General healthcare personal use	Bacteria	E1174	EN1499	3	*Serratia marcescens* ATCC 14756
					If ASTM: *Escherichia coli* ATCC 11229
			EN1500		If CEN: *Escherichia coli* K12 NCTC 10538
	Mycobacteria	E1174	EN1499	3	*Mycobacterium terrae* ATCC 15755
			EN1500		*Mycobacterium avium* ATCC 15769
	Fungi	E2613	Not applicable	2	*Candida albicans* ATCC 10231
					Aspergillus niger ATCC 16404
	Viruses	E2011	Not applicable	2	Hepatitis A VR1402
					Human adenovirus type 5 VR1516
					Human rotavirus Wa VR2018
					Murine norovirus
					Rhinovirus type 37 or 14 VRI147 or VR284
Surgical handscrubs used with or without water	Bacteria	E1115	EN12791	ASTM: 3 CEN: not significantly worse than reference	Perform *in situ* on hands against volunteer's indigenous flora
	Fungi	E2613	Not applicable	2	*Canada albicans* ATCC 10231
					Aspergillus niger ATCC 16404
Patient preoperative skin preparations used with or without water	Bacteria	E1173	Not applicable	2-$\log_{10}$/cm^2 (dry skin site) 3-$\log_{10}$/cm^2 (moist skin site)	Perform *in situ* against volunteer's indigenous flora
	Fungi	E2613	Not applicable	2	Same as general healthcare personnel claim
$\log_{10}$ or percent reduction	Bacteria Mycobacteria Fungi Viruses	This labeling claim is allowed if testing for the specified healthcare category desired is performed, the product meets the efficacy requirement for acceptable $\log_{10}$ reduction stated for each claim, and if multiple indications are sought, efficacy outcomes must meet the most stringent criteria for each category			This labeling claim is allowed if testing for the specific healthcare category desired is performed and if multiple indications are sought, efficacy outcomes must meet the most stringent criteria for each category
Organism-specific	Bacteria Mycobacteria Fungi Viruses	This labeling claim is allowed if testing for the specific healthcare category desired is performed and if multiple indications are sought, efficacy outcomes must meet the most stringent criteria for each category			Evaluate organisms highlighted in food handler use product label
Persistence	Bacteria	E1115	EN12791	ASTM: 3 CEN: not significantly worse than reference	Perform *in situ* against volunteer's indigenous flora

used to make claims of bactericidal, fungicidal, mycobactericidal or virucidal activity on product labels.

If an applicant desires claims for healthcare personal use, surgical handscrub, skin prepping prior to injection or patient preoperative skin prepping, *in vivo* studies must be performed, and the results must meet the efficacy requirements described in Tables 13.2 or 13.5 for Health Canada and the FDA, respectively. Interestingly, Health Canada recommends *in vivo* methods for assessing products and substantiating claims not only for specific healthcare uses, but also for claims of organism-specific $\log_{10}$ or percent reduction and/or antimicrobial persistence (Table 13.2). The FDA only allows claims for specific healthcare uses, as described in Table 13.5. Although the FDA provides a protocol in its reference document, it also incorporates by reference the

ASTM methods described in Table 13.5; these ASTM methods are used to assess effectiveness of antiseptics for submission of antiseptic new drug applications (NDAs).

For the *in vitro* and *in vivo* tests described in Tables 13.1 and 13.2, the test results must demonstrate $\log_{10}$ reductions greater than or equal to the lower boundary of the 95% confidence interval on the mean when a power of 80% and an α of 5% are used. In addition, if a leave-on product requires more than 30 s or a product used with water requires more than 1 min to achieve the required $\log_{10}$ reduction for a specified indication, the product will not be approved for marketing in Canada. For the *in vivo* tests described in Table 13.5, the FDA requirements are dependent on the indication sought, but these are currently being reconsidered as a result of an FDA Advisory Committee meeting [33]. The

Table 13.3 United States Food and Drug Administration *in vitro* testing requirement to assess the *in vitro* minimum inhibitory concentration of test antiseptics against specified genera and species (adapted from [12] and personal communications with the Division of Nonprescription Clinical Evaluation, US FDA).

In vitro test method	Test group	Test microorganism
CLSI M7-A8	Gram-negative organisms	*Acinetobacter* spp.
		Bacteroides fragilis
		Enterobacter spp.
		Escherichia coli, including ATCC 11229 and 25922
		Haemophilus influenzae
		Klebsiella spp., including *K. pneumoniae*
		Pseudomonas aeruginosa, including ATCC 15442 and 27853
		Proteus mirabilis
		Serratia marcescens, including ATCC 14756
	Gram-positive organisms	Coagulase-negative *Staphylococcus* spp., including *S. epidermidis* ATCC 12228
		Staphylococcus spp., including *S. aureus* ATCC 6538 and 29213
		Staphylococcus hominis
		Staphylococcus haemolyticus
		Staphylococcus saprophyticus
		Micrococcus luteus, including ATCC 7468
		Enterococcus faecalis, including ATCC 29212
		Enterococcus faecium
		Streptococcus pyogenes
		Streptococcus pneumoniae
None recommended	Fungi	*Candida* spp.
		Candida albicans

Table 13.4 United States Food and Drug Administration *in vitro* testing requirement to assess the time-kill kinetics of test antiseptics against specified genera and species (adapted from [12] and personal communications with the Division of Nonprescription Clinical Evaluation, US FDA).

In vitro test method	Test group	Test microorganism
Method not specified, but general principles of study design articulated	Gram-negative organisms	*Escherichia coli*, including ATCC 11775 and 25922
		Klebsiella pneumoniae ATCC 13883 and ATCC 27736
		Pseudomonas aeruginosa, including ATCC 15442 and 27853
		Serratia marcescens, including ATCC 14756 and 8100
		Burkholderia cepacia ATCC 25416 and 25608
	Gram-positive organisms	*Enterococcus faecalis* ATCC 19433 and 29212
		Vancomycin-resistant *Enterococcus faecalis* ATCC 51299 and 51575
		Enterococcus faecium ATCC 19434 and 51559
		Staphylococcus aureus ATCC 6538 and 29213
		Methicillin-resistant *Staphylococcus aureus* ATCC 33591 and 33592
		Staphylococcus epidermidis ATCC 12228
		Methicillin-resistant *Staphylococcus epidermidis* ATCC 51625
		Streptococcus pneumoniae ATCC 6303 and 49619
		Streptococcus pyogenes ATCC 14289 and 19615
	Fungi	*Candida albicans* ATCC 18804 and 66027

Table 13.5 United States Food and Drug Administration *in vivo* testing requirement to assess the efficacy of test antiseptics (adapted from [12] and personal communications with the Division of Nonprescription Clinical Evaluation, US FDA).

In vivo claim for professional healthcare use product		Accepted *in vivo* test method (ASTM)	Acceptable ≥ log10 reduction requirement	Surrogate test microorganism
General healthcare personal use	Bacteria	E1174	Wash 1: 2-log$_{10}$ per hand Wash 10: 3-log$_{10}$ per hand	*Serratia marcescens* ATCC 14756
Surgical handscrubs used with or without water	Bacteria	E1115	Day 1: 1-log$_{10}$ Day 2: 2-log$_{10}$ Day 5: 3-log$_{10}$	Perform *in situ* on hands against volunteer's indigenous flora
Patient preoperative skin preparations used with or without water	Bacteria	E1173	2-log$_{10}$/cm^2 dry skin site 3-log$_{10}$/cm^2 moist skin site	Perform *in situ* on study site against volunteer's indigenous flora
Pre-injection	Bacteria	E1173	1-log$_{10}$/cm^2 dry skin site	Perform *in situ* on study site against volunteer's indigenous flora

Table 13.6 Phase of development and standard test methods used to assess efficacy for marketing of biocidal drug products in Member Countries of the EU.

Phase/step	Reference number	Title
1	BS EN1040:2005	Chemical disinfectants and antiseptics – Quantitative suspension test for the evaluation of basic bactericidal activity of chemical disinfectants and antiseptics – Test method and requirements
	BS EN1275:2005	Quantitative suspension test for the evaluation of basic fungicidal or basic yeasticidal activity of chemical disinfectants and antiseptics – Test method and requirements
	PrEN WI 216003 (under development)	Chemical disinfectants and antiseptics – Basic sporicidal activity – Test method and requirements
2/1	BS EN12054:1995	Chemical disinfectants and antiseptics – Quantitative suspension test for the evaluation of bactericidal activity of products for hygienic and surgical handrub and handwash used in human medicine – Test method and requirements
	BS EN14348:2005	Chemical disinfectants and antiseptics – Quantitative suspension test for the evaluation of mycobactericidal activity of chemical disinfectants in the medical area including instrument disinfectants – Test methods and requirements
	BS EN14476:2005	Chemical disinfectants and antiseptics – Virucidal quantitative suspension test for chemical disinfectants and antiseptics used in human medicine – Test method and requirements
	CEN WI 216039	Chemical disinfectants and antiseptics – Quantitative suspension test for the evaluation of fungicidal activity of products for hygienic and surgical handrub and handwash used in human medicine – Test methods and requirements
	CEN WI 216023 (under development)	Chemical disinfectants and antiseptics in the medical field – Fungicidal activity – Test method and requirements
2/2	BS EN1499:1997	Chemical disinfectants and antiseptics – Hygienic handwash – Test methods and requirements
	BS EN1500:1997	Chemical disinfectants and antiseptics – Hygienic handrub – Test methods and requirements
	PrEN 12791:2009	Chemical disinfectants and antiseptics – Surgical handrub and wash – Test method and requirements

directions for use of antiseptics submitted for approval by the FDA must be the same as those used to perform the *in vivo* clinical studies for assessment of effectiveness.

European Union Perspective

The primary objective of the European Biocidal Products Directive is to assure submission of data relevant to substantiating claims made on product labels for PT1 biocides [13, 14]. The regulatory strategy used in the EU for PT1 biocides is assessment of the effectiveness of the investigational antiseptic by *in vitro* test methods (screening tests), and if data are acceptable, further assessment in clinical trials (simulation tests) [14]. Appendices to Chapter 7 of the *TNsG on Product Evaluation* recommends, but does not require, the use of the CEN Technical Committee 216 (TC216) standard methods developed to assess efficacy of PT1 biocides. Efficacy assessment of PT1 biocides is based on a three-level matrix. Phase 1 (P1) suspension testing performed with the diluted product in the absence of organic or inorganic soil is used to support basic labeling claims (Table 13.6). These P1 evaluations are designed to assess the basic bactericidal, fungicidal, yeasticidal and sporicidal activity of the antiseptic under specified test conditions by measuring decimal $\log_{10}$ reductions from a pre-established baseline population. Phase 2 (P2) is a two-step process: step 1 evaluates the activity of the biocide in a simulated use suspension test using practical use conditions and an additional select battery of challenge microorganisms appropriate for a product's intended use. P2 step 1 tests are quantitative suspension tests requiring 4–5-$\log_{10}$ reductions as a demonstration of efficacy under specified test conditions. P2 step 2 methods

evaluate antiseptic products simulating practical use conditions and measuring reductions of transient flora from the fingertips of test subjects. Antiseptic handwashes evaluated using EN1499 must exhibit a significantly greater mean $\log_{10}$ reduction than that produced by an unmedicated soap control and meet the performance criteria described in EN12054. If the antiseptic is a handrub, EN1500 is used to evaluate efficacy, and the antiseptic must demonstrate reductions that are not significantly smaller than produced by the control, propan-2-ol 60% (w/v), and also must meet the criteria described in EN12054. EN12791 may also be used to assess handrub and handwash efficacy; one of two analyses of the data is performed, depending on labeling claims. In the first, the antiseptic is required to demonstrate a mean $\log_{10}$ reduction for immediate effect, and the 3 h effect must not be inferior to that achieved by 60% propan-1-ol, the control antiseptic. If the company desires a claim of "sustained effect", the mean $\log_{10}$ reduction for the 3 h effect must be superior to that achieved by the control antiseptic. Phase 3 requires field testing performed under practical use conditions, but is not a requirement for PT1 biocides.

Conclusions

The standardized *in vitro* and *in vivo* reference methods used by regulatory agencies are surrogates for in-use clinical trials. These *in vitro* and *in vivo* methods are limited in that the methods are not validated as surrogates, and the results cannot be used to predict a successful clinical outcome in actual-use conditions.

Nonetheless, the extrapolation of effectiveness observed by the application of these *in vitro* and *in vivo* test methods in the regulatory arena is logical. Regulatory agencies assume that if specific efficacy objectives are achieved using relevant test methods and an antiseptic is capable of reducing test organisms by statistically significant degrees, such reductions decrease the probability of transmission of pathogens under use conditions and, subsequently, the risk of infection or illness. The supposition that reduction of the flora of the skin or hands results in the reduction of disease, although intuitive to healthcare professionals, has not been supported by adequate and well-controlled clinical studies, as has been hotly debated in at least one meeting of the FDA Non-Prescription Products Advisory Committee meeting [33].

References

1 Semmelweis, I.P. (1995) The etiology, concept, prevention of childbed fever. Originally published 1861, reprinted in *American Journal of Obstetrics and Gynecology*, **172**, 236–237.

2 Holmes, O.W. (1843) The contagiousness of puerperal fever. *New England Quarterly Journal of Medicine and Surgery*, **1**, 503–530.

3 Kuchenmeister, G.F.H. (1860) On disinfecting action in general, carbolic acid and its therapeutic application in particular. *Deutsche Klinik*, **12**, 123.

4 Lister, J. (1867) On the topical antimicrobial drug product principle in the practice of surgery. *Lancet*, **2**, 353–356.

5 Kroing, B. and Paul, T.L. (1897) The chemical foundation of the study of disinfection and the action of poisons. *Zeitschrift fur Hygiene und Infektionskrankheiten, medizinische Mikrobiologie, Immunologie und Virologie*, **25**, 1–112.

6 Rideal, S. and Walker, J.T.A. (1903) The standardization of disinfectants. *Journal of the Royal Sanitary Institute (Great Britain)*, **24**, 424–441.

7 Chick, H. and Martin, C.J. (1908) The principles involved in the standardization of disinfectants and the influences of organic matter upon germicidal value. *Journal of Hygiene*, **8**, 654–697.

8 Anon. (1998) *Annual Book of Standards*, section II, vol. 11.05, E35.15, ASTM International, West Conshohocken, PA.

9 European Committee for Standardization (2009) *What is CEN?*, http://www.cen.eu/cen/AboutUs/Pages/default.aspx (accessed May 29, 2012).

10 Anon. (2012) *Food and Drugs Act, Part C Drugs. Divisions 1 and 8*, http://laws.justice.gc.ca/eng/C.R.C.-C.870/page-2.html#anchorbo-ga:l_C (accessed May 29, 2012).

11 US Code of Federal Regulations (2011) *Procedures for Classifying OTC Drugs as Generally Recognized as Safe and Effective and Not Misbranded, and for Establishing Monographs*, Part 330.10, http://www.accessdata.fda.gov/scripts/cdrh/cfdocs/cfcfr/CFRSearch.cfm?fr=330.10 (accessed May 29, 2012).

12 US General Services Administration (1994) Topical antimicrobial drug products for over-the-counter use – tentative final monograph for health-care antiseptic drug products. *Federal Register*, **59**, 31402–31452.

13 Anon. (1992) Treaty of the European Union signed in Maastricht. *Official Journal of the European Communities*, **35**, 1–115.

14 Anon. (1998) Directive 98/8/EC of the European Parliament and of the Council. *Official Journal of the European Communities*, **L123**, 1–63.

15 Anon. (2008) *Technical Guidance Document in Support of the Directive 98/8/EC Concerning the Placing of Biocidal Products on the Market (ECB February 2008). Guidance on Data Requirements for Active Substances and Biocidal Products*, http://ecb.jrc.ec.europa.eu/documents/Biocides/TECHNICAL_NOTES_ FOR_GUIDANCE/TNsG_DATA_REQUIREMENTS/TNsG-Data-Requirements.pdf (accessed May 29, 2012).

16 Anon. (2009) *Technical Notes for Guidance. In Support of Annex VI of Directive 98/8/EC of the European Parliament and Council. Concerning the Placing of Biocidal Products on the Market. Common Principles and Practical Procedures for the Authorization and Registration of Products*, http://ecb.jrc.ec.europa.eu/documents/Biocides/TECHNICAL_NOTES_FOR_GUIDANCE/TNsG_PRODUCT_EVALUATION/TNsG-Product-Evaluation.pdf (accessed May 29, 2012).

17 Anon. (2009) *Technical Notes for Guidance. Revision of Chapter 6.2 (Common Principles and Practical Procedures for the Authorisation and Registration of Products) of the TNsG on Product Evaluation, and a Revision of Chapter 101 (Assessment for the Potential for Resistance to the Active Substance) of the TNsG on Annex I Inclusion*, http://ecb.jrc.ec.europa.eu/documents/Biocides/TECHNICAL_NOTES_FOR_GUIDANCE/TNsG_PRODUCT_EVALUATION/TNsG_Product_Evaluation_Annex_I_Inclusion_Chapter_Resistance.pdf (accessed May 29, 2012).

18 Bauer, T.M. *et al.* (1990) An epidemiological study assessing the relative importance of airborne and direct contact transmission of microorganisms in a medical intensive care unit. *Journal of Hospital Infection*, **15**, 301–309.

19 Pittet, D. *et al.* (2000) Effectiveness of a hospital-wide programme to improve compliance with hand hygiene. *Lancet*, **356**, 1307–1312.

20 Pittet, D. *et al.* (1999) Bacterial contamination of the hands of hospital staff during routine patient care. *Archives of Internal Medicine*, **139**, 821–826.

21 Boyce, J.M. *et al.* (1990) A common-source outbreak of *Staphylococcus epidermidis* infections among patients undergoing cardiac surgery. *Journal of Infectious Diseases*, **161**, 493–499.

22 Widmer, A.F. *et al.* (1993) Outbreak of *Pseudomonas aeruginosa* infections in a surgical intensive care unit: probable transmission via hands of a health care worker. *Clinical Infectious Diseases*, **16**, 372–376.

23 Boyce, J.M. *et al.* (1993) Spread of methicillin-resistant *Staphylococcus aureus* in a hospital after exposure to a health care worker with chronic sinusitis. *Clinical Infectious Diseases*, **17**, 496–504.

24 Jarvis, W.R. (1991) Nosocomial outbreaks: the Centers for Disease Control's Hospital Infections Program experience, 1980–1990. *American Journal of Medicine*, **91**, 101–106.

25 Maki, D.G. (1989) The use of antiseptics for hand washing by medical personnel. *Journal of Chemotherapy*, **1**, 3–11.

26 Larson, E. (1988) A causal link between handwashing and risk of infection? Examination of the evidence. *Infection Control and Hospital Epidemiology*, **9**, 28–36.

27 Mangram, A.J. *et al.* (1999) Guideline for prevention of surgical site infection. Centers for Disease Control and Prevention (CDC) Hospital Infection Control Practices Advisory Committee. *Infection Control and Hospital Epidemiology*, **20**, 250–278.

28 Altemeier, W.A. *et al.* (1968) Surgical considerations of endogenous infections – sources, types, and methods of control. *Surgical Clinics of North America*, **48**, 227–240.

29 Reichman, D.E. and Greenberg, J.A. (2009) Reducing surgical site infections: a review. *Reviews in Obstetrics and Gynecology*, **2**, 212–221.

30 Larson, E.L. *et al.* (2000) An organizational climate intervention associated with increased handwashing and decreased nosocomial infections. *Behavioral Medicine*, **26**, 14–22.

31 Rotter, M. (2004) Special problems in hospital antiseptics, in *Russell, Hugo and Ayliffe's Principles and Practice of Disinfection, Preservation & Sterilization*, 4th edn (eds A. Fraise, P.A. Lambert and J.-Y. Maillard), Blackwell Publishing, Oxford, pp. 540–562.

32 Health Canada (2009) *Guidance Document: Human-Use Antiseptic Drugs*, http://www.hc-sc.gc.ca/dhp-mps/prodpharma/applic-demande/guide-ld/antiseptic_guide_ld-eng.php (accessed May 29, 2012).

33 Nonprescription Drugs Advisory Committee (2005) Notice of meeting. *Federal Register*, **70**, 8376–8377.

14.1

Legislation Affecting Disinfectant Products in Europe: the Biocidal Products Directive and the Registration, Evaluation and Authorization of Chemicals Regulations

Jennifer A. Hopkins

Bayer SAS Environmental Science, Lyon, France

Introduction

What is disinfection? A search on the internet brings up all kinds of definitions such as "treatment to destroy harmful organisms" and "the destruction of pathogenic and other kinds of microorganisms by physical or chemical means", some being entirely inaccurate such as "to sterilize by the use of a cleaning agent such as bleach". The development of legislation in Europe to encompass the use of disinfection will obviously bring about its own definition. This chapter focuses on the European legislation used to control the placing on the market of products used for the purposes of disinfection.

The biocidal products directive

Development of the legislation

In 1991 the European Community published a piece of legislation to control the placing on the market of plant protection products (Directive 91/414/EEC [1]). During the discussion in the European Council it was noted that there was no harmonized approach within the European Community for non-agricultural pesticides (now called biocides). This discussion led to the development of a piece of legislation to control the placing on the European Union (EU) market of biocides (non-agricultural pesticides). This legislation is called the Biocidal Products Directive (BPD; 98/8/EC [2]).

Definitions and scope

So, the first consideration is whether a given product is a biocidal product and therefore falls within the scope of the legislation. The BPD defines biocidal products as:

> . . . active substances and preparations containing one or more active substances, put up in the form in which they are supplied to the user, intended to destroy, deter, render harmless, prevent the action of, or otherwise exert a controlling effect on any harmful organism by chemical and biological means.

Therefore the use of a product for disinfection, preservation or sterilization will be considered to be within the scope of the BPD if it meets the above definition and is covered by product types 1–5 (outlined in Table 14.1.1). The exhaustive list of all 23 product types covered by the BPD is also included in Table 14.1.1.

How does the BPD work?

The BPD operates a two-step procedure for ensuring that biocidal products placed on the EU market offer a high level of protection for humans, animals and the environment. The first step of the process is to examine the active substances used in biocidal products and then the biocidal products themselves.

Active substances

In order to carry out the evaluation of active substances Member States first need to know what active substances were on the

Russell, Hugo & Ayliffe's: Principles and Practice of Disinfection, Preservation and Sterilization, Fifth Edition. Edited by Adam P. Fraise, Jean-Yves Maillard, and Syed A. Sattar.

Table 14.1.1 Biocidal product types and their descriptions.

Product type number	Product type name	Description
Main group 1: Disinfectants and general biocidal products		
These product types *exclude* cleaning products that are not intended to have a biocidal effect, including washing liquids, powders and similar products		
1	Human hygiene biocidal products	Products in this group are biocidal products used for human hygiene purposes
2	Private area and public health area disinfectants and other biocidal products	Products used for the disinfection of air, surfaces, materials, equipment and furniture which are not used for direct food or feed contact in private, public and industrial areas, including hospitals, as well as products used as algaecides
		Usage areas include swimming pools, aquariums, bathing and other waters; air conditioning systems; walls and floors in health and other institutions; chemical toilets, wastewater, hospital waste, soil or other substrates (in playgrounds)
3	Veterinary hygiene biocidal products	Biocidal products used for veterinary hygiene purposes including products used in areas in which animals are housed, kept or transported
4	Food and feed area disinfectants	Products used for the disinfection of equipment, containers, consumption, utensils, surfaces or pipework associated with production, transport, storage or consumption of food, feed or drink (including drinking water) for human and animals
5	Drinking water disinfectants	Products used for the disinfection of drinking water (for both humans and animals)
Main group 2: Preservatives		
6	In-can preservatives	Products used for the preservation of manufactured products, other than foodstuffs or feeding stuffs, in containers by the control of microbial deterioration to ensure their shelf-life
7	Film preservatives	Products used for the preservation of films or coatings by the control of microbial deterioration in order to protect the initial properties of the surface of the materials or objects such as paints, plastics, sealants, wall adhesives, binder, papers and art works
8	Wood preservatives	Products used for the preservation of wood, from and including the saw-mill stage, or wood products by the control of wood-destroying or wood-disfiguring organisms
9	Fiber, leather, rubber and polymerized materials preservatives	Products used for the preservation of fibrous or polymerized materials, such as leather, rubber or paper or textile products and rubber by the control of microbiological and algal attack
10	Masonry preservatives	Products used for the preservation and remedial treatment of masonry or other construction materials other than wood by the control of microbiological and algal attack
11	Preservatives for liquid-cooling and processing systems	Products used for the preservation of water or other liquids used in cooling and processing systems by the control of harmful organisms such as microbes, algae and mussels
		Products used for the preservation of drinking water are not included in this product type
12	Slimicides	Products used for the prevention or control of slime growth on materials, equipment and structures, used in industrial processes, e.g. on wood and paper pulp, porous sand strata in oil extraction
13	Metalworking fluid preservatives	Products used for the preservation of metalworking fluids by the control of microbial deterioration
Main group 3: Pest control		
14	Rodenticides	Products used for the control of mice, rats and/or other rodents
15	Avicides	Products used for the control of birds
16	Molluskicides	Products used for the control of mollusks
17	Piscicides	Products used for the control of fish; these products exclude products for the treatment of fish diseases
18	Insecticides, acaricides and products to control other arthropods	Products used for the control of arthropods (e.g. insects, arachnids, crustaceans)
19	Repellents and attractants	Products used to control harmful organisms (invertebrates such as fleas, vertebrates such as birds), by repelling or attracting, including those that are used for human or veterinary hygiene either directly or indirectly
Main group 4: Other biocidal products		
20	Preservatives for food or feedstocks	Products used for the preservation of food or feedstocks by the control of harmful organisms
21	Antifouling products	Products used to control the growth and settlement of fouling organisms (microbes and higher forms of plant or animal species) on vessels, aquaculture equipment or other structures used in water
22	Embalming and taxidermist fluids	Products used for the disinfection and preservation of human or animals corpses, or parts thereof
23	Control of other vertebrates	Products used for the control of vermin

market at the time the legislation came into force. Therefore, manufactures/users/importers were asked to "identify" active substances used in biocidal products. Approximately 950 different active substances were identified. Identification was a very simple process and required companies to provide details such as the name of the substance and its CAS (Chemical Abstract System) number. Identifying a substance did not mean that you were committed to provide any data on the safety or efficacy of these substances.

At the same time as the identification process was underway manufactures/users/importers of biocidal active substances were also asked to "notify". This meant that they were notifying their intention to support these active substances for a review and subsequent inclusion into Annex I of the Directive. Approximately 400 of the 950 active substances that were identified were also notified to the review program for evaluation of their safety and efficacy and subsequent inclusion into Annex I. Those 550 substances that were identified only (i.e. were not notified for review of their safety and efficacy) were lost from the market in 2006.

As the process has developed over time further notified substances have been lost (as dossiers were not submitted by individual companies or task forces). It is currently expected that around 200 active substances will remain after the end of the evaluation period for reviewing existing active substances in 2014 (Figure 14.1.1) (the review programme will be extended until 2024). These 200 active substances represent approximately 700 submissions because many active substances will be used in more than one product type (see below).

If an active substance is included in the review program, then products containing it can remain on the market according to the specific national rules of the individual Member State until the outcome of the review is known. So, for example, in the UK the majority of disinfectant products are not currently authorized. This will remain the case until disinfectant actives are included on Annex I.

Each biocidal active substance was notified for review for use in a particular product type (PT; see Table 14.1.1). For example, the active substance formaldehyde was originally notified for review in PTs 1–6, 9, 11–13, 18 and 20–23. A decision was taken to review active substances by product types and therefore manufacturers/users/importers had to submit a dossier of information on the safety and efficacy of the substance on its own and within a representative product to a Member State. Formaldehyde could, therefore, potentially be included in Annex I 15 times to cover all the relevant PTs. There was a series of deadlines per product type to submit the dossier of information and these were:

- For PTs 8 and 14: March 28, 2004.
- For PTs 16, 18, 19 and 21: April 30, 2006.
- For PTs 1–6 and 13: July 31, 2007.
- For PTs 7, 9–12, 15, 17, 20, 22 and 23: October 31, 2008.

An evaluation of an active substance by a Member State should take a minimum of 15 months. A 3-month period is taken by the Member State to check that the dossier contains all the relevant data (which would include toxicology and ecotoxicology data). Then a period of 12 months is needed for the evaluation of the data, production of the risk assessments and finalizing their own Member State report. Following finalization of the Member State report all Other Member States (OMSs) discuss the dossier and decide on its acceptance for inclusion into Annex I. These discussions take place both on a technical and political level. Each active substance can be discussed more than once at each of the Technical (for technical discussions) and Competent (for political discussions) Authority meetings.

Once the dossier on the active substance has been thoroughly evaluated and proven to be safe to humans, animals and the environment then there would be a vote at the Standing Committee on Biocides to include it in Annex I (or IA for low-risk active substances). Once the vote has been taken to include an active substance in Annex I then the decision is published in the *Official Journal* of the European Union. This process normally takes 3 months after the vote. Once it is published in the *Official Journal* then the inclusion comes into effect a total of 2 years later.

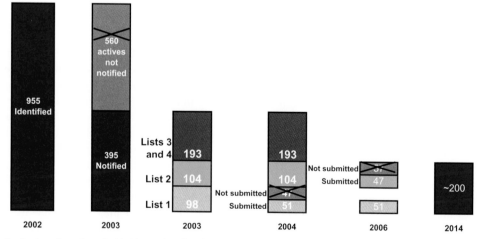

Figure 14.1.1 Loss of active ingredients from the biocides market after the introduction of the Biocidal Products Directive.

Currently an evaluation of an active substance dossier through the whole process from submission by the applicant, through evaluation by Member States, to inclusion into Annex I or IA is taking on average more than 6 years. An example timeline is shown below:

• Dossier submitted for review: July 31, 2007.
• Agreement on the active substance at a technical and political level: May 2011.
• Vote at the Standing Committee on Biocides: July 2011.
• Publication of the decision in the *Official Journal*: October 2011.
• Substance included in Annex I: October 2013.

As of July 2012, there are 56 active substances included or voted for inclusion in Annex I covering product types 2, 8, 12 (a new active substance), 14, 18 and 19. Three active substances are included in more than one product type. At present, only hydrochloric acid has been voted for inclusion in Annex I for use in PT2. This and other inclusion decisions (or decisions on non-inclusions) of active substances for use in disinfectant products will occur after 2014.

Biocidal products

Following the inclusion of the active substance into Annex I formulators can apply for authorization of their products in Member States of the EU (this is step 2 of the process). Like the dossier submited for inclusion of the active substance, the dossier for the biocidal product (disinfectant product) for which authorization is sought should include data to show the product is safe, when used in accordance with the label instructions, for humans (in an industrial setting, by professionals and/or by consumers), for animals (including domestic animals) and the environment. Once a substance is included in Annex I then the process of authorizing the product in each Member State where it is to be sold begins.

The dossier for showing that the biocidal product is safe and efficacious needs to be submitted by the date that the active substance is included in Annex I (i.e. October 2013 if we use our example from earlier). Therefore, by October 2013 the dossier needs to be submitted to one Member State who will evaluate the dossier on behalf of all the others. The OMSs need to be informed that mutual recognition in their Member State will be sought in the future. The OMSs are informed of this by using the R4BP (Register for Biocidal Products) [3] system, which is an internet system run by the Commission for applying for biocidal products across the EU. Each OMS where mutual recognition is sought will also require a copy of the dossier submitted to the first Member State.

The authorizing Member State will then carry out a completeness check (3 months) and the evaluation (12 months). Once the first Member State has granted authorization the individual companies then have 2 months to formally apply for mutual recognition in each Member State. The OMSs then have 120 days to grant (or refuse) the mutual recognition. All Member States should have authorized (or refused authorization) the product a total of 2 years after the date of inclusion in Annex I (if we use the same example as previously this would mean by January 1, 2015).

At the time of writing few substances have been through the authorization and mutual recognition processes. Possibly because of the limited experience that the industry and Member States have with the process, there have not been many mutual recognition product applications that have been granted within the 120-day time period. However, it is hoped with time and experience gained by Member States working with the system that timelines will be met more often.

Legislation evolves

The BPD will be repealed on September 1, 2013 by the Biocidal products regulation (BPR) (528/2012) [4], which entered into force in June 2012. The general principles of the new text remain the same as previously but there are some new features.

1. The European Chemicals Agency (ECHA) is responsible for administering the legislation.

2. The text will include "exclusion criteria" for active substances. These are hazard-based criteria; that is, if a substance carries a classification such as a carcinogen category 1A or 1B it will not be approved (instead of included). These are the same as seen in the new legislation for plant protection products (1107/2009 [5]) that has repealed Directive 91/414. However, there are derogations to these "exclusion criteria", which means an active substance can be approved if it is essential to prevent a serious danger to public health or the environment.

3. Active substances could also be defined as candidates for substitution. If a product contains an active which is a candidate then it will be subject to comparative assessment.

4. Product authorization – as in the BPD there is the opportunity to seek national authorisation followed by mutual recognition. However, an applicant can also seek union authorization providing that conditions of use are similar across the EU. This means that one authorization would allow the product to be made available on the market in all Member States without the need to seek mutual recognition. Disinfectant products can take advantage of this feature from September 1, 2013 for PTs 1, 3, 4 and 5 and from January 1, 2017 for those products in PT2.

5. The text attempts to address the 'free-rider' issue (companies who continued to sell their active substance because another had provided data as part of the review programme) that was a part of the BPD. As of September 1, 2013 all those supplying active substance on the EU market must submit the relevant information. If data are not submitted, then by September 1, 2015 biocidal products cannot be placed on the EU market.

6. There is no specific requirement for a Sustainable Use Directive for biocidal products in the same way as for plant protection products (Sustainable Use Directive (2009/129/EC [6]). However, a report needs to be prepared to show how the regulation, in particular for professional users, reduces the risks posed by biocides.

Registration, evaluation, authorization and restriction of chemicals (REACH)

Development of the legislation

REACH (1907/2006) [7] was the most complex piece of legislation ever to come out of Europe when it finally became law in December 2006 [8]. REACH aims to address the production and use of chemical substances, and their potential impacts on both human health and the environment. It is 849 pages long (with its annexes) and took 7 years to pass. It is the strictest law to date regulating chemical substances and affects not just the chemical industry but other industries (e.g. the car industry) also.

Definitions and scope

The aim of the regulation, like that for biocidal products, is to ensure a high level of protection for human health and the environment as well as the free circulation of substances on the internal EU market. In addition, REACH aims to promote alternative methods for assessment of hazards of substances and to enhance competitiveness and innovation. The regulation is based on the principle that it is for manufacturers, importers and downstream users to ensure that they manufacture, place on the market or use substances (i.e. a chemical element and its compounds in the natural state or obtained by any manufacturing process, including any additive necessary to preserve its stability and any impurity deriving from the process used, but excluding any solvent which may be separated without affecting the stability of the substance or changing its composition) that do not adversely affect human health or the environment. It covers a chemical substance used on its own, in a preparation (i.e. a mixture or solution composed of two or more substances) or in an article (i.e. an object that during production is given a special shape, surface or design which determines its function to a greater degree than does its chemical composition).

It is important to know in REACH where you are in the supply chain because the responsibilities you have may vary. In REACH terms you can be a manufacturer of a substance in the EU, an importer of a substance into the EU or a downstream user. A downstream user is a person or company that uses the substance on its own or in a preparation, in the course of industrial or professional activities. Therefore, if you use a substance to formulate disinfectant products then you are a downstream user. If you work as a professional operator disinfecting a hospital, in REACH terms, you are also considered to be a downstream user.

How does REACH work?

REACH is based on the principle of "no data, no market". That is, a chemical substance should not be manufactured in the EU or placed on its market unless it has been registered (the first "R" of REACH). So, in essence, every manufacturer or importer who manufactures or imports a substance into the EU will need a registration.

Registration

For registration, REACH works on the principle that it is those who manufacture or import a chemical substance into the EU who know that substance best. It is therefore their responsibility to show that the chemical is safe to human health and the environment. Therefore, if a manufacturer or importer makes or brings into the EU >1 tonne per annum (tpa) of substance (on its own, in a preparation or in an article with an intended release) then they must register that substance with the ECHA in Helsinki (echa.europa.eu).

REACH uses tonnage as a surrogate for risk and therefore the more that is manufactured or imported of a substance, the sooner the registration dossier needs to be supplied to the ECHA (REACH effectively comes into force over a 10-year period). If the substance already carries a certain classification then the timelines vary and are less dependent on the tonnage threshold. To make use of these phased-in deadlines the pre-registeration had to be made before December 1, 2008 (Figure 14.1.2).

For a phase-in substance that was placed on the market after June 1, 2007 (date of entry into force of the legislation), the registration dossiers on each of the substances have to be submitted in accordance with the timelines in Figure 14.1.2. If the substance was not placed on the market, then the registration dossiers have to be submitted prior to it being placed on the market within the EU. As discussed earlier, REACH uses tonnage as a surrogate for risk. Therefore, the higher the tonnage of a substance manufactured or imported, the more data that are needed in the registration dossier.

All substances (>1 tpa manufactured or imported) must have a technical dossier, which should include information on the identity of the substance, the classification and labeling of the substances and the uses for which it can be used (e.g. in disinfectant formulations). If the substance is manufactured or imported in quantities of >10 tpa then a chemical safety report (CSR) also needs to be submitted. A CSR must detail the human health and environmental hazard assessment. If the assessment shows that the substance is hazardous (carries a classification), then the CSR must also include an exposure assessment and risk characterization that shows the safe use of that substance. The CSR must include all the areas where the substance may be used, for example in disinfectant products for use by professional operators and in disinfectant products for use by amateur (or consumer) operators. A shorter version of the exposure assessment and any risk mitigation measures (e.g. wear appropriate and suitable gloves) will be then detailed in the Annex to the safety data sheet (SDS) that is sent to downstream users.

Registration requirements do not apply to active substances used in biocidal products. This is because the active substance is thoroughly evaluated for inclusion in Annex I of the BPD (or approval under BPR) – the amount of data needed to support an Annex I inclusion under the BPD is (probably) greater than that needed to support a >1000 tpa substance in REACH. Therefore, in REACH an active substance already in the biocides review program or in Annex I of the BPD is already considered

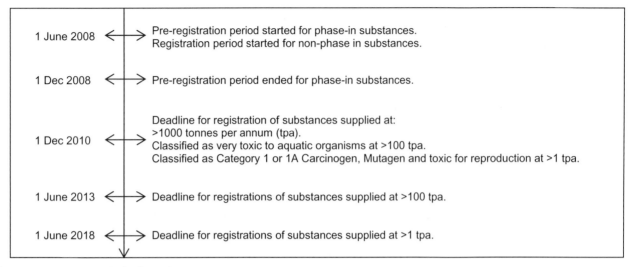

Figure 14.1.2 Registration timeline for REACH.

registered. However, the registration requirements are applicable (if within the scope of REACH) to all other components (e.g. solvents, thickeners) within the disinfectant formulation. Therefore, it is important that those making biocidal products are in constant discussion with their suppliers on when the registration dossiers will be submitted and that the use of the disinfectant is covered in any CSR.

Evaluation

Evaluation is a process undertaken by Member States. There are two types of evaluation:

1. Compliance check of evaluations: a minimum of 5% of the dossiers submitted to the ECHA for registration purposes will be checked to ensure that they are in compliance with the requirements of REACH.

2. Substance evaluation: every 3 years from December 1, 2011 a Community Rolling Action Plan will be developed that will specify the substances that will be evaluated by the ECHA or a Member States in each year of the plan. A substance will be included in the plan if there is evidence (from the registration dossier or an appropriate source) that it constitutes a risk to human health or the environment.

Authorization

If a substance meets one of the following criteria then it may be subject to authorization:

• Classification as a category 1A or 1B carcinogen, mutagen or toxic by reproduction.
• The substance is persistent, bioaccumulative and toxic (PBT).
• The substance is very persistent and very bioaccumulative (vPvB).
• Substances that have endocrine disrupting properties.

Once it is agreed that a substance meets the above criteria it is considered to be a substance of very high concern (SVHC). The substance is moved to the candidate list for authorization (the so

called "black list") of substances. Once a substance is classified as an SVHC then it will at some point move from the candidate list of substances onto Annex XIV of REACH. Only when the substance is included in Annex XIV of REACH does one need an authorization to *use* it.

However, substances that are used in biocidal products, such as disinfectant products, do not need a separate authorization under REACH for this use. This is because the use as a biocidal product is already considered when the product is authorized by Member States in accordance with Directive 98/8 or Regulation 528/2012.

Restriction

If there is an unacceptable risk to human health and/or the environment across the European Community that arises from the manufacture, use or placing on the market of a substance then it will be restricted. Therefore, if an individual substance is restricted for use in professional products only it cannot therefore be used in a consumer disinfectant formulation; that is the product will not be approved for this use by the authorities in charge of biocidal products in Member States.

A list of substances and the restriction applied (e.g. not to be used in consumer formulations) is available in Annex XVII of the REACH legislation.

Downstream users

A downstream user (e.g. formulator, disinfectant user) of substances also has responsibilities within REACH. They are responsible for passing information up and down the supply chain on how the substance is used (e.g. the substance is added to formulate disinfectant products) throughout the supply chain. A downstream user can also prepare their own CSR for any use which is outside the conditions covered in the exposure scenario by the manufacturer or importer.

A downstream user (e.g. a professional user of a disinfectant product) should follow the risk mitigation measures proposed in the CSR and communicated in the SDS. It is important that those manufacturing disinfectant products (which can contain numerous individual substances) examine all risk mitigation measures for the individual substances and combine these with those identified when the biocidal product is authorized so information is more easily communicated to those further down the supply chain.

Safety data sheets

As discussed earlier in the chapter, a SDS needs to be provided for a substance if it carries a classification as dangerous, is PBT or vPvB, or is on the candidate list for authorization. A SDS for a preparation must be provided on request if certain other conditions are met, for example if it contains a substance for which there is a European Community workplace exposure limit. A SDS does not need to be supplied where dangerous substances or preparations are offered or sold to the general public providing they are given sufficient information to enable them to take the necessary measures to protect human health, safety and the environment.

The SDS will look slightly different than it has in the past. For example, the sections on hazard identification (which in the old format was heading 3 but is now heading 2) and composition/information on ingredients have switched. In addition, if a CSR had to be prepared then the relevant exposure scenarios (including use and exposure categories) have to be placed in an annex to the SDS covering the identified uses (i.e. where the substance is used in the supply chain). The addition of these exposure scenarios as an annex to the SDS (known as extended-SDS or e-SDS) will certainly increase the length and complexity of the information provided.

If a SDS does not need to be provided there is still a responsibility to provide the registration number of the substance, if the substance is subject to authorization, any restrictions imposed, plus any information that is necessary to enable appropriate risk mitigation measures to be applied during use of the substance.

Legislation evolves

By June 1, 2012 the European Commission is required to undertake a review of how the scope of the REACH regulation has worked since it came into force. The specific aim of the review is to examine whether or not to amend the scope of REACH to avoid overlaps with other Community legislation. For example, if there are overlaps between REACH and BPD/BPR, then it is possible that REACH will be amended to remove the overlap and ambiguity in the legal texts.

References

1 Anon. (1991) *Council Directive 91/414/EC Concerning the Placing of Plant Protection Products on the Market*, http://eur-lex.europa.eu/LexUriServ/LexUriServ.do?uri=CONSLEG:1991L0414:20070201:EN:PDF (accessed May 30, 2012).

2 Anon. (1998) *Directive 98/8/EC of the European Parliament and the Council of the 16 February 1998 Concerning the Placing of Biocidal Products on the Market*, http://eur-lex.europa.eu/LexUriServ/LexUriServ.do?uri=OJ:L:1998:123:0001:0063:EN:PDF (accessed May 30, 2012).

3 Community Register for Biocidal Product portal: https://webgate.ec.europa.eu/env/r4bp/user.language.cfm?CFID=80283&CFTOKEN=850cccb916170c49-4C83B0A5-E084-7E06-59AB6D7335526811&jsessionid=57084b0864ca622c101bTR (accessed May 30, 2012).

4 Anon (2012) Regulation (EU) No 528/2012 of the European Parliament and of the Council of 22 May 2012 concerning the making available on the market and use of biocidal products, http://eur-lex.europa.eu/LexUriServ/LexUriServ.do?uri=OJ:L:2012:167:0001:0123:EN:PDF (accessed July 23, 2012).

5 Anon. (2009) *Regulation (EC) No. 1107/2009 of the European Parliament and of the Council of 21 October 2009 Concerning the Placing of Plant Protection Products on the Market and Repealing Council Directives 79/117/EC and 91/414/EC*, http://eur-lex.europa.eu/LexUriServ/LexUriServ.do?uri=OJ:L:2009:309:0001:0050:EN:PDF (accessed May 30, 2012).

6 Anon. (2009) *Directive 2009/128/EC of the European Parliament and of the Council of 21 October 2009 Establishing a Framework for Community Action to Achieve the Sustainable Use of Pesticides*, http://eur-lex.europa.eu/LexUriServ/LexUriServ.do?uri=OJ:L:2009:309:0071:0086:EN:PDF (accessed May 30, 2012).

7 Documents portal: *Regulation (EC) No. 1907/2006 of the European Parliament and of the Council of 18 December 2006 Concerning the Registration, Evaluation, Authorisation and Restriction of Chemicals (REACH), Establishing a European Chemicals Agency, Amending Directive 1999/45/EC and Repealing Council Regulation (EEC) No. 793/93 and Commission Regulation (EC) No. 1488/94 as well as Council Directive 76/769/EEC and Commission Directives 91/155/EEC, 93/67/EEC, 93/105/EC and 2000/21/EC*, http://eur-lex.europa.eu/LexUriServ/LexUriServ.do?uri=CELEX:32006R1907:EN:NOT (accessed May 30, 2012).

8 EUobserver.com (2007) EU's REACH chemicals law begins life in Helsinki, http://euobserver.com/9/24169 (accessed May 30, 2012).

14.2   Regulatory Authorization of Hard Surface Disinfectants in Canada

Andre G. Craan[1], Ian A. Chisholm[2] and Shannon C. Wright[3]

[1] Biotechnology Section, Marketed Biologicals, Biotechnology and Natural Health Products Bureau, Marketed Health Products Directorate, Health Canada, Ottawa, Ontario, Canada

[2] AIDS and Viral Diseases Division, Bureau of Gastroenterology, Infection and Viral Diseases, Therapeutic Products Directorate, Health Canada, Ottawa, Ontario, Canada

[3] Disinfectants Unit, Bureau of Gastroenterology, Infection and Viral Diseases, Therapeutic Products Directorate, Health Canada, Ottawa, Ontario, Canada

Introduction

Hard surface disinfectants belong to a class of products that contain antimicrobial ingredients for use on hard, non-porous inanimate objects. Table 14.2.1 provides additional classes and examples of products containing such ingredients, along with their corresponding legislative framework. Such variety of antimicrobial uses makes it necessary to clearly define hard surface disinfectants that are regulated in Canada as "drugs", with a view to distinguishing them from the other classes of products, such as pesticides. This is a key reason why Health Canada, in September 2001, introduced regulatory amendments enabling the Therapeutic Products Directorate (TPD) to become the sole regulatory authority responsible for the premarket review of applications for products classified as disinfectant drugs. This legislative measure eliminated a pre-existing regulatory overlap for disinfectant products between the TPD and the Pest Management Regulatory Agency (PMRA). This was done through the consolidation of the administration of hard surface disinfectants and disinfectant drugs with sanitizer claims on the label, within a single window at TPD and under the Food and Drugs Act (F&DA) and Food and Drug Regulations (F&DR). The PMRA continues to regulate products intended for controlling plant pathogens and other pests, for example disinfectants to control plant pathogens such

as those used in greenhouses, swimming pool disinfectants and non-food contact sanitizers.

On January 1, 2004, the Natural Health Product Regulations (NHPR) came into effect under the F&DA; thus, the Natural Health Products Directorate is responsible for the regulatory authorization of natural health products (NHPs) in Canada. While NHPs are classified as "drugs" under the F&DA, the NHPR describe which substances are marketable as NHPs and which are not. In terms of disinfectants, these are excluded from the NHPR and thus TPD continues to regulate them under the F&DA and F&DR.

The focus of this chapter is on hard surface disinfectants that are regulated as drugs; when marketed, these products are required to be labeled with a drug identification number (DIN), as assigned by Health Canada. Table 14.2.2 provides a list of abbreviations and corresponding terms that appear in the chapter.

Disinfectants versus sanitizers

Health Canada's *Guidance Document: Disinfectant Drugs* defines a hard surface disinfectant as an antimicrobial agent capable of destroying pathogenic and potentially pathogenic microorganisms on environmental surfaces and inanimate objects [1]. Disinfectants are considered to include bactericides, fungicides,

Russell, Hugo & Ayliffe's: Principles and Practice of Disinfection, Preservation and Sterilization, Fifth Edition. Edited by Adam P. Fraise, Jean-Yves Maillard, and Syed A. Sattar.

Table 14.2.1 Products that contain antimicrobial ingredients for use on inanimate objects.

Product class	Legislation and regulatory body	Example
Disinfectant drugs	Food and Drugs Act and Regulations (F&DA and F&DR)	Hard surface disinfectants Toilet bowl disinfectant cleaners
Pesticides	Therapeutic Products Directorate, Health Canada	Contact lens disinfectants
	Pest Control Products Act and Regulations (PCPA and PCPR)	Plant pathogen disinfectants (greenhouse) Swimming pool/spa disinfectants
	Pest Management Regulatory Agency, Health Canada	Pest control sanitizers Material preservatives, e.g. wood
Food sanitizers	Food and Drugs Act and Regulations (F&DA and F&DR) Food Directorate, Health Canada	Food contact surface sanitizers
WHMIS "controlled products"	Hazardous Products Act (HPA) Consumer Product Safety Directorate, Health Canada	Cleaning agents
Consumer products	Canada Consumer Product Safety Act (CCPSA) Consumer Product Safety Directorate, Health Canada	

Table 14.2.2 List of abbreviations.

Term	Abbreviation
Consumer Chemicals and Containers Regulations, 2001	CCCR, 2001
Canada Consumer Product Safety Act	CCPSA
Canadian General Standards Board	CGSB
Chemistry and manufacturing	C&M
Certified Product Information Document	CPID
Controlled Products Regulations	CPR
Drug identification number	DIN
Food and Drugs Act	F&DA
Food and Drug Regulations	F&DR
Good manufacturing practices	GMP
Hazardous Products Act	HPA
Health Products and Food Branch	HPFB
Health Products and Food Branch Inspectorate	HPFBI
Marketed Health Products Directorate	MHPD
Natural Health Product	NHP
Natural Health Products Regulations	NHPR
New Drug Letter	NDL
New Drug Submission	NDS
Notice of Compliance	NOC
Notice of Deficiency/Withdrawal	NOD/W
Notice of Non-compliance/Withdrawal	NON/W
Not Satisfactory Notice	NSN
Pest Control Products Act	PCPA
Pest Control Products Regulations	PCPR
Post-DIN changes	PDCs
Pest Management Regulatory Agency	PMRA
Quality Overall Summary	QOS
Screening Rejection Letter	SRL
Therapeutic Products Directorate	TPD
Workplace Hazardous Materials Information System	WHMIS

virucides, mycobactericides, sporicides and sterilants or combinations of these. This guidance document also provides the various levels of disinfection that correspond to product classes, such as high-level, intermediate-level or low-level disinfectants. In contrast, a sanitizer is a product that reduces the level of microorganisms present by significant numbers, for example a 3-$\log_{10}$ reduction (99.9%) or more.

Disinfectants that are associated with the additional purpose of sanitization are recognized by the TPD as disinfectant-sanitizers [1]. They are characterized by two use types, two contact times and two directions for use. As noted in Table 14.2.1, these antimicrobials are regulated under the F&DA and F&DR and thus fall under the jurisdiction of TPD by virtue of their disinfection claim.

Whether an antimicrobial product is classified as a disinfectant or a sanitizer is dependent on the efficacy data submitted to the appropriate regulatory agency. In general, two key factors determine which regulatory agency is responsible for the authorization of a product: (i) its intended use; and (ii) the surface or object to which it is applied. As an example, sanitizers that are intended for food contact purposes are regulated by the Food Directorate under the F&DA and F&DR and those intended for non-food contact are regulated by the PMRA under the Pest Control

Products Act (PCPA) and Pest Control Products Regulations (PCPR), as seen in Table 14.2.1 [2–4].

Cleaning products that have no disinfectant or sanitization claims, as described above, require no premarket review. However, inspectors monitor and enforce their compliance through postmarket regulatory activities under the purview of Health Canada's Consumer Product Safety Directorate. These products fall under one of the two following pieces of legislation: (i) the Hazardous Products Act (HPA) if they are for use in the workplace; or (ii) the Canada Consumer Product Safety Act (CCPSA) if they are intended for non-commercial purposes, including domestic, recreational and sports activities [5, 6]. In the first instance, they are referred to as WHMIS (Workplace Hazardous Materials Information System) "controlled products" and are subject to the material safety data sheet and labeling requirements of sections 13 and 14 of the HPA, as further developed in the Controlled Products Regulations (CPR). In the second instance, the products must comply with the labeling requirements set out in the Consumer Chemicals and Containers Regulations, 2001. The CCPSA came into force on June 20, 2011 [6]. On that date,

Part I of and Schedule I to the HPA, which related primarily to consumer products including cleaning agents, were repealed, rendering the HPA a stand-alone WHMIS legislation [5].

Legislative and regulatory authority

In Canada, hard surface disinfectants are regulated as drugs under the F&DA and F&DR. This legislation provides Health Canada with the statutory authority to regulate the safety, efficacy and quality of therapeutic products, which include disinfectant drugs as specified in Section 2 of the F&DA. In addition to the legislation, the TPD has published guidance documents that describe the regulatory approval process for disinfectant drugs.

To receive market authorization, a sponsor must provide the TPD with scientific evidence that takes into account the requirements described in the applicable guidance documents. These are meant to provide assistance to stakeholders such as manufacturers and/or DIN applicants, on how to comply with the governing statutes, regulations and, when applicable, relevant and acceptable standards. This evidence is reviewed to determine whether the risks associated with the product are acceptable in light of its potential benefits. If they are, and if the product has been proven to be effective under the proposed conditions of use, it is authorized for sale in Canada and is assigned a DIN.

This section further expands on how the legislative and regulatory authority, guidance documents and standards, as depicted in Figure 14.2.1, are utilized during the regulatory review process of hard surface disinfectants.

The food and drugs act

Section 2 of the F&DA defines "drug" to include any substance or mixture of substances manufactured, sold or represented for use in: (i) the diagnosis, treatment, mitigation or prevention of a disease, disorder or abnormal physical state, or its symptoms, in human beings or animals; (ii) restoring, correcting or modifying organic functions in human beings or animals; or (iii) disinfection in premises where food is manufactured, prepared or kept [2]. Therefore, based on this definition, a disinfectant product is classified as a drug.

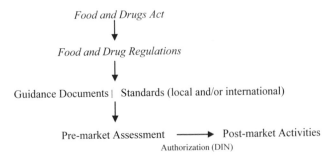

Figure 14.2.1 General overview of the regulatory authorization process for marketing hard surface disinfectants in Canada.

The food and drug regulations

The F&DR further develop the purpose and application of the F&DA and provide the TPD with the regulatory authority to assign DINs to disinfectants that are intended for use on hard, non-porous inanimate surfaces and objects [3].

Division 1 of Part C of the F&DR outlines the requirements such as labeling for attaining market authorization of drugs, including disinfectants. Division 1A refers to establishment licenses and provides the regulatory oversight for activities performed at specific sites, such as the manufacture, distribution, testing and importation of drugs, including disinfectants, whereas Division 2 outlines good manufacturing practices (GMPs). Both Division 1A and GMP regulatory requirements fall under the purview of the Health Products and Food Branch Inspectorate (HPFBI).

While high-level disinfectants and chemosterilants (i.e. products with the capacity to destroy spore-forming bacteria) are regulated under both Divisions 1A and 2, low-level disinfectants (e.g. virucides, fungicides, bactericides) are exempt. Further information can be obtained from the Health Products and Food Branch (HPFB) Inspectorate Guide 0049 entitled *Standard for the Fabrication, Control and Distribution of Antimicrobial Agents for Use on Environmental Surfaces and Certain Medical Devices* [7].

Division 8 of Part C of the F&DR refers to new drugs and includes disinfectants that have not been sold in Canada for sufficient time and in sufficient quantity to establish their safety and effectiveness under the conditions of use recommended in the labeling. Products authorized for sale under Division 8 receive a Notice of Compliance (NOC) in addition to a DIN. An example of a submission that could be subject to Division 8 includes a disinfectant product that contains a novel active ingredient.

Premarket review process

The focus of this section is limited to the premarket review requirements for hard surface disinfectants regulated under the F&DA and F&DR, and evaluated by the TPD. Health Canada has published several guidance documents related to the premarket review requirements and process for drug products, including disinfectants. As stated above, these publications provide assistance to stakeholders, such as manufacturers/sponsors, on how to comply with governing statutes and regulations. They also help Health Canada staff implement its regulatory mandates and objectives in a fair, consistent and effective manner.

When preparing an application for a disinfectant drug, applicants should familiarize themselves with the following guidance documents and standards:

1. Health Canada's *Guidance Document: Disinfectant Drugs* [1].
2. Health Canada's *Frequently Asked Questions Related to Health Canada's Guidance Document: Disinfectant Drugs* [8].
3. Health Canada's *Guidance to Industry: Management of Drug Submissions* [9].

4. Canadian General Standards Board (CGSB) Document CGSB-2.161-97, which refers to the microbicidal efficacy test standards [10].

5. Health Products and Food Branch (HPFB) Inspectorate Guide 0049 for low-level disinfectants [7].

6. The good manufacturing practices as indicated in Division 2 of the Food and Drug Regulations for higher-level disinfectants.

Pre-submission meeting

Sponsors may request a pre-submission meeting in order to deliver a presentation about their proposed product prior to filing a New Drug Submission (NDS). The purpose of such a meeting is to discuss the information required in the submission to support the safety, effectiveness and quality of the product intended for the Canadian market. In addition, such a meeting provides sponsors with the following opportunities.

1. To familiarize TPD staff with the forthcoming submission prior to its filing and discuss the included data to facilitate the premarket review.

2. To uncover any major unresolved problems or potential issues and propose options to settle disputes prior to submitting the application.

3. To identify and discuss studies that a particular sponsor considers to be adequate and well controlled in establishing the effectiveness of the disinfectant drug.

4. To discuss details of the submission with the TPD and obtain feedback regarding any areas of concern based on current experience and regulatory requirements.

5. To gain a better understanding of the submission review process and labeling requirements.

6. To allow the TPD to realign resources, if necessary, with a view to accommodating the arrival of the submission.

Section 14.2.5.1 of Health Canada's *Guidance for Industry: Management of Drug Submissions* offers more detailed information relating to pre-submission meetings, including the data package that sponsors should prepared in advance of such a meeting [9].

DIN authorization

The authorization process for obtaining a DIN is initiated by the receipt of a drug submission by the TPD. Depending on the application type, a submission is assessed under one of the following four streams:

1. Category IV Monograph.

2. Administrative submission.

3. Full DIN submission.

4. New drug submission.

Application streams 1–3 are subject to the requirements set forth in Division 1 of Part C of the F&DR whereas stream 4 is subject to both Division 1 and Division 8 of Part C of the F&DR. In addition, although safety and quality data are not required at the time of submitting a disinfectant drug application for streams 1–3, the TPD may request such information along with additional efficacy, or alterations to the proposed product labeling, during the review process.

Category IV Monograph

Category IV Monographs were developed for disinfectants that utilize chemicals which have characterized safety and efficacy profiles under specific conditions of use. They outline the permitted conditions of use and labeling requirements, such as the minimal use dilution, intended use, directions for use, warnings, active ingredients and combinations thereof. Health Canada has published Category IV Monographs for the following products:

• Hard surface disinfectants.
• Toilet bowl disinfectants.
• Contact lens disinfectants.

An applicant may reference a Category IV Monograph when a disinfectant drug product and its labeling are consistent with the information set out in the document. Category IV Monograph applications are subject to an abbreviated review period of 45 days.

The monographs apply only to products considered to be low-level disinfectants. However, not all low-level disinfectants are eligible for DIN approval through the Category IV Monograph process due to the type of active ingredient(s) in the product and/or the listing of specific claims. As an example, a Category IV Monograph disinfectant may be labeled as a bactericide, fungicide, virucide, disinfectant or disinfectant-cleaner, but claims against specific microorganisms are not permitted through this process.

Administrative submission

There are three types of administrative submissions that are applicable for disinfectants:

1. Product name change.

2. Manufacturer's name change.

3. Licensing agreement.

The first two administrative submission types are only applicable to products that are currently authorized with a DIN. Licensing agreement submissions allow a sponsor to copy the label of a disinfectant product, authorized with a DIN, through a signed arrangement with the DIN holder. A separate DIN is assigned to the copy product.

Full DIN submission

If a disinfectant product does not meet the criteria for DIN authorization through the Category IV Monograph process, a full DIN application will be required. The application must contain the appropriate efficacy data to support the proposed labeling claims.

Prior to review, the application undergoes a 45-day screening period to ensure that it contains the necessary elements for the review process. Once the screening period is complete, the DIN application is subject to a review period of either 180 or 210 days depending on the type of efficacy data received. Additional information related to the period allocated for the review process is provided in the *Guidance for Industry: Management of Drug Submissions* [9].

New drug submission

Under Division 8 of the F&DR, a drug that includes an active or inactive ingredient, indication and/or condition of use and has not been sold in Canada for sufficient time and in sufficient quantity to establish its safety and efficacy, may be considered a new drug. When a disinfectant is defined as a new drug, it will be assessed under Division 8 of the F&DR, and will require an NDS. The application must contain the appropriate safety, efficacy and quality data to support its indicated use, in addition to the necessary administrative and labeling information.

The required safety information for an NDS could include one of more of the following:
- Toxicity and/or hazard assessment of the formulation proposed for marketing.
- Exposure assessment with data, models or scenarios, including any indications of a tolerable acute, daily, subchronic and/or chronic exposure when available.
- Assessment of any risk to the user, including consideration of sensitive populations.
- Relevant epidemiological information.

The quality/chemistry and manufacturing (C&M) part of an NDS is expected to be filed in accordance with quality or C&M guidance, which includes completing the Quality Overall Summary (QOS) and the Certified Product Information Document (CPID). The C&M-related guidance and the QOS and CPID templates are available on Health Canada's website [11–13]. Considering the nature and intended use of hard surface disinfectants, which are distinct from other therapeutic products regulated under the F&DR, not all sections in these templates may be applicable. Nonetheless, the onus is on the sponsor to provide Health Canada with satisfactory scientific rationales justifying why a particular requirement does not need to be fulfilled.

Prior to review, the application undergoes a 45-day screening period to ensure that it contains the necessary elements for the review process. Once the screening period is complete, the NDS submission is subject to a 300-day review period.

As noted above, submission sponsors should consider requesting a pre-submission meeting prior to filing an NDS. During the course of such a meeting, sponsors could discuss any new information regarding a proposed claim and how they have addressed a particular concern based on these data. As an example, data gathered from pharmacovigilance and market history have allowed the identification of microbiocidal requirements that are specific to contact lens disinfectants. As a result, an NDS for these products may have to include proof of efficacy against such fungi as *Fusarium* spp. [14].

Regulatory decision

Upon completing the evaluation of a submission, the TPD provides a regulatory decision to the sponsor as to whether they have the authorization to sell a disinfectant drug product on the Canadian market. Section 14.2.5.5 of Health Canada's *Guidance for Industry: Management of Drug Submissions* provides additional information related to the evaluation process, which includes the various types of regulatory decisions [9]. The regulatory decision of granting authorization for sale of a disinfectant regulated under Division 1 of the F&DR is communicated to the sponsor using a DIN letter; submissions considered as an NDS and regulated under Division 8 of the F&DR are issued an NOC.

The TPD utilizes established processes and procedures to request additional information that could help address deficiencies during premarket screening and review. Provided below are some of the most common deficiencies encountered in disinfectant drug submissions.
- Non-conformance to a Category IV Monograph.
- Inadequate data to support efficacy claims.
- Labeling of products for use on inappropriate surfaces or media.
- Label indicating more than one contact time and use dilution varying with targeted pathogens.

The *Frequently Asked Questions Related to Health Canada's Guidance Document: Disinfectant Drugs* provides additional examples of the types of enquiries that the TPD's Disinfectant Unit has responded to since the posting of the *Guidance Document: Disinfectant Drugs* [1, 8].

Reconsideration process

The reconsideration of final decisions process is a formal conflict resolution approach that applies to disputes arising between Health Canada and sponsors of drug submissions. It is intended to be initiated when informal mechanisms have failed to resolve the issue(s). For example, sponsors may file a Request for Reconsideration following the issuance of a final decision such as one of the following.
- A Screening Rejection Letter (SRL).
- A New Drug Letter (NDL).
- A Notice of Deficiency – Withdrawal Letter (NOD/W).
- A Notice of Non-compliance – Withdrawal Letter (NON/W).
- A Not Satisfactory Notice (NSN).

Additional information related to the reconsideration process is available in Health Canada's guidance document titled *Reconsideration of Final Decisions Issued for Human Drug Submissions* [15].

Post-DIN changes

After receiving a DIN authorization to market a disinfectant drug, a sponsor may wish to make changes to the product, or the information associated with it. Examples of post-DIN changes (PDCs) and the related submission requirements are provided in the *Guidance Document on Post-Drug Identification Number (DIN) Changes* [16]. Prior to submitting a PDC, applicants should ensure that they have met the relevant requirements of this document and of Health Canada's *Guidance Document: Disinfectant Drugs*.

Disinfectants that have been approved through the NDS process under Division 8 of the F&DR and have received an NOC are not eligible for PDCs. Alternatively, Health Canada's guidance document titled *Post-Notice of Compliance (NOC) Changes: Safety and Efficacy* should be followed [17].

Postmarket regulatory activities

Postmarket regulatory activities regarding disinfectant drugs are conducted by two parts of Health Canada:
1. The Health Products and Food Branch Inspectorate (HPFBI).
2. The Marketed Health Products Directorate (MHPD).

The HPFBI is responsible for compliance monitoring and enforcement activities related to therapeutic products, including disinfectants. These activities are conducted to verify that regulatory requirements are being appropriately adhered to, and could include industry inspections and product compliance and verification. In some instances, the inspectorate could require the relevant program area to conduct a health risk assessment prior to determining the appropriate compliance strategy. In the case of hard surface disinfectants, such requests are handled by the TPD.

The MHPD works to assure that HPFB programs take a consistent approach to post-approval safety surveillance and trends, signal assessment and risk communications concerning all regulated marketed health products.

In utilizing a "life cycle" management approach to hard surface disinfectants, several opportunities exist that require both the pre- and postmarket areas to work together. For instance, when dealing with a non-compliance issue, the inspectorate could require input from the TPD and MHPD. Moreover, the TPD, MHPD and HPFBI utilize a common risk management model, known as Health Canada's *Decision-Making Framework for Identifying, Assessing, and Managing Health Risks*. This document provides the elements of a decision-making process that is comparable with other risk management frameworks [18].

Emerging pathogens

As the regulatory body responsible for the authorization of hard surface disinfectants in Canada, the TPD is required to assess the nature of various emerging pathogens on a case-by-case basis, and could consider the development and issuance of specific guidance in a timely manner. The development of such guidance takes into consideration the evidence available, and may include input from both internal and external consultations, for example industry, other regulatory bodies such as the US Environmental Protection Agency, stakeholder organization groups, etc. A recent example of the development and issuance of a specific guidance is the *Notice to Sponsors: Requirements for Efficacy Claims against the 2009 (H1N1) Pandemic Influenza A Virus for Hard Surface Disinfectant Drug Products* in relation to the pandemic 2009 (H1N1) influenza A virus [19].

Additional sources of information

The following sources provide additional information that could be applicable to hard surface disinfectant drugs:

1. Health Canada's Drug Product Database: this is an online tool containing product-specific information on drugs, including hard surface disinfectants, authorized for use in Canada. The database is managed by Health Canada and contains approximately 15,000 products which companies have notified Health Canada as being marketed [20].
2. *Access to Therapeutic Products: the Regulatory Process in Canada*: this publication describes how therapeutic products in Canada make their way from the laboratory to the marketplace. It explains how Canada's regulatory system facilitates access to safe drugs, including hard surface disinfectants [21].

Acknowledgments and disclaimer

The authors recognize the contributions of Yadvinder Bhuller, Lisa Lange and Karin Hay, as well as the assistance of Thea Mueller and Hema Gupta in reviewing the manuscript.

The content of this chapter represents a collation of information that is available on Health Canada's website, as well as from both current and former members of the TPD's Disinfectants Unit. It does not create or confer any rights for or on any person, and does not operate to bind Health Canada or the public.

References

1 Health Canada (2007) *Guidance Document: Disinfectant Drugs*, http://www.hc-sc.gc.ca/dhp-mps/prodpharma/applic-demande/guide-ld/disinfect-desinfect/index_e.html (cited May 2010).

2 Justice Canada (2010) *Food and Drugs Act*, http://laws.justice.gc.ca/PDF/Statute/F/F-27.pdf (cited May 2010).

3 Justice Canada (2010) *Food and Drug Regulations*, http://laws.justice.gc.ca/PDF/Regulation/C/C.R.C.,_c._870.pdf (cited May 2010).

4 Justice Canada (2006) *Pest Control Products Act*, http://laws-lois.justice.gc.ca/PDF/P-9.01.pdf (cited July 2011).

5 Justice Canada (2011) *Hazardous Products Act*, http://laws-lois.justice.gc.ca/PDF/H-3.pdf (cited July 2011).

6 Justice Canada (2011) *Canada Consumer Product Safety Act*, http://laws-lois.justice.gc.ca/PDF/C-1.68.pdf (cited July 2011).

7 Health Canada (2006) *Standard for the Fabrication, Control and Distribution of Antimicrobial Agents for Use on Environmental Surfaces and Certain Medical Devices, Version 2 (Guide-0049)*, http://www.hc-sc.gc.ca/dhp-mps/compli-conform/gmp-bpf/pol/gui_49-eng.php (cited May 2010).

8 Health Canada (2010) *Frequently Asked Questions related to Health Canada's Guidance Document: Disinfectant Drugs*, http://www.hc-sc.gc.ca/dhp-mps/prodpharma/applic-demande/guide-ld/disinfect-desinfect/notice_faq_disinfec_avis_faq-eng.php (cited May 2010).

9 Health Canada (2011) *Management of Drug Submissions*, http://www.hc-sc.gc.ca/dhp-mps/alt_formats/hpfb-dgpsa/pdf/prodpharma/mands_gespd-eng.pdf (cited July 2011).

10 Canadian General Standards Board (1997) *Assessment of Efficacy of Antimicrobial Agents for Use on Environmental Surfaces and Medical Devices (CAN/CGSB: 2-161-97)*. Available from Minister of Public Works and Government Services, Ottawa.

11 Health Canada (2001) *Draft Quality (Chemistry and Manufacturing) Guidance: New Drug Submissions (NDSs) and Abbreviated New Drug Submissions (ANDSs)*, http://www.hc-sc.gc.ca/dhp-mps/prodpharma/applic-demande/guide-ld/ctd/qual_ndsands_pdnpadn_07-01-eng.php (cited May 2010).

12 Health Canada (2004) *Quality Overall Summary (QOS) Templates*, http://www.hc-sc.gc.ca/dhp-mps/prodpharma/applic-demande/templates-modeles/qoscendsands_sgqecpdnpadn-eng.php (cited May 2010).

13 Health Canada (2004) *Certified Product Information Document (CPID) Template*, http://www.hc-sc.gc.ca/dhp-mps/prodpharma/applic-demande/templates-modeles/cpidce_dcipec-eng.php (cited May 2010).

14 Centers for Disease Control and Prevention (CDC) (2006) Fusarium keratitis, 2005–2006: United States. *MMWR. Morbidity and Mortality Weekly Report*, **55**, 563–564.

15 Health Canada (2006) *Guidance for Industry: Reconsideration of Final Decisions Issued for Human Drug Submissions*, http://www.hc-sc.gc.ca/dhp-mps/prodpharma/applic-demande/guide-ld/revision-final/decisions_hum_drug_drogue-eng.php (cited May 2010).

16 Health Canada (2009) *Guidance Document on Post-Drug Identification Number (DIN) Changes*, http://www.hc-sc.gc.ca/dhp-mps/prodpharma/applic-demande/guide-ld/change_din-eng.php (cited May 2010).

17 Health Canada (2009) *Post-Notice of Compliance (NOC) Changes: Safety and Efficacy*, http://www.hc-sc.gc.ca/dhp-mps/prodpharma/applic-demande/guide-ld/postnoc_change_apresac/noc_pn_saf_ac_sa_inn-eng.php (cited May 2010).

18 Health Canada (2000) *Health Canada Decision-Making Framework for Identifying, Assessing, and Managing Health Risks – August 1, 2000*, http://hc-sc.gc.ca/ahc-asc/alt_formats/hpfb-dgpsa/pdf/pubs/risk-risques-eng.pdf (cited May 2010).

19 Health Canada (2009) *Notice to Sponsors: Requirements for Efficacy Claims against the 2009 (H1N1) Pandemic Influenza A Virus for Hard Surface Disinfectant Drug Products*, http://www.hc-sc.gc.ca/dhp-mps/prodpharma/applic-demande/guide-ld/disinfect-desinfect/notice_avis_disinfectant_h1n1_ld-eng.php (cited May 2010).

20 Health Canada (2011) *Drug Product Database*, http://www.hc-sc.gc.ca/dhp-mps/prodpharma/databasdon/index-eng.php (accessed May 30, 2012).

21 Health Canada (2006) *Access to Therapeutic Products: the Regulatory Process in Canada*, http://hc-sc.gc.ca/ahc-asc/alt_formats/hpfb-dgpsa/pdf/pubs/access-therapeutic_acces-therapeutique-eng.pdf (cited May 2010).

14.3

United States Regulation of Antimicrobial Pesticides

Sally Hayes

Scientific and Regulatory Consultants, Inc., Columbia City, IN, USA

Introduction

The Federal Insecticide, Fungicide and Rodenticide Act (FIFRA) outlines the registration requirements for antimicrobial pesticides in the United States. This law, administered by the Environmental Protection Agency (EPA), is not the only law governing antimicrobial pesticides. There are numerous variables and issues that an applicant must understand to ensure that the antimicrobial product is in compliance with all applicable laws, regulations and policies.

The FIFRA provides the overall framework for the federal pesticide registration program and requires pesticide products be registered by the EPA before distribution or sale in the United States [1]. The Office of Pesticide Programs (OPP) within the EPA is responsible for registering or licensing pesticide products. The EPA mission is to protect not only the environment, but also public health. Pesticide registration decisions are based on a detailed assessment of the potential effects of a product on human health and the environment, when used according to label directions, and any required efficacy data.

Pesticide history

The primary federal laws that regulate antimicrobial pesticides are FIFRA and the Federal Food, Drug and Cosmetic Act (FFDCA) [2]. FFDCA limits pesticide residues on food. The two most important amendments to FIFRA are the Food Quality Protection Act (FQPA) [3] and the Pesticide Registration Improvement Act (PRIA).

Pesticide laws have been in existence since the early 1900s. The early laws, administered by the US Department of Agriculture (USDA), focused on labeling and consumer protection. In 1947, the first Federal Insecticide, Fungicide, Rodenticide Act was passed. It was not until 1970 that the EPA was formed as a central repository of all laws impacting the environment.

In 1996, substantive changes to FIFRA were enacted with the passage of FQPA. This law formally recognized that antimicrobial products were uniquely different from other pesticide products. A separate definition for antimicrobial pesticides was provided and the Antimicrobial Division (AD) was created within the OPP for regulating antimicrobial pesticides. The

Russell, Hugo & Ayliffe's: Principles and Practice of Disinfection, Preservation and Sterilization, Fifth Edition. Edited by Adam P. Fraise, Jean-Yves Maillard, and Syed A. Sattar.

FQPA also required the EPA take into account the unique nature of antimicrobial pesticides when registering non-food antimicrobial pesticides.

The FQPA strengthened the health-based safety standard for pesticide residues in all foods. It uses a "reasonable certainty of no harm" as the general safety standard for food uses. The FQPA requires the EPA to consider all non-occupational sources of exposure, including drinking water and residential exposure. It requires evaluation of exposure to other pesticides with a common mechanism of toxicity when setting tolerances [4]. The FQPA also changed how the OPP conducted risk assessments. Emphasis is now placed on the sensitivity of infants and children to pesticides. The OPP can also group chemicals that have common mechanisms of toxicity but must also look at non-pesticide as well as pesticide uses when determining risk.

Pesticides used on food or food contact surfaces must meet the requirements of FIFRA as well as certain portions of FFDCA. Before pesticides are allowed in materials used in manufacturing, packing, packaging, transporting or holding food, the Food and Drug Administration (FDA) must determine that there is a "reasonable certainty of no harm" presented. Once known as "indirect food additives", FDA now refers to these materials as "food contact substances" and evaluates safety through the food contact notification process. EPA then determines whether a tolerance, that is a maximum permissible pesticide residue on a particular food/feed commodity, is needed, or if the pesticide can be exempted from a tolerance.

Environmental protection agency structure

The OPP at the EPA administers the registration aspects of FIFRA. Within the OPP there are three divisions that handle the registration activities for all pesticides: the Antimicrobial Division (AD), Biopesticides and Pollution Prevention Division (BPPD) and Registration Division (RD).

The AD is responsible for antimicrobial pesticides, such as disinfectants and sanitizers. Antimicrobial pesticides: (i) disinfect, sanitize, reduce or mitigate growth or development of microbiological organisms; or (ii) protect inanimate objects (e.g. floors, walls), industrial processes or systems, surfaces, water or other chemical substances from contamination, fouling or deterioration caused by bacteria, viruses, fungi, protozoa, algae or slime [5]. Antimicrobial pesticides do not include liquid chemical sterilant products (including any sterilant or subordinate disinfectant claims on such products) for use on critical or semicritical medical device products. These products are regulated by the FDA's Center for Devices and Radiological Health (CDRH). Antimicrobial pesticides used on non-critical medical device products are jointly regulated by the EPA and FDA. The FDA has exempted these general purpose disinfectants from premarket notification but they are still subject to the Quality System Regulation, Part 820.

The BPPD is responsible for pesticides derived from natural materials such as animals, plants, bacteria and certain minerals. Biopesticides fall into three major classes:
1. Microbial pesticides consist of a microorganism (e.g. bacteria, fungi, virus or protozoa) as the active ingredient.
2. Plant-incorporated protectants (PIPs) are pesticidal substances that plants produce from genetic material that has been added to the plant.
3. Biochemical pesticides are naturally occurring substances that control pests by non-toxic mechanisms.

The RD handles conventional pesticides that are generally synthetic materials which directly kill or inactivate the pest. These include herbicides, rodenticides, molluskides, insecticides, etc.

The EPA also has ten regional offices. Each region is responsible for executing EPA programs within the respective states and territories assigned to the region. Federal EPA has delegated authority to the regions for certain activities including import/export regulations and initiation of enforcement actions.

Antimicrobial pesticides overview

The EPA categorizes antimicrobial pesticides based on the type of efficacy claim(s). Public health products are intended to control microorganisms in any inanimate environment is of public health concern. Examples are disinfectants used in hospitals, swimming pool disinfectants and sanitizers used in food-handling establishments. Non-public health products are used against microorganisms not considered to be of public health concern. Examples are algae, odor-causing bacteria, bacteria which cause spoilage, deterioration or fouling of materials, and microorganisms infectious only to animals.

The EPA requires submission of efficacy data to support each public health claim. Submission of data for non-public health organisms is generally not required but must be on file with the registrant. The EPA retains the right to require submission of non-public health data on a case-by-case basis.

More than 5000 antimicrobial end use pesticide products are currently registered with EPA. There are over 275 active ingredients used in antimicrobial products [6]. The resulting product may be marketed in a variety of forms including wipes, sprays, liquids, powders and gases. Nearly 60% of antimicrobial products are registered to control microorganisms of public health concern in hospitals and other healthcare environments [4].

Public health antimicrobial pesticide categories
Public health categories are organized by the degree of effectiveness. The efficacy achieved determines the label claims and use sites allowed for the antimicrobial pesticide.

Sterilants represent the highest or most efficacious level of antimicrobial pesticide. Sterilants destroy or eliminate all forms of bacteria and fungi, including their spores, and viruses. Since spores are the most difficult form of a microorganism to kill, the EPA considers the term "sporicide" synonymous with sterilant.

Disinfectants destroy or irreversibly inactivate bacteria, fungi and/or viruses but not their spores. There are three levels of disinfectants [7]:

1. *Hospital disinfectants*: these are capable of killing both Gram-negative and Gram-positive bacteria. The EPA has identified three organisms that a hospital disinfectant must be effective against: *Pseudomonas aeruginosa*, *Staphylococcus aureus* and *Salmonella enterica*. Claims against additional bacteria, viruses or fungi are allowed if supported with data. Products intended for use in patient care areas of healthcare facilities including hospitals, surgery centers, dental suites and nursing homes must achieve this efficacy profile.

2. *General or broad-spectrum disinfectants*: these are capable of killing both Gram-negative (*S. enterica*) and Gram-positive (*S. aureus*) bacteria but are not required to be effective against *P. aeruginosa*. Claims against additional bacteria, viruses or fungi are allowed if supported with data. Label claims for use in patient care areas of healthcare facilities are not allowed.

3. *Limited disinfectants*: these are capable of killing either Gram-negative (*S. enterica*) or Gram-positive (*S. aureus*) bacteria. Claims against additional bacteria are allowed, but only in the category in which the product showed effectiveness. Label claims for use in patient care areas of healthcare facilities are not allowed.

Sanitizers reduce, but do not necessarily eliminate, microorganisms from the inanimate environment. There are two types of sanitizers [7]:

1. *Non-food contact sanitizers*: these must demonstrate a 99.9% reduction against Gram-positive (*S. aureus*) and Gram-negative bacteria (*Klebsiella pneumoniae* or *Enterobacter aerogenes*) over a parallel untreated control in ≤5 min. EPA policy does not allow virucidal, tuberculocidal or fungicidal sanitizing claims.

2. *Food contact sanitizers*: these must demonstrate a 99.999% reduction against Gram-positive (*S. aureus*) and Gram-negative bacteria (*Escherichia coli*) over a parallel control in 30 s. Though the EPA requires effectiveness to be demonstrated in 30 s, existing policy limits the contact time stated on the label to 60 s. EPA policy does not allow virucidal, tuberculocidal or fungicidal sanitizing claims.

Emerging pathogens

The EPA generally requires the submission of efficacy data to support all public health claims. However, with emerging pathogens this is not always possible due to unavailability of the wild strain, biosafety concerns, incompatibility with disinfection test methods, etc. An emerging pathogen is a newly appearing infectious organism that is "capable of causing disease in humans under natural transmission conditions" [8]. The EPA has developed a policy to help identify products effective against emerging viral pathogens [9]. Before the guidance can be used by a registrant, the Centers for Disease Control and Prevention (CDC) must identify and publish the emerging virus taxonomy.

The guidance, applicable only to viruses, uses a hierarchal approach based on viral structure which imparts a given viral family with its susceptibility profile. From Klein and DeForest, viral strains are categorized into three clusters based on their structure or inactivation susceptibility [10]. To make a claim for the emerging pathogen, the EPA must have reviewed and accepted a successful study against a virus in the same or higher cluster (i.e. a more difficult to inactivate virus) thus predicting the product's effectiveness against the emerging pathogen.

Information regarding the emerging pathogen cannot be added to the product's marketing label. However, the guidance contains provisions that allow effectiveness against the emerging pathogen to be provided on websites, technical literature or through other means. No submission to the EPA is required as long the registrant adheres to the guidance.

Determining whether a product is a pesticide

A pesticide is any substance or mixture of substances intended for preventing, destroying, repelling or mitigating any pest. Pests can be insects, mice and other animals, unwanted plants (weeds), fungi or microorganisms like bacteria and viruses. The term pesticide applies to insecticides, antimicrobials, herbicides, fungicides and various other substances used to control pests. Under US law, a pesticide is also any substance or mixture of substances intended for use as a plant regulator, defoliant or desiccant. The intended use of a product, expressed or implied, is the main determinate of its pesticide status. If a product is represented in any manner (written or verbal) to have pesticidal properties then it is considered a pesticide by the FPA whether or not it is registered [11].

A product is also classified as a pesticide if it contains an ingredient that has no other commercially viable use except as a pesticide or the person distributing or selling the product has actual or constructive knowledge that the product will be used as pesticide [12]. The definition of pesticides is broad, but certain products are excluded from the definition [13]:

• Liquid chemical sterilants intended and labeled only for use on critical or semicritical medical devices; these are regulated by the FDA.

• Drugs used to control fungi, bacteria, viruses or other microorganisms in or on living humans or animals; these are regulated by the FDA.

• Fertilizers, nutrients and other substances used to promote plant survival and health are not considered plant growth regulators and thus are not pesticides.

• Biological control agents, except for certain microorganisms, are exempted from regulation by the EPA.

• Cleaners, deodorizers and bleaches making no pesticidal claims. Other products are pesticides but have been exempted from FIFRA regulation. These include:

• Items containing a pesticide to protect the article itself from deterioration; that is article preservatives commonly known as "treated articles". Certain conditions must be met for a treated article to be eligible for the FIFRA exemption [14].

• Minimum-risk pesticides containing certain low-risk ingredients, such as garlic and mint oil, meeting certain conditions are exempt from EPA registration [1]. State regulatory requirements may still apply.

A device used to "trap, destroy, repel or mitigate" a pest is regulated as a pesticide but is exempt from EPA registration. Pesticide devices use only physical or mechanical action to control pests.

Obtaining a pesticide registration

Once a company has determined it wants to market a pesticide product there are three avenues for obtaining a registration: (i) file for a registration; (ii) supplementally register an existing EPA registered product; or (iii) purchase an existing registration.

File a registration
Each applicant for registration must file:
• Various administrative forms.
• Proposed product labeling.
• Statement of formula.
• Technical and scientific data that meet the data requirements related to the proposed product.
• Statement of whether any data compensation requirements apply.

Supplemental registration process
Section 3(e) of FIFRA allows pesticide registrants to distribute or sell a registered pesticide product under a different name instead of or in addition to their own. Such distribution and sale is termed "supplemental distribution" and the product is termed a "distributor product". The EPA requires the company that owns the EPA registration, that is the "basic registrant", to submit a Notice of Supplemental Distribution when they enter into an agreement with a second company that will distribute their product under the second company's name and product name.

The distributor is considered an agent of the basic registrant for all intents and purposes under the Act, and both the registrant and the distributor may be held liable for violations pertaining to the distributor's product. Therefore, the longest part of the supplemental registration process is usually obtaining the basic registrant's approval of the supplemental label.

The distributor label must be the same as the basic registrant's EPA-accepted label except for allowances to identify the distributor product and company name, distributor EPA number and place of manufacture. The distributor cannot add claims, additional sites or organisms but can choose to omit claims that are on the EPA-registered label as long as required language – that is precautionary statements, signal words, etc. – remains.

Purchase an existing registration
Purchasing an existing registration allows a prospective registrant to avoid the time and cost of filing for a registration. FIFRA does not expressly provide for the transfer of registrations but the EPA has historically allowed transfers. Transferring a registration is accomplished by submitting a document, signed by authorized representatives of the companies, stating that the transfer is unconditional and irrevocable. The company owning the registration, that is the "transferor", also must provide a notarized statement certifying that the person signing the transfer agreement is authorized to bind the transferor; that no court order prohibits the transfer; and that the transfer is authorized under federal, state and local laws, and relevant corporation charters, bylaws or partnership agreements.

The registration process

The EPA must determine that a product is safe and efficacious prior to granting market approval. This requires the EPA to evaluate both the active ingredient(s) and each non-pesticidal ingredient (referred to as inert ingredients) in the context of the application site and the rate of application.

The EPA evaluates the chemistry, toxicology, environmental and ecological fate profile of the active ingredient to determine there are no undue risks for the intended use site. The data required vary depending upon whether the product is used directly or indirectly on food, or is used indoors, outdoors or in aquatic settings. The EPA uses this information to determine the risk to humans, the environment and non-target species.

A new use of an active ingredient may trigger the need for additional risk assessments. For example, if an active ingredient has been evaluated for indoor, non-food uses and an applicant applies for an indoor, food use, the EPA will consider this a new use requiring an additional risk assessment. This assessment may determine that data gaps exist that must be fulfilled before a registration can be granted.

The EPA performs a similar evaluation for each inert; that is, formulation components that do not have pesticidal activity. For inerts used in non-food settings, the EPA typically does not expect an applicant to conduct new studies. Supporting information can be supplied from publically available literature and summaries of existing data. The EPA will also accept structural activity relationship (SAR) data with a scientific rationale explaining the relevancy of the surrogate to the proposed inert. New inerts for use in direct or indirect food settings are approved through petitioning the EPA for the establishment of a tolerance or exemption from tolerance. Along with the information described above for non-food inerts, a discussion of anticipated dietary (from food and drinking water), residential (dermal, inhalation and incidental oral) and occupational exposures from the proposed and existing pesticidal uses of the chemical is required. All filings are published in the Federal Register for 30-day public comment. After the EPA's review is completed, a Final Rule is published in the Federal Register allowing use of the inert under the appropriate use pattern.

Registration of end use products (EPs) requires the EPA to evaluate chemistry, acute toxicology and, where required, efficacy data. The label is a critical component of the registration as the proposed claims will determine what efficacy data must be generated to support the product. FIFRA and the Code of Federal Regulations (CFR) include specific requirements for label language and format and, therefore, govern what must (and what cannot) appear on the label [15]. It is often said that "the label is the law" when referring to EPA-registered pesticide products.

Fulfilling data requirements

Registrants must address all data required to support the use patterns and label claims made for a proposed product. This can be done by:

- Conducting data studies.
- Citing data from the EPA's existing database.
- Requesting a waiver.

Conducting data studies

Studies may be conducted by the applicant or by third party laboratories. All studies must be conducted in accordance with 40 CFR paragraph 160 good laboratory practice (GLP) standards. The GLP standards prescribe three possible statements that describe how the study complies with GLP. The GLP compliance statement is required in all final study reports. It is important to note if the EPA audits a study and finds GLP deviations not noted in the final report compliance statement, the applicant, not the laboratory, is responsible for any civil and/or criminal penalties that may result.

Testing of unregistered products or new uses of registered products may require testing under conditions of use, for example swimming pool disinfectants. This testing must be evaluated to determine if an experimental use permit (EUP) is required. In general, EUPs are issued for pesticides containing any active ingredient, or combination of active ingredients, that have not been included in any previously registered pesticide and new uses of active ingredients. Testing performed in laboratories is generally exempt but it is important to note that testing of unregistered disinfectants under actual use conditions is subject to EUPs. The state and local area in which the test is conducted may also require EUPs to be issued.

In 2006, the EPA enacted a rule that extended the Federal Policy for the Protection of Human Subjects of Research (the Common Rule) to cover all third-party intentional dosing studies submitted to the OPP in support of a pesticide registration. Pregnant or nursing women and children are not allowed to participate in any pesticide studies that involve intentional dosing. The EPA has established a Human Studies Review Board (HSRB) to review all protocols and human studies for pending pesticide actions. These human studies are also posted for public comment. Once this process is completed, EPA will then decide whether the human study can be used to support a proposed registration. Swimming pool and spa studies are exempt from this requirement.

Citing data

Applicants are allowed to cite any data in the EPA's files to support their proposed registration. The data cited must be from a substantially similar product. If an applicant chooses to provide some or all of the required data in this manner, they must comply with the data compensation obligations provided in FIFRA. Except for exclusive-use data, an applicant is allowed to cite data without the permission of the data holder. In exchange, the applicant must notify the registrant of the data used and offer reasonable compensation for use of the data. The applicant must certify to the EPA that compensation offers have been made to all potential data owners.

If the applicant and data holder cannot reach an agreement regarding compensation, FIFRA provides a binding arbitration process. The finding of the arbitrator is final and cannot be overturned except in the case of fraud, misrepresentation or similar actions. Data that is 15 years or older is considered by the EPA to be in the public domain and therefore not compensable. These data can be cited by an applicant without an offer of compensation.

Data submitted to support a new active ingredient, a new combination of active ingredients or a new use for an existing active, is extended additional data rights. These data are granted exclusive-use protection for 10 years after the date of initial registration. Any follow-on applicant must have written authorization to use the data.

Waiver requests

An applicant can request waivers for data requirements they feel are not applicable to their product; for example a flammability waiver request for products that contain no combustible or flammable material. A written scientific justification must be provided for EPA consideration.

EPA review process

A separate application is needed for each pesticide product. The EPA also does not allow directions for an end use product to be on the same label as a product used for formulating other products such as a manufacturing use product. When the EPA receives an application, it undergoes a "front-end" review to determine that all required elements have been submitted. The EPA has 21 days to complete this review. Any deficiencies identified during this period must be addressed by the applicant or the package will be returned. During this period, if the applicant does not already have an EPA company number, the EPA will assign a number.

During the front-end review, the EPA assigns a file symbol and master record identification number(s) (MRID) for the data submitted. A file symbol consists of the company's EPA number and a series of letters, for example 123-RE. The letters will be converted to numbers when the registration is granted. MRID numbers are a series of eight unique numbers used to identify a specific study.

Under PRIA, each division of the OPP has established timelines and fees for various registration actions. After the 21-day review, the PRIA review clock begins. If it is determined during the review period that additional data or other information must be supplied, a PRIA extension can be requested to allow the applicant to gather the requested information and for the EPA to review the new data.

Once the EPA determines a product does not present an unreasonable risk, a registration is granted with the condition that the registrant submit any additional information that may be requested by the EPA in the future. Thus, EPA registrations are termed "conditional". This condition is placed on each registration, except pesticides with human dietary exposure undergoing Special Review or certain pesticides used on food or feed crops.

Changes to registrations

After a registration has been granted by the EPA, amendments to the label, formula, packaging or manufacture of the product can be made through an amendment or notification process. The EPA has outlined minor changes that may be filed as notifications or non-notifications in Pesticide Registration Notice (PRN) 98-10. All other modifications must be made through the amendment process with any required supporting information or data.

Labels

FIFRA defines labels as "the written, printed, or graphic matter on, or attached to, the pesticide or device or any of its containers or wrappers", and labeling as "all labels and all other written, printed, or graphic matter (a) accompanying the pesticide or device at any time; or (b) to which reference is made on the label" [16]. The information on pesticide labels provides information to the consumer on how to safely use the pesticide product. In addition, the label content is critical to the EPA's determination of data requirements and risk assessments needed to support the intended use of the pesticide. The following information is required on EPA pesticide labels: the brand name, the name and amount of the pesticide (active) ingredient, EPA registration and establishment number, child hazard statement, signal word, net contents, precautionary and first aid statements, physical and environmental hazards, directions for use, and storage and disposal instructions.

The EPA has authority to review all language, both pesticidal and non-pesticidal, on a label. When the EPA grants registration of a product, a label with an accepted stamp is provided. The EPA stamped label contains all accepted uses and claims. No product marketing label is allowed to make claims that are not on the master label. Any non-mandatory language, either pesticidal or non-pesticidal, is not required to be on the marketing label. Any marketing literature or advertisements must be consistent with the terms of the registration; that is the master label.

Labeling that bears any statement, design or graphic that is false or misleading is "misbranded" [17]. The EPA's regulations detail specific examples that constitute misbranding including

comparative and safety claims [18]. The EPA has issued additional guidance in the *Label Review Manual*, PRN 93-6 and the EPA's label consistency website [15, 19, 20]. It is unlawful to distribute or sell a misbranded pesticide [21].

Registrant obligations

The registrant is the company that owns the EPA-registered pesticides. A registrant must produce the product at an establishment listed with the EPA using product containers with EPA-accepted labeling. The product must contain the declared amount of active "up to the expiration time indicated on the label" [22] or to the "date of use" [23] if there is no expiration date. A registrant must also report adverse effects, including efficacy failures, associated with the pesticide, maintain production, disposal and import/export records, file yearly pesticide producer's reports and register each product name in the state or US territory it will be offered for sale.

Antimicrobial testing program

The Antimicrobial Testing Program (ATP) began in 1991 with hospital sterilants. The program continues today with testing of hospital disinfectants and tuberculocides. The EPA collects samples from manufacturers or from the marketplace for testing. The purpose of the testing is to ensure that products in the marketplace meet the registered efficacy claims. If a product fails testing, it is subject to enforcement and possible stop to sales or recall. If the failure cannot be refuted through additional testing or test method issues, the registrant may need to modify label claims, remove claims, reformulate or cancel the registration in response to an ATP failure.

State pesticide registration

Following federal EPA approval, pesticide products must be registered in each state where the product will be sold, manufactured, distributed or transported. State laws, state fees and the state agencies regulating pesticides differ from state to state. After initial state approval, the product registration must be maintained through annual renewals.

Treated articles

Treated articles are articles or products that are treated with a pesticide to protect the article or product themselves. For example, paints often contain a fungicide that protects the dried paint film from degradation from algae. These articles are exempted from all aspects of FIFRA if certain conditions are met. To meet the treated articles exemption, the treatment must be intended to protect the article or product itself and only non-public health claims may be made. In addition, the pesticide used to treat the article must be registered with the EPA for this use.

Devices

A pesticidal device is any instrument or contrivance (other than a firearm) intended for trapping, destroying, repelling or mitigating any pest. The regulations exempt "ultraviolet light systems, certain water and air filters, or ultrasonic devices that make claims that the device kills, inactivates, entraps, or suppresses growth of fungi, bacteria, or viruses in various sites" [24]. The premise of a device is that it works by a mechanical or physical means to control pests. If a chemical substance is included and the "device" does not produce its intended effect without it, then it is classified as a pesticide and not a pesticide device. For example, a filter that uses pore size only to trap microorganisms is a pesticide device; however, a filter that is treated with a chemical to capture or kill microorganisms is a pesticide.

Pesticide devices are exempt from EPA registration but are still subject to labeling requirements. Pesticide device labels cannot have false or misleading statements and must list the pesticide establishment number. While pesticide devices are exempt from EPA registration, several states require registration. These states have varying requirements for registration.

Minimum risk pesticides

The EPA has determined that pesticides containing certain active and inert ingredients have a sufficiently safe profile that allow exemption from EPA registration. These are classified as minimum risk pesticides. They are often called 25(b) products since this is the FIFRA section addressing these products.

To qualify as a minimum risk pesticide, specific conditions must be met. The product can contain only actives that are identified in the regulations, only inerts identified as "inert ingredients of minimal concern", all ingredients must be listed on the label, and public health claims are not allowed [25]. While minimum risk pesticides are exempt from EPA registration, several states require registration. These states have varying requirements for registration.

Nanotechnology

Nanotechnology has been in existence for quite some time. There is not a uniformly standard definition but generally the particles are classified as nanoparticles if they are 1–100 nm in size. The OPP defines nanomaterial as "An ingredient that contains particles that have been intentionally produced to have at least one dimension that measures between approximately 1 and 100 nanometers" [26]. Nanomaterials may exhibit different physical properties than larger-sized materials. Thus, it is believed that nanomaterials may present different health and environmental hazards. The EPA is in the process of determining whether additional or new data requirements will be required for nanomaterials.

OECD antimicrobial efficacy methods

The EPA efficacy requirements currently rely upon methods that are largely unique to the USA. The EPA is actively participating in an Organization for Economic Cooperation and Development (OECD) process of developing internationally harmonized antimicrobial efficacy methods. The goal is to create validated, reproducible, quantitative methods that will be accepted in all OECD member countries. While each country may be able to establish its own performance criteria, label claims, test conditions, replication, etc., the development of harmonized methods should facilitate the sharing of data and review across OECD regulatory agencies.

Conclusions

Antimicrobial pesticides are primarily regulated by the EPA under FIFRA. The laws are complex and the interpretations are evolving as new technologies and emerging health issues arise. The EPA must constantly balance its mission of protecting the public health and the environment with evolving science and public policy. Registrants must remain aware of these changes to ensure that their products are efficacious and in compliance with current regulations and policy.

References

1 Federal Insecticide, Fungicide, and Rodenticide Act, amended (7 U.S.C., 136 et. seq.) Section 3(a), http://agriculture.senate.gov/Legislation/Compilations/Fifra/FIFRA.pdf (accessed June 18, 2012).

2 Federal Food, Drug, and Cosmetic Act, as amended through December 31, 2004, http://www.fda.gov/regulatoryinformation/legislation/federalfooddrugand cosmeticactfdcact/default.htm (accessed June 18, 2012).

3 The Food Quality Protection Act, 1996, http://www.epa.gov/endo/pubs/fqpa.pdf (accessed June 18, 2012).

4 Environmental Protection Agency (n.d.) *Pesticides Frequent Questions*, http://pesticides.supportportal.com/ics/support/default.asp?deptID=23008 (accessed June 18, 2012).

5 Federal Insecticide, Fungicide, and Rodenticide Act, amended (7 U.S.C., 136 et. seq.) Section 2 (mm), http://agriculture.senate.gov/Legislation/Compilations/Fifra/FIFRA.pdf (accessed June 18, 2012).

6 Environmental Protection Agency (n.d.) *Pesticides: Topical and Chemical Fact Sheets*, http://www.epa.gov/pesticides/factsheets/antimic.htm (accessed June 18, 2012).

7 Environmental Protection Agency (n.d.) *What are Antimicrobial Pesticides?*, http://www.epa.gov/oppad001/ad_info.htm (accessed June 18, 2012).

8 Woolhouse, M.E.J. and Gowtage-Sequeria, S. (2005) Host range and emerging and reemerging pathogens. *Emerging Infectious Diseases*, **11** (12), 1842–1847.

9 Environmental Protection Agency (n.d.) *Antimicrobial Policy and Guidance Documents: Disinfection Hierarchy and Emerging Pathogens Guidance*, http://www.epa.gov/oppad001/regpolicy.htm (accessed June 18, 2012).

10 Klein, M. and DeForest, A. (1983) Principles of viral inactivation, in *Disinfection, Sterilization, and Preservation*, 3rd edn (ed. S. Block), Lea & Febiger, Philadelphia, pp. 422–434.

11 Environmental Protection Agency (revised as of July 1, 2011) *40 CFR §162.4(a)*, EPA.

12 Environmental Protection Agency (revised as of July 1, 2011) *40 CFR §152.15*, EPA.

13 Environmental Protection Agency (revised as of July 1, 2011) *40 CFR §152.6*, EPA.

14 Environmental Protection Agency (revised as of July 1, 2011) *40 CFR §152.25(a)*, EPA.

15 Environmental Protection Agency (n.d.) *Label Review Manual*, http://www.epa.gov/oppfead1/labeling/lrm/ (accessed June 18, 2012).

16 Federal Insecticide, Fungicide, and Rodenticide Act, amended (7 U.S.C., 136 et. seq.) Section 2 (p), http://agriculture.senate.gov/Legislation/Compilations/Fifra/FIFRA.pdf (accessed June 18, 2012).

17 Federal Insecticide, Fungicide, and Rodenticide Act, amended (7 U.S.C., 136 et. seq.) Section 2(q)(1)(A), http://agriculture.senate.gov/Legislation/Compilations/Fifra/FIFRA.pdf (accessed June 18, 2012).

18 Environmental Protection Agency (revised as of July 1, 2011) *40 CFR §156.10(a)(5)*, EPA.

19 Environmental Protection Agency (1993) *Pesticide Registration Notice 93-6: False or Misleading Statements Related to Efficacy; Revision of PR Notice 91-7*, http://www.epa.gov/PR_Notices/#1993 (accessed June 18, 2012).

20 Environmental Protection Agency (n.d.) *Pesticide Labeling Consistency*, http://www.epa.gov/pesticides/regulating/labels/label_review.htm (accessed June 18, 2012).

21 Federal Insecticide, Fungicide, and Rodenticide Act, amended (7 U.S.C., 136 et. seq.) Section 12(a)(1)(E), http://agriculture.senate.gov/Legislation/Compilations/Fifra/FIFRA.pdf (accessed June 18, 2012).

22 Environmental Protection Agency (revised as of July 1, 2011) *40 CFR §156.10(g)(6)(ii))*, EPA.

23 Environmental Protection Agency (revised as of July 1, 2011) *40 CFR §158.30*, EPA.

24 Federal Government (1976) *Federal Register*, 51065–51066, http://www.epa.gov/compliance/resources/policies/monitoring/devicepolicy.pdf (accessed June 18, 2012).

25 Environmental Protection Agency (revised as of July 1, 2011) *40 CFR §152.25(f)*, EPA.

26 Jordan, W. (2010) *Nanotechnology and Pesticides*, Pesticide Program Dialogue Committee, Environmental Protection Agency, http://www.epa.gov/pesticides/ppdc/2010/april2010/session1-nanotec.pdf (accessed June 18, 2012).

15.1   Heat Sterilization

Charles O. Hancock

Charles O. Hancock Associates, Inc., Fairport, NY, USA

Introduction

"Sterilization" is an absolute term meaning the ability to destroy all life forms. Sterilization, by its very nature, damages or alters the materials subjected to the process. Heat is the most widely recognized agent for sterilization. From the beginning of recorded history, humans have been concerned with the transmission of disease. Mosaic law incorporated the use of fire and water as purifying agents.

Early investigators focused their efforts on the study of fermentation and putrefaction. The work of Pasteur, Tyndall and Cohn resulted in a model of the heat resistance of bacteria that serves to differentiate moist heat and dry heat as major considerations today. Tyndall is perhaps best known and generally recognized as the originator of the method of fractional sterilization by discontinuous (intermittent) heating.

Heat is now the major sterilization method in use worldwide employing pressurized steam. Heat has also been used in combination with other microbicidal agents, including chemicals and ionizing radiation [1, 2]. First, the principles underlying thermal processing will be considered. Subsequent parts of this chapter will examine the response of bacterial spores to moist and dry heat, and applications of thermal processes in the medical field and in the food industry. Reviews that provide additional information can be found in references [2–23] including a more recent review [24].

Kinetics of heat inactivation

Bigelow and Esty [25] made the first mathematical evaluation of heat sterilization, and Ball [26] built on this to derive "methods of calculations for determining the time necessary to process canned foods". Many new approaches have since been proposed [27], and processes are now set using elegant software programs and are delivered by computer-controlled retorts. However, the original studies provided a sound foundation for most of the subsequent publications that underpin modern thermal process technologies.

The goal of thermal processing for sterilization is to deliver sufficient heat to inactivate all of the organisms that might be present. While this is the ultimate objective, as a result of the inactivation kinetics of microorganisms by heat (see below), a more accurate definition is to reduce the probability of survival of microorganisms to an acceptably low level. The rationale of

Russell, Hugo & Ayliffe's: Principles and Practice of Disinfection, Preservation and Sterilization, Fifth Edition. Edited by Adam P. Fraise, Jean-Yves Maillard, and Syed A. Sattar.

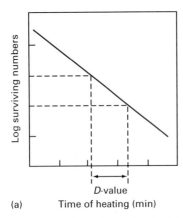
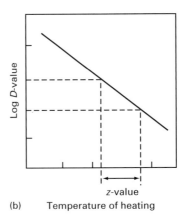

Figure 15.1.1 Idealized heat-inactivation curves of bacterial spores showing: (a) exponential decline in numbers of survivors during heating at constant temperature and the derivation of the *D*-value; and (b) exponential decline in the *D*-value with rise in temperature and derivation of the *z*-value. Esty, J.R. & Meyer, K.E. (1922) The heat resistance of the spores of B. botulinus and allied anaerobes. XI. *Journal of Infectious Diseases*, 31, 650–663. With permission from Oxford University Press.

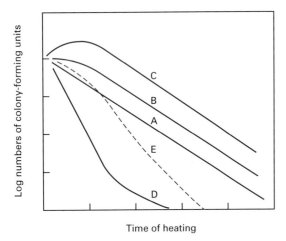

Figure 15.1.2 Varieties of experimentally derived heat-inactivation curves (B–E) that differ from the idealized kinetics (A) summarized in Figure 15.1.1. For proposed explanations see text (from [6]).

what is an acceptably low level developed over many years, following the original studies of Esty and Meyer [28] on the thermal inactivation kinetics of spores of proteolytic strains of *Clostridium botulinum*.

Process calculations assume exponential inactivation kinetics of spores held at constant temperature (Figure 15.1.1), and this relationship remains the basis of effective thermal processing, although many reports have been made of non-exponential kinetics (Figure 15.1.2). Various explanations for deviations from linearity have been proposed [3, 6, 29, 30]. For example, it has been suggested that survivor curves with shapes like curve B in Figure 15.1.2 result from multihit processes [29]. Alternatively, the presence of large numbers of clumps of cells in a suspension may result in a delay before the numbers of colony-forming units begin to fall. An initial rise in count (curve C) or a shoulder may result from a requirement of the spores to be heat-activated before they are able to germinate. Tailing (curve D) is often seen

and may result from the presence of small numbers of large clumps in the suspension, from a variation in the heat resistances of individual spores within the population [30, 31] or from an increase in spore heat resistance occurring during the heating process itself (heat adaptation, [32]). A mixture of these effects will be expected to lead to the commonly observed sigmoid type of curve (curve E).

At the very high temperatures of ultraheat treatment (UHT) processing, when inactivation rates are quite high, accurate data are difficult to obtain. Consequently, extrapolations have been made to small values of *D*, assuming constant *z* over the whole temperature range (Figure 15.1.1b). Experiments using spores of *C. botulinum* at temperatures in excess of 140°C have indicated that inactivation kinetics are close to those that would be expected by extrapolation from lower temperatures [33]. The most confidently acquired data therefore suggest that there has not been an underestimate of required heat processes, and theoretical considerations indicate that any deviations within the practicably useful range of temperatures should be small [34].

If the vegetative forms of bacteria are heated at sublethal temperatures, their resistance to subsequent heating at higher temperatures may increase, due to the phenomenon of heat adaptation, or the heat-shock response. This is part of a complex series of stress responses that many types of microorganism, plant and animal cells undergo [35, 36]. The extent to which the synthesis of heat-shock proteins that occurs within the stressed cells, and the consequent thermal adaptation, are important in practical processing is arguable. This is because most practical uses of heat, in sterilization and pasteurization procedures, involve relatively rapid heating rates, so that the opportunity for adaptation does not arise. However, some slow heating procedures are used, for example for large-bulk products, and cooking in the home may sometimes involve long, slow heating. It has therefore been suggested that heat adaptation may be significant in a limited number of cases (e.g. with respect to the survival of organisms such as *Salmonella*), which contaminate many foods of animal origin and in which the effect can be quite large.

Despite these reported variations in inactivation kinetics, the generally observed efficacy of sterilization processes, and the lack of major problems when the procedures are properly carried out, has provided evidence over many years that the basic rationale, however derived, is sound and cautious.

The three most important terms used to characterize thermal inactivation are the D-value, the z-value and the F-value:

1. The D-value (decimal reduction time (DRT)), is defined as the time in minutes at a particular constant temperature to reduce the viable population by 1-$\log_{10}$, that is to 10% of the initial value, or by 90%.

2. The z-value is defined as the temperature (°C) to bring about a 10-fold reduction in D-value; it is obtained from the slope of the curve in which the D-value on a logarithmic scale is plotted against temperature on an arithmetic scale.

3. The F-value expresses a heat treatment at any temperature as equivalent to that effect produced by a certain number of minutes at 121°C; F_0 is the F-value when z is 10°C.

An F_0 of 2.45 min thus delivers a 12-$\log_{10}$ inactivation of spores of proteolytic *C. botulinum*, which have a D-value of 0.2 min at 121°C; this is regarded as the minimum F_0 necessary to ensure the safety of low-acid canned foods. In fact, most foods are heated at higher F_0 than this, in order to control spoilage by more resistant organisms, particularly thermophiles such as *Geobacillus stearothermophilus* and *Clostridium thermosaccharolyticum* if the food is to be distributed in tropical environments. The *British Pharmacopoeia* (2010) generally requires a minimum F_0-value of 8 from a steam-sterilization process. As pointed out by Denyer and Hodges [22], the temperature–time combination of 121°C for 15 min equates to an F_0-value of 15, but this relates to the sterilization of material that may contain large numbers of thermophilic bacterial spores. They add that an F_0 of 8 is appropriate when the bioburden is low, mesophilic spores are likely to be present, and the process has been validated microbiologically. The F_0-values can be calculated graphically or can be calculated from the equation

$$F_0 = A_t \sum 10^{(T-121)/z}$$

in which A_t is the time interval between temperature measurements, T is the product temperature at time t and z is assumed to be 10°C.

Microbial susceptibility to heat

Microorganisms show wide variation in their response to moist heat. Non-sporulating bacteria are usually destroyed at temperatures of 50–60°C, although enterococci are more resistant [10, 37]. The vegetative forms of yeasts and molds show a similar response to most vegetative bacteria [9]. Many viruses are sensitive to moist heat at 55–60°C [38, 39], but Gardner and Peel [10] point out that boiling or autoclaving is recommended for the inactivation of viruses in association with blood and tissues (e.g. human immunodeficiency virus (HIV) and hepatitis B virus

(HBV)), although HIV in small amounts of blood will still be inactivated at recommended temperatures, such as 70°C for 3 min. Although the vegetative cells (trophozoites) of amoebae, such as *Acanthamoeba polyphaga*, are sensitive to temperatures of 55–60°C, the cyst forms survive for long periods and higher temperatures are needed to inactivate them [40]. Low-temperature steam (dry, saturated steam) at 73°C for not less than 10 min is a disinfection process that inactivates vegetative microorganisms and heat-sensitive viruses [17]. Boiling water inactivates non-sporulating microbes, fungi, viruses and some mesophilic spores [17]. Of the common microorganisms, spores of thermophilic bacteria are the most resistant [3], with some having enormous resistances; for example, *Desulfotomaculum nigrificans* has been reported to have a $D_{121°C}$-value of well over 10 min [41].

Prions are highly resistant to moist heat [42]. The limited data available indicate a heat resistance for the agents of bovine spongiform encephalopathy and variant Creutzfeld–Jakob disease similar to that of scrapie [43], which showed non-exponential inactivation kinetics [44]. Casolari [45] used these and other data to conclude that current thermal processes would deliver little inactivation of these prions. These observations have been supported by Oberthur *et al.* [46] (see also Chapter 10).

Moist heat

Sterilization in an autoclave using moist heat is optimal in saturated steam at the phase boundary between the steam and condensate at the same temperature. Steam at any point on the phase boundary has the same temperature as the boiling water from which it was produced but holds an extra load of latent heat, which, without drop in temperature, is available for transfer when it condenses on to a cooler surface. Superheated steam is hotter than dry saturated steam at the same pressure but is less efficient, becoming equivalent to dry heat (see below). Superheated steam behaves as an ideal gas and only slowly yields its heat to cooler objects. A small degree of superheating (maximum 5°C), is permitted, that is the steam temperature must not be greater than 5°C higher than the phase boundary temperature at that particular pressure (see Table 15.1.1 for relationships between temperature and pressure in steam sterilization).

Table 15.1.1 Temperature and pressure relationships in steam sterilization. Esty, J.R. & Meyer, K.E. (1922) The heat resistance of the spores of B. botulinus and allied anaerobes. XI. *Journal of Infectious Diseases*, 31, 650–663. With permission from Oxford University Press.

Temperature (°C)	Steam pressure	
	kPa	psi
121	103	15
126	138	20
134	207	30

Table 15.1.2 Time–temperature relationships in thermal sterilization processes.

Process	Temperature (°C)	Holding period (min)
Moist heat (autoclaving)	121	15
	126	10
	134	3
Dry heat	Minimum of 160	Not less than 120
	Minimum of 170	Not less than 60
	Minimum of 180	Not less than 30

Table 15.1.3 Uses of moist heat as a sterilization process. Gardner, J.F. & Peel, M.M. (1991) Principles of heat sterilization. In *Introduction to Sterilization, Disinfection and Infection Control*, pp. 47–59. Edinburgh: Churchill Livingstone.

Product or equipment	Comment
Metal instruments (including scalpels)	Dry heat preferred method; cutting edges to be protected from mechanical damage
Rubber gloves	Gamma-radiation preferred method; if autoclave used, care with drying at end of process (little oxidative damage when high-vacuum autoclave used)
Respirator parts	Recommended method; if disinfection is required, low-temperature steam or hot water at 80°C to be used
Surgical dressings	Choice of sterilization method depends upon stability of dressings material to stress applied and nature of dressings components
Parenteral products	Autoclaving is the approved method for sterilization of thermostable products
Non-parenteral sterile fluids	Sterile fluids suitable for clinical use; autoclaving process wherever possible
Ophthalmic solutions (eye drops)	Autoclaving is approved method for sterilization of thermostable products

When air is present in a space with steam, the air will carry part of the load, so that the partial pressure of the steam is reduced. The temperature achieved in the presence of air will thus be less than that associated with the total pressure recorded, although large volumes of air trapped in an autoclave load are not necessarily associated with reduced temperatures. However, the heating-up period will be prolonged. Such times are considerably reduced when an efficient air-removal system is used [47]. The removal of air is thus important in ensuring efficient autoclaving; the presence of air in packages of porous materials, such as surgical dressings, or within lumens comprising endoscopic devices, hinders the penetration of steam, thereby reducing the efficacy of the sterilization process [48].

For the sterilization of healthcare products, the International Organization for Standardization (ISO) documents ISO 17665-1 and 2 *Sterilization of Health Care Products – Moist Heat* [49, 50] should be used for requirements and guidance. The UK's National Health Service Estates has a substantial body of Health Technical Memoranda (HTMs) [51] for the accomplishment of that objective. HTMs give comprehensive advice and guidance on the design, installation and operation of equipment for use in the delivery of healthcare.

A number of time–temperature relationships are authorized by the *British Pharmacopoeia* (1998) (Table 15.1.2). The lethality of the process includes not only the holding period but also the heating-up and cooling-down periods The F_0-value is used to express the lethality of the whole process as an equivalent holding period at 121°C. At the higher temperatures presented in Table 15.1.2, the lethal effect is considerably greater, calculated F_0-values at 121°C (15 min), 126°C (10 min) and 134°C (3 min) being 15, 31 and 59, respectively [49]. At 115°C for 30 min, the calculated F_0-value is 8.1 [7].

In the food area, there is a wide range of methods available for the delivery of heat to products. Some of them, such as domestic cooking, are important from the standpoint of public health but are not under strict control. On the other hand, the various commercial processes for delivering heat to foods are tightly controlled [21, 23]. Still retorts (non-agitating, non-continuous) have been used for more than 100 years for the processing of low-acid foods (foods with pH values above 4.5), but in many canning operations these have been replaced by continuous agitating retorts that improve heat transfer to the product. In agitating, discontinuous, pressure processing machines, the containers of product are held within some type of basket which rotates within the retort, increasing the rate of heat transfer and shortening the process. Altogether, these actions reduce unwanted overheating of the product, and therefore result in higher quality. In continuous, hydrostatic, pressure cooker–cooler systems, the system is open – there are no valves or locks. A single chain conveyor with can-carrying flights is continuous throughout the entire system. Steam pressures of 6, 10 or 138 kPa, necessary for sterilizing at 115.5, 121, or 127°C respectively, are balanced by hydrostatic water head pressures in the heating and cooling legs. Net water heads of 7, 10.5 and 14 m are necessary to produce pressures of 6, 10 and 138 kPa. The efficiency of these systems is illustrated by a hydrostatic sterilizer reported to have replaced 33 retorts and processed 35,000 cans per hour with savings of steam, water, labor and floor space [52].

Table 15.1.3 covers the different uses of moist heat in the sterilization process.

Parenteral products

Whenever possible, injectable liquids are terminally sterilized by autoclaving, the exception being products containing heat-labile drugs. Pharmacopoeial methods in Europe recommend moist-heat sterilization at a minimum temperature of 121°C maintained throughout the load during a holding period of 15 min. Other combinations of time and temperature can be used, but the crucial requirement is that the cycles deliver an adequate level of "lethality" to the product. In practice, many manufacturers apply the F_0 principle (see above), an F_0 of 8 being the usual minimum lethality acceptable. However, in some instances of poor heat tolerance of a product, an F_0-value as low as 4 can be employed.

It is essential in all cases to ensure a low pre-sterilization bioburden and the absence of spores with high resistance to heat, especially when the F_0 approach is employed. In addition to the requirement for sterility, all parenteral products must be free from excessive numbers of particles and be non-pyrogenic (see [53] and the *Pharmaceutical Codex*, 1993).

Small-volume injection preparations of heat-stable drugs are distributed into, and sterilized in, glass or plastic ampoules. The most critical operation during the preparation of glass ampoules is the ampoule-sealing process [54]. To detect leakage, the most convenient method is to immerse ampoules in a heat-stable dye solution during autoclaving. Any seal failure will lead to loss of air from the ampoule during heating up and consequent ingress of dye during cooling, which is easily seen on inspection. For a detailed analysis of leak testing, see reference [55]. Injections can also be manufactured in polyethylene or polypropylene ampoules, using blow–fill–seal technology, for example the Rommelag process, in which the ampoule is formed, filled, sealed and heat sterilized in one continuous process [56].

A small number of injections are still required in multidose containers, comprising glass vials with an aluminum ring holding the rubber closure tightly on the bottle neck. Multidose injections must include a preservative unless the drug is intrinsically antimicrobial [57]. However, none of the multidose injections that remain acceptable to licensing authorities, such as insulin, some vaccines and heparins, are heat sterilized.

It is possible to prepare a stable fat emulsion for parenteral administration, which is sterilized by autoclaving. Such emulsions consist of 10–20% oil in water, stabilized by lecithin. The droplet size is in the range 0.2–0.4 μm diameter.

Thermostable drugs prepared in anhydrous vehicles intended for parenteral administration are sterilized by dry heat, using a cycle of 180°C for 30 min, or its equivalent time/temperature combination [58].

Large-volume aqueous injections (100 ml) have a variety of clinical uses. These include restoration of electrolyte balance (e.g. saline or glucose infusion), fluid replacement, large-volume infusions containing a therapeutic agent (e.g. chlormethiazole) and concentrated solutions of amino acids used in parenteral nutrition. Such preparations are prepared in glass or plastic containers. The manufacturing process for large-volume parenterals (LVPs) is designed to ensure that a particle- and pyrogen-free solution with low microbial content is filled into clean containers.

Rigid containers manufactured from borosilicate glass were widely used for large-volume sterile fluids in the past, but have now been largely superseded by plastic containers. However, glass bottles are still used for some products, such as amino acid infusions, some blood substitutes and agents such as the hypnotic, chlormethiazole. Such products are sterilized by autoclaving. Borosilicate glass is more resistant to thermal and chemical shock.

Bottles are closed using a rubber (elastomer) plug secured by an aluminum ring, which holds the rubber plug tightly on to the bottle rim. The major microbial risk to a product autoclaved in a glass bottle sealed with a rubber plug results from seal failure under the physical stress exerted on the closure during the autoclaving cycle. For a typical glass infusion container, the combined effect of steam under pressure and air at 121°C, together with the compression of the head-space due to water expansion, creates a pressure in the bottle of approximately 290 kPa (2.9 bar, 42 psi) greater than the chamber pressure. This internal pressure exerts considerable stress on the rubber closure, already softened by the high temperature. Seal failure can occur because of poor manufacturing tolerances of the bottle neck or rim, inadequate torque applied to the rubber plug by the aluminum cap, incorrect hardness of the rubber, or poor closure design. The consequence of seal failure is air loss from the bottle during the heating-up stage of autoclaving [59] and subsequent ingress of water during spray-cooling [60]. The entry of spray-cooling water poses the greatest risk, since it may contain viable microorganisms [61]. Even if the spray-cooling water is sterile, it remains contaminated with particulate matter, trace metals and pyrogens. The incidence of closure failure may be reduced by improved closure design [62]. Glass containers are no longer considered the most suitable container for parenterals, especially as plastic containers provide a product more cheaply, with less risk of contamination and lower particulate levels.

The choice of a suitable plastic to package LVPs is largely governed by the thermal stability of the material [63]. However, a number of factors must be considered. These include the ease of production of a suitable design which is particle- and pyrogen-free, is easily filled under clean-room conditions and does not impart significant quantities of extractables, leached from the material of the container itself to the contents. For example, it is well recognized that plasticizers in polyvinyl chloride (PVC), such as phthalate salts, can leach from poor-quality film into aqueous solutions [64]. Plastic containers can be formed into a completely sealed pouch or bottle before autoclaving. Therefore, there is no danger of spray-cooling water or air entering the contents during autoclaving provided there is no seam failure or pinholing (these faults are normally detected by leakage of the contents). Because plastic films become more flexible on heating, the pressure increase in the container during autoclaving is far less than in a rigid container. However, in order to prevent flexible plastic containers from bursting, it is essential that autoclaving be conducted in an air–steam mixture to counterbalance pressure differences [65]. Plastic LVP containers are discussed by Petrick and others [66–68]. The most commonly used plastics for sterile products are PVC, polyethylene, polypropylene and non-PVC-containing laminates. The relative merits of each are discussed by Hambleton and Allwood [62] and Turco and King [67]. One significant point of relevance to sterilization is that PVC-fabricated packs can be placed in an outer wrap before autoclaving. Also, PVC is able to withstand higher temperatures (up to 115–117°C) than polyethylene (112–114°C).

Non-parenteral products

Sterile fluids suitable for clinical use (see Table 15.1.3) include non-injectable water (for use in theaters and wards when sterile fluids are required to wash open wounds or for peritoneal dialysis), fluids for antiseptic solutions in ready-to-use dilution in critical risk areas, and for diluents for drugs used in nebulizers. All of these applications require the sterile fluid to be packaged in such a way that it can be used without becoming contaminated. For example, non-injectable water is required in a rigid bottle that allows pouring of a sterile liquid; antiseptic solutions should be transferable to a sterile container at the bedside without contamination. Peritoneal fluids must be packaged in order to allow convenient delivery into the peritoneum via suitable administration sets. This requires a flexible-walled container that collapses on emptying.

Most producers manufacture non-injectable water in rigid polypropylene bottles. The bottle may be sealed using a screw cap, with tear-off hermetic overseal, or with a snap-break closure of a fully molded container. Peritoneal dialysis fluids are packaged in flexible PVC pouches or rigid polypropylene bottles. Smaller-volume antiseptic solutions and nebulizer solutions may be packaged in plastic ampoules, PVC or laminate sachets. All these preparations should be autoclavable (Table 15.1.3).

Traditionally, eye drops have been prepared in glass containers (see below), although it is now far more common to use plastic. Single-dose packs are available in which the solutions can be sterilized by autoclaving in air-ballasted autoclaves. These solutions can therefore be formulated without a preservative. Eye drops are sterilized by autoclaving whenever the stability of the therapeutic agent permits. Multidose preparations must contain an antimicrobial preservative to prevent proliferation of contaminants during use and to support the maintenance of sterility. Examples of preservatives are phenylmercuric nitrate or acetate (0.002% w/v), chlorhexidine acetate (0.01% w/v) or benzalkonium chloride (0.01% w/v). Choice is to some extent dependent upon the active ingredient and the formulation. Preservatives can, however, migrate into both plastic and rubber components of the packaging [68]. Most types of rubber absorb preservatives [69]. It is therefore necessary to compensate for this loss by pre-equilibrating rubber closures with the particular preservative in the formulation. Benzalkonium chloride may be incompatible with natural rubber [70] and therefore synthetic rubber teats should be substituted, silicone rubber being recommended. However, moisture loss through silicone rubber occurs rapidly during storage, thus limiting the shelf-life of such a package [71]. This is sometimes overcome by supplying the dropper separately from the bottle, the dropper being applied to the bottle immediately before use. Eye drops are also commonly prepared in plastic dropper bottles, using filter-sterilized solutions and aseptic processing into pre-sterilized containers.

The sealing of eye dropper bottles during autoclaving can be improved by substituting metal for bakelite caps [72]. Other suggestions have been made for improving this type of packaging [73]. Similar problems relate to containers for eye lotions, except that the closure does not incorporate a rubber teat. Eye lotions are normally treated as single-dose items and a preservative is not included. In contrast, contact lens solutions, as well as being prepared as sterile preparations, preferably terminally sterilized by autoclaving, contain antimicrobial combinations to act as preservatives since they are multidose preparations [74].

Dressings

Traditionally, gravity (downward-displacement) autoclaves have been used to sterilize dressings [75–77]; however, this technology is now considered obsolete and high-vacuum, porous-load steam sterilizers are the method of choice [78]. In both cases, the essential requirements are for total removal of air from the load and the prevention of excessive condensation within the dressing packs during the cycle. If air is not removed, sterilizing conditions throughout the load will not be attained. If excessive condensation occurs, the dressing will become unusable. Condensation may also interfere with heat penetration. Porous-load autoclaves for dressing sterilization are described in European Committee for Standardization (CEN) Standard EN285.

The essential difference between the traditional downward-displacement systems and pre-vacuum dynamic air removal is the use of a far greater vacuum applied in the chamber to remove almost all of the air in the air space and trapped within the dressing packs. It is essential that air leaks into the chamber are prevented [79]. This vacuum must be below 20 mmHg absolute, which will remove more than 95% of the air in the chamber and load. The depth of vacuum and rapidity of pulsing will determine the amount of time required for air removal and steam penetration of the load. As the initial pressure is very low, steam is less likely to condense on the load material during the initial heating-up phase. This also depends on packing, and will vary in mixed loads; in fact, to ensure complete air removal from the load, it is usual to employ a rapid-pulsing evacuation procedure before the final heating-up stage, taking 6–8 min in all. The minimum holding time of 3 min at 134–138°C, a saturated-steam pressure equivalent to 220 kPa (2.2 bar, 32 psi), is followed by steam removal, by condenser or vacuum, and drying, which can be shortened to 3–4 min for most loads packaged in paper or linen. Therefore, the total cycle time is about 28–35 min.

Another means of air removal/steam penetration by dynamic means is the steam-flush pressure-pulse [80, 81] control, which may be found in both healthcare sterilizers for reprocessing reusable medical devices and in some smaller table-top sterilizers. Steam-flush pressure-pulse sterilizers use a repeated sequence consisting of a steam flush and a pressure pulse system that removes air from the sterilizing chamber and processed materials using steam at above atmospheric pressure (no vacuum is required). Like a pre-vacuum sterilizer, a steam-flush pressure-pulse sterilizer rapidly removes air from the sterilizing chamber and wrapped items; however, the system is not susceptible to air leaks because air is removed with the sterilizing chamber pressure at above atmospheric pressure. Typical operating temperatures are 121–123, 132–135 and 141–144°C.

Whichever equipment is used it is essential to ensure that the steam is dry and saturated, containing 5% or less by weight of water as condensed droplets. If the steam is too wet, it will soak porous items, causing them to trap air. The other danger to be avoided is superheating. This can be caused by the lagging of reducing valves, by exothermic reactions related to grease in valves, etc., by too high a jacket temperature, or by retention of air in the load. Superheating can also occur within the load from the heat of hydration of very dry (1% moisture content) cotton fabrics [82–84]. This can be avoided by allowing fabrics to equilibrate with normal levels of humidity (50% relative humidity) before sterilization.

Most porous wrapped packs are sterilized by moist heat. The nature of the packaging must allow complete steam penetration into the dressing, as well as post-sterilization drying, and must be designed to allow the item to be removed aseptically. In general, all porous items are double-wrapped so that items can be taken through a contamination barrier into a clean area, during which the porous item and its immediate packaging remain sterile. Also, items are usually packed individually or in porous item kits (all the required items for one procedure are packed into one outer wrapping [85]). Fortunately, packaging developments have proceeded apace with improvements in autoclave technology. Improvements in the design of the autoclave cycle have allowed the use of improved packaging materials and methods of packaging. Thus, introduction of dynamic air-removal autoclave cycles has not only provided a much shorter cycle period and improved sterilization performance, but also provided greater flexibility in the use of packaging techniques.

Any packaging material must allow steam and air to penetrate but still maintain its resistance to heat and breakage, especially when wet [86]. It should be an adequate barrier in preventing entry of dust or microorganisms during storage. There is a considerable choice of material available, including metal, rigid polymers, muslin, cardboard, paper and plastic films. It is now common practice to pack each item in a paper/plastic pouch, and then overwrap it in paper or fabric; alternatively, they may be placed in rigid sterilization containers, although other packaging materials are also available. In general, steam- and air-permeable packs are relatively easily sterilized, either by gravity or dynamic air-removal steam control. In addition, the wrapping material is cheap and readily disposed of, and each pack is sealed with self-adhesive autoclave tape. Fabrics such as muslin are suitable for gravity-steam penetration and the material often proves to be a reasonably effective air filter. However, fabrics are less resistant to bacterial penetration than paper [87]. They are reusable but require laundering. Some plastic-film materials can be employed provided the material is steam penetrable. The method of packing is often critical, especially in gravity-displacement autoclaves. Packs must be arranged so that the critical steam flow is not impeded between packs. The use of dynamic air-removal cycles largely overcomes the problem of steam penetration, provided the packing is sufficiently loose to allow good air and steam circulation inside and between packs and packaging material.

Dynamic air-removal sterilizers are used for sterilizing wrapped goods, lumened devices and porous materials. Air removal is vital and this is achieved by providing a driving force to exhaust air

Table 15.1.4 Types of steam sterilizers (based on [7] and [17]). Dewhurst, E. & Hoxey, E.V 2002, *Guide to microbiological control in pharmaceuticals* with permission from Taylor and Francis.

Type of steam sterilizer	Sterilization conditions	Use
Porous load	134–138°C, 3 min	Unwrapped instruments, dressings and utensils
Fluid cycle	121°C, 15 min	Fluids in sealed containers, e.g. injections in ampoules
Unwrapped instruments	134–138°C, 3 min	Unwrapped instruments and utensils
LTSF[a]	73°C, 3 h	Heat-sensitive equipment

[a] Doubts have been expressed about the efficiency of low-temperature steam with formaldehyde (LTSF) as a sterilization process.

and inject steam. The pre-vacuum procedure (if used) is monitored routinely with the Bowie–Dick test [88, 89]; the basis of evaluating the efficacy of the air removal and steam penetration is a uniform color change of a temperature-sensitive indicator. An air detector may be used to independently ensure the absence of air in the sterilizer.

Gravity-displacement (instrument and utensil) sterilizers rely upon downward displacement of air by steam admitted from a separate steam source or generated within the sterilizing chamber. Despite the terminology, steam generated within the chamber by heating water may, in fact, cause upward displacement of air through a temperature-actuated electrically-operated valve [7].

The sterilizers described above rely on direct contact between steam and the product being sterilized. In contrast, bottled-fluids sterilizers act in a different manner; here, steam condenses on the surface of the containers, followed by heat transfer across the container walls, so that the contents are raised to the sterilizing temperature. The pressure within the sealed container will rise; this may be counteracted by the strength of the container and the pressure of steam within the chamber. The chamber pressure may be increased by the addition of sterile air (air ballasting) to prevent breakage of glass containers or deformation of polymeric ones. After the holding period has been completed, the cooling period can be accelerated by spray-cooling with water (sterile, to prevent the possibility of contamination).

Further information about the uses of these types of sterilizers is provided in Table 15.1.4.

Validation of steam sterilizers is achieved by determining the inactivation of heat-resistant spores [90–92], for example *Geobacillus stearothermophilus* (D_{121}-value 1.5 min, z-value 10°C). When employing ISO 176665-2A, biological indicators have no role in monitoring steam sterilization. Functional performance tests involving physical (thermometric) measurement of the conditions, as described in the reference Annex, must be met. Chemical indicators may provide a visual indication that a process has been undertaken, but provide no guarantee as to sterility.

Lumened devices

Endoscopes are lumened devices used to diagnose and treat numerous medical conditions. Although endoscopes represent a valuable diagnostic and therapeutic tool in modern medicine and the incidence of infection associated with their use reportedly is very low (about one in 1.8 million procedures) [93] more healthcare-associated outbreaks have been linked to contaminated endoscopes than to any other medical device [94–96]. In order to prevent the spread of healthcare-aassociated infections, all endoscopes (e.g. gastrointestinal endoscopes, bronchoscopes, nasopharygoscopes) must be properly cleaned and, at a minimum, subjected to high-level disinfection after each use. High-level disinfection can be expected to destroy all microorganisms, although when high numbers of bacterial spores are present, a few spores might survive.

Because of the body cavities they enter, flexible endoscopes acquire high levels of microbial contamination (bioburden) during each use [97]. For example, the bioburden found on flexible gastrointestinal endoscopes after use has ranged from 10^5 to 10^{10} cfu/ml, with the highest levels found in the suction channels [97–100]. The average load on bronchoscopes before cleaning was 6.4×10^4 cfu/ml. Cleaning can reduce the level of microbial contamination by 4–6-$\log_{10}$ [101, 102].

Flexible endoscopes are particularly difficult to clean and disinfect/sterilize [103] and easy to damage because of their intricate design and delicate materials [104]. Meticulous cleaning must precede any sterilization or high-level disinfection of these instruments. Failure to perform good cleaning can result in sterilization or disinfection failure, and outbreaks of infection can occur. Lumened devices are particularly difficult to inspect for cleanliness, especially for lumens which are single (dead) ended lumens. Many endoscopic devices, in the past, have been designed for liquid chemical reprocessing.

Since steam sterilization is perceived to be the most economic method of sterilization for reuseable, reprocessable medical devices, some endoscope manufacturers have redesigned their devices for compatibility with steam sterilization. Such redesigned lumened devices present a sterilization challenge which may or may not be adequately addressed by the current sterilizer control systems. For example, the porous-load sterilizers intended to deal with dressings (as described above) can be challenged with the Bowie–Dick test pack; the air removal/steam penetration challenge may be significantly different from the challenge presented by a complex, multilumened endoscope with small (<1 mm) lumens and intricate, complex mechanisms. The dynamics of air removal from a wrapped fabric pack are different from those of a long, narrow lumen where air removal, sterilant penetration and the presence of moisture may be in conflict.

Thermal processing of foods

Thermal processing for the sterilization of high pH (low acid), high water activity (A_w) foods for ambient stability aims to inactivate the spore forms of all those bacteria that could otherwise grow in these products. Pasteurization processes aim to inactivate mainly vegetative spoilage or pathogenic microorganisms, with subsequently limited product shelf-life – or with longer shelf-life if the growth of any surviving microorganisms is inhibited, for example by low-temperature storage, by the addition of preservatives or due to the intrinsic properties of a particular food.

If an otherwise unpreserved food is to be stable during indefinite storage at ambient temperatures, all microorganisms capable of growth in that food must be eradicated and reinfection from extraneous sources prevented. If the ambient temperatures expected during the life of the food include those typical of tropical conditions, the thermal process must be sufficient to inactivate spores of those organisms able to grow at high temperatures (thermophiles), such as *Geobacillus stearothermophilus* and *Clostridium thermosaccharolyticum*. Such thermophilic bacteria produce the most resistant types of spores, so the required processes are severe. On the other hand, if the food is destined for temperate regions, complete eradication of thermophiles is not necessary, since they cannot grow at the lower temperatures, and milder thermal processes are adequate. Such foods therefore need not be sterile. However, they must be heated sufficiently to be free from the spores of spoilage and toxigenic microorganisms that are capable of growth under temperate ambient conditions. This is sometimes referred to as "commercial sterility". Special attention is given to the eradication of any spores of proteolytic strains of *C. botulinum* that may be present, because these are the most heat resistant of the toxigenic spores and their survival and growth can result in particularly severe food poisoning.

If foods are formulated in such a way that spoilage and toxigenic spore-formers are inhibited from growing, for instance by reduction in pH value or A_w or by the addition of preservatives, then it may be unnecessary to inactivate the spores. Milder pasteurization processes may then be adequate to ensure stability and safety. Finally, for some foods that are unpreserved and yet stored for limited periods of time or at well-controlled low temperatures, pasteurization may likewise be sufficient. Requirements for sterilization are therefore clearly defined (see below), whereas requirements for pasteurization vary according to product characterists and intended storage life.

In order to determine the correct conditions for foods thermally processed in sealed containers, temperatures are usually measured using thermocouples during heating and cooling at the slowest heating point within containers in the retort. The F_0-value delivered is calculated from the lowest integrated time–temperature curve registered, and the required minimal treatment is based on this. A consequence of using the minimum-heat point is that most of the food in a batch is usually substantially overprocessed. Biological indicators (e.g. spores of *G. stearothermophilus*, [105]) have sometimes been used to check the validity of processes.

Guidelines for setting processes are covered in several standard texts [106–109]. All rely on integration to determine the total

F-value of the process, having chosen the values of *D* and *z*, and there are a variety of ways of doing this. In the graphical method, the lethal rate per minute, at a particular temperature, is represented by length on the vertical axis of "*F*-reference paper". Time is plotted linearly on the horizontal axis. The area beneath the curve is then a measure of the *F*-value, and can be calculated by multiplication by the appropriate scale factor. In the addition method, the lethal rate per minute at each specific temperature is read from a table, and the F_0-value calculated from the sum of the lethal effects (rates) multiplied by the appropriate time factor in minutes.

The precision of the two basic methods is similar and has been further improved by the availability of user-friendly software, allowing quicker and more confident computer-aided integration of lethality [110, 111]. Changing the *z*-values and reference temperatures allows the programs to be used for pasteurization processes.

Process control has likewise become increasingly precise with the use of modern temperature recorder–controllers, which have been developed to the point where they are complete process controllers themselves [112].

Combination treatments

The combination of other factors with thermal processes can allow a reduction in the degree of heating necessary to achieve product stability. The most widely employed is the combination with acidification, such that foods with pH values below 4.5 do not require a full "botulinum cook". This is because any spores of *C. botulinum* that may be present and survive in such "acid-canned" foods cannot grow at such a low pH.

Combinations with reduced A_w, with or without pH reduction, were first shown by Braithwaite and Perigo [113] to lead to a variety of options for combinations of pH, A_w and F_0 that ensure stability. Some of these options are now widely used for the preservation of ambient or long-chill-stored products. Particularly successful examples include the shelf-stable products (SSPs) – meat-based and other products promoted by the "hurdle technology" concept of Leistner and his colleagues [114–116]. These pH- and A_w-adjusted products, some with additional preservation due to the presence of nitrite or other adjuncts, receive mild heat treatments in sealed packs. They contain surviving spores. These slowly germinate during storage, but they are unable to grow and therefore die, steadily reducing in numbers as time passes (auto-sterilization [117]).

Combinations of heating with chill storage are widely employed to extend the shelf-life of mildly heated, high-quality food products. Much attention has been given to determining the level of heating necessary to control pathogens in such foods. There is now general agreement that the safety of mildly heated products that are intended to have a short shelf-life, and that are otherwise unpreserved, can be assured by a minimum heat treatment and a tight restriction of shelf-life [118]. Such products are therefore given heat treatments sufficient to inactivate vegetative pathogens, for example in excess of a 10^6-fold reduction in numbers of *Listeria monocytogenes*, which can be achieved by 70°C for 2 min or a heat process of equivalent lethality assuming a *z*-value between 6 and 7.4°C [119], or in excess of 10^8-fold, achieved by a 72°C, 2-min process [120]. However, these processes are insufficient to inactivate spores of psychrotrophic strains of *C. botulinum*, some of which are able to grow slowly at temperatures as low as 3.3°C. The processes are therefore acceptable only if the temperatures of storage are sufficiently low and the storage times sufficiently short to prevent growth from any of these spores that may be present [118].

There is general agreement that, for products intended to have a long shelf-life, and which are otherwise unpreserved, heat processing must be more severe. It must be sufficient to achieve a large, that is 106-fold, reduction of spores of psychrotrophic *C. botulinum* if storage below 3.3°C cannot confidently be assured [121]. It is generally agreed that a temperature–time combination of 90°C for 10 min or a process of equivalent lethality will achieve this, although it is recognized that additional data are still required [122–124]. These chilled food products, which have been mildly heated in hermetically sealed packages, or heated and packaged without recontamination, include refrigerated processed foods of extended durability (REPFEDs) [125, 126]: "sous vide" products [127] and other products with pasteurization and preservation combinations that deliver extended shelf-lives under chill storage [128]. "Sous vide" refers to a process in which foods are vacuum packed prior to cooking for long periods of time at relatively low pasteurization temperatures, so as to deliver high quality with respect to texture and retention of flavor.

A combination of mild heat processing with high hydrostatic pressure is being suggested as a further means of reducing heat damage to foods. While this combination works well, it is still not sufficiently effective to match the safety requirements of traditional thermal processing for long-ambient-stable foods (see Chapter 13).

Low-temperature steam (LTS) at subatmospheric pressure was developed originally for disinfecting heat-sensitive materials. At 80°C, LTS was found to be much more effective than water at the same temperature, and the addition of formaldehyde to LTS to produce LTSF achieved a sporicidal effect [128–132]. As a sterilization procedure, LTSF has been reviewed a number of times [7, 9, 22, 39, 133].

Generally, LTSF operates in a temperature range of 70–80°C, with a formaldehyde concentration per sterilization chamber volume of c. 14 mg/l. The design of an LTSF sterilizer is similar to that of a porous-load steam sterilizer (see above), the main differences being its operation at subatmospheric pressure and the injection of formaldehyde gas. Further detailed information can be found in Chapter 12.

Wright [134] reported that LTSF-treated spores of *Geobacillus stearothermophilus* could be revived by a postexposure heat shock, so that spores may not, after all, be inactivated by LTSF. Some doubt has thus been cast on the efficacy of this combined treatment.

The activity of a chemical agent is normally increased when the temperature at which it acts is raised. At ambient temperatures, the chlorinated phenol, chlorocresol, and the organomercurials, phenylmercuric nitrate (PMN) and phenylmercuric acetate (PMA), are sporistatic rather than sporicidal [4, 135]. At elevated temperatures, however, they are sporicidal, a property that suggested to Berry [136] that these agents might find usage in sterilization procedures. They accordingly proposed a new method of "heating with a bactericide" (chlorocresol or PMN) for the sterilization of some types of parenteral products, which was incorporated into the fourth addendum to the 1932 *British Pharmacopoeia*. The underlying procedure was also invoked as one that was allowed officially in the UK for the sterilization of eye drops – the bactericides being PMN, PMA, chlorhexidine diacetate and benzalkonium chloride. It is interesting to note that relatively low numbers of *Bacillus subtilis* spores were found to survive heating with chlorocresol [137] or PMN [138]. It must, however, be pointed out that the containers used in these experiments consisted of screw-capped bottles with rubber liners; both chlorocresol and, to a greater extent, PMN are absorbed into rubber, thereby reducing their concentration and efficacy [83]. Heating with a microbicidal agent is no longer permitted as an official method of sterilization of injectables or eye drops in the UK.

Inactivation of vegetative microorganisms by moist heat has been practiced for many years. For example, the pasteurization of milk is based upon Louis Pasteur's observations that spoilage of wines could be prevented by heating at temperatures of 50–60°C. Likewise, the inactivation of bacteria in killed bacterial vaccines may be achieved by similar temperatures, although generally an agent such as phenol is nowadays employed [139].

Disinfection with LTS is achieved by using an automatically controlled disinfector under conditions that ensure the removal of air and subsequent exposure to subatmospheric, dry, saturated steam at 73°C for not less than 10 min. Details of the equipment, monitoring procedure, uses and monitoring are provided by BS 3970 (1990, Parts 1 and 5) [16, 140] and HTM 2010 (1994) [50]. The process kills most vegetative microorganisms and viruses.

Disinfection may also be achieved by means of soft-water boiling at normal atmospheric pressure at 100°C for 5 min or more. Articles to be disinfected in this manner must be pre-cleaned. Details of the equipment required and its operation and maintenance, together with the disadvantages of the process, are described by the Medical Devices Directorate [17].

Washer disinfectors achieve disinfection by a combination of physical cleaning and thermal effects [141, 142]. A temperature of about 80°C is employed and the process inactivates all microorganisms except bacterial spores. The Medical Devices Directorate [17] provides additional information. Babb [140] considers the process options, using moist-heat temperatures of 65–100°C for various implants. *Enterococcus faecalis* may be employed as a biological indicator of thermal disinfection.

While a "12D" process for inactivation of spores of proteolytic strains of *C. botulinum* has become regarded as the minimum process requirement for safety of thermally processed low-acid foods, lesser inactivation factors have been proposed for pasteurized foods. An example is a "7D" process proposed to ensure safety with respect to the inactivation of salmonellae during the cooking of meat [143]. This formed the basis of a US Department of Agriculture (USDA) requirement for this level of inactivation in the cooking of roast beef, and a "5D" process was required for salmonellae in ground beef and for *Escherichia coli* O157 in fermented sausages. Similarly, "6D" processes [118] or "7D" processes [120] were proposed to ensure safety with respect to the survival of *Listeria monocytogenes* in mildly-heated, in-pack pasteurized, chill-stored foods.

Alternative means for heat delivery and control

Recent developments in the thermal processing of foods have targeted improvements in product quality through: (i) reducing heat-induced damage by aiming for high-temperature short-time (HTST) processing, particularly through aseptic processing; (ii) using new forms of packaging that allow more rapid and more uniform heat transfer into and out of packed foods during processing; (iii) delivering heat in new ways (e.g. ohmic, microwave; see below); and (iv) controlling processes more tightly so as to achieve minimal processing and so avoid the extreme over-processing that often occurs within batches of conventionally thermally-processed foods.

Progress with aseptic processing has been substantial. The high-temperature treatments are normally delivered to foods in plate or tubular heat exchangers if the products are liquid or viscous, or in scraped-surface heat exchangers if the products tend to congeal on the exchanger surfaces or contain particulates (which can be up to about 1.5 cm in diameter). Typically, temperatures are in the range 135–145°C and holding times are less than 5 s. It is not possible to measure continuously the temperature within a food particle as it moves through a heat exchanger, so the F_0 delivered must be estimated from the thermal properties of the food materials and the kinetics, residence times, etc., within the system. The process can then usefully be verified using biological methods [144]. Such methods have involved the use of "biological thermocouples", consisting of spores sealed into small glass bulbs [145] or entrained within gel particles, such as beads of calcium alginate [146].

Most of the filling systems in aseptic processes make use of hot hydrogen peroxide to sterilize packs or webs of packaging material prior to dosing the sterilized (or pasteurized) product. These procedures can regularly achieve inactivation of spores on packaging by factors in excess of 10^8-fold. However, rigorous control of the whole system is essential. This is illustrated by the statistics quoted by Warwick [147], who found, in a survey of 120 users of aseptic systems in Europe, that nearly 50% of installations experienced more than one non-sterile pack per 10,000, and that these resulted from contamination not from failure of the thermal process per se.

The major changes in packaging that allow improved, more uniform, heat penetration into products have involved the development of new flexible pouches and polypropylene rigid containers. Cartons and thermoformed containers are the most-used forms of packaging for aseptically processed foods, but any kind of pack that can be hermetically sealed can be used. Materials now include tin-free steel, aluminum, aluminum foil and a wide variety of foil–plastic combinations in addition to glass and tin plate [148]. Packs that do not have the strength of conventional cans or jars require special handling techniques to avoid damage and are often retailed in overwraps or carton outers to protect them and avoid recontamination during distribution [149, 150].

New heat-delivery systems include a number of alternatives to steam heating, including direct application of flame to containers, heating by passing alternating electric currents through products (ohmic heating) prior to aseptically packaging them, and heating using microwave energy. In particular, much development work has been undertaken on electrical-resistance heating procedures and commercial developments have been tested and applied in some countries [151]. Electrical-resistance heating allows liquids and contained particulates to heat at the same rate and very rapidly, giving the potential for minimal thermal damage and high product quality. The physical basis of the process is complex but well understood, so that results are closely predictable from first principles [152]. Microwave processing also has the advantage over conventional thermal processing that heat can be delivered very rapidly, and to solid food products, and volumetrically, so that heat transfer within the food can be much faster than processes that rely on conduction [153]. The slow take-up of microwaves for commercial food sterilization reflects technical barriers to confident large-scale control of heat distribution, as well as marketing constraints.

Dry heat

Sterilization by dry heat is less efficient than by moist heat. Definitions of D-value and z-value given for moist heat above apply equally here. The F-value concept utilized in steam-sterilization processes has an equivalent in dry-heat sterilization, although its application has been limited[21]. This equivalent, FH, describes the lethality in terms of the equivalent number of minutes at 170°C. Russell [2, 3] has demonstrated that higher D-values and z-values are found with dry heat than with moist heat and in dry-heat calculations a z-value of 20°C is considered to be suitable. Bacterial spores are the most resistant organisms to dry heat [2]. Resistance depends on the degree of dryness of the cells [154]. A variety of methods can be used to achieve dry-heat sterilization. They include the most widely employed procedure (hot air) and sterilizing tunnels, which utilize infrared irradiation to achieve heat transfer [155].

Dry heat as a means of sterilization is reserved for those products and materials that contain little or no water and cannot be saturated with steam during the heating cycle (Table 15.1.5). It

Table 15.1.5 Uses of dry heat as a sterilization process.

Product or equipment[a]	Comment
Syringes (glass)[b]	Dry heat is preferred method using assembled syringes
Needles (all metal)	Preferred method
Metal instruments (including scalpels)	Preferred to moist heat
Glassware	Recommended method
Oils and oily injections	Autoclaving clearly unsuitable
Powders	One of four methods (others are ethylene oxide, γ-radiation, filtration) recommended by *British Pharmacopoeia* (1993)

[a] Dry heat may also be used at high temperatures (200°C) for the depyrogenation of glassware.
[b] Now mainly replaced by disposable syringes sterilized by γ-radiation (see Chapter 12).

is used for dry powdered drugs, heat-resistant containers (but not rubber items), certain terminally-sterilized preparations, and some types of surgical dressings and surgical instruments. The instruments include metal scalpels, other steel instruments and glass syringes (although most syringes now consist of plastic and are disposable). The advantage offered by dry-heat sterilization of syringes is that they can be sterilized fully assembled in the final container [156]. The difficulties associated with autoclaving syringes include lack of steam penetration, enhanced by the protective effect of lubricant, and the need to assemble them after sterilization. Examples of pharmaceutical products subjected to dry-heat sterilization include implants [157], eye ointment bases, oily injections (usually sterilized in ampoules) and other oily products (e.g. silicone used for catheter lubrication, liquid paraffin, glycerin). Dressings sterilized by dry heat include paraffin gauze and other oily-impregnated dressings.

The recommended treatment is maintenance of the item at 160°C for 2 h. This may be limited by the heat stability of the particular item and therefore some dispensation is accepted (e.g. human fibrin foam is sterilized at 130°C for 3 h). Sutures may be sterilized at 150°C for 1 h in a non-aqueous solvent. However, after this treatment, the suture material must be transferred to aqueous tubing fluid to render the material flexible and restore its tensile strength. Ionizing radiation is now the preferred method of sterilization of sutures as it minimizes the loss of tensile strength.

A hot-air oven is usually employed to effect dry-heat sterilization. The sterilizer consists of an insulated, polished, stainless steel chamber, which contains perforated shelving to permit circulation of hot air. Sterilization depends upon heat transfer from a gas (hot air) to cooler objects and it is essential that even temperature distribution throughout the sterilization chamber is achieved. In practice, this is done by the inclusion of a fan unit at the rear of the oven, which ensures forced air circulation. The items that are to be sterilized must be cleaned and dried before commencement of the process. Further information is to be found in BS 3970 [17, 140], the Medical Devices Directorate [17] and HTM. 2010 [51], as well as in useful discourses on dry-heat sterilization by Gardner and Peel [11] and Wood [15, 16].

Infrared heaters have also been used to achieve dry-heat sterilization. Infrared rays are characterized by long wavelengths and very low levels of radiant energy. They depend upon the fact that the radiant energy is converted to heat when it is absorbed by solids or liquids. Infrared rays have the ability to raise rapidly the surface temperature of objects that they strike, with the interior temperature raised by conduction.

Microwave radiations are also characterized by long wavelengths and very low levels of radiant energy. Although microwave radiation has been considered for sterilization purposes [158–160], the major problem with its use has been the uneven heating achieved. It has also been applied to the inactivation of microorganisms in suspension [161–163] and in infant formula preparations [164], although the microwaves are not operating here, of course, as a source of dry heat. *Mycobacterium bovis* dried on to scalpel blades was destroyed after 4 min of microwave exposure [165]. Microwaves have also been used for the disinfection of contact lenses and urinary catheters [166]. The problems associated with the use of infrared and microwave radiations were discussed by Gardner and Peel [11] and by Mullin [153].

Validation of dry-heat processes can be achieved by determining the inactivation of a suitable dry-heat-resistant organism, such as spores of a non-toxigenic *Clostridium tetani* strain. As with steam sterilization, routine monitoring is undertaken by thermometric measurement. Chemical indicators provide a visual check that a process has taken place, but give no guarantee of sterility.

Lyophilization

Lyophilization is a process more commonly known as freeze-drying. The word is derived from Greek, and means "made solvent-loving". Lyophilization is a way of drying something that minimizes damage to its internal structure. Because lyophilization is a relatively complex and expensive form of drying, it is limited to those materials that are sensitive to heat and have delicate structures and substantial value. The preferred method of preservation in the biotechnology industry, lyophilization is regularly used to preserve vaccines, pharmaceuticals and other proteins. Freeze-drying is also used to preserve special food products, eliminating the need for refrigeration. Lyophilization is used by botanists to preserve flower samples indefinitely. Because the process of freeze-drying removes most of the water from the sample, freeze-dried materials become highly absorbent, and merely adding water can restore the sample to something close to its original state.

The energy and equipment costs of lyophilization are around 2–3 times higher than those of other drying methods. The drying cycle is also longer, about 24 h. First, the temperature of the sample is lowered to near freezing point. Then, the sample is inserted into a vacuum chamber. The more energetic molecules escape, lowering the temperature further, while the extremely low pressure causes water molecules to be drawn out of the sample. Attached to the vacuum chamber is a condenser, which converts the airborne moisture into liquid and siphons it away. Great care is taken throughout the process to ensure that the structure of the sample remains constant. For instance, the sample could merely be frozen by the vacuum rather than being frozen under atmospheric pressures, but that would cause shrinkage in the sample, damaging its structure irreversibly.

Mechanisms of microbial inactivation

It is highly unlikely that thermal inactivation results from a single event in a vegetative cell or a spore. There are several potential target sites in non-sporulating bacteria, ranging from the outer membrane of Gram-negative bacteria to the cytoplasmic membrane, ribonucleic acid (RNA) breakdown and protein coagulation [2, 6, 167, 168]. Virtually all structures and functions can be damaged by heat but repair to non-deoxyribonucleic acid (DNA) structures can occur only if DNA remains functional, thereby providing the necessary genetic information. A considerable body of evidence implicates the involvement of DNA in heat damage, probably as a result of enzymatic action after thermal injury [6, 169].

Brannen [170] presented experimental evidence in favor of the assumption that the principal mechanism for moist-heat inactivation of spores is DNA denaturation, whereas the *British Pharmacopoeia* [58], suggested that the site of injury is the spore structure destined to become the cell membrane or cell wall. In bacterial spores, thermal injury has, in fact, been attributed also to denaturation of vital spore enzymes, impairment of germination and outgrowth, membrane damage (leading to leakage of calcium dipicolinate), increased sensitivity to inhibitory agents, structural damage (as demonstrated by electron microscopy) and damage to the spore chromosome (shown by mutations or DNA strand breaks [2]). Effects on DNA are much more pronounced during dry heating, which generates a high level of mutants in spore populations by depurination of nucleotides [171].

Deficiencies in DNA repair mechanisms render spores more heat sensitive [171]. Thus, the ability to repair DNA after heating must be an important aspect of heat tolerance. Likewise, *B. subtilis* spores pretreated with ethidium bromide are rendered heat sensitive, the reason being an inability of the cells to repair heat-damaged DNA during outgrowth [172].

The germination system itself may, however, be a key target for heat inactivation [6]. Heated spores may be unable to initiate germination; with heated spores of some strains of clostridia, the presence of lysozyme in the recovery media aids revival, inducing germination by hydrolyzing cortex peptidoglycan. "Artificial" germinants, such as calcium dipicolinate, have similar effects, sometimes aiding the recovery of heated spores.

Considering the strong influence of A_w on the dry-heat resistance of spores, a possible explanation of dry-heat inactivation could be the removal of bound water, critical for maintaining the helical structure of proteins. This belief is stressed in investigations that show that a certain level of water is necessary for the maintenance of heat stability in spores. If the spores were strongly desiccated by high-vacuum drying, they would be sensitized to heat [173]. Furthermore, it has been shown that *B. subtilis* spores heated at lower A_w are inactivated in accordance with a constant *z*-value (23°C) over the temperature interval of 37–190°C [174]. Thus, in a dry environment the spores were inactivated at growth temperature (D_{37}-value 44 days) and this inactivation followed the same inactivation model as the one valid at high temperatures (140–190°C).

Mechanisms of spore resistance to heat

Improved means for spore inactivation would probably be facilitated if more was known about the mechanisms by which spores achieve their enormous resistances. Early theories about the possible mechanisms of spore resistance to thermal processes were discussed by Molin [175], Roberts and Hitchins [3, 14] and Gould [6].

The resistance of spores to moist heat can be manipulated over several orders of magnitude by exposure to extreme pH values or cationic-exchange treatment (respectively, the H or Ca form [176–178]). The content and location of water in the spore core have an important role to play, but spore coats do not contribute to thermal resistance. Spores have a low internal water content and Gould and colleagues [6, 179] found that resuspension of newly germinated spores in high concentrations of non-permeating solutes (sucrose or NaCl, but not glycerol) restored resistance to heat, presumably by osmotic dehydration. An osmoregulatory mechanism was proposed, by which the cortex would control the water content of the spore protoplast essentially by osmosis. An alternative theory to account for this was the "anisotropic swollen cortex by enzymatic cleavage" hypothesis put forward by Gould and Dring [180, 181]. There is abundant evidence, most recently from studies of mutants with defective peptidoglycan structure, that the peptidoglycan that makes up the cortex plays a major role in maintaining a low water content in the enclosed protoplast [182]. Peptidoglycan breakdown is one of the earliest events accompanying the return of heat sensitivity that occurs during spore germination [183].

Atrih *et al.* [184] proposed three types of mechanisms which would contribute to protein stability in spores, namely: they could be intrinsically stable; substances might be present which could help in stabilizing them; and the removal of water could alter their stability. The role of calcium dipicolinate in heat resistance has yet to be fully determined [6]. Several spore properties, however, are now known to be important for the heat resistance of spores. These include dehydration, but also mineralization, thermal adaptation and cortex function [185–190]. Small acid-soluble proteins (SASPs), found in the spore core [191], help to stabilize DNA. Spores lacking SASPs are more thermosensitive than wild-type spores, implicating DNA damage in spore inactivation [191] though heat resistance during sporulation is attained well after their synthesis. SASPs are thus not a major determinant of spore resistance to moist heat.

Conclusions

The various developments that aim to minimize heat damage to the components of foods and pharmaceuticals, while at the same time ensuring that the correct F_0 is delivered, will probably remain the most important targets in the near future. These will include the further exploitation of the newer heat delivery and packaging systems, but also improved, tighter control of conventional processes. Combination treatments, in which the thermal process is reduced and yet compensated for by other "hurdles", are already employed and probably set to find wider use as confidence in the procedures grows. Finally, radically new approaches, such as some of those summarized in Chapter 13, will probably continue to be more widely exploited in growing niche markets.

Acknowledgments

The author acknowledges the work of Grahame W. Gould for his development of the original text of this chapter which forms the basis for this revision.

References

1 Russell, A.D. *et al.* (1997) Synergistic sterilization. *PDA Journal of Pharmaceutical Science and Technology*, **51**, 174–175.

2 Russell, A.D. (1998) Microbial sensitivity and resistance to chemical and physical agents, in *Topley and Wilson's Microbiology and Microbial Infections, vol. 2, Systematic Bacteriology*, 9th edn, (eds A. Balows and B.I. Duerden), Arnold, London, pp. 149–184.

3 Russell, A.D. (1982) *The Destruction of Bacterial Spores*, Academic Press, London.

4 Russell, A.D. (1991) Fundamental aspects of microbial resistance to chemical and physical agents, in *Sterilization of Medical Products*, vol. V (eds R.F. Morrissey and Y.I. Prokopenko), Polyscience Publications, Morin Heights, Canada, pp. 22–42.

5 Russell, A.D. (1993) Theoretical mechanisms of microbial inactivation, in *Industrial Sterilization* Technology (eds R.F. Morrissey and G.B. Phillips), Van Nostrand Reinhold, New York, pp. 3–16.

6 Gould, G.W. (1989) Heat-induced injury and inactivation, in *Mechanisms of Action of Food Preservation Procedures* (ed. G.W. Gould), Elsevier Applied Science, London, pp. 11–42.

7 Dewhurst, E. and Hoxey, E.V. (1990) Sterilization methods, in *Guide to Microbiological Control in Pharmaceuticals* (eds S.P. Denyer and R.M. Baird), Ellis Horwood, Chichester, pp. 182–218.

8 Haberer, K. and Wallhaeusser, K.-H. (1990) Assurance of sterility by validation of the sterilization process, in *Guide of Microbiological Control in Pharmaceuticals* (eds S.P. Denyer and R.M. Baird), Ellis Horwood, Chichester, pp. 219–240.

9 Soper, C.J. and Davies, D.J.G. (1990) Principles of sterilization, in *Guide to Microbiological Control in Pharmaceuticals* (eds S.P. Denyer and R.M. Baird), Ellis Horwood, Chichester, pp. 156–181.

10 Taylor, D.M. (1999) Inactivation of prions by physical and chemical means. *Journal of Hospital Infection*, **43** (Suppl. 1), S69–S76.

11 Gardner, J.F. and Peel, M.M. (1991) Sterilization by dry heat, in *Introduction to Sterilization, Disinfection and Infection Control*, Churchill Livingstone, Edinburgh, pp. 60–69.

12 Rees, J.A.G. and Bettison, J. (eds) (1991) *Processing and Packaging of Heat Preserved Foods*, Blackie & Sons Ltd, Glasgow.

13 Richards, R.M.E., Fletcher, G. and Norton, D.A. (1963) Closures for eye drop bottles. *Pharmaceutical Journal*, **191**, 655–660.

14 Roberts, T.A. and Hitchins, A.D. (1969) Resistance of spores, in *The Bacterial Spore* (eds G.W. Gould and A. Hurst), Academic Press, London, pp. 611–670.

15 Wood, R.T. (1991) Dry heat sterilization, in *Sterilization of Medical Products*, vol. V (eds R.F. Morrissey and Y.I. Prokopenko), Polyscience Publications, Morin Heights, Canada, pp. 365–375.

16 Wood, R.T. (1993) Sterilization by dry heat, in *Sterilization Technology* (eds R.F. Morrissey and G.B. Phillips), Van Nostrand Reinhold, New York, pp. 81–119.

17 Medical Devices Directorate (1993) *Sterilization, Disinfection and Cleaning of Medical Equipment*, HMSO, London.

18 Owens, J.E. (1993) Sterilization of LVPs and SVPs, in *Sterilization Technology* (eds R.F. Morrissey and G.B. Phillips), Van Nostrand Reinhold, New York, pp. 254–285.

19 Young, J.H. (1993) Sterilization with steam under pressure, in *Sterilization Technology* (eds R.F. Morrissey and G.B. Phillips), Van Nostrand Reinhold, New York, pp. 120–151.

20 Brown, K.L. (1994) Spore resistance and ultra heat treatment processes. *Journal of Applied Bacteriology*, **76** (Suppl.), 67–80.

21 Holdsworth, S.D. (1997) *Thermal Processing of Packaged Foods*, Blackie Academic & Professional, London.

22 Denyer, S.P. and Hodges, N.A. (1998) Principles and practice of sterilization, in *Pharmaceutical Microbiology*, 6th edn (eds W.B. Hugo and A.D. Russell), Blackwell Scientific Publications, Oxford, pp. 385–409.

23 Pflug, I.J. and Gould, G.W. (2000) Heat treatment, in *The Microbiological Safety and Quality of Food* (eds B.M. Lund *et al.*), Aspen Publishers, Gaithersburg, MD, pp. 36–64.

24 Rutala, W.A., Weber, D.J. and HICPAC (2008) *Guidelines for Disinfection and Sterilization in Healtcare Facilities*, CDC, Atlanta, GA, pp. 58–61.

25 Bigelow, W.D. and Esty, J.R. (1920) Thermal death point in relation to time of typical thermophilic organisms. *Journal of Infectious Diseases*, **27**, 602–617.

26 Tucker, G.S. (1991) Development and use of numerical techniques for improved thermal process calculations and control. *Food Control*, **2**, 15–24.

27 Esty, J.R. and Meyer, K.E. (1922) The heat resistance of the spores of *B. botulinus* and allied anaerobes. XI. *Journal of Infectious Diseases*, **31**, 650–663.

28 Pflug, I.J. and Holcomb, R.G. (1977) Principles of thermal destruction of micro-organisms, in *Disinfection, Sterilization and Preservation* (ed. S.S. Block), Lea & Febiger, Philadelphia, pp. 933–994.

29 Moats, W.A. *et al.* (1971) Interpretation of non-logarithmic survivor curves of heated bacteria. *Journal of Food Science*, **36**, 523–526.

30 Cerf, O. (1977) Trailing of survival of bacterial spores. *Journal of Applied Bacteriology*, **42**, 1–19.

31 Sharpe, K. and Bektash, R.M. (1977) Heterogeneity and the modelling of bacterial spore death: the cause of continuously decreasing death rate. *Canadian Journal of Microbiology*, **23**, 1501–1507.

32 Han, Y.W. *et al.* (1976) Death rates of bacterial spores: mathematical models. *Canadian Journal of Microbiology*, **22**, 295–300.

33 Brown, K.L. and Gaze, J.E. (1988) High temperature resistance of bacterial spores. *Dairy Industries International*, **53** (10), 37–39.

34 McKee, S. and Gould, G.W. (1988) A simple mathematical model of the thermal death of micro-organisms. *Bulletin of Mathematical Biology*, **50**, 493–501.

35 Schlessinger, M.J. *et al.* (eds) (1982) *Heat Shock: from Bacteria to Man*, Cold Spring Harbor Laboratory Press, Cold Spring Harbor, NY.

36 Storz, G. and Hengge-Aronis, R. (eds) (2000) *Bacterial Stress Responses*, American Society for Microbiology, Washington, DC.

37 Bradley, C.R. and Fraise, A.P. (1996) Heat and chemical resistance of enterococci. *Journal of Hospital Infection*, **34**, 191–196.

38 Russell, A.D. and Hugo, W.B. (1987) Chemical disinfectants, in *Disinfection in Veterinary and Farm Animal Practice* (eds A.H. Linton *et al.*), Blackwell Scientific Publications, Oxford, pp. 12–42.

39 Alder, V.G. and Simpson, R.A. (1992) Heat sterilization. A. Sterilization and disinfection by heat methods, in *Principles and Practice of Disinfection, Preservation and Sterilization*, 2nd edn (eds A.D. Russell *et al.*), Blackwell Scientific Publications, Oxford, pp. 483–498.

40 Kilvington, S. (1989) Moist heat disinfection of pathogenic *Acanthamoeba* cysts. *Letters in Applied Microbiology*, **9**, 187–189.

41 Donnelly, L.S. and Busta, F.F. (1980) Heat resistance of *Desulfotomaculum nigrificans* spores in soy protein infant preparations. *Applied and Environmental Microbiology*, **40**, 712–724.

42 Taylor, D.M. (1987) Autoclaving standards for Creutzfeldt–Jakob disease agent. *Annals of Neurology*, **22**, 557–558.

43 Taylor, D.M. (1994) Decontamination studies with the agents of bovine spongiform encephalopathy and scrapie. *Archives of Virology*, **139**, 313–326.

44 Brown, P. *et al.* (1986) Newer data on the inactivation of scrapie virus and Creutzfield–Jacob disease virus in brain tissue. *Journal of Infectious Diseases*, **153**, 1145–1148.

45 Casolari, A. (1998) Heat resistance of prions and food processing. *Food Microbiology*, **15**, 59–63.

46 Oberthür, M. et al. (2006) *Ligand–Substrate Communication in Group 4 Aminopyridinato Complexes*, pp. 787–794.

47 Scruton, M.W. (1989) The effect of air with steam on the temperature of autoclave contents. *Journal of Hospital Infection*, **14**, 249–262.

48 Alder, V.G. and Gillespie, W.A. (1961) Disinfection of woollen blankets in steam at subatmospheric pressure. *Journal of Clinical Pathology*, **14**, 515–518.

49 ISO (2006) *17665-1:2006. Sterilization of Health Care Products – Moist Heat – Part 1: Requirements for the Development, Validation and Routine Control of A Sterilization Process for Medical Devices*, International Organization for Standardization, Geneva.

50 ISO/TS (2009) *17665-2:2009. Sterilization of Health Care Products – Moist Heat – Part 2: Guidance on the Application of ISO 17665-1*, International Organization for Standardization, Geneva.

51 NHS Estates/Department of Health (1994) *Health Technical Memorandum, HTM 2010. Sterilization*, British Standards Institute, London.

52 Ryan, J.P. *et al.* (1976) 3 in 1 hydrostatic cooker replaces 33 retorts. *Food Processing*, **37**, 54–56.

53 Groves, M.J. (1973) *Parenteral Products*, Heinemann, London.

54 Brizell, I.G. and Shatwell, J. (1973) Methods of detecting leaks in glass ampoules. *Pharmaceutical Journal*, **211**, 73–74.

55 Anon. (1992) *The Prevention and Detection of Leaks in Ampoules, Vials and Other Parenteral Containers*, Technical Monograph No. 3, Pharmatec.

56 Sharpe, J.R. (1988) Validation of a new form-fill-seal installation. *Manufacturing Chemist and Aerosol News*, **59**, 22, 23, 27, 55.

57 Allwood, M.C. (1998) Sterile pharmaceutical products, in *Pharmaceutical Microbiology*, 6th edn (eds W.B. Hugo and A.D. Russell), Blackwell Scientific Publications, Oxford, pp. 410–425.

58 Anon. (1998) *British Pharmacopoeia*, HMSO, London.

59 Allwood, M.C. *et al.* (1975) Pressure changes in bottles during sterilization by autoclaving. *Journal of Pharmaceutical Sciences*, **64**, 333–334.

60 Beverley, S. *et al.* (1974) Leakage of spray cooling water into topical water bottle. *Pharmaceutical Journal*, **213**, 306–308.

61 Coles, J. and Tredree, R.L. (1972) Contamination of autoclaved fluids with cooling water. *Pharmaceutical Journal*, **209**, 193–195.

62 Hambleton, R. and Allwood, M.C. (1976) Evaluation of a new design of bottle closure for non-injectable water. *Journal of Applied Bacteriology*, **14**, 109–118.

63 Wickner, H. (1973) Hospital pharmacy manufacturing of sterile fluids in plastic containers. *Svensk Farmaceutisk Tidskrift*, **77**, 773–777.

64 Hambleton, R. and Allwood, M.C. (1976) Containers and closures, in *Microbiological Hazards of Infusion Therapy* (eds L. Phillips *et al.*), MTP Press, Lancaster, pp. 3–12.

65 Schuck, L.J. (1974) Steam sterilization of solutions in plastic bottles. *Developments in Biological Standards*, **23**, 1–5.

66 Petrick, R.J. *et al.* (1977) Review of current knowledge of plastic intravenous fluid containers. *American Journal of Hospital Pharmacy*, **34**, 357–362.

67 Turco, S. and King, R.E. (1987) *Sterile Dosage Forms*, 3rd edn, Lea & Febiger, Philadelphia.

68 Allwood, M.C. (1990) Package design and product integrity, in *Guide to Microbiological Control in Pharmaceutical* (eds S. Denyer and R. Baird), Ellis Horwood, Chichester, pp. 341–355.

69 Allwood, M.C. (1978) Antimicrobial agents in single- and multi-dose injections. *Journal of Applied Bacteriology*, **44**, Svii–Sxiii.

70 Anon. (1966) *Pharmaceutical Society Laboratory Report P/66/7*.

71 Shaw, S. *et al.* (1972) Eye drop bottles. *Journal of Hospital Pharmacy*, **April**, 108.

72 Richards, R.M.E. *et al.* (1963) Closures for eye drop bottles. *Pharmaceutical Journal*, **191**, 655–660.

73 Norton, D.A. (1962) The properties of eye-drop bottles. *Pharmaceutical Journal*, **189**, 86–87.

74 Davies, D.J.G. (1978) Agents as preservatives in eye drops and contact lens solutions. *Journal of Applied Bacteriology*, **44** (Suppl.), xix–xxxiv.

75 Anon. (1959) *Medical Research Council, Report by Working Party on Pressure-Steam Sterilization*, HMSO, London.

76 Fallon, R.J. and Pyne, J.R. (1963) The sterilization of surgeons' gloves. *Lancet*, **i**, 1200–1202.

77 Knox, R. and Pickerill, J.K. (1964) Efficient air removal from steam sterilized dressing without the use of high vacuum. *Lancet*, **i**, 1318–1321.

78 Anon. (1993) *Sterilisation, Disinfection and Cleaning of Medical Equipment: Guidance on Decontamination*, Microbial Advisory Committee to Department of Health Medical Devices Directorate, HMSO, London.

79 Fallon, R.J. (1961) Monitoring of sterilization of dressing in high vacuum pressure-steam sterilizers. *Journal of Clinical Pathology*, **14**, 666–669.

80 Hancock, C.O. (1997) Steam sterilizer: sterilizer operation, in *Sterilization Technology for the Health Care Facility* (eds M. Reichert and J.H. Young), Aspen Publishers, Gaithersburg, MD, pp. 134–145.

81 Hancock, C.O. *et al.* (1994) Steam Sterilization, in *Central Service Technical Manual* (ed. C. Fluke *et al.*), International Association of Healthcare Central Service Material Management, Chicago, pp. 99–106.

82 Bowie, J.H. (1961) The control of heat sterilisers, in *Sterilization of Surgical Materials* (eds J.H. Bowie *et al.*), Pharmaceutical Press, London, pp. 109–142.

83 Sykes, G. (1958) The basis for "sufficient of a suitable bacteriostat" in injections. *Journal of Pharmacy and Pharmacology*, **10**, 40T–45T.

84 Sykes, G. (1965) *Disinfection and Sterilization*, 2nd edn, E. & F.N. Spon, London.

85 Hopkins, S.J. (1961) Central sterile supply in Cambridge hospitals, in *Sterilization of Surgical Materials* (eds J.H. Bowie *et al.*), Pharmaceutical Press, London, pp. 153–166.

86 Hunter, C.L.F. *et al.* (1961) Packaging papers as bacterial barriers, in *Sterilization of Surgical Materials* (eds J.H. Bowie *et al.*), Pharmaceutical Press, London, pp. 166–172.

87 Standard, P.G. *et al.* (1973) Microbial penetration through three types of double wrappers for sterile packs. *Applied Microbiology*, **26**, 59–62.

88 Bowie, J.H. *et al.* (1963) The Bowie and Dick autoclave tape test. *Lancet*, **i**, 586–587.

89 Schneider, P.M. *et al.* (2005) Performance of various steam sterilization indicators under optimum and sub-optimum exposure conditions. *American Journal of Infection Control*, **33** (5 Suppl. 2), S55–S67.

90 Swenson, D. *et al.* (2009) Steam sterilization validation for implementation of parametric release at a healthcare facility. *Biomedical Instrumentation and Technology*, **44** (2), 166–174.

91 Cantrell, S. (2005) Indicators of sterility: mechanical, chemical, biological. *Hospital Purchasing News*, http://www.hpnonline.com/inside/January%2005/0501biological.html (accessed June 12, 2012).

92 Williamson, J.E. (2005) Sterility Assurance Capabilities Elevated With Improved Products. *Hospital Purchasing News*, http://www.hpnonline.com/inside/October%2005/0510ProductsServices.html (accessed June 12, 2012).

93 Schembre, D.B. (2000) Infectious complications associated with gastrointestinal endoscopy. *Gastrointestinal Endoscopy Clinics of North America*, **10**, 215–232.

94 Spach, D.H. *et al.* (1993) Transmission of infection by gastrointestinal endoscopy and bronchoscopy. *Annals of Internal Medicine*, **118**, 117–128.

95 Weber, D.J. and Rutala, W.A. (2001) Lessons from outbreaks associated with bronchoscopy. *Infection Control and Hospital Epidemiology*, **22**, 403–408.

96 Weber, D.J. *et al.* (2002) The prevention of infection following gastrointestinal endoscopy: the importance of prophylaxis and reprocessing, in *Gastrointestinal Diseases: an Endoscopic Approach* (eds A.J. DiMarino, Jr. and S.B. Benjamin), Slack Inc., Thorofare, NJ, pp. 87–106.

97 Chu, N.S. and Favero, M. (2000) The microbial flora of the gastrointestinal tract and the cleaning of flexible endoscopes. *Gastrointestinal Endoscopy Clinics of North America*, **10**, 233–244.

98 Alfa, M.J. and Sitter, D.L. (1994) In-hospital evaluation of orthophthalaldehyde as a high level disinfectant for flexible endoscopes. *Journal of Hospital Infection*, **26**, 15–26.

99 Vesley, D. *et al.* (1999) Microbial bioburden in endoscope reprocessing and an in-use evaluation of the high-level disinfection capabilities of Cidex PA. *Gastroenterology Nursing*, **22**, 63–68.

100 Chu, N.S. *et al.* (1998) Natural bioburden levels detected on flexible gastrointestinal endoscopes after clinical use and manual cleaning. *Gastrointestinal Endoscopy*, **48**, 137–142.

101 Rutala, W.A. and Weber, D.J. (1995) FDA labeling requirements for disinfection of endoscopes: a counterpoint. *Infection Control and Hospital Epidemiology*, **16**, 231–235.

102 Rutala, W.A. and Weber, D.J. (2004) Reprocessing endoscopes: United States perspective. *Journal of Hospital Infection*, **56**, S27–S39.

103 Merighi, A. *et al.* (1996) Quality improvement in gastrointestinal endoscopy: microbiologic surveillance of disinfection. *Gastrointestinal Endoscopy*, **43**, 457–462.

104 Bond, W.W. (1998) Endoscope reprocessing: problems and solutions, in *Disinfection, Sterilization, and Antisepsis in Healthcare* (ed. W.A. Rutala), Polyscience Publications, Champlain, NY, pp. 151–163.

105 Pflug, I.J. *et al.* (1980) Measuring sterilization values in containers. *Journal of Food Protection*, **43**, 119–123.

106 Stumbo, C.R. (1973) *Thermobacteriology and Food Processing*, 2nd edn, Academic Press, New York.

107 Hersom, A.C. and Hulland, E.D. (1980) *Canned Foods: Thermal Processing and Microbiology*, 7th edn, Churchill Livingstone, London.

108 Pflug, I.J. (1982) *Textbook for an Introductory Course in the Microbiology and Engineering of Sterilization Processes*, Environmental Sterilization Laboratory, Minneapolis.

109 Pflug, I.J. (1982) *Selected Papers on the Microbiology and Engineering of Sterilization*, 4th edn, Environmental Sterilization Laboratory, Minneapolis.

110 Tucker, G.S. and Clark, P. (1989) *Computer Modelling for the Control of Sterilization Processes.*, Technical Memorandum No. 529, Campden Food and Drink Research Association, London.

111 Tucker, G.S. (1990) Evaluating thermal processes. *Food Manufacture*, **65** (6), 39–40.

112 Hamilton, R. (1990) Heat control in food processing. *Food Manufacture*, **65** (6), 33–36.

113 Braithwaite, P.J. and Perigo, J.A. (1971) The influence of pH, water activity and recovery temperature on the heat resistance and outgrowth of *Bacillus* spores, in *Spore Research 1971* (eds A.N. Barker *et al.*), Academic Press, London, pp. 189–302.

114 Leistner, L. (1995) Use of hurdle technology in food: recent advances, in *Food Preservation by Moisture Control: Fundamentals and Applications* (eds G.V. Barbosa-Canovas and G. Welti-Chanes), Technomic Publishing, Lancaster, PA, pp. 377–396.

115 Leistner, L. *et al.* (1981) Microbiology of meat and meat products in high and intermediate-moisture ranges, in *Water Activity: Influences on Food Quality*

(eds L.B. Rockland and G.F. Stewart), Academic Press, New York, pp. 855–916.

116 Leistner, L. and Gould, G.W. (2002) *Hurdle Technologies: Combination Treatments for Food Stability, Safety and Quality*, Kluwer Academic/Plenum Publishers, New York.

117 Leistner, L. (1995) Principles and applications of hurdle technology, in *New Methods of Food Preservation* (ed. G.W. Gould), Blackie Academic & Professional, Glasgow, pp. 2–21.

118 Anon. (1989) *Chill and Frozen: Guidelines on Cook–Chill and Cook–Freeze Catering Systems*, HMSO, London.

119 Gaze, J.E. *et al.* (1989) Heat resistance of *Listeria monocytogenes* in homogenates of chicken, beef steak and carrot. *Food Microbiology*, **6**, 251–259.

120 Mossel, D.A.A. and Struijk, C.A. (1991) Public health implications of refrigerated pasteurized ("sous-vide") foods. *International Journal of Food Microbiology*, **13**, 187–206.

121 ACMSF (1992) *Report on Vacuum Packaging and Associated Processes*, HMSO, London.

122 Notermans, S. *et al.* (1990) Botulism risk of refrigerated processed foods of extended durability. *Journal of Food Protection*, **53**, 1020–1024.

123 Lund, B.M. and Peck, M.W. (1994) Heat resistance and recovery of spores of non-proteolytic *Clostridium botulinum* in relation to refrigerated, processed foods with an extended shelf life. *Journal of Applied Bacteriology*, **76** (Suppl.), 115–128.

124 Gould, G.W. (1999) Sous vide foods: conclusions of ECFF Botulinum Working Party. *Food Control*, **10**, 47–51.

125 Mossel, D.A.A. *et al.* (1987) Human listeriosis transmitted by food in a general medical-microbiological perspective. *Journal of Food Protection*, **50**, 894–895.

126 Livingston, G.E. (1985) Extended shelf life chilled prepared foods. *Journal of Foodservice Systems*, **3**, 221–230.

127 Brown, M.H. and Gould, G.W. (1992) Processing, in *Chilled Foods: a Comprehensive Guide* (eds C. Dennis and M.F. Stringer), Ellis Horwood, London, pp. 111–146.

128 Alder, V.G. *et al.* (1966) Disinfection of heat-sensitive material by low-temperature steam and formaldehyde. *Journal of Clinical Pathology*, **19**, 83–89.

129 Alder, V.G. *et al.* (1971) Disinfection of cystoscopes by subatmospheric steam and formaldehyde at 80°C. *British Medical Journal*, **iii**, 677–680.

130 Line, S.J. and Pickerill, J.K. (1973) Testing a steam formaldehyde sterilizer for gas penetration efficiency. *Journal of Clinical Pathology*, **26**, 716–720.

131 Gibson, G.L. (1977) Processing urinary endoscopes in a low-temperature steam and formaldehyde autoclave. *Journal of Clinical Pathology*, **30**, 269–274.

132 Alder, V.G. (1987) The formaldehyde/low temperature steam sterilizing procedure. *Journal of Hospital Infection*, **9**, 194–200.

133 Hoxey, E.V. (1991) Low temperature steam formaldehyde, in *Sterilization of Medical Products*, vol. V (eds R.F. Morrissey and Y.I. Prokopenko), Polyscience Publications, Morin Heights, Canada, pp. 359–364.

134 Wright, A.M. *et al.* (1997) Biological indicators for low temperature steam formaldehyde and sterilization: effect of variations in recovery conditions on the response of spores of *Bacillus stearothermophilus* NCIMB 8224 to low temperature steam and formaldehyde. *Journal of Applied Microbiology*, **82**, 552–556.

135 Russell, A.D. (1991) Bacterial spores and chemical sporicidal agents. *Clinical Microbiology Reviews*, **3**, 99–119.

136 Berry, H. *et al.* (1938) The sterilization of thermolabile substances in the presence of bactericides. *Quarterly Journal of Pharmacy and Pharmacology*, **11**, 729–735.

137 Davies, G.E. and Davison, J.E. (1947) The use of antiseptics in the sterilization of solutions for injection. Part I. The efficiency of chlorocresol. *Quarterly Journal of Pharmacy and Pharmacology*, **20**, 212–218.

138 Davison, J.E. (1951) The use of antiseptics in the sterilization of solutions for injection. Part II. The efficiency of phenylmercuric nitrate. *Journal of Pharmacy and Pharmacology*, **3**, 734–738.

139 Sheffield, F.W. (1998) The manufacture and quality control of immunological products, in *Pharmaceutical Microbiology*, 6th edn (eds W.B. Hugo and A.D. Russell), Blackwell Scientific Publications, Oxford, pp. 304–320.

140 Babb, J.R. (1993) Methods of cleaning and disinfection. *Zentralblatt Sterilization*, **1**, 227–237.

141 Anon. (1993) *BS 2745 – 1: Washer-Disinfectors for Medical Purposes. Specification for General Requirements*, British Standards Institute, London.

142 Anon. (1995) *HTM 2030 – Washer-Disinfectors*, British Standards Institute, London.

143 Angelotti, R. (1978) Cooking requirements for cooked beef and roast beef. *Federal Register*, **43**, 30791–30793.

144 Dignan, D.M. *et al.* (1989) Safety considerations in establishing aseptic processes for low-acid foods containing particulates. *Food Technology*, **43** (3), 112–118, 131.

145 Hersom, A.C. and Shore, D.T. (1981) Aseptic processing of foods comprising sauce and solids. *Food Technology*, **35**, 53–62.

146 Dallyn, H. *et al.* (1977) Method for the immobilization of bacterial spores in alginate gel. *Laboratory Practice*, **26**, 773–775.

147 Warwick, D. (1990) Aseptics: the problems revealed. *Food Manufacture*, **65**, 49–50.

148 Bean, P.G. (1983) Developments in heat treatment processes for shelf-stable products, in *Food Microbiology: Advances and Prospects* (eds T.A. Roberts and F.A. Skinner), Academic Press, London, pp. 97–112.

149 Turtle, B.I. and Alderson, M.G. (1971) Sterilizable flexible packaging. *Food Manufacture*, **45**, 23, 48.

150 Aggett, P. (1990) New niche for processables. *Food Manufacture*, **65**, 43–46.

151 Goddard, R. (1990) Developments in aseptic packaging. *Food Manufacture*, **65** (10), 63–66.

152 Fryer, P. (1995) Electrical resistance heating of foods, in *New Methods of Food Preservation* (ed. G.W. Gould), Blackie Academic & Professional, Glasgow, pp. 205–235.

153 Mullin, J. (1995) Microware processing, in *New Methods of Food Preservation* (ed. G.W. Gould), Blackie Academic & Professional, Glasgow, pp. 112–134.

154 Ababouch, L.H. *et al.* (1995) Thermal inactivation kinetics of *Bacillus subtilis* spores suspended in buffer and in oils. *Journal of Applied Bacteriology*, **78**, 669–676.

155 Molin, G. and Östlund, K. (1975) Dry heat inactivation of *Bacillus subtilis* spores by means of infra-red heating. *Antonie van Leeuwenhoek/Journal of Microbiology and Serology*, **41**, 329–335.

156 Anon. (1962) *The Sterilization, Use and Care of Syringes*, MRC Memorandum No. 14, HMSO, London.

157 Cox, P.H. and Spanjers, F. (1970) The preparation of sterile implants by compression. *Overdurk Mit Pharmaceutisch Weekblad*, **105**, 681–684.

158 Rohrer, M.D. and Bulard, R.A. (1985) Microwave sterilization. *Journal of the American Dental Association*, **110**, 194–198.

159 Lohmann, S. and Manique, F. (1986) Microwave sterilization of vials. *Journal of Parenteral Science and Technology*, **40**, 25–30.

160 Jeng, D.K.H. *et al.* (1987) Mechanism of microwave sterilization in the dry state. *Applied and Environmental Microbiology*, **53**, 2133–2137.

161 Latimer, J.M. and Masten, J.M. (1977) Microwave oven irradiation as a method for bacterial decontamination in a clinical microbiology laboratory. *Journal of Clinical Microbiology*, **6**, 340–342.

162 Fujikawa, H. *et al.* (1992) Kinetics of *Escherichia coli* destruction by microwave irradiation. *Applied and Environmental Microbiology*, **58**, 920–924.

163 Fujikawa, H. and Ohta, K. (1994) Patterns of bacterial destruction in solutions by microwave irradiation. *Journal of Applied Bacteriology*, **76**, 389–394.

164 Kindle, G. *et al.* (1996) Killing activity of microwaves in milk. *Journal of Hospital Infection*, **33**, 273–278.

165 Rosaspina, S. *et al.* (1994) The bactericidal effect of microwaves on *Mycobacterium bovis* dried on scalpel blades. *Journal of Hospital Infection*, **26**, 45–50.

166 Douglas, C. *et al.* (1990) Microwave: practical cost-effective method for sterilizing urinary catheters in the home. *Urology*, **35**, 219–222.

167 Allwood, M.C. and Russell, A.D. (1970) Mechanisms of thermal injury in non-sporulating bacteria. *Advances in Applied Microbiology*, **12**, 89–119.

168 Russell, A.D. (1984) Potential sites of damage in microorganisms exposed to chemical or physical agents, in *The Revival of Injured Microbes*, Society for Applied Bacteriology Symposium Series No. 23 (eds M.H.E. Andrew and A.D. Russell), Academic Press, London, pp. 1–18.

169 Pellon, J.R. and Sinskey, A.J. (1984) Heat-induced damage to the bacterial chromosome and its repair, in *The Revival of Injured Microbes,* Society for Applied Bacteriology Symposium Series No. 12 (eds M.H.E. Andrew and A.D. Russell), Academic Press, London, pp. 105–125.

170 Brannen, J.P. (1970) On the role of DNA in wet heat sterilisation of microorganisms. *Journal of Theoretical Biology,* **27**, 425–432.

171 Flowers, R.S. and Adams, D.M. (1976) Spore membrane(s) as the site of damage within heated *Clostridium perfringens* spores. *Journal of Bacteriology,* **125**, 429–434.

172 Kadota, H. *et al.* (1978) Heat-induced DNA injury in spores and vegetative cells of *Bacillus subtilis,* in *Spores,* vol. VII (eds G. Chambliss and J.C. Vary), American Society for Microbiology, Washington, DC, pp. 115–137.

173 Hanlin, J.H. *et al.* (1985) Heat and UV light resistance of vegetative cells and spores of *Bacillus subtilis* Rec mutants. *Journal of Bacteriology,* **163**, 774–774.

174 Soper, C.J. and Davies, D.J.G. (1973) The effects of rehydration and oxygen on the heat resistance of high vacuum treated spores. *Journal of Applied Bacteriology,* **36**, 119–130.

175 Molin, G. (1977) Inactivation of *Bacillus* spores in dry systems at low and high temperatures. *Journal of General Microbiology,* **101**, 227–231.

176 Russell, A.D. (1971) The destruction of bacterial spores, in *Inhibition and Destruction of the Microbial Cell* (ed. W.B. Hugo), Academic Press, London, pp. 451–612.

177 Alderton, G. and Snell, N. (1963) Base exchange and heat resistance in bacterial spores. *Biochemical and Biophysical Research Communications,* **10**, 139–143.

178 Alderton, G. and Snell, N. (1969) Chemical states of bacterial spores: dry heat resistance. *Applied Microbiology,* **19**, 565–572.

179 Alderton, G. *et al.* (1980) Heat resistance of the chemical resistance forms of *Clostridium botulinum* 62A spores over the water activity range 0 to 0.9. *Applied and Environmental Microbiology,* **40**, 511–515.

180 Gould, G.W. and Dring, G.J. (1975) Role of expanded cortex in resistance of bacterial endospores, in *Spores VI* (eds P. Gerhardt *et al.*), American Society for Microbiology, Washington, DC, pp. 541–546.

181 Warth, A.D. (1977) Molecular structure of the bacterial spore. *Advances in Microbial Physiology,* **17**, 1–45.

182 Warth, A.D. (1978) Relationship between the heat resistance of spores and the optimum and maximum growth temperatures of *Bacillus* species. *Journal of Bacteriology,* **124**, 699–705.

183 Popham, D.L. *et al.* (1996) Muramic lactam in peptidoglycan of *Bacillus subtilis* spores is required for spore outgrowth but not for spore dehydration or heat resistance. *Proceedings of the National Academy of Sciences of the United States of America,* **93**, 15405–15410.

184 Atrih, A. *et al.* (1998) Peptidoglycan structural dynamics during germination of *Bacillus subtilis* 168 endospores. *Journal of Bacteriology,* **180**, 4603–4612.

185 Warth, A.D. (1985) Mechanisms of heat resistance, in *Fundamental and Applied Aspects of Bacterial Spores* (eds G.J. Dring *et al.*), Academic Press, London, pp. 209–225.

186 Murrell, W.G. (1981) Biophysical studies on the molecular mechanisms of spore heat resistance and dormancy, in *Sporulation and Germination* (eds H.S. Levinson *et al.*), American Society for Microbiology, Washington, DC, pp. 64–77.

187 Beaman, T.C. and Gerhardt, P. (1986) Heat resistance of bacterial spores correlated with protoplast dehydration, mineralization, and thermal adaptation. *Applied and Environmental Microbiology,* **52**, 1242–1246.

188 Beaman, T.C. *et al.* (1988) Heat shock affects permeability and resistance of *Bacillus stearothermophilus* spores. *Applied and Environmental Microbiology,* **54**, 2515–2520.

189 Beaman, T.C. *et al.* (1989) Low heat resistance of *Bacillus sphaericus* spores correlated with high protoplast water content. *FEMS Microbiology Letters,* **58**, 1–4.

190 Gerhardt, P. and Marquis, R.E. (1989) Spore thermo-resistance mechanisms, in *Regulation of Procaryotic Development* (eds I. Smith *et al.*), American Society for Microbiology, Washington, DC, pp. 17–63.

191 Marquis, R.E. *et al.* (1994) Molecular mechanisms of resistance to heat and oxidative damage. *Journal of Applied Bacteriology,* **76** (Suppl.), 40–48.

15.2   Radiation Sterilization

Peter A. Lambert

School of Life and Health Sciences, Aston University, Birmingham, UK

Introduction

Ionizing radiation in the form of γ-rays from radioactive isotopes (e.g. cobalt-60) or high speed electron beams (E-beams) produced by particle accelerators is widely used as an alternative to gaseous sterilization for the terminal sterilization of pharmaceutical or medical products. Advantages of the radiation process are high intrinsic process safety, fast throughput, parametric release of treated products, immediate usability without further testing, treatment in whole boxes (E-beam) or pallets (γ), treatment through dense packaging materials, easy process documentation and validation, cold process, and suitability for heat-sensitive goods. Disadvantages are that transport is required to and from the facility, and materials have to be qualified for the process. Radiation sterilization is mostly performed with medical devices, packaging materials, labware, raw materials, and some cosmetic and pharmaceutical goods. Approximately half of the medical devices that are sterilized today employ irradiation technology using γ-radiation produced by cobalt-60 radioactive sources. Issues such as the fluctuating cost, availability, transport and disposal of radioactive sources have led medical device manufacturers to evaluate alternative sterilization technologies such as X-rays. Although X-ray sterilization of medical products was first proposed over 40 years ago, its adoption has been slow because of the low output power of the early electron accelerators used to generate X-rays. Recent availability of high-power accelerators permits generation of high-energy X-rays suitable for sterilization processing; these are now becoming available through specialized commercial facilities.

Unlike γ-rays, electron beams and X-rays, ultraviolet (UV) light is not an ionizing radiation. It causes excitation of atoms within molecules, promoting electrons within their atomic orbitals, but does not remove them to produce ions. UV radiation has little penetrative power through solids and is extensively absorbed by glass and plastics. Sterilization of pharmaceutical and medical products would be achieved only by use of impracticably high irradiation levels [1, 2]. UV radiation does find some applications in disinfection rather than in sterilization procedures. For example, it has been employed in the disinfection of drinking water [3, 4], the production of pyrogen-free water [5] and especially in air disinfection (in combination with air filtration), notably in hospital wards and operating theaters, in aseptic laboratories and in safety cabinets designed for handling dangerous microorganisms [6]. It is important to emphasize that such UV radiation is an effective addition to other measures such as air filtration, but not a replacement, stand-alone technology for air sterilization [7].

This chapter will concentrate upon the most important features of γ-ray, X-ray and E-beam sterilization, including the nature and sources of radiation, mechanisms of microbial killing and resistance, choice of dose, control procedures and

Russell, Hugo & Ayliffe's: Principles and Practice of Disinfection, Preservation and Sterilization, Fifth Edition. Edited by Adam P. Fraise, Jean-Yves Maillard, and Syed A. Sattar.

Table 15.2.1 Properties of electromagnetic and particulate radiation.

Type of radiation	Example	Properties
Electromagnetic	γ-Rays	Short-wavelength ionizing radiation, high energy and penetrating power
	X-rays	Short-wavelength ionizing radiation, high energy and penetrating power
	Ultraviolet light	Excitation of electrons, non-ionizing radiation
	Infrared	Long wavelength, very low levels of radiant energy
	Microwaves	Long wavelength, very low levels of radiant energy
Particulate	α-Rays	Helium nuclei, charged and heavy, little penetrating power
	β-Rays	Electrons: when accelerated to very high speeds, gain energy and penetrating power

applications. Brief accounts will be given of UV radiation (mechanisms and applications) and the potential applications of the newer technologies.

Radiation energy

Types of radiation

Radiation can be classified into two groups, electromagnetic and particulate (Table 15.2.1). Electromagnetic radiation includes γ-rays, X-rays, UV and visible light, infrared rays and microwave energy. Particulate radiation includes α-rays, β-rays (high-speed electrons), neutrons and protons. In practice, only γ-rays and high-speed electrons have found usage as sterilization methods. Infrared radiation and microwaves raise the temperature of objects and therefore kill organisms by thermal effects, although the heating effect of microwaves can be uneven (see also Chapter 12).

X-rays and γ-rays are very short wavelength radiations. X-rays are produced by the direction of high-energy electron beams onto metal targets; γ-rays are emitted naturally from radioactive sources such as cobalt-60 (^{60}Co) and cesium-137 (^{137}Cs). High-speed electrons were originally produced from radioactive isotopes but had little penetrative power; subsequently, various machines were developed that accelerated atomic particles, thereby giving them the energies for penetrating materials more deeply [2, 8–10].

Units of nuclear radiation

Because nuclear radiation has an energy that is very high relative to the energies of chemical reactions, absorption of nuclear radiation by matter causes many chemical reactions to take place. When the target is living cells (including microbes), these chemical reactions cause serious injury or death. Quantitative measurement of nuclear radiation involves two types of units, those that measure physical nuclear radiation itself and those that measure the biological effect of nuclear radiation. Physical radiation units measure the activity of a source of radiation. The SI unit of physical nuclear radiation is the becquerel (Bq). A radiation source with an activity of 1 Bq has 1 nuclear disintegration per second.

Biological radiation units measure the effect of nuclear radiation on living tissue. The SI unit of biological radiation effect is the gray (Gy); 1 Gy corresponds to the transfer of 1 J of energy to 1 kg of living tissue. The older unit of rad (radiation absorbed dose) is equivalent to the transfer of 100 ergs to 1 g (0.01 J/kg) of tissue; 1 Gy is equal to 100 rad, so 25 kGy (the usual sterilizing dose) is equivalent to 2.5 Mrad.

Radiation sources

The properties required of a radioisotope as a source of γ-rays suitable for sterilization include: availability of the isotope in large quantity; provision of γ-rays with sufficient energy to penetrate deeply into packages; and a half-life sufficiently long to maintain a reasonably steady processing rate [11, 12]. Only ^{137}Cs and ^{60}Co have met these requirements and been found to be suitable for sterilization by γ-rays [13]. Most radionucleide sterilization facilities use ^{60}Co that is produced in a nuclear reactor by exposure of the naturally occurring element ^{59}Co to neutrons. ^{60}Co emits two γ-rays (photons) with energies of 1.33 and 1.17 MeV and one electron. With a half-life of 5.3 years, the radiation reduces by about 10% per year. ^{137}Cs is a fission product recovered from spent fuel elements in nuclear reactors. Its radiation comprises one photon (0.66 MeV) and one electron, with a half-life of approximately 30 years.

Irradiation of a product is carried out in a batch operation or, more commonly, as a continuous process. The irradiation source is shielded with concrete to protect personnel and the environment. In a batch procedure, the product is placed close to the radiation source and its position changed at intervals. In the continuous process, items are loaded onto a mechanical conveyer which passes them through the irradiation chamber, shifting the position of the product relative to the radiation source to obtain even exposure. The intensity of the radiation decreases as it penetrates the product, 10 cm of material with a density of 1 g/cm^3 reduces the intensity of radiation from ^{60}Co by 50%. Industrial γ-radiation plants use a ^{60}Co source of $1–4 \times 10^{16}$ Bq that is reloaded regularly to allow for the 10% annual reduction due to the radioactive decay of the source.

High-energy X-rays are high frequency, short wavelength electromagnetic photons. They are emitted when high-energy electrons impact upon a material that has a high atomic number. X-ray photons are produced by the electron interaction with orbital electrons; bremsstrahlung photons are produced by the interaction with the nucleus of the atom. These high-energy bremsstrahlung X-rays are a highly penetrating form of ionizing radiation. With X-ray energies of 5 and 7 MeV, product penetration is greater than that provided by γ-rays from an uncollimated

^{60}Co source. High-energy X-rays are ideal for sterilizing large packages and pallet loads of medical devices. In contrast to γ-rays, which are emitted in all directions from a ^{60}Co source, high-energy X-rays are concentrated in the direction of the incident electron beam, and their dispersion decreases as the electron energy increases [14].

Accelerators producing electron beams with energies of 5–10 MeV are suitable for radiation sterilization [15, 16]. High-intensity electron beams provide short exposure times with minimal degradation of product materials, but the beam is less penetrating than with γ-rays. Electron beams penetrate approximately 1 cm of material of density 1 g/cm^3 for each MeV. One advantage of electron beams over γ-rays is that the sources can be turned off and the beams are directional. As for γ-radiation plants, the electron beam source is shielded with concrete. This protects personnel and the environment from Röntgen rays that are generated when the electron beam strikes material of high density. Products are mechanically conveyed through the plant and irradiated from one or two sides; exposure times are much shorter than in γ-radiation plants. Details of the design aspects of each type of radiation sterilization facility are given in the review of radiation of healthcare products produced by the International Atomic Energy Agency (IAEA) [17].

Sensitivity and resistance of microorganisms to radiation

General aspects

As with other methods of sterilization, irradiation requires a compromise between inactivation of the contaminating microorganisms and damage to the product and container being sterilized. Ionizing radiations remove electrons from the atoms of the material through which they pass. The chemical and biological effects that kill contaminating organisms are produced by these electrons and through generation of highly reactive free radicals. Clearly these active species can also exert unwanted damaging effects on both the pharmaceutical product and the container materials.

Table 15.2.2 lists the relative sensitivities of microorganisms to ionizing radiation. Bacterial spores are generally the most resistant bacterial types to radiation, although *Deinococcus radiodurans* is the most resistant organism known [22], other than prions. Among the clostridial spores, *Clostridium botulinum* types A and B are the most resistant, with type E being highly sensitive. Among *Bacillus* spp., *Bacillus pumilus* E601 is probably the most resistant [23].

In general, multicellular organisms are more sensitive to radiation than are unicellular organisms. Gram-negative bacteria are more sensitive than Gram-positive ones. The most radiation-resistant fungi are about as resistant as those bacterial spores having moderate radiation resistance, and viruses in general are more resistant than bacteria. Some viruses exhibit high resistance to radiation with *D*-values (see below) around 5 kGy [24] while prions (containing no nucleic acid) are extremely resistant. The scrapie agent has a *D*-value of about 50 kGy [25]. It should be noted that the lethal dose for humans is 10 Gy or less.

Table 15.2.2 Radiation sensitivities of microorganisms to ionizing radiation.

Radiation response (D-value)^a	Examples
Sensitive (0.2 kGy)	Gram-negative bacteria
Moderately resistant (0.5–0.6 kGy)	Molds, yeasts and aerobic Gram-positive sporulating bacteria (e.g. *Bacillus subtilis*)
Resistant (2.2–3.3 kGy)	Spores of anaerobic Gram-positive bacteria (*Clostridium botulinum, Clostridium tetani*)
	Enterococcus faecium (dried from serum broth)
	Deinococcus radiodurans
	Most viruses
Highly resistant (4.5–50 kGy)	Foot-and-mouth disease virus, prions (bovine spongiform encephalopathy)

^{a}D-value denotes the radiation dose (kGy) necessary to reduce the viable cell number by 90%.
Table based on values from Thornley [18]; Russell [19]; Phillips [9]; Gardner and Peel [2]; Taylor [20]; and Farkas [21].

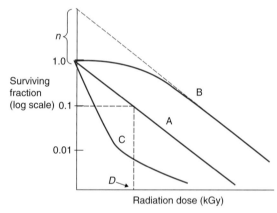

Figure 15.2.1 Different shapes of dose–response curve (A–C) that can be obtained when microorganisms are exposed to ionizing radiations. *D* represents the *D*-value, the radiation dose necessary to reduce the initial microbial population by 90% for an exponential death curve (A). Curve B represents the curve obtained for single hit killing with multiple targets in an organism, and *n* is the number of targets. Curve C represents results obtained for a population containing a small number of organisms with some resistance to radiation.

Microorganisms with a low resistance will not survive an exposure to a dose of radiation efficient enough to have a measurable influence on a very resistant microorganism, even when the number of sensitive cells is high. It must, however, be noted that enzymes, pyrogens, toxins and antigens of microbial origin are in general very radiation resistant compared with living cells. Therefore, the number of microorganisms present prior to radiation sterilization is of importance when dealing with medical products, regardless of the radiation resistance of the contaminating population.

Dose–response aspects

Figure 15.2.1 illustrates the different shapes of dose–response curve that can be obtained when microorganisms are exposed to ionizing radiations. Curve A represents an exponential rate of inactivation, which has been reported with some bacterial spores and several types of non-sporulating bacteria [18, 19, 26, 27]. The type A curve is represented by the equation:

$$N_t/N_0 = e^{-kD}$$

where N_0 and N_t are the numbers of viable cells at time zero and t respectively, after an absorbed dose of radiation D, and k is the inactivation rate constant.

Curve B is a more common type of response, in which an initial shoulder on the curve is followed by an exponential death rate. This pattern is found with various types of spores and with *D. radiodurans*, and under certain conditions with *Enterococcus faecium* [2, 19, 28–31]. The type B response can be represented by the following equation, which is derived on the basis that a single hit is necessary on more than one target to achieve cell inactivation:

$$N_t/N_0 = 1-\left(1-e^{-kD}\right)^n$$

where n is the number of targets. Equations have also been derived on the basis that more than one hit, that is multihits, on a single susceptible target is necessary to achieve cell inactivation [32].

The type C response, in which an exponential rate of kill is followed by a decreasing rate of spore inactivation, is encountered less frequently, although such "tailing-off" phenomena have been observed for sporing and non-sporulating bacteria [19]. The reasons for such an effect are unknown, but it may result from the production of radiation-resistant mutants or from non-homogeneous resistance in the microbial population. For practical sterilization purposes, the type C response is considered to be atypical.

Terminology

The D-value (kGy) is the radiation dose necessary to reduce the initial microbial population by 90% for an exponential death curve (e.g. curve A in Figure 15.2.1). It can be read directly from the dose–survival curve, or from the following equation:

$$D\text{-value} = \text{radiation dose}/\log N_0 - \log N$$

where N_0 and N represent a 1-log difference in viable numbers. The D_{37}-value is the radiation dose that reduces the microbial population to 37% of its original value. This term is based on the halfway point of a $\log_{10}$ scale (0.5) and equates to 37% survival.

The inactivation factor (IF) is the initial number of viable cells divided by the final number. It can also be calculated from the following equation:

$$IF = \text{radiation dose}/D\text{-value}$$

The degree of sterility can be calculated from:

IF/average number of organisms per article sterilized

Factors influencing sensitivity of irradiated microorganisms

Several factors affect the sensitivity of microorganisms to ionizing radiation [19, 21, 23]. As with other sterilization methods, the number of organisms present in the product being sterilized (the bioburden) determines the effective sterilizing dose. There are considerable differences in sensitivity of organisms within the same species. Pre-irradiation treatment also affects the susceptibility. Freeze-drying in the presence of sugars can exert a protective effect on subsequent radiation. Similarly, organisms dried from serum broth are much more resistant to radiation [28]. The presence of other agents can affect the response to radiation treatment. Oxygen present during or after irradiation increases sensitivity, as does hydrogen peroxide and ketones such as acetone and acetophenone (reviewed in [25]). The effect is presumably related to the generation of free radicals, including the hydroxyl radical, OH˙, and hydride radical, H˙, since the addition of radical scavengers eliminates the radiosensitization [33].

Mechanisms of lethal action
Microbial target site

In the case of radiation sterilization, microbial inactivation occurs either through direct ionization of a vital cellular molecule (DNA, key enzyme, etc.) or indirectly through the reaction of the free radicals produced in the cellular fluid. The main target sites of ionizing radiation in microorganisms are nucleic acids, principally DNA, but also RNA in RNA viruses. Additional damage may be caused to cell membranes and enzymes involved in nucleic acid repair [22, 29–31].

An exponential rate of kill (Figure 15.2.1, curve A), indicates that a single "hit" on the sensitive target site, DNA, is responsible for cell death. An initial lag period before an exponential rate of kill (Figure 15.2.1, curve B) suggests that multiple hits on DNA are needed to inactivate DNA, or that DNA repair mechanisms protect the organism (see below).

DNA damage

Ionizing radiations induce structural damage in microbial DNA, which, unless repaired, will inhibit DNA synthesis or cause some error in protein synthesis, leading to cell death [34]. Ionizing radiation produces highly reactive, short-lived hydroxyl radicals (OH˙) in water within microorganisms that cleave phosphodiester bonds in DNA, resulting in single-strand breaks (SSBs) or double-strand breaks (DSBs). Damage to the sugars and bases may also occur, for example the production of 5,6-dihydroxy-5,6-dihydrothymine from thymine (see Figure 15.2.3).

DNA repair

Mechanisms involved in DNA repair involve excision of modified bases and sealing SSB and DSB damage through recombination with undamaged daughter strands [19, 22, 31, 35–38].

Double-stranded breaks are more difficult to repair than SSBs. Very few DSBs are tolerated in organisms such as *Escherichia coli*, but they are much more likely to occur in radiation-resistant bacteria, such as *Deinococcus radiodurans*, with recombination being involved in the repair of a multiplicity of DSBs [39–41].

Although the group of small acid-soluble proteins (SASPs) present in bacterial spores play an important role in conferring heat resistance and UV resistance, they appear not to be involved in γ-radiation resistance [42–44]. Repair enzymes may be present in an inactive state in dormant spores and become activated during germination [45].

Choice of radiation dose
Dose to achieve a sterility assurance level
Sterilization is defined as a validated process that renders a product free from viable microorganisms. Because the killing process is described by an exponential function, the presence of viable microorganisms remaining on the individual item can only be expressed in terms of probability. While the probability may be reduced to a very low number by the sterilization process, it can never be reduced to zero. The probability can be expressed as a sterility assurance level (SAL), the probability of a viable microorganism being present on the product unit after sterilization.

The delivery of a radiation dose of 25 kGy (2.5 Mrad) is generally accepted as providing adequate assurance of sterility. The choice of a radiation dose of 25 kGy is based on the presterilization microbial contamination, the bioburden. The bioburden is an important factor influencing radiation efficacy. The lower the bioburden, the more effective the process will be. A dose of 25 kGy is sufficient provided that the bioburden does not exceed 100 microorganisms per item and that the organisms are not more resistant than *B. pumilus* [2]. In practice, a dose of 25 kGy has been found to be perfectly acceptable [46–49]. However, for some applications, sterilization doses below 25 kGy are required to avoid radiation damage to the product. This is particularly relevant for some polymers used in medical devices and human tissue such as bone, tendon and soft tissue allografts. These are discussed in the following section.

Effect of radiation dose upon the product
The radiation dose employed for sterilization should have no harmful effect on the product. This is difficult to achieve in practice since the mechanisms whereby ionizing radiation inactivates organisms also damage drug molecules [50], polymers [51] and tissues [52]. Although studies using radioprotective excipients (free radical scavengers) and cryo-irradiation demonstrate the feasibility of radiosterilization of drugs in aqueous solutions [53, 54], regulatory bodies require proof that the drug's potency is unaffected by the process, and proof that degradation products are not harmful [50]. Irradiation should not replace traditional methods of sterilization for common, large-volume parenterals, but can be considered seriously to sterilize powders for injection and small-volume parenterals that are sterilized by non-terminal processes.

Particular problems arise through adverse effects upon polymeric materials used for medical devices or containers [55, 56]. Acetabular cups used in prosthetic joints have shown changes in surface crystallinity caused by irradiation rather than mechanical friction during *in vitro* tests [57]. The mechanical toughness of polyethylene that has been sterilized by γ-irradiation in air decreases after a long shelf-life [58].

The potential for transmission of human immunodeficiency virus (HIV) type 1 has created serious concern for the continued clinical use of bone and soft tissue allografts. Studies on the γ-irradiation of frozen human bone transplants showed that a dose of 34 kGy is necessary for the sterilization of frozen bone transplants to achieve a reduction factor for viral infectivity titers of at least $4\text{-}\log_{10}$ [59]. However, these levels of irradiation are known to produce an unacceptable reduction in the mechanical integrity of bone [60, 61] and tendon allografts [62–64]. Validation of lower doses (e.g. 15 and 11 kGy) has been carried out for frozen bone allografts [65, 66]. The IAEA has produced recommendations for the radiation sterilization of tissue allografts [67, 68]. This code of practice sets out the requirements of a process for ensuring that the radiation sterilization of tissues produces standardized sterile tissue allografts suitable for safe clinical use. The approach is not applicable if viral contamination is identified and it is emphasized that the human donors of the tissues must be medically and serologically screened.

Standards and control procedures
ISO 11137 [49], produced by the International Organization of Standardization, is the key standard for validation and quality control of the process of radiation sterilization of healthcare products using γ-rays, X-rays and E-beams. It is published in three sections that discuss radiation sterilization, establish the sterilization dose for radiation sterilization, and cover dosimetric aspects of radiation sterilization [69–71]. Explanatory notes to clarify selected aspects of ISO 11137-1 [69] have been provided by the Microbiology Sub Group of the Panel on Electron and Gamma Irradiation [72]. Although this standard is limited to medical devices, it specifies requirements and provides guidance that may be applicable to other products and equipment. Most regulatory authorities expect radiation sterilization doses to be selected according to one of the methods described in ISO 11137. Revision of these standards is planned to accommodate and base them on the general standard for sterilization of healthcare products, ISO 14937 [73].

Radiation sterilization doses are selected according to one of the methods described in ISO 11137-2 [70]. Method 1, the most common method used, requires the average microbial contamination of representative samples of the product to be determined. The sterilizing dose needed for the average bioburden per sample and the desired SAL for the product is then determined. Method 2 does not require measurement of the bioburden of the product. It involves a series of experiments at increasing radiation doses to establish at which dose one in 100 samples will be non-sterile (i.e. an SAL of 10^{-2}). A sterilization dose is then established by extrapolation using a dose-resistance factor calculated from the incremental-dose experiments reflecting the remaining microbial resistance. An alternative method, the verification dose (VD$_{max}$) method, has been devised to substantiate use of a 25 kGy dose [47]. This method involves determination of the bioburden and a verification dose experiment. In substantiating the 25 kGy dose, the VD$_{max}$ method confirms that the bioburden on the product is less radiation resistant than a microbial population of maximal resistance, consistent with an SAL of 10^{-6} at 25 kGy. ISO 11137-2 also allows 25 kGy doses to be substantiated using methods 1 and 2. All methods require periodic audits to be carried out to confirm the appropriateness of the sterilization dose.

Biological indicators are not used for routine monitoring of the radiation sterilization process. The control of the irradiation plant must ensure that the recommended dose is delivered to all points within the product being sterilized. Radiation is accurately monitored by exposure of dosimeters within the load. ISO 11137-3 gives useful guidance on dosimetry used in the measurement of absorbed dose during radiation sterilization. Mathematical modeling may be used to estimate doses in certain applications. Calculations are performed to optimize the irradiation geometry to achieve the desired throughputs and dose homogeneity. Mathematical modeling can also be used to determine the radiation performance of the irradiator when filled with homogeneous product and to ensure that a sufficient number of dosimeters are distributed in the expected zones for minimum and maximum doses during irradiator dose mapping studies.

Uses of ionizing radiation

The major uses of ionizing radiation are for the sterilization of thermolabile medical items, as demonstrated in Table 15.2.3. Radiation sterilization has thus proved to be an invaluable industrial procedure. However, it must be pointed out that deleterious changes may occur in irradiated products, especially preparations in aqueous solutions where radiolysis of water contributes to the damage. For these reasons, radiation sterilization is usually reserved for articles in the dried state. Use of radioprotective excipients has been investigated for radiation sterilization of certain aqueous pharmaceuticals [53, 74]. Glass or plastic, such as polypropylene, can also be damaged.

The use of radiation for sterilizing foodstuffs is gaining recognition but remains a contentious issue. In the early 1980s, the World Health Organization (WHO) and the Food and Agriculture Organization (FAO) approved the use of radiation for the treatment of food with doses lower than an average of 10 kGy [75, 76]. The FAO estimate that 25% of all food production is lost to insects, bacteria and rodents after harvesting. Radiation has the potential to improve this situation in a number of ways: low-dose irradiation (1 kGy) causes sprout inhibition, delays ripening, inactivates parasites and aids insect disinfestation. Medium doses (1–10 kGy) reduce the number of spoilage organisms and pathogens in food, while high dosage (>10 kGy) reduces the numbers to sterility. These potential advantages of irradiation of foods have been likened to those of milk pasteurization. However, concerns remain over the destruction of vitamins, formation of lipid oxides imparting off-odours and tastes, and the generation of other radiolytic products from carbohydrates, proteins and lipids. Furthermore, food irradiation does not inactivate dangerous toxins that have already been produced by bacteria prior to irradiation. In some cases, such as *C. botulinum*, it is the toxin produced by the bacterium, rather than the bacterium itself, which poses the health hazard. Bacterial spores, viruses and prions can also survive the doses used to irradiate food [20, 77, 78], therefore simply destroying the bacteria does not guarantee that the food is safe. Summaries on radiation microbiology relative to food irradiation have been published [79–81].

In the USA, irradiation has been approved by the Food and Drug Administration (FDA) for the purpose of microbial disinfestation of meat, poultry, fresh fruits, vegetables and spices [82]. In Europe, the Framework Directive 1999/2/EC lays down general and technical aspects of food ingredients treated with ionizing radiation [83]. The Scientific Committee on Food advises the European Commission on key aspects of food irradiation. They have concluded that specific irradiation doses and food classes should only be endorsed in cases for which adequate toxicological, nutritional, microbiological and technical data are available [84]. Although there is an agreement among international committee experts that food is safe and wholesome for consumption after irradiation up to a dose of 10 kGy, there is no approval for irradiation of all foods up to this limit in any country. Most countries approve food irradiation on a case-by-case basis [85].

Ultraviolet radiation

Ultraviolet light encompasses light with wavelengths shorter than the violet end of the visible spectrum. Generally, light with wavelengths between 200–400 nm is considered to be UV light.

Table 15.2.3 Actual and potential uses of radiation sterilization procedures.

Type of product	Ionizing radiation suitable for
Medical and pharmaceutical	Disposable syringes, labware, culture media Sutures Tissue grafts (cartilage, tendon, skin, heart valves, bone) Some types of powders Adhesive and other dressings Intravenous infusion sets
Foodstuffs and animal feeds	Ionizing radiation widely used in USA but currently forbidden in EU except for dried herbs, spices and seasonings

The division into three ranges is connected with the human skin's sensitivity to ultraviolet light. The UVA range (315–400 nm) causes changes in the skin that lead to sun tanning, the UVB range (280–315 nm) causes sun burning, while the UVC range (200–280 nm) can lead to cell mutations and/or cell death. UVC is also called the germicidal range, since it is very effective at inactivating bacteria, viruses and some protozoan oocysts [86–88]. Most commercial UV lamps (i.e. low-pressure mercury arc lamps) emit UV light around 254 nm, which corresponds to the maximum absorbance of the bases in DNA [29, 86]. Commercially available UV light-emitting diodes (LEDs) emitting light in the 250–270 nm range have useful potential in water disinfection [89, 90] and those operating in the UVA range (365 nm) have been shown to be effective [91]. Because UV light cannot penetrate solid, opaque, light-absorbing objects, its main use is to disinfect surfaces, air and other materials such as water [2, 23]. Despite these limitations UVC is effective in the sterilization of platelet concentrates [92]. It is also used to destroy trace amounts of contaminating DNA in cabinets and apparatus used to handle DNA for manipulation by the polymerase chain reaction.

Survival curves following ultraviolet radiation

Survival curves of bacteria or bacterial spores exposed to UV light are generally of two types (Figure 15.2.2): a straight-line response against UV dose (line A), or an initial shoulder, followed by exponential death (curve B). The shoulder represents the action of effective DNA repair mechanisms in the irradiated organism. Many organisms have the ability to repair UV damage to their DNA. This activity is most pronounced in *Deinococcus radiodurans*, which is highly resistant to UV as well as to ionizing radiation.

Sensitivity to ultraviolet radiation

Bacterial spores are generally more resistant to UV radiation than are vegetative cells [43, 44, 86, 93, 94], although the degree

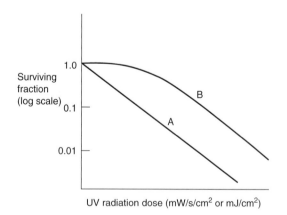

Figure 15.2.2 Survival curves for UV-exposed bacteria: (A) some non-sporulating bacteria (e.g. *Salmonella typhimurium*), and (B) bacterial spores and *Deinococcus radiodurans*.

of sporulation can influence the sensitivity. Some viruses are also inactivated by UV light; they are less resistant than bacterial spores but are often more resistant than non-sporulating bacteria [1]. Avian influenza virus H5N1 is inactivated by UV light in water [95] Rotaviruses are among the most resistant waterborne enteric viruses to UV disinfection [96]. Unenveloped viruses are more resistant to UV light than enveloped ones [97], but conventional virus types are considerably more susceptible than are prions. The Creutzfeldt–Jakob disease agent is highly resistant to UV radiation [98]; the agents of scrapie, kuru and BSE are likewise insusceptible [20, 99, 100]. Cysts of waterborne protozoa such as *Giardia lamblia* and *Cryptosporidium parvum* are more UV resistant than non-sporulating bacteria [101, 102]. The required UV light dose for a 2-$\log_{10}$ reduction in infectivity (99% inactivation) of *C. parvum* oocysts is approximately 1.0 mW/s/cm^2 (mJ/cm^2) at 20°C with an extremely high dose of 230 mW/s/cm^2 for a similar reduction in excystation [102].

Target site and inactivation

The major target site for UV radiation is DNA. Several types of damage have been found to occur in UV-treated bacteria. The most important event is the accumulation of photoproducts (Figure 15.2.3), particularly dimers between adjacent thymine residues in the same DNA strand [31, 103]. Low numbers of phosphodiester strand breaks, DNA intrastrand cross-links and nucleic acid–protein cross-links are also induced at high UV doses, but their significance in microbial inactivation is uncertain. Another type of photoproduct (5,6-dihydroxy-5,6-dihydrothymine; Figure 15.2.3) is found in *Deinococcus radiodurans*. In bacterial spores, a different photoproduct, 5-thyminyl-5,6-dihydrothymine, TDHT; Figure 15.2.3) is also induced.

Repair mechanisms

Unless removed, the photoproducts resulting from UV radiation form non-coding lesions in DNA, and cell death occurs. There are a number of repair mechanisms that operate after UV-induced damage to DNA.

1. Photoreactivation (light repair) is specific for pyrimidine dimers formed by UV. It uses high-wavelength UV light (near UV) and a photolyase enzyme to break the pyrimidine dimers and restore the wild-type sequence. Because this mechanism removes or replaces nucleotides, it is error-free.

2. Nucleotide excision repair (dark repair) also works on base dimers and any other base damage that results in distortion of the DNA. This mechanism involves a repair endonuclease (uvrABC) that removes the thymine dimer or modified bases along with some bases on either side of the lesion. The resulting single-stranded gap, about 12 nucleotides long, is filled by the action of DNA polymerase I and sealed by DNA ligase.

3. Recombination repair (or post-replication repair) is another form of dark repair that operates on damaged regions of DNA where bases are missing or there is damage on both strands. The

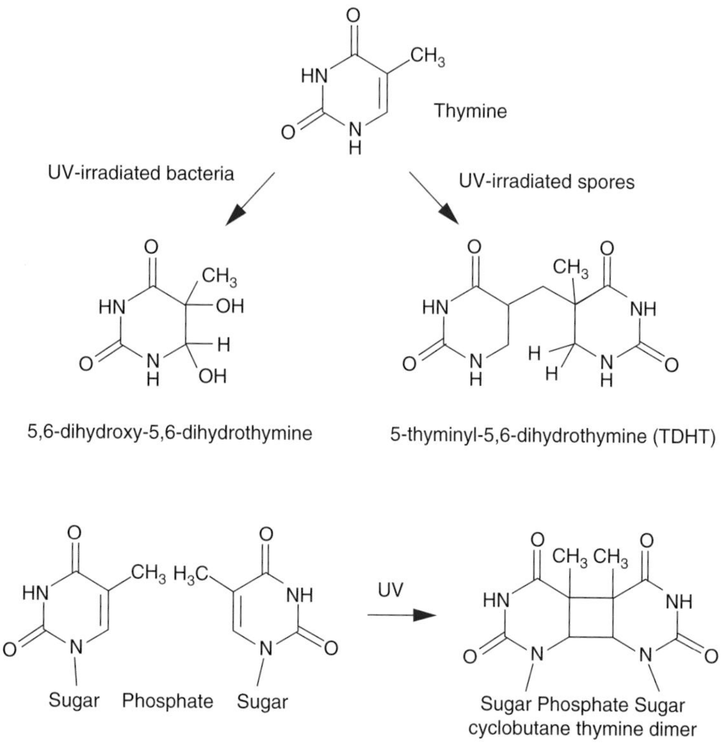

Figure 15.2.3 Formation of thymine dimmer and other photoproducts in irradiated DNA in bacteria and spores.

recA protein cuts a piece of DNA from a sister molecule (present in the same cell after chromosomal replication) and uses it to fill the gap or replace a damaged strand.

4. SOS repair is induced by single-stranded gaps and/or the presence of DNA degradation products. It operates when the DNA damage is extensive and can rapidly repair major damage caused by UV radiation. The recA protein binds to single-stranded DNA with adenosine triphosphate (ATP), forming recA nucleoprotein filaments. These trigger the action of DNA polymerase V, a low fidelity DNA polymerase that repairs DNA opposite thymine dimer sites by inserting any base. This error-prone process, called translesion DNA synthesis, causes the very broad spectrum of mutations following UV radiation [104].

Effect of ultraviolet radiation on bacterial spores
Inactivation and repair

Bacterial spores are more resistant than vegetative bacteria to UV radiation, and at certain times during germination spores become much more resistant. When bacterial spores are irradiated, thymine-containing photoproducts such as TDHT accumulate which are different from the thymine-containing cyclobutane dimers (Figure 15.2.3) produced in vegetative cells [42–44]. In spores, these non-cyclobutane photoproducts do not disappear after a photoreactivation process, but are eliminated from DNA by a light-independent spore photoproduct lyase, an iron–sulfur protein that uses *S*-adenosylmethionine to catalyze repair without strand breakage [105].

Role of small acid-soluble proteins

Some 10–20% of the protein in the core of the dormant spore occurs in the form of a group of SASPs [43, 44, 93]. These SASPs comprise α,β-types, which are associated with DNA and γ-types, which are not associated with any macromolecule. They are important because of their relationship to spore resistance to UV radiation and sodium hypochlorite. During germination, SASPs are rapidly degraded and are thus not found in vegetative cells of spore-forming species.

The α,β-type SASPs appear to coat the DNA in wild-type spores of *B. subtilis*. Spores (α⁻,β⁻) lacking such SASPs are significantly more sensitive to UV light [106], even more so than vegetative cells [107]. The reason for the increased sensitivity of α⁻,β⁻ spores is the reduced generation of spore photoproduct but the production of significant levels of thymine dimers.

During sporulation, UV resistance is acquired in parallel with α,β-type SASPs. The fore spores are, in fact, more UV resistant than the dormant spores. A possible reason for this is because dipicolinic acid (DPA), which sensitizes spore DNA to UV [108], is synthesized later in sporulation. Spores lacking DPA are resistant to UV [109]. During spore germination, DPA is lost well before SASP degradation occurs. Thus, during the first few minutes of germination, UV resistance increases above the level found in dormant spores. Subsequently, as α,β-type SASPs are degraded, UV sensitivity ensues. During germination, SASP degradation is initiated by a germination endoprotease (GPR), which cleaves SASP. If a mutation occurs in GPR, α,β-type SASP degradation is slowed, so that the hyper-resistance to UV radiation persists for a longer period during germination [110].

Ultraviolet radiation and hydrogen peroxide

Although bacterial spores are more resistant to UV light and to hydrogen peroxide than non-sporulating bacteria, simultaneous treatment of spores with far-UV radiation and peroxide produces a greatly enhanced rate of kill [111–113]. The most effective wavelength is around 270 nm, and it has been postulated that the action of the UV radiation in the combination is not directly on spore DNA but rather on the production of hydroxyl radicals from hydrogen peroxide [111].

One mechanism of sporicidal action of hydrogen peroxide is the generation of hydroxyl radicals, which cleave the DNA backbone [114]. The α,β-type SASPs saturate the spore chromosome and protect the DNA backbone against hydroxyl–radical cleavage. The α^-,β^- spores are much more sensitive than wild-type spores to peroxide [115].

Practical uses of ultraviolet radiation

Because it has little penetrative power through solids and is extensively absorbed by glass and plastics, UV radiation is not used for sterilization [2]. However, it is employed in the disinfection of drinking water [3, 88, 116] and air disinfection, notably in hospitals [6, 7], aseptic laboratories, aseptic isolator units, ventilated safety cabinets for handling dangerous microorganisms [1], as a bioterrorism countermeasure [117] and in food-handling premises. In air disinfection of rooms, UV irradiation is directed towards the upper portion of the room to protect any personnel working in these areas [118]. In contrast to this indirect irradiation, continuous irradiation from wall- or ceiling-fixed UV lamps can be employed, but any personnel present must wear protective clothing and adequate eye shields. Pulsed UV light has the potential for inactivation of bacterial pathogens in milk [119] and soft fruit [120]. The use of intense, short-duration pulses of broad-spectrum light has potential for food decontamination. The germicidal effect appears to be due to both photochemical and photothermal effects of the pulsed light [121]. Combinations of pulsed white light with UV or mild heat treatment have some potential to prevent fungal spoilage of soft fruit [122].

Other forms of radiation used in disinfection and sterilization

Heating through microwave irradiation has some potential for exploitation in the reduction of bioburden and disinfection. Although microwave irradiation offers a rapid means of energy transfer, uneven heating of the load remains a problem for sterilization purposes. Despite these restrictions a number of applications of microwave radiation for sterilization have been pursued. These include a continuous microwave system for sterilization of ampoules [123–125], a microwave-powered sterilizable port allowing aseptic access to a bioreactor [126] and a non-incineration microwave-assisted device for disposal of clinical waste [127]. Patient-operated microwave disinfection of soft contact lenses has also been evaluated [128, 129] and has shown to be an effective and cheap method for keeping contact lens cases free from *Acanthamoeba* [130]. Microwave treatment of whole dentures has been evaluated for denture disinfection, particularly as treatment of oral candidiasis [131] and denture stomatitis in immunocompromised patients [132, 133]. Microwaves have been considered for their ability to generate UV light *in situ* in containers [134] and to power electrode-less UV lamps for water disinfection [135].

Radiant heating through infrared irradiation has been investigated as a method for thermal sterilization [136]. Although effective in achieving a 10^{-6} SAL with *B. subtilis* spores, its application would be limited to heat-resistant instruments [137].

Another form of radiation evaluated for sterilization is high-intensity, broad-spectrum, pulsed light [121, 138]. These systems might be of use in surface decontamination of foods such as removal of *Salmonella* from egg shells [139, 140].

Cold oxygen plasma generated by subjecting air to high-energy UV radiation has been investigated for the removal of airborne respiratory viruses [141].

Conclusions

Commercial radiation sterilization has been used for more than 50 years; there are currently around 160 commercial ^{60}Co irradiators for radiation sterilization operating in 47 countries worldwide. Items sterilized in this way include: syringes, surgical gloves, gowns, masks, sticking plasters, dressings, artificial joints, food packaging, raw materials for pharmaceuticals and cosmetics. An increasing number of E-beam accelerators are also being operated. Commercial high-volume processing of medical devices sterilized with X-rays is expected to expand following the introduction of X-radiation sterilization facilities.

Irradiation of foodstuffs has met with much public resistance but may gradually be accepted in Europe as it has been in the USA. Acceptance of irradiation as a tool for food preservation is increasing but good manufacturing practices in all aspects of food production are still essential in order to produce safe food. Not all pathogenic spores and viruses will be destroyed by irradiation and, if food is not handled properly after irradiation, it can become contaminated. However, irradiation is a safe and effective means of destroying many foodborne pathogens and it should be useful in contributing to a safe food supply. Although UV light is much less useful as a sterilizing/disinfecting agent than ionizing radiation, it is nevertheless of value in air and water disinfection, especially for the control of waterborne protozoans.

References

1 Morris, E.J. (1972) The practical use of ultraviolet radiation for disinfection purposes. *Medical Laboratory Technology*, **29**, 41–47.

2 Gardner, J.F. and Peel, M.M. (1991) *Introduction to Sterilization, Disinfection and Infection Control*, 2nd edn, Churchill Livingstone, Edinburgh.

3 Angehrn, M. (1984) Ultraviolet disinfection of water. *Aqua*, **2**, 109–115.

4 Cook, A.M. and Saunders, L. (1962) Water for injection by ion-exchange. *Journal of Pharmacy and Pharmacology*, **14**, 83T–86T.

5 Lidwell, O.M. (1994) Ultraviolet radiation and the control of airborne contamination in the operating room. *Journal of Hospital Infection*, **28**, 245–248.

6 Reed, N.G. (2010) The history of ultraviolet germicidal irradiation for air disinfection. *Public Health Reports*, **125** (1), 15–27.

7 Memarzadeh, F. *et al.* (2010) Applications of ultraviolet germicidal irradiation disinfection in health care facilities: effective adjunct, but not stand-alone technology. *American Journal of Infection Control*, **38** (5, Suppl. 1), S13–S24.

8 Stewart, J.C. and Hawcroft, D.M. (1977) *A Manual of Radiobiology*, Sedgwick & Jackson, London.

9 Phillips, J.E. (1987). Physical methods of veterinary disinfection and sterilization, in *Disinfection in Veterinary and Farm Animal Practice* (eds A.H. Linton *et al.*), Blackwell Scientific Publications, Oxford, pp. 117–143.

10 Silverman, G.J. (1991) Sterilization and preservation by ionizing radiation, in *Disinfection, Sterilization and Preservation*, 4th edn (ed. S.S. Block), Lea & Febiger, Philadelphia, pp. 566–579.

11 Herring, C.M. and Saylor, M.C. (1993) Sterilization with radioisotopes, in *Sterilization Technology* (eds R.F. Morrissey and G.B. Phillips), Van Nostrand Reinhold, New York, pp. 196–217.

12 Jacobs, G.P. (1992) Gamma radiation sterilization, in *Encyclopedia of Pharmaceutical Technology*, vol. 6 (eds J. Swarbrick and J.C. Boylan), Marcel Dekker, New York, pp. 303–332.

13 Beers, E. (1990) Innovations in irradiator design. *Radiation Physics and Chemistry*, **35**, 539–546.

14 Meissner, J. (2008) X-ray sterilisation. *Medical Device Technology*, **19** (2), 12–14.

15 Cleland, M.R. and Beck, J.A. (1992) Electron beam sterilization, in *Encyclopedia of Pharmaceutical Technology*, vol. 5 (eds J. Swarbrick and J.C. Boylan), Marcel Dekker, New York, pp. 105–136.

16 Cleland, M.R. *et al.* (1993) Sterilization with accelerated electrons, in *Sterilization Technology* (eds R.E. Morrissey and G.B. Phillips), Van Nostrand Reinhold, New York, pp. 218–253.

17 International Atomic Energy Agency (2008) *Trends in Radiation Sterilization of Health Care Products*, IAEA, Vienna.

18 Thornley, M.J. (1963) Radiation resistance among bacteria. *Journal of Applied Bacteriology*, **26**, 334–345.

19 Russell, A.D. (1982) *The Destruction of Bacterial Spores*, Academic Press, London.

20 Taylor, D.M. (1991) Inactivation of BSE agent. *Developments in Biological Standardization*, **75**, 97–102.

21 Farkas, J. (1994) Tolerance of spores to ionizing radiation: mechanisms of inactivation, injury and repair. *Journal of Applied Bacteriology*, **76** (Suppl.), 81–90.

22 Moseley, B.E.B. (1989) Ionizing radiation: action and repair, in *Mechanisms of Action of Food Preservation Procedures* (ed. G.W. Gould), Elsevier Applied Science, London, pp. 43–70.

23 Russell, A.D. (1998) Microbial susceptibility and resistance to chemical and physical agents, in *Topley and Wilson's Microbiology and Microbial Infections*, vol. 2, 9th edn (eds A. Balows and B.I. Duerden), Edward Arnold, London, pp. 149–184.

24 Sullivan, R. *et al.* (1971) Inactivation of thirty viruses by gamma radiation. *Applied Microbiology*, **22**, 61–65.

25 Gibbs, C.F. *et al.* (1978) Unusual resistance to ionizing radiation of the viruses of kuru, Creutzfeldt–Jakob disease and scrapie. *Proceedings of the National Academy of Sciences of the United States of America*, **75**, 6268–6270.

26 Halls, N. (1992) The microbiology of irradiation sterilization. *Medical Device Technology*, **6**, 37–45.

27 Goldblith, S.A. (1971) The inhibition and destruction of the microbial cell by radiations, in *Inhibition and Destruction of the Microbial Cell* (ed. W.B. Hugo), Academic Press, London, pp. 285–305.

28 Christensen, E.A. and Kjems, E. (1965) The radiation resistance of substrains from *Streptococcus faecium* selected after irradiation of two different strains. *Acta Pathologica et Microbiologica Scandinavica. Section B, Microbiology*, **63**, 281–290.

29 Bridges, B.A. (1976) Survival of bacteria following exposure to ultraviolet and ionizing radiations, in *The Survival of Vegetative Microbes*, 26th Symposium of the Society for General Microbiology (eds T.G.R. Gray and J.R. Postgate), Cambridge University Press, Cambridge, pp. 183–208.

30 Moseley, B.E.B. and Williams, E. (1977) Repair of damaged DNA in bacteria. *Advances in Microbial Physiology*, **14**, 99–156.

31 Moseley, B.E.B. (1984) Radiation damage and its repair in non-sporulating bacteria, in *The Revival of Injured Microbes*, Society for Applied Bacteriology Symposium Series No. 12 (eds M.H.E. Andrew and A.D. Russell), Academic Press, London, pp. 147–174.

32 Soper, C.J. and Davies, D.J.G. (1990) Principles of sterilization, in *Guide to Microbiological Control in Pharmaceuticals* (eds S.P. Denyer and R.M. Baird), Ellis Horwood, Chichester, pp. 156–181.

33 Tallentire, A. and Jacobs, G.P. (1972) Radiosensitization of bacterial spores by ketonic agents of different electron affinities. *International Journal of Radiation Biology*, **21**, 205–213.

34 Hutchinson, F. (1985) Chemical changes induced in DNA by ionizing radiation. *Progress in Nucleic Acid Research and Molecular Biology*, **32**, 115–154.

35 Van Houten, B. and McCullough, A. (1994) Nucleotide excision repair in *E. coli*. *Annals of the New York Academy of Sciences*, **726**, 236–251.

36 Kuzminov, A. (1999) Recombinational repair of DNA damage in *Escherichia coli* and bacteriophage lambda. *Microbiology and Molecular Biology Reviews*, **63**, 751–813.

37 Kuzminov, A. (2001) DNA replication meets genetic exchange: chromosomal damage and its repair by homologous recombination. *Proceedings of the National Academy of Sciences of the United States of America*, **98**, 8461–8468.

38 Goosen, N. and Moolenaar, G.F. (2008) Repair of UV damage in bacteria. *DNA Repair (Amsterdam)*, **7** (3), 353–379.

39 Minton, K.W. (1994) DNA repair in the extremely radioresistant bacterium *Deinococcus radiodurans*. *Molecular Microbiology*, **13**, 9–15.

40 Battista, J.R. (1997) Against all odds: the survival strategies of *Deinococcus radiodurans*. *Annual Review of Microbiology*, **51**, 203–224.

41 Cox, M.M. *et al.* (2010) Rising from the ashes: DNA repair in *Deinococcus radiodurans*. *PLoS Genetics*, **6** (1), e1000815.

42 Setlow, P. (2001) Resistance of spores of *Bacillus* species to ultraviolet light. *Environmental and Molecular Mutagenesis*, **38**, 97–104.

43 Setlow, P. (2006) Spores of *Bacillus subtilis*: their resistance to and killing by radiation, heat and chemicals. *Journal of Applied Microbiology*, **101** (3), 514–525.

44 Setlow, P. (2007) I will survive: DNA protection in bacterial spores. *Trends in Microbiology*, **15** (4), 172–180.

45 Farkas, J. (1998) Irradiation as a method for decontaminating food. A review. *International Journal of Food Microbiology*, **44**, 189–204.

46 Lambert, B.J. and Hansen, J.M. (1998) ISO Radiation Sterilization Standards. *Radiation Physics and Chemistry*, **52** (1–6), 11–14.

47 Kowalski, J.B. and Tallentire, A. (2000) VDmax. A new method for substantiating 25 kGy. *Medical Device Technology*, **11** (4), 22–25.

48 Morrissey, R.F. and Herring, C.M. (2002) Radiation sterilization: past, present and future. *Radiation Physics and Chemistry*, **63** (3–6), 217–221.

49 International Organization for Standardization (ISO) (2006) *Sterilization of Health Care Products – Radiation, Part 1: Requirements for Development, Validation and Routine Control of a Sterilization Process for Medical Devices. Part 2: Establishing the Sterilization Dose. Part 3: Guidance on Dosimetric Aspects*, ISO 11137, ISO, Geneva.

50 Jacobs, G.P. (1995) A review of the effects of gamma radiation on pharmaceutical materials. *Journal of Biomaterials Applications*, **10** (1), 59–96.

51 Masefield, J. and Brinston, R. (2007) Radiation sterilisation of advanced drug-device combination products. *Medical Device Technology*, **18** (2), 12–14, 16.

52 Kamiński, A. *et al.* (2009) Mechanical properties of radiation-sterilised human bone-tendon-bone grafts preserved by different methods. *Cell and Tissue Banking*, **10** (3), 215–219.

53 Maquille, A. *et al.* (2008) Radiosterilization of drugs in aqueous solutions may be achieved by the use of radioprotective excipients. *International Journal of Pharmaceutics*, **349** (1–2), 74–82.

54 Maquille, A. *et al.* (2008) Cryo-irradiation as a terminal method for the sterilization of drug aqueous solutions. *European Journal of Pharmaceutics and Biopharmaceutics*, **69** (1), 358–363.

55 Ishigaki, I. *et al.* (1991) Radiation effects on polymeric materials, in *Sterilization of Medical Products*, vol. V (eds R.F. Morrissey and Y.I. Prokopenko), Polyscience Publications, Morin Heights, Canada, pp. 308–321.

56 Woo, L. and Purohit, K.S. (2002) Advancements and opportunities in sterilisation. *Medical Device Technology*, **13**, 12–17.

57 Affatato, S. *et al.* (2002) Effects of the sterilisation method on the wear of UHMWPE acetabular cups tested in a hip joint simulator. *Biomaterials*, **23**, 1439–1446.

58 McGovern, T.F. *et al.* (2002) Rapid polyethylene failure of unicondylar tibial components sterilized with gamma irradiation in air and implanted after a long shelf life. *Journal of Bone and Joint Surgery, American Volume*, **84**, 901–906.

59 Pruss, A. *et al.* (2002) Effect of gamma irradiation on human cortical bone transplants contaminated with enveloped and non-enveloped viruses. *Biologicals*, **30**, 125–133.

60 Currey, J.D. *et al.* (1997) Effects of ionizing radiation on the mechanical properties of human bone. *Journal of Orthopaedic Research*, **15**, 111–1117.

61 Akkus, O. and Rimnac, C.M. (2001) Fracture resistance of gamma radiation sterilized cortical bone allografts. *Journal of Orthopaedic Research*, **19**, 927–934.

62 Schwartz, H.E. *et al.* (2006) The effect of gamma irradiation on anterior cruciate ligament allograft biomechanical and biochemical properties in the caprine model at time zero and at 6 months after surgery. *American Journal of Sports Medicine*, **34** (11), 1747–1755.

63 McGilvray, K.C. *et al.* (2010) Effects of (60)Co gamma radiation dose on initial structural biomechanical properties of ovine bone-patellar tendon-bone allografts. *Cell and Tissue Banking*, **12**, 89–98.

64 Hoburg, A.T. *et al.* (2010) Effect of electron beam irradiation on biomechanical properties of patellar tendon allografts in anterior cruciate ligament reconstruction. *American Journal of Sports Medicine*, **38** (6), 1134–1140.

65 Nguyen, H. *et al.* (2008) Validation of 15 kGy as a radiation sterilisation dose for bone allografts manufactured at the Queensland Bone Bank: application of the VDmax 15 method. *Cell and Tissue Banking*, **9** (2), 139–147.

66 Nguyen, H. *et al.* (2010) Validation of 11 kGy as a radiation sterilization dose for frozen bone allografts. *Journal of Arthroplasty*, **26** (2), 303–308.

67 Anon. (2007) *Radiation Sterilization of Tissue Allografts: Requirements for Validation and Routine Control, a Code of Practice*, International Atomic Energy Agency, Vienna.

68 Hilmy, N. *et al.* (2007) Experiences using IAEA Code of Practice for radiation sterilization of tissue allografts: validation and routine control. *Radiation Physics and Chemistry*, **76** (11–12), 1751–1755.

69 International Organization for Standardization (ISO) (2006) 11137-1. *Sterilization of Health Care Products – Radiation – Part 1: Requirements for Development, Validation and Routine Control of a Sterilization Process for Medical Devices*, ISO, Geneva.

70 International Organization for Standardization (ISO) (2006) 11137-2. *Sterilization of Health Care Products – Radiation – Part 2: Establishing the Sterilization Dose*, ISO, Geneva.

71 International Organization for Standardization (ISO) (2006) 11137-3. *Sterilization of Health Care Products – Radiation – Part 3: Guidance on Dosimetric Aspects*, ISO, Geneva.

72 Panel on Gamma and Electron Irradiation (2010) *Explanatory Notes and Experience in Implementation of ISO11137-1 Interpretation of and experiences in the implementation of ISO11137-1: 2006*, Microbiology Group of the Panel on Electron and Gamma Irradiation, London.

73 International Organization for Standardization (ISO) (2009) 14937. *Sterilization of Health Care Products – General Requirements for Characterization of a Sterilizing Agent and the Development, Validation and Routine Control of a Sterilization Process for Medical Devices*, ISO, Geneva.

74 Terryn, H. *et al.* (2007) Irradiation of human insulin in aqueous solution, first step towards radiosterilization. *International Journal of Pharmaceutics*, **343** (1–2), 4–11.

75 World Health Organization (WHO) (1994) *Safety and Nutritional Adequacy of Irradiated Food*, WHO, Geneva.

76 Food and Agriculture Organization (FAO) and World Health Organization (WHO) (1984) *Codex General Standard for Irradiated Foods and Recommended International Code of Practice for the Operation of Radiation Facilities Used for the Treatment of Goods*. Codex Alimentarius Commission, vol. XV, 1st edn, FAO/WHO, Rome.

77 Maxcy, R.B. (1983) Significance of residual organisms in foods after substerilizing doses of gamma radiation: a review. *Journal of Food Safety*, **5** (4), 203–211.

78 Weissmann, C. *et al.* (2002) Transmission of prions. *Journal of Infectious Diseases*, **186** (Suppl. 2), 157–165.

79 Venugopal, V. *et al.* (1999) Radiation processing to improve the quality of fishery products. *Critical Reviews in Food Science and Nutrition*, **39**, 391–440.

80 Lado, B.H. and Yousef, A.E. (2002) Alternative food-preservation technologies: efficacy and mechanisms. *Microbes and Infection*, **4**, 433–440.

81 Morehouse, K.M. and Komolprasert, V. (2004) Irradiation of food and packaging: an overview, in *Irradiation of Food and Packaging*, ACS Symposium Series 875 (eds V. Komolprasert and K.M. Morehouse), American Chemical Society; Washington, DC, pp. 1–11.

82 Anon. (2010) *Code of Federal Regulations 21 CFR 179.26 – Ionizing Radiation for the Treatment of Food*, United States Government Printing Office, New York.

83 Anon. (1999) Directive 1999/2/EC of the European Parliament and of the Council of 22 February 1999 on the approximation of the laws of the Member States concerning foods and food ingredients treated with ionising radiation. *Official Journal of the European Communities*, 1999L0002-EN-20.11.2003-001. 001-1-12.

84 Anon. (2003) *Revision of the Opinion of the Scientific Committee on Food on the Irradiation of Food*, SCF/CS/NF/IRR/24, European Commission Health and Consumer Protection Directorate-General, Brussels.

85 Anon. (2009) List of Member States' authorisations of food and food ingredients which may be treated with ionising radiation. *Official Journal of the European Union*, **52**, C283/5.

86 Coohill, T.P. and Sagripanti, J.L. (2008) Overview of the inactivation by 254 nm ultraviolet radiation of bacteria with particular relevance to biodefense. *Photochemistry and Photobiology*, **84** (5), 1084–1090.

87 McDevitt, J.J. *et al.* (2007) Characterization of UVC light sensitivity of vaccinia virus. *Applied and Environmental Microbiology*, **73** (18), 5760–5766.

88 Hijnen, W.A. *et al.* (2006) Inactivation credit of UV radiation for viruses, bacteria and protozoan (oo)cysts in water: a review. *Water Research*, **40** (1), 3–22.

89 Vilhunen, S. *et al.* (2009) Ultraviolet light-emitting diodes in water disinfection. *Environmental Science and Pollution Research International*, **16** (4), 439–442.

90 Chatterley, C. and Linden, K. (2010) Demonstration and evaluation of germicidal UV-LEDs for point-of-use water disinfection. *Journal of Water and Health*, **8**, 479–486.

91 Hamamoto, A. *et al.* (2007) New water disinfection system using UVA light-emitting diodes. *Journal of Applied Microbiology*, **103** (6), 2291–2298.

92 Mohr, H. *et al.* (2009) Sterilization of platelet concentrates at production scale by irradiation with short-wave ultraviolet light. *Transfusion*, **49** (9), 1956–1963.

93 Moeller, R. *et al.* (2009) Roles of small, acid-soluble spore proteins and core water content in survival of *Bacillus subtilis* spores exposed to environmental solar UV radiation. *Applied and Environmental Microbiology*, **75** (16), 5202–5208.

94 Coohill, T.P. and Sagripanti, J.L. (2009) Bacterial inactivation by solar ultraviolet radiation compared with sensitivity to 254 nm radiation. *Photochemistry and Photobiology*, **85** (5), 1043–1052.

95 Lénès, D. *et al.* (2010) Assessment of the removal and inactivation of influenza viruses H5N1 and H1N1 by drinking water treatment. *Water Research*, **44** (8), 2473–2486.

96 Gerba, C.P. *et al.* (2002) Comparative inactivation of enteroviruses and adenovirus 2 by UV light. *Applied and Environmental Microbiology*, **68**, 5167–5169.

97 Li, D. *et al.* (2009) UV inactivation and resistance of rotavirus evaluated by integrated cell culture and real-time RT-PCR assay. *Water Research*, **43** (13), 3261–3269.

98 Rappaport, E.B. (1987) Iatrogenic Creutzfeldt–Jakob disease. *Neurology*, **37**, 1520–1522.

99 Latarjet, R. (1979) Inactivation of the agents of scrapie, Creutzfeldt–Jakob disease and kuru by radiations, in *Slow Transmissible Diseases of the Nervous System*, vol. 2 (eds S.B. Prusiner and W.J. Hadlow), Academic Press, London, pp. 387–407.

100 Bellinger-Kawahara, C. *et al.* (1987) Purified scrapie prions resist inactivation by UV irradiation. *Journal of Virology*, **61** (1), 159–166.

101 Linden, K.G. *et al.* (2002) UV disinfection of *Giardia lamblia* cysts in water. *Environmental Science and Technology*, **36**, 2519–2522.

102 Morita, S. *et al.* (2002) Efficacy of UV irradiation in inactivating *Cryptosporidium parvum* oocysts. *Applied and Environmental Microbiology*, **68**, 5387–5393.

103 Sinha, R.P. and Häder, D.P. (2002) UV-induced DNA damage and repair: a review. *Photochemical and Photobiological Sciences*, **1** (4), 225–236.

104 Patel, M. *et al.* (2010) A new model for SOS-induced mutagenesis: how RecA protein activates DNA polymerase V. *Critical Reviews in Biochemistry and Molecular Biology*, **45** (3), 171–184.

105 Donnellan, J.E. and Stafford, R.S. (1968) The ultraviolet photochemistry and photobiology of vegetative cells and spores of *Bacillus megaterium*. *Biophysical Journal*, **8**, 17–28.

106 Mason, J.M. and Setlow, P. (1986) Essential role of small, acid-soluble spore proteins in resistance of *Bacillus subtilis* spores to UV light. *Journal of Bacteriology*, **167**, 174–178.

107 Setlow, P. (1992) I will survive: protecting and repairing spore DNA. *Journal of Bacteriology*, **174**, 2737–2741.

108 Douki, T. *et al.* (2005) Photosensitization of DNA by dipicolinic acid, a major component of spores of *Bacillus* species. *Photochemical and Photobiological Sciences*, **4** (8), 591–597.

109 Paidhungat, M. *et al.* (2000) Characterization of spores of *Bacillus subtilis* which lack dipicolinic acid. *Journal of Bacteriology*, **182** (19), 5505–5512.

110 Sanchez-Salas, J.-L. and Setlow, P. (1993) Proteolytic processing of the protease which initiates degradation of small, acid-soluble, proteins during germination of *Bacillus subtilis* spores. *Journal of Bacteriology*, **175**, 2568–2577.

111 Waites, W.M. *et al.* (1988) The destruction of spores of *Bacillus subtilis* by the combined effects of hydrogen peroxide and ultraviolet light. *Letters in Applied Microbiology*, **7**, 139–140.

112 Rutherford, G.C. *et al.* (2000) Method to sensitize bacterial spores to subsequent killing by dry heat or ultraviolet irradiation. *Journal of Microbiological Methods*, **42** (3), 281–290.

113 Reidmiller, J.S. *et al.* (2003) Characterization of UV-peroxide killing of bacterial spores. *Journal of Food Protection*, **66** (7), 1233–1240.

114 Imlay, J.A. and Linn, S. (1988) DNA damage and oxygen radical toxicity. *Science*, **240**, 1302–1309.

115 Setlow, P. (1994) Mechanisms which contribute to the long-term survival of spores of *Bacillus* species. *Journal of Applied Bacteriology*, **76** (Suppl.), 49–60.

116 Rose, J.B. *et al.* (2002) Risk and control of waterborne cryptosporidiosis. *FEMS Microbiology Reviews*, **26**, 113–123.

117 Brickner, P.W. *et al.* (2003) The application of ultraviolet germicidal irradiation to control transmission of airborne disease: bioterrorism countermeasure. *Public Health Reports*, **118** (2), 99–114.

118 Nardell, E.A. *et al.* (2008) Safety of upper-room ultraviolet germicidal air disinfection for room occupants: results from the Tuberculosis Ultraviolet Shelter Study. *Public Health Reports*, **123** (1), 52–60.

119 Krishnamurthy, K. *et al.* (2007) Inactivation of *Staphylococcus aureus* in milk using flow-through pulsed UV-light treatment system. *Journal of Food Science*, **72** (7), M233–M239.

120 Bialka, K.L. and Demirci, A. (2008) Efficacy of pulsed UV-light for the decontamination of *Escherichia coli* O157:H7 and *Salmonella* spp. on raspberries and strawberries. *Journal of Food Science*, **73** (5), M201–M207.

121 Elmnasser, N. *et al.* (2007) Pulsed-light system as a novel food decontamination technology: a review. *Canadian Journal of Microbiology*, **53** (7), 813–821.

122 Marquenie, D. *et al.* (2003) Combinations of pulsed white light and UV-C or mild heat treatment to inactivate conidia of *Botrytis cinerea* and *Monilia fructigena*. *International Journal of Food Microbiology*, **85** (1–2), 185–196.

123 Sasaki, K. *et al.* (1996) Microwave continuous sterilization of injection ampoules. *PDA Journal of Pharmaceutical Science and Technology*, **50**, 172–179.

124 Sasaki, K. *et al.* (1998) Evaluation of high-temperature and short-time sterilization of injection ampules by microwave heating. *PDA Journal of Pharmaceutical Science and Technology*, **52**, 5–12.

125 Sasaki, K. *et al.* (1999) Validation of a microwave sterilizer for injection ampules. *PDA Journal of Pharmaceutical Science and Technology*, **53**, 60–69.

126 Atwater, J.E. *et al.* (2001) A microwave-powered sterilizable interface for aseptic access to bioreactors that are vulnerable to microbial contamination. *Biotechnology Progress*, **17**, 847–851.

127 Veronesi, P. *et al.* (2007) Non-incineration microwave assisted sterilization of medical waste. *Journal of Microwave Power and Electromagnetic Energy*, **40** (4), 211–218.

128 Crabbe, A. and Thompson, P. (2001) Effects of microwave irradiation on the parameters of hydrogel contact lenses. *Optometry and Vision Science*, **78**, 610–615.

129 Crabbe, A. and Thompson, P. (2004) Testing of a dual-mode microwave care regimen for hydrogel lenses. *Optometry and Vision Science*, **81** (6), 471–477.

130 Hiti, K. *et al.* (2001) Microwave treatment of contact lens cases contaminated with *Acanthamoeba*. *Cornea*, **20**, 467–470.

131 Banting, D.W. and Hill, S.A. (2001) Microwave disinfection of dentures for the treatment of oral candidiasis. *Special Care in Dentistry*, **21**, 4–8.

132 Ribeiro, D.G. *et al.* (2009) Denture disinfection by microwave irradiation: a randomized clinical study. *Journal of Dentistry*, **37** (9), 666–672.

133 Sanitá, P.V. *et al.* (2009) Growth of *Candida* species on complete dentures: effect of microwave disinfection. *Mycoses*, **52** (2), 154–160.

134 Devine, D.A. *et al.* (2001) Ultraviolet disinfection with a novel microwave-powered device. *Journal of Applied Microbiology*, **91**, 786–794.

135 Bergmann, H. *et al.* (2002) New UV irradiation and direct electrolysis – promising methods for water disinfection. *Chemical Engineering Journal*, **85**, 111–117.

136 Sawai, J. *et al.* (2006) Characteristics of the inactivation of *Escherichia coli* by infrared irradiative heating. *Biocontrol Science*, **11** (2), 85–90.

137 Mata-Portuguez, V.H. *et al.* (2002) Sterilization of heat-resistant instruments with infrared radiation. *Infection Control and Hospital Epidemiology*, **23**, 393–396.

138 Wallen, R.D. *et al.* (2001) Sterilization of a new medical device using broad-spectrum pulsed light. *Biomedical Instrumentation and Technology/Association for the Advancement of Medical Instrumentation*, **35**, 323–330.

139 Hierro, E. *et al.* (2009) Inactivation of *Salmonella enterica* serovar Enteritidis on shell eggs by pulsed light technology. *International Journal of Food Microbiology*, **135** (2), 125–130.

140 Keklik, N.M. *et al.* (2010) Pulsed UV light inactivation of *Salmonella enteritidis* on eggshells and its effects on egg quality. *Journal of Food Protection*, **73** (8), 1408–1415.

141 Terrier, O. *et al.* (2009) Cold oxygen plasma technology efficiency against different airborne respiratory viruses. *Journal of Clinical Virology*, **45** (2), 119–124.

15.3 Gaseous Sterilization

Jean-Yves Dusseau[1], Patrick Duroselle[2] and Jean Freney[3]

[1] Unité d'Hygiène, CHI Annemasse-Bonneville, Annemasse; Unité d'Hygiène, Hôpitaux du Léman, Thonon-les-Bains, France
[2] Sète, France
[3] Institut des Sciences Pharmaceutiques et Biologiques, UMR 5557 – CNRS Ecologie Microbienne, Bactéries pathogènes Opportunistes et Environnement, Université Lyon 1, Lyon, France

Introduction

One of the oldest references regarding gas disinfection was reported by Homer in song XXII of the *Odyssey*. When Ulysses returned to his palace in Ithaca after killed all his wife's suitors, and following his coronation, he asked his old servant Euryclea to disinfect the banquet room by burning sulfur. This process was also used in patients' rooms during the Great Plague epidemic of the 14th century. During the same period, the burning of juniper branches was also recommended.

Louis-Bernard Guyton de Morveau (1737–1816), one of the greatest chemists of all time, was a pioneer of the disinfection of hospitals and prisons. During the hard winter of 1773, it was impossible to bury cadavers in the cemeteries of Burgundy (France). The corpses were placed in the cathedral of Saint Etienne in Dijon. The decomposition of the corpses produced a horrible odor which led Guyton de Morveau to propose combating it using chlorine gas. This was produced by heating sulfuric acid (vitriol) and sea salt. After 2 days, the bad odors disappeared. This process was then used to disinfect prisons in a town where an epidemic took place. Later, the method was modified by replacing chlorhydric acid with chlorine.

At the end of the 19th century, rooms occupied by infectious patients were disinfected with formaldehyde. A major step forward in sterilization was taken by Charles Chamberland (a close co-worker of Louis Pasteur) who invented the first steam sterilizers. This process is fast, efficient, easy to use and inexpensive and has remained until today the main method used to sterilize reusable medical devices [1, 2].

In recent decades, medical practice in developed countries has been influenced by numerous modifications of medical/surgical devices used in diagnostic and therapy with a rapid proliferation of minimally invasive approaches; a good example here is endoscopic surgery. Indeed, many such devices are not only heat and moisture sensitive but are also increasingly complex and fragile with several narrow lumens and channels (see also Chapter 19.3). Concurrently, the number of immunocompromised patients is on the rise. These factors together are catalyzing a general and rapid evolution in methods for disinfecting and sterilizing medical/surgical devices between patients. This is being achieved by refining old technologies and introducing new ones [3–7].

Before discussing procedures for low-temperature gaseous sterilization, "disinfection" and "sterilization" must be clearly defined. While "sterility" is a state of being free from all living microorganisms, in practice it is a probability function, such as the probability of a microorganism surviving being one in a million [8]. Infections linked to an incorrect treatment of reusable medical devices shows the importance of the choice of the procedure and of its strict application. In all such procedures, thorough pre-cleaning is always essential.

Suitable alternatives to conventional autoclaving are essential when fragile devices are to be reprocessed on a regular basis. Gaseous sterilization with ethylene oxide is one such alternative,

Russell, Hugo & Ayliffe's: Principles and Practice of Disinfection, Preservation and Sterilization, Fifth Edition. Edited by Adam P. Fraise, Jean-Yves Maillard, and Syed A. Sattar.
© 2013 Blackwell Publishing Ltd. Published 2013 by Blackwell Publishing Ltd.

which was in wide use following the studies by Charles R. Phillips and Saul Kaye at the US Army Chemical Corps (Fort Detrick, MD) in 1949 [9]. Recent years have seen a reduction in the use of ethylene oxide due to concerns with toxicity to humans and the environment, escalating costs and tighter regulations [10–14]. Formaldehyde sterilization also has drawbacks with its use now being permitted in only certain countries [15]. Other methods of low-temperature sterilization are based on hydrogen peroxide, peracetic acid, ozone and chlorine dioxide [1, 3, 6, 7], and also the use of cold plasma obtained from certain molecules mentioned above. A major limitation of low-temperature technologies remains their performance validation [7].

General principles

Characteristics of an ideal low-temperature gaseous sterilizing agent

While the properties of an ideal gas for sterilization are numerous [1, 5, 7, 13, 16, 17] no sterilizing chemical possesses all of those characteristics (Table 15.3.1):
• Broad-spectrum microbicidal activity: bactericidal, tuberculocidal, virucidal, fungicidal and sporicidal.
• Rapid activity: achieve sterilization quickly and below 65°C.
• Resistance to organic and inorganic materials: withstand a reasonable amount of soil without loss of microbicidal activity.

Table 15.3.1 Characteristics of an ideal low-temperature gaseous sterilizing agent.

Characteristic	Comments
Broad-spectrum microbicidal activity	Bactericidal, tuberculocidal, virucidal, fungicidal and sporicidal
Rapid activity	Achieve sterilization quickly and below 65°C
Resistance to organic and inorganic materials	Withstand a reasonable level of soil without loss of microbicidal activity
Strong penetrability	Penetrate common medical device packaging materials and also into device lumens
Materials compatibility	Compatible with a wide range of products and materials (no change in their appearance or function even after repeated processing)
Non-toxic for both operators and patients	Present no health risk to the operator as a toxic gas and no health risk to patients through any toxic residues in the processed devices
Environmental emission	Should be non-hazardous to the environment
Monitoring capability	Allow easy and accurate monitoring using physical, chemical and biological means
Ease of use	Permit safe and effective sterilization on a routine basis without need for extensive knowledge and training in operational procedures
Adaptability	Be suitable for large or small hospitals
Cost-effectiveness	Should be reasonable in cost for installation and routine operations

• Strong penetrability: penetrate common medical device packaging materials and also into device lumens.
• Materials compatibility: compatible with a wide range of products and materials (no change in their appearance or function even after repeated processing).
• Non-toxic for both operators and patients: present no health risk to the operator.as a toxic gas and no health risk to patients through any toxic residues in the processed devices.
• Environmental emission: should be non-hazardous to the environment.
• Monitoring capability: allow easy and accurate monitoring using physical, chemical and biological means.
• Ease of use: permit safe and effective sterilization on a routine basis without need for extensive knowledge and training in operational procedures.
• Adaptability: be suitable for large or small hospitals.
• Cost-effectiveness: should be reasonable in cost for installation and routine operations.

Types of gaseous sterilizing agent and mechanisms of action

There are two main categories of sterilizing agents, which are distinguished by their microbicidal action: alkylating and oxidizing (Table 15.3.2).

Alkylating agents

Alkylating gases are highly reactive and can react with amino, sulphydryl and hydroxyl groups in proteins and/or purine bases of nucleic acids in microbial cells. The most commonly used alkylating agents are ethylene oxide and formaldehyde, but propiolactone, methylbromide and propylene oxide are also important. Propylene oxide is used mainly in the food industry [16].

Oxidizing agents

Oxidation is characterized by the transfer of electrons from the target (oxidized) molecule to the oxidizing molecule, which plays the role of the electron acceptor. Low-temperature oxidizing agents include chlorine compounds such as chlorine dioxide and

Table 15.3.2 Summary of properties of gaseous sterilants [13].

Sterilants	Chemical formula	Molecular weight	Boiling point (°C)
Alkylating agents			
Ethylene oxide	C_2H_4O	44.05	10.8
Formaldehyde	CH_2O	30.03	−19.1
Oxidizing agents			
Hydrogen peroxide	H_2O_2	34.02	150.2
Peracetic acid	CH_3COOH	76.05	110
Ozone	O_3	48	−111.35
Chlorine dioxide	ClO_2	67.45	11
Hydrogen peroxide gas plasma	H_2O_2	–	–

superoxides and peroxides such as ozone, hydrogen peroxide and peracetic acid. The plasma phase of the last two compounds may also be used as oxidizing agents.

Principal features of sterilizing equipment

Basically, gaseous sterilizers consist of a leak-proof enclosure including a thermoregulation system, an evacuation system, an automatic or computerized driving unit, a gas generator, a steam generator and a front panel which comprises some parameter-recording systems. A demineralized water supply is also required [13, 16].

Validation

Any sterilizer must be properly validated before use. Validation is done in two steps, comprising the installation qualification of the apparatus followed by a performance qualification. During the installation qualification phase, two requirements must be checked: conformity of the device with nominal specifications of the type and conformity of its implementation to specifications. An important aspect of installation qualification for a gaseous sterilization process is the determination of the temperature in the empty sterilizer chamber.

In the second phase, performance qualification must demonstrate experimentally that processed products will be acceptable when the apparatus has been correctly used, leading to "true" sterilization. This procedure can be further divided in two stages: physical and microbiological qualifications. During physical qualification, several probes measuring parameters such as temperature or humidity are incorporated into the enclosure. Microbiological qualification uses microbiological indicators. Both results are useful for the operation or qualification. Physical and microbiological qualifications must be conducted again after any maintenance operation on the apparatus or change in the nature of the load. There are no standards specifying requirements for validation or control of low-temperature gas sterilization processes; one must refer to the European and International Standard Organization (ISO) EN14937 [18, 19].

Load release

Parametric load releases are not suitable for gaseous sterilization. Biological indicators placed in the bulk of the load must complete the physical parameter recordings. The load will only be released after completion of the incubation period of biological indicators [13, 16].

Biological indicators

Standardized samples of specially chosen spores are used as biological indicators. The choice of spore-forming microorganisms is based on several criteria: resistance to the type of process used, absence of pathogenicity and ease of culture. They are characterized by the species, the source, the number of viable spores and the decimal reduction time (D-value). Indicator samples consist of filter paper strips, glass slides, plastic tubes or sealed vials. Some include a vial of culture medium directly placed in the packaging

of the indicator. The packaging must allow penetration of the gas. It also must prevent alteration or contamination of the microorganism and avoid adsorption of the sterilizing gas. It must include an expiry date [13, 16, 20].

Residues of gas sterilants

An international standard dealing with gas residues is currently under discussion [21]. It deals mainly with gases with high penetration power, such as ethylene oxide.

Alkylating agents

Ethylene oxide
Background

Devices using ethylene oxide first appeared in hospitals in the 1960s. Once considered an alternative to steam sterilization, ethylene oxide has now fallen out of favor because of its human and environmental toxicity as well as cost constraints [10–14]. However, some still value the strong microbicidal activity as a highly desirable attribute of the gas despite its known drawbacks [5, 16].

Properties
Physical and chemical properties

Ethylene oxide (also called epoxyethane or oxyrane) is a small molecule whose formula is C_2H_4O, molecular weight is 44.05 and boiling point is 10.8°C. Its industrial production is based on oxidation of ethylene with air and oxygen, and it can be provided as pure liquid in compressed-gas cylinders. It occurs in gaseous form at room temperature. It is therefore necessary to protect it from the cold, especially in pipes, to keep it in a gaseous state. With a density of 1.52 compared with air, it does not mix easily with air in static conditions. Its solubility is good in water as well as in organic solvents. Colorless, it has a light ethereal odor, with its olfactive threshold being about 700 ppm. The small size of the molecule as well as its very weak polarity gives it a high penetration power in narrow spaces. Its chemical structure is responsible for a high chemical reactivity. Its very inflammable gaseous state can form an explosive mixture in air from concentrations of 3%. In contact with water, it can transform into ethylene glycol and, in the presence of chlorine compounds, into ethylene chlorohydrin. It irreversibly polymerizes, producing inactive compounds. This polymerization is catalyzed by light, heat or metal particles. On the other hand, ethylene oxide is not corrosive for metals. It can spontaneously decompose, with the formation of methane, ethane and carbon dioxide. This decomposition is facilitated in special conditions such as the presence of air, temperature, pressure and some catalysts [12–14, 16, 22].

Microbicidal activity

Ethylene oxide has bactericidal, fungicidal, virucidal and sporicidal properties. Activity against the protozoan, *Cryptosporidium parvum* has also been shown [23]. It reacts as an alkylating agent upon hydroxyl, sulphydryl, carboxyl and amino groups converting them to the hydroxyethyl adducts. The main alkylation actions are as follows:

$$R-OH+C_2H_4O \rightarrow R-O-CH_2-CH_2-OH$$

$$R-SH+C_2H_4O \rightarrow R-S-CH_2-CH_2-OH$$

$$R-COOH+C_2H_4O \rightarrow R-COO-CH_2-CH_2-OH$$

$$R-NH_2+C_2H_4O \rightarrow R-NH-CH_2-CH_2-OH$$

These reactions lead to modifications of microbial metabolism and denaturation of proteins, enzymes and nucleic acids.

Apart from the prions, against which ethylene oxide has no activity, bacterial spores are the most resistant to it [24]. The resistance is, however, only 2–10 times greater than that of the corresponding vegetative forms. *Bacillus atrophaeus*, in its spore form, has been chosen as the reference due to its very high resistance [10]. Nevertheless, some have reported vegetative bacteria such as enterococci to be more resistant than bacterial spores, in particular the spores of *B. atrophaeus* [25]. Endotoxins are resistant to ethylene oxide.

Factors affecting microbicidal activity
Alkylation is a first-order chemical reaction, water being the indispensable catalyst to facilitate opening of the ethylene oxide ring. Moreover, the degree of hydration of the microbes can play an important role in their destruction by ethylene oxide. This fact is particularly demonstrated by dehydrated bacterial spores, which are more resistant than the corresponding vegetative cells [13, 26]. At a constant temperature, the inactivation rate is approximately proportional to the concentration of ethylene oxide in the range of 400–1600 mg/l. As for sporicidal activity of saturated steam, the inactivation of spores by ethylene oxide follows a logarithmic law, allowing the definition of a decimal reduction value time (*D*-value). This value for *B. atrophaeus* spores is 2.7 min at 50°C. The alkylation rate increases with temperature according to the Arrhenius law: the rate doubling for every 10°C rise in temperature.

Many studies have reported the influence of organic residues and salt crystals on the activity of ethylene oxide. Sodium chloride salts at 0.65% w/v are responsible for a bigger decrease in activity than bovine serum at 10% w/v. This inactivation is more apparent when pathogenic agents are in contact with interfering substances in a device with a lumen, and ethylene oxide in its pure form is more sensitive than in a mixture with a carrier gas [27–31].

Compatibility
Ethylene oxide is compatible with most medical devices [1]. Surface-state modifications of nickel-titane biomaterials induced by ethylene oxide have been reported by Thierry *et al.* [32], while Lerouge *et al.* [33] noticed slight alkylation phenomena on surfaces of polyurethane devices. Due to its small size, ethylene oxide can be adsorbed by plastics and the factors affecting this are the type of material, the dimensions of the device and its packaging, as well as the sterilization parameters.

Type of material
Some studies have been carried out on this subject [10]. For a standard cycle of a 3 h exposure with 600 mg/l ethylene oxide at 54°C and a 40% relative humidity, the following results have been found in terms of residual ethylene oxide [12]:
1. *Dimensions of the device*: the thicker the surface is, the greater the adsorption will be.
2. *Conditioning*: the conditioning material and its affinity for ethylene oxide can play a role; also polyamides and/or polyvinyl chlorides are not compatible.
3. *Sterilization parameters*: the adsorption is directly proportional to exposure time and concentration, and reversibly proportional to the temperature. Relative humidity has a beneficial role in the penetration of ethylene oxide.

Toxicity
Because of its high reactivity, ethylene oxide reacts with all living tissues. Carcinogenic risks have been shown with many animal species with, for example, a lethal dose of 200 mg/kg in mice. The toxic risks in humans are linked to ethylene oxide and its derivatives, ethylene glycol and ethylene chlorohydrin, which can be formed during the sterilization process. The toxicity concerns both the staff working on sterilization and the patients. There are two kinds of toxicity: acute and chronic.

The exposure to ethylene oxide vapors can produce allergic reactions, headaches, dizziness, nausea and irritation of ocular and respiratory mucosa. At a high concentration, risks include severe coughing and dyspnea and neurological damage caused by a depressing effect on the central nervous system. In the liquid state, ethylene oxide can induce skin irritation and burns. The appearance of cataracts, polyneuropathies and memory impairment has been attributed to prolonged exposure to ethylene oxide. Many epidemiological studies have been carried out on the carcinogenic risk in humans. Some of them showed a higher incidence of stomach cancers, leukemia and Hodgkin's disease in exposed workers. Other studies showed an increase in spontaneous abortion in women exposed to ethylene oxide [10, 12].

Ethylene oxide has been classified as a carcinogen since 1994 by the International Cancer Research Agency [34]. This classification was linked to the observation of genetic mutations among hospital staff accidentally exposed to high concentrations or to prolonged low concentrations. Patient toxicity is related to the amount of residual gas present in the sterilized material. Problems have been observed during the introduction of devices where the gas has not been evacuated, for example from the outside body circuit. These problems are essentially blood abnormalities such as thrombopenia, fibrinolysis, allergic phenomenon, respiratory problems and cardiovascular attacks [10, 12–14, 34].

Sterilization process
Conditioning of ethylene oxide

Ethylene oxide is used in sterilization either as a pure gas or mixed with a gas carrier. In spite of the polymerization phenomenon, pure gaseous ethylene oxide can exist in a stable state at very high concentrations, but can be extremely dangerous because it is highly flammable and explosive nature. That is why in hospitals, pure ethylene oxide is used in the form of small 100 g aluminum cartridges [1].

To avoid the aforementioned risk, ethylene oxide can be mixed with an inert carrier gas. The use of chlorofluorocarbon (CFC) is now prohibited to preserve the ozone layer. Some countries have also forbidden the use of hydrochlorofluorocarbon (HCFC), the final ban at the international level is set for 2030. On the other hand, the use of carbon dioxide is still possible. It is an inexpensive product whose low concentration in ethylene oxide must be taken into account in determining the length of contact time for sterilization [1]. The mixture of 10% ethylene oxide and 90% carbon dioxide (by weight) is supplied in liquid form in metal bottles pressurized to 0.5 kPa (50 bars). These bottles are made of special steel and undergo a treatment to eliminate all irregularities which could be a source of polymerization. They also have to be kept out of heat to avoid polymerization. They have a shelf-life of only 3 months. The prevention of polymerization is also important due to the physical form of the polymer whose density increases with the degree of polymerization; initially oily, the polymer rapidly becomes solid, blocking filters and valves inside the sterilizers.

Apparatus

Sterilizations have been carried out in closed stainless steel chambers with either single or double openings. These chambers have a thermoregulation system (heated water, air or electrical), a vacuum pump allowing evacuation during start and end phases of the cycle, a steam generator supplied with demineralized water and an microbicidal filter in the air flow. Ethylene oxide can be eliminated from the chamber through different systems: a catalytic converter, an acid scrubber or other elimination systems. The system includes an automatic controller and a recorder collecting data of the process such as temperature and pressure.

The CEN (Comité Européen de Normalization) European Standard EN1422 [35] specifies the minimum construction and performance specifications of a sterilizer. Conformity to this norm allows autocertification and CE "medical device" labeling. This norm includes six appendices:

1. Quality test of the water vapor (neither too dry nor wet).
2. Thermal test of the chamber (this test checks the homogeneity of the temperature in the chamber).
3. Test for acoustic pressure.
4. Test for leak proofing of the gas in the chamber (this test is carried out in a vacuum enclosure and under pressure and must demonstrate a volume of leakage less than 0.1 kPa/min).
5. Test of biological performance.
6. Recording equipment for measuring temperature during the tests.

The European Standard EN550 [36] has been obsolete since 2009 but the European and International Standard EN ISO 11135-1 [37, 38] has the same requirements concerning the validation and routine control of industrial ethylene oxide sterilization. After installation of the sterilizer, this standard also states that physical and microbiological performance qualifications must be done. These must be repeated after each intervention on the apparatus or modification to the composition of the load. It proposes different methods for the microbiological performance qualification. The half-cycle method is described in the information section of the standard.

Sterilization parameters

As stated above, the microbicidal activity depends on different parameters, which have to be controlled to guarantee good results.

• *Relative humidity.* The optimal humidity is 35%. In practice, it must be between 40% and 80% due to the absorption phenomenon caused by the conditioning. Besides its role as a catalyst of the alkylation reaction, the humidity facilitates the penetration of ethylene oxide through the conditioning. On the other hand, the formation of inactive ethylene glycol must be avoided.

• *Gas concentration.* Usually, concentrations between 400 and 1000 mg/l are used for sterilization. Higher concentrations create greater toxicity problems, requiring longer desorption time even though better penetration of the gas is achieved in these conditions.

• *Temperature.* The average temperature is usually between 40 and 50°C and the thermosensibility of medical devices must be considered.

• *Duration.* Other parameters being fixed, the efficacy will depend on the duration of the exposure, which will vary from 30 min to 10 h according to the circumstances.

Typical cycles

There are different cycles for processes performed in a vacuum and those performed under pressure.

• *Vacuum cycle.* After an evacuation of the chamber, an essential phase is the "pretreatment", which includes preheating and humidification of the load using short steam injections followed by evacuation. Ethylene oxide, pure or mixed with carbon dioxide, is then injected. The contact between the load and the gas occurs at a pressure lower than atmospheric pressure. After an exposure time of one to several hours, the cycle is ended by repeated evacuations followed with filtered fresh air draining at a constant sterilization temperature. High-efficiency particulate air (HEPA) filtered fresh air injection allows recovery of atmospheric pressure.

• *Pressurized cycle.* In this process, ethylene oxide is always mixed. Depending on the pressure, the exposure lasts from 30 min to 2 h. The pressure is always higher than atmospheric pressure.

The vacuum process has the advantage of avoiding any leak of ethylene oxide. The advantages of the pressurized cycles are that they are shorter and fire hazards are eliminated. It should be noted that in the pharmaceutical industry, pretreatment takes place in an auxiliary chamber so as not to interrupt the operation of the sterilizer.

Desorption

Repeated draining at the end of a cycle is not sufficient to achieve the correct desorption of ethylene oxide. For safe recovery, this desorption can be performed by simple storage in a ventilated room or by the use of special desorption enclosures where air ventilation is provided along with temperature regulation, because temperature is the most important factor. These special enclosures are especially interesting when one considers that for desorption a polyethylene device has to stay for 15 days at room temperature. The devices are loaded into baskets in order to ease ventilation of filtered warmed air, which is pumped into the lower part of the enclosure and exhausted from the upper part [12, 39]. Some sterilizers are able to perform the desorption process in the sterilization enclosure [10].

Sterilization management
Preparation
The medical devices processed must be compatible with ethylene oxide. As with any other sterilization processes, thorough cleaning and drying of devices are essential requirements, especially for devices with lumens.

Packaging of medical devices
Packaging requirements for ethylene oxide sterilization are specified in the CEN European Standards EN868-6 and EN868-7 [40, 41]. The packaging paper is composed of primary-use bleached cellulose fibers. The mechanical strength of these fibers is reinforced by polymers. These packages are usually sheaths or wrappings of standardized dimensions composed of polyethylene polyester sheeting. These materials are air permeable and their mesh is finer than the steam sterilization papers as the small size of the ethylene oxide molecule allows easier penetration.

Sterilization controls and load release
The load release conditions differ between industrial and hospital sterilization requirements. In industry, parametric release is routine practice. This is based on the performance qualification of the sterilizer and of the load, and on the control of all the parameters; in particular, ethylene oxide concentration must be evaluated using a direct method (e.g. gas phase chromatography or infrared spectrometry). Microwave spectroscopy has been noted to be a very valuable technique in measuring ethylene oxide by some authors [42]. In hospital sterilization the usual release procedure additionally takes into account biological indicators, since loads are characterized by their heterogeneity.

In field use, hospital staff must ensure correct loading, adequate parameters and cycle selection, and the proper processing.

Release of a load requires an examination of the following parameters: graphic recording, process indicators and biological indicators. The graphic recording includes pressure and temperature as a function of time and must be similar to the nominal recording of the sterilizer. Process indicators use color-changing ink and are directly printed on the packaging or adhesive tapes. The indicators on sterilized and non-sterilized devices have to be distinguished easily. Other indicators use the progressive modification of colored ink through the concentration of ethylene oxide, correct temperature and humidity rate. They are placed on each package or randomly disposed in the load; in this last case at least five indicators are used for each load.

The European and International Standard EN ISO 11138-2 [43, 44] specifies the absolute need for biological indicators in each cycle. These indicators are usually paper strips or ready-to-use tubes containing a culture medium vial with a colorimetric indicator. A biological indicator contains at least 10^6 *Bacillus atrophaeus* spores. It must be placed in a critical part of the chamber and allows a true measure of the effect of the cycle on a known number of organisms introduced together with the load. As for process indicators, biological indicators must be properly qualified. As the incubation time is similar to the duration of desorption, their use is not a limiting factor. Some biological indicators that are readable after only 4 h of incubation time have been described [17]. They use an enzymatic activity to reveal the presence of viable spores and also to detect the production of acid metabolites. These indicators have been cleared by the US Food and Drug Administration (FDA) and can be used to monitor pure and mixed ethylene oxide (HCFC) sterilization cycles. They have not been tested in carbon dioxide mixture sterilization cycles.

Desorption control
The European and International Standard EN ISO 10993-7 [45, 46] specifies the maximum threshold of ethylene oxide residues and their evaluation methods in medical devices. This evaluation includes ethylene oxide as well as ethylene chlorohydrin. Ethylene glycol evaluation is not required when the ethylene oxide rate is controlled. The acceptable thresholds take into account the patient/device contact time; the contact is classified as: (i) permanent, when it exceeds 30 days; (ii) long, for a contact of between 1 and 30 days; and (iii) limited, when less than 24 h. The use of several devices must be considered in the toxicity evaluation as well as its potential use on newborn children. The evaluation rate is performed after recovery and protection of a device placed in a bulk of the load. The dosage method uses gas chromatography and enables a desorption curve of the residues to be established.

Safe conditions for staff
Due to the many risks linked to ethylene oxide use, several countries have imposed national rules for its safe utilization [1, 16, 47–50]. The goal of some of these regulations is to limit ethylene oxide use on the following bases [47]:

• Ethylene oxide processing should only be used when no other process is available.
• Easy maintenance is required.
• Staff need to be qualified in its use.
• Radiation sterilization of plastic devices should be banned.
• Emergency sterilization should be banned because of the required desorption phase.

The sterilization site must have controlled access and a clear warning sign notifying the presence of ethylene oxide and its related risks. It must have appropriate ventilation to ensure air renewal. Natural ventilation is sufficient if there is no gas bottle or if bottles are placed in a tight, ventilated enclosure; it is also sufficient if low-volume cartridges are used. In other cases, mechanical ventilation is required.

A continuous control of the atmosphere is achieved using specific sensors in the lower part of the site. These sensors trigger a sound alarm if the concentration exceeds 5 ppm. The long-term exposure limit (LTEL) (8 h time-weighted average) is 1 ppm and the short-term exposure limit (STEL) (15 min reference period) is 5 ppm [49, 50]. Storage rooms must be ventilated in the same way. Furthermore, the quantity of gas stored is limited and no other gas storage is allowed. The location must be a distance from any heat source or electrical installation. Staff must be properly educated and protected, and must pass a medical check-up. It must be noticed that the Occupational Safety and Health Administration (OSHA) has established a permissible exposure limit (PEL) of 5 ppm for ethylene chlorohydrin in the workplace.

Formaldehyde
Background
In 1939 Gunnar Nordgren established the scientific uses of formaldehyde [51]. In his landmark study, he showed with a sample of 70 different bacterial types that the majority of bacteria were killed by a 20–50 min exposure in an atmosphere containing 1 mg of formaldehyde per liter of air. He also showed that the efficiency depended on the microorganism and also on the humidity of the atmosphere. He concluded that formaldehyde is a strong bactericidal agent but that its efficiency is dramatically reduced at low temperature. It also requires a reduced pressure to allow the penetration of the agent through narrow orifices.

The production of wet vapor containing formaldehyde gas was obtained from liquid formalin. In 1956, Kaitz proposed a process that allows formaldehyde depolymerization from the polymer para-formaldehyde, enabling the production of dry formaldehyde gas to sterilize surfaces and other areas [52, 53].

Formaldehyde is used either in liquid form or as a gas. In 1966, it was shown that the addition of water vapor to formaldehyde gave a sporicidal mixture [54]. This combination, called LTSF (low-temperature steam formaldehyde), was cheap, efficient and easy to control. It was then used in automated sterilization processes and largely in medical centers, especially in Scandinavian countries, Germany, France and the UK. Sterilization using formaldehyde should not be confused with disinfection [55]. Nowadays, two methods of sterilization based on formaldehyde gas

are used: LSTF sterilization and high-temperature formaldehyde-alcohol sterilization [56].

Properties
Physical and chemical properties
Formaldehyde comes from the Latin *formica*, meaning ant (ants produce formic acid as a natural defense). Formaldehyde (methanal), also called formic aldehyde, is a small-molecule monoaldehyde whose formula is CH_2O and molecular weight is 30.03. It can exist in three states: gaseous, liquid and solid.

Dry and pure, formaldehyde is a colorless monomeric gas characterized by a pungent odor, easily detectable from 0.1 to 0.5 ppm. This extremely strong smell at very low concentration tends to prevent exposure to higher concentrations. It is stable at atmospheric pressure only at temperatures above 800°C or at room temperature if the concentration is very low (less than 1.75 mg/l). At a higher concentration and at room temperature, it polymerizes to produce a polyoxymethylene $(CH_2O)_n$ film. An equilibrium curve of the concentration of the solid, liquid and gas phases related to temperature was described by Veyre in 2001 [57].

One of the major drawbacks of formaldehyde gas sterilization is its spontaneous polymerization and its condensation on any available surfaces as a thin white film. This film is composed of *para*-formaldehyde (hydrated polymers) and of polyoxymethylenes (anhydric polymers) such as trioxymethylene.

Formaldehyde is highly soluble in water, resulting in the production of hydrates. This solubility explains its easy elimination from the chamber after a sterilization cycle. It is also soluble in alcohol and ether but insoluble in hydrocarbons. Its boiling point is *c.* 19.1°C. In the liquid state, the diluted water solution is stable until its concentration reaches 35%. At a higher concentration, it shows spontaneous polymerization [58].

Microbicidal activity
The spectrum of formaldehyde activity is particularly wide. It is bactericidal [59], fungicidal and virucidal [60, 61]. It is also active on insects and other animal life [53]. Although Phillips showed that bacterial spores were 2–15 times more resistant to formaldehyde than vegetative forms [62], the activity on spores is interesting. Tulis showed, for example, that 10^5 *Bacillus subtilis* var. *niger* spores placed on filter paper were killed in 40 min, 10^6 in 55 min and 10^7 in 60 min in the presence of a formaldehyde concentration of 3.5 mg/l, at a temperature of 28°C and a relative humidity of 84% [53]. However, it was noticed that spores treated with liquid formaldehyde or by a mixture of LTSF were still alive. It has been possible after an appropriate thermal treatment to revive formaldehyde-treated spores [63]. This could explain some discrepancies found in different studies [64]. Lastly, formaldehyde is inactive against prions and strongly fixes the residual infectivity of prions. The comparison of the sensitivities of various organisms versus formaldehyde on the basis of published data is difficult due to the variations in exposure conditions and experimental methods used [65].

Formaldehyde is a potent alkylating agent. It is generally considered to be not very active as a microbicidal agent. It reacts very slowly and its lethal effects are linked to the alkylation of nucleic acids, leading to inhibition of the germination process [66]. However, the revival of spores treated with LTSF by post-processing heat treatment suggests that the mechanisms of action of alkylating agents is complex, and the precise mode of action remains unexplained [65]. Formaldehyde interacts with proteins, RNA and DNA, the interaction with the latter probably explaining its mutagenic activity [13, 67, 68].

Factors affecting microbicidal activity

The activity of gaseous formaldehyde is markedly influenced by the concentration of the gas, the temperature, the water content of the microorganisms and the duration of exposure. There is a complex interrelationship between these factors [65]. Formaldehyde is used mainly as a surface sterilizing agent because, unlike ethylene oxide, it does not penetrate deeply. This low penetrability necessitates pre-evacuation of the sterilizer chamber and operation of the LTSF cycles at pressures between 10 kPa (100 mbar) and 40 kPa [65]. The following factors are important to consider:

1. *Temperature.* Temperature is one of the major factors influencing the sterilizing activity of formaldehyde gas. Microbial inactivation increases with temperature up to 70–80°C. The temperature must not be lower than 18°C [60]. In practice, two temperatures are used during sterilization: either 80°C, which allows more rapid cycles, or 55–56°C, which often represent the maximum temperature accepted by the material.

2. *Relative humidity.* Relative humidity is also an essential factor. Relative humidity must always exceed 50%, its optimum being situated between 80% and 90% [60]. Humidity is usually controlled to maintain a rate of 75–100%, while steam condensation must be avoided. These conditions are difficult to obtain in practice. In this case, temperature and humidity are the two indispensable parameters to control in order to prevent condensation of steam in water [16].

3. *Concentration.* Likewise, the inactivation efficiency increases with formaldehyde concentration. The usual concentration of formaldehyde gas used ranges between 6 and 50 mg/l according to the apparatus, with an average close to 20 mg/l; a threshold around the latter concentration has been reported and further increases have little effect [16, 65, 69]. Concentration falls in the atmosphere of an enclosure by 2 mg/l per hour [70]. In LTSF cycles a formaldehyde concentration of 8–16 mg/l is generated at an operating temperature of 70–75°C [17].

4. *Vacuum.* The better the vacuum obtained, the higher the penetration of the gas into the materials to be sterilized. The vacuum, usually between 5 and 50 mmHg [5], also modifies vapor pressure and increases the concentration of formaldehyde in the gas phase.

5. *Nature of the material.* This can influence the efficiency of the sterilization. Tulis, for example, obtained large differences in sporicidal activity by using either a paper or stainless steel support; the efficiency was much better on the latter [53].

6. *Organic materials.* Formaldehyde's action is greatly diminished by organic materials, the implication being to treat only pre-cleaned items [57].

There are also large differences of penetration according to the products. Thus polyethylene sheets are much more permeable to formaldehyde than cellophane [53]. The permeability of materials, the affinity with formaldehyde and the properties of the surface could all influence the amount of residual formaldehyde following LTSF sterilization. Kanemitsu *et al.* [71] measured the amount of residual formaldehyde on different plastic materials and medical devices and proved that this amount varies according to the material used. For example, it was higher on polyamide-6, polyurethane, natural rubber and polyacetal than that left on the filter paper used as a control. It is necessary to confirm that formaldehyde residues remain below certain levels. Evidence that sterilization has been achieved and that the functional integrity of the equipment is not affected also needs to be provided. At present, there are no standardized safety criteria regarding the level of formaldehyde residues on sterilized medical equipment.

Toxicity

Formaldehyde is toxic for humans when it penetrates into the respiratory or digestive tracts, or through the skin. It is irritating for the eyes, nose and throat as soon as it reaches a concentration in the air of "some parts per million". It also has a necrotizing action at a high concentration or following prolonged exposure. Allergic reactions to formaldehyde have also been reported [72]. In 2004, the US Environmental Protection Agency (EPA) and the International Agency for Research on Cancer [34] declared formaldehyde as a carcinogen (mainly nasopharyngeal and leukemia cancers). Nonetheless, the most modern LTSF sterilization systems use solutions containing formaldehyde at low concentrations (2%), which are supplied in disposable bags that do not require staff handling during the loading of materials [73].

The permissive exposure limit of formaldehyde in work areas is 0.75 ppm measured as an 8 h time weighted average (TWA). The OSHA have established a LTEL of 0.75 ppm [1]. Other values have been stated in various countries. For example, in France, the LTEL is 0.5 ppm and the STEL is 1 ppm [57].

Formaldehyde gas is flammable and explosive when it is mixed with air with a concentration ratio of 7% v/v or more. However, the usual concentration of formaldehyde used in the sterilization process is well below the explosive concentrations and there is no ignition risk.

Sterilization process and management
Production and storage

Gaseous formaldehyde is not commercially available. Because of its properties, formaldehyde gas cannot be stored in bottles or containers. However, it is easy to prepare extemporaneously by heating a 35–40% stabilized formalin solution [16]. For example, the LTSF sterilizer GEF 449 (Getinge AB, Getinge, Sweden) has a 185 l chamber in which 34–38% formalin is injected during

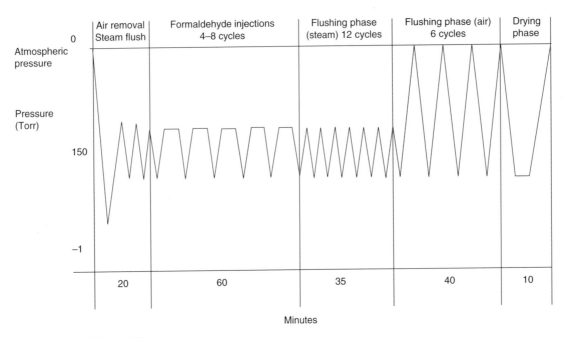

Figure 15.3.1 Illustration of an LTST cycle [57].

operation. Formalin solution is evaporated before entering the chamber. Formaldehyde can also be obtained by sublimation of *para*-formaldehyde. However, evaporation is the most usual process. The raw material is cheap and easy to obtain.

Apparatus

The "low-temperature steam" (or steam under vacuum) concept highlighted in the LTSF sterilization process provides both humidity and temperature control during the procedure [56]. This process must be reserved for devices that cannot withstand temperature over 80°C such as with high-pressure steam. A sterilizer using formaldehyde can be used in two modes: as a steam sterilizer alone (operating above atmospheric pressure at the usual temperatures for steam sterilization) or as a combined steam/formaldehyde sterilizer (operating at subatmospheric pressure and 55–80°C) [57]. As all parameters (formaldehyde concentration, humidity, temperature, process duration) are interdependent, it is impossible to determine a general guideline.

The Harvey Chemiclave (Barnstead/Thermolyne Corporation, Dubuque, IA) system developed for dental practice combines the microbicidal activity of high-temperature formaldehyde and alcohol. A mixture of formaldehyde (0.23%), alcohol (72% ethanol and <4% methanol) and distilled water (VapoSteril) is vaporized under pressure (138 kPa) by heating it to 132°C in a dedicated sterilizer [56].

Typical cycles

In the LTSF sterilizer GEF 449, the sterilization cycle consisted of six phases: pre-vacuum; pre-pulses of steam, formaldehyde feeding, sterilization, washing pulses and air pulses (Figure 15.3.1). Air is eliminated from the chamber during the pre-vacuum period, and then subatmospheric steam is added repeatedly to the humid hot chamber during the pre-pulsing period [74]. Careful checking of the correct injection of the steam–formaldehyde mixture as well as sterilization indicators is necessary.

In the study by Kanemitsu *et al.* [30], the sterilization phases employed were performed with a program using steam at 60°C and a 2% concentration of formaldehyde, the sterilization processes being carried out at 12.3 kPa (123 mbar) for 120 min. They found that the LTSF sterilizer was equivalent to an ethylene oxide gas (EOG) sterilizer and was better than a hydrogen peroxide gas plasma sterilizer. Moreover, the LTSF sterilizer had some advantage compared with the EOG sterilizer, including little impact on the environment, cost effectiveness and shorter processing times.

Sterilization controls and load release

As for ethylene oxide, the sterilization process must be routinely checked at different stages. First, hospital staff must make sure of correct loading, of the right parameters and cycle selection, and of proper processing. Then, release of the load requires examination of the following parameters: graphic recording, process indicators and biological indicators. The graphic recording includes pressure and temperature as a function of time. Process indicators based on color-changing ink (adhesive tapes on the packaging) allow sterilized and non-sterilized devices to be distinguished. Other indicators reflect the concentration of gas, relative humidity, cycle length and temperature [75].

Sterilization monitoring can be performed according to International and European Standard EN14180. In their study, Mariscal *et al.* [73] used the monitoring system Attest TM (3M,

Minneapolis, MN), containing spores of *Geobacillus stearothermophilus* (ATCC 7953) as a biological indicator. The manufacturer of the LTSF sterilizer (Albert Browne Ltd, Leicester, UK) recommends three types of indicators that can be used as chemical controls.

The detection of formaldehyde residuals is done by using filter paper [71]. Mariscal *et al.* [73] have developed a microtiter plate toxicity test based on fluorescence to determine the residual concentration of formaldehyde on medical items after LTSF sterilization.

Since the LTSF sterilization process is mainly used for narrow lumen and optical instruments, a special challenge test has been developed to simulate a complex instrument. The challenge test unit proposed for the Getinge LTSF sterilizer consists of a narrow (2 mm inside diameter), one-aperture lumen, 1.5 m long, with an indicator at the closed end of the tube.

Advantages and drawbacks

Sterilization using formaldehyde can find its place in the central sterilization unit as a complement to sterilization using ethylene oxide. It can also provide a unique means of sterilization in small or average structures, where it can be used either as a low-temperature sterilization process or for classic steam sterilization [57].

The main advantages are easy detection of low concentrations due to odor (0.2–0.6 ppm) compared with ethylene oxide and no ignition or explosion risk. Moreover, its cost is lower than ethylene oxide and, as there is no desorption problem, the yield is increased [11, 55].

The fact that formaldehyde is only a surface sterilizing agent means that it does not have the permeation capabilities necessary to sterilize occluded locations sealed within plastic materials [16]. Sterilizing porous materials can be difficult as a result of polymer formation inhibiting further sterilant access. Formaldehyde exhibits very strong corrosion on certain materials. It must not be applied either to cellulose-made materials (diapers, bandages) or to any material suspected of carrying prions. There is no specific wrapping for this sterilization process, which represents a major drawback. It is also very unstable and therefore difficult to manage. It is difficult to use with products sensitive to high humidity and with products that are not clean because gas may not penetrate organic and inorganic soil [65]. The problem of residual formaldehyde in the apparatus after sterilization must be considered. A high number of washing pulses may be necessary to reduce formaldehyde residues; the European Standard EN14180 suggests residues of <200 μg per filter paper [74].

Its use for sterilization has been almost abandoned in the USA, Canada, France and Australia. The formaldehyde steam sterilization system has not been cleared by the FDA for use in healthcare facilities [17]. In France, formaldehyde sterilizers are no longer used due to lack of activity against prions. Some health centers in northern Europe (Scandinavia, Germany, UK) [17] continue to use them because of a long sterilizing tradition of reusable medical devices [51] such as endoscopes, laparoscopes and

optic-fiber materials [13]. For example, Getinge AB (Sweden) proposes the use of LTSF sterilizers for heat-sensitive goods, especially plastic and hollow instruments (e.g. rigid and flexible endoscopes), which may be damaged by the high temperatures of a conventional steam sterilizer. Recently, Kanemitsu *et al.* [76], using an LTSF sterilizer, demonstrated the potential of this method for sterilizing endoscopes.

Sterilization process norms

In order to limit short-term and environmental risks, these processes are tightly regulated through various norms. Their purpose is to ensure the safety of the sterilization process by evaluating several essential parameters. These norms include:

• European and International Standard EN ISO 10993-17-2002: *Biological Evaluation of Medical Devices. Part 17. Establishment of Allowable Limits for Leachable Substances.*
• European and International Standard EN ISO 14180-2003: *Sterilizers for Medical Purposes – Low Temperature Steam and Formaldehyde Sterilizers – Requirements and Testing.*
• European Standard EN15424-2007: *Sterilization of Medical Devices. Low Temperature Steam and Formaldehyde. Requirements for Development, Validation and Routine Control of a Sterilization Process for Medical Devices.*
• International Standard ISO 11138-5-2006: *Sterilization of Health Care Products – Biological Indicators – Part 5: Biological Indicators for Low-Temperature Steam and Formaldehyde Sterilization Process for Medical Devices.*
• International Standard ISO 14937-2009: *Sterilization of Medical Devices – General Requirements for Characterization of Sterilizing Agent and the Development, Validation and Routine Control of a Sterilization Process.*

Oxidizing agents

Hydrogen peroxide gas
Background

Hydrogen peroxide was discovered by the French chemist Thénard in 1818 while trying to produce chloride from the reaction of hydrochloric acid on barium dioxide. He was surprised to find that oxygen was generated in the glass apparatus [77]. After further studies, he discovered a new combination of hydrogen and oxygen, which he named *eau oxygénée*. This was at first translated into English as "oxidized water" but it is now known as hydrogen peroxide.

In 1858, the English physician Richardson noted the ability of this substance to combat bad smells, considered, at the time, to be the manifestation of infection [77]. It became a very popular antiseptic for a time, though it was considered to have limited applications (due to its instability at low concentration and the peroxidase activity of living tissues). As it seemed very safe, it was used as a disinfectant in the food industry. For example, it has been used since 1913 for the preservation of milk and water as well as fruit juices and is approved in many countries for this purpose. Nevertheless, development of hydrogen peroxide vapor devices did not occur until the 1990s.

Properties

Physical and chemical properties

Hydrogen peroxide is a colorless liquid with a nitrous smell. It has a marked viscosity and its density is 1.465 at 4°C while it solidifies at *c.* 0.89°C into a quadratic crystal system. It has a natural tendency to decompose when heated at atmospheric pressure but it boils at 85°C under a pressure of 70 mmHg, which means that its theoretical boiling point should be about 150°C.

The chemical formula of hydrogen peroxide is H_2O_2, which can be represented as H–O–O–H, with the characteristic peroxide bridge –O–O–. X-ray spectrometry indicates that the two O–H bonds are not linear but in two orthogonal planes [77].

Production and storage

The Thénard process, based on barium dioxide decomposition using dilute mineral acid, is still in use, despite its cost. This process was used to produce 1600 t/year of 35% solution for V2 rocket propellant during World War II. Nowadays, electrolytic H_2SO_4 decomposition processes combined with hydrolysis of the by-products enable mass production. Further distillation results in high-concentration commercial products (up to 50%).

Hydrogen peroxide formation from water is an endothermic reaction, thus explaining its easy decomposition:

$$H_2O_2(liquid) \rightarrow H_2O(liquid) + O_2(gas) + 23\ kcal$$

Decomposition is rather slow at high dilution or for the pure product, if stored in a perfectly clean flask, protected from light. But many substances can act as catalysts and accelerate this decomposition. Platinum moss or pumice stone induce spontaneous explosions in concentrated solutions. This decomposition is also encouraged by dissolved salts. Colloidal or viscous substances such as glycerin inhibit decomposition [77]. Since the work of Schumb *et al.* [78], the discovery of factors that cause catalytic decomposition led to the development of highly efficient stabilization processes without significant diminution of hydrogen peroxide's disinfection power [77].

Gaseous hydrogen peroxide is generated by evaporation or vaporization. Hydrogen peroxide vapor may be obtained through evaporation of a heated stock solution. It is a slow process. At first glance, such a process seems very simple; nevertheless, this evaporation must take into account the fact that water in the solution is more volatile than the hydrogen peroxide itself. So, in order to obtain the required peroxide gas concentration, steam must be partially eliminated prior to the gas injection into the sterilization chamber. In order to obviate such a problem, a new method to generate hydrogen peroxide vapor from a non-aqueous organic hydrogen peroxide complex instead of a stock solution has been proposed [79] and a dual-circuit generator designed which should also minimize this problem. Vaporization instantaneously forms a peroxide–water gas in the same proportions as the initial liquid concentrations. Flash vaporization can be performed by dropping peroxide onto a heated surface (>100°C) or by passing it through a heated cylinder [56]. Meanwhile, new families of hydrogen peroxide concentration sensors, one based on near-infrared absorption [80] and the other on a special transistor [81], should allow proper concentration monitoring. Significant hydrogen peroxide generation has been demonstrated *in situ* on the electroplated coating of medical devices [82].

Microbicidal activity and factors affecting microbicidal activity

Many studies have been performed on the microbicidal activity of hydrogen peroxide in solution. Hydrogen peroxide is active against bacteria, fungi, yeast, spores and viruses. This activity is a function of concentration and contact time but seems to be rather independent of pH in the range from 2 to 10. As with ozone, the microbicidal activity is greater against Gram-negative than against Gram-positive bacteria. The presence of catalase or other peroxidases allows increased tolerance, due to enzymatic degradation. Its sporicidal activity is greatly improved by increased concentration (25–60%) and temperature but does not seem to be affected by organic matter or salts. *Geobacillus stearothermophilus* spores are accepted as being the most resistant to gaseous hydrogen peroxide.

The microbicidal activity of hydrogen peroxide gas is much greater at lower concentration than that of the liquid form [6]. However, in the vapor phase its activity seems to be greatly affected by water condensation on the target, which results in a lower local concentration. This means that previous evacuation and drying is required before vapor injection [7]. The maximal activity seems to occur at the start of the condensation process, that is at the dew point, as reported by Bardat *et al.* [83] and Marcos-Martin *et al.* [84] for other vapors. Activity is also affected by decomposition due to catalytic action and absorption by porous cellulosic materials such as paper [7].

Its efficacy against *Cryptosporidium* and *Giardia* in the gaseous form at concentration of 1–6 mg/l, and against parasites eggs [56], has been described. In addition, it has been shown that gaseous peroxide inactivates prions in both *in vitro* and *in vivo* assays. In contrast, liquid peroxide is not effective [85]. Finally, gaseous peroxide also reduces surface contamination with endotoxins and proteinaceous exotoxins [56].

The main mechanism of action seems to be the local formation of hydroxyl radicals, OH˙, which are among the strongest oxidants known. These radicals could be produced under the action of superoxide ions by the reaction:

$$O_2^- + H_2O_2 \rightarrow OH^\bullet + OH^- + O_2$$

Another reaction uses the presence of non-toxic metal salt ions in the medium or in the cell itself in the following reaction:

$$H_2O_2 + Fe^{2+} \rightarrow OH^\bullet + OH^- + Fe^{3+}$$

Such highly active hydroxyl radicals are believed to react with membrane lipids, DNA and double bonds of essential cell components.

The roles of O˙ and OH˙ radicals in the mechanism of activity do not seem to differ much from those involved in other micro-bicide oxidants based on oxygen, such as ozone and peracetic acid. This is why much research is currently being undertaken to enhance formation of these radicals, for example by use of cold plasmas of hydrogen peroxide or peracetic acid.

Synergism with hydrogen peroxide

Much research is currently being conducted into cold plasma techniques in order to increase the yield of free radicals, and many alternative techniques to achieve this have been described. These techniques are currently referred to as advanced oxidation processes (AOPs). As far back as 1930, Dittmar used cupric and ferric ions. More recently, Bayliss and Waites [86] used UV radiation for the same purpose and dramatically enhanced the activity of low-concentration hydrogen peroxide solutions, but the draw-back of this process is the weak penetration of UV radiation and its absorption by hydrogen peroxide at high concentrations. More recently, the combination of ozone and hydrogen peroxide (Peroxone) has been described for tapwater treatment [87], but further studies revealed that Peroxone activity was decreased in raw water [88].

Behr and co-workers established that the sporicidal activity of ozone in the vapor phase was increased by over 35% by a low concentration of hydrogen peroxide vapor, even in the presence of a fair amount of organic material [89].

Toxicity

Direct-contact toxicity is low at usual concentrations, including the vapor phase, which causes temporary irritation. At higher concentrations (35–50%) burns can occur. Its effect is more acute on mucous membranes and the cornea, while ingestion of a small quantity of a 35% solution can lead to lethal brain ischemia [90]. No carcinogenic activity has been established in humans. The LTEL is 1 ppm [7].

Sterilization process and management

The urgent need for faster low-temperature processes, which are less harmful than ethylene oxide for the operators and the environment, has encouraged investigators and manufacturers to concentrate their efforts on finding a chemical that would breakdown into benign by-products such as oxygen and water. Vapor hydrogen peroxide (VHP) technology has for a long time been employed in the food industry. In this technology, a deep vacuum pulls hydrogen peroxide solution through a heated vaporizer. Vapor is injected into the sterilization chamber. An additional vacuum enhances gas penetration. This sequence is repeated several times, according to need. After sterilization is completed, the whole device is vented through a catalytic converter which breaks down the remaining hydrogen peroxide into oxygen and water, allowing the safe recovery of sterile

product. In practice, the processing occurs at a temperature of 35–49°C and the concentration of hydrogen peroxide is established around 10 mg/l. This concentration is obtained from a 35% solution.

VHP technology has potential applications in the sterilization of endoscopes and dental sterilizers and for surface disinfection of isolators [7,91]. Steris® developed such a process: the AMSCO® V-PRO 1. This system is intended for use in terminal sterilization of thoroughly cleaned, rinsed and dried reusable metallic and non-metallic medical devices used in healthcare. The sterilizer vaporizes the correct amount of liquid hydrogen peroxide from the multiple-cycle VAPROX® cartridge (59% solution). Standard cycle duration is 55 min. Exposure to numerous cycles does not significantly affect the appearance or functionality of most medical instruments. Biological indicators used are composed of *Geobacillus stearothermophilus* spores. The V-PRO 1 process conforms to starndard EN ISO 14937 [18, 19] and is CE-labeled and FDA approved. Some refinement of the VHP process had been tested by Taizo *et al.* [81] to sterilize centrifuges coupled to a standard generator, which was monitored through a new transistor sensor.

It must be noted that only certain synthetic packaging materials and containers allowing the penetration of peroxide can be used as they limit absorption of the sterilizing agent. More recently, a very efficient isolator and room decontamination unit has been developed. The Clarus C™ generator (Bioquell Inc., Hampshire, UK) is linked to special high-velocity dispensers of peroxide vapor and to several monitoring sensors, including an original condensation monitor, and is now widely marketed. These features linked to a dual drying and evaporation circuit seem to ensure accurate parametric control of the whole process. In other studies, hydrogen peroxide vapor decontamination has been found to be an effective method of eradicating methicillin-resistant *Staphylococcus aureus* (MRSA), *Serratia marcescens* and *Clostridium difficile* spores from rooms, furniture, surfaces and equipment [17, 92–98].

Peracetic acid
Background

Although the microbicidal activity of peracetic acid in water solution has been known since the beginning of the 20th century [99], it has only been used since the 1950s [100]. Like hydrogen peroxide, this oxidative agent is not a gas but a liquid at room temperature. Microbicidal properties of the aqueous solutions have been used as well as its vapors, the former being more frequently used [101].

Its corrosive nature had limited its use in sterilization until recently. The main applications are in the food industry and for disinfecting sewage sludge [77]. Liquid peracetic acid has been used in healthcare in recent years for the reprocessing of kidney dialysis machines and for the sterilization of immersed surgical instruments [7]. One of the major advantages of peracetic acid is that its degradation products (oxygen, acetic, water) do not present any environmental impact.

Properties
Physical and chemical properties
Peracetic acid (peroxide of acetic acid or peroxyacetic acid), whose formula is CH_3COOOH, has a molecular weight of 76.05 and a boiling point of 110°C. Its flash point is 46°C. The solution is in equilibrium between peracetic acid, acetic acid, hydrogen peroxide and water according to the following equation:

$$CH_3COOH + 2H_2O_2 \leftrightarrows CH_3COOOH + 2H_2O$$

As the reaction is a reversible equilibrium, strong acidic stabilizers are used to orientate the reaction in the right direction.

Peracetic acid is a colorless liquid with a pungent and offensive smell. It is totally soluble in water and polar organic solvents. Peracetic acid is more soluble in lipids than hydrogen peroxide. It explodes violently at about 110°C or at room temperature if the concentration rises above 56% [58]. From a 5% concentration, solutions are corrosive and flammable, and they release oxygen when they decompose.

It is usually produced industrially by the reaction of acetic acid or acetic anhydride with hydrogen peroxide in the presence of a catalyst, usually sulfuric acid. To avoid the reverse reaction, solutions are supplemented with acetic acid and hydrogen peroxide and a catalyst is added to chelate metal traces which would accelerate the decomposition. Peracetic acid can also be obtained from a generator of acetyl radicals in the presence of hydrogen peroxide:

$$CH_3COR + H_2O_2 \rightarrow CH_3COOOH + RH$$

This reaction is not in equilibrium and avoids the need for stabilizers such as strong acids. The thermodynamic stability of solutions of peracetic acid is average. Slow decomposition of the solutions produces acetic acid and oxygen. For a peracetic acid solution of 0.2% in distilled water at 20°C, the amount of peracetic acid decreases by 0.1% in 4 weeks, although its half-life is 2.5–3 weeks at 25°C [102]. Increasing temperature accelerates this degradation. It is thus necessary to store it at low temperatures. It is commercially available as an aqueous solution at concentrations reaching 40%. Vapor-phase peracetic acid is generated by heating a solution of peracetic acid [13].

Peracetic acid is a strong oxidizing agent which reacts in an explosive way with acetic anhydrid, ether solvents, chlorides (potassium, calcium) and organic materials. Decomposition of highly concentrated aqueous solutions is strongly enhanced in the presence of metallic residues (iron, copper, manganese). Peracetic acid can remove surface contaminants (primarily proteins) on endoscope tubings [17].

Microbicidal activity
Its disinfectant action was reported for the first time by Greenspan and MacKellar [103]. It is bactericidal, tuberculocidal, sporicidal, virucidal and fungicidal [104–106]. It is one of the most active microbicides, its microbicidal power being stronger than that of hydrogen peroxide. Its action is comparable to that of sodium hypochlorite but it has the advantage of not producing fixed residues because its degradation products are all volatile (acetic acid, hydrogen peroxide, oxygen, water) [58].

Peracetic acid is a strong oxidizing agent. It is a weak acid that reacts more at low pH, but it is also active in high pH conditions at higher concentrations. Its lethal action seems to be due to the formation of hydroxyl radicals. It must also be noted that a strong synergy occurs with hydrogen peroxide.

Sprossig et al. showed that peracetic acid in the gaseous phase at 22°C and under pressure of around 12 mmHg was active against all the vegetative bacteria tested and also on spores of *Bacillus cereus* and *Bacillus mesentericus* in 20 min at a concentration of 40% [107]. Peracetic acid demonstrates a greater stability and higher penetration power than other gaseous oxidizing agents, with a better penetration of paper and porous materials [56].

Peracetic acid is an oxidizing agent that attacks the protein components of the microbial cell, including vital enzymes. It not only reacts with the proteins of the cell wall, but it also penetrates as a slightly dissociated acid into the interior of the cell [7]. A partial activity has been shown by Taylor [108] in the brains of mice infected with the ME strain of scrapie agent.

Factors affecting microbicidal activity
In the vapor phase, sporicidal activity of peracetic acid was shown at a relative humidity between 40% and 80% with maximum activity at 80%. However, at 20%, the inactivation power was considerably reduced [104]. Due to its good solubility in lipids and its lack of inhibition by enzymes such as catalases and peroxidases [109], its action is not much altered by interfering substances such as blood. Its activity is not modified by organic materials.

Toxicity
The toxicity appears in local irritation during deep and repeated inhalation. Exposure to vapor-phase peracetic acid may irritate the skin, the upper respiratory tract and eyes. The severity increases with the concentration. Its toxicity is considered to be weak for the skin (irritating at a concentration of 0.4–2%), for the eyes (irritating at 0.4%) and by inhalation (acute toxicity level of 520 mg/m^3); the tolerance level is 1 mg/m^3 with stinging in the eyes and nostrils, while the olfactive perception level is 0.005 mg/m^3 [110]). The LTEL of peracetic acid has not been determined but the LTEL of acetic acid is 10 ppm [7]. It is not allergenic and probably not carcinogenic. Finally, it is environmentally friendly.

Care should be taken to ensure that peracetic acid and other toxic residuals which can form on surfaces during sterilization are adequately vented to remove the risk of adverse reactions, particularly for critical surgical devices [56].

Sterilization process and management
Apparatus
Peracetic acid gas can be produced by vaporization of liquid peracetic acid–water solution at 35–45%. Peracetic acid solutions are supplied in solution with water, hydrogen peroxide and acetic

acid. Probably due to its corrosive nature, the applications of peracetic acid for sterilization are not numerous [104]. Malchelsky in 1993 proposed a system using peracetic acid for the disinfection of endoscopes [106]. Though many systems using the liquid phase have been described and commercialized, few use the gas phase [111]. United States Patent No. 5 008 079 and European Patent No. 0 109 352 describe a system using peracetic acid in the gas phase for the sterilization of heat-sensitive medical devices [7]. In this system, a 40% peracetic acid solution is converted into gas in a heated vaporizer and delivered to an evacuated, preheated chamber. The system is designed to operate optimally within a temperature range of 40–50°C (higher temperatures may cause the rapid breakdown of the gas and loss of efficacy) and a peracetic acid chamber concentration of approximately 10 mg/l. Total cycle time is about 60 min [112].

To our knowledge, it seems that only one device working in the vapor phase has been commercialized – the Sterivap®. This apparatus is designed for "disinfection–sterilization" of isolators, to which it is linked during the process and then disconnected. This apparatus heats a solution to 45°C and propels the evaporated gas using compressed air. At the end of the cycle, an automatic cleaning with compressed air allows the evacuation of gas outside. Heating of peracetic acid is carried out at 45°C and allows its evaporation. The evaporated volume is 40–50 ml/h. Contact time varies from 4 to 6 h.

Sterilization controls and load release
There are no standard procedures to validate and control the activity of peracetic acid in the vapor phase [13]. For each step, validation and routine control protocols have been established.

Advantages and drawbacks
Peracetic acid is remarkably efficient. It reacts quickly and, moreover, it has a depyrogenic effect [113]. It is efficient even in the presence of organic matter. It is highly soluble in water and it does not produce toxic residues.

Despite its very low toxicity, its use is limited by its instability, its low penetration power and its very low flash point with correlative difficulties in handling and storage. Moreover, its smell is pungent. It is very corrosive for certain materials. Thus, steel, iron, copper or brass are damaged even if they are painted or plated with nickel and chrome. It is also corrosive towards many polymers, particularly polyurethane, cement and other construction materials. Rubber degrades to varying extents depending on its quality and the frequency of the disinfection process. Aluminum alloys are not damaged if the exposure time is less than 20 min and if the temperature is less than 30°C. Stainless steel, porcelain, Teflon, earthenware, polyethylene and polypropylene are not damaged by peracetic acid.

Gaseous ozone
Background
The "electric substance smell" was first described by van Marum in 1781 and it was considered as a simple body by Schönbein in 1840, who suggested naming it ozone from the Greek *ozein* meaning "which emits an odor". The composition of this gas, a tri-atomic allotrope of oxygen, was finally determined by Ott in 1899. It was only in 1922 that Riesenfeld and Schwab were able to produce pure ozone [114].

Ozone's disinfectant activity was suspected at the very end of the 19th century, and it was used for the first time in a drinking water treatment plant in 1893 at Oudshourn in the Netherlands [16]. Calmette and Roux in France gave government approval for this technology and the first French water treatment plant started operating in 1906 in Nice [115]. Since this period, many studies have been performed to improve a process which is nearly universal in developed countries, and from these works many other applications using ozone in the liquid phase were developed, such as paper pulp bleaching, wastewater treatment, the disinfection of swimming pools or aquaculture waters, and the sterilization of mineral water bottles or blood transfusion pouches. It is now also used in the treatment of water for industrial heat exchangers [16, 116, 117].

It is amazing to note that this chemical species, which is gaseous in normal conditions, has been used and studied in aqueous solution for over a century while techniques for using the gas phase are, comparatively, rather primitive. The need for low-temperature sterilization techniques has spurred research into this area over the last decade, leading to some promising new technologies.

Properties
Physical and chemical properties
Ozone is a tri-atomic allotrope of oxygen commonly referred to as to O_3. It is a highly unstable gas in the thermodynamic conditions of the earth's surface. It has, at a low concentration, a pleasant "clean" smell originally described as the "thunder smell" by the Greek poet Homer, while at higher concentrations it is deeply irritating. At high concentrations, its color is dark blue. Its density compared with air is 1.657 and it solidifies at a temperature of *c.* 192°C. Its boiling point at atmospheric pressure is *c.* 112°C.

The molecule is far more unstable when dissolved in water (half-life: 4 min at 20°C) than in air (half-life: 14 h at 20°C). It is important to know, for further discussion, that its solubility decreases as temperature increases, from 1400 mg/l at 0°C to nil at 70°C.

The formula is usually written as O_3 but in fact the third oxygen atom orbits around the molecular oxygen di-atomic structure. This means that the bond link of the third atom to the molecule structure is a very weak one and this explains why the molecule is so highly reactive. It also explains the easy decomposition of the molecule and recombination of its constituents into more stable molecular oxygen [114]:

$$2O_3 \rightarrow 2O_2 + 2O \rightarrow 3O_2$$

This recombination in molecular oxygen can be induced, for instance, by increasing the temperature, which enhances the probability of intermolecular collisions. In this way, all the ozone molecules recombine into molecular oxygen when the gas temperature exceeds 300°C, whatever the initial concentration. Recombination can also be obtained at far lower temperatures thanks to the catalytic action of substances such as platinum, palladium or silicon and many organic or inorganic materials. A very fast destruction of the ozone molecule also occurs thanks to its extreme reactivity in the oxidation of environmental material. This recombination into non-toxic molecular oxygen avoids the need for long venting periods before the safe recovery of materials submitted to ozone.

Production

Since it liquefies at a very low temperature and its decomposition is highly exothermic, storage of liquid ozone is impossible. Its relatively short half-life at atmospheric pressure decreases dramatically as pressure increases, rendering bottled storage useless. However, there was a proposal some decades ago to bottle a low concentration solution of ozone in liquid Freon [115]. This means that ozone must be produced immediately prior to use. It can be obtained at low concentration by UV radiation but the main production technique is based on the corona discharge effect, which produces a glowing cold plasma [114]. Such a corona discharge is produced in neon lights and also in the aurora borealis.

Microbicidal activity

Ozone is bactericidal, mycobactericidal and sporicidal. It is also active against yeast, fungi, amoebae and viruses. *Geobacillus stearothermophilus* spores are considered to be the most resistant microorganism to its action. Its use for disinfecting water has been documented for nearly a century [16, 114, 118–120]. Studies dealing with its microbicidal activity in the gas or vapor phases are not so numerous. Furthermore, varying experimental methods combined with difficulties in controlling the parameters, lead to some discrepancies in the results.

One of the first attempts to develop a gaseous ozone sterilization chamber was carried out by German *et al.* in 1966 [115]. With concentrations maintained by continuous gassing and varying from 0.2 to 20 mg/l, they obtained sterilization of *Staphylococcus* strains in 30 min at 20 mg/l and in 300 min at 0.2 mg/l. The sterilization of sporulated *Bacillus atrophaeus* strains required an exposure time of 45 min at 20 mg/l, but a sterilization rate of 50% was only reached with a contact of 720 min at a concentration of 0.2 mg/l. This initial study clearly showed that spores are far more resistant to ozone than vegetative bacteria.

Ishizaki *et al.* [121] tested several strains of *Bacillus* spores. They emphasized the role of humidity, stating that, for an ozone concentration of 3.0 mg/l, no sporicidal activity occurred if the relative humidity was 50% and that efficient activity required at least 80% relative humidity. Other studies revealed that Gram-positive bacteria seemed to be more sensitive to ozone than Gram-negatives and that *Candida albicans* was more resistant than bacteria. One study has demonstrated that MRSA is more ozone resistant than methicillin-sensitive *S. aureus* (MSSA) [122].

Most studies dealing with the virucidal activity of ozone have been performed in water. They have covered many species of non-enveloped and enveloped viruses including human immunodeficiency virus (HIV) type 1. Behr *et al.* [123, 124] presented good data with combined ozone–hydrogen peroxide vapor used against poliovirus type 1, human hepatitis A virus (non-enveloped) and herpes simplex virus type 1 (enveloped) (see also Chapter 9). Ozone is active against endotoxins and preliminary studies revealed a potential action against prions [125].

Ozone produces its microbicidal activity by directly oxidizing organic substances, especially at double bonds within the molecule, leading to the formation of ozonide functional groups. Ozone can also act as a catalyst, inducing swift fixation of diatomic oxygen on substances which are, in normal conditions, slowly self-oxidizing. The main mechanism involved in its microbicidal activity is the formation of free radicals (O˙ and OH˙) from ozone decomposition. In the gas phase activity could be due to the O˙ radicals, but these would only exist at a minimum relative humidity; reaction of O˙ radicals with water to produce OH˙ radicals would present a far stronger oxidation potential. Such a view is reinforced by the sporicidal synergism observed between ozone and hydrogen peroxide in the vapor phase and in solution [89].

Factors affecting microbicidal activity

Several factors can alter ozone's microbicidal activity, such as temperature, pH and relatively humidity, which have been mentioned elsewhere (see Chapter 3). Biological fluids, proteins, fats or salts decrease the microbicidal activity of most chemical disinfectants; these substances are classically referred to as interfering substances. The same is likely to be true for gaseous ozone, though there are few data available from studies dealing with ozonated air.

From a practical point of view, a very crucial factor limiting the activity of ozone is its self-recombination into stable molecular oxygen through the catalytic action of organic substances, thus limiting the activity of free radicals. This is clearly illustrated in Figure 15.3.2 where the two curves show the variation of ozone concentration in a BOX03™ infectious waste decontamination system [126]. In such a device, pressurized ozonated air is cyclically injected into a previously evacuated chamber containing ground-up heterogeneous organic waste. After each injection, ozone concentration dramatically drops in a loaded chamber (Figure 15.3.2b) while the concentration remains at a high level, until the following evacuation, in the absence of organic material (Figure 15.3.2a). It is important to note that, if ozone from the same generator is injected as a continuous flow into the same apparatus without previous accumulation, then no signal is readable and there is no microbicidal activity since the minimum effective concentration is never reached, even for an exposure time exceeding several hours.

This immediate self-recombination limits, for instance, ozone's activity inside packaging materials such as paper or polyethylene. This is because partial recombination occurs when gas passes

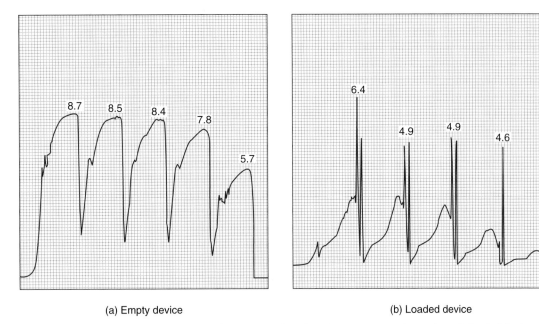

(a) Empty device   (b) Loaded device

Figure 15.3.2 Catalytic recombination of ozone by inorganic substances. Recordings show the ozone concentration on the vertical scale following sequential injections of ozone into (a) an empty and (b) a loaded device (recordings made from right to left).

through the barrier despite the small size of the molecule, which should allow easy penetration. Such a spontaneous recombination could explain why ozone should be considered only for the decontamination of surfaces.

Synergism

Synergy of activity between ozone and hydrogen peroxide has been achieved in water (Peroxone). When studying the sporicidal activity of gaseous ozone, Behr et al. [123] noticed the same synergy in the BOX03 system. An exposure time of 66 min was necessary to kill 10^6 Bacillus atrophaeus spores and 10^5 Geobacillus stearothermophilus spores when only ozonated air was used, while the same result was achieved in 40 min when a non-active low concentration of evaporated hydrogen peroxide was added. It has been shown that most of the classic interfering substances did not alter sporicidal activity of the ozone–hydrogen peroxide mixture.

Another very promising synergism may be by combining ozone–hydrogen peroxide–acetic acid, first used by Bardat et al. [83].

Compatibility

As for any chemical producing O˙ and OH˙ free radicals, ozone is highly corrosive, especially against casting alloys containing iron and zinc. Nevertheless, most types of stainless steel and some zinc-free aluminum alloys are resistant, even at very high concentrations, low pH and high relative humidity. Free radicals also induce fast de-reticulation of butadiene or artificial rubbers and depolymerization of nylon, polystyrene and, at a lower rate, polypropylene. Most silicones, viton, polycarbonate and rigid polyvinyl chloride resist ozone well. Latex, Kraton (synthetic latex),

cellulose and ether-based polyurethanes are not compatible. It must also be noted that ozone alters a number of organic staining substances.

Toxicity

Ozone is a toxic gas. One can smell it at concentrations as low as 0.02–0.04 ppm. The toxicity threshold is around 0.4 ppm. This means that the presence of ozone can be detected at concentrations 10 times below its minimum toxicity level; this represents an important safety factor as compared with ethylene oxide gas. Occupational regulations in most countries have settled the maximum threshold of concentration for permanent exposure to a level of 0.1 ppm. This relates to electrical devices such as photocopiers or laser printers. At higher concentrations, ozone induces ocular and respiratory irritation which may be irreversible if exposure exceeds 24 h at concentrations exceeding 1 ppm. No carcinogenic effect of ozone has been described thus far.

Sterilization process and management

Since the 1980s many teams focused their attention on gas-phase ozone [127–129] without any sterilization devices reaching the market. More recently, a Canadian company, TSO3 Inc., studied and developed a sterilizer of 125 l capacity named Sterizone® [17, 125]. The main innovation brought by this technology is the monitoring of the humidity and dew point in order to avoid condensation on the load and enclosure surface, while maintaining a high humidity level of 80–100% [130].This is achieved through a multistep cycle. After loading, the closed chamber is warmed in order to establish a homogeneous temperature of all surfaces; this is called the conditioning phase. Then, the sterilization cycles comprises the four following steps:

1. Evacuation to a pressure value of 133 kPa (1 Torr).

2. Humidification. The combination of homogeneous temperature and very low pressure avoids condensation on the load and chamber surfaces. Local conditions are over the dew point despite a temperature that does not exceed 35°C.

3. Injection of ozone produced from hospital-grade pure oxygen. The generator, included in the sterilizer, is cooled to 6°C, thus increasing its yield and lowering the rate of recombination into molecular oxygen.

4. Exposure time during which ozone reacts with vapor to form O˙ and OH˙ radicals as the sterilant. During the entire process, temperature never exceeds 35°C inside the sterilization chamber. Thus, the Sterizone process seems to occur at the lowest temperature for any new-generation sterilizer.

This cycle is repeated twice and is followed by a draining of the chamber medium, exhaust gas being composed of water and molecular oxygen, with no noxious by-products being ejected. Furthermore, the whole process being conducted at a temperature under 38°C, the load can be immediately released. The entire process takes about 4.5 h, but on-going developments may further reduce processing times. This innovative apparatus is already approved for sale in Canada and the USA, and is under review in Europe. The whole process is monitored and recorded by a digital device, but parametric release is not yet allowed; the use of classic biological indicators is still needed. The load is conditioned in special pouches or placed in anodized aluminum boxes equipped with cellulose filters.

A wide variety of surgical and medical instruments can be processed in this sterilizer, subject to materials compatibility with ozone and size; the diameter of rigid endoscopes must also be considered, which may comprise several channels [131]. At this stage, flexible endoscopes cannot be processed in this device.

As ozone is generated inside the apparatus, exposure of the staff to the gas is eliminated. Ozone at the catalyst exhaust, as determined by the manufacturer, showed concentrations lower than 0.02 ppm during the critical phases of the cycle. It is, nevertheless, stipulated that the device should be installed in a room with an air exchange rate of 10 times per hour. At the end of 2009, TSO3 Inc. was granted another patent for shorter processing cycles as well as the possibility of sterilizing multichanneled flexible endoscopes.

Chlorine dioxide
Background
Chlorine dioxide has been used especially for drinking water disinfection and as a bleaching agent for paper pulp. When treating drinking water, it can remove phenolic taste and odor. It has also been used in the food industry as a hard surface sanitizer [7]. It was only at the beginning of the 1980s that the sporicidal activity of gaseous chlorine dioxide was reported [132, 133].

Properties
Physical and chemical properties
Under standard pressure, chlorine dioxide (ClO_2) freezes at a temperature of c. 59°C and boils at 11°C; thus, it is a gas at room temperature [134]. Its yellow color is darker than that of chlorine, with a similar pungent odor. The odor threshold is around 0.1 ppm [13]. It is soluble in water, giving a stable solution in the dark, but it decomposes slowly under the action of light to a mixture of chlorous acid and chloric acid:

$$2ClO_2 + H_2O \rightarrow HClO_2 + HClO_3$$

Chlorine dioxide is relatively unstable and explosive when heated or at concentrations above 10% v/v in air [13]. It is non-inflammable and non-explosive at concentrations used for sterilization. Due to its unstable nature, chlorine dioxide must be generated on site in the same way as ozone [7]. It is produced by the action of gaseous chlorine on sodium chlorite or of hydrochloric acid on sodium chlorite in solution [13]:

$$Cl_2 + 2NaClO_2 \rightarrow 2ClO_2 + 2NaCl$$

$$4HCl + 5NaClO_2 \rightarrow 4ClO_2 + 5NaCl + 2H_2O$$

Microbicidal activity
Chlorine dioxide has a broad spectrum of action. It is active against bacteria, viruses, protozoa, fungi, algae and prions [134]. It is also sporicidal. According to Jeng and Woodworth, chlorine dioxide gas would be 1075 times more potent than ethylene oxide at a temperature of 30°C and similar relative humidity [135]. Chlorine dioxide is a mild oxidizing agent, which reacts with proteins but not nucleic acids [7]. The reactivity of chlorine dioxide is very selective and different from that of chlorine and most of the other oxidizing agents [7].

Factors affecting microbicidal activity
The sporicidal activity of chlorine dioxide is related to its concentration and relative humidity; a 70–75% relative humidity is necessary for effective sterilization [13]. It is compatible with most plastics and soft metals but must be carefully used with polycarbonates, carbon steel and uncoated aluminum foils [7].

Toxicity
Chlorine dioxide produces no cumulative health effects, is non-carcinogenic and is not a reproductive hazard. However, one should note that most of these studies have been carried out on liquid chlorine dioxide in treating water for drinking and not on its gaseous form [7]. Chlorine dioxide gas is a mucous irritant at a concentration of 5 ppm, but this effect is reversible and dose dependent; the LTEL is 0.1 ppm and the STEL 0.3 ppm [7, 50].

Sterilization process and management
Apparatus
A gaseous chlorine dioxide sterilization device was developed at the end of the 1980s by Scopas Technology Co., Inc., New York [136], and the rights were acquired by Johnson and Johnson in 1991. In the Scopas system, dry sodium chlorite reacts with chlorine gas in a nitrogen gas carrier to produce chlorine dioxide gas.

The process operates at 25–30°C, with 70–80% relative humidity, and the concentration of chlorine dioxide is between 10 and 50 mg/l. The cycle time is 1–1.5 h with no or minimal aeration required [7].

This type of device was used for the sterilization of polymethylmethacrylate intraocular lenses. The sterilizing power of chlorine dioxide was equivalent to that of ethylene oxide. Chlorine dioxide is broken down into chlorite, chlorate and chloride compounds, which are considered to be non-toxic. Actually, no gaseous chlorine dioxide system is currently FDA cleared [17].

Sterilization controls and load release

There is no specific standard for the validation and routine control of sterilization by gaseous chlorine dioxide. Most of the protocols follow the general requirements [13, 19].

Advantages and drawbacks

Chlorine dioxide is effective at non-explosive, low concentrations and at atmospheric pressure or below [134]. The spectrophotometric measurement of gas concentration during the sterilization cycle coupled with appropriate process controls enables the parametric validation for the release of sterilized products [134]. Chlorine dioxide gas is able to penetrate packed material such as polyvinyl chloride tubes or rigid polyvinyl chloride medical-device containers (about 0.03 mm thickness).

Plasma sterilization

Background

Ninety-nine per cent of material in the universe is in the plasma state. Physicists call plasma the fourth state of matter, after the solid, liquid or gaseous states. Basically, plasma is composed of gas molecules that have been dissociated by an energy input. Gases can be converted into the plasma form using a radiofrequency electromagnetic field. Atoms and molecules submitted to shocks by high-energy electrons form various chemical species including ions, electrons, free radicals and excited molecules. For sterilization purposes, only cold plasma is used. This is generated under comparatively low temperature and pressure, as in the aurora borealis or in neon lights. This must be differentiated from the hot plasma occurring in the sun or the stars [2, 13, 137, 138].

Many modern medical devices are thermo- and hydrosensitive. Given the drawbacks and limitations of other low-temperature processes as described above, plasma sterilization could represent a valuable alternative. The first patent dealing with plasma sterilization was published in 1968 [139] while the first practical application was developed in 1972 [140]; it used halogen gas plasma and was intended to sterilize contaminated surfaces. Since then, many have worked on this subject [141–149].

Comparative studies of the sporicidal activity of various gas plasmas have shown that hydrogen peroxide plasma is the most efficient. Currently, the only device marketed is based on plasma derived from this molecule: the Sterrad® technology (Advanced Sterilization Products, ASP; Johnson and Johnson, Irvine CA) [150–152]. Furthermore, the other FDA-approved technology, the

Plazlyte® process [153], was withdrawn from the market in 1998 following several cases of irreversible corneal lesions after ophthalmic surgery devices were sterilized by this process [2, 31, 154]. These lesions seemed to be due to copper and zinc splintering from instruments [155, 156]. The Plazlyte process was based on a two-phase cycle. In the first step, liquid peracetic acid was evaporated in the sterilization chamber; in the second phase, a low-temperature plasma of a gas mixture composed of hydrogen, oxygen and argon was generated in a separate chamber and flowed continuously into the sterilization chamber through a dispenser. The duration and number of cycles varied, depending on the type of device which had to be sterilized and the kind of packaging.

This chapter will focus on the Sterrad technology. The most recent studies on other technologies will be considered later.

Properties of the sterrad process

Physical and chemical properties

The Sterrad process is not strictly a cold-plasma process as it is based on hydrogen peroxide, first in the gas phase and then in plasma form [154]. After an evacuation of the sterilization chamber, producing a deep vacuum, a small quantity of liquid hydrogen peroxide is injected into the chamber and immediately evaporated. The vapor diffuses through the load to be sterilized. In the second step, hydrogen peroxide vapor is energized to plasma, leading to the production of hydroxyl and hydroperoxyl free radicals:

$$\frac{1}{2}O_2 + H-O-H \xrightarrow{e^-} OH^\cdot + OH^\cdot$$

$$\frac{1}{2}O_2 + OH^\cdot + H-O-H \xrightarrow{1-10eV} H_2O + O-O-H^\cdot$$

$$H-O-O-H \xrightarrow{e^-} H-O-O-H'$$

$$H-O-O-H' \rightarrow H-O-O-H + radiation \text{ (visible or UV)}$$

where $OH^\cdot$ is a hydroxyl free radical, $OOH^\cdot$ is a hydroperoxyl free radical and H_2O_2' is excited hydrogen peroxide with a high-energy level electron. H_2O_2' molecules revert to a more stable state by emitting visible and UV radiation. When the glow stops, the active components recombine into stable molecules such as H_2O and O_2 [157].

Microbicidal activity

The microbicidal activity of this process has been extensively documented [16, 151]. The activity of the whole process is made up from the intrinsic activity of each element of the cycle: hydrogen peroxide vapor, free radicals and UV radiation, which may or may not be involved according to the different phases of the cycle.

The whole process activity has been studied using shortened cycles with lowered hydrogen peroxide concentrations and decreased diffusion times in the true vapor phase or plasma periods. Field isolates of hospital pathogens or strains known for their resistance to hydrogen peroxide were inoculated onto sterile paper strips placed in sealed Tyvex®/Milar packaging [2]. These pathogens represented vegetative bacteria as well as spores, mycobacteria, enveloped and non-enveloped viruses, yeast and fungi. These studies revealed that *Geobacillus stearothermophilus* spores were the most resistant. Similar studies and studies using animal models showed activity of the process against hepatitis A virus, HIV, duck hepatitis B virus (a model of human B hepatitis) as well as *Cryptosporidium parvum* oocysts [23, 158–161]. Recently, Rutala and Weber [162] reported efficacy of the process versus emerging pathogens such as *Helicobacter pylori*, *Escherichia coli* O157:H7, antibiotic-resistant bacteria, potential bioterrorism agents (*Bacillus anthracis*) and hepatitis C virus. The intrinsic activity of hydrogen peroxide is well known and extensively documented [7, 13, 16, 77, 91].

Three basic mechanisms are involved in the plasma inactivation of microbes as described by Moisan *et al.* [163]. These are: (i) direct destruction by UV irradiation of the genetic material of microorganisms; (ii) erosion of microorganisms atom by atom through intrinsic photodesorption by UV radiation to form volatile compounds combining atoms intrinsic to the microorganisms; and (iii) erosion of microorganisms atom by atom, through etching, to form volatile compounds as a result of slow combustion using oxygen atoms or radicals emanating from the plasma. In some cases, etching is further activated by UV photons, thus increasing the elimination rate of microorganisms [163, 164].

From a practical point of view, it is interesting to note that some studies attribute the microbicidal activity of the Sterrad process to the hydrogen peroxide vapor phase alone; the hydrogen peroxide plasma phase playing only (according to the manufacturer) a detoxification role of gaseous residues [165].

To close this discussion on the microbicidal activity of such a process, we have to mention the paper of Tessarolo *et al.* [166], which suggests its activity against endotoxins, and the recent publication of Rogez-Kreuz *et al.* [167], which studies its efficacy versus prions. In the latter study, the *in vivo* tests have been completed by *in vitro* ones that showed that the last-generation sterilizer Sterrad® NX is among the most effective process, even outperforming the 134°C/18 min autoclave cycle, and the soda/autoclaving procedure (Advanced Sterilization Product, ASP) [168].

Factor affecting microbicidal activity

Many factors have been described that affect the microbicidal activity of plasma sterilization (see Chapter 3). However, for some of them, for instance plasma inducing electromagnetic field power, precursor gas concentration and temperature, there are some discrepancies in the data [13]. One must keep in mind that a free radical's life is shortened when the pressure is increased. In the same way, free radical activity decreases when the distance between the plasma generator and the device to be sterilized increases [2].

In addition, the microbicidal activity of the Sterrad process is lowered in the presence of interfering substances, as with other chemical sterilization processes. Sodium chloride 0.65% seems to decrease this activity more than proteins [27, 169, 170]. Some studies evaluated sporicidal activity, using germ carriers contaminated with *Geobacillus stearothermophilus* spores placed in small-diameter metal or plastic tubes [30, 31, 171]. These studies revealed a more irregular sporicidal activity; Sterrad devices of the last generation show the most regular activity.

Compatibility

Plasma is compatible with fewer materials than ethylene oxide [1]. Material decay can be caused by hydrogen peroxide, vacuums and the electric energy of the plasma generator. Generally there is a good compatibility with metals such as aluminum, stainless steel and alloys or polymers such as polypropylene, polyethylene, polyvinyl chloride, silicone, polyurethane, vinyl acetate, polycarbonate and Teflon. However, expanded polystyrene presents a major risk of desegregation [138]. Compatibility with glass is good, including optic-fibers [138]. According to the study of Feldmann and Hui [172], 95% of medical devices tested did not reveal abnormalities after sterilization even though in 5% of cases cosmetic alteration was noticed. It was also noticed that the process had a good compatibility with electronic devices and microsurgical instruments, which retained their functionality. Nevertheless, several other investigators have pointed out that independent studies are rare [33, 154]. As a matter of fact, the oxidizing action of hydrogen peroxide necessarily leads to modifications of devices during sterilization. Some complementary studies disclosed noticeable surface modifications of plastic devices containing polyethylene, polyvinyl chloride and polyurethane. These were single devices that were sterilized 1–10 times. Another recent study demonstrated modification of the nominal tensile strength of latex, silicone or polyurethane devices [173].

Before deciding whether a device is compatible, users must take into account the chemical composition of any newly-acquired device as well as its manufacturing process. They should also ask the manufacturer for their recommended sterilization procedure as well as a certificate of compatibility. Advanced Sterilization Products, in collaboration with manufacturers, has established a list of compatible and non-compatible medical devices. This list is periodically updated and is available to customers from Advanced Sterilization Products.

Even if not considered as incompatible, some other materials are not well suited to the Sterrad process including cellulose, viscose, cotton, liquid, powders and foam devices. For instance, hydrogen peroxide is absorbed by cellulose, preventing the normal cycle to occur; in the same way, the presence of liquid interferes with proper vacuum formation. Heavy orthopedic instruments must not be processed in this device either.

Toxicity and biocompatibility

Liquid hydrogen peroxide is well known as an irritating agent for the skin and eyes, and in its vapor phase it is an irritant for the upper respiratory tract. Respiratory irritation ceases after short exposures, but ocular lesions can be irreversible. It is worth noting that the latest generations of sterilizers prevent staff from being in contact with hydrogen peroxide. Hydrogen peroxide is conditioned in sealed cassettes of different volumes according to the apparatus. These are packed in a plastic film with a chemical color indicator for detecting leaks. A color change warns medical staff of defects, preventing exposure to hydrogen peroxide. Once in place in the devices, the cassettes are automatically processed until their elimination. Some tests of the environment around working devices showed that the surrounding hydrogen peroxide concentration was lower than 1 ppm [2]; such a value has been stated as the LTEL [7]. Peniston and Choi [174] in a recent publication showed that the rate of hydrogen peroxide absorbed by polymers tested was very low. However, some studies found more significant hydrogen peroxide concentrations in the environment, especially at the end of the sterilization cycle after the door opening, and from medical devices within an hour of being removed from the sterilizer [1]. During observation of hydrogen peroxide leakages linked to some filter failures, the manufacturer reiterated the necessity to place the devices in suitably ventilated rooms with 10 air volume changes per hour [125].

Numerous biocompatibility tests performed on raw materials as well as on medical devices did not reveal any toxicity risks. These tests included cytotoxicity tests, acute systemic toxicity tests, ocular and cutaneous irritation tests, hemolysis tests and complement activation tests. Since there is no toxic residue, there is no need for a desorption period. At this time, no data are available on hydrogen peroxide's mutagenic, carcinogenic or antifertility activities [175].

A long-term hazard from radiowaves has been suggested, but manufacturers certify that devices are in accordance with electromagnetic compatibility norms.

Sterilization process of the sterrad process
Apparatus
The first commercial apparatus available in Europe (1992) was the Sterrad® 100. The commercial range has since diversified to include the Sterrad® 100S, Sterrad® 50, Sterrad® 200, Sterrad® 100NX and Sterrad® NX. At the present time four different Sterrad systems are available: the 100S, 200, 100NX and NX. Another device has also been developed for industrial sterilization, the Sterrad® 100S/I GMP [2]. Such a diversification occurred in parallel with process improvements, including shorter cycles, an adjustable volume of the sterilizer chamber according to users' needs, dual doors and a new vaporization system. The new system removes most of the water from the hydrogen peroxide, resulting in an improved diffusion of the peroxide into lumens of devices.

Basically, except for the dual-doored Sterrad 200, all devices include the following characteristics: a cylindrical or parallelipedic sterilization chamber including two electrodes (one being the chamber body itself and the other one being a perforated metal cylinder placed a few centimeters from the chamber walls); an evacuation system producing a high vacuum; a thermostatic system; a 13.56 MHz plasma generator; a numeric instrumenta-

tion unit; an active filter for destroying hydrogen peroxide residues in the chamber in the case of process failure; and a HEPA filter to sterilize injected air. The NX generation devices include a built-in monitoring system that allows recording of critical parameters. They are also equipped with a direct control of hydrogen peroxide during all cycles. An optional external system can be retrofitted to 100S generation devices [168]. Installation only requires a standard electric power supply [176].

The sterilization of devices incorporating long and narrow lumens can be unreliable. To reduce these risks, an adapted booster is commercially available for 100S generation apparatus. This comprises a 59% hydrogen peroxide capsule that can be fixed to one end of the device. However, one-end-closed devices cannot be processed.

Typical cycles
The Sterrad 50 and 100S (Table 15.3.3, Figure 15.3.3) were the first devices equipped with a double hydrogen peroxide injection concept. A typical sterilization cycle includes two analogous half cycles following a pretreatment phase (evacuation followed by an injection of air plasma in order to eliminate residual humidity of the load). The Sterrad 100S offers a single program lasting 55 min and a concentration level of 6 mg/l is reached in the chamber.

The cycles of the Sterrad 200 last 75 min. The greater volume of the chamber tends to lengthen some phases of the cycles. The pretreatment phase is also characterized by multiple repetitions of a 5 min evacuation phase, followed by atmospheric pressure

Table 15.3.3 Steps of hydrogen peroxide gas plasma sterilization cycles in the Sterrad 100S [138].

Steps of the processes	Sterrad 100S short cycle time (min)
Pretreatment drying phase	
Vacuum stage, pressure 700 mTorr[a]	10
Low-temperature air plasma then ventilation	10
Sterilization A	
Vacuum stage, pressure 400 mTorr	5
Injection, pressure 6–14 Torr	6
Diffusion, pressure 760 Torr	2
Vacuum stage	5
Hydrogen peroxide gas plasma	2
Sterilization B	
Vacuum stage, pressure 400 mTorr	0.1
Injection, pressure 6–14 Torr	6
Diffusion, pressure 760 Torr	2
Vacuum stage	5
Hydrogen peroxide gas plasma	2
Aeration	0.3
Total	55

[a] 1 Torr = 133 Pa = 1 mmHg.

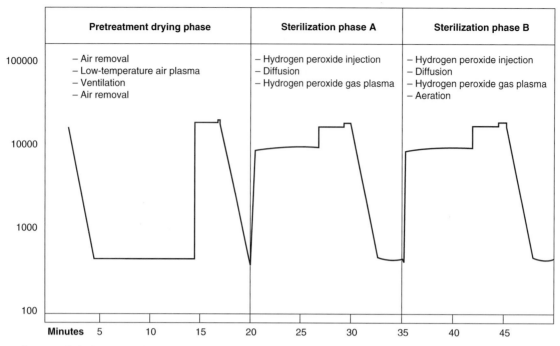

Pretreatment drying phase	Sterilization phase A	Sterilization phase B
– Air removal – Low-temperature air plasma – Ventilation – Air removal	– Hydrogen peroxide injection – Diffusion – Hydrogen peroxide gas plasma	– Hydrogen peroxide injection – Diffusion – Hydrogen peroxide gas plasma – Aeration

Figure 15.3.3 Illustration of a hydrogen peroxide gas plasma sterilization cycle in the Sterrad 100S [138].

recovery. The volume of the hydrogen peroxide cassette is 2.1 ml, which provides a concentration inside the chamber of 9.3 mg/l.

The Sterrad 100NX and NX devices include a new hydrogen peroxide vaporization system. Two optional cycles are available. The first one, devoted to most surgical instruments, lasts 47 min for the Sterrad 100NX and 28 min for the Sterrad NX. The second optional cycle is devoted to monochannel, flexible endoscopes and lasts, respectively, 42 and 38 min. In the Sterrad 100NX, a concentration level of 6 mg/l is reached in the chamber.

Regulation

The four aforementioned Sterrad devices have been approved by the FDA for commercialization. However, the use of the booster is not approved by the FDA. These devices are also CE labeled in accordance with European Directive 93/42 CEE Annexe 2 (class IIA), and in accordance with basic requirements of the European and International Standard EN ISO 14937 [18, 19].

Sterilization management of the sterrad process
Preparation

Preliminary processing is the same as for any other sterilization process but the final drying step is essential for the Sterrad process.

Packaging of medical devices

Articles have to be placed in packages that allow free penetration of hydrogen peroxide in order to ensure a contact with them while still providing an efficient sterile barrier. Some rigid containers and various packaging have been evaluated. As cellulose

is highly absorbent for hydrogen peroxide, all cellulose papers or their derivatives must be avoided for packaging. Some pouches or sheaths with unwoven treated polyethylene (Tyvek®) and one translucent plastic sheath have been developed as well as unwoven polypropylene or polycarbonate/polystyrene material.

Sterilization controls and load release

In order to verify that a load has been correctly sterilized, the parameters are verified using a series of indicators:
• Printing of the sterilization parameters (pressure, phase duration).
• Recovery of colored indicators (strips or adhesive tape).
• Verification of the analogy of the load with a validated analogous load.
• Reading the biological indicators after 48 h (since 1999, *Geobacillus stearothermophilus* spores have been recognized as the standard biological indicator).

In France, the Agence Française de Sécurité Sanitaire des Produits de Santé (AFSSAPS) published in 2007 [176] a document that authorizes parametric release under specific conditions:
• The sterilization unit must be equipped with an independent monitoring system allowing recording of critical parameters of the cycles.
• True validation according to norm NF EN ISO 14937 (*Qualification d'Installation, Opérationnelle et des Performances*).
• Strict observation of manufacturer indications with respect to the load and the nature of instruments to be treated (constitutive materials and dimensions, with special attention to the internal lumen and channels).

Other processes

In recent years, many studies have shown the great value of plasma sterilization and possible market opportunities [177–185]. These studies have dealt with plasmas obtained from argon, nitrogen, oxygen or mixtures of oxygen–argon, nitrogen–oxygen, helium–oxygen and hydrogen peroxide–oxygen. Some of these studies evaluated the efficacy of these plasmas versus various pathogens and spores: such as *S. aureus*, *E. coli*, *Bacillus atrophaeus*, *Geobacillus stearothermophilus* spores and *Saccharomyces cerevisiae*. Others focused on the activity of plasmas versus polypeptides, prions, enzymes, endotoxins and nucleic acids from bacteria and viruses.

Conclusions

From this general survey of gas and low-temperature sterilization, it seems very clear that the ideal process is still to be found (Table 15.3.4). Nevertheless, some aspects of the matter can be identified. Firstly, irrespective of the process chosen, the quality of the pre-cleaning is a fundamental prerequisite to achieve sterilization. This is why sterilizer and medical device manufacturers must cooperate. Secondly, gas sterilization appears to be one useful approach to low-temperature sterilization. Other processes exist for the same purpose, such as those based on radiation, but they are mainly used for industrial sterilization of single-use devices. Liquid peracetic acid is also widely used for the sterilization of reusable devices but it does not maintain sterile conditions for the object. Thirdly, as shown, gaseous sterilization processes are various. Neither the newly developed nor the more classic technologies can satisfy the ideal criteria for these processes. If it seems easy to argue in favor of the withdrawal of the ethylene oxide sterilization process, it is not always easy to completely avoid it in field practice [125, 187]. Microbiological efficacy, operational costs or incompatibility of materials do not appear to be sufficient criteria for choosing a suitable system. In fact, even if the various technologies are effective, insufficient and unreliable data relating to their operational cost are available. Furthermore, each technology has some incompatibility of materials.

Safety, short cycle duration and easy set up and maintenance are the main criteria to consider. It should be noted that the choice must be made according to the specific needs of each establishment. As a result, a combination of several processes could be the correct response to local needs, finance considerations included.

Table 15.3.4 Comparison of common low-temperature sterilants [1, 5, 186].

Properties	Ethylene oxide	Gas plasma H_2O_2	Low-temperature formaldehyde
High efficacy (against all forms of microbial life including spore-formers)	Yes	Yes	Yes
Rapid activity	No	Yes	Yes
Organic material resistance (effective even when exposed to organic material residue)	No	No	No
Penetrability:			
Packaging	Yes	Yes[a]	Yes
Lumens and inner spaces of medical devices	Yes	Yes, but with restrictions	Needs to be validated; based on lumen size efficacy has been questioned for some devices
Material compatibility	Compatible with most materials and not compatible with liquids packaging	Compatible with stainless steel and plastics that have been validated; not compatible with cellulose material, liquids[b]	Compatible with most materials and packaging; steel and plastics that have been validated; not compatible with cellulose material, liquids[b]
Toxicity (low toxicity and minimal exposure risks to operator and environment)	Toxic, but well-established safeguards are readily available	Risks not clear, but appear available	Toxic, but safeguards are to be minimal
Monitoring capability (monitored easily and accurately with physical, chemical and biological process monitors)	Yes	Yes	Yes
Potential for misapplication	No, automated	No, automated	No, automated
Cost-effectiveness (reasonable cost for installation and for routine operation)	Initial cost of the sterilizer is high, operating costs are low	Initial cost of the sterilizer is high, operating costs are low	Cost of sterilizer and operating costs are low

[a] Requires synthetic packaging and special container tray.
[b] Several investigators pointed out that independent studies are rare [154].

Sterrad sterilizers are nowadays used worldwide, probably because of agreed parametric load clearance standards and demonstrated activity against prions. The more recent Sterizone ozone sterilizer seems able to reach the market with success, especially if shorter cycles are validated. This process is manufactured by the American firm 3M.

Most new processes are based on the efficacy of free radicals, especially O˙ and OH˙, whatever the procedure used to produce them. The main challenge is to obtain the maximum concentration of these short-life radicals and to manage their penetration inside all parts of complex devices such as an endoscope's channels, despite their length and small diameter. A promising solution is described by Fournier [188] for dual-aperture channels. Basically, this consists of connecting one aperture to a tight vessel of sufficient volume; the whole device is then placed in the sterilization chamber with a direct link between the free end of the endoscope and the chamber. After evacuation, and when pressure equilibrium between the vessel and the chamber is established, a pressure gradient exists during injection of the gas, which produces a rapid flow through the narrow channel until a new equilibrium of the pressure is established.

Finally, one should keep in mind that the abrupt commercial withdrawal of Plazlyte for safety reasons demonstrates the absolute need for accurate validation of any new process.

References

1 Anon. (1999) Choosing a low-temperature sterilization technology. *Health Devices*, **28**, 430–455.

2 Jacobs, P.T. and Lin, S.M. (2001) Sterilization processes utilizing low-temperature plasma, in *Disinfection, Sterilization and Preservation*, 5th edn (ed. S.S. Block), Lippincott Williams & Wilkins, Philadelphia, pp. 747–763.

3 Hurell, D.J. (1998) Recent developments in sterilization technology. *Medical Plastics and Biomaterials*, **5**, 26–37.

4 Rutala, W.A. and Weber, D.J. (1996) Low-temperature sterilization technologies: do we need to redefine "sterilization"? *Infection Control and Hospital Epidemiology*, **17**, 87–91.

5 Rutala, W.A. and Weber, D.J. (1998) Clinical effectiveness of low-temperature sterilization technologies. *Infection Control and Hospital Epidemiology*, **19**, 798–804.

6 Rutala, W.A. and Weber, D.J. (2001) New disinfection and sterilization methods. *Emerging Infectious Diseases*, **7** (Suppl.), 348–353.

7 Schneider, P.M. (1998) Emerging low temperature sterilization technologies (non-FDA approved), in *Disinfection, Sterilization and Antisepsis in Health Care* (ed. W.A. Rutala), Polyscience Publications, Champlain, NY, pp. 79–92.

8 Block, S.S. (2001) Definition of terms, in *Disinfection, Sterilization and Preservation*, 5th edn (ed. S.S. Block), Lippincott Williams & Wilkins, Philadelphia, pp. 19–28.

9 Phillips, C.R. and Kaye, S. (1949) The sterilizing action of gaseous ethylene oxide. I. Review. *American Journal of Hygiene*, **50**, 270–279.

10 Galtier, F. (1996) La stérilisation par les gaz alkylants: oxyde d'éthylène et aldéhyde formique, in *La Stérilisation* (ed. F. Galtier), Arnette Blackwell, Paris, pp. 121–140.

11 Adler, S. *et al.* (1998) Costs of low-temperature plasma sterilization compared with other sterilization methods. *Journal of Hospital Infection*, **40**, 125–134.

12 Thiveaud, D. (1998) Stériliserà l'oxyde d'éthylène. *Hygiène en Milieu Hospitalier*, **9**, 21–28.

13 Hoxey, E.V. and Thomas, N. (1999) Gaseous sterilization, in *Disinfection, Preservation and Sterilization*, 3th edn (eds A.D. Russell *et al.*), Blackwell Science, Oxford, pp. 703–732.

14 Mazeaud, P. and Pidoux, H. (2001) Stérilisation par les gaz, in *La Stérilisation en Milieu Hospitalier*, 3rd edn (ed. Collège d'Enseignement Pharmaceutique Hospitalier), CEPH, Cahors, France, pp. 239–270.

15 Hoffman, R.K. (1971) Toxic gases, in *Inhibition and Destruction of the Microbial Cell* (ed. W.B. Hugo), Academic Press, London, pp. 225–258.

16 Joslyn, L.J. (2001) Gaseous chemical sterilization, in *Disinfection, Sterilization and Preservation*, 5th edn (ed. S.S. Block), Lippincott Williams & Wilkins, Philadelphia, pp. 337–359.

17 Rutala, W.A. and Weber, D.J. (2008) *Guideline for Disinfection and Sterilization in Healthcare Facilities*, CDC, Atlanta, GA.

18 Comité Européen de Normalisation (European Committee for Standardization, CEN) (2009) EN: 14937: 2009. *Sterilization of Healthcare Products – General Requirements for Characterization of a Sterilizing Agent, and the Development, Validation and Routine Control of a Sterilization Process*, CEN, Brussels.

19 International Standards Organization (ISO) (2009) *ISO 14937. Sterilization of Healthcare Products – General Requirements for Characterization of a Sterilizing Agent, and the Development, Validation and Routine Control of a Sterilization Process*, ISO, Geneva.

20 Goullet, D. (2001) Pharmacopée française, Pharmacopée européenne, in *La Stérilisation en Milieu Hospitalier*, 3rd edn (ed. Collège d'Enseignement Pharmaceutique Hospitalier), CEPH, Cahors, France, pp. 43–56.

21 International Standards Organization (ISO) (1997) *ISO DIS 14538. Method for the Establishment of Allowable Limits for Residues in Medical Devices using Health-Based Risk Assessment*, ISO, Geneva.

22 Goullet, D. *et al.* (1996) Fiches de stérilisation no. 12: Stérilisation par l'oxyde d'éthylène. *Hygiènes*, **12**, 1–209.

23 Barbee, S.L. *et al.* (1999) Inactivation of *Cryptosporidium parvum* oocyst infectivity by disinfection and sterilization processes. *Gastrointestinal Endoscopy*, **49**, 605–611.

24 Darbord, J.C. (1999) Inactivation of prions in daily medical practice. *Biomedecine and Pharmacotherapy*, **53**, 34–38.

25 Lundholm, M. and Nyström, B. (1994) Validation of low temperature sterilizers. *Zentral Sterilisation*, **2**, 370–374.

26 Russell, A.D. (1991) Chemical sporicidal and sporostatic agents, in *Disinfection, Sterilization, and Preservation*, 4th edn (ed. S.S. Block), Lea & Febiger, Philadelphia, pp. 365–376.

27 Alfa, M.J. *et al.* (1996) Comparison of ion plasma, vaporized hydrogen peroxide, and 100% ethylene oxide gas sterilizer to the 12/88 ethylene oxide gas sterilizer. *Infection Control and Hospital Epidemiology*, **17**, 92–100.

28 Alfa, M.J. *et al.* (1998) Comparison of liquid chemical sterilization with peracetic acid and ethylene oxide sterilization for long narrow lumens. *American Journal of Infection Control*, **26**, 469–477.

29 Goveia, V.R. *et al.* (2007) Low-temperature sterilization and new technologies. *Revista Latino-Americana de Enfermagem*, **15**, 373–376.

30 Kanemitsu, K. *et al.* (2005) A comparative study of ethylene oxide gas, hydrogen peroxide gas plasma and low-temperature steam formaldehyde sterilization. *Infection Control and Hospital Epidemiology*, **26**, 486–489.

31 Rutala, W.A. *et al.* (1998) Comparative evaluation of the sporicidal activity of new low-temperature sterilization technologies: ethylene oxide, 2 plasma sterilization systems, and liquid peracetic acid. *American Journal of Infection Control*, **26**, 393–398.

32 Thierry, B. *et al.* (2000) Effects of sterilization processes on NiTi alloy: surface characterization. *Journal of Biomedical Materials Research*, **49**, 88–98.

33 Lerouge, S. *et al.* (2000) Plasma-based sterilization: effect on surface and bulk properties and hydrolytic stability of reprocessed polyurethane electrophysiology catheters. *Journal of Biomedical Materials Research*, **52**, 774–782.

34 International Agency for Research on Cancer (IARC) (1994) *Ethylene Oxide*, IARC Monograph, World Health Organization, Geneva.

35 Comité Européen de Normalisation (European Committee for Standardization, CEN) (2009) EN 1422: 2009. *Sterilizers for Medical Purposes – Ethylene Oxide Sterilizers*, CEN, Brussels.

36 Comité Européen de Normalisation (European Committee for Standardization, CEN) (1994) EN 550: 1994. *Sterilization of Medical Devices – Validation and Routine Control of Sterilization by Ethylene Oxide*, CEN, Brussels.

37 Comité Européen de Normalisation (European Committee for Standardization, CEN) (2007) *EN 11135 1: 2007. Sterilization of Health Care Products – Part 1: Requirements for Development, Validation and Routine Control of a Ethylene Oxide Sterilization Process for Medical Devices*, CEN, Brussels.

38 International Standards Organization (ISO) (2007) *ISO 11135 1. Sterilization of Health Care Products – Part 1: Requirements for Development, Validation and Routine Control of a Ethylene Oxide Sterilization Process for Medical Devices*, ISO, Geneva.

39 Nakata, S. *et al.* (2000) Aeration time following ethylene oxide sterilization for reusable rigid sterilization containers: concentration of gaseous ethylene oxide in containers. *Biomedical Instrumentation and Technology*, **34**, 121–124.

40 Comité Européen de Normalisation (European Committee for Standardization, CEN) (2009) *EN 868-6: 2009. Packaging for Terminally Sterilized Medical Devices – Part 6: Paper for Low Temperature Sterilization Processes. Requirements and Test Methods*, CEN, Brussels.

41 Comité Européen de Normalisation (European Committee for Standardization, CEN) (2009) *EN 868-7: 2009. Packaging for Terminally Sterilized Medical Devices – Part 7: Adhesive Coated Paper for Low Temperature Sterilization Processes. Requirements and Test Methods*, CEN, Brussels.

42 Matthews, I.P. *et al.* (1998) Parametric release for EtO sterilization. *Medical Device Technology*, **6**, 22–26.

43 Comité Européen de Normalisation (European Committee for Standardization, CEN) (2006) *EN 11138-2: 2006. Sterilization of Health Care Products. Biological Indicators – Part 2: Biological Indicators for Ethylene Oxide Sterilization Processes*, CEN, Brussels.

44 International Standards Organization (ISO) (2006) *ISO 11138-2. Sterilization of Health Care Products. Biologica Iindicators – Part 2: Biological Indicators for Ethylene Oxide Sterilization Processes*, ISO, Geneva.

45 Comité Européen de Normalisation (European Committee for Standardization, CEN) (2008) *EN 10993-7: 2008. Biological Evaluation of Medical Devices – Part 7: Ethylene Oxide Sterilization Residuals*, CEN, Brussels.

46 International Standards Organization (ISO) (2008) *ISO 10993–7. Biological Evaluation of Medical Devices – Part 7: Ethylene Oxide Sterilization Residuals*, ISO, Geneva.

47 Ministère de la Santé et de la Sécurité Sociale (1980) Circulaire ministérielle no.93 du 7/12/1979 relative à l'utilisation de l'oxyde d'éthylène pour la stérilisation. *Journal Officiel*, **January 10**, NC 307–309.

48 Ministère de l'Intérieur – Direction de la Sécurité Sociale (1980) Instruction technique du 24/07/1980 concernant l'emploi de l'oxyde d'éthylène prise en application du réglement de sécurité contre les risques d'incendie et de panique dans les établissements recevant du public. *Journal Officiel*, **August 22**, NC 7659–7662.

49 Ministère du Travail (1993) Circulaire DRT no.93–18 du 12/07/1993 concernant les valeurs admises pour les concentrations de certaines substances dangereuses dans l'atmosphère des lieux de travail.

50 Weber, D.J. and Rutala, W.A. (1998) Occupational risks associated with the use of selected disinfectants and sterilants, in *Disinfection, Sterilization and Antisepsis in Health Care* (ed. W.A. Rutala), Polyscience Publications, Champlain, NY, pp. 211–226.

51 Nordgren, G. (1939) Investigations on the sterilization efficacy of gaseous formaldehyde. *Acta Pathologica et Microbiologica Scandinavica*, Suppl. XL, 1–165.

52 Kaitz, C. (1961) *Poultry and Egg Fumigation Process*, US Patent 2, 993, 832.

53 Tulis, J.J. (1973) Formaldehyde gas as a sterilant, in *Industrial Sterilization: International Symposium, Amsterdam 1972* (eds B.G. Phillips and W.S. Miller), Duke University Press, Durham, NC, pp. 209–238.

54 Adler, V.G. *et al.* (1966) Disinfection of heat sensitive material by low temperature steam and formaldehyde. *Journal of Clinical Pathology*, **19**, 83–89.

55 Goullet, D. *et al.* (1996) Fiches de stérilisation no. 13: Stérilisation par le formaldéhyde. *Hygiènes*, **12**, 1–209.

56 McDonnell, G.E. (2007) *Antisepsis, Disinfection, and Sterilization*, ASM Press, Washington, DC.

57 Veyre, M.-C. (2001) Stérilisation par le formaldéhyde, in *La Stérilisation en Milieu Hospitalier*, 3th edn (ed. Collège d'Enseignement Pharmaceutique Hospitalier), CEPH, Cahors, France, pp. 271–284.

58 Chaigneau, M. (1977) *Stérilisation et Désinfection par les Gaz*, Maisonneuve, Sainte Ruffine, France.

59 Rubbo, S.D. *et al.* (1967) Biological activities of glutaraldehyde and related compounds. *Journal of Applied Bacteriology*, **30**, 78–87.

60 Sykes, G. (1965) Sterilization by gases and vapors, in *Disinfection and Sterilization*, 2nd edn (G. Sykes), E. & F.N. Spon, London, pp. 202–227.

61 Spicher, G. and Peters, J. (1976) Microbial resistance to formaldehyde I. Comparative quantitative studies in some selected species of vegetative bacteria, bacterial spores, fungi, bacteriophages and viruses. *Zentralblatt für Bakteriologie, Parasitenkunde, Infections-Krankheiten und Hygiene, I, Abteilung Originale Reihe B*, **163**, 486–508.

62 Phillips, C.R. (1952) Part IX. Relative resistance of bacterial spores and vegetative bacteria to disinfectants. *Bacteriological Reviews*, **16**, 135–138.

63 Wright, A.M. *et al.* (1997) Biological indicators for low temperature steam formaldehyde sterilization: effect of variations in recovery conditions on the response of spores of *Bacillus stearothermophilus* NCIMB 8224 to low temperature steam formaldehyde. *Journal of Applied Bacteriology*, **82**, 552–556.

64 Russell, A.D. (1990) Bacterial spores and chemical sporicidal agents. *Clinical Microbiology Reviews*, **3**, 99–119.

65 Denyer, S.P. and Baird, R.M. (2007) *Guide to Microbiological Control in Pharmaceuticals and Medical Devices*, CRC Press, Boca Raton, FL.

66 Trujillo, R. and David, T.J. (1972) Sporostatic and sporicidal properties of aqueous formaldehyde. *Applied Microbiology*, **23**, 618–622.

67 Bedford, P. and Fox, B.W. (1981) The role of formaldehyde in methylene dimethansulphonate-induced DNA cross-links and its relevance to cytotoxicity. *Chemico-Biological Interactions*, **38**, 119–126.

68 Russell, A.D. and Chopra, I. (1996) *Understanding Antibacterial Action and Resistance*, Ellis Horwood, Chichester.

69 Hoxey, E.V. (1991) Low temperature steam formaldehyde, in *Sterilization of Medical Products* (eds R.F. Morrissey and Y.I. Prokopenko), Polyscience, Morin Heights, Canada, pp. 359–364.

70 Kanemitsu, K. *et al.* (2005) Residual formaldehyde on plastic materials and medical equipment following low-temperature steam and formaldehyde sterilization. *Journal of Hospital Infection*, **59**, 361–364.

71 Phillips, C.R. (1954) Gaseous sterilization, in *Antiseptics, Disinfectants, Fungicides and Physical Sterilization* (ed. G.F. Reddish), Lea & Febiger, Philadelphia, pp. 638–654.

72 Hendrick, D.J. and Lane, D.J. (1975) Formalin asthma in hospital staff. *British Medical Journal*, **1**, 607–608.

73 Mariscal, A. *et al.* (2005) A fluorescence bioassay to detect residual formaldehyde from clinical materials sterilized with low-temperature steam and formaldehyde. *Biologicals*, **33**, 191–196.

74 Kanemitsu, K. *et al.* (2003) Evaluation of a low-temperature steam and formaldehyde sterilizer. *Journal of Hospital Infection*, **55**, 47–52.

75 International Standards Organization (ISO) (2006) *ISO 11138-1. Sterilization of Health Care Products. Biological Indicators – Part 1: General Requirements*, ISO, Geneva.

76 Kanemitsu, K. *et al.* (2005) Validation of low-temperature steam with formaldehyde sterilization for endoscopes, using validation device. *Gastrointestinal Endoscopy*, **62**, 928–932.

77 Block, S.S. (2001) Peroxygen compounds, in *Disinfection, Sterilization and Preservation*, 5th edn (ed. S.S. Block), Lippincott Williams & Wilkins, Philadelphia, pp. 185–204.

78 Schumb, W.C. *et al.* (1955) *Hydrogen Peroxide*, Van Nostrand Rheinhold, New York, pp. 813–816.

79 Lin, S.M. *et al.* (1997) *Vapor Sterilization Using a non-Aqueous Source of Hydrogen Peroxide*, US Patent 5, 674,450.

80 Corveleyn, S. *et al.* (1997) Near-infrared (NIR) monitoring of H_2O_2 vapor concentration during vapor hydrogen peroxide (VHP) sterilisation. *Pharmaceutical Research*, **14**, 294–298.

81 Taizo, I. *et al.* (1998) Application of a newly developed hydrogen peroxide vapor phase sensor to HPV sterilizer. *Journal of Pharmaceutical Science and Technology*, **52**, 13–18.

82 Zhao, Z.H. *et al.* (1998) Toxicity of hydrogen peroxide produced by electroplated coating to pathogenic bacteria. *Canadian Journal of Microbiology*, **44**, 441–447.

83 Bardat, A. *et al.* (1996) Condensable chemical vapors for sterilization of freeze dryers. *Journal of Pharmaceutical Science and Technology*, **50**, 83–88.

84 Marcos-Martin, M.A. *et al.* (1996) Sterilization by vapor condensation. *Pharmaceutical Technology Europe*, **8**, 24–32.

85 Fichet, G. *et al.* (2007) Prion inactivation using a new gaseous hydrogen peroxide sterilization process. *Journal of Hospital Infection*, **67**, 278–286.

86 Bayliss, C.E. and Waites, W.M. (1979) The combined effect of hydrogen peroxide and ultra-violet light irradiation on bacterial spores. *Journal of Applied Bacteriology*, **47**, 263–269.

87 McGuire, M.J. and David, M.K. (1998) Treating water with Peroxone: a revolution in the making. *Water Engineering Management*, **135**, 42–49.

88 Wolfe, R.L. *et al.* (1989) Disinfection of model indicator organisms in a drinking water pilot plant by using peroxone. *Applied and Environmental Microbiology*, **55**, 2230–2241.

89 Behr, H. *et al.* (1997) Program abstract. Comparative sporicidal effects of vapor phase ozone alone and hydrogen peroxide alone and in combination. *97th Annual Meeting of American Society of Microbiology, Miami, May 4–8, 1997*, Abstract Q9.

90 Ashdown, B.C. *et al.* (1998) Hydrogen peroxide poisoning causing brain infarction: neuroimaging findings. *American Journal of Roentgenology*, **170**, 1653–1655.

91 Galtier, F. (1996) La stérilisationà basse température (T < 60°C) par d'autres agents chimiques gazeux, in *La Stérilisation* (ed. F. Galtier), Arnette Blackwell, Paris, pp. 141–148.

92 Barbut, F. *et al.* (2009) Comparaison of the efficacy of a hydrogen peroxide dry-mist disinfection system and sodium hypochlorite solution for eradication of *Clostridium difficile* spores. *Infection Control and Hospital Epidemiology*, **30**, 507–514.

93 Bates, C.J. and Pearse, R. (2005) Use of hydrogen peroxide vapor for environmental control during a *Serratia* outbreak in a neonatal intensive care unit. *Journal of Hospital Infection*, **61**, 364–366.

94 Boyce, J.M. (2009) New approaches to decontamination of rooms after patients are discharged. *Infection Control and Hospital Epidemiology*, **30**, 515–517.

95 French, G.L. *et al.* (2004) Tackling contamination of the hospital environment by methicillin-resistant *Staphylococcus aureus* (MRSA): a comparaison between conventional terminal cleaning and hydrogen peroxide vapor decontamination. *Journal of Hospital Infection*, **57**, 31–37.

96 Marty, N. *et al.* (2007) La désinfection par brouillard sec. *Hygiènes*, **4**, 317–320.

97 Otter, J.A. and French, G.L. (2009) Survival of nosocomial bacteria and spores on surfaces and inactivation by hydrogen peroxide vapor. *Journal of Clinical Microbiology*, **47**, 205–207.

98 Otter, J.A. *et al.* (2009) Feasibility of routinely using hydrogen peroxide vapor to decontaminate rooms in a busy United States hospital. *Infection Control and Hospital Epidemiology*, **30**, 574–577.

99 Freer, P.C. and Novy, F.G. (1902) On the formation, decomposition and germicidal action of benzoylacetyl and diacetyl peroxides. *American Chemical Journal*, **27**, 161–193.

100 Hutchings, I.J. and Xenozes, H. (1949) Comparative evaluation of the bactericidal efficiency of peracetic acid, quaternaries and chlorine containing compounds. In *49th Annual Meeting of American Society of Microbiology, Cincinnati, 1949*.

101 Jones, L.A. *et al.* (1967) Sporicidal activity of peracetic acid and beta-propriolactone at subzero temperatures. *Applied Microbiology*, **15**, 357–362.

102 Mücke, H. (1970) Properties of peracetic acid. *Wissenschaftliche Zeitschrift der Universität, Roostock. Mathematisch-naturwissenschaftliche Reihe*, **19**, 267–270.

103 Greenspan, F.P. and MacKellar, D.G. (1951) The application of peracetic acid germicidal washes to mold control of tomatoes. *Food Technology*, **5**, 95–97.

104 Portner, D.M. and Hoffman, R.K. (1968) Sporicidal effect of peracetic acid vapor. *Applied Microbiology*, **16**, 1782–1785.

105 Leaper, S. (1984) Influence of temperature on the synergistic sporicidal effect of peracetic plus hydrogen peroxide on *Bacillus subtilis* (SA 22). *Food Microbiology*, **1**, 199–230.

106 Malchesky, P.S. (1993) Peracetic acid and its application to medical instrument sterilization. *Artificial Organs*, **17**, 147–152.

107 Sprössig, M. *et al.* (1974) Experiments and considerations on the sterilization of thermolabile materials with peracetic acid. *Die Pharmazie*, **29**, 132–137.

108 Taylor, D.M. (1991) Resistance of the ME7 scrapie agent to peracetic acid. *Veterinary Microbiology*, **27**, 19–24.

109 Klopotek, B.B. (1998) Peracetic acid methods of preparation and properties. *Clinica Oggi*, **16**, 33–37.

110 Goullet, D. *et al.* (1995) Désinfection en pratique hospitalière, in *Antisepsie et Désinfection* (eds J. Fleurette *et al.*), ESKA, Paris, pp. 511–596.

111 Malchesky, P.S. (2001) Medical application of peracetic acid, in *Disinfection, Sterilization and Preservation*, 5th edn (ed. S.S. Block), Lippincott Williams & Wilkins, Philadelphia, pp. 979–996.

112 Wulzler, P. *et al.* (1991) *Apparatus and Method for Sterilizing or Disinfecting Objects*, US Patent 5, 008, 079.

113 Darbord, J.C. *et al.* (1992) Biofilm model for evaluating hemodialyzer reuse processing. *Dialysis and Transplantation*, **21**, 644–650.

114 Weavers, L.K. and Wickramanayake, G.B. (2001) Disinfection and sterilization using ozone, in *Disinfection, Sterilization and Preservation*, 5th edn (ed. S.S. Block), Lippincott Williams & Wilkins, Philadelphia, pp. 205–214.

115 German, A. *et al.* (1966) Essais de stérilisation par l'ozone. *Annales Pharmaceutiques Françaises*, **24**, 693–701.

116 Baticos, J. *et al.* (1981) Etude et réalisation d'un nouveau type d'ozoneur alimenté sous tension continue. *Environmental Technology Letters*, **2**, 67–74.

117 Rice, R.G. (1999) Ozone in the United States of America state-of-the-art. *Ozone: Science and Engineering*, **21**, 99–118.

118 Hudson, J.B. *et al.* (2007) Inactivation of Norovirus by ozone gas in conditions relevant to healthcare. *Journal of Hospital Infection*, **66**, 40–45.

119 Sharma, M. and Hudson, J.B. (2007) Ozone gas is an effective and practical antibacterial agent. *Infection Control and Hospital Epidemiology*, **36**, 559–563.

120 Wickramanayake, G.B. (1991) Disinfection and sterilization by ozone, in *Disinfection, Sterilization, and Preservation*, 4th edn (ed. S.S. Block), Lea & Febiger, Philadelphia, pp. 182–190.

121 Ishizaki, K. *et al.* (1986) Inactivation of *Bacillus* spores by gaseous ozone. *Journal of Applied Bacteriology*, **60**, 67–72.

122 Berrington, A.W. and Pedler, S. (1998) Investigation of gaseous ozone for MRSA decontamination of hospital side-rooms. *Journal of Hospital Infection*, **40**, 61–65.

123 Behr, H. *et al.* (1999) Program abstract. Effects of acetic acid adding to ozone–hydrogen peroxide complex. A comparative study of inactivation of vegetative forms, bacterial spores and yeasts. *99th Annual Meeting of American Society of Microbiology, Chicago, 30 June–3 July 1999*, Abstract Q126.

124 Behr, H. *et al.* (1999) Program abstract. Evaluation of virucide activity of BOX03™ device against coated and naked viruses. *99th Annual Meeting of American Society of Microbiology, Chicago, 30 June–3 July 1999*, Abstract Q125.

125 Agence d'Evaluation des Technologies et des Modes d'Intervention en Santé (2009) *Note informative du 25/02/2009. Evaluation de solutions de rechange à l'oxyde d'éthylène en stérilisation: plasma de peroxyde d'hydrogène et ozone*, Quebec.

126 Coronel, B. *et al.* (2001) *In situ* decontamination of medical wastes using oxidative agents: a 16-month study in a polyvalent intensive care unit. *Journal of Hospital Infection*, **50**, 207–212.

127 Masuda, S. (1988) *Method for Sterilizing Objects to be Sterilized and Sterilizing Apparatus*, European Patent 0, 281, 870.

128 Karlson, E.L. (1989) Ozone sterilization. *Journal of Healthcare Material Management*, **7**, 43–45.

129 Stoddart, G.M. (1989) Ozone as a sterilizing agent. *Journal of Healthcare Material Management*, **7**, 42–43.

130 Robitaille, S. *et al.* (2003) *Method and Apparatus for Ozone Sterilization*, Canadian Patent CA2466307.

131 Dufresne, S. *et al.* (2007) Relationship between lumen diameter and length sterilized in the 125L ozone sterilizer. *Infection Control and Hospital Epidemiology*, **36**, 291–297.

132 Orcutt, R.P. *et al.* (1981) Alcide™: an alternative sterilant to peracetic acid, in *Recent Advances in Germfree Research. Proceedings of the VIIth International Symposium on Gnotobiology* (eds S. Sasaki *et al.*), Tokai University Press, Tokyo, pp. 79–81.

133 Rosenblatt, D.H. *et al.* (1985) *Use of Chlorine Dioxide as a Chemosterilizing Agent*, US Patent 4, 504, 442.

134 Knapp, J.E. and Battisti, D.L. (2001) Chlorine dioxide, in *Disinfection, Sterilization and Preservation*, 5th edn (ed. S.S. Block), Lippincott Williams & Wilkins, Philadelphia, pp. 215–227.

135 Jeng, D.K. and Woodworth, A.G. (1990) Chlorine dioxide gas sterilization under square wave conditions. *Applied and Environmental Microbiology*, **56**, 514–519.

136 Morrissey, R.F. (1996) Changes in the science of sterilization and disinfection. *Biomedical Instrumentation and Technology/Association for the Advancement of Medical Instrumentation*, **30**, 404–406.

137 Thiveaud, D. (1998) Stérilisation par gaz-plasma. *Hygiène en Milieu Hospitalier*, **7**, 19–23.

138 Cariou, S. and Hermelin-Jobet, I. (2001) Stérilisation en phase plasma, in *La Stérilisation en Milieu Hospitalier*, 3rd edn (ed. Collège d'Enseignement Pharmaceutique Hospitalier), CEPH, Cahors, pp. 285–300.

139 Menashi, W.P. (1968) *Treatment of Surfaces*, US Patent 3, 383, 163.

140 Ascham, L.E. and Menashi, W.P. (1972) *Treatment of Surfaces with Low Pressure Plasmas*, US Patent 3, 701, 628.

141 Fraser, S. *et al.* (1974) *Sterilizing and Packaging Process Utilizing Gas Plasma*, US Patent 3, 851, 436.

142 Fraser, S. *et al.* (1974) *Sterilizing and Packaging Process Utilizing Gas Plasma*, US Patent 3, 948, 601.

143 Tensmeyer, L.G. (1976) *Method of Killing Micro-organisms in the Inside of a Container Utilizing a Laser Beam Induced Plasma*, US Patent 3, 955, 921.

144 Boucher, R.R. (1980) *Seeded Gas Plasma Sterilization Method*, US Patent 4, 207,286.

145 Tensmeyer, L.G. *et al.* (1981) Sterilization of glass containers by laser initiated plasmas. *Journal of Parenteral Science and Technology*, **35**, 93–96.

146 Bithell, R.M. (1982) *Packaging and Sterilizing Process for Same*, US Patent 4, 321,232.

147 Bithell, R.M. (1982) *Plasma Pressure Pulse Sterilization*, US Patent 4, 348, 357.

148 Peeples, R.E. and Anderson, N.R. (1985) Microwave coupled plasma sterilization and depyrogenation I. Systems characteristics. *Journal of Parenteral Science and Technology*, **39**, 2–8.

149 Peeples, R.E. and Anderson, N.R. (1985) Microwave coupled plasma sterilization and depyrogenation II. Mechanisms of action. *Journal of Parenteral Science and Technology*, **39**, 9–15.

150 Jacobs, P.T. and Lin, S. (1987) *Hydrogen Peroxide Plasma Sterilization System*, US Patent 4, 643, 876.

151 Addy, T.O. (1989) Low-temperature plasma: a new sterilization technology for hospital application, in *Sterilization of Medical Products* (eds R.F. Morrissey and Y.I. Prokopenko), Polyscience Publications, Morin Heights, Canada, pp. 80–95.

152 Addy, T.O. (1991) Low-temperature plasma: a new sterilization technology for hospital application, in *Sterilization of Medical Products* (eds R.F. Morrissey and Y.I. Prokopenko), Polyscience Publications, Morin Heights, Canada, pp. 89–95.

153 Caputo, R.A. *et al.* (1992) *Plasma Sterilizing Process with Pulsed Microbicidal Agent*, US Patent 5, 084, 239.

154 Lerouge, S. *et al.* (2002) Safety of plasma-based sterilization: surface modifications of polymeric medical devices induced by Sterrad® and Plazlyte® processes. *Bio-medical Materials and Engineering*, **12**, 3–13.

155 Duffy, R.E. *et al.* (2000) An epidemic of corneal destruction caused by plasma gas sterilization. *Archives of Ophthalmology*, **118**, 1167–1176.

156 Smith, C.A. *et al.* (2000) Unexpected corneal endothelial cell decompensation after intracellular surgery with instruments sterilized by plasma gas. *Ophthalmology*, **107**, 1561–1566.

157 Spry, C. (1998) Low-temperature hydrogen peroxide gas plasma – atomic age sterilization technology. *Today's Surgical Nurse*, **20**, 25–28.

158 Roberts, C. and Antanoplus, P. (1998) Inactivation of human immunodeficiency virus type 1, hepatitis A virus, respiratory syncitial virus, vaccinia virus, herpes simplex virus type 1, and poliovirus type 2 by hydrogen peroxide gas plasma sterilization. *American Journal of Infection Control*, **26**, 94–101.

159 Vassal, S. *et al.* (1998) Hydrogen peroxide gas plasma sterilization is effective against *Cryptosporidium parvum* oocysts. *American Journal of Infection Control*, **26**, 136–138.

160 Rulata, W.A. *et al.* (1999) Sporicidal activity of a new low-temperature sterilization technology: the Sterrad 50 sterilizer. *Infection Control and Hospital Epidemiology*, **20**, 514–516.

161 Vickery, K. *et al.* (1999) Inactivation of duck hepatitis B virus by a hydrogen gas plasma sterilization system: laboratory and "in-use" testing. *Journal of Hospital Infection*, **41**, 317–322.

162 Rutala, W.A. and Weber, D.J. (2004) Disinfection and sterilization in health care facilities: what clinicians need to know. *Clinical Infectious Diseases*, **39**, 702–709.

163 Moisan, M. *et al.* (2001) Low-temperature sterilization using gas plasmas: a review of the experiments and an analysis of the inactivation mechanisms. *International Journal of Pharmaceutics*, **226**, 1–21.

164 Lerouge, S. *et al.* (2000) Effect of gas composition on spore mortality and etching during low-temperature plasma sterilization. *Journal of Biomedical Materials Research*, **51**, 128–135.

165 Krebs, M.C. *et al.* (1998) Gas-plasma sterilization: relative efficacy of the hydrogen peroxide phase compared with that of the plasma phase. *International Journal of Pharmaceutics*, **160**, 75–81.

166 Tessarolo, F. *et al.* (2006) Sterility and microbiological assessment of reused single-use cardiac electrophysiology catheters. *Infection Control and Hospital Epidemiology*, **27**, 1385–1392.

167 Rogez-Kreuz, C. *et al.* (2009) Inactivation of animal and human prions by hydrogen peroxide gas plasma sterilization. *Infection Control and Hospital Epidemiology*, **30**, 769–777.

168 Advanced Sterilization Products (ASP) (2008) Etudes sur l'inactivation des prions par les systèmes de sterilisation Sterrad®. *Hygienes*, **3**, 205.

169 Alfa, M.J. *et al.* (1998) New low temperature sterilization technologies: microbicidal activity and clinical efficacy, in *Disinfection, Sterilization and Antisepsis in Health Care* (ed. W.A. Rutala), Polyscience Publications, Champlain, NY, pp. 67–78.

170 Penna, T.C.V. *et al.* (1999) The presterilization microbial load on used medical devices and the effectiveness of hydrogen peroxide gas plasma against *Bacillus subtilis* spores. *Infection Control and Hospital Epidemiology*, **20**, 465–472.

171 Okpara-Hofmann, J. *et al.* (2005) Comparison of low-temperature hydrogen peroxide gas plasma sterilization for endoscopes using various Sterrad™ models. *Journal of Hospital Infection*, **59**, 280–285.

172 Feldman, L.A. and Hui, H.K. (1997) Compatibility of medical devices and materials with low-temperature hydrogen gas plasma. *Medical Device and Diagnostic Industry*, **19**, 57–62.

173 Brown, S.A. *et al.* (2002) Effects of different disinfection and sterilization methods on tensile strength of materials used for single-use devices. *Biomedical Instrumentation and Technology*, **36**, 23–27.

174 Peniston, S.J. and Choi, S.J. (2007) Effect of sterilization on the physicochemical properties of molded poly(L-lactic acid). *Journal of Biomedical Materials Research. Part B, Applied Biomaterials*, **80**, 67–77.

175 Institut National de Recherche et de Sécurité (INRS) (2007) *Peroxyde d'hydrogène et solutions aqueuses*, Fiche Toxicologique No. 123, INRS, Paris.

176 Goullet, D. *et al.* (1996) Fiches de stérilisation no. 15: Stérilisation en phase plasma. *Hygiènes*, **12**, 1–209.

177 Baxter, H.C. *et al.* (2005) Elimination of transmissible spongiform encephalopathy infectivity and decontamination of surgical instruments by using radio-frequency gas-plasma treatment. *Journal of General Virology*, **86**, 2393–2399.

178 Boscariol, M.R. *et al.* (2008) Sterilization by pure oxygen plasma and by oxygen-hydrogen peroxide plasma: an efficacy study. *International Journal of Pharmaceutics*, **353**, 170–175.

179 Hong, Y.F. *et al.* (2009) Sterilization effect of atmospheric plasma on *Escherichia coli* and *Bacillus subtilis* endospores. *Letters in Applied Microbiology*, **48**, 33–37.

180 Lakhssassi, N. *et al.* (2006) Dégradation de l'ADN bactérien par de l'azote atomique produit par plasma. Apport de la détection par PCR en temps réel. *Pathologie et Biologie*, **54**, 482–487.

181 Lee, K. *et al.* (2006) Sterilization of bacteria, yeast, and bacterial endospores by atmospheric-pressure cold plasma using helium and oxygen. *Journal of Microbiology*, **44**, 269–275.

182 Seong-Mi, K. and Jong-Il, K. (2006) Decomposition of biological macromolecules by plasma generated with helium and oxygen. *Journal of Microbiology*, **44**, 466–471.

183 Shintani, H. *et al.* (2007) Inactivation of microorganisms and endotoxins by low-temperature nitrogen gas plasma exposure. *Biocontrol Sciences*, **4**, 131–143.

184 Thiveaud, D. (2008) La stérlisation basse température. *Hygiène en Milieu Hospitalier*, **91**, 15–27.

185 Yu, Q.S. *et al.* (2007) Bacterial inactivation using a low-temperature atmospheric plasma brush sustained with argon gas. *Journal of Biomedical Materials Research. Part B, Applied Biomaterals*, **80**, 211–219.

186 Rutala, W.A. and Weber, D.J. (1999) Infection control: the role of disinfection and sterilization. *Journal of Hospital Infection*, **43** (Suppl.), 43–55.

187 Vincent, I. *et al.* (2003) Problématique liée à la disparition des procédés de stérilisation à basse température en milieu hospitalier: expérience de l'hôpital Haut-Lévêque. *Techniques Hospitalières*, **58**, 21–24.

188 Fournier, S. (2002) *Method for Sterilizing an Endoscope*, US Patent 6, 365,103.

15.4 Gas Plasma Sterilization

Gerald McDonnell

Research and Technical Affairs, STERIS Ltd, Basingstoke, UK

Introduction

From a chemical perspective, matter can be defined as any living or non-living thing that takes up space. It can be made of single elements (such as with hydrogen, oxygen and nitrogen) or a combination of elements (such as water, H_2O, and hydrogen peroxide, H_2O_2). In all cases they can exist in three energy states: solids, liquids and gases. The simplest example is with water; at low temperatures/pressures it can be present in a solid form (ice) but as energy is added (in the form of heat) it becomes a liquid (water) and eventually a gas (steam). Plasma (or gas plasma) are considered as a fourth state of matter. They are essentially gases that are energized to cause ionization of the molecules present into equal numbers of positively- and negatively-charged particles. These particles, depending on the source liquid/gas, have potential microbicidal effects as they can be very reactive with any molecules they meet such as proteins and lipids. Plasmas are naturally occurring, for example as lightening and as part of the sun/other stars. They are used for a variety of industrial applications in different forms, such as in televisions, fluorescent lights, surface modifications and for microfabrication (e.g. circuit boards).

Plasma can be classified in many ways, for example using the source gas (oxygen or nitrogen gas plasma) or as being of "high"

or "low" temperature. The temperature has a direct impact on the extent of ionization, where higher temperatures are required to fully ionize the gas and lower temperatures for partial ionization. However, in some industrial applications, "cold" plasma can be at significantly high temperatures (>1000°C). For decontamination applications we are primarily concerned with cold plasma applications. Plasma can be generated by the application of sufficient energy, in the form of temperature or an electromagnetic field, to a gas. Typical methods used to generate low-temperature plasma from their source gases include the use of microwaves, direct current or radiofrequency waves. They are more commonly generated under deep vacuum (low pressure), although atmospheric plasmas that operate at low temperatures have also been described [1]. Overall, the life-times of any reactive species present on plasma generation are short-lived (in particular when the energy source is removed), but under atmospheric conditions they are much shorter than for plasma generated under vacuum. The generation of temperature during these processes can also be a concern; therefore, some investigators have suggested that atmospheric or partial vacuum conditions using plasma pulsing may be a useful compromise [2]. Vacuum conditions are not only important in the consideration of optimum plasma generation but also in the removal of interfering air/gases that can limit the penetration of any plasma reactive species to a given load for sterilization (similar to steam and low-temperature sterilization processes, discussed in Chapters 15.1 and 15.3, respectively). However, it should also be remembered that air itself is a mixture of gases (primarily nitrogen and oxygen) that could itself be activated by plasma generation as a microbicidal process or for the treatment of air.

Plasmas have been investigated for a variety of decontamination applications including cleaning, disinfection and sterilization. The term "plasma" can be used to describe a variety of processes that use plasma directly or indirectly for its cleaning and/or microbicidal effects. In its pure sense, the direct use of plasma (either under atmospheric or vacuum conditions) has been investigated for its cleaning [3, 4] and microbial inactivation (see, for example, [5–7]) benefits. Investigations have focused on studying the microbicidal effects against various pathogens and, in particular, bacterial spores (as the key target for achieving the minimum criteria in the development of a sterilization process) [1, 8, 9]. There are even more applications that describe the indirect use of plasma in a variety of ways, such as for the removal of residuals from gas-exposed surfaces [10, 11] and for the "activation" of water (or other liquids) to generate various active species (such as ozone and hypochlorite ions) that are actually the true source of microbicidal activity rather than the plasma itself [12].

In this chapter, direct and indirect methods of plasma sterilization are of specific interest, with some brief consideration given to cleaning and disinfection methods. Emphasis is placed on the direct use of plasma as a microbicide and the differences observed in the use of various source gases used to generate the plasma. These investigations have led to some interesting proposals regarding the mode of action of various types of gas plasma. Perspectives on the future development of gas plasma as true sterilization techniques are further discussed.

Applications of gas plasma for decontamination

Decontamination, in the context of this chapter, can be defined as any physical or chemical means to render a surface or item safe for handling, use or disposal. From a microbicidal point of view, this can include the physical removal of contamination (or cleaning) and/or the inactivation of microorganisms on a surface (disinfection and sterilization). Various types of plasma have been investigated for all these forms of application, either on their own on in combination with other technologies.

Plasma cleaning has been recently developed in laboratory-scale applications for the detailed removal of proteins and other molecules (including lipopolysaccharides such as endotoxins) from surfaces [4], with a particular application for the removal of prion proteins associated with infectivity at low detectable concentrations [3]. Particular investigations have focused on the use of argon–oxygen gas mixture plasma [3]. In these studies, the authors found that low levels of soil, below visual detection limits, remained on device surfaces following their routine cleaning. Surfaces that were pre-wetted with water and then treated with argon–oxygen plasma showed excellent soil removal when analyzed by scanning electron microscopy and by energy-dispersive analysis of X-ray (EDX). Organic material was more efficiently removed than inorganic soil deposits. Similar results had been reported with plasma cleaning of dental instruments [4]. It was suggested that routine cleaning (with detergents) could be used to remove gross soil, followed by detailed cleaning with plasma. This has particular medical significance when considering prion contamination, as prions are infectious, hydrophobic proteins that can be difficult to physically remove from surfaces [13] (also see Chapter 10). Industrial applications that may also have rigorous requirements for protein or other biomolecule residue removal from surfaces may similarly benefit from considering this technology. Plasma methods have been recommended as alternative cleaning methods due to their ability to degrade biological molecules, including proteins. Such processes require further investigation for practical implementation in various cleaning applications.

Numerous patents and publications describe the use of plasma in microbicidal methods for at least the past 20 years (e.g. describing hydrogen peroxide gas plasma [14, 15]; using peracetic gas plasma [16]) and have been reviewed [5, 10]. These processes can be considered for disinfection (to reduce the levels and types of microorganisms that may be present on a given surface or in the air) as well as for sterilization applications (defined as the complete inactivation of all microorganisms on a surface or in the air, to achieve sterility or being free of viable microorganisms). Particular plasmas of interest include those based on hydrogen peroxide, peracetic acids, oxygen, nitrogen, nitric oxide and aldehydes such as formaldehyde and glutaraldehyde. The first truly commercialized patents focused on the use of oxidizing agent gases (such as hydrogen peroxide [14] and peracetic acid [16]). However, the subsequent development of sterilization processes using these technologies has generally used plasma as only part of the overall cycle. The most notable of these processes are the Sterrad® family of hydrogen peroxide gas plasma sterilizers. Patents around this process initially described the introduction of hydrogen peroxide to the load and then applying an energy source to generate the plasma for sterilization purposed [14], while a subsequent patent described the use of plasma to remove residual levels of hydrogen peroxide that could remain within the load [15].

The Sterrad and other similar sterilizer designs that have been subsequently developed are described in further detail later in this chapter. For all these cases, the plasmas are actually only generated in part of the process for residual removal, with the true microbicidal effects primarily achieved using hydrogen peroxide gas (itself a powerful microbicidal agent) [11, 12, 17, 18]. In these systems, the gas is allowed to contact the sterilizer load under vacuum for a given period of time, most of the gas is then evacuated and any residual of gas/liquid peroxide is then removed by plasma application. Although the plasma could have some microbicidal activity, in practical use little to no contributory microbicidal effect has been observed in the presence or absence of the plasma [11]. In these cases, the main role of the plasma is for the adequate removal of any gas (in particular condensed liquid) residuals that may be present in the load following gas exposure.

In other cases, plasmas have been used as a source of energy to generate the oxidizing agent gas from a liquid source. Other applications have been described that similarly use plasma indirectly as energy or activation sources as part of a microbicidal process. These include air and liquid applications. Air disinfection systems have been described, where air is passed through an electric field to generate "plasma". It is suggested that the observed microbicidal effects are due to the localized generation of reactive oxygen species that are present in plasma, but this may equally be due to the localized generation of ozone (a particularly effective agent at low concentrations against bacteria) as the true mechanism of action. Similar systems have been described for liquid (particularly water systems) and are often referred to as "activated" or "plasma-activated" water. Again, in these cases the activity observed may not be due to any true plasma effects but may be due to the production of ozone or, in particular, the hypochlorite ion (OCl^-), being one of the main active species in a chlorine solution [12].

More recent investigations have focused on the direct use of plasma as microbicidals, such as those based on oxygen, nitrogen, other noble gases and mixtures thereof [1]. These have been primarily studied for their direct microbicidal properties, with particular emphasis on their use as alternative low-temperature sterilization processes to steam sterilization. The potential use of these technologies at low temperature, as well as their ability not only to show broad-spectrum microbicidal activity against "traditional" microorganisms such as bacteria (including endospores), viruses and fungi, but also to neutralize toxic (endotoxin) or transmissible (prion) molecules, has made them attractive alternatives to traditional heat- and chemical-based sterilization methods. Similar applications could also be used for lower-level disinfection or sanitization uses, such as for device, general surface, dental, tissue, food and air treatment methods. These include the particular use of atmospheric, non-thermal plasma jets [19–21].

Overall, plasmas can be applied in various applications in two general ways: (i) directly, where the plasma is directly generated at the site of application (e.g. where the gas is allowed to diffuse over an area and then the plasma activated); or (ii) indirectly, where the plasma is generated at a remote site and transferred to a site of use. The latter system may be useful when the surface to be treated is exposed to the plasma directly, not requiring significant penetration. It has been concluded during initial studies with plasma, particularly for sterilization applications requiring penetration through packaging materials (used to store the materials under sterile conditions until used), that gas plasmas were not particularly penetrating [10, 14]; while plasmas tested could demonstrate microbicidal activity on exposed surfaces, little to no activity was observed in packaged materials. In this case, the authors concluded that the gas should be allowed to diffuse through the packaging materials prior to plasma activation in order to optimize plasma sterilization efficiency. In disinfection applications – such as on foods, skin, wound and general hard surfaces – direct application of low-temperature, non-thermal plasma could be practically used by generation of the plasma remotely and applying to a surface [19, 20].

Sterilization systems that use gas plasma

Hydrogen peroxide gas plasma sterilization

Hydrogen peroxide is one of the most widely used microbicides, both in liquid and in gas form [12] (see Chapters 2 and 15.3). This is primarily due to its broad-spectrum microbicidal activity (dependent on its concentration and use), reasonably good safety profile, and lack of significant environmental concerns (rapidly degrading into water and oxygen). It is therefore used as a potent antiseptic, disinfectant and sterilization agent. It has been known for some time (since the 1970s) that hydrogen peroxide gas is a more efficient microbicidal at dramatically lower concentrations than in liquid form [17]. Hydrogen peroxide gas sterilization systems can be considered in two groups: those that use plasma during the process and those that do not. The non-plasma-containing systems were initially used for efficient room disinfection applications [18] and more recently for sterilization. Sterilization applications using hydrogen peroxide gas alone include their use under atmospheric conditions in high-speed packaging systems (at temperatures in the 40–60°C range) that allow the use of high concentrations of peroxide gas with or without condensation [22] and under vacuum conditions for package device sterilization [23, 24]. Overall, hydrogen peroxide gas is itself a widely accepted sterilization agent. These processes are described elsewhere in further detail [12](see also Chapter 15.3) but further consideration is given to the use of hydrogen peroxide plasma sterilization systems within the context of this chapter.

A variety of hydrogen peroxide plasma sterilizers have been marketed worldwide (Figure 15.4.1). The most widely used hydrogen peroxide plasma sterilization systems in use today are the Sterrad series of sterilizers. However, in recent years many similar sterilizer designs have become available. With some system-specific differences, these sterilizers all work by the same basic mechanism and are similar in design. For the purpose of this chapter, the particular processes used in the Sterrad series are described in further detail.

The first commercial sterilizer in the range was the Sterrad® 100 and was introduced in the early 1990s [10]. The sterilizer, with a chamber size of 75 l, was limited in the capacity of the load that could be sterilized per cycle, requiring the use of non-cellulose-based packaging materials and limitations in the ability to sterilize devices that contained internal channels (3 mm internal diameter by ≤400 mm length). For longer-lumened, opened-ended devices, an accessory known as a "booster" could be used that itself contained a 59% liquid hydrogen peroxide source and was attached to one end of the lumen to directly deliver peroxide

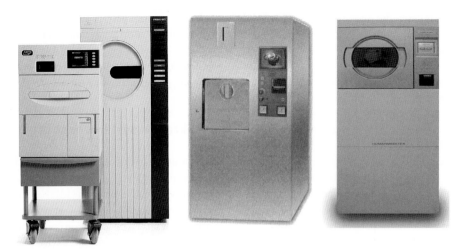

Figure 15.4.1 Examples of various different low-temperature sterilizers that use plasma indirectly as part of their sterilization processes: the Sterrad 50 (shown on a cart) and Sterrad 100S sterilizers on the left.

gas during the process. However, this accessory only received regulatory approval and has only been commercialized in certain geographic regions. The original Sterrad 100 sterilization cycle consisted of drawing a deep vacuum in the sterilization chamber, the vaporization of 59% liquid hydrogen peroxide (41% water) in the chamber (to give a saturated gas concentration of c. 6 mg/l in a non-loaded chamber), allowing the gas to diffuse to elicit its microbicidal activity, redrawing the deep vacuum, generating a plasma and then venting to atmospheric pressure to allow access to the chamber [10]. The plasma is this case was generated by applying radiofrequency energy (400 W) to any remaining hydrogen peroxide within the chamber. In this case, any peroxide residuals could be safely degraded to non-toxic by-products such as water and oxygen. The process was validated to be effective against bacteria (Gram-positive and Gram-negative), mycobacteria, bacterial spores, yeast, fungi, viruses (enveloped and non-enveloped) and protozoal oocysts [10]. Hydrogen peroxide gas itself is rapidly effective against these organisms and several studies have confirmed that *Geobacillus stearothermophilus* endospores are the most resistant organism, in contrast to the spores of *Bacillus atrophaeus* being the most resistant to liquid hydrogen peroxide [17, 18]. Hydrogen peroxide gas is an effective sporicidal agent even at concentrations as low as 0.1 mg/l (with a typical *G. stearothermophilus* spore D-value of c. 10 min at this concentration). Initial studies by the manufacturer of the process demonstrated a significant microbicidal effect, depending on the peroxide gas concentration, diffusion time and power of plasma generation. However, the true contribution of the plasma to the microbicidal activity of the process was subsequently shown to be at best minor in comparison to the direct effects of the peroxide gas alone [11]. The process (in addition to a further peracetic acid gas plasma process, the Plazlyte®) was also shown to be very sensitive to the presence of residual organic and/or inorganic soil [25].

The Sterrad 100 process was subsequently updated and released in 1997 as the Sterrad® 100S [26]. This provided a different, more efficient sterilization cycle. This was also the basis of the development of smaller (Sterrad® 50, with a capacity of 44 l) and larger (Sterrad® 200, with a capacity of 150 l) sterilizers. The exact cycle (or cycles) programmed vary depending on the specific design, in particular due to the size of the sterilizer chamber and regulatory approvals. In general, this Sterrad series (100S, 200 and 50 sterilizers) have similar cycle conditions, consisting of three basic phases: preconditioning, sterilization and venting. During the Sterrad 100S cycle (Figure 15.4.2), the chamber walls are maintained at c. 45°C during the whole cycle, essentially to maintain ambient conditions during the cycle.

For preconditioning, the aluminum chamber is evacuated to c. 0.09 kPa (0.7 Torr) pressure, a plasma is generated (by applying radiofrequency energy) in any remaining air (or water that maybe present) for 10 min, and the chamber is returned to atmospheric pressure (c. 101 kPa or 760 Torr). The preconditioning cycle is used to remove some moisture from the load, which will interfere with the sterilization process due to the lack of penetration of peroxide gas into liquids, as well as allowing for some pre-heating of the load. The sterilization phase is in two identical pulse cycles. In each pulse, the chamber pressure is reduced to 0.05 kPa (0.4 Torr), and 59% liquid hydrogen peroxide (41% water) is injected, vaporized and allowed to diffuse for about 6 min (to give a typical concentration in an empty chamber of c. 7 mg/l hydrogen peroxide gas, although this concentration will be significantly less in the presence of a chamber load). The chamber is then allowed to diffuse to atmospheric pressure for 2 min and is re-evacuated over a minimum of 5 min to 0.065 kPa (0.5 Torr). It is during this stage that the majority of the remaining peroxide gas is removed from the chamber. Only then is the plasma initiated for a total time of 2 min. The second pulse begins by further reducing the pressure from 0.065 kPa (0.5 Torr) to 0.05 kPa and

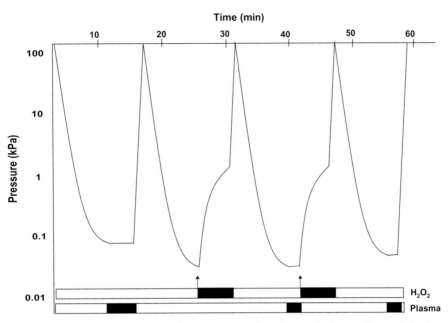

Figure 15.4.2 The Sterrad 100S sterilization cycles. The exposure time, for this particular cycle is about 55 min. Pressure changes during the cycle are shown in a log_{10} scale. During the cycle, exposures to hydrogen peroxide gas (injection of gas indicated by arrows) and times of plasma generation are shown (black bars). Note that atmospheric pressure is 101.35 kPa or 760 mmHg (760 Torr).

repeating the rest of the pulse (peroxide injection, diffusion, re-evacuation and plasma generation) as described above. The chamber is then simply vented to atmospheric pressure to allow access to the load. Unlike other traditional low-temperature gaseous sterilization methods (based on the use of humidified ethylene oxide or formaldehyde), no further aeration is required and any materials are immediately ready for use.

Overall, the minimum cycle time in this case is about 55 min, although longer cycle times will result in the presence of larger chamber loads due to variations in the times for evacuation to low pressure levels during the cycle. Each sterilizer may have specific cycles defined and claims regarding restrictions on lumen lengths/diameters, the specifics of which are detailed in the manufacturer's instructions. The Sterrad 200 for example has been used for hospital as well as industrial applications, where unique cycles can be developed to address specific load requirements industrially. In recent years, the Sterrad 100S process has been tested against prions. Although hydrogen peroxide gas has been shown to inactivate the infectivity associated with prions [27, 28], the 100S process has not been shown to be effective against prions following single or multiple cycles [29, 30]. These results highlight specific differences in safety and efficacy that can be result from different cycle conditions.

A new series of Sterrad sterilizers have become available recently, known as the NX series (the Sterrad® NX and Sterrad® 100NX). This has presented a new sterilizer process distinct from the older 100S process. The major difference with the NX technology is a patented vaporization system that concentrates hydrogen peroxide by removing most of the water [31]. This is achieved

by taking advantage of the differences in vapor pressure between peroxide and water gas; 59% liquid peroxide (in 41% water) is vaporized to generate a mixture of peroxide and water gas in a separate chamber. By reducing the temperature in the chamber, concentrated liquid peroxide condenses out leaving water in gas phase, which can then be removed from the chamber. The concentrated peroxide (at 90–95%) is then re-vaporized for use in the main chamber for sterilization. The concentration stage is performed while the pressure in the main chamber is being reduced to allow for the subsequent introduction of peroxide gas, diffusion, reapplying the vacuum and initiating plasma production on any residuals. This is repeated for a total of two pulses.

The Sterrad NX is a smaller sterilizer (with a claimed useable chamber of 30 l) with, at the time of writing, two alternative sterilization cycles using the new concentrated process [32]. It is used for metal and non-metal device sterilization, including diffusion-restrictive instruments such as the hinged parts of scissors and forceps. The "standard" cycle has an estimated cycle time of 28 min and can be used for various devices, including single-channeled stainless steel lumens with an internal diameter of ≥1 mm and length of ≤150 mm or ≥2 mm diameter and length of ≤ 400 mm. An additional "advanced" cycle (38 min cycle time) may be used for longer, stainless steel, lumened devices (≥1 mm and length of ≤500 mm) and certain single-channeled flexible devices (≥1 mm and length of ≤850 mm). These cycles do not require the use of boosters, as previously described for the older-generation Sterrad sterilizers. In addition to the use of a higher concentration of peroxide gas, the plasma power generated is higher at 500 W in comparison to the older-generation sterilizers.

The Sterrad 100NX uses a similar sterilization cycle principle but with a larger chamber (claimed usable volume of *c.* 100 l, and >25% larger than the 100S sterilizer chamber), with a standard cycle of 47 min and a "flex" cycle of 42 min [33, 34]. Independent testing of these cycles and lumen claims have supported efficacy (under full cycle test conditions), although there have been reports of device incompatibility, in particular related to the effects on surface finishes and adhesives [35]. The microbicidal efficacy in the NX process is supported by previous investigations with the older Sterrad series, to include bactericidal, sporicidal, virucidal, fungicidal and mycobactericidal activities. In addition, a sterility assurance level (SAL) of 10^{-6} has been demonstrated for the process [33]. It is of interest to note that the NX process has been shown to be effective against prions in contrast to previous reports on the effectiveness of the 100S process [30]. This may be due to the higher concentrations of peroxide used or other differences in process conditions such as reducing the risk of peroxide condensation [28].

Other hydrogen peroxide gas plasma sterilizers (such as the Human Mediteck HMTS series, Belimed Plasmater™ series, Shinva PS™ series and the CISA SPS™ series) all essentially use the same processes as described for the Sterrad 100S, although they differ in cycles times, temperatures, concentration of peroxide liquid to generate the sterilant, final concentration of gas in the chamber, presence of saturated or unsaturated gas, methods and extent of plasma generation, vacuum levels employed throughout the cycle, and number/types of vacuum pulses during the cycle. In all cases they use plasma as a method to degrade peroxide residues within the chamber (either directly within the chamber or adjacent to it) and the contribution to microbicidal efficacy is considered negligible (or not to date demonstrated otherwise). However, in some designs, plasma is used to generate the peroxide gas (as an alternative to heat or hot-plate vaporization) itself but not at sufficient energy levels to generate any true gas plasma. At the time of writing there have been few independent data published on or comparing the range of hydrogen peroxide gas plasma sterilizers available.

Other oxidizing agent-based plasma systems

Similar peracetic acid gas plasma sterilizers have been described and developed. These systems include the use of peracetic acid gas plasma directly as the microbicide, or the use of the gas as the sterilant, followed by removal of gas residuals using plasma, as described for the hydrogen peroxide systems above. Caputo and co-workers described the use of peracetic acid gas (*c.* 0.5 mg/l) along with plasma for sterilization [16]. Peracetic acid itself, in liquid or gas form, is a powerful microbicide at low concentrations due to its oxidizing agent activity [36, 37]. At the same time, the liquid form can be very aggressive on certain types of surface materials if not correctly formulated [37]. The gas has been considered to be less aggressive when used at lower concentrations for sporicidal activity, although this requires further investigation.

A sterilization process developed in the USA, the AbTox Plazlyte™ sterilization system, used humidified peracetic acid gas exposure followed by plasma generation in multiple, pulsing cycles [38, 39]. Specific cycles were defined for various hospital and industrial applications, such as in hospitals for porous loads and for endoscopic, lumened devices. Despite some successful use of the process in such applications, in 1998 the US Food and Drug Administration (FDA) issued a safety alert on one of the hospital-based devices based on an investigation of toxicity associated with Plazlyte-sterilized ocular devices following surgery. The product was at that time withdrawn from use and circulation. Investigations with a similar system demonstrated good microbicidal effects but potential problems with device compatibility and toxicity [40].

Similar processes have been proposed with peracetic acid, chlorine dioxide and ozone-based plasma sterilization processes, both using the respective gas plasma directly for disinfection/sterilization purposes or indirectly as part of the process (including residue neutralization and load preconditioning).

Sterilization with gas plasma

There has been particular interest over the last 10 years in the investigation of microbicidal properties and sterilization process development with gas plasma. This has been encouraged by advances in the development of plasma technologies (low temperature, atmospheric plasma as an example), the increasing development of temperature-sensitive reusable devices that require rapid sterilization turnaround times, and the proposed benefits of plasma over existing technologies (such as broad-spectrum microbicidal activity, lack of toxic residues, ease and safety of generation, etc.). An emphasis of these studies has been to study and maximize the microbicidal effects of gas plasma against bacterial spores, which are generally considered the most resistant types of microorganisms to inactivation, and the associated requirement of international standards (see, for example, [41] and Chapter 6.2). Many of these studies have produced encouraging results, not only showing the ability of various types of gas plasma to be effective against various microorganisms (e.g. endospores, viruses, bacteria), and other agents such as endotoxins (which are not neutralized by steam sterilization) and prions [1]. Various types of gases, as sources for plasma production, and plasma generation methods have been discussed [5, 42] (E. Comoy, personal communication). These investigations have highlighted important differences in the observed microbicidal activity, safety and materials compatibility in the choice of gas and generation systems. For example, heat generation is an important consideration. Further, many of these applications have been investigated under limited laboratory situations initially and require further investigations for practical application as routine sterilization techniques [24].

Oxygen

Oxygen (O_2) is probably the most widely investigated gas as a plasma sterilization method. During plasma generation, a variety of potent active species can be generated and detected, including various radicals such as ˙OH, ˙OOH and ˙O [7, 43]. The hydroxyl radical, in particular, is predicted to contribute significantly to the microbicidal activity of oxygen gas plasma. Sporicidal activity has been investigated in some detail and at various levels of oxygen gas concentration [7, 43, 44]. Plasmas generated in oxygen alone were more effective as sporicidal agents than those generated in nitrogen or oxygen–nitrogen mixtures. At the same time, lower concentrations of oxygen in nitrogen (N_2O) mixtures appear effective through the production of UV light [45]. By studying the microscopic appearance of oxygen plasma-treated endospores, the spore structures appeared to collapse or shrink; the extent of shrinkage increased at higher concentrations of oxygen gas, correlating with increased sporicidal activity [7, 44]. Interestingly, these effects were not observed with nitrogen gas, although sporicidal activity was observed, suggesting that differences in mechanisms of action may exist depending on the source of gas plasma. It has been proposed that active oxygen species can penetrate into the spore core to elicit a direct effect on essential components (such as the core DNA molecule [46]).

Hydrogen peroxide and peracetic acid

The microbicidal effects of hydrogen peroxide and peracetic acid in gas plasma have been discussed above. The optimal way to apply these gas plasma processes appears to be by allowing the microbicide in gas form to diffuse within a given load and then to generate the plasma to elicit maximal microbicidal effects [1]. Indeed, initial patents with plasma-phase microbicides claimed greater activity than with the gas microbicide itself [14, 16]. The kill kinetics of hydrogen peroxide gas plasma have been discussed [1]. It was suggested that significant sporicidal effects of hydrogen peroxide gas alone have been difficult to differentiate from those observed on plasma generation at the same concentration. For this reason, lower concentrations of peroxide gas (1–3 mg/l) were tested to differentiate the direct gas effects from those of plasma generation. Despite this, in these experiments, the impact of plasma generation was minimal; the typical *Geobacillus stearothermophilus* endospore *D*-value for peroxide gas at 1 mg/l is about 1 min, while the estimated *D*-value in the presence of plasma (at 300 W) at the same concentration was 5 min [1]. Supporting this, the gas diffusion time prior to plasma generation was important for the increased sporicidal effect observed, suggesting that the gas alone was responsible for the majority of microbicidal activity. At even lower test conditions (0–0.25 mg/l peroxide gas), some minor effects of sporicidal activity were observed over the period of plasma generation. Overall, the limitations in the sporicidal activity observed may reflect the lack of penetration of the various plasma species generated, as theoretically the increased production of reactive species within the plasma should be significant but short-lived. Similar results with peracetic acid, although less studied than hydrogen peroxide gas, have shown it was difficult to differentiate the contribution of the plasma phase to microbicidal (in particular sporicidal) activity

in comparison with controls and under the test methods utilized [16]. Overall, these effects are easier to demonstrate with gases that have little to no intrinsic sporicidal activity, such as observed with oxygen and nitrogen gas in contrast to their respective plasma forms.

Nitrogen

Nitrogen gas alone (or in combination with oxygen gas) has been shown to be a particularly effective sporicide in the plasma phase [1, 47, 48]. Although the broad-spectrum activity has not been studied in detail, some experiments have shown effects against bacteria, viruses and some fungi. To date, studies have particularly focused on bacterial spores, as being one the most resistant forms of microorganisms to disinfection and sterilization [5, 45]. For consideration as a true sterilization technique, these effects need to be confirmed. It is interesting to note that, unlike oxygen plasma (showing direct shrinkage of endospore structures), spores appeared intact or had been ruptured following exposure to nitrogen plasma and were unviable [7]. It has been suggested that this may reflect a difference in mechanism of action between gas plasma and oxygen, and may be linked to differences in difficulty in ionization of nitrogen gas in comparison with oxygen [1]. As N_2 the molecule has a triple bond, and the required energy to dissociate the molecule into its plasma form is significantly higher than that for oxygen (9.91 eV compared to 5.21 eV, respectively). The reactive ions subsequently produced may be particularly microbicidal (or have specific targets different to oxygen plasma) and may be linked to differences in localized heat production.

In addition, the effects of voltage application may be linked to the generation of particular wavelengths of UV light that may contribute to microbicidal activity. UVC (*c.* 254 nm) is known to be particularly bactericidal but is not expected to be present at the required amount to be sporicidal. Vacuum UV (V-UV; <200 nm) has been proposed to be involved, but this remains to be tested and confirmed [1]. Similar results have been reported for N_2–O_2 plasma gas mixtures [5, 45, 46]. The observed microbicidal effects appear to be due to the chemically reactive N and O species, as well as UV light (emitted from NO excited molecules). The UV light appears to be the dominant activity, where the concentration of O_2 on plasma generation has been optimized to provide the maximum light intensity [45]. Attempts to balance the microbicidal effects of O_2–N_2 mixtures with minimal damage to material surfaces (such as polymers) have recently been described [47]. Based on maximizing the UV intensity during the process, 0.6% O_2 (at a pressure of 266 Pa (2 Torr)) was found to be optimal, while interestingly the authors reported that damage to polymer materials was greater in the absence of O_2. Overall, it should be remembered that N_2, O_2 and N_2–O_2 mixture plasma all show microbicidal effects (with some synergistic activity being reported under controlled heat conditions [48]), but appear to use different mechanisms. These effects may be further optimized to achieve a unique balance for microbicidal effects but with minimal surface damage.

Other gases

Other gas plasmas have been investigated for their microbicidal and macromolecule degradation activities, in particular those based on the rare or noble gases such as argon, helium, xeon and neon. It is unknown at this time the exact species that may be responsible for observed microbicidal effects, but it is likely due to various electrons, ions, radicals and potential radiation (UV) produced during exposure. Similar to that described with nitrogen, these gases are often considered in combination with oxygen, such as helium–oxygen gas mixtures [6, 46]. The direct effects of helium gas plasma appear to be similar to those described for nitrogen. Under atmospheric pressure and low-temperature conditions, helium–oxygen plasma generated a low level of UV light in combination with various reactive species that were bactericidal/sporicidal and had specific damaging effects to internal cell components such as proteins and DNA [46, 49]. In one study, the optimum concentration of oxygen in helium was found to be 0.2% at a radiofrequency of c. 13.5 MHz [49]. Helium gas plasma alone has also been shown to be effective against oral bacteria and yeasts [20].

Argon has been particularly well studied, alone [44, 50] and in combination with oxygen [3]. Argon–oxygen plasma has been shown to be effective in cleaning processes, particularly in the physical removal and inactivation of prion (protein) contamination [3]. It is interesting to note from these experiments that while the plasma tested was effective for organic material removal, it was not as effective for inorganic (salt crystal) materials. Direct bacterial inactivation has also been shown on dental instruments [51]. Further studies have observed microbicidal effects of a variety of low-pressure plasmas, including mixtures of argon, oxygen, nitrogen and hydrogen, against various pathogens [52]. These results have also confirmed the unique antiprion effects of argon–oxygen mixtures, but not with argon–nitrogen or argon–hydrogen mixtures. These effects appear to be due to etching (physical removal) rather than direct inactivation by various active species [13].

In addition to microbicidal investigations, various types of gas plasma have been investigated for a variety of medical applications such as for antisepsis, wound healing, surgery and chemotherapy [53, 54].

Mechanisms of action

The mode of action of plasma is most likely due to a variety of microbicidal effects. In some cases this may be a combination of intrinsic microbicidal activity of the source gas (as is the case with the current commercially available hydrogen peroxide gas plasma sterilization systems), while in others the effects are specifically due to the various types of active species generated on plasma activation [12]. Theoretically, many types of generated active species will contribute to the overall microbicidal effects of gas plasma (Figure 15.4.3). They can include various types of ions, electrons, radicals, electromagnetic radiation (UV light), electrical fields, etc. It is also important to consider that these active species may be present in different proportions or have different combined effects depending on the source gas and even the method used to generate the plasma. This has been shown experimentally in investigations of differences in the mechanisms of action of plasma on bacterial endospores [1] and in their activity against prions [13] (E. Comoy, personal communication).

Excluding the use of gas plasma as part of the disinfection/sterilization process and associated microbicidal processes (see above), investigations of the microbicidal effects of gas plasma have shown remarkable differences in their mechanisms of action. Hydrogen peroxide and oxygen gas plasma, for example, may be expected to form various free radicals (such as $^{\cdot}OH$) and other reactive species that contribute to the overall microbicidal activity of the plasma. These may include $HO^{\cdot}$, $^{\cdot}OH$, HOH, $^{\cdot}OOH$, $^{\cdot}O$, $^{\cdot}H$ and UV light, which recombine on loosing energy to form stable compounds such as water (H_2O_2) and oxygen (O_2). These various species are highly reactive with various

Plasma generation

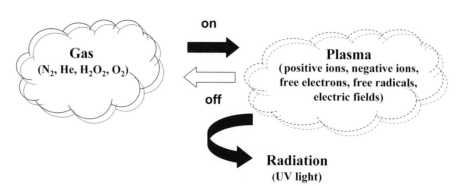

Figure 15.4.3 Generation of plasma and various active species, including ions, electrons and radiation. The specific types and quantities of active species that can be present will depend on the initial gas/gases present and the energy applied to generate the plasma.

macromolecules such as proteins and DNA, and may be expected to damage these molecules, culminating in loss of structure and functions that are necessary for viability [12]. There is some evidence to confirm this hypothesis [10, 46, 49]. This primarily appears to be due to oxidation and reduction effects on these macromolecules.

Differences in the mechanisms of action have been proposed and observed between oxygen-based plasma in comparison to gases such as nitrogen, argon and helium [1]. Direct observation has been made of the effects of various gas plasmas on bacterial spore structures [43, 45, 55]. In some cases, as observed with oxygen gas plasma, the effects appear to be dominant (at least initially) at the spore surface, with observed etching or spore shrinkage. There is a direct correlation between the concentration of oxygen and the extent of spore shrinkage observed [7, 43]. These observations may be explained by initial oxidation–reduction reactions on various surface molecules (such as proteins) and then subsequent cross-linking, the effects of which culminate in spore death. In contrast, nitrogen plasma-treated spores did not show shrinkage effects, but breaks/cracks on the surface of the spores over time have been reported [1, 2]. These differences may be due to the difficulty in ionizing gases like nitrogen, argon and helium, as compared with oxygen, so that the major efficacy effects may be due to the effects of UV radiation rather than ions, radicals, etc. Further, the effects of oxygen gas plasma appear to penetrate deeper into the spore structure than observed with nitrogen plasma. The relative efficacy of combined gas plasma (particularly nitrogen–oxygen and argon–oxygen) may combine these effects to optimize the microbicidal properties. Although the mechanisms of action have not been directly studied on other microorganisms, it would seem likely that given their respective surface and internal structures that the culmination of damage to macromolecules will lead to loss of viability of cells/viruses.

Future perspectives

Despite much research regarding the microbicidal effects of gas plasma, there is yet to be commercialized any true decontamination processes (atmospheric or vacuum). The microbicidal properties of plasma have been known since the 1970s, with many subsequent research reports, reviews and patents. Despite these reports, the only processes developed to date are not true plasma microbicidal processes, as they only use plasma generation for primarily non-microbicidal effects (such as the widely used hydrogen peroxide gas plasma sterilization systems described in this chapter). Studies with these systems have shown little to no effect of plasma during the microbicidal process [11], but plasma generation appears to primarily play a role in removing residues following the use of peroxide liquid/gas. There has been a resurgence of interest in this field over the last 10 years, not only for the potential microbicidal benefits of plasma but also due to many other medical and industrial applications. Plasmas are

unique as microbicidal agents as they are generally associated with no residues following surface treatment (unlike other microbicides such as glutaraldehyde and ethylene oxide) and are relatively easy to generate. They have been shown to inactivate microorganisms and can also be used to neutralize/remove contaminating macromolecules which can be associated with adverse effects in patients (e.g. toxicity, irritation, prion infectivity, pyrogenicity). Balancing these benefits with surface compatibility is a key part of the successful development of plasma processes [24, 47]. A further consideration is safety in applications, which can be achieved by applying existing engineering designs and safety standards. The choice of gas or mixture of gases is an important part of defining optimized processes from a safety and efficacy point of view. With this in mind, the decontamination applications may include cleaning processes and disinfection/sterilization of air, gases, liquids and surfaces [54].

References

1 Sakudo, A. and Shintani, H. (2010) *Sterilization and Disinfection by Plasma: Sterilization Mechanisms, Biological and Medical Applications*, NOVA Science, Hauppauge, NY.

2 Shintani, H. *et al.* (2007) Inactivation of microorganisms and endotoxins by low temperature nitrogen gas plasma exposure. *Biocontrol Science*, **12**, 131–143.

3 Baxter, H.C. *et al.* (2005) Elimination of transmissible spongiform encephalopathy infectivity and decontamination of surgical instruments by using radio-frequency gas-plasma treatment. *Journal of General Virology*, **86**, 2393–2399.

4 Whittaker, A.G. *et al.* (2004) Plasma cleaning of dental instruments. *Journal of Hospital Infection*, **56**, 37–41.

5 Moisan, M. *et al.* (2001) Low-temperature sterilization using gas plasmas: a review of the experiments and an analysis of the inactivation mechanism. *International Journal of Pharmaceutics*, **226**, 1–21.

6 Lee, K. *et al.* (2006) Sterilization of bacteria, yeast, and bacterial endospores by atmospheric-pressure cold plasma using helium and oxygen. *Journal of Microbiology (Seoul, Korea)*, **44**, 269–275.

7 Rossi, F. *et al.* (2006) Decontamination of surfaces by low pressure plasma discharges. *Plasma Processes and Polymers*, **3**, 431–442.

8 Shintani, H. *et al.* (2010) Gas plasma sterilization of microorganisms and mechanisms of action. *Experimental and Therapeutic Medicine*, **1**, 731–738.

9 Boudam, M.K. and Moisan, M. (2010) Synergy effect of heat and UV photons on bacterial-spore inactivation in an N2-O2 plasma-afterglow sterilizer. *Journal of Physics D: Applied Physics*, **43**, 1–17.

10 Jacobs, P.T. and Lin, S.-M. (2001) Sterilization processes utilizing low-temperature plasmas, in *Disinfection, Sterilization and Preservation*, 5th edn (ed. S.S. Block), Lippincott Williams & Wilkins, Philadelphia, pp. 747–765.

11 Krebs, M.C. *et al.* (1998) Gas plasma sterilization: relative efficiency of the hydrogen peroxide phase as compared to that of the plasma phase. *International Journal of Pharmaceutics*, **160**, 75–81.

12 McDonnell, G. (2007) *Antisepsis, Disinfection, and Sterilization: Types, Action and Resistance*, ASM Press, Washington DC.

13 McDonnell, G. and Comoy, E. (2010) Inactivation of prions, in *Sterilization and Disinfection by Plasma: Sterilization Mechanisms, Biological and Medical Applications* (eds A. Sakudo and H. Shintani), Nova Science, Hauppauge, NY, pp. 61–73.

14 Jacobs, P.T. and Lin, S.-M. (1987) *Hydrogen Peroxide Plasma Sterilization System*, US Patent 4, 643, 876.

15 Jacobs, P.T. and Lin, S.-M. (1988) *Hydrogen Peroxide Plasma Sterilization System*, US Patent 4, 756, 882.

16 Caputo, R.A. *et al.* (1992) *Plasma Sterilizing Process with Pulsed Antimicrobial Agent*, US Patent 5, 084, 239.

17 Block, S.S. (1991) Peroxygen compounds, in *Disinfection, Sterilization and Preservation*, 4th edn (ed. Block, S.S.), Lippincott Williams & Wilkins, Baltimore, MD, pp. 167–181.

18 Antloga, J.E. *et al.* (2005) Area fumigation with hydrogen peroxide vapor. *Applied Biosafety*, **10** (2), 91–100.

19 Perni, S. *et al.* (2008) Cold atmospheric plasma disinfection of cut fruit surfaces contaminated with migrating microorganisms. *Journal of Food Protection*, **71**, 1619–1625.

20 Rupf, S. *et al.* (2010) Killing of adherent oral microbes by a non-thermal atmospheric plasma jet. *Journal of Medical Microbiology*, **59**, 206–212.

21 Burts, M.L. *et al.* (2009) Use of atmospheric non-thermal plasma as a disinfectant for objects contaminated with methicillin-resistant *Staphylococcus aureus*. *American Journal of Infection Control*, **37**, 729–733.

22 Hultman, C. *et al.* (2007) The physical chemistry of decontamination with gaseous hydrogen peroxide. *Pharmaceutical Engineering*, **27**, 22–32.

23 Vogel, D.B. (2004) Bringing sterilization inside. *Medical Design Technology*, **12**, 24–27.

24 McDonnell, G. (2010) Current and future perspectives of gas plasma for decontamination, in *Sakudo and Shintani Sterilization and Disinfection by Plasma: Sterilization Mechanisms, Biological and Medical Applications* (eds A. Sakudo and H. Shintani), Nova Science, Hauppauge, NY, pp. 99–109.

25 Alfa, M.J. *et al.* (1996) Comparison of ion plasma, vaporized hydrogen peroxide and 100% ethylene oxide sterilizers to the 12/88 ethylene oxide gas sterilizer. *Infection Control and Hospital Epidemiology*, **17**, 92–100.

26 Rutala, W.A. *et al.* (1998) Comparative evaluation of the sporicidal activity of new low-temperature sterilization technologies: ethylene oxide, 2 plasma sterilization systems and liquid peracetic acid. *American Journal of Infection Control*, **26**, 393–398.

27 Fichet, G. *et al.* (2004) Novel methods for disinfection of prion-contaminated medical devices. *Lancet*, **364** (9433), 521–526.

28 Fichet, G. *et al.* (2007) Prion inactivation using a new gaseous hydrogen peroxide sterilisation process. *Journal of Hospital Infection*, **67**, 278–286.

29 Yan, Z.X. *et al.* (2004) Infectivity of prion protein bound to stainless steel wires: a model for testing decontamination procedures for transmissible spongiform encephalopathies. *Infection Control and Hospital Epidemiology*, **25**, 280–283.

30 Rogez-Kreuz, C. *et al.* (2009) Inactivation of animal and human prions by hydrogen peroxide gas plasma sterilization. *Infection Control and Hospital Epidemiology*, **30**, 769–777.

31 Lin, S.-M. *et al.* (2010) *Rapid Sterilization System*, US Patent 7, 670, 550.

32 Advanced Sterilization Products (2009) *STERRAD® NX™ Datasheet AD-52368-01-US_D*. Advanced Sterilization Products, Irvine, CA.

33 Advanced Sterilization Products (2008) *STERRAD® 100NX™ Datasheet AD-55299-001_A*. Advanced Sterilization Products, Irvine, CA.

34 Advanced Sterilization Products (2009) *STERRAD® 100NX™ Sterilization System Technical Information AD-54083-001Rev B*. Advanced Sterilization Products, Irvine, CA.

35 Heeg, P. *et al.* (2009) Comparison of the microbiology efficacy and practical application of three alternative types of low temperature sterilization processes based on hydrogen peroxide. *Central Sterilization*, **17**, 183–190.

36 McDonnell, G. *et al.* (2009) Amsco V-PRO 1: a new low temperature sterilization system. *Central Sterilization*, **17**, 108–113.

37 Malchesky, P.S. (2001) Medical applications of peracetic acid, in *Disinfection, Sterilization, and Preservation*, 5th edn (ed. S.S. Block), Lippincott Williams & Wilkins, Philadelphia, pp. 979–996.

38 Gaspar, M.C. *et al.* (1995) Preliminary study on the efficacy of sterilization with AbTox system: comparison with ethylene oxide. *Medicina Preventiva*, **1**, 1–6.

39 Bryce, E.A. *et al.* (1997) An evaluation of the AbTox Plazlyte™ sterilization system. *Infection Control and Hospital Epidemiology*, **18**, 646–653.

40 Sadahiko, F. *et al.* (2000) Sterilization with low temperature gas plasma and vapor of peracetic acid and hydrogen peroxide. *Japanese Association for Operative Medicine*, **21**, 140–144.

41 International Standards Organization (ISO) (2009) *EN ISO 14937. Sterilization of Health Care Products: General requirements for characterization of a sterilizing agent and the development, validation and routine control of a sterilization process for medical devices*. ISO, Geneva.

42 Calpo, P. *et al.* (2008) Plasma sources and reactor configurations, in *Advanced Plasma Technology* (eds. R. d'Agostino *et al.*), Wiley-VCH, Weinheim, Germany, pp. 17–34.

43 Rossi, F. *et al.* (2008) Mechanisms of sterilization and decontamination of surfaces by low-pressure plasma, in *Advanced Plasma Technology* (eds. R. d'Agostino *et al.*), Wiley-VCH, Weinheim, Germany, pp. 319–340.

44 Deng, X. *et al.* (2006) Physical mechanisms of inactivation of *Bacillus subtilis* spores using cold atmospheric plasmas. *IEEE Transactions on Plasma Science*, **34**, 1310–1316.

45 Boudam, M.K. *et al.* (2006) Bacterial spore inactivation by atmospheric-pressure plasmas in the presence or absence of UV photons as obtained with the same gas mixture. *Journal of Physics D: Applied Physics*, **39**, 3494–3507.

46 Kim, S.M. and Kim, J.I. (2006) Decomposition of biological macromolecules by plasma generated with helium and oxygen. *Journal of Microbiology (Seoul, Korea)*, **44**, 466–471.

47 Boudam, M.K. *et al.* (2007) Characterization of the flowing afterglows of an N2-O2 reduced-pressure discharge: setting the operating conditions to achieve a dominate late afterglow and correlating the NO2 UV intensity variation with the N and O atom densities. *Journal of Physics D: Applied Physics*, **40**, 1694–1711.

48 Benedikt, J. *et al.* (2008) BIODECON – European project on plasma inactivation of bacteria and biomolecules. *GMS Krankenhaushygiene Interdisziplinär*, **11**, 3.

49 Hong, Y.F. *et al.* (2009) Sterilization effect of atmospheric plasma on *Escherichia coli* and *Bacillus subtilis* endospores. *Letters in Applied Microbiology*, **48**, 33–37.

50 Yu, Q.S. *et al.* (2007) Bacterial inactivation using a low-temperature atmospheric plasma brush sustained with argon gas. *Journal of Biomedical Materials Research. Part B, Applied Biomaterials*, **80B**, 211–219.

51 Baier, R.E. *et al.* (1992) Radiofrequency gas plasma (glow discharge) disinfection of dental operative instruments, including handpieces. *Journal of Oral Implantology*, **18**, 236–242.

52 von Keudell, A. *et al.* (2010) Inactivation of bacteria and biomolecules by low-pressure plasma discharges. *Plasma Processes and Polymers*, **11**, 1–35.

53 Kong, M.G. *et al.* (2009) Plasma medicine: an introductory review. *New Journal of Physics*, **11**, 1–35.

54 McCombs, G.B. and Darby, M.L. (2010) New discoveries and directions for medical, dental and dental hygiene research: low temperature atmospheric pressure plasma. *International Journal of Dental Hygiene*, **8**, 10–15.

55 Purevdorj, D. *et al.* (2003) Effect of feed gas composition of gas charge plasmas on Bacillus pumillus spore mortality. *Letters in Applied Microbiology*, **37**, 31–34.

15.5 Filtration Sterilization

Susannah E. Walsh[1] and Stephen P. Denyer[2]

[1] School of Pharmacy, Microbiology, De Montfort University, Leicester, UK
[2] Cardiff School of Pharmacy and Pharmaceutical Sciences, Cardiff University, Cardiff, Wales, UK

Historical introduction

Early attempts to purify water were made by allowing it to percolate through beds of sand, gravel or cinders and a complex ecosystem developed on these filters. An increasing knowledge of bacteriology and an awareness of the involvement of waterborne bacteria, pathogenic protozoa and worms in disease and epidemics, eventually led to a more thorough study of filtration devices.

Chamberland, a colleague of Louis Pasteur, invented a thimble-like vessel, made by sintering a molded kaolin and sand mix. These so-called Chamberland candles were the first fabricated filters and represent another example of the inventive output from the Pasteur school [1]. Later to be made by the English firm of Doulton and other ceramic manufacturers, they were essentially of unglazed porcelain. These filters enjoyed a great vogue in the pharmaceutical industry until the advent of membrane filters rendered them practically obsolete in this area.

Filtration media

The ideal filter medium to remove microorganisms from solutions destined for parenteral administration should offer the following characteristics: efficient removal of particles above a stated size; acceptably high flow rate; resistance to clogging; steam sterilizable; flexibility and mechanical strength; low potential to release fibers or chemicals into the filtrate; low potential to sorb materials from the liquids being sterilized; non-pyrogenic; and biologically inert.

Additionally, when such a medium is mounted in a holder or support, it must be amenable to *in situ* sterilization and integrity testing. The medium most frequently employed, and which most nearly approaches the ideal, is the polymeric membrane, usually in the format of a flat disk or a pleated cartridge (see below). As a consequence this medium is by far the most important in current use, but several other filter media have been used in the past, which are deficient in one or more of the above qualities and yet retain limited and specialized applications.

Filters of diatomaceous earth

Diatomaceous earth, added to liquid products to form a suspended slurry, has been widely used as a filter aid in the pharmaceutical industry. The slurry is deposited on porous supports and the liquid then passes through, leaving coarse particulate matter entrained within the retained filter cake. Such an approach has been employed in rotary-drum vacuum filters [2], as used in antibiotic manufacture for instance, where the drum rotates within the slurry, pulling filtered liquid through the retained cake under vacuum and leaving the cell debris behind.

Russell, Hugo & Ayliffe's: Principles and Practice of Disinfection, Preservation and Sterilization, Fifth Edition. Edited by Adam P. Fraise, Jean-Yves Maillard, and Syed A. Sattar.
© 2013 Blackwell Publishing Ltd. Published 2013 by Blackwell Publishing Ltd.

Fibrous pad filters

Originally constructed of asbestos fibers, until the toxicity of asbestos was recognized, microfibers of borosilicate glass are now employed to create these filters. They have found widespread application in filter presses and as pre-filters for clarification of pharmaceutical solutions. It is usual to employ such filters with a membrane filter (see below) downstream to collect any shed fibers. Other materials used in the construction of this type of filter include paper, nylon, polyester and cellulose-acetate fibers.

Sintered or fritted ware

This type of filter was made by taking particles of glass or metal (stainless steel or silver), assembling them in suitable holders and subjecting them to a heat process, so that the particles melted or softened on their surfaces and, on cooling, fused together. It is clear that a complete melting would defeat the object of the technology and this partial melting, followed by surface fusion, was called sintering or frittering. Such a process will give rise to a porous sheet of material, which can then act as a filter [3]. This process differs from the sintering process used in the manufacture of unglazed porcelain, in that the latter contains several components and the process is accompanied by chemical changes in the constituents.

Membrane filters

Membrane filter technology has had over 80 years in which to develop, since the first description, by Zsigmondy and Bachmann in 1918 [4], of a method suitable for producing cellulose membrane filters on a commercial scale. The full potential of membrane filters was not recognized until their successful application in the detection of contaminated water supplies in Germany during World War II [5]. Following their commercial exploitation in the 1950s and 1960s, a number of large international companies evolved which now offer a wide array of filters and associated equipment from which to choose. Undoubtedly, the role played by membrane filters continues to expand, both in the laboratory and in industry, and they are now routinely used in water analysis and purification, sterility testing and sterilization. Their future is assured, at least in the pharmaceutical industry, unless other, as yet undiscovered, techniques emerge, since they represent the most suitable filtration medium currently available for the preparation of sterile, filtered parenteral products to a standard accepted by all the various regulatory authorities.

Methods of manufacture

There are four major methods of membrane filter manufacture currently employed on an industrial scale. These involve either a gelling and casting process, an irradiation–etch process, an expansion process or a procedure involving the anodic oxidation of aluminum. Each method produces membranes with their own particular characteristics.

Gelling and casting process

This is perhaps the most widely used process, and all the major filter manufacturers offer filters prepared by this method. Cast polymeric membranes, as they are known, are principally derived from pure cellulose nitrate, mixed esters of acetate and nitrate or other materials offering greater chemical resistance, for example nylon 66 [6], polyvinylidine fluoride (PVDF) or polytetrafluoroethylene (PTFE) [5].

In essence, the process still utilizes the principles outlined by Zsigmondy and Bachmann in 1918 [4], where the polymer is mixed with a suitable organic solvent or combination of solvents and allowed to gel [7]. In the modern process, a minute quantity of hydrophilic polymer may be present as a wetting agent, ethylene glycol may be added as a "pore former" and glycerol is often included to afford flexibility to the finished membrane. The mixture is then cast on to a moving, perfectly smooth, stainless steel belt, to give a film 90–170 µm thick (Figure 15.5.1). By carefully controlling the temperature and relative humidity, the solvents are slowly evaporated off, leaving a wet gel of highly porous, three-dimensional structure, which dries to give a membrane of considerable mechanical strength (Figure 15.5.2). Pore size and other membrane characteristics are determined by the initial concentration of the polymer, the mixing process, including the solvents added, and the environmental drying conditions.

Track–etch (irradiation–etch) process

Developed from the method of Fleischer *et al.* [8] and originally patented with the Nuclepore Corporation, this process is operated in two stages. First, a thin film (5–10 µm thick) of polycarbonate or polyester material is exposed to a stream of charged particles in a nuclear reactor; this is followed by a second stage, where the fission tracks made through the film are etched out into round, randomly dispersed cylindrical pores (Figure 15.5.3). Pore density and pore size are controlled by the duration of exposure of the film within the reactor and by the etching process, respectively. The finished track-etched membranes are thin, transparent, strong and flexible (Figure 15.5.4).

Expansion process

Stretching and expanding of fluorocarbon sheets, for example PTFE, along both axes is sometimes undertaken to provide porous, chemically inert membranes. A support of polyethylene or polypropylene is usually bonded to one side of the membrane to improve handling characteristics. Their hydrophobic nature ensures that these filters are widely employed in the filtration of air and non-aqueous liquids.

An alternative method of production for PTFE filters is by a process that forms a continuous mat of microfibers, fused together at each intersection to prevent shedding into the filtrate. These filters usually have no supporting layer to reduce their chemical resistance.

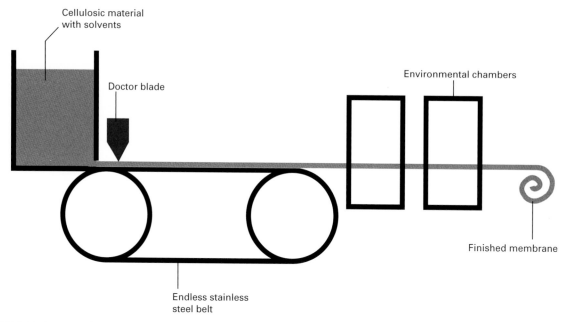

Cellulosic material with solvents

Doctor blade

Environmental chambers

Finished membrane

Endless stainless steel belt

Figure 15.5.1 Membrane manufacture: the casting process.

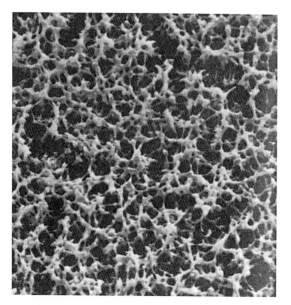

Figure 15.5.2 Scanning electron micrograph (4000×) of the surface of a 0.22 μm pore size cast cellulose membrane filter.

Anodic oxidation of aluminum

This procedure is employed to produce ultrathin membranes, with a honeycomb-pore structure, in which the pores have a narrow size distribution [9]. These membranes are hydrophilic and offer several advantages over polymeric membranes, including very high temperature stability (up to 400°C) and minimal levels of extractable materials, because monomers, plasticizers and surfactants are not used in the production process.

Other methods of filter construction

Other methods of manufacture include solvent leaching of one material from a cast mixture leaving pores, the production of bundles of hollow fibers, and deposition and etching of sacrificial layers of silicon [10].

Mechanisms of membrane filtration

Membrane filters are often described as "screen" filters and are thereby contrasted directly with filter media that are believed to retain particles and organisms by a "depth" filtration process. By this simple definition, filters made from sintered glass, compressed fiber or ceramic materials are classified as depth filters, while membranes derived from cast materials, stretched polymers and irradiated plastics are classified as screen filters. In essence, during depth filtration, particles are trapped or adsorbed within the interstices of the filter matrix, while screen filtration involves the exclusion (sieving out) of all particles larger than the rated pore size.

Unfortunately, classification of membrane filters is not nearly as simple as this scheme might suggest. For example, some manufacturers use the terms screen filter and depth filter, respectively, to describe membranes with capillary-type pores, that is track-ûetch membranes, and those possessing tortuous interlinked pores made by gel casting. It is now recognized that the filtration characteristics of many membrane filters cannot be accounted for in terms of the sieve retention theory alone. In 1963, Megaw and Wiffen [11] pointed out that, although membrane filters would be expected to act primarily by sieve retention, they did possess the property of retaining particles that were much smaller than the membrane pore size, larger particles being trapped by impaction in the filter pores. (This aspect is discussed in more detail

Stage 1

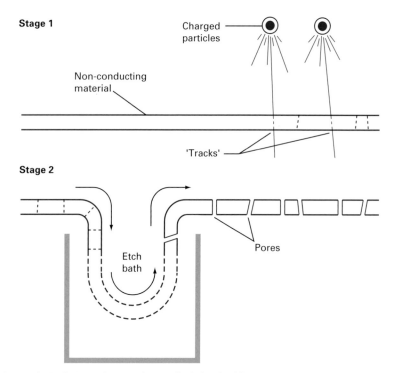

Stage 2

Charged particles

Non-conducting material

'Tracks'

Etch bath

Pores

Figure 15.5.3 Membrane manufacture: the irradiation–etch process (see text for further details).

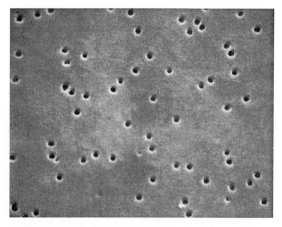

Figure 15.5.4 Scanning electron micrograph (10,000×) of the surface of a 0.2 μm pore size polycarbonate track-etched membrane filter.

below.) A more precise classification might be expected to take into consideration the considerable variation in membrane filter structure (see above) and the subsequent influence that this may have on the mechanism of filtration.

Influence of membrane filter structure on the filtration process
Several studies have reported a marked difference between the pore structure of the upper and lower surfaces of polymeric membrane filters. Of particular note are the works of Preusser [12], Denee and Stein [13] and Marshall and Meltzer [14]. These workers have all shown one surface to have a greater porosity than the other. This phenomenon can be used to advantage in

filtrations, since it confers a depth-like filtration characteristic on the membranes when used with the more open side upstream. Particles can now enter the interstices of the filter, increasing the time to clogging. The variation in flow rate and total throughput resulting from the different directions of flow can exceed 50%. Most filter manufacturers recognize the asymmetry of their membranes; indeed, several emphasize it in their technical literature and ensure that all disk filters are packed in the preferred flow direction (top to bottom). Highly anisotropic membranes, with superior filtration characteristics to those of conventional mixed-ester membranes, have been described [15, 16]. Exactly the same principle is applied in the manufacture of depth filters where increased filter life and dirt-holding capacity are achieved when the density of the filter medium increases from the upstream direction. The improved dirt retention is particularly useful when depth filters are used as a pre-filter for a sterilizing-grade screen membrane.

A membrane filter can be further characterized by its pore size distribution and pore numbers. Manufacturers have traditionally given their membranes either an "absolute" or "nominal" pore size rating, usually qualified by certain tolerance limits. There has been increasing recognition, however, that the designation "absolute" is misleading. Complete removal of all suspended material can only be assured when a sieving mechanism is operative and all the particles are larger than the largest pore in the membrane, but the situation rarely prevails in which the diameters of the smallest particle and the largest pore are known with certainty. Even if this situation were known to exist, an "absolute" filter could only be expected to remove all suspended material for a limited

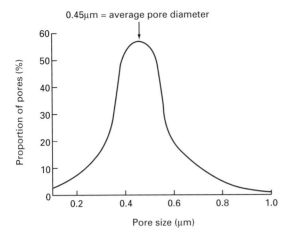

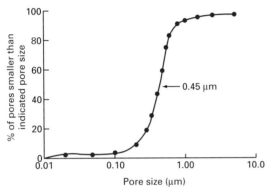

Figure 15.5.5 Typical pore size distribution curves for 0.45 μm-rated cellulose membranes obtained from mercury intrusion tests.

Table 15.5.1 Pore size characteristics of three nominal 0.2 μm membranes from different manufacturers.

Filter supplier	Minimum pore size (μm)	Average pore size (μm)	Maximum pore size (μm)
1	0.16	0.225	0.33
2	0.195	0.264	0.388
3	0.203	0.269	0.367

Jacobs [19] first described the distribution of pore diameters in graded ultrafilter membranes and discussed the maximum pore diameters and average pore diameters of various commercially available membranes. Subsequently, other workers were unable to confirm a pore size distribution of ±0.03 μm about a mean value, as is claimed for certain 0.45 μm filters [14, 20]. While it has long been established that track-etched filters normally possess a greater uniformity than cast polymeric membranes, it is, nevertheless, clear that track-etched filters may not be entirely free from irregularities in pore size and shape [20, 21]. A broader pore size distribution within a membrane filter is not necessarily considered a failing, since it offers resistance to early clogging occasioned by too close a match between the dominant pore size and the prevailing particle size.

Cellulosic filters (available in a range of pore sizes from around 12 μm down to 0.025 μm) possess between 10^7 and 10^{11} pores/cm², the number increasing as the pore size decreases. This contrasts with the 10^5 to 6×10^8 pores/cm² offered by a similar size range of track-etched filters. The number of pores and their size distribution will contribute to the overall porosity (void volume) of the filter system, which is considered to be approximately 65–85% for cellulose filters (decreasing with decreasing pore size) and only 5–10% for the track-etched product. Overall fluid-flow characteristics are similar for both types of filter [22]; however, the greater thickness of cellulose filters ($\simeq$150 μm) and their tortuous pore system afford approximately 15 times more resistance to flow than the 10 μm-thick track-etched filter.

There appears little justification for assuming a uniform pore structure, at least within the cast polymeric membranes, and the simple capillary pore model does not describe correctly the typical membrane filter. Duberstein [23] states that the bacterial removal efficiency of membrane filters depends on the membrane pore size distribution and on the thickness of the membrane; the latter is in disagreement with the sieve theory (see below), which relies solely on retention associated with the pore size of the surface pores. Furthermore, these two factors are not the only ones that have a bearing on the bacterial removal efficacy; both the tortuosity of the pores through the membrane and its chemical composition (and hence its surface charge) will influence the extent of removal. The characteristics of the fluid being filtered (pH, ionic strength, presence of surfactants, etc.), the character of the suspended organism or particle and the differential pressure across the membrane [24] are additional factors that all have a

time, because on prolonged use there is the possibility of microorganisms growing through the membrane. "Nominal" pore size implies that a certain percentage of contamination above that size is retained. Graphs depicting pore size distribution have been offered by several filter manufacturers (Figure 15.5.5). It must be remembered that the techniques used to establish pore size vary from manufacturer to manufacturer, and the values obtained are not necessarily comparable. Indeed, not only are manufacturers not obliged to measure pore size by a standardized method, but they are also under no obligation to give any details of the particle size distribution (although this may be available on request). If these facts are considered together with the observation that pore size measurements based upon bubble-point determinations (see below) may be influenced by membrane thickness and the nature of the membrane polymer [17], it is not surprising that membranes having the same labeled pore size display substantial differences. Table 15.5.1 shows that the largest pores measured in the 0.2 μm membrane of one manufacturer were, in fact, almost twice that dimension, and the average pore size in another membrane was 35% greater than the labeled value [18]. It is apparent from these data that the designated pore size should not be regarded as absolute, but would be better interpreted as a label indicating the likely suitability for a particular purpose.

bearing on the efficiency of particle retention. Indeed, the extent to which particle retention efficiency is dependent upon such physicochemical parameters gives an indication of the relative contributions of sieving and adsorption to the particle removal process.

For the thin track-etched membrane, the contribution made by the thickness of the filter towards the retention process may be considered small, especially in the light of their relatively uncomplicated pore structure, and the term screen filter may adequately described this type of membrane [25]. The thicker cast polymeric membranes, as exemplified by the cellulose filters, however, offer characteristics between those of a true depth filter and those of a true screen filter and may best be described as membrane depth filters. With these filters, very small particles will be retained by adsorption, but a point must be reached beyond which the smallest particle confronting any filter is larger than that filter's largest pore, in which case the sieve mechanism can adequately describe the filtration phenomenon.

Removal of microorganisms from liquids by filtration

If terminal sterilization is not possible, filtration through a bacteria-retentive filter can be used. Sterile filtration is usually considered to be the absolute removal of bacteria, yeasts and mold, but for biological products of animal or human origin, the removal or inactivation of viruses may also be required [26]. It should by definition be able to deliver a sterile effluent independently of the challenge conditions, even when these are severe [27]. In practice, this can be achieved by means of a 0.22 (or 0.2) μm filter, although various authors have, in fact, shown that this filter is not absolute. Bowman *et al.* [28] described the isolation of an obligate aerobe (cell diameter <0.33 μm), then termed *Pseudomonas* sp. ATCC 19146 (now *Brevundimonas diminuta*), which could pass through a 0.45 μm membrane filter (see below); this poses a severe challenge to sterilization by filtration. The idea that sterile filtration is independent of the challenge condition is untenable. One of the prerequisites for successful filtration is an initial low number of organisms; as the number of *B. diminuta* in the test challenge increases, the probability of bacteria in the filtrate increases [29]. An early report [30] had likewise shown that a filter's ability to retain organisms decreased as the number of test organisms (in this case, *Serratia marcescens*) increased and as the filter's pore size rating increased. Approximately 0–20 *Pseudomonas* organisms can pass through even so-called absolute filters [31]; the extent of the passage of *B. diminuta* through membrane filters is encouraged by increasing pressures [32].

Leptospira species, together with other waterborne bacteria, have also been reported in the filtrate of well water that had passed through a 0.2 μm-rated membrane [33], and even the larger cells of *S. marcescens* can also pass through a 0.2 μm filter, although to a much smaller extent than *B. diminuta* [31]. Mycoplasmas, which lack rigid cell walls and consequently have a more plastic structure than bacteria, can pass through 0.22 μm filters [34], and such an organism, *Acholeplasma laidlawii*, has been used to validate 0.1 μm-rated sterilizing filters [35]. The variety of organisms that have now been reported as capable of penetrating 0.2 (0.22) μm membranes is substantial. In addition to those mentioned above, Sundaram *et al* [36] have identified reports of filter transmission of bacterial L-forms, several genera of water-borne bacteria, spirochaetes, Gram-negative opportunist pathogens like *Ralstonia pickettii*, corynebacteria and streptomycetes. While the early reports were confined to specific membrane types, high bacterial challenge levels and non-pathogens that were unlikely to arise in pharmaceutical materials, the more recent ones demonstrated that this was not invariably the case. This has led to the same authors strongly supporting the proposal first put forward by Robinson [37] that the 0.2 (0.22) μm membranes should no longer be regarded as the routine sterilizing grade, but replaced with 0.1 μm membranes for this purpose [38–40]. This is by no means the consensus view, however, and several observers consider there to be no need to consider an industry-wide change in this respect. Rather, they contend that thorough validation studies (see below) using realistic bioburden isolates are likely to ensure a satisfactory level of sterility assurance [17, 18, 41, 42]. There is general agreement, however, that the circumstances in which 0.1 μm membranes are appropriate for sterilization include the following: (i) when there is evidence of mycoplasmas present in the normal bioburden; (ii) when the product is, or contains, serum; and (iii) when manufacturing water for injection or pharmacopoeial purified water from a source likely to contain small bacteria (since many organisms are known to minimize their surface to volume ratio and become smaller in conditions of nutrient deprivation).

Wallhausser [31] emphasizes the pore size distribution of filter materials, which may be heterogeneous in form and composition, and the fact that pore size itself cannot be taken as an absolute yardstick for sterile filtration. It is to be expected, therefore, that two filters with the same nominal pore size can have markedly different filtration efficiencies, not only because the number, tortuosity and sorption characteristics of the channels within them may vary, but also because they have been characterized using different methods. Clearly, therefore, care must be exercised in selecting a filter, particularly in an industrial setting, when there are several alternatives of the same nominal grade to choose from. There are dangers in attempting to select on the basis of price alone.

The reduction in bacterial concentration used as a parameter of filter efficiency is normally termed the titer reduction value (Tr). Because it is the ratio of the number of organisms challenging the filter to the number of organisms that pass through, the production of a sterile filtrate will, axiomatically, give a Tr of infinity. Under these circumstances, convention places ">" in front of the challenge number, so that a sterile filtrate resulting from a challenge of 10^7 is represented as a Tr of $>10^7$. The Tr may also be represented as its logarithmic value, that is 7, when it is called a log removal factor or log reduction value (LRV).

The foregoing thus suggests that sieve retention is only one mechanism responsible for sterile filtration. Other contributing factors include van der Waals forces and electrostatic interactions

[34]. Tanny *et al.* [43] showed that many *B. diminuta* cells could be removed from suspension by adsorptive sequestration, using a 0.45 μm membrane filter, and postulated that an organism could actually enter the pore but be retained there by this mechanism.

The retention mechanisms operating during membrane filtration are elegantly illustrated in the scanning electron micrographs of Todd and Kerr [44], where the screen filter action of a track-etched filter is clearly contrasted with the depth filter characteristics of a cellulose membrane filter. Similarly, Osumi *et al.* [45] published scanning electron micrographs clearly showing that many of the pores in a 0.2 μm-rated membrane were much larger than the *B. diminuta* cells that were entrapped within them, and that the bacteria were usually retained by the membrane within the first 30 μm of the filter depth. The dominance of adsorptive effects during the filtration of plasma proteins and influenza vaccine through 0.22 and 0.45 μm membrane filters, respectively, has been recognized [46, 47]. Track-etched filters show few adsorptive properties and this can be attributed to their thinness, lack of tortuous channels and hence purely sieve-like properties. Adsorptive sequestration is not an inherent quality of a filter, but rather describes the ability of that filter to capture organisms of a given size [48, 49]. Depth-type filters, with a broad distribution of pore sizes, are believed to retain organisms largely by adsorption [49]. Bobbit and Betts [50] compared bacterial retention at a range of pore sizes on both screen-type polycarbonate membranes and cellulose-ester membranes. They observed that the former exhibited a much more distinct size threshold at which no further cells would pass through the membrane, and so had greater potential for the selective removal of bacteria from suspension according to size.

Thus, sieve retention may yet be the most important mechanism whereby sterile filtration is achieved, but it is unlikely to be the sole contributory factor. Although many membrane filters can no longer be considered to act simply as sieves, their thinness and greater uniformity of pore size give them several advantages over conventional depth filters, a fact that is widely exploited in filtration technology.

Cross-flow filtration

The traditional mode of filtration (sometimes termed normal filtration) is that in which the liquid approaches the filter perpendicularly, and all of it passes through as a result either of upstream pressure or, less commonly, downstream vacuum. A problem that often arises using this form of filtration is that the filter membrane becomes blocked with suspended solids. Such blockage is minimized in cross-flow filtration where the liquid to be filtered is pumped in a direction parallel with the membrane surface and the filtrate (also called permeate) passes through the membrane as a result of a pressure differential – the transmembrane pressure (Figure 15.5.6). The principle of cross-flow membrane filtration can be applied not only to suspended solids of microscopic dimensions – where it is termed microfiltration, but also to the separation of dissolved molecules from the solvent. Ultrafiltration is the term applied to the separation of solutes having molecular weights of the order of 10,000–100,000, while nanofiltration and reverse osmosis describe similar separations of progressively smaller molecules. The term tangential flow is also used to describe cross-flow filtration, although, in reality, it is a misnomer because the liquid does not approach the membrane at a tangent.

In cross-flow microfiltration the speed at which the fluid passes over the surface is critical; it is usually 1–6 m/s, and if reduced below this range the tendency to blockage of the membrane pores is much increased. Just as in any other form of filtration the rate at which the suspending medium is separated from the solids is increased as the surface area of the membrane increases. Although the membrane can be flat, a tubular form is also common, and it is beneficial to design a system with maximum tube circumference and minimum cross-sectional area. This means that it is more efficient to have tubes that have in-foldings so they are star-shaped in cross-section, or multiple small-bore tubes rather than a single tube of large diameter. Small lumens result in high pressures within the tube (typically 70–240 kPa (10–35 psi)) and require powerful pumps to achieve the required velocity; on an industrial scale this may mean significant energy costs. The high costs, however, are offset by the fact that the membrane is less inclined to block than a traditional screen or depth filter, and in

(a)

(b)

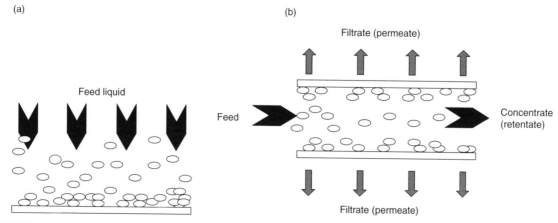

Figure 15.5.6 Comparison between (a) normal and (b) cross-flow filtration.

situations where the filter may be reused it is easier to clean by back-washing.

Not all of the suspending medium or solvent in the feed liquid passes through the membrane, and that which is retained, the retentate (concentrate), has an increased concentration of suspended solid or solute; it may be recirculated via a holding tank. The ratio of permeate to feed volume is termed the recovery, and recovery values up to 80% or more may be achieved under optimized conditions. The membranes used in cross-flow systems are highly asymmetrical with the surface facing the feed liquid having a fine and carefully controlled pore size; this surface may be formed as a film approximately 0.1–5.0 μm deep on a much more porous support up to 50 μm or more thick. Multiple pairs of flat membranes can be mounted into cassettes with porous separators between each pair; alternatively, cross-flow membranes may be coated onto the inside wall of a tubular element having a typical diameter of approximately 0.6–2.5 cm. Several such elements can be mounted together in the filter device to produce modules having from three to more than 100 elements. As part of an extensive review of the process, Dosmar and Brose [51] give a well-illustrated account of the various designs of cross-flow filtration devices that are currently available.

The filter membrane itself can be manufactured from the various polymers that are used for traditional perpendicular (normal) flow filtration systems, but ceramic or metallic membranes are also available, and all can achieve the 0.1–10 μm pore size range typical of clarifying and sterilizing membranes used in traditional filtration systems. Ceramic membranes are usually made from alumina, and although more expensive, afford better heat resistance than polysulfone membranes (a common alternative) without any loss of chemical resistance. Cross-flow filtration systems employing flexible textile supports are used for water purification; here the filter membrane is formed by deposition of the suspended material as a thin film on the inner surface of the tube. If the quantity of suspended material in the feed liquid is insufficient to form the membrane, a filter aid may be added initially to the feed water.

Membrane filters used for sterilization

The most suitable pore size for a sterilizing-grade filter is chosen, in part, by considering the minimum dimension (frequently less than 1 μm) of the microorganism to be retained. The efficient removal of all bacteria from contaminated solutions may sometimes require a 0.1 μm-rated membrane filter (see above). However, under normal pharmaceutical good manufacturing practice (GMP) conditions, the sterilization of products can be assured by their passage through a membrane filter with a nominal pore size of 0.22 μm or less [26, 52]. The integrity of the sterilizing filter must be verified before use and checked after use. Sterility testing of a suitable sample of each batch of product is required [26]. It must be noted that filtration is not sufficient if sterilization of a product in the final container is possible; consideration should be given to some degree of heat treatment if feasible [53].

Table 15.5.2 Effect of filter diameter on filtration volumes.

Filter diameter (mm)	Effective filtration area[a] (cm²)	Typical batch volume[b] (l)
13	0.8	0.01
25	3.9	0.05–0.1
47	11.3	0.1–0.3
90	45	0.3–5
142	97	5–20
293	530	20

[a] Taken from one manufacturer's data and to some extent dependent on the type of filter holder used. Values may well vary from manufacturer to manufacturer.
[b] For a low-viscosity liquid.

Filters with larger pore sizes may be considered sufficient for some processes, for example the removal of yeast during the stabilization of beers and wines can be effected by a 0.6 μm membrane filter. In general, however, such filters are only employed in systems where a reduction in bacterial numbers and not sterilization is demanded. An ideal example of this is the routine filtration through a 0.45 μm-rated filter of parenteral solutions that are later to be terminally sterilized. This reduces the likelihood of bacterial growth and pyrogen production prior to autoclaving.

Sterilizing membrane filters are available in disks ranging from 13 to 293 mm in diameter and their filtrative capacities make them the ideal choice for the small- and medium-scale processes normally encountered in the laboratory or hospital pharmacy (Table 15.5.2).

The flow rate of a clean liquid through a membrane filter (volume passed per unit time) is a function of that liquid's viscosity, the pressure differential across the filter and the filtration area, and is given by:

$$Q = C(AP/V)$$

where Q is the volumetric flow rate, A the filtration area, V the viscosity of the liquid, P the pressure differential across the membrane and C the resistance to fluid flow offered by the filter medium, governed in part by the size, tortuosity and number of pores.

The industrial manufacturer of sterile fluids needs to filter very large volumes and, as a consequence, demands a flow rate far beyond the capabilities of the largest available membrane disk. To provide the filtration area needed, multiple-plate filtration systems have been employed, where up to 60 flat filter disks of 293 mm diameter, separated by screens and acting in parallel, can be used to provide a total surface area of 3.0 m². A typical multiple-plate filtration system is illustrated in Figure 15.5.7.

A second approach can be to use cartridge filters [54]. These are essentially hollow cylinders formed from a rigid perforated plastic core, around which the membrane filter, supported by a

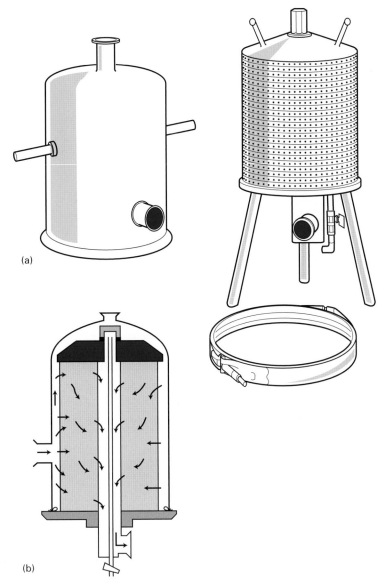

(a)

(b)

Figure 15.5.7 (a) A typical multiple-plate filtration system. (b) The fluid flow path during filtration.

suitable mesh and sometimes protected by a pre-filter, is wound. An outer perforated plastic sleeve provides protection against back-pressure and is held in place by bonded end-caps. The cartridge filter combines the advantages of increased filtration area with ease of handling. Since the filter is no longer in the form of a fragile disk, it can be easily installed in special holders. Multiple cartridge units are available, which may contain, for example, up to twenty 79 cm filter tubes (of 5.7 cm diameter), giving a maximum filtration area of approximately 2.4 m^2.

The most common filter format for use in large-scale filtration systems is the pleated-membrane cartridge. Early devices were manufactured from a flexible acrylic polyvinylchloride copolymer membrane, incorporating a nylon web support [55]. Other membranes have now evolved, which can also be pleated without

damage [56], and the range of materials includes cellulose esters, PVDF, PTFE, nylon, acrylic and polysulphone. The pleated configuration of the membrane ensures a far greater surface area for filtration than a normal cartridge filter of similar dimensions. For comparison, a single standard-pleated polycarbonate membrane cartridge of 24.8 cm length and 6.4 cm diameter, such as that illustrated in Figure 15.5.8, can offer a filtration area approaching 1.7 m^2, approximately 30 times that afforded by a typical 293 mm membrane disk; the effective area can be increased even further by connecting these cartridges in series. Pleated cartridges are also manufactured as units in sealed plastic capsules, which are disposable and convenient to use, but relatively expensive. Figure 15.5.9 shows the diverse range of cartridges and capsules available.

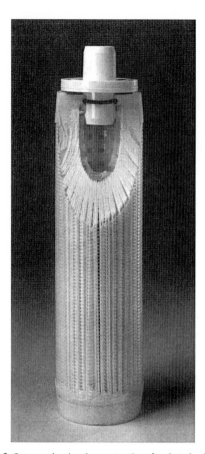

Figure 15.5.8 Cutaway showing the construction of a pleated polycarbonate membrane cartridge filter.

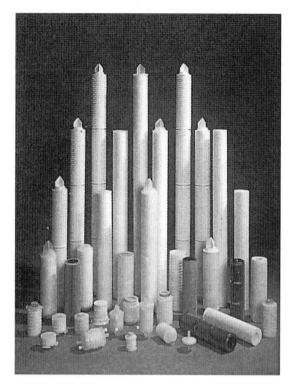

Figure 15.5.9 A selection of cartridge and capsule filters, which illustrate the variety available from a major manufacturer.

To ensure the widest application for their filters, manufacturers offer their membranes in a wide variety of constituent materials and formats (Figure 15.5.9). This permits the selection of a suitable filter type for use with most of the commonly encountered solvent systems [5, 57]. Extensive chemical compatibility lists are included in the catalogs of most manufacturers and further guidance can often be obtained through their technical support services. Subtle changes in filter structure do occur, however, when processing mixtures of liquids, the complex fluid presenting entirely different solvent properties to the membrane from what could be predicted from compatibility studies involving the individual liquid components. In a number of instances, these changes have resulted in filter failure, and compatibility tests should always be undertaken when mixed-solvent systems are to be processed [58]. It is as well to remember, also, that any system is only as compatible as its least resistant component, and attention must be paid to the construction materials of the filter holder, seals, tubing and valves. Table 15.5.3 describes the properties of polymers commonly used in membrane construction.

Hydrophobic filters (e.g. PTFE) are available for the sterile aeration of holding tanks and fermentation vessels in the beverage and biotechnology industries, for the supply of fermentation tanks with sterilized gas, for the filtration of steam and for the removal of water droplets from an oily product. They can be used to filter aqueous solutions by first wetting the membrane with a low molecular weight alcohol, such as ethanol. Hydrophobic-edged filters, derived from cellulose nitrate or acetate, whose rims have been impregnated to a width of 3–6 mm with a hydrophobic agent can also be obtained. These find wide application in filtrations requiring that no residual solution remains trapped under the sealing ring of the filter holder, for example during the sterility testing of antibiotics. They also have the advantage that air or gas trapped behind a filter can escape through the rim and thus prevent airlocks or dripping during a filtration process.

To ensure the production of a sterile filtrate, the final filter and its holder, together with any downstream distribution equipment, must be sterilized. To minimize aseptic manipulations, it is customary to sterilize the membrane filter after mounting it in the filter holder. The sterilization method is usually selected from among the following: autoclaving, in-line steaming, dry heat, ethylene oxide and γ-irradiation. The choice depends largely on the heat resistance of the filter and its ancillary equipment, and, before embarking upon any sterilizing procedure, it is first necessary to confirm their thermal stability.

Most filter types will withstand autoclaving conditions of 121°C for 20–30 min and, as a result, the routine autoclaving of assembled small-scale filtration equipment is common practice. Similarly, in-line steaming (sterilization in place) is a widely used process, in which moist steam is forced through the assembled filter unit (and often the entire filtration system) under

Table 15.5.3 Properties of polymers used in filter membrane construction.

Material	Cellulose esters	Polyvinylidene fluoride (PVDF)	Polypropylene	Nylon 66	Polytetrafluoro-Ethylene (PTFE)	Polysulphone/Polyether-sulphone	Polycarbonate	Polyamide
Typical minimum pore size (μm)	0.025	0.1	0.2	0.04	0.1	0.04	0.05	0.2
Autoclavable at 121°C?	Yes	Yes	Yes	Yes	Yes	Yes	Yes	Yes
Solvent resistance	Poor to moderate	Limited	Good	Good	Good	Limited	Good	Good
Extractables	Varies with grade	Low	Low	Very low	Low	Low	Very low	Low
Wettability	Hydrophilic	Naturally hydrophobic but available as hydrophilic	Hydrophobic	Hydrophilic	Normally hydrophobic, but hydro-philic available	Hydrophilic	Hydrophilic but available as hydrophobic	Hydrophobic
Protein binding	Acetate low, but nitrate and mixed esters high	Hydrophobic high; hydrophilic very low	Low	Very low binding grades available	Hydrophobic high; hydrophilic low	Low	Low	High
Special properties	Good strength and heat resistance but may be brittle	Not brittle Grades having good virus removal available	Flexible and strong	Positively charged grades enhance endotoxin removal	Tolerance of pH extremes, solvents and high temperatures	Polyethersulphone membranes having high flow rates are available	Usually track-etched membranes of high tensile strength	Tolerant of solvents and bases
Uses	Sterilization of aqueous solutions	Sterilization of aqueous solutions; hydrophobic membranes for gases	As an alternative to PTFE in many applications	Sterilization of aqueous solutions	Filtration of acids, bases, gases and solvents	Sterilization of tissue culture media and protein solutions	Microscopical observation of particles on filter surface	Highly alkaline solutions

conditions sufficient to ensure an adequate period of exposure at 121°C or other appropriate temperature [52, 59, 60]. This method is of particular value in large systems employing cartridge filters. It has the added advantage that the complete system can be sterilized, thereby lowering the bacterial contamination upstream from the final bacteria-proof filter. Voorspoels *et al.* [61] undertook temperature mapping and process-lethality determinations at different locations within assembled cartridge filters, and their findings are particular pertinent to the design of *in situ* sterilization validation protocols. If the sterilization temperature or time exceeds the limits which are imposed by the manufacturer, "pore collapse" may occur, with a subsequent reduction in membrane porosity. Frequently, cartridge filters are validated for a fixed number of re-sterilizations, for example four exposures, each of 15 min at 121°C. For this reason, dry-heat sterilization is rarely used, since the conditions employed are often too severe. For convenience, certain membrane filters may be obtained in a pre-sterilized form, either individually packed or ready-assembled into filter holders, as single-use devices. Sterility is, in this case, usually achieved by ethylene oxide treatment or γ-irradiation.

Advantages and disadvantages of membrane filters

Membrane filters have several advantages over conventional depth-filtration systems, a conclusion emphasized by the technical literature supplied by the major membrane filter companies. Table 15.5.4 summarizes the more important characteristics of membrane filters and compares them with conventional depth filters. Several features require further discussion, since they have considerable bearing on the quality of the final filtered product.

Table 15.5.4 Characteristics of membrane and depth filters.

Characteristic	Membrane	Depth
Filtration (retention efficiency for particles > rated pore size	100%	<100%
Speed of filtration	Fast	Slow
Dirt-handling capacity	Low	High
Duration of service (time to clogging)	Short	Long
Shedding of filter components (media migration)	No	Yes
Grow-through of microorganisms	Rare (see text)	Yes
Fluid retention	Low	High
Solute adsorption	Low	High
Chemical stability	Variable (depends on membrane)	Good
Mechanical strength	Considerable (if supported)	Good
Sterilization characteristics	Good	Good
Ease of handling	Generally poor	Good
Disposability	Yes	Not all types
Leaching of extractables	Variable (depends on membrane)	Unlikely

A problem usually associated only with conventional depth filters is that of "organism grow-through". If a bacterial filter is used over an extended period of time, bacteria lodged within the matrix can reproduce and successive generations will penetrate further into the filter, eventually emerging to contaminate the filtrate. The extent of this phenomenon will be a function of, at least in part, the nutritional status of the medium being filtered and the nutritional requirements of the contaminant. This problem is no longer considered to be exclusive to conventional depth filters and has been recognized to occur with some 0.45 μm membrane "depth" filters [62] (see above). For this reason, it is recommended that the duration of filtration be as short as possible and the same filter should not be used for more than one working day unless such use has been validated [49, 53, 63].

Solute adsorption by filter is rarely a major problem in large-scale industrial processes, but it can be of greater consequence in the filtration of small volumes containing medicaments at high dilution. Conventional depth filtration media have been implicated in the adsorption of antibiotics from solution [64], while the thinner membrane filters appear to suffer less from this disadvantage [65]. Bin *et al.* [66] observed between 116 and 429 μg benzalkonium chloride adsorption per 47 mm diameter disk, with the higher values arising on hydrophobic or anionic membranes. S. P. Denyer (unpublished results) has observed a similar loss (38%) of tetradecyltrimethylammonium bromide after filtration of 10 ml of a 0.001% w/v solution through a 0.22 μm cellulose membrane filter. Drug sorption has been reported by De Muynck *et al.* [67], and a method for its control suggested by Kanke *et al.* [68]. Presumably, adsorption sites are rapidly saturated in these thin membranes, and the passage of additional solution would probably occur without further loss. Nevertheless, it emphasizes the need to select the most compatible filter material and to discard, if at all possible, the first few milliliters of solution run through any filtration system. Flushing through to remove downstream particles is often an integral part of the filtration process anyway.

Care should be taken in the choice of filter in special operations, particularly where the loss of high-value material could be of significant economic importance. For instance, proteins (in particular those of high molecular weight) are readily removed from solution on passage through cellulose–nitrate and mixed ester filters, and nylon [46, 69, 70]. This is not so evident for fluorocarbon and cellulose–acetate filters, which would therefore be more suitable for the filtration of pharmaceutical protein preparations [71]. The conformational changes elicited in proteins by filtration through filter media have been highlighted by Truskey *et al.* [72].

A further problem associated with some membrane filters is the leaching of extractives, some of which may be potentially toxic [57, 73]. Surfactants, glycerol and other extractable materials added during the manufacturing process may leach from these filters during use, and limited flushing beforehand has been recommended [74]. As an alternative to flushing, a leaching process has been suggested, which requires boiling the new filter for 5–10 min in two changes of apyrogenic water. The level of extractable material ranges from 0% to 15% of the filter weight and varies according to filter type and filter manufacturer. Kao *et al.* [75] have shown proton nuclear magnetic resonance spectroscopy to be a convenient means of characterizing extractables. Special low-water-extractability filters, for example those constructed of anodized aluminum [9], are available for use in highly critical applications involving sensitive biological systems, such as tissue-culture work, or very small volumes of filtrate. Track-etched membranes yield no leachable material and need not be treated before use.

One problem associated with membrane filters of all types, and of considerable economic importance, is the rapidity with which they clog when a large volume of solution or highly contaminated fluid is processed. To overcome this, it is possible to introduce a depth filter, as a pre-filter, into the system, the high "dirt"-handling capacity of which will remove many of the initial solids and complement the filtering efficiency of the final (sterilizing) membrane filter [76]. Such a pre-filter is generally constructed of bonded borosilicate glass fiber and is available from most manufacturers in sizes and grades compatible with their membrane filters. For use on a large scale, pre-filters are often supplied as cartridges. In the critical area of parenteral product filtration, cellulose-webbing pre-filters that do not shed particles are available. By selecting the correct grade of pre-filter, the throughput characteristics for any membrane-filtration assembly can be improved significantly (Figure 15.5.10).

The correct matching or pre-filter grade with membrane pore size rating does not, on its own, provide the most economical and efficient system. Consideration must also be given to the pre-filter membrane surface : area ratio, since too small a pre-filter area will result in premature plugging with useable life still remaining in the membrane. Conversely, if the area of the pre-filter is too large, it will be left only partly used when the membrane becomes blocked. The ideal ratio will make for the most economic filtration and must be determined for each new system.

Removal of viruses, prions and endotoxins by filtration

Despite sterilizing filtration still being defined by the removal of "most bacteria and molds", but not all viruses or mycoplasmas, via a retentive membrane [26, 53], there has, nevertheless, been an increased interest in recent years in the subject of virus removal or reduction by filtration. This has stemmed in part from the rise in numbers of biotechnology products and from a greater awareness of the potential of plasma products to act as vectors of viral transmission [77, 78]. These developments, combined with the improved characterization of bacteriophages and mammalian viruses to act as size markers, have led to more detailed guidelines for the validation of virus removal from biotechnology and other vulnerable products [79, 80].

Mammalian viruses vary in size from about 300 nm (e.g. vaccinia) down to about 20–25 nm (e.g. polio and parvoviruses), so those at the top of this range approximate in size to small bacteria (*Brevundimonas diminuta* is 300×700 nm and *Acholeplasma* species about 300 nm in diameter). It is to be expected, therefore,

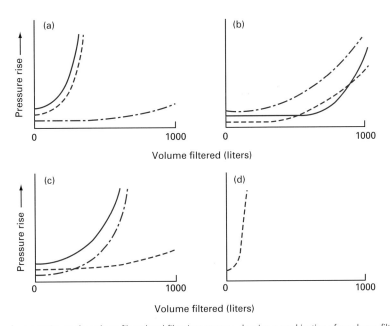

Figure 15.5.10 Effect of prefilter characteristics on the volume filtered and filtration pressure, showing a combination of membrane filter and pre-filter (– – –), the pre-filter alone (——) and the membrane filter alone (– - – - –). (a) If the pre-filter is too coarse, there is insufficient pre-separation, the membrane filter clogs rapidly and the pressure rises rapidly. (b) If the pre-filter is too fine, the pre-filter clogs faster than the membrane filter and there is poor effective filter life. (c) With the correct pre-filter, the pre-filter and membrane filter exhaust themselves approximately simultaneously, with the optimum effective filter life. (d) In a membrane filter without pre-filter there is a rapid rise in pressure and short effective filter life.

that sterilizing filters rated at 0.22 μm are likely to effect a reduction in concentration of some viral species by size exclusion, but the majority of viruses could only be removed by adsorptive mechanisms operating within such membranes. Because the efficiency of adsorption as a removal mechanism is much influenced by process-related factors like flow rate, pH and ionic strength of the fluid, pressure differential and temperature of the filter itself, it is considered less desirable to rely on adsorption-based filtration systems than size exclusion (sieving) ones. For that reason several of the major manufacturers have produced virus-retentive membranes with pore sizes in the ultrafiltration range, but these provide a confusing array of nominal ratings. Some are, or were originally, rated on the basis of exclusion of polymers, usually dextrans or proteins of known hydrodynamic diameters, others are rated on average pore size, and yet others on the basis of the log reduction values that result from challenges with viruses of known dimensions. Despite the intention that virus-retentive membranes should operate on the basis of size exclusion rather than adsorption, Bechtel et al. [81] reported that a membrane with virus-sized pores was unable to discriminate between three viral species of significantly different dimensions, producing approximately the same log reduction for each species. Such a finding would not be expected if a sieving mechanism were operative. This failure was attributed to mechanical imperfections inherent in ultrafiltration membranes that result in the creation of a small fraction of exceptionally large pores that may have a disproportionately large impact on virus retention. Testing of virus-retentive membranes is inherently limited by the difficulty in detecting low viral concentrations. Due to this, a statistical approach is adopted and more than one approach may be required to establish the safety of a product. Confidence in a process may be derived from demonstration of a purification regime's capability to remove/inactivate viruses as well as from direct testing for infectious virus in the final product [82].

The virus-retentive membranes available are commonly manufactured from PVDF or polyethersulfone (PES) although regenerated cellulose is also used, and they are available for direct-flow and cross-flow filtration systems in the usual range of flat disks, capsules and pleated cartridges. Because pores of a size sufficient to retain small viruses also retard the passage of large polymer molecules, several of the virus filters are rated according to their molecular weight cut-off. In selecting a filter therefore, it is particularly important to know the size of the viruses to be removed and the molecular weights of the protein(s) that need to pass into the filtrate in order to achieve optimal filter performance. A typical specification for a virus-retentive membrane is currently a log reduction value of approximately 6 for larger viruses (HIV, influenza and human T-cell leukemia viruses all at approximately 100 nm) with a LRV of 3 for parvoviruses while permitting >95% recovery of proteins up to 150 kDa; use of filters in series permits an LRV of approximately 6 even for small viruses [83]. Levy et al. [84] and Aranah [77] have compiled comprehensive tabulations of LRVs published for a wide range of viruses and the filters of the major manufacturers.

The concerns about serum-derived products acting as vectors for the spread of viral infection are equally valid in respect of prions. These agents of transmissible spongiform encephalopathies are resistant to heat, radiation and chemical methods of sterilization yet capable of transmission via residues on surgical instruments and in therapeutic products manufactured from human tissues [84, 85]. Virus removal filters having a pore size of 9 nm were shown to achieve over 5-log reductions of scrapie agent ME7 in artificially contaminated albumin solutions, but performance was much reduced by the presence of detergents and by increase in pore size to 35 nm [86]. A study by Yunoki et al. [87] reported that although a 15 nm filter can remove prion protein effectively, this removal is not complete. A low molecular weight and/or soluble form of the prion did pass through the 15 nm filter and caused disease in a hamster model [87].

Many sterile medicinal products must also satisfy pharmacopoeial limit tests for endotoxins (bacterial lipopolysaccharide), so the ability to remove or retain such material is a desirable property in a filter membrane. Just as membranes designed specifically to effect viral removal have been introduced in recent years, so, too, have membranes intended for endotoxin removal. Because lipopolysaccharides are negatively charged, the filters by which they are most effectively removed are treated to exhibit a positive charge so that removal is achieved by adsorption; size exclusion pays no part in the removal process since the endotoxin molecules are much smaller than the membrane pores. Hydrophilic PVDF is the material most commonly used in membrane manufacture, although positively charged nylon filters can also be effective [88]. On a research rather than production basis, it has been shown that immobilization of polymyxin B, deoxycholate and other materials onto polymer membranes can achieve such high affinity that endotoxin levels may be reduced below those required for parenteral products with residence times of only 6 s [89]. Although non-polymer membranes have been introduced successfully in other filtration applications, membranes made of either ceramics or aluminum were shown by Bender et al. [90] to be unsuitable for endotoxin removal.

Because the removal mechanism is adsorption there is a finite amount of endotoxin that can be retained on each membrane, and the maximum weight of pure endotoxin that can be adsorbed per unit area of membrane (ng/cm^2) should be the least ambiguous way of expressing filter performance. Despite this, some manufacturers make claims for endotoxin removal in terms of log reduction values without specifying the volume and concentration of endotoxin in the solution with which the filter is challenged.

The performance of a filter membrane is influenced by the physical conditions under which the filtration occurs and the nature of the fluid being filtered. Vanhaecke et al. [88] found endotoxin retention by nylon filters was much reduced when sodium chloride was added to 5% glucose solution compared with the value for glucose alone, although Brown and Fuller [91] noted that retention improved with increasing molarity and decreasing pH. Because the extent of endotoxin removal is markedly affected by the nature of the fluid passing through the membrane and the possibility of competitive adsorption of other negatively charged molecules, thorough validation of the process is necessary before filtration can be relied upon as a means of endotoxin removal. Furthermore, the efficiency of adsorption might be reduced at high flow rates, so it is necessary to specify maximum pressure differentials in order to achieve satisfactory removal. Because of these constraints, a strategy of avoiding endotoxin accumulation in the process fluid in the first place is generally preferred to one of attempting to remove it at the end.

Applications and limitations of filtration

Filtration "sterilization"

Sterilization by filtration is widely used industrially and in hospitals, although the term air "sterilization" has not been used since the 1990s as a 0.3 μm filter might be inadequate to retain small microorganisms. In brief, it may be employed for the sterilization of thermolabile solutions and soluble solids, as well as in the "sterilization" of air and other gases. Air filtration is of particular importance in areas involving the aseptic production of many pharmaceutical products [92–94], in surgical theaters and in hospital wards specially designed for patients with a low resistance to infection. It would, however, be erroneous to imply that filtration sterilization has no disadvantages or limitations, and these will be considered where appropriate.

Sterilization of liquids

Wherever possible, solutions should be sterilized by heating in an autoclave, because this eliminates the contamination risks associated with the transfer of filtered liquid to sterilized containers. Some solutions are unstable when heated and consequently an alternative sterilizing procedure has to be sought. Ionizing radiation has been studied extensively, but, unfortunately, many substances that can be sterilized by this process in the solid state are unstable when irradiated in solution. Filtration is an obvious choice, although it must be added that another alternative for substances which are thermostable in the solid form but unstable in solution (even at ambient temperatures) is to sterilize the solid by dry heat and prepare the solution aseptically immediately before use.

Filtration cannot, in fact, be regarded as a true sterilization process. Admittedly, it will remove microorganisms (see above for a discussion of the possible mechanisms of filtration), but the filtration process must then be followed by an aseptic transference of the sterilized solution to the final containers, which are then sealed, and recontamination at this stage remains a possibility.

Sterility assurance levels for products that have been filter-sterilized and aseptically filled are typically of the order of 10^{-3} [95], and it is for this reason that such products are much more heavily reliant on tests for sterility than heat-processed ones, which have sterility assurance levels of, at least, 10^{-6} and usually much better than this. Persuasive arguments, based on a statistical appraisal of the information conventional sterility tests can supply, have been put forward for their abandonment as a means of monitoring thermal sterilization processes. In the case of terminally sterilized products, physical proofs which are based on biology and automatically documented are of greater assurance than sterility tests, and parametric release may therefore be considered appropriate [96]. Nevertheless, although there might be much scientific merit in their abandonment, they do form an additional defense in the case of litigation following trauma from a suspected contaminated product, and sterility testing should always be carried out on samples of any batch prepared by an aseptic method. This would mean, in essence, that a solution that can be sterilized rapidly by filtration should ideally not be used until the test sample has passed the sterility test, which may take several days. In an emergency, however, it may well be that clinical judgment has to come down in favor of a hospital-prepared product which has not yet passed a test for sterility, if failure to use it poses a greater risk to the patient.

Despite these criticisms, filtration sterilization is performed on a wide range of liquid preparations [97, 98] and routinely on liquid parenteral products (including sera) and on ophthalmic solutions. It is often the only method available to manufacturers of products that cannot be sterilized by thermal processes. Information as to the actual procedures may be found in the *United States Pharmacopeia*, *British Pharmacopoeia* and other national and international pharmacopoeias. It must be emphasized that membrane filters are almost exclusively used in this context and that filtration with a filter of 0.22 (or 0.2) μm pore size, rather than one of 0.45 μm, is required for this purpose.

Membrane filters find an equally important application in the small-scale intermittent preparation of sterile radiopharmaceuticals and intravenous additives. As a result of the special circumstances surrounding the preparation and use of such products, disposable, sterile filters attached to a syringe are generally used. Preparation of these products is best performed under laminar air flow (LAF) conditions (see below).

The use of sterilizing-grade filters in parenteral therapy is not confined to the production stage alone. In-line terminal membrane filtration has been widely advocated as a final safeguard against the hazards associated with the accidental administration of infusion fluids contaminated with either particles or bacteria [60, 97, 99, 100]. These filtration units, generally of 0.22 μm rating, may comprise an integral part of the administration set or form a separate device for introduction proximal to the cannula. In addition to affording some protection against particles and microorganisms introduced during the setting up of the infusion or while making intravenous additions [101], terminal filters also reduce the risk of an air embolism from air bubbles or when an intravenous infusion runs out (a wetted 0.22 μm membrane filter will not pass air at a pressure below 379 kPa (55 psi)). The properties of a wetted membrane filter have been further exploited in infusion-burette devices, where they act as an air shut-off "valve", designed to operate following administration of the required volume.

Although conventional wisdom formerly suggested that membrane filtration cannot be employed successfully in the sterilization of emulsions [97], reports have since shown this not to be so, and parenteral emulsions [102], liposome suspensions [103] and nanoparticle suspensions [104] have all been sterilized by this method.

Sterilization of solid products

The *British Pharmacopoeia* [26] lists four methods that may be used to sterilize powders: ionizing radiation, dry heat, ethylene oxide and filtration. The principle of the filtration process is that the substance to be sterilized is dissolved in an appropriate solvent, the solution is filtered through a membrane filter and the sterile filtrate collected. The solvent is removed aseptically by an appropriate method (evaporation, vacuum evaporation, freeze-drying) and the sterile solid transferred into sterile containers, which are then sealed. Such a method was originally used in the manufacture of sterile penicillin powder.

It appears likely that the probability of contamination occurring during the post-filtration (solid recovery) stage is higher than that described above for sterilizing solutions.

"Sterilization" of air and other gases

Air is, of course, the most common gas which is required in a sterile condition, although there is a less frequent, but nevertheless significant, requirement for other sterile gases, for example nitrogen for sparging the head-space above oxidation-prone liquids and oxygen administered to patients with breathing difficulties. Filters intended to sterilize air are employed in a variety of industrial applications, often as part of a venting system on fermenters, centrifuges, autoclaves and lyophilizers [105], or in hospitals to supply filter air in operating theaters or through respirators to patients vulnerable to infection. In both the indus-

trial and hospital settings, very clean air is also required for "clean rooms" used for aseptic manufacturing or testing.

Many aspects of liquid filtration have direct parallels in the filtration of gases, although there are certain features specific to the latter. Prominent among these is the fact that particles suspended in a gas are exposed to Brownian motion, as a result of bombardment by the gas molecules. This phenomenon, which operates to an insignificant degree in liquids, means that particles suspended in the gas occupy an effective volume greater than that which would be expected from their real size, and so a filter with a given pore structure will remove much smaller particles from a dry, unwetted gas than it will from a liquid (provided that it is not wetted during use). Filters of up to 1.2 μm pore size have been found suitable for the provision of sterile air. Nevertheless, at these larger pore sizes occasional problems with moisture condensation and subsequent grow-through of bacteria can occur, and GMP regulations generally require a 0.2–0.22 μm filter for air "sterilization".

Air filters may be made of cellulose, glass-wool or glass-fiber mixtures, or of PTFE with resin or acrylic binders [106]. Depth filters, such as those made from fiberglass, are believed to achieve very clean air because of the tortuous passage through which the air passes, ensuring that any microorganisms present are trapped not only on the filter surface, but also within the interior. The removal of microorganisms from air occurs as a result of interception, sedimentation, impaction, diffusion and electrostatic attraction [107]. However, reproduction of microorganisms on the filter and their subsequent release into the atmosphere is one cause of "sick building syndrome" [108].

The quality of moving air is described by the maximum level of particles permitted. The International Standards Organization (ISO) published classifications for clean rooms and associated environments in 1999 [109]. The standard (BS EN ISO 14644-1) is currently being updated, but in the new draft version the maximum allowable concentrations remain largely unchanged [110]. Airborne particle limits are summarized in Table 15.5.5. The rules governing medicinal products in the

Table 15.5.5 Clean room classifications based on airborne particulates.

System	EU GMP grade				A/B		C	D
	ISO 14644-1 class	3	4	5	6	7	8
Performance specifications for the	0.1 μm	1,000	10,000	100,000	1,000,000	–	–
control of airborne particulates	0.2 μm	237	2,370	23,700	237,000	–	–
defined as limits on the number of	0.3 μm	102	1,020	10,200	102,000	–	–
particles of given size (μm) that may	0.5 μm	35	352	3,520	35,200	352,000	3,520,000
be present in a cubic meter of air	1.0 μm	8[a]	83	832	8,320	83,200	832,000
	5.0 μm	–	–	29[b]	293	2,930	29,300

[a]Omitted from draft of updated BS EN ISO 14644-1 as sampling and statistical limitations for particles in low concentrations make classification inappropriate.
[b]Omitted from draft of updated BS EN ISO 14644-1 as sample collection limitations for both particles in low concentrations and sizes greater than 1 μm make classification inappropriate, due to potential particle losses in the sampling system.

European Union set limits for particles when environments A–D are "in operation" and "at rest". Grade A is the local zone for high-risk activities, which is equivalent to ISO class 5 (dictated by the limit for particles ≥5 µm), and is normally an area with LAF or an isolator. Grade B is also equivalent to ISO class 5 when at rest, but has higher limits for particles when in use (ISO class 7). For grade C areas, the airborne particle classification is ISO class 7 at rest and ISO class 8 during operation. The lowest grade of clean room involved in the manufacture of sterile pharmaceutical products is grade D, which has equivalency to ISO class 8 when at rest [53]. Aseptic filling normally takes place in a grade A zone with a grade B background, but if an isolator is being utilized a lower grade background may be permitted.

Microbial monitoring is required in clean room areas. During operation <1 cfu/m³ is permitted in a grade A area by each of the following methods: air sampling, settle plates, contact plates and glove prints. Further information about limits for other grades of clean room can be found by consulting the rules governing the medicinal products in the European Union [53].

High-efficiency particulate air (HEPA) filters are available that remove particles of 0.3 µm or larger [111] and, indeed, for strict aseptic conditions. Phillips and Runkle [112] state that such filters will remove particles much smaller than this. Passage of phage particles (0.1 µm diameter) through ultrahigh-efficiency filters is remarkably low and it is considered that these filters provide excellent protection against virus aerosols [113].

An important type of air filtration incorporates the principle of laminar air flow (LAF). This was introduced by Whitfield in 1961 [114–116] and is defined as unidirectional air flow within a confined area moving with uniform velocity and minimum turbulence. Close control of airborne contamination may be a difficult problem, partly because of the non-uniform nature of the air flow patterns in a conventional clean room, partly because they do not carry particulate matter away from critical work areas and partly because airborne contamination is not removed as quickly from the room as it is brought in [98, 114, 117]. Whitfield [114] concluded that a uniform air flow pattern was needed to carry airborne contamination away from the work area. LAF was designed originally to remove dust particles from air by filtration, but it will also remove bacteria [118]. It was employed initially in the electronics and aerospace industries for the purpose of producing air with low particulate levels, necessary to prevent instrument and circuitry malfunction, but is now widely used by the pharmaceutical, cosmetic and other industries.

Laminar air flow can be used in the form of:
1. LAF rooms with wall or ceiling units, the air flow originating through one wall or ceiling and exiting at the opposite end, to produce a displacement of air.
2. LAF units (see below) suitable for small-scale operations, such as the LAF bench used for aseptic processing and sterility testing [98, 108].

Thus, airborne contamination is controlled in the work space, and any generated by manipulations within that area is swept away by the laminar air currents [119]. Nevertheless, there are limitations to the use of LAF, namely it will not sterilize a contaminated product or area [111]. LAF controls only airborne particulate contamination and does not remove surface contamination [120, 121]. Correct techniques must be used, since poor aseptic technique can nullify LAF, and holes in the HEPA filter or air leaks in the system may allow contaminated air to enter the aseptic area [117, 122].

Filters that are used in LAF devices are HEPA filters, mentioned above. These have been designed with a bacterial removal efficiency of greater than 99.99% [98, 108, 117] and often possess particle removal efficiencies in the order of 99.9997% against 0.3 µm particles, a standard sufficient for even the most exacting pharmaceutical purposes. Their life can be prolonged by employing low-efficiency filters upstream to intercept most of the larger particles and some smaller ones before they reach the expensive HEPA filters. HEPA filters are most efficient when air passes through them at an average velocity of 0.5 m/s (c. 100 ft/min) [53, 119].

Laminar air flow is the term applied to very clean air that has been forced through a HEPA filter so that it flows non-turbulently in one direction. In clean rooms, grade A areas can be provided by fitting the entire or part of the ceiling or wall of the clean room with HEPA filters or via a purpose-built laminar flow cabinet. LAF rooms or cabinets differ from conventional turbulent clean rooms in that the air flow is linear and any potential microbial or particulate contamination is swept away by displacement rather than by dilution. A LAF cabinet can be used to provide extra protection for the product (and the operator if a total exhaust or filtered system is used depending on the application) within a conventional turbulent clean room [123, 124].

LAF units providing ISO class 5 (grade A) clean air are of two types, horizontal and vertical, depending upon the direction of the air flow. In vertical LAF (Figure 15.5.11), a supply fan passes air down through an ultrahigh-efficiency filter into the work area, and the air exhausts through a grated work surface, often with the aid of a second fan. A slight negative pressure is maintained by adjusting the fans to exhaust more air than is supplied; this causes ambient air to move from the operator towards the external periphery of the work area, so that a protective curtain of air is created [123, 125]. A vertical LAF of 0.5 m/s maintains a grade A condition, whereas 0.3 m/s (60 ft/min) does not [126]. In horizontal LAF (Figure 15.5.12), air passes from back to front through a HEPA filter at an average velocity of 0.5 m/s, travels horizontally with minimum turbulence and exits as the front of the unit [127, 128].

LAF units have three general areas of usefulness: (i) for product protection, for example in sterility testing or aseptic filling; for these purposes, a standard horizontal LAF is suitable; (ii) for personal protection, that is protection of personnel processing infectious material, where a horizontal LAF is obviously unsuitable;

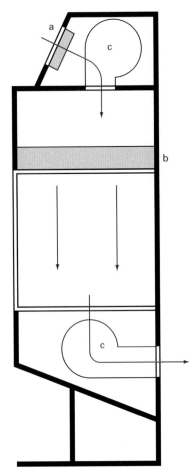

Figure 15.5.11 Vertical laminar air flow unit: (a) pre-filter, (b) HEPA filter and (c) fan.

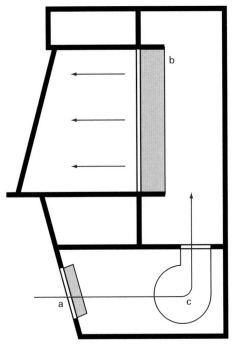

Figure 15.5.12 Horizontal laminar air flow unit: (a) pre-filter, (b) HEPA filter and (c) fan.

here, a vertical LAF is essential; and (iii) for product and personnel protection, in which case a vertical LAF must be used.

LAF rooms have found additional uses, including:

1. In conferring protection to patients undergoing bone-marrow transplants. In this procedure, LAF, in conjunction with a strict aseptic technique, produces maximum protection against microbial contamination from the environment [129].

2. In conferring protection from the environment upon leukemic patients undergoing immunosuppressive (radiomimetic) and anticancer drug therapy. Results suggest that the incidence of infection of leukemic patients in LAF rooms is substantially less than for those treated elsewhere [130].

3. For preventing cross-contamination in germ-free mice [131].

4. For aiding in the treatment of burns [132].

On a smaller scale, the sterile filtration of air (and other gases) for venting, aeration or pressuring purposes can often be accomplished through membrane filters. In line, these filters can also ensure the clarification and sterilization of medical gases. Mechanical patient ventilators may incorporate bacteria-proof filters commonly constructed from hydrophobic glass-fibers [133], although Das and Fraise [134] have questioned their value

in reducing cross-infection. Most membranes used are deliberately of the hydrophobic type, so that they will resist wetting by entrained water droplets, which might otherwise cause an airlock. Hydrophobic filters of 0.2 μm have been used to replace the conventional airways needed with rigid infusion and irrigation containers. The hydrophobic material will support the solution but allow filtered sterile air to enter as the fluid is used.

Microbiological safety cabinets

Microbiological safety cabinets are of three types: class III, which provides the highest degree of containment for handling category 4 pathogens; class II (laminar-flow recirculating cabinet), which protects both the work and the operator from contamination; and class I (exhaust protective cabinet), which protects the worker against bacterial aerosols possibly generated when handling pathogenic material [135]. The cabinets employ HEPA and pre-filters, and further information can be obtained by consulting references [136, 137].

Non-sterilizing uses of membrane filtration

Apart from their use, described above, as a method of "sterilization", filters – and especially membrane filters – have wide applications in other microbiological areas. Membrane filtration in the sterility testing of antibiotics was first described by Holdowsky [138] and this method is now commonly employed in sterility testing generally. See the *United States Pharmacopeia*, *European Pharmacopoeia* and *British Pharmacopoeia* for more information [139].

One method of determining the numbers of colony-forming units in bacterial suspensions or in fluids that may be contaminated by microorganisms is by means of membrane filtration. Basically, this procedure consists of filtering a suitable dilution of the suspension through a membrane filter, which retains the organisms and which is then transferred to the surface of an appropriate solid medium. This method has been used for the bacterial examination of water [140] and for the determination of bioburden in parenteral solutions prior to heat sterilization [141] and is routinely employed for evaluating bacterial retention of other sterilizing-grade filters [26]. Suitable adaptations have been made to this procedure for determining the numbers of cells surviving treatment with or in formulations containing antibiotics [139, 142] or disinfectants/preservatives [139, 143, 144]. The amounts of disinfectants, for example benzalkonium chloride, phenylmercuric borate or chlorhexidine gluconate, adsorbed on to most types of membrane filters are apparently small [145, 146]. The *British Pharmacopoeia* [147] recommends the use of membrane filtration in preservative efficacy tests when the preservative cannot be readily inactivated by dilution or specific neutralizing agents. Membrane filtration combined with epifluorescent microscopy (known as the direct epifluorescent filtration technique (DEFT)) has been employed for the rapid enumeration of contaminating microorganisms in the water industry [148], dairy and food products [149], ultrapure water [150, 151] and parenteral pharmaceutical products [152, 153], and as a rapid method in preservative evaluation [154].

A further analytical application for membrane filters is in the bacteriological sampling of moist surfaces, using a simple contact technique [155]. In this method, the sterile membrane (3–5 μm pore size) is placed in direct contact with a contaminated surface for 5 s and then removed, incubated in the conventional manner on the surface of a solid nutrient medium and the resultant colonies counted. A comparison with traditional contact sampling techniques indicates that the membrane filter method can be successfully employed for the quantitative bacteriological examination of contaminated clinical surfaces [155].

Membrane filtration has been adapted, by means of tangential-flow filter systems, to provide an alternative to centrifugation for the small-scale harvesting of cultures [57, 156, 157]. These filtration devices combine normal fluid flow through the membrane with a washing action, and as a result manage to keep the majority of filtered material in suspension, thereby preventing rapid clogging of the filter [158]. The technique is reported to have little effect on cell viability and offers a recovery efficiency of up to 75% [156]. For the concentration of particularly delicate organisms, a "reverse-flow" filtration system has been developed [57, 157]. Other applications of tangential filtration have been described by Genovesi [159].

Ultrafilter membranes have been used in the purification of water by reverse osmosis [160]. This process may be defined as a reversal of the natural phenomenon of osmosis. If a solution of dissolved salts and pure water is separated by a semipermeable membrane, water will pass through the membrane into the salt solution. This is osmosis itself. Solutes dissolved in the water diffuse less easily and, if their molecular weight is greater than 250, they do not diffuse at all. To reverse the process of osmosis, a pressure in excess of the osmotic pressure of the salt solution is applied and water is thereby forced out of this solution through the membrane in the reverse direction. Since the typical reverse osmosis membrane has pores approaching 2 nm in diameter, this process will remove bacteria, viruses and pyrogens and the purified water produced will be sterile and apyrogenic. It must, however, be added that contamination could occur after production. Ultrafiltration membranes are also exploited in hemodialysis.

Testing of filters

Confidence in the integrity and suitability of a filter for its intended task is of paramount importance in filtration sterilization, and this must ultimately rely on stringent testing.

The list of desirable properties that a filter medium should possess (see above) gives a guide to the parameters that are controlled during manufacture and the specifications of the finished product. Each manufactured batch of filters should conform to specifications regarding their release of particulate materials, mechanical strength, chemical characteristics, including for example oxidizable materials and the leaching of materials which may cause a pH shift when flushed with water, and their pyrogenicity. However, filtration performance is of paramount interest, and this, basically, can be tested in two ways. A challenge test is the only true measure of what a filter is capable of removing from suspension, but this is a destructive test and so it cannot be applied to each individual unit in the manufactured batch. What can be, and is, normally applied to each cartridge filter is an integrity test, and the data it provides can be correlated with those from a challenge test in order to assess the validity of the non-destructive procedure as a substitute. The tests described below are most frequently applied to membrane filters but the underlying principles will apply equally well in the validation of most other filtration media.

Filters used in liquid sterilization

The challenge test, which is the most severe and direct test to which a bacteria-proof filter can be subjected, involves filtration of a bacterial suspension through a sterile filter assembly, with subsequent collection into a nutrient medium and incubation of the filtrate [28]. In the absence of passage of organisms, no growth should be visible.

In the filter industry, such tests are employed for validation purposes [161]. They generally use *Serratoa marcescens* (minimum dimensions approximately 0.5 μm) and *Saccharomyces cerevisiae* to challenge 0.45 and 0.8 μm pore size filters, respectively, while a more rigorous challenge is applied to the 0.2–0.22 μm-rated and 0.1 μm-rated sterilizing filters. Such filters are defined as being capable of removing completely from suspension *Brevundimonas diminuta* ATCC 19146, NCIMB 11091 or CIP 103020 (minimum dimension *c.* 0.3 μm) [26] or *Acholeplasma laidlawii*, respectively. Guidelines on testing procedures have been produced by a number of regulatory and professional bodies including the American Society for Testing and Materials (ASTM), the Health Industry Manufacturers Association (HIMA), the United States Food and Drug Administration (FDA), the Parenteral Drug Association (PDA) and the European and United States Pharmacopoeias. Both Waterhouse and Hall [17] and Carter and Levy [162] have reviewed these methods and the latter authors have tabulated comparisons between them. Technical report 26 (available from the PDA) provides much practical guidance on the conduct of filter validation tests in general.

Bacterial retention determinations are undertaken as part of the validation process of filter sterilizing a product, but they cannot be conducted using the normal manufacturing facilities because they would entail introducing microorganisms into an area from which they should be excluded. If the manufacturer conducts the tests at all, they would be undertaken using a scaled down testing plant, but more commonly they are undertaken in the testing laboratories of filter manufacturers. A typical protocol involves exposure of a sterile filter at a pressure of 207 kPa (30 psi) to a volume of culture medium containing 10^7/ml *B. diminuta* cells to result in a total challenge of approximately 10^9 organisms (the British Pharmacopoeia [26] recommends that a challenge of at least 10^7 cfu/cm^2 of active filter surface is used). The filtrate is either passed through a second 0.22 μm membrane disk, which is then placed on an agar plate and incubated for 2 days, or the effluent itself is collected in a sterile flask and incubated for up to 5 days. Any sign of growth would result in failure of the filter. Griffiths *et al.* [163] have shown that the 48 h incubation period can be halved by use of bioluminescent and fluorescent recombinant strains of *B. diminuta*. A satisfactory filter would be expected to have a Tr of $\geq 10^7$ [45]. In addition to more obvious factors like membrane thickness, transmembrane pressure and filtration rate, the ability of a filter to retain *B. diminuta* will be influenced by the physical characteristics of the liquid in which the bacteria are suspended, and the size, charge and aggregation potential of the bacterial cells as determined by their growth conditions [164–166]. Consequently, the bacteria are preferably grown in a lactose broth rather than a tryptone soya broth in order to achieve individual cells of consistently small size, and they should be suspended in the process liquid that is to be sterilized; if this liquid proves inimical to the bacteria a surrogate (placebo) fluid may be used. Ensuring that the substitute is as realistic as possible is particularly important since it has been shown that the fluid composition may influence not just the size of the bacteria but also the size of the pores in the membrane [167].

Regulatory guidelines for aseptic manufacture of pharmaceuticals recommend the validation of sterilizing filters by bacterial challenge under "worst-case" conditions; a validation protocol applicable to the filter sterilization of high-viscosity fluids at high differential pressures has been described by Aranah and

Meeker [168]. Meltzer [169] has pointed out, however, that the need to test under worst-case conditions only applies for filters that act by adsorptive retention rather than by sieving. It is possible to determine the extent to which these two mechanisms contribute to particle retention by flow decay studies (plotting flow rates as a function of time), and if it were shown that a filter acts solely by sieve retention, that would suffice to validate the filter for all pharmaceutical filtrations and eliminate the need for individual validation for each product and operating condition.

The bacterial retention tests described above are destructive tests and could not be used by the manufacturers of parenteral products to substantiate the efficacy and integrity of the membrane before and after use, as required by a number of regulatory authorities [170]. Similarly, the physical method of mercury intrusion, frequently used to determine pore size distribution [14], does not offer a satisfactory in-process test. What is required is a simple, rapid, non-destructive test that can be performed under aseptic conditions on sterile membranes to ensure the integrity of the membrane and the use of the correct pore size [171]. With this aim in mind a considerable proportion of the industry's research effort has been directed towards validating existing indirect tests and establishing new ones.

The oldest and perhaps most widely used non-destructive test is the bubble-point test [172], which is the subject of BS 1752 [173]. To understand the principles behind this test, it is necessary to visualize the filter as a series of discrete, uniform capillaries, passing from one side to the other. When wetted, the membrane will retain liquid in these capillaries by surface tension, and the minimum gas pressure required to force liquid from the largest of these pores is a measure of the maximum pore diameter (*d*) given by:

$$d = (K\sigma\cos\theta)/P$$

where *P* is bubble-point pressure, σ is surface tension of the liquid, θ is liquid to capillary wall contact angle and *K* is the experimental constant. The pressure (*P*) will depend in part upon the characteristics of the wetting fluid, which, for hydrophilic filters, would be water but, for hydrophobic filters, may be a variety of solvents (e.g. methanol, isopropanol).

To perform the test, the pressure of gas upstream from the wetted filter is slowly increased and the pressure at which the largest pore begins to pass gas is the first bubble point (Figure 15.5.13). In practice, this value is frequently taken as the lowest pressure required to produce a steady stream of bubbles from an immersed tube on the downstream side. The bubble point for a water-wet 0.22 μm-rated filter is 379 kPa (55 psi). An automated method for bubble-point testing has been developed [174].

The inadequacies of the capillary pore model for describing the membrane structure have already been discussed. The bubble-point test is unlikely, therefore, to provide an exact indication of pore dimensions [48, 56] and it does not, in itself, indicate how

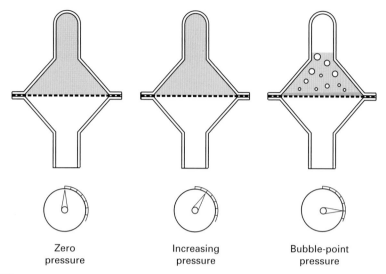

Figure 15.5.13 Stages in the bubble-point test.

efficient the filter is. Instead, its value lies in the knowledge that experimental evidence has allowed the filter manufacturer to correlate bacterial retentivity with a particular bubble point. Thus, any sterilizing-grade filter having a bubble point within the range prescribed by the manufacturer has the support of a rigorous bacterial challenge test regime to ensure confidence in its suitability. In the words of one manufacturer, "An observed bubble point which is significantly lower than the bubble point specification for that particular filter indicates a damaged membrane, ineffective seals, or a system leak. A bubble point that meets specifications ensures that the system is integral."

Small volumes of fluid are often sterilized by passage through a filter unit attached to a hypodermic syringe. The following approximation to the bubble-point test can be applied to such a system to confirm its integrity after use. If the syringe is part-filled with air, then any attempt to force this air through the wet filter should meet appreciable resistance (the bubble-point pressure). Any damage to the membrane would be immediately indicated by the unhindered passage of air.

The bubble-point test has been criticized because it involves a certain amount of operator judgment and is less precise when applied to filters of large surface area [171, 175, 176]. Johnston and Meltzer [177] recognized an additional limitation to the accuracy of this test: commercial membranes often include a wetting agent (see "Methods of manufacture" above), which may well alter the surface tension characteristics of water held within the filter pores and hence the pressure at which bubbles first appear. This wetting agent is frequently extracted from the membrane during aqueous filtrations, rendering invalid any attempt to make an accurate comparison between before and after bubble-point values [177]. These authors have proposed an additional test based on the flow of air through a filter at pressures above the bubble point. The robust air flow test examines the applied

pressure–air flow rate relationship and is amenable to both single-point and multiple-point determinations. This test is described as convenient to use and would, if several readings were taken at different applied air pressures, be more accurate than the single-point bubble-point determination.

The passage of a gas through a wetted filter is not confined solely to bulk flow at applied pressures in excess of the bubble point; it can also occur at lower-pressure values by a molecular diffusion process. With filters of small surface area, this flow is extremely slow, but it increases to significant levels in large-area filters and provides the basis for a sensitive integrity test [27]. This test finds its widest application in large-volume systems, where the need to displace a large quantity of downstream water before the detection of bubbles makes the standard bubble-point test impracticable. To perform this diffusion test, gas under pressure is applied at 80% of the bubble-point pressure [27, 74] for that particular wetted filter and the volumetric gas flow rate determined by measuring either the rate of flow of displaced water or the volume of gas passed in a specified time [175]. A marked increase in gas flow seen at lower pressures than would normally be expected for that filter type indicates a breakdown in the integrity of the system.

Jornitz et al. [167, 178] have advocated the use of multipoint diffusive testing rather than testing at a single pressure because it can more rapidly detect a pending product failure due to gradual filter deterioration. In such a multipoint test, the gas flow rate is related to pressure in a manner similar to that shown in Figure 15.5.14. Impending filter failure may be indicated by an increase in slope of the early portion of the plot corresponding to diffusional flow. This approach can be used to assess pore size distribution; a narrow distribution would be indicated by a significant rise in gas flow at applied pressures only marginally above the bubble point, while a wide distribution would cause a more gradual increase in gas flow.

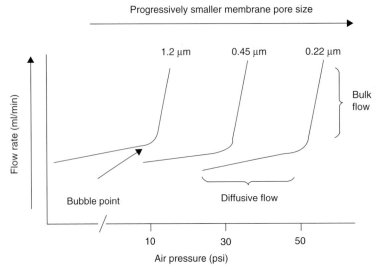

Figure 15.5.14 The relationship between air pressure and flow rate in diffusive flow filter testing.

Virus-retentive filters pose particular problems with respect to validation because their pore sizes correspond to wet bubble-point pressures of the order of 2070 kPa (300 psi). These cannot easily be achieved in conventional testing equipment, so diffusive flow integrity testing is the preferred procedure. There is the possibility of destructive filter testing using a viral challenge analogous to the testing of bacterial filters with *Brevundimonas diminuta*. The problems that exist with bacterial integrity testing with respect to ensuring uniformity of cell size and non-aggregation of the test organism are also seen with viral testing. While the sizes of many common pathogenic viruses are now well defined, using these as challenge organisms may pose unacceptable infection risks to the operators and problems of enumeration, since plaque counts in cell monolayers are not particularly easy or precise. For these reasons Aranha-Creado and Brandwein [179] have advocated the use of appropriately sized bacteriophages as a safe, economical and effective method of filter testing. However, even bacteriophages do not present problem-free alternatives to human viruses because they, like bacteria, display the potential to aggregate and so form unrealistically large particles of variable and unknown dimensions. Parks *et al.* [180] quoted LRVs of the order of 9 for MS-2 coliphages during the operating of air filters, but the phages were generated as aerosols, and the authors acknowledged that the droplets were likely to be much greater than the dimensions of the individual phage particles (23 nm).

All the major suppliers of cartridge filters have developed and supply to their customers integrity-testing instrumentation, which can evaluate the diffusive flow characteristics of the filters at any time during their working life. The testing procedures tend to be named differently by the various manufacturers, for example "pressure decay test", "pressure hold test", "forward flow test" or "diffusive flow test", but they all operate on similar principles. A review of integrity tests performed by US pharmaceutical manufacturers showed that diffusive flow and bubble-point tests were undertaken by 63% and 87%, respectively, of the companies responding [181].

Filters used in gas "sterilization"

The bubble-point and diffusive flow tests described in the previous section are also applicable, with modifications, to membrane filters used for gas "sterilization" in venting systems. The major difference is that air filters are hydrophobic, so it is necessary to use a liquid with a lower surface tension than water in order to achieve adequate wetting; isopropyl alcohol mixed with water is most commonly used for this purpose. Water-based testing procedures have been developed for use in situations where alcohol is undesirable, and these are similar in principle to the bubble-point procedure [182]. In these so-called water-intrusion tests, the parameter measured is the pressure required to cause water to be forced through a hydrophobic filter, rather than air to be passed through a wetted filter.

The continuous production of high-quality filtered air by any HEPA filtration system (see above) can be assured by the application of rigorous efficiency tests to the filter, both at the time of installation and at intervals throughout its service life. The original test method developed to quantify particles passing through a HEPA filter was the dioctylphthalate (DOP) smoke test [183, 184]. Due to concerns about the potential carcinogenicity and teratogenicity of dioctylphthalate, the chemical used has been changed to a synthesized mineral oil. The process is still referred to as the DOP test, but now this signifies "dispersed oil particulate" [185].

In this test, the oil is heated upstream of the filter to produce an aerosol of particles which can be detected in the filtered air using a suitable photoelectric device [186]. For efficiency testing by the filter manufacturer, DOP smoke should be thermally generated, to give mono-sized particles of approximately 0.3 μm diameter, but cold DOP aerosols of larger poly-disperse droplet size [187] have been recommended for detecting small flaws and leaks that may develop in a filter during use [184]. The passage of DOP particles is best examined in a LAF unit by using a small probe to scan the filter surface closely in an overlapping pattern [183]. This will detect any areas of particular weakness, such as pinholes or poor seals [188]. A HEPA filter is expected to have an overall minimum retention efficiency of 99.97% to hot DOP [184], this value being increased to 99.999% for ultra-HEPA filters [189]. Mika [190] has suggested that filtration efficiency is at a minimum for airborne particles of 0.2–0.3 μm diameter, and the bacterial-retention properties of a HEPA filter may well be underrated by this test.

Alternatively, filters can be examined using the sodium-flame test [191], in which a minimum retention efficiency of 99.995% is expected of all HEPA filters used to prepare air to grade A standard [191]. An aerosol is produced from a sodium chloride solution, upstream of the filter, and rapid evaporation of these droplets then ensures that the air arriving at the filter contains minute particles of sodium chloride. Retention efficiency is evaluated by downstream sodium-flame photometry. Other testing methods involve discoloration by atmospheric dust or weight gain during filtration, and are generally confined to filters of a coarser grade.

A bacterial aerosol challenge test has been developed to study the filtration efficiency of air and gas filters [192]. Other workers [190, 193, 194] have suggested using phage particles, vegetative organisms and spores as a suitable challenge for HEPA filters.

Designing a filtration system for the preparation of medicinal products

Sterilization and clarification by filtration are routinely applied to a variety of liquids, which often differ markedly in their filtration characteristics. The first stage in designing any filtration system, therefore, is to classify the fluid to be processed according to the ease with which it can be filtered. The majority of aqueous solutions for intravenous, ophthalmic and irrigation purposes pass easily through a sterilizing-grade membrane filter, while, at the other end of the spectrum, oils and fluids with a high particulate or protein content (e.g. vaccine, serum, plasma and tissue culture media) will, without exception, require some form of pretreatment before final processing. The early methods of pretreatment, which included centrifugation and settling, have largely been replaced by extensive pre-filtration (see Figure 15.5.10) or by sequential filtration through a series of membrane filters of progressively smaller pore size. Often, this series consists of a stack of membrane disks, separated by a support mesh, assembled together in a single filter holder. For ease of handling, it is advisable to arrange the stack of filters in a separate holder from the final sterile, 0.22 μm sterilizing filter. The serial filters can then be replaced when they become clogged

without jeopardizing the sterility of the final filter. The successive filtration of serum through various grades of pre-filter, followed by passage through 1.2, 0.8, 0.45 and 0.22 μm membranes, provides a typical example of serial filtration. The pore size of the final filter is dictated by the need to provide a sterile product.

Small-volume parenteral, ophthalmic and other hospital-produced products are routinely passed through single-disk filter systems capable of processing batches in the region of 500 l. Bulk industrial production, however, with its larger volumes and attendant high capital investment, requires a more sophisticated approach to system design. Invariably, this will demand a pilot study, where results obtained from flow-decay tests performed on approximately 0.1 % of the batch volume or with small-capacity filters, can be used to provide sufficient information for the scaling-up operation [56]. Major filter firms may offer an on-site analysis program, culminating in a computer-assisted appraisal of the filtration process. Any system finally chosen must attempt to optimize total fluid throughput, flow rate and filter and pre-filter life.

The ancillary equipment required for an evolving filtration system is determined, at least in part, by the scale of the process. Large industrial systems will make many individual demands for specialized equipment, which may include pumps, holding tanks, cartridge filter holders and extensive stainless steel plumbing. This combination of components is rarely found in small-scale hospital units.

Accumulated expertise has now clearly demonstrated that, when selecting equipment for assembly into any filtration system, no matter what its size, the following important points must be taken into consideration:

1. Is filtration to be performed under positive or negative pressure? Vacuum filtration is well suited for small-scale analytical processes, such as sterility testing, but should not be used for production purposes. Positive pressure, provided by syringe, pump or nitrogen gas under pressure, offers the important advantages of high flow rates and easier bubble-point testing, and also protects against the ingress of unsterile air and solvent evaporation. Equipment should be designed, therefore, to withstand the pressures employed during the filtration process.
2. Is filtration to be a batch or continuous process? In a continuously operating large-scale system, provision must be made to allow filter changes without interrupting the process. To do this, a valve must be included to switch flow over to another unit fitted with a fresh filter.
3. The system must be amenable to regular maintenance and cleaning. If not, the filters may well be exposed to challenge levels in excess of their capabilities.
4. The amount of particulate contamination within a system is directly proportional to the number of valves, joints and junctions. It is considered advisable, therefore, to keep any system as simple as possible.
5. All valves shed particles during use and must be placed upstream of the final filter.

6. It is axiomatic that the final membrane filter must be placed at the last possible point in the system.

A system that pays attention to all these points should be capable of providing parenteral products of a standard acceptable to all the regulatory authorities. As a final cautionary word, however, the quality of the finished product does not depend solely upon the design and efficiency of the filtration system; it will also owe a great deal to the standard of the production environment, containers used and personnel employed and must, therefore, depend ultimately upon the continued observance of all pharmaceutical GMP requirements [53, 123].

Acknowledgments

We are indebted to the Nuclepore Corporation, who originally supplied the photographs for Figures 15.5.1–15.5.4 and 15.5.8, to Pall Corporation for Figure 15.5.9 and to Schleicher and Schull GMBH for Figure 15.5.10. We also thank Norman A. Hodges who co-wrote the original chapter in the last edition, on which this one is based.

References

1 Chamberland, C. (1884) Sur un filtre donnant de l'eau physiologiquement pure. *Compte Rendu Hebdomadaire des Séances de l'Académie des Sciences*, **99**, 247–552.

2 Dahlstrom, D.A. and Silverblatt, C.E. (1986) Continuous vacuum and pressure filtration, in *Solid/Liquid Separation Equipment Scale-up* (eds D.B. Purchase and R.J. Wakeman), Uplands Press and Filtration Specialists, London, pp. 510–557.

3 Smith, I.P.C. (1944) Sintered glassware: its manufacture and use. *Pharmaceutical Journal*, **152**, 110–111.

4 Zsigmondy, R. and Bachmann, W. (1918) Über neue Filter. *Zeitschrift für Anorganische und Allgemeine Chemie*, **103**, 119–128.

5 Gelman, C. (1965) Microporous membrane technology: part 1. Historical development and applications. *Analytical Chemistry*, **37**, 29A–37A.

6 Kesting, R.E. *et al.* (1983) Nylon microfiltration membranes: state of the art. *Journal of Parenteral Science and Technology*, **37**, 97–104.

7 Ehrlich, R. (1960) Application of membrane filters. *Advances in Applied Microbiology*, **2**, 95–112.

8 Fleischer, R.L. *et al.* (1964) Novel filter for biological materials. *Science*, **143**, 249–250.

9 Jones, H. (1990) Inorganic membrane filter for biological separation applications. *International Labmate*, **15**, 57–58.

10 Desai, T.A. *et al.* (1999) Characterization of micromachined silicon membranes for immunoisolation and bioseparation applications. *Journal of Membrane Science*, **159**, 221–231.

11 Megaw, W.J. and Wiffen, R.D. (1963) The efficiency of membrane filters. *International Journal of Air and Water Pollution*, **7**, 501–509.

12 Preusser, H.J. (1967) Elektronenmikroskopische Untersuchungen an Oberflachen von Membranfiltern. *Kolloidzeitschrift und Zeitschrift für Polymere*, **218**, 129.

13 Denee, P.B. and Stein, R.L. (1971) An evaluation of dust sampling membrane filters for use in the scanning electron microscope. *Powder Technology*, **5**, 201–204.

14 Marshall, J.C. and Meltzer, T.H. (1976) Certain porosity aspects of membrane filters: their pore-distribution and anisotropy. *Bulletin of the Parenteral Drug Association*, **30**, 214–225.

15 Kesting, R. *et al.* (1981) Highly anisotropic microfiltration membranes. *Pharmaceutical Technology*, **5**, 53–60.

16 Wrasidlo, W. and Mysels, K.J. (1984) The structure and some properties of graded highly asymmetrical porous membranes. *Journal of Parenteral Science and Technology*, **38**, 24–31.

17 Waterhouse, S. and Hall, G.M. (1995) The validation of sterilizing grade microfiltration membranes with *Pseudomonas diminuta*. *Journal of Membrane Science*, **104**, 1–9.

18 Kawamura, K. *et al.* (2000) Absolute or sterilizing grade filtration – what is required? *PDA Journal of Pharmaceutical Science and Technology*, **54**, 485–492.

19 Jacobs, S. (1972) The distribution of pore diameters in graded ultrafilter membranes. *Filtration and Separation*, **September/October**, 525–530.

20 Pall, D.B. (1975) Quality control of absolute bacteria removal filters. *Bulletin of the Parenteral Drug Association*, **29**, 192–204.

21 Alkan, M.H. and Groves, M.J. (1978) The measurement of membrane filter pore size by a gas permeability technique. *Drug Development and Industrial Pharmacy*, **4**, 225–241.

22 Ballew, H.W. and the Staff of Nuclepore Corporation (1978) *Basics of Filtration and Separation*, Nuclepore Corporation, Pleasanton, CA.

23 Duberstein, R. (1979) Filter Validation Symposium. II. Mechanisms of bacterial removal by filtration. *Journal of the Parenteral Drug Association*, **33**, 251–256.

24 Lee, K.Y. *et al.* (1998) The effect of vacuum pressure in membrane filtration systems for the efficient detection of bacteria from natural mineral water. *Journal of Microbiology and Biotechnology*, **8**, 124–128.

25 Heidam, N.Z. (1981) Review: aerosol fractionation by sequential filtration with Nucleopore filters. *Atmospheric Environment*, **15**, 891–904.

26 British Pharmacopoeia (2011) British Pharmacopoeia. *Appendix XVIII Methods of Sterilisation*, HMSO, London.

27 Reti, A.R. (1977) An assessment of test criteria for evaluating the performance and integrity of sterilizing filters. *Journal of Parenteral Drug Association*, **31**, 187–194.

28 Bowman, F.W. *et al.* (1967) Microbiological methods for quality control of membrane filters. *Journal of Pharmaceutical Sciences*, **56**, 222–225.

29 Wallhausser, K.H. (1976) Bacterial filtration in practice. *Drugs Made in Germany*, **19**, 85–98.

30 Elford, W.J. (1933) The principles of ultrafiltration as applied in biological studies. *Proceedings of the Royal Society*, **112B**, 384–406.

31 Wallhausser, K.H. (1979) Is the removal of microorganisms by filtration really a sterilization method? *Journal of the Parenteral Drug Association*, **33**, 156–170.

32 Reti, A.R. and Leahy, T.J. (1979) Filter Validation Symposium. III. Validation of bacterially retentive filters by bacterial passage testing. *Journal of the Parenteral Drug Association*, **33**, 257–272.

33 Howard, G. Jr. and Duberstein, R. (1980) A case of penetration of 0.2 μm rated membrane filters by bacteria. *Journal of the Parenteral Drug Association*, **34**, 95–102.

34 Lukaszewicz, R.C. and Meltzer, T.H. (1979) Filter Validation Symposium. I. A co-operative address to current filter problems. *Journal of the Parenteral Drug Association*, **33**, 247–249.

35 Bower, J.P. and Fox, R. (1985) Definition and testing of a biologically retentive 0.1 micron pore size membrane filter. Presented at the Society of Manufacturing Engineers Conference "Filtration in Pharmaceutical Manufacturing", Philadelphia, 26–28 March 1985.

36 Sundaram, S. *et al.* (1999) Application of membrane filtration for removal of diminutive bioburden organisms in pharmaceutical products and processes. *PDA Journal of Pharmaceutical Science and Technology*, **53**, 186–201.

37 Robinson, J.P. (1984) The great filter rating debate (Editorial). *Journal of Parenteral Science and Technology*, **38**, 47.

38 Sundaram, S. *et al.* (2001) Retention of water-borne bacteria by membrane filters part II. Scanning electron microscopy (SEM) and fatty acid methyl ester (FAME) characterisation of bacterial species recovered downstream of 0.2/0.22 micron rated filters. *PDA Journal of Pharmaceutical Science and Technology*, **55**, 87–113.

39 Sundaram, S. *et al.* (2001) Retention of water-borne bacteria by membrane filters part III. Bacterial challenge tests on 0.1 micron rated. *PDA Journal of Pharmaceutical Science and Technology*, **55**, 114–126.

40 Sundaram, S. *et al.* (2001) Retention of water-borne bacteria by membrane filters part I. Bacterial challenge tests on 0.2 and 0.22 micron rated filters. *PDA Journal of Pharmaceutical Science and Technology*, **55**, 65–86.

41 Bardo, B. *et al.* (2001) Letter to the editor. *PDA Journal of Pharmaceutical Science and Technology*, **55**, 207–208.

42 Levy, R.V. (2001) Sterilizing filtration of liquids, in *Filtration in the Biopharmaceutical Industry* (eds T.H. Meltzer and M.W. Jornitz), Marcel Dekker, New York, pp. 399–412.

43 Tanny, G.B. *et al.* (1979) Adsorptive retention of *Pseudomonas diminuta* by membrane filters. *Journal of the Parenteral Drug Association*, **33**, 40–51.

44 Todd, R.L. and Kerr, T.J. (1972) Scanning electron microscopy of microbial cells on membrane filters. *Applied Microbiology*, **23**, 1160–1162.

45 Osumi, M. *et al.* (1991) Bacterial retention mechanisms of membrane filters. *Pharmaceutical Technology (Japan)*, **7**, 11–16.

46 Hawker, R.J. and Hawker, L.M. (1975) Protein losses during sterilization by filtration. *Laboratory Practice*, **24**, 805–807.

47 Tanny, G.B. and Meltzer, T.H. (1978) The dominance of adsorptive effects in the filtrative purification of a flu vaccine. *Journal of the Parenteral Drug Association*, **32**, 258–267.

48 Lukaszewicz, R.C. *et al.* (1978) Membrane filter characterizations and their implications for particulate retention. *Pharmaceutical Technology*, **2** (11), 77–83.

49 Lukaszewicz, R.C. and Meltzer, T.H. (1979) Concerning filter validation. *Journal of the Parenteral Drug Association*, **33**, 187–194.

50 Bobbit, J.A. and Betts, R.P. (1992) The removal of bacteria from solutions by membrane filtration. *Journal of Microbiological Methods*, **16**, 215–220.

51 Dosmar, M. and Brose, D. (1998) Crossflow ultrafiltration, in *Filtration in the Biopharmaceutical Industry* (eds T.H. Meltzer and M.W. Jornitz), Marcel Dekker, New York, pp. 493–532.

52 Sharp, J. (2000) Sterile products: basic concepts and principles, in *Quality in the Manufacture of Medicines and Other Healthcare Products* (ed. J. Sharp), Pharmaceutical Press, London, pp. 333–360.

53 Eudralex (2008) Annex 1: manufacture of sterile medicinal products, in *EU Guidelines to Good Manufacturing Practice Medicinal Products for Human and Veterinary Use*, vol. 4, European Commission, Enterprise and Industry Directorate-General, Brussels.

54 Cole, J.C. *et al.* (1979) Cartridge filters, in *Filtration: Principles and Practice, Part II* (ed. C. Orr), Marcel Dekker, New York, pp. 201–259.

55 Conacher, J.C. (1976) Membrane filter cartridges for fine particle control in the electronics and pharmaceutical industries. *Filtration and Separation*, **May/June**, 1–4.

56 Meltzer, T.H. and Lukaszewicz, R.C. (1979) Filtration sterilization with porous membranes, in *Quality Control in the Pharmaceutical Industry*, vol. 3 (ed. M.S. Cooper), Academic Press, London, pp. 145–211.

57 Brock, T.D. (1983) *Membrane Filtration: a Users' Guide and Reference Manual*, Science Tech, Madison, WI.

58 Lukaszewicz, R.C. and Meltzer, T.H. (1980) On the structural compatibilities of membrane filters. *Journal of the Parenteral Drug Association*, **34**, 463–474.

59 Kovary, S.J. *et al.* (1983) Validation of the steam-in-place sterilization of disc filter housings and membranes. *Journal of Parenteral Science and Technology*, **37**, 55–64.

60 Chrai, S.S. (1989) Validation of filtration systems: considerations for selecting filter housings. *Pharmaceutical Technology*, **13**, 85–96.

61 Voorspoels, J. *et al.* (1996) Validation of filter sterilization and autoclaves. *International Journal of Pharmaceutics*, **133**, 9–15.

62 Rusmin, S. *et al.* (1975) Consequences of microbial contamination during extended intravenous therapy using in-line filters. *American Journal of Hospital Pharmacy*, **32**, 373–377.

63 US Department of Health and Human Services Food and Drug Administration (2004) *Guidance for Industry: Sterile Drug Products Produced by Aseptic Processing – Current good manufacturing practice*. Food and Drug Administration, Silver Spring, MD.

64 Wagman, G.H. *et al.* (1975) Binding of aminoglycoside antibiotics to filtration materials. *Antimicrobial Agents and Chemotherapy*, **7**, 316–319.

65 Rusmin, S. and Deluca, P.P. (1976) Effect of in-line intravenous filtration on the potency of potassium penicillin G. *Bulletin of the Parenteral Drug Association*, **30**, 64–71.

66 Bin, T. *et al.* (1999) Adsorption of benzalkonium chloride by filter membranes: mechanisms and effect of formulation and processing parameters. *Pharmaceutical Development and Technology*, **4**, 151–165.

67 De Muynck, C. *et al.* (1998) Binding of drugs to end-line filters: a study of four commonly administered drugs in intensive care units. *Journal of Clinical Pharmacy and Therapeutics*, **13**, 335–340.

68 Kanke, M. *et al.* (1983) Binding of selected drugs to a "treated" inline filter. *American Journal of Hospital Pharmacy*, **40**, 1323–1328.

69 Olson, W.P. *et al.* (1977) Rapid delipidation and particle removal from human serum by membrane filtration in a tangential flow system. *Preparative Biochemistry*, **7**, 333–343.

70 Akers, M.J. *et al.* (1993) Sterility testing of antimicrobial-containing injectable solutions prepared in the pharmacy. *American Journal of Hospital Pharmacy*, **48**, 2414–2418.

71 Pitt, A.M. (1987) The non-specific protein binding of polymeric microporous membranes. *Journal of Parenteral Science and Technology*, **41**, 110–113.

72 Truskey, G.A. *et al.* (1987) The effect of membrane filtration upon protein conformation. *Journal of Parenteral Science and Technology*, **41**, 180–193.

73 Kristensen, T. *et al.* (1985) Micropone filters for sterile filtration may leach toxic compounds affecting cell cultures (HL-60). *Experimental Hematology*, **13**, 1188–1191.

74 Olson, W.P. *et al.* (1980) Aqueous filter extractables: detection and elution from process filters. *Journal of the Parenteral Drug Association*, **34**, 254–267.

75 Kao, Y.H. *et al.* (2001) Characterization of filter extractables by proton NMR spectroscopy: studies on intact filters with process buffers. *PDA Journal of Pharmaceutical Science and Technology*, **55**, 268–277.

76 Lukaszewicz, R.C. *et al.* (1981) Prefilters/final filters: a matter of particle/pore/size distribution. *Journal of Parenteral Science and Technology*, **35**, 40–47.

77 Aranah, H. (2001) Viral clearance strategies for biopharmaceutical safety, part 2: filtration for viral clearance. *Biopharm*, **14**, 32–43.

78 Wickramasinghe, S.R. *et al.* (2010) Understanding virus filtration membrane performance. *Journal of Membrane Science*, **365**, 160–169.

79 Anon. (1998) Guidance on viral safety evaluation of biotechnology products derived from human cell lines of human or animal origin. *Federal Register*, **63**, 51074–51084.

80 EMEA (2006) *Guidelines on Virus Safety Evaluation of Biotechnological Investigational Medicinal Products*, Evaluation of Medicines for Human Use, Doc. Ref. EMEA/CHMP/BWP/398498/2005-corr, European Medicines Agency, London.

81 Bechtel, M.K. *et al.* (1998) Virus removal or inactivation in haemoglobin solutions by ultrafiltration or detergent/solvent treatment. *Biomaterials, Artificial Cells and Artificial Organs*, **16**, 123–128.

82 EMEA (1997) *Quality of Biotechnological Products: Viral safety evaluation of biotechnology products derived from cell lines of human or animal origin*, ICH Topic Q5A (R1), CPMP/ICH/295/95, European Medicines Agency, London.

83 Abe, H. *et al.* (2000) Removal of parvovirus B19 from hemoglobin solution by nanofiltration. *Artificial Cells Blood Substitutes and Immobilization Biotechnology*, **28**, 375–383.

84 Levy, R.V. *et al.* (1998) Filtration and the removal of viruses from biopharmaceuticals, in *Filtration in the Biopharmaceutical Industry* (eds T.H. Meltzer and M.W. Jornitz), Marcel Dekker, New York, pp. 619–646.

85 Taylor, D.M. (1999) Transmissible degenerative encephalopaties: inactivation of the unconventional causal agents, in *Principles and Practice of Disinfection, Preservation and Sterilization*, 3rd edn (eds A.D. Russell *et al.*), Blackwell, London, pp. 222–236.

86 Tateishi, J. *et al.* (2001) Scrapie removal using Planova virus removal filters. *Biologicals*, **29**, 17–25.

87 Yunoki, M. *et al.* (2010) Infectious prion protein in the filtrate even after 15 nm filtration. *Biologicals*, **38**, 311–313.

88 Vanhaecke, E. *et al.* (1989) Endotoxin removal by end-line filters. *Journal of Clinical Microbiology*, **12**, 2710–2712.

89 Anspach, F.B. and Petsch, D. (2000) Membrane adsorbers for selective endotoxin removal from protein solutions. *Process Biochemistry*, **35**, 1005–1021.

90 Bender, H. *et al.* (2000) Membranes for endotoxin removal from dialysate: considerations on feasibility of commercial ceramic membranes. *Artificial Organs*, **24**, 826–829.

91 Brown, S. and Fuller, A.C. (1993) Depyrogenation of pharmaceutical solutions using submicron and ultrafilters. *PDA Journal of Pharmaceutical Science and Technology*, **47**, 285–288.

92 Hargreaves, D.P. (1990) Good manufacturing practice in the control of contamination, in *Guide to Microbiological Control in Pharmaceuticals* (eds S. Denyer and R. Baird), Ellis Horwood, Chichester, pp. 68–86.

93 Sharp, J. (2005) Sterile products manufacture: basic principles, in *Good Pharmaceutical Manufacturing Practice: Rationale and Compliance* (ed. J. Sharp), CRC Press, London, pp. 329–370.

94 Denyer, S.P. (1998) Factory and hospital hygiene and good manufacturing practice, in *Pharmaceutical Microbiology*, 6th edn (eds W.B. Hugo and A.D. Russell), Blackwell Scientific Publications, Oxford, pp. 426–438.

95 Gilbert, P. and Allison, D. (1996) Redefining the "sterility" of sterile products. *European Journal of Parenteral Sciences*, **1**, 19–23.

96 British Pharmacopoeia (2011) *SC IV P. Guidelines for using the Test for Sterility*, HSMO, London.

97 McKinnon, B.T. and Avis, K.E. (1993) Membrane filtration of pharmaceutical solutions. *American Journal of Hospital Pharmacy*, **50**, 1921–1936.

98 Avis, K.E. (1997) Assuring the quality of pharmacy-prepared sterile products. *Pharmacopoeial Forum*, **23**, 3567–3576.

99 Maki, D.G. (1976) Preventing infection in intravenous therapy. *Hospital Practice*, **11**, 95–104.

100 Lowe, G.D. (1981) Filtration in IV therapy. Part 1: clinical aspects of IV fluid filtration. *British Journal of Intravenous Therapy*, **2**, 42–52.

101 Holmes, C.J. and Allwood, M.C. (1979) A review: the microbial contamination of intravenous infusions during clinical use. *Journal of Applied Bacteriology*, **46**, 247–267.

102 Hosokawa, T. *et al.* (2002) Formulation development of a filter-sterilizable lipid emulsion for lipophilic KW-3902, a newly synthesised adenosine A1 receptor antagonist. *Chemical and Pharmaceutical Bulletin*, **50**, 87–91.

103 Goldbach, P. *et al.* (1995) Sterile filtration of liposomes – retention of encapsulated carboxyfluorescein. *International Journal of Pharmaceutics*, **117**, 225–230.

104 Konan, Y.N. *et al.* (2002) Preparation and characterization of sterile and freeze-dried sub 200 nm nanoparticles. *International Journal of Pharmaceutics*, **233**, 239–252.

105 Ljungqvist, B. and Reinmuller, B. (1998) Design of HEPA filters above autoclaves and freeze dryers. *PDA Journal of Pharmaceutical Science and Technology*, **52**, 337–339.

106 Underwood, E. (1998) Ecology of microorganisms as it affects the pharmaceutical industry, in *Pharmaceutical Microbiology*, 6th edn (eds W.B. Hugo and A.D. Russell), Blackwell Scientific Publications, Oxford, pp. 339–354.

107 White, P.J.P. (1990) The design of controlled environments, in *Guide to Microbiological Control in Pharmaceuticals* (eds S.P. Denyer and R. Baird), Ellis Horwood, Chichester, pp. 87–124.

108 Kelly-Wintenberg, K. *et al.* (2000) Air filter sterilization using a one atmosphere uniform glow discharge plasma (the Volfilter). *IEEE Transactions on Plasma Science*, **28**, 64–71.

109 British Standards Institution (BSI) (1999) *BS EN ISO 14644-1. Cleanrooms and Associated Controlled Environments – part 1: Classification of Air Cleanliness*, BSI, London.

110 British Standards Institution (BSI) (2010) *Draft BS EN ISO 14644-1, DPC: 10/30152865 DC. Cleanrooms and Associated Controlled Environments – part 1: Classification of Air Cleanliness by Particle Concentration*, BSI, London.

111 Wayne, W. (1975) Clean rooms – letting the facts filter through. *Laboratory Equipment Digest*, **December**, 49.

112 Phillips, G.B. and Runkle, R.S. (1972) Design of facilities, in *Quality Control in the Pharmaceutical Industry*, vol. 1 (ed. M.S. Cooper), Academic Press, New York, pp. 73–99.

113 Harstad, J.B. *et al.* (1967) Air filtration of submicron virus aerosols. *American Journal of Public Health*, **57**, 2186–2193.

114 Whitfield, W.J. (1967) Microbiological studies of laminar flow rooms. *Bulletin of the Parenteral Drug Association*, **21**, 37–45.

115 Soltis, C. (1967) Construction and use of laminar flow rooms. *Bulletin of the Parenteral Drug Association*, **21**, 55–62.

116 Whitfield, W.J. and Lindell, K.F. (1969) Designing for the laminar flow environment. *Contamination Control*, **8**, 10–21.

117 Neiger, J. (1997) Life with the UK pharmaceutical isolator guidelines: a manufacturer's viewpoint. *European Journal of Parenteral Sciences*, **2**, 13–20.

118 Coriell, L.L. and McGarrity, G.J. (1967) Elimination of airborne bacteria in the laboratory and operating room. *Bulletin of the Parenteral Drug Association*, **21**, 46–51.

119 Coriell, L.L. (1975) Laboratory applications of laminar air flow, in *Quality Control in Microbiology* (eds J.E. Prior *et al.*), University Park Press, Baltimore, pp. 41–46.

120 Phillips, G.B. and Brewer, J.H. (1968) Recent advances in microbiological control. *Development in Industrial Microbiology*, **9**, 105–121.

121 Brewer, J.H. and Phillips, G.B. (1971) Environmental control in the pharmaceutical and biological industries. *CRC Critical Reviews in Environmental Control*, **1**, 467–506.

122 Stockdale, D. (1987) Clean rooms for aseptic pharmaceutical manufacturing, in *Aseptic Pharmaceutical Manufacturing Technology for the 1990s* (eds W. Olson and M.J. Groves), Interpharm Press, Prairie View, TX, pp. 151–160.

123 Sharp, J. (2000) Assurance of quality in the manufacture of sterile products, in *Quality in the Manufacture of Medicines and Other Healthcare Products* (ed. J. Sharp), Pharmaceutical Press, London, pp. 361–406.

124 Sharp, J. (2005) GMP and quality assurance in sterile products manufacture, in *Good Pharmaceutical Manufacturing Practice: Rationale and Compliance* (ed. J. Sharp), CRC Press, London, pp. 371–403.

125 Favero, M.S. and Berquist, K.R. (1968) Use of laminar airflow equipment in microbiology. *Applied Microbiology*, **16**, 182–183.

126 Loughhead, H. and Vellutato, A. (1969) Parenteral production under vertical laminar air flow. *Bulletin of the Parenteral Drug Association*, **23**, 17–22.

127 Coriell, L.L. and McGarrity, G.J. (1968) Biohazard hood to prevent infection during microbiological procedures. *Applied Microbiology*, **16**, 1895–1900.

128 Corriell, L.L. and McGarrity, G.J. (1970) Evaluation of the Edgegard laminar flow hood. *Applied Microbiology*, **20**, 474–479.

129 Solberg, C.O. *et al.* (1971) Laminar airflow protection in bone marrow transplantation. *Applied Microbiology*, **21**, 209–216.

130 Bodey, G.P. *et al.* (1969) Studies of patients in a laminar air flow unit. *Cancer*, **24**, 972–980.

131 Van der Waaij, D. and Andres, A.H. (1971) Prevention of airborne contamination and cross-contamination in germ-free mice by laminar flow. *Journal of Hygiene, Cambridge*, **69**, 83–89.

132 Anon. (1975) Clean areas aid treatment of burns. *Laboratory Equipment Digest*, **December**, 51–52.

133 Nielsen, H.J. *et al.* (1996) Comparative study of the efficiency of bacterial filters in long-term mechanical ventilation. *Anaesthetist*, **45**, 814–818.

134 Das, I. and Fraise, A. (1998) How useful are microbial filters in respiratory apparatus? *Journal of Hospital Infection*, **37**, 263–272.

135 Clark, R.P. (1980) Microbiological safety cabinets. *Medical Laboratory World*, **March**, 27–33.

136 British Standards Institution (BSI) (2000) *BS EN 12469. Biotechnology – Performance Criteria for Microbiological Safety Cabinets*, BSI, London.

137 British Standards Institution (BSI) (2005) *BS 5726. Microbiological Safety Cabinets – Information to be Supplied by the Purchaser to the Vendor and to the Installer, and Siting and Use of Cabinets – Recommendations and Guidance*, BSI, London.

138 Holdowsky, S. (1957) A new sterility test for antibiotics: an application of the membrane filter technique. *Antibiotics and Chemotherapy*, **7**, 49–54.

139 British Pharmacopoeia (2011) *Appendix XVI A. Test for Sterility*, HMSO, London.

140 British Standards Institution (BSI) (2000) *BS EN ISO 9308-1. Water Quality – Detection and Enumeration of Escherichia coli and Coliform Bacteria. Part 1: Membrane Filtration Method*, BSI, London.

141 Boom, F.A. *et al.* (1991) Microbiological aspects of heat sterilization of drugs. 3. Heat resistance of spore-forming bacteria isolated from large-volume parenterals. *Pharmaceutisch Weekblad – Scientific Edition*, **13**, 130–136.

142 Meers, P.D. and Churcher, G.M. (1974) Membrane filtration in the study of antimicrobial drugs. *Journal of Clinical Pathology*, **27**, 288–291.

143 Prince, J. *et al.* (1975) A membrane filter technique for testing disinfectants. *Journal of Clinical Pathology*, **28**, 71–76.

144 British Pharmacopoeia (2011) *Appendix XVI B. Microbiological Examination of Non-sterile Products*, HMSO, London.

145 Van Ooteghem, M. and Herbots, H. (1969) The adsorption of preservatives on membrane filters. *Pharmaceutica Acta Helvetiae*, **44**, 610–619.

146 Naido, H.T. *et al.* (1972) Preservative loss from ophthalmic solutions during filtration sterilization. *Australian Journal of Pharmaceutical Sciences*, **NS1**, 16–18.

147 British Pharmacopoeia (2011) *Appendix XVI C. Efficacy of Antimicrobial Preservation*, HMSO, London.

148 Hobbie, J.E. *et al.* (1977) Use of Nucleopore filters for counting bacteria by fluorescence microscopy. *Applied and Environmental Microbiology*, **33**, 1225–1228.

149 Pettipher, G.L. (1983) *The Direct Epifluorescent Filter Technique for the Rapid Enumeration of Microorganisms*, Research Studies Press, Letchworth.

150 Mittelman, M.W. *et al.* (1983) Epifluorescence microscopy: a rapid method for enumerating viable and non-viable bacteria in ultra-pure water systems. *Microcontamination*, **1**, 32–37.

151 Mittelman, M.W. *et al.* (1985) Rapid enumeration of bacteria in purified water systems. *Medical Device and Diagnostics Industry*, **7**, 144–149.

152 Denyer, S.P. and Lynn, R. (1987) A sensitive method for the rapid detection of bacterial contaminants in intravenous fluids. *Journal of Parenteral Science and Technology*, **41**, 60–66.

153 Newby, P.J. (1991) Analysis of high quality pharmaceutical grade water by a direct epifluorescent filter technique microcolony method. *Letters in Applied Microbiology*, **13**, 291–293.

154 Connolly, P. *et al.* (1993) A study of the use of rapid methods for preservative efficacy testing of pharmaceuticals and cosmetics. *Journal of Applied Bacteriology*, **75**, 456–462.

155 Craythorn, J.M. *et al.* (1980) Membrane filter contract technique for bacteriological sampling of moist surfaces. *Journal of Clinical Microbiology*, **12**, 250–255.

156 Tanny, G.B. *et al.* (1980) Improved filtration technique for concentrating and harvesting bacteria. *Applied and Environmental Microbiology*, **40**, 269–273.

157 Kempken, R. *et al.* (1996) *Dynamic Membrane Filtration in Cell Culture Harvest, Technical Report*, Pall Europe, Portsmouth.

158 Lukaszewicz, R.C. *et al.* (1981) Functionality and economics of tangential flow micro filtration. *Journal of Parenteral Science and Technology*, **35**, 231–236.

159 Genovesi, C.S. (1983) Several uses for tangential-flow filtration in the pharmaceutical industry. *Journal of Parenteral Science and Technology*, **37**, 81–86.

160 Pohland, H.W. (1980) Seawater desalination by reverse osmosis. *Endeavour (New Series)*, **4**, 141–147.

161 Wallhausser, K.H. (1982) Germ removal filtration, in *Advances in Pharmaceutical Sciences* (eds H.S. Bean *et al.*), Academic Press, London, pp. 1–116.

162 Carter, J.R. and Levy, R.V. (2001) Microbial retention testing in the validation of sterilizing filtration, in *Filtration in the Biopharmaceutical Industry* (eds T.H. Meltzer and M.W. Jornitz), Marcel Dekker, New York, pp. 577–604.

163 Griffiths, M.H. *et al.* (2000) Rapid methods for testing the efficacy of sterilization-grade filter membranes. *Applied and Environmental Microbiology*, **66**, 3432–3437.

164 Mittelman, M.W. *et al.* (1998) Bacterial cell size and surface charge characteristics relevant to filter validation studies. *PDA Journal of Pharmaceutical Science and Technology*, **52**, 37–42.

165 Levy, R.V. (2001) Sterile filtration of liquids and gases, in *Disinfection, Sterilization and Preservation*, 5th edn (ed. S.S. Block), Lippencott, Williams & Wilkins, Philadelphia, pp. 795–822.

166 Lee, S.H. *et al.* (2001) Changes in cell size and buoyant density of *Pseudomonas diminuta* in response to osmotic shocks. *Journal of Microbiology and Biotechnology*, **11**, 326–328.

167 Jornitz, M.W. *et al.* (2002) Considerations in sterile filtration – part I: the changed role of filter integrity testing. *PDA Journal of Pharmaceutical Science and Technology*, **58**, 4–10.

168 Aranah, H. and Meeker, J. (1995) Microbial retention characteristics of 0.2-microns-rated nylon membrane filters during filtration of high viscosity fluids at high differential pressure and varied temperature. *Journal of Pharmaceutical Science and Technology*, **49**, 67–70.

169 Meltzer, T.H. (1995) The significance of sieve-retention to the filter validation process. *PDA Journal of Pharmaceutical Science and Technology*, **49**, 188–191.

170 Olson, W. (1980) LVP filtration conforming with GMP. Communication prepared for the Sartorius Symposium 50 Jahre Sartorius Membranfilter held on 7 October 1980 at the Holiday Inn, Frankfurt.

171 Springett, D. (1981) The integrity testing of membrane filters. *Manufacturing Chemist and Aerosol News*, **February**, 41–45.

172 Bechold, H. (1908) Durchlässigkeit von Ultrafiltern. *Zeitschrift für Physikalische Chemie*, **64**, 328–342.

173 British Standards Institution (BSI) (1983) *BS 1752. Laboratory Sintered or Fritted Filters including Porosity Grading*, BSI, London.

174 Sechovec, K.S. (1989) Validation of an automated filter integrity tester for use in bubble point testing. *Journal of Parenteral Science and Technology*, **43**, 23–26.

175 Trasen, B. (1979) Filter Validation Symposium, IV Non-destructive tests for bacterial retentive filters. *Journal of the Parenteral Drug Association*, **33**, 273–279.

176 Johnston, P.R. *et al.* (1981) Certain imprecisions in the bubble point measurement. *Journal of Parenteral Science and Technology*, **35**, 36–39.

177 Johnston, P.R. and Meltzer, T.H. (1980) Suggested integrity testing of membranes filters at a robust flow of air. *Pharmaceutical Technology*, **4** (11), 49–59.

178 Jornitz, M.W. *et al.* (1998) Experimental evaluations of diffusive airflow integrity testing. *PDA Journal of Pharmaceutical Science and Technology*, **52**, 46–49.

179 Aranha-Creado, H. and Brandwein, H. (1999) Application of bacteriophages as surrogates for mammalian viruses: a case for use in filter validation based on precedents and current practices in medical and environmental virology. *PDA Journal of Pharmaceutical Science and Technology*, **53**, 75–82.

180 Parks, S.R. *et al.* (1996) A system for testing the effectiveness of microbiological air filters. *European Journal of Parenteral Sciences*, **1**, 75–77.

181 Madsen, R.E. and Meltzer, T.H. (1998) An interpretation of the pharmaceutical industry survey of current sterile filtration practices. *PDA Journal of Pharmaceutical Science and Technology*, **52**, 337–339.

182 Dosmar, M. *et al.* (1992) The water pressure integrity test for hydrophobic membrane filters. *Journal of Parenteral Science and Technology*, **46**, 102–106.

183 Gross, R.I. (1976) Laminar flow equipment: performance and testing requirements. *Bulletin of the Parenteral Drug Association*, **30**, 143–151.

184 Gross, R.I. (1978) Testing of laminar flow equipment. *Journal of the Parenteral Drug Association*, **32**, 174–181.

185 Japuntich, D. (1995) DOP testing: history and perspective. *3M JobHealth Highlights*, **13**, 1–5.

186 Huberty, J. (1995) Laboratory filtration tests for particulate respirators: do they relate to the workplace. *3M JobHealth Highlights*, **13**, 5–7.

187 Caldwell, G.H. Jr. (1978) Evaluation of high efficiency filters. *Journal of the Parenteral Drug Association*, **32**, 182–187.

188 McDade, J.J. *et al.* (1969) Principles and applications of laminar flow devices, in *Methods in Microbiology*, vol. 1 (eds D.W. Ribbons and J.R. Norris), Academic Press, London, pp. 137–168.

189 Groves, M.J. (1973) *Parenteral Products*, William Heinemann Medical Books, London.

190 Mika, H. (1971) Clean room equipment for pharmaceutical use. *Pharmaceutica Acta Helvetiae*, **46**, 467–482.

191 British Standards Institution (BSI) (1969) *BS 3928. Method for Sodium Flame Test for Air Filters (Other than for Air Supply to I.C. Engines and Compressors)*, BSI, London.

192 Duberstein, R. and Howard, G. (1978) Sterile filtration of gases: a bacterial aerosol challenge test. *Journal of the Parenteral Drug Association*, **32**, 192–198.

193 Harstad, J.B. and Filler, M.E. (1969) Evaluation of air filters with submicron viral aerosols and bacterial aerosols. *American Industrial Hygiene Association Journal*, **30**, 280–290.

194 Regamey, R.H. (1974) Application of laminar flow (clean work bench) for purifying the atmosphere. *Developments in Biological Standards*, **23**, 71–78.

16 New and Emerging Technologies

Peter A. Burke[1] and Gerald McDonnell[2]

[1] STERIS Corporation, Mentor, OH, USA

[2] Research and Technical Affairs, STERIS Ltd, Basingstoke, UK

Introduction

Microbicidal practices are hundreds of years old, including the preservation and disinfection of foods/water for consumption, which developed over time to the disinfection/sterilization of reusable medical/dental devices and many other types of materials in healthcare, industrial and research settings. For example, Lister in 1867 discovered that simple carbonic acid (phenol), in its own right significantly reduced surgical site infections. Although phenol itself is not practically used for such applications (the limitations of phenol were described by Lister himself), different types of phenolic compounds remain in wide use today as antiseptics and disinfectants [1, 2]. Many types of physical, chemical and combination technologies are in use today as microbicidal agents. Our objective here is to explore the new and emerging technologies in this area. It is worth noting here that many of the basic microbicidal methods in use have not changed much except for certain improvements in their microbicidal activity, delivery of the active, in surface compatibility as well as in enhanced safety for patients, staff and the environment. This applies to physical agents such as heat and also to a wide variety of microbicidal chemicals.

A microbicide can be described as any single chemical or mixture of chemicals used for the purpose of preservation, disinfection, antisepsis or sterilization. Properly formulating such a chemical or mixture of chemicals with other inert ingredients (sometimes referred to as "excipients") is the key to the success of a given product for its intended use. The microbicide can either be placed directly in/on the target or released into the air for space decontamination. The main types of chemicals with broad-spectrum microbicidal activity are listed in Table 16.1 [1].

Since the 1950s the introduction of truly new microbicidal agents has been limited mainly due to ever-escalating developmental costs coupled with increasingly strict regulations on human safety and ecotoxicity. However, examples of relatively recently introduced microbicides include triclosan, octenidine, ortho-phthaldehyde and the newer generations of phenolics and quaternary ammonium compounds (QACs).

A microbicidal agent must have a wide spectrum of activity against harmful organisms (dependent on its desired application), be rapid in its action with high materials compatibility while being as safe as possible for humans and the environment. Though these key criteria are obvious, the ability of such chemicals to be properly formulated is very crucial and merits further comment. Most microbicidal agents (with the exception of gases

Table 16.1 Commonly used microbicidal agents.

Microbicidal agents	Microbicidal use	Date of introduction
Alcohols (ethanol, isopropanol, n-propanol)	Antisepsis, disinfection	Alcohols have been described and used for millennia, though not necessarily for their disinfectant qualities. In modern times the first true chemical description was in 865 AD and in 1763 was reportedly used as an antiseptic
Chlorhexidine digluconate	Antisepsis	1954
Ethylene oxide	Disinfection, sterilization	1936
Glutaraldehyde	Disinfection, sterilization	1957
Halogens (iodine, iodophors, chlorine or chlorine-releasing agents such as hypochlorites, related compounds)	Antisepsis, disinfection, sterilization	Chlorine discovered in 1744; iodine in the 1800s
Hydrogen peroxide	Antisepsis, disinfection, sterilization	Discovered in 1818, used in medicine since 1891
Mercury, mercuric chloride	Antisepsis	Middle Ages
Peracetic acid	Disinfection, sterilization	1955
Phenols	Antisepsis, disinfection	Mid-1800s
Quaternary ammonium compounds	Antisepsis, disinfection	1916
Silver, silver complexes, silver sulfadiazine	Antisepsis, disinfection	Use for water applications as far back as 450 BC

used for space decontamination and some halogens used for disinfection of water) are formulated with various excipients for specific applications. For example, most liquid disinfectants or sterilants contain surfactants, chelating agents, anticorrosive agents and other ingredients to enhance stability and to optimize activity in the presence of soils.

It should be noted, for example, that formulation effects can actually increase or decrease efficacy as well as toxic effects [3, 4]. In rare cases, synergistic effects between chemical microbicides and/or formulation excipients can be observed, where the microbicidal agent(s) alone has less activity than when mixed together in formulation. This is not only true with liquid chemicals, but also important in optimizing the effects of gas or physical microbicides. An important example is the effect of water (humidity) content and temperature in the microbicidal activities of ethylene oxide (EtO), ozone and chlorine dioxide. Clinical or other field testing may often have to meet defined criteria for microbial reduction (e.g. the US Food and Drug Administration (FDA) [5], and as proposed by the European Union (EU) EN Phase 3 microbicidal tests [6]).

The development and introduction of a new microbicidal formulation can be quite complex and costly, often taking a decade or more for safety/compatibility testing and regulatory approval. In the USA, human-use antiseptic drugs and most medical device disinfectants/sterilants come under the purview of the US FDA, while the US Environmental Protection Agency (EPA) reviews and approves for sale microbicidal products to be used on environmental surfaces and for aerial decontamination of indoor spaces. The ultimate environmental fate of such chemicals is reviewed not only by federal government but also by those states that have their own environmental requirements. This is also true in the EU under the Biocides Directive (98/8/EC); in this case, an initial review of the safety and efficacy of various microbicides in use today has been made for inclusion in the directive,

with the result that soon the use of many existing microbicides will no longer be allowed in the EU. Also, the inclusion of any new chemicals in the list will be a lot more demanding, in particular, for gases.

General considerations

Process optimization
The most widely described and used method for killing microorganisms is heat, both "dry" and "wet". Heat can also enhance the microbicidal activity of chemicals. Examples of improvements in applying direct heat include the methods of heat generation (e.g. the use of microwaves), heat distribution (alternatives to fans and optimized pressure/vacuum combinations in steam sterilization processes) and, for food or other liquid applications, other factors such as osmotic pressure, surface tension modifiers and oxygen levels in combination with heat treatment. Other advances in this area relate to the development of alternatives to heat due to the growing use of heat-sensitive materials and devices requiring reprocessing, and to improve organoleptic perceptions in the food and beverage industry. Such physical methods include E-beam radiation, hydrostatic pressure, high-voltage electric discharges, high-intensity lasers, high magnetic field pulses and nano-thermosonication, some of which are further discussed in this chapter. Optimization of process conditions has also been an important development in the use of chemical microbicides. The control of variables such as temperature, pH, concentration, etc., has been successful in the optimization of disinfection and sterilization applications with microbicides. This has been shown with formulated chemistries such as those based on peracetic acid [7] or peracid generational systems [8], as well as for chemical gas sterilization methods such as EtO [9], formaldehyde [10] and ozone [11] where defined temperature ranges, humidity levels

and exposure times need to be tightly controlled for optimal microbicidal effects.

Particular advances over the past decade have been in methods of ozone generation ([11] and associated patents), the use of UV light [12] and various proposed synergistic methods (such as UV and ozone and/or hydrogen peroxide gas).

Formulation optimization, including synergism

It is outside the scope of this chapter to describe the various types of formulation effects that have or could be used to enhance the activity of a microbicide. In short, a variety of effects can be combined to demonstrate optimized activity, stability, tolerance of variable water quality (with dilutable products), and synergism between chemicals; many of these effects have been successfully patented. A novel, recent example is the description of a liquid formulation including 0.2% sodium dodecyl sulfaate (SDS) and 0.3% NaOH in 20% n-propanol that was shown to be effective against surface prion contamination [13]. In addition, such formulations also showed significant inactivation of viruses (poliovirus, hepatitis A virus and caliciviruses), bacteria (*Enterococcus faecium*, *Mycobacterium avium*) and fungi (*Aspergillus brasiliensis*). Alkali are known to be effective microbicidal and anti-prion agents, but generally at relatively higher concentrations (e.g. 1 M NaOH is widely used for both purposes), although recent evidence would suggest that such high concentrations are not required for activity against prions and that formulation concentrations can have a dramatic impact even against these agents [14]. Similarly, concentrations of alcohols are known to enhance the activity of aldehydes such as glutaraldehyde in high-level disinfectant applications [15].

Direct synergism between microbicides is often a debatable point [16]. Synergism in this context is defined as two or more microbicides that work together so the combined microbicidal effect is greater than the sum of the individual microbicides alone. With this in mind, many have claimed to observe synergistic benefits with combinations of microbicides but have not excluded the cumulative effects of the individual components [16, 17]. Despite this, many synergistic effects can be observed. A common example is in the use of chelating agents such as ethylenediamine tetraacetic acid (EDTA; a weak microbicide but some preservative qualities) with triclosan, other chelating agents and some QACs. These effects are limited to certain types of bacteria and appear to be from destabilization of the cell wall/membrane, allowing the microbicide access to its target site(s) [18]. Another example is the acidification of hydrogen peroxide for increased mycobactericidal effects, possibly due to the disruption of the highly lipophilic cell wall structure of these bacteria.

The reported synergistic effects between hydrogen peroxide and peracetic acid in formulation may be primarily due to preservation of the peracetic acid concentration (known to be a much more potent microbicidal at lower concentration than peroxide) as such solutions are always in equilibrium. Although these are also known microbicides, their contribution to the activity in formulation is debatable. The formulation of

hydrogen peroxide itself is of interest due to its latent microbicidal activity; complex stabilized formulations known as "accelerated" hydrogen peroxide (AHP) have been developed as hard surface disinfectants (Virox Corporation). The formulations can range in peroxide concentration (e.g. 0.5–7%), but have much greater microbicidal activity when mixed with peracetic acid than comparable concentrations of peroxide alone. Similarly, synergistic reactions between hydrogen peroxide gas and ozone have been proposed, although little evidence of the true effects of each active alone and/or in combination has been published to date.

Ultrahigh pressure and supercritical fluids

The inactivation of vegetative bacteria by ultrahigh pressure (also known as ultrahigh pressure homogenization (UHPH)) is not new, with initial reports demonstrating some effects at or above 100 MPa for over 100 years. As a reference, atmospheric pressure is 101.35 kPa (14.7 psi, 1 bar or 760 mmHg (or Torr) at sea level) and a typical steam sterilization process operates at 204–308 kPa. Therefore, these pressures are quite significant and are proposed for various types of foods and vaccines. The extent of microbicidal activity was found to be limited, with bacterial spores, for example, being shown to be much more resistant, surviving pressures higher than 1200 MPa [19]. Practical limitations of high-pressure technology prevented commercial use for food preservation until recently, but applications now include the treatment of jams, fruit juices, meat and an expanding variety of other foodstuffs [20–22]. The effects of high pressure (and therefore changes in volume) are essentially derived from LeChatelier's principle on any system in equilibrium, where a change in pressure (as well as other variables such as concentration, temperature, etc.) will cause a shift to counteract the change and establish a new equilibrium. Such dramatic changes in biological vegetative systems that are essentially in equilibrium will lead to a variety of detrimental effects, such as the unfolding of protein and lipid structures, increases in the ionization of dissociable molecules due to "electrostriction", etc. [23, 24]. Such changes may be expected to culminate in cellular death or at least inhibition of growth [25]. Effects on gene expression, protein synthesis, nucleic acids, ribosomes, specific proteins, maintenance of cytoplasmic pH and tran-membrane pH gradients have all been observed [26], although none are expected to be key targets during pressure-induced inactivation. Of interest to the food industry, low molecular weight flavor and odor compounds in foods tend to survive pressure treatment unchanged, with quality advantages in some types of products in comparison with heat treatment. Overall, these effects may be limited from a microbicidal point of view as kinetic studies have shown some examples of exponential inactivation of cells held at constant pressure (e.g. *Escherichia coli* [27]), but the majority of the studies have reported "tails" on survivor curves, that is a decreasing death rate with increasing treatment time (Figure 16.1) [28].

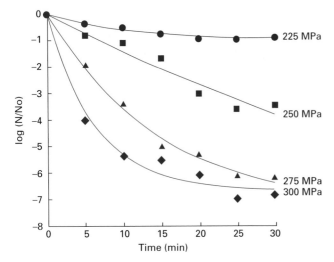

Figure 16.1 Hydrostatic pressure–survivor curves of *Yersinia enterocolitica* in pH 7 phosphate buffered saline at 20°C showing the effect of increasing pressure and the non-linearity of survivor[28].

It has been proposed that at higher temperatures (e.g. in the case of *E. coli*, 40°C and above at 250 MPa) inactivation is near first order, whereas at lower temperatures (e.g. 30°C for *E. coli*) it is nearer second order, and that membrane lipid changes may account for these differences [29]. Temperature may play an important role in these effects, with such pressures shown to be more effective in inactivating vegetative bacteria at the lower (<0°C) than the higher (>10°C) temperatures [30]. Indirect effects from pressure changes may be important; for example, pressure increases ionization that can lead to a reduction in pH. Many vegetative bacteria are known to be quite sensitive and others resistant to acidic pH [1]. pH effects may also have benefits in combination with various microbicides, for example in the activity of sorbic acid against *Saccharomyces bailii* [31]. Further, such effects may be specific to the material being treated, as shown with foods. *Salmonella enterica* serotype Typhimurium was inactivated more efficiently in pork in 10 min at 300 MPa, than in baby food at 350 MPa [32]. The spectrum of antibacterial activity may be limited in such cases, as strain-to-strain variability in sensitivity to pressure is greater than with other inactivation techniques, such as heat [28]. Exponential-phase bacteria are more pressure sensitive than when in the stationary phase [33] and Gram-positive bacteria are more pressure tolerant than Gram-negatives [34]; overall, these generalizations will vary depending on the target/resident bacteria and the food product under investigation. Despite these variations, a number of successful applications have been published, such as against a wide range of bacteria and fungi in fruit juices at 100, 200 and 300 MPa, and at 2 and 4°C [35], with similar results in milk [36].

Although bacterial spores are known to be pressure tolerant, under certain conditions inactivation of the spores proceeded more successfully at lower pressures [37]. This may be explained by the inactivation of spores in two stages. First, increased

pressure can cause spores to initiate germination and further pressure increases can then inactivate the vegetative forms. This has led to further studies on the synergistic effects with factors such as temperature [37] and low-dose irradiation [38] to achieve a higher level of spore inactivation. Such effects have been confirmed for a wide range of spore types, although the effectiveness of the combination varies greatly in magnitude for different spores [39, 40]. *Bacillus cereus* spores, for example, are considered relatively sensitive to pressure, while those of others such as *Geobacillus stearothermophilus* and *Clostridium botulinum* are quite resistant [21]. This may change with the development of presses that operate at higher temperature–pressure combinations, or the development of other effective combination techniques. The fact that high-pressure application can directly lead to temperature increases, for example by about 3°C per 100 MPa for water, and as an opposite effect of cooling, allows pressure to be used to heat/cool various products very rapidly. For example, the application of pressure at 800 MPa may raise the temperature of products, without any need for time/energy-consuming conduction or convection, very quickly by about 25°C and, most importantly, reduce the temperature by the same amount as the pressure is reduced at the end or treatment, perhaps within a few seconds. Such rapid temperature changes could be very useful in gaining much tighter control over thermal processes, with reduced heat-induced damage, and consequent benefits in product quality [41]. Optimization of such processes will have benefits to certain applications, particularly in food production.

A further application of high pressure is in the use of "supercritical" (or dense) liquids as disinfecting/sterilizing agents for surfaces and/or materials. Supercritical fluids are defined physically as any substance that is above its critical point, where the phase boundary between a solid, liquid and gas no longer exists. Essentially, any matter can exist as a solid, liquid or gas depending on the pressure and temperature. A typical example is with water that forms a solid (ice) below 0°C, when heated assumes its liquid phase (water) and at higher temperatures (>100°C) forms a gas (steam). Equally, as the pressure is changed, the phase can change (due to the relationship between temperature and pressure described in the gas laws), where, for example, water can be maintained in a liquid form at temperatures above 100°C by changing the pressure. Therefore, at increased temperatures and pressures, typical examples such as water and carbon dioxide cross the phase boundaries of being a liquid/gas to become supercritical fluids. By controlling very high pressure levels, the temperatures can be maintained at low levels for more sensitive applications.

As an example, supercritical carbon dioxide can be generated above the critical temperature (*c.* 31°C) and pressure (*c.* 7.4 MPa); under such conditions it assumes the properties of both a gas and a liquid. Supercritical fluids are used industrially for a variety of purposes, such as water for power generation and carbon dioxide for dry cleaning, decaffeination and oil extraction (often used for their intrinsic microbicidal properties). Supercritical carbon dioxide itself has been described for its direct microbicidal properties. The microbicidal effects were first described in the 1950s, but have been particularly studied and applied to various industrial applications in the last 20 years [42]. Typical conditions apply to carbon dioxide at 20–70 MPa, 40–100°C for 30 min to 6 h of contact; for example disinfection (pasteurization) activity can be demonstrated at 20 MPa, 40°C for 15 min [42, 43]. Overall, there are mixed reports in the literature regarding sporicidal activity; however, recent advances have been made to enhance sporicidal activity as the basis for sterilization process development. For example. little to no activity against *G. stearothermophilus* and *Bacillus atrophaeus* spores was observed at low temperatures and cycle times [44]. At higher temperatures (*c.* 100°C) and pressures (20 MPa) a 6-log reduction in the viability of the spores was observed within 25 min. Similar enhancements of sporicidal activity at elevated but traditionally non-sporicidal temperatures have been described by others [45]. It has also been reported that the addition of low concentrations of water or hydrogen peroxide had some synergistic effects, with 100 ppm of hydrogen peroxide being particularly effective at 40°C for 1 h [44]. The addition of various chemical modifiers at low concentrations appears to enhance sporicidal activity. *Bacillus pumilus* spores were inactivated at 45–50°C and 10 MPa of supercritical carbon dioxide in the presence of hydrogen peroxide, formic acid, Triton X-100 and mixtures thereof [46]. Similar effects have been reported with low concentrations of peracetic acid, water and surfactants [43]. It may be expected that the microbicidal effects of supercritical carbon dioxide are due to the same effects on vegetative microorganisms as described above, with a variety of direct (e.g. oxidative agent) and indirect (permeabilization) action on the outer and inner structures of bacterial spores that culminate in spore death. Initial diffusion of carbon dioxide (and other chemicals) into the cell may be expected to have dramatic effects on metabolism, with changes in intracellular pH and further effects on microbial surface layers. Microbicidal applications for supercritical carbon dioxide to date have included various disinfection/sterilization-sensitive materials such as human/animal tissues, protein preparations and drug–device combinations.

High-voltage electric pulses

While the direct application of electricity to heat materials has become well established (e.g. in food applications [22]), the use of electric pulses for non-thermal inactivation of certain vegetative microorganisms has been investigated [47]. Such techniques using lower, non-lethal voltage gradients are widely used for the introduction of genetic material into recipient cells (predominantly bacteria) in a process known as electroporation; presumably, this process allows for the temporary permeabilization of the cell wall/membrane to permit uptake but without bacterial inactivation. Studies have demonstrated the inactivation of bacteria and yeasts by a variety of electrical parameters [48]. For bactericidal activity, field strengths shown to be effective have ranged

from about 10 to 100 kV/cm, with very short pulses (micro- or millisecond ranges) in repeated delivery to obtain the desired inactivation. The rate and duration of electric pulsing can prevent excessive increases in the temperature created [49]. In some applications, limiting any unwanted thermal effects are important (e.g. food processing) but in others this may be less of a concern. While the effects of high-voltage fields on microorganisms are not understood at the molecular level, the gross effects and the mechanisms that cause them are well described. Significant effects result from the permeabilization of the cell wall/membrane [50]. Gross structural effects occur when the potential difference across the membrane exceeds about 1 V – not surprisingly considering the electrical balances across bacterial cell membranes that are important for cell metabolism and outer cell structures. This was rapidly followed by massive leakage of the cytoplasm, culminating in cell death. Microscopical examination of electrically-treated cells has shown an initial thinning of the membrane, followed by hole formation and leaking of the cytoplasm.

Electric pulse inactivation has been reported to have a limited effect on vegetative bacteria, yeasts and molds, including *E. coli*, *Salmonella* spp., *Staphylococcus aureus*, *Listeria monocytogenes*, *Saccharoomyces cerevisiae* and *Candida albicans* [49, 51]. Considering their structures and dormancy, bacterial spores [52] and yeast ascospores [53] are a greater challenge and appear to be resistant, even at very high-voltage gradients (i.e. above 30 kV/cm). There may be some benefits in applying low concentrations of chemical microbicides in combination with such electric pulses to enhance sporicidal activity. Indeed a number of intrinsic and extrinsic factors have already been shown to influence the effectiveness of the electrical treatments. Inactivation increased greatly with elevations in temperature, pH variations and osmotic pressure of the surrounding media [54]. For example, in a skimmed milk application, a reduction in pH (from 6.8 to 5.7) led to a doubling for observed *E. coli* reduction. It may be expected from these results that the growth phase of the target organism will also be important, a phenomenon not usual in disinfection studies or in genetic electroporation experimentation.

Some other potentially useful synergistic reactions have been described. For example, electroporated cells of *E. coli*, *L. monocytogenes* and *S. enterica* serovar Typhimurium were more sensitive than untreated cells to microbicidal peptides such as nisin and pediocin [55]. These results suggest that the greater peptide penetration is achieved through electrically-treated cells to access internal cell targets of these actives.

Electric pulse treatments have been applied to a number of liquid foods as an alternative to cold pasteurization methods against vegetative bacteria and yeasts. For example, treatment of apple juice at temperatures below 30°C, with fewer than 10 pulses in a continuous treatment chamber, gave a greater than 10^6 reduction in *S. cerevisiae* populations at a voltage gradient of 35 kV/cm; lower voltage pulses (22 kV/cm) gave a respectively lower reduction of about 10^2 [54]. Applications for the use of pulsed electric field technology to treat liquid foods have included fruit juices, milk and liquid egg [49]. Field intensities employed range from

12 to 25 kV/cm, with treatment times from 1 to 100 ms over multiple pulsing cycles depending on the level of disinfection desired. Electric fields may be delivered in a variety of ways, but the most economic method to date involves raising the field strength as high as possible, while reducing the duration of the pulses, without reducing pulse energy.

On the other hand, the use of very high field strengths demands more complex and expensive engineering. As a result of these competing requirements, most modern pulse-field devices employ field strengths from about 20 up to about 70 kV/cm, with pulse durations between 1 and about 5 ms. Repetition rates are typically from 1 up to 30 s or so at the higher voltages in order to minimize rises in temperature. While applications to date have focused on the use of electric pulses for pasteurization applications in foods, further applications can be envisioned in other liquid preparations and may be further enhanced (in particular with the addition of other microbicides) to increase observed microbial reduction rates and spectrum of activity.

Other physical processes

High-intensity light

Various non-ionizing (ultraviolet wavelength range) and ionizing (γ) radiations are traditionally used for disinfection and sterilization [1]. High-intensity laser and light in the visual wavelength range ("white light") are also known to inactivate microorganisms under certain conditions [53]. The wavelengths of light generally applied range in wavelengths from near UV (c. 200 nm) to the infrared (c. 1500 nm) range. White light (sunlight) is not considered a microbicide per se, but when the intensity of the light is increased (e.g. in the energy range of 0.01–50 J/cm^2) microbicidal effects have been reported. Although test results vary depending on the lamps used and doses applied, the technology has been shown to be bactericidal, fungicidal (against yeasts and molds), virucidal, sporicidal and cysticidal. Similar to that described for electrical and high-pressure systems, during high-intensity light treatment the light source is pulsed to limit any unwanted heat generation; the number, intensity and extent of pulses will depend on the application and desired microbicidal level. The exact microbicidal effects and extent may vary depending on the choice of lamp used and light wavelengths/ intensities produced for a given application. For these reasons, the degree of microbicidal activity can vary considerably from low-level disinfection to sterilization. The delivery of light to packaging materials, food surfaces and transparent liquid products, in short pulses of high intensity, has been shown to inactivate vegetative and spore forms of microorganisms [56, 57]. Further, applications have included medical and dental instruments [58, 59] and antiseptic applications for the control of acne [60].

Commercially available systems for treating exposed surfaces of foods, materials and medical devices have been described [61]. Many use broad-spectrum light (across the visible light range and most often including part of the UV wavelength spectrum) with pulse durations from 10^{-6} to 10^{-1} s and with energy densities from about 0.1 to 50 J/cm^2. Different spectral distributions and energies are selected for different applications. For example UV-rich light, in which about 30% of the energy is at wavelengths shorter than 300 nm, is recommended for treatment of packaging materials, water or other transparent fluids. In contrast, for food surfaces, where high intensities of UV may accelerate lipid oxidation or cause color loss, etc., the shorter wavelengths are filtered out and the killing effects are largely considered thermal. The advantage of delivering heat in this manner is that a large amount of thermal energy is transferred to a very thin layer of product surface very quickly, while the temperature rise within the bulk of the product can be very small [61]. Significant effects of pulsed UV have been reported [62], including activity against a broad range of viruses [63] and protozoan oocysts [64]. Some synergistic reactions have been reported in combination with other chemicals, such as the microbicidal peptide nisin [56], although these and other true synergistic reactions remain to be confirmed.

Pulsed light is very sensitive to and has significantly reduced activity in the presence of any interfering factors such as surfaces not directly exposed to the light source and any porous surface (due to restricted penetration). Despite these initial limitations, some applications have been shown to be successful in reducing foodborne pathogens such as *Salmonella* [57]. The benefits include no process residuals, rapid cycle times and generally good compatibility (particularly with limited temperature increases). The mechanisms of action appear similar to other non-ionizing radiation sources, including direct effects on DNA, proteins and lipids [1]. Overall, high-intensity light treatments appear to be effective due to localized heat and/or similar effects to UV treatments, with some advantages for industrial and clinical applications [53].

Magnetic fields

Exposure to oscillating magnetic fields has been reported to have a variety of effects on vegetative cells, ranging from selective inactivation of malignant eukaryotic cells [65] to the inactivation of prokaryotes (bacteria) on packaging materials and in foods [66]. Treatment times tested have been relatively short, ranging from 2 to 25 ms and high field strengths (typically from 0.26 to 13.3 kPa (2–100 Torr) at frequencies between about 5 and 500 kHz). However, the findings of the limited number of studies conducted on magnetic fields so far show the overall microbicidal effects to be limited. For example a 10^2 reduction of vegetative bacteria, yeasts and molds inoculated into milk (*Streptococcus thermophilus*), orange juice (*Saccharomyces*) or bread rolls (mold spores) was observed in one study, but no effects were observed with bacterial spores [66]. Based on these results, the practical potential for the technique on its own, as it has been developed so far, appears to be limited although it may deserve further investigation [53, 67]. It has been suggested that the mechanism of action could involve alteration of ion fluxes across the cell membrane in target microorganisms, but this has not been confirmed. Potential synergistic effects may be explored in combination with chemical microbicides to test for greater uptake or direct effects to enhance microbicidal activity. To date this has not been widely reported, although similar potentiation effects have been described in biofilm disruption and in improving the activity of antibiotics against biofilm-resident bacteria [68].

Sonication

Sonication is a method widely used for a variety of cleaning applications, but has also been reported to have some microbicidal effects. The use of sonication (or the generation of ultrasound waves in a liquid) to inactivate microorganisms was first reported in the 1920s. The mechanism of action derives from the rapidly alternating compression and decompression zones generated in a liquid (for surface application or for direct effects within the liquid itself) leading to cavitations. Cavitations involve the formation and collapse of small bubbles, generating shock waves often associated with very high temperatures and pressures, which can be sufficiently intense to catalyze chemical reactions and disrupt animal, plant and microbial cells [69, 70]. Liquid products are easily sonicated, but in solids the structure and high viscosity severely impede efficacy. Generally, the larger the cells, the more susceptible they are to such cavitation effects. The cell structure also seems to affect efficacy, with rod-shaped bacteria being reportedly more sensitive than cocci [71] and Gram-positive bacteria more sensitive than Gram-negative [72]. Bacterial spores and many fungal spores are essentially resistant in studies to date [72].

Although the direct use of sonication may have limited microbicidal effects alone, potential synergistic effects have been reported. Combinations with heat and pressure have shown advantages for the inactivation of bacterial spores (*B. cereus* and *Bacillus licheniformis* [73]), thermoresistant streptococci [74], *S. aureus* and other vegetative microorganisms [74–76]. In studies with spores, as the temperature was raised, the potentiating effect of ultrasound became less and less, and had essentially no effect near the boiling point of water. Increased pressure–temperature effects may have further optimization potential [77]. The combination procedure was reported to generally have the effect of reducing the apparent heat resistance of microorganisms by about 5–20°C or so, depending on the temperature, the organism and its z-value. Since sonication can generate, locally, very high temperatures, it has been difficult to disentangle the influence of heat and specific ultrasonic effects. Nevertheless, nano-thermosonication has been claimed to operate in some liquid foods [77], and requires further investigation.

Observed indirect effects of sonication have been shown in wastewater applications to be simply due to the disruption of larger microbial particles (clumped microorganisms in the presence/absence of soils) into smaller particles and improvements in efficacy in the presence of UV light [78] and presumably other chemical microbicides.

Microwaves

Microwave energy is a source of non-ionizing radiation within the wavelength range of 0.1–0.001 mm and an equivalent energy level of 2×10^{-24} to 2×10^{-22} J. It is generally accepted that microwaves have little to no direct microbicidal effects from studies to date, in comparison to other irradiation sources at higher energy levels [1]. Despite this, significant microbicidal activity has been attributed to microwave energy, predominantly due to direct heating effects of water molecules associated with target surfaces/solutions. Activity has been described against bacteria, fungi and viruses, with little to no activity against thermoresistant bacterial spores (e.g. *Geobacillus stearothermophilus* spores). Sporicidal activity can be achieved in some applications; for example 2.0 kW microwave applications led to breakdown of *B. licheniformis* spore coat and inner membrane structures, as indicated by the leakage of internal spore proteins/DNA [79]. Because the primary effects are due to localized heating of water, microbial contamination on wet surfaces is more rapidly inactivated than on dry surfaces (e.g. as shown with yeast inactivation studies [80]).

Microwaves have the benefit of being conveniently produced in widely available and electrically-operated ovens. The microbicidal activity observed is essentially equivalent to the temperatures produced; although some investigations have reported enhanced activity with microwaves this may be due to localized heat production in the test medium rather than direct effects of the wavelength on microbial components [81]. Microwaves have been primarily used as flash disinfection methods for a variety of applications including tissues (e.g. heart valves [82]), medical devices [83], catheters [84] and other materials. A typical application includes treatment of biomedical waste that is shredded, sprayed with water, heated by microwave to *c.* 95°C and held for the desired decontamination time [85].

Gas plasma

The applications of gas plasmas for microbicidal, particularly sterilization, purposes are detailed in Chapter 15.4 and are, therefore, only briefly touched upon in this section. Plasma is essentially an excited or energized liquid or gas. In consideration of the gas laws, matter can assume any of the three essential states (solid, liquid, gas) depending on the temperature and pressure applied. Energy can be applied, for example in the case of water and temperature as described earlier in this chapter, to form a gas but when the gas is further energized it can form the so-called fourth state of matter, plasma. In a true plasma generation model, the gas molecules become ionized to form a variety of active and potentially microbicidal species such as ions, radicals, etc. In such forms, potent microbicidal activity has been reported [86]. Plasmas naturally occur in space, but for microbicidal purposes artificial plasmas can be created by the application of a strong energy source (such as electromagnetic fields and/or temperatures) to a variety of gases or liquids such as oxygen, nitrogen, helium, water and hydrogen peroxide.

There is often confusion in the literature regarding the use of the term "plasma". Many patents and publications erroneously describe certain disinfection/sterilization processes as being plasmas, and direct applications of plasmas have been limited so far to laboratory investigations for their microbicidal purposes. Optimal activities of such experiments have been shown with argon/oxygen, nitrogen/oxygen and hydrogen peroxide plasmas (as discussed in Chapter 15.4) [86]. For example, various types of microbicides including hydrogen peroxide, peracetic acids, nitric oxide and aldehydes such as formaldehyde and glutaraldehyde have been investigated to try and increase their activity. Initial patents focused on the use of oxidizing gases such as hydrogen peroxide [87] and peracetic acid [88]; however, these studies have already highlighted limitations in the practical application of plasma technologies, in particular limited penetration for packaged materials. The optimum use, in these cases, was to allow the gas to distribute first within the load and then apply the required energy to generate the plasma locally at the required sites of activity. However, most of these investigations included the use of gaseous oxidizing agents with intrinsic microbicidal activity and it was therefore difficult to differentiate the true contribution of plasma generation to microbicidal activity. Subsequent investigations have focused on the use of what may be referred to as inert gases, such as oxygen, nitrogen, argon, helium, xeon and neon, both on their own and particularly in various mixtures. Unlike previous investigations, these gases have little to no intrinsic microbicidal activity until activated into the plasma form. Particular success has been reported with N/O and Ar/O gas mixtures in various proportions (see Chapter 15.4). In addition to traditional microbicidal effects (against bacterial spores, fungi, viruses, etc.), some studies have shown activity in neutralizing endotoxin and infectious proteins (prions) (see Chapter 10).

Further developments are required to bring these technologies, including cleaning, disinfection and sterilization applications, to commercial use. It is important to not only focus on the optimization of the desired microbicidal effects but also on limiting any negative effects such as overheating and damage to materials and on ensuring uniformity in applying the plasma process to a target load [89].

To date, most plasma processes that have seen commercial success are actually indirect. For example, the plasma may be generated in a gas or liquid at a remote site and then transferred to the point of use. In this case, the true plasma will only be maintained when the energy applied is constant and it may be expected that the initial plasma activation allows for reassociation/generation of other microbicides that are actually responsible for the observed microbicidal effects. A typical example is found in processes using nitrogen and oxygen, where both gases are essentially inert but when activated by plasma formation and then allowed to reassociate will theoretically lead to the generation of a variety of microbicidal molecules such as ozone and nitric oxide. A further example is the activation of water, where a variety of microbicidal chemicals can be generated on energization, not unlike those described for "activated" or electrolysed water processes that are primarily microbicidal due to the production of hypochlorous ions [1]. Similar effects may be observed in plasma generation of air (containing a significant proportion of nitrogen and oxygen) for various applications. Such processes could be used for a variety of microbicidal purposes, including food, skin, wound care, air and general hard surface applications [90, 91].

A notable indirect use of plasma is in hydrogen peroxide plasma sterilization processes, such as the Sterrad® sterilizers. Initial patents around this process described the distribution of hydrogen peroxide gas in an evacuated chamber and the subsequent generation of the plasma for sterilization [87], as well as the use of plasma to remove residual levels of hydrogen peroxide liquid/gas remaining following sterilization with peroxide gas [92]. Hydrogen peroxide gas is a powerful microbicidal agent in its own right [93] and the Sterrad processes developed so far have used peroxide liquid/gas exclusively for sterilization, while only using plasma generation either as a heating/drying mechanism prior to gas introduction or following gas evacuation to remove any remaining residuals of liquid/gas (see Chapter 15.4). Essentially, gas plasma is not used for any true microbicidal benefit in these cases. Although the plasma may have a theoretical effect on microbicidal activity in such processes, studies have confirmed that they are insignificant from a microbicidal point of view [94], but necessary in the design of these particular processes for safe residual removal/aeration.

Vapor-phase oxidants

Oxidizing agents such as hydrogen peroxide, peracetic acid and chlorine dioxide have been widely used as antiseptics, disinfectants and sterilants. Until recently, the major uses of these microbicides were primarily in liquid form, either on their own (as in the case of chlorine dioxide for water treatment or hydrogen peroxide on skin/wounds [1]) or in formulation with other excipients. Over the last 15 years, further research and applications have been described in the use of these microbicides in vapor (or gas phase). The most widely and successfully used to date is hydrogen peroxide gas (often referred to under its trademarked name as VHP®, for vaporized hydrogen peroxide). The terms "gas" and "vapor" can be alternatively used in this case; chemically, a vapor is a gas but can also exist in the liquid (or solid) form below the critical temperature of the substance. Essentially, depending on the concentration of peroxide and its temperature/pressure it may be readily present as a gas, a liquid or liquid/gas ("fog") mixture. This point is often underestimated in consideration of vapor-phase oxidants.

Hydrogen peroxide in its liquid form is a powerful microbicide, but has limitations in sporicidal, cysticidal and even virucidal activity at relatively high concentrations. Its microbicidal (particularly sporidical/cysticidal) activity is dramatically increased and different to liquid activity in the gaseous phase. As an example, 1 mg/l gaseous peroxide demonstrates equivalent sporicidal activity to *c.* 400 mg/l liquid peroxide [95, 96]; the most resistant organism to peroxide gas is *G. stearothermophilus* spores, in comparison to liquid peroxide preparations where the most resistant organism is *B. atrophaeus* spores [93, 97]. Concentrations as low as 0.1 mg/l gas peroxide retain appreciable sporicidal activity, with estimated *D*-valves (time for a $\log_{10}$ reduction of bacterial spore populations) decreasing exponentially from about 10 min at 0.1 mg/l to 1 min at 1 mg/l and <0.1 min at 10 mg/l. For these reasons, gas peroxide has been successfully used for disinfection [93] and sterilization [98] purposes in industrial, pharmaceutical, research and healthcare applications. Examples include fumigation of rooms/buildings (as an alternative to formaldehyde) and for sterilization of reusable, thermosensitive devices (as more rapid alternatives to ethylene oxide and formaldehyde sterilizers). In addition to potent microbicidal effects, peroxide gas has also been shown to be effective in the inactivation of prions [99, 100], endotoxins and cytotoxic drugs [101]. Recent studies on the mechanisms of action of gas and liquid peroxide have shown that, at least for activity against proteins and peptides, gas peroxide targets the peptide bonds that hold together the amino acids in protein structures, while liquid peroxide targets amino acid side-chains [102]. Unlike older reports in the literature, the gas has been found to be reactive with but can tolerate high levels of soiling (depending on the application [93]), but also has important advantages in materials compatibility and a reasonable safety profile (e.g. breaking down rapidly into water and oxygen in the environment).

Gas peroxide is generated by heating, typically by flash vaporization of liquid peroxide applied directly onto a hot surface [103]. However, the commercial applications of gas peroxide can vary significantly with various terms being used including VHP, hydrogen peroxide vapor (HPV), dry mists, etc. [104]. These systems can all use hydrogen peroxide as a microbicide but in different ways; some may generate and apply the gas in an unsaturated (gas) form, others in a saturated (liquid/gas or condensed gas) form and, finally, simply dispensing a liquid peroxide formulation in a given area over surfaces to be treated. The safety and efficacy of such processes can vary [103, 104]. To date, not much has been published on the impact of various process conditions such as humidity, temperature and concentration on the microbicidal activity of peroxide gas. From some studies, peroxide does not require high humidity levels to be effective in comparison with other gaseous microbicides, including formaldehyde, ethylene and chlorine dioxide. Typically, gas is generated from peroxide solutions in water (35–60% v/v in water); therefore, a humidity level is always present and can affect the saturation level of peroxide at a given temperature. For 35% peroxide, humidity levels are typically in the range of 40% although this level will increase as the peroxide degrades into oxygen and water vapor. For this reason, regeneration (closed) systems have been developed that constantly release peroxide gas into a given area but also remove peroxide/water vapor from a treated area. Other systems release an initial bolus of peroxide/water vapor into a given area and allow this to naturally degrade over time. Overall, the key

parameters for microbicidal activity are peroxide concentration, temperature and distribution of the peroxide to ensure contact with all target surfaces. Humidity levels can be important at close to saturation concentrations (increasing the risk of peroxide/water condensation), although the direct impact on the activity of peroxide gas deserves further study.

Gas-based systems have also been described for chlorine dioxide, a newer generation of ozone processes and peracetic acid [1]. In contrast to hydrogen peroxide gas, all of these systems are dependent on high humidity conditions for optimal microbicidal activity. Gaseous peracetic acid has not been widely utilized, primarily due to compatibility concerns; disinfection and sterilization (in combination with plasma [105]) have been described but have seen little new development. On the other hand, gaseous chlorine dioxide and ozone processes have seen some recent developments. Chlorine dioxide is a water-soluble gas that has been widely used for liquid disinfection (e.g. water and surface disinfection) and can be generated by a variety of chemical reactions such as acidification of sodium chlorate ($NaClO_3$) [1, 106]. Examples include the reaction of sodium chloride and citric acid to form chlorine dioxide or by passing chlorine gas over sodium chloride under high humidity conditions [107–109]. To be more specific, the humidity needs to be between 85% and 90%, which is thought to be a prerequisite for optimal microbicidal action. Gaseous applications have been described for sterilization and disinfection (fumigation) use, although its primary use today is for laminar flow cabinet, room and building fumigation [109]. Fumigation applications as of yet are limited, in comparison to formaldehyde or hydrogen peroxide gas. Chlorine dioxide has some reported negative attributes such as being highly toxic via inhalation and causing ocular damage at low concentrations and dermal irritation, as well as being very corrosive to steel and aluminum. Despite this, it has been successfully used for various fumigation applications. The anthrax attack of the Washington, DC Senate mail building system was remediated with multiple rounds of chlorine dioxide gas, which after reaching a minimum of 90% relative humidity has also proved effective as a sporicidal agent. Chlorine dioxide gas is more effective at lower concentrations (with typical use concentrations varying from 0.5 to 30 mg/l), but is more dependent on high humidity levels for activity (>65% relative humidity), with broad-spectrum (including sporicidal) microbicidal activity. Mobile and fixed generator systems that can control the humidification, gas generation and aeration process are commercially available. Applications have also been described directly on foods, to prevent fungal spoilage, at 10 ppm of ClO_2 at 95% relative humidity, with fungicidal activity reported against *Candida*, *Saccharomycetes* and *Penicillin* [110]. Although sterilization processes have been patented [109], such systems have yet to be successfully commercialized.

From an antiseptic perspective, a blend of 0.1% sodium chloride and 0.5% mandelic acid has been used as a preoperative preparation [110, 111]. A triple approach was theorized as the mechanism of microbicidal action via the formation of chlorous acid and chlorine dioxide as well as residual mandelic acid [112]. Periodontal preparations have been described for gingivitis treatment using chlorine dioxide as the active microbicidal agent.

Ozone is well described as one of the most effective oxidizing microbicides, but recent advances in the generation and maintenance of ozone concentrations allow for further practical uses of the technology, and in particular for medical device sterilization applications [1, 11, 113]. Ozone can be readily generated by applying energy (e.g. UV light or an electric charge) to oxygen (pure gas or as present in air), but close control of humidity levels is required for optimal microbicidal activity. Typical processes (fumigation or sterilization) consist of three phases: humidification (to 70–80% relative humidity), ozone concentration/humidification maintenance for a defined time, and aeration to remove any residual levels to below a safe level (generally reported as 0.1 ppm). Newer ozone-based sterilization systems have been developed for medical device applications including the TSO_3 sterilizer [11, 113]. This vacuum-based process humidifies the sterilizer load during preconditioning, followed by two identical stages of humidification (85–100%) and ozone diffusion (85 mg/l) at 30–36°C followed by ventilation, for a cycle time in the range of 4–6 h. Similar, ozone disinfection technologies have been described for laundry reprocessing as alternatives to heat-based methods. Humidified ozone is a powerful microbicidal, but can be limited in use with certain types of plastics and metal surfaces, including aluminum, brass, polyurethanes and rubber materials. Similar to other gaseous oxidants, specific process conditions may be defined or used with ozone for the disinfection of liquids and cellulose-based materials (due to their reactive and absorbing nature to the microbicide). There has been a recent resurgence of interest in the use of ozone for environmental space decontamination, with a variety of generation systems commercially available for miscellaneous applications.

Nitric oxide and nitrogen dioxide

Nitric oxide (NO, nitrogen monoxide) and nitrogen dioxide (NO_2) gases have both been investigated for their microbicidal activities. NO is an important, naturally occurring, reactive biological molecule expressed in cells as a signaling molecule, for protection of tissue damage, particularly during inflammation, and as part of the immune response; over- or continuous expression can lead to cell damage and a variety of tissue toxicity effects [114]. It is rapidly oxidized in air to form NO_2, a brown-colored gas that is also cytotoxic. Both molecules are considered effective microbicides and have been particularly studied for their effects against bacteria. Mechanisms of action are primarily referred to as being fragmentation of DNA, although investigations have shown a variety of cellular effects (from investigations with bacteria that can also be extrapolated to proposed effects on viruses and other microorganisms) such as enzyme inactivation, lipid modifications (affects cell membrane structures) and protein nitrification as well as DNA fragmentation [115, 116].

Sterilization systems that describe the use of NO and NO_2 have been patented, with the emphasis on NO_2 as the major microbicide [117]. It provides many advantages as a sterilant, including few aeration requirements following exposure (unlike ethylene oxide), it is not believed to generate toxic residues, it is non-explosive and has a reasonable materials compatibility profile. Typical sterilization conditions proposed include 0.25–3% NO_2 at 70–90% humidity, 18–30°C and 30–60 min of exposure. Similar to other such processes, air removal is important but various processes based on vacuum, pressurized and atmospheric pressure conditions can be envisioned. A typical sterilization process could include conditioning (for humidity/air removal), introduction and holding of gas/humidity (for the required number of pulsing phases to achieved sterilization) and aeration to release the load for safe handling/use. Other applications have included use in antiseptic creams [118] and as a general disinfectant, including food applications [119].

In addition to these forms, nitrous oxide (N_2O; more commonly known as laughing gas) may also be proposed as a microbicide as it is a known oxidizing agent, but it has yet to be investigated for this purpose. N_2O is a non-flammable, colorless gas with a slightly sweet odor. Its primary use today is as an anesthetic/analgesic.

Bacteriophages and other biological substances

The idea of using bacteriophages and microbicidal peptides as alternatives to conventional antimicrobials is not new. Bacteriophages ("phages"), ubiquitous viruses that prey upon bacteria, are experiencing a renewed interest as therapeutic alternatives to antibiotics, especially to counter multidrug-resistant bacterial pathogens [120–122]. The highly bacterial host-specific nature of phages, their ability to multiply *in situ* and safety for humans are added advantages over antibiotics and conventional microbicides. However, and unlike many microbicidal chemicals, the need for phages to infect and multiply in their respective hosts inevitably produces a lag of several hours between application and the desired level of activity. This is not necessarily an impediment in wound care where a single type of phage or a group of carefully selected phages can be applied as a preventive or therapeutic measure without the need for instantaneous action.

Microbicidal peptides have been identified from a wide variety of eukaryotes and prokaryotes [123, 124]. From a microbicidal perspective, and similar to bacteriophages, their microbicidal applications are generally limited as alternatives to antibiotics for specific antiseptic, disinfectant and/or preservative uses. Such peptides, which are produced naturally for host defense often in response to injury [125], show not only microbicidal effects but may also be effective in wound care, reducing inflammation reactions, and even in cancer therapy [124, 126]. As compared with antibiotics, they are considered broad spectrum with antimicrobial activity against a wide range of bacteria (including mycobacteria), fungi, protozoa and some enveloped viruses, depending on

Table 16.2 Examples of microbicidal peptides.

Structural subgroup	Example	Primary (amino acid) sequence
α-Helical	Magainin	GIGKFLHSAKKFGKAFVGEIMNS
β-Sheet	Lacteroferrin	FKCRRWQWRMKKLGAPSITCVRRAF
	α-Defensin	ACYCRIPACIAGERRYGTCIYQGRLWAFCC
Loop-structured	Microcin J25	GGAGHVPEYFVGIGTPISFYG
Extended	Indolicidin	ILPWKWPWWPWRR

the specific peptide under investigation. Many such peptides with specific antimicrobial properties are now known [127]. For example, a database updated in 2008 lists 1228 entries including 76 antiviral, 327 antifungal and 944 antibacterial peptides [128]. Structurally, most of them comprise of 1250 amino acid residues, although larger ones (>100 amino acids) also exist. Examples are shown in Table 16.2.

In general, their amino acid composition, hydrophobic nature, size and charge allow them to assume structures that can bind to and interact with the outer surface of microbes as their primary site of action. Others, such as microcidin J25, can interact with bacterial RNA polymerase as well as other intracellular targets [129]. A further example is a series of peptidoglycan recognition peptides (PRPs; [130]). For those cationic, amphiphilic peptides, cell membrane insertion is observed but the exact mechanisms leading to disruption of cell metabolism and death require further investigation [131]; it may be simply due to gross disruption of the structure/function of the cell membrane but could also be due to pore formulation, inhibition of specific membrane-associated metabolic functions or a variety of other effects. Interestingly, similar to antibiotics, the development of bacterial resistance to peptides has been described and a variety of mechanisms have been elucidated [130].

Nisin has been one of the most widely investigated antimicrobial peptides and has been used for over 50 years as a food preservative [132]. Typical concentrations of it can range from 1 to 25 ppm. It is produced commercially from *Lactococcus lactis* as a 34-amino acid chain that contains some unusual amino acids such as lanthionine and methylanthionine. Nisin is particularly active against Gram-positive bacteria including *Staphylococcus* spp. and is sporistatic against *Bacillus* and *Clostridium* spp. It has also been used in combination with other chemicals (e.g. chelating agents) to enhance activity against Gram-negative bacteria, predominantly to increase the penetration of the peptide into the cell membrane. The structure of nisin varies in aqueous solution, but assumes an amphiphilic and β-sheet structure when associated with lipid membranes and therefore in its active form [133].

Other peptides investigated for clinical applications such as pexiganan, iseganan, omiganan and the PGLYRP series have yielded mixed success [130]. Of note, the PGLYRP series have been described to be peptidoglycan-recognition peptides and,

therefore, target peptidoglycan as their site of action. Synergistic reactions have also been described with other cationic, amphiphilic peptides [130].

While it is envisioned that phages and antimicrobial peptides may offer certain benefits over conventional microbicidal chemicals, their particular promise to date (with the notable exception of nisin) is as alternatives to antibiotics.

Glucoprotamines

Glucoprotamines are a group of chemicals that can be generated by condensation of N-substituted propylene diamines with 2-aminoglutaric compounds [134]. The first described microbicide was produced from reacting L-glutamic acid and cocopropylene-1,3-diamine to give a wax-like substance that can be dissolved in water [135]. In initial investigations, these non-sensitizing and readily biodegradable chemicals showed broad-spectrum activity against vegetative bacteria (including mycobacteria), fungi and viruses [135]. In addition, clinical investigations with soiled medical instruments demonstrated good bactericidal activity [136]. Longer contact times (15 min at 2500 ppm glucoprotamine) were required to inactivate 4-$\log_{10}$ of atypical mycobacteria, although a glutaraldehyde-resistant strain of *Mycobacterium chelonae* was also cross-resistant to glucoprotamine [137]. In these studies, up to 2200 ppm for 60 min or 5000 ppm for 15 min were required to be effective against that strain, suggesting that available surface proteins may be a key target for the initial mycobactericidal activity of glucoprotamine [138]. The development of resistance may be unique to mycobacterial strains, as a further study of clinical and reference bacterial and fungal strains with two glucoprotamine-containing disinfectants demonstrated rapid activity [139].

Microbicidal surfaces

Recent years have seen much interest in producing microbicide-coated or impregnated materials (see Chapters 20.1 and 20.2) for environmental surfaces in healthcare settings and food-handling establishments, catheters and other device surfaces, textiles, and air and water filters. Common substances used to confer such microbicidal activity are triclosan, QACs and metals such as silver and copper. These and other novel means are reviewed below [140, 141].

Copper and silver
The metals silver and copper are well recognized for their microbicidal potential on their own and in formulation, and have been receiving increasing interest as microbicidal surfaces. While copper is widely used as a microbicide, particularly in agriculture, water treatment and as a preservative [1], copper-containing surfaces have been the focus of more recent investigations in hospitals and other environments in reducing contamination

with nosocomial pathogens on frequently-contacted surfaces such as bed rails, door handles and bedside tables. One study examined the levels of bacterial contamination on copper and non-copper surfaces (toilet seats, tap handles, door push plates) and found the counts of viable bacteria to be statistically significantly lower on the copper ones [142]. Another study showed similar results and lower re-contamination rates over time [143]. Similar studies have shown benefits in other applications such as the control of *E. coli* on food-handling surfaces [144] and in controlling fungal contamination on polyester fibers [145]. Laboratory studies have also shown similar effects against the vegetative form of *Clostridium difficile* over a 3 h contact time and in the presence/absence of soil in comparison with stainless steel [146]. The authors also suggested a reduction in the viability of the spores, although copper under these conditions is expected to have sporistatic attributes. More detailed studies showed that copper alloy surfaces with a copper content of >70% provided a significant reduction of both vegetative and spore forms of *C. difficile* [147].

In addition to direct copper alloy surfaces, other applications have been proposed using copper oxide nanoparticles that contain copper ions [148]. Such particles could be used in a variety of suspension and surface applications; in suspension studies bactericidal activity could be further enhanced in combination with silver nanoparticles. It has often been assumed that copper and silver have similar mechanisms of action, but recent evidence suggests that this may not be so.

Silver is also being used to confer microbicidal attributes to environmental surfaces and, in particular, wound dressings and indwelling devices such as catheters [140]. Traditional sources for silver have been silver nitrate and silver sulfadiazine, but silver itself (or as silver nitrate or silver oxide) can be directly integrated into a variety of materials such as polymers. Similar to copper, further advanced methods of presentation have included nanoparticles or crystalline silver [149, 150]. The benefits of these applications have been the subject of much debate and have been particularly described in situations requiring long contact times (such as larger wounds and long-term indwelling catheters). Despite these reports, a careful review of the literature shows little evidence to support the benefits of such applications in preventing infections with short-term implantable devices [140]. In contrast, others have reported improved microbicidal efficacy of silver nanoparticle-based technologies, in particular as alternatives to antibiotic use [151].

The integration of surface microbicides, or indeed other materials or surface modifications, may play an important role in preventing the initial attachment and subsequent colonization of surfaces, as the first stages in biofilm development are often associated with such devices [152]. The benefit of the widespread use of silver and copper for such microbicidal applications has been the subject of some debate, with many suggesting little role in reducing the rates of healthcare-acquired infections and the potential risks of microbial resistance development. These arguments should be considered further. For example Gram-positive

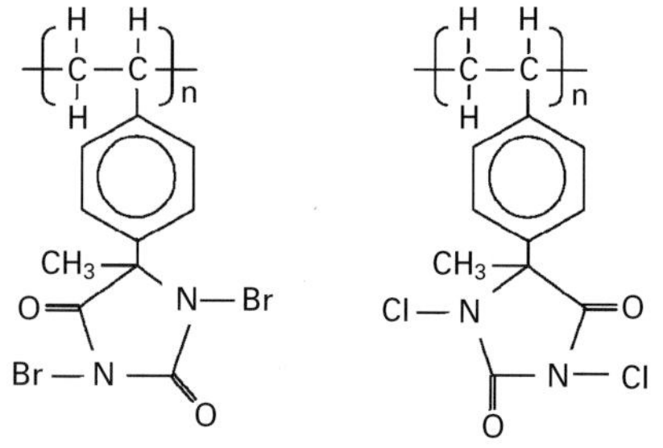

Figure 16.2 Examples of polymeric *N*-halamine chemical structures. The free chlorine (Cl) or bromine (Br) groups are responsible for microbicidal activity.

and Gram-negative strains of bacteria with intrinsic or acquired resistance to copper have been described; interestingly, such resistance was observed only under dry conditions and not when the inoculum was still wet [153]. Chromosomal and plasmid-mediated resistance mechanisms have been described in *E. coli* [1]. Plasmid-mediated tolerance to silver has already been well described in *Salmonella* and silver tolerance is emerging in methicillin-resistant *S. aureus* (MRSA) [154], although the clinical relevance of such levels of resistance is currently unknown.

N-halamines

N-halamines are a novel class of halogen-releasing agents (Figure 16.2). They are available as a range of monomeric and polymeric microbicides for both suspension and surface applications [123, 155, 156]. Such applications include the treatment of filters and textiles, and the disinfection of liquids, environmental surfaces and electron-spun fibers [157, 158].

The basis for the microbicidal activity of *N*-halamine is the anchoring of free (and therefore microbicidal) chlorine or bromine to nitrogen-containing compounds such as imidazolidins, oxazolidinones and modified polymers. On microbial contact, the halogens are released to elicit their microbicidal effects, but can also be constituted by the addition of halogen-containing liquids into the suspension or directly onto the surface. Due to the relatively low concentrations of the microbicide present, these preparations generally have a low odor, are considered stable and, being able to be reconstituted, have benefits over other impregnated microbicidal surfaces [157, 159–161]. The specific microbicidal activity depends on the *N*-halamine structure and its applications. Examples include the use of chlorine- and bromine-based *N*-halamines against bacteriophages (as a test model for other viruses) and in reducing toxins (with the bromine-based compounds showing superior activity [162]), fecal bacteria and coliphages in sewage-contaminated water [163]. A recent study with chlorinated, polymeric *N*-halamine in the form of *N*-chloro-2,2,6,6-tetramethyl-4-piperidinyl methacrylate showed persistent broad-spectrum activity over a year and rechargeable activity against bacteria (*S. aureus*, *E. coli*, *Enterococcus*), fungi (*Candida*, *Stachybotrys*) and a model phage (MS2) in microbicidal paint applications [164]. A recent patent has described methods for optimizing the generation of active polymers [165].

Titanium dioxide

Titanium dioxide (TiO_2; also known as titania), is a commonly-used white pigment for a variety of commercial applications (such as in paints, sunscreens, paper, etc.). It is also used for its photocatalytic activity under UV light, where surface radicals and other oxidizing agents are produced. This is used industrially for the oxidation of organic/inorganic contaminants as well as for its direct microbicidal purposes. Such applications include odor control, water disinfection, preservation, air treatment and on microbicidal (e.g. painted) surfaces. Reports of microbicidal activity vary in the literature and most investigated the activity under laboratory conditions. Recent studies have looked at more practical applications. For example, a continuous-flow water treatment pilot application has shown some success and stability using titania with solar activation [166] and silver/titanium dioxide photocatalysis showed particular use in the disinfection of air in medical settings [167]. Overall, such applications provide a low level (particularly bactericidal) of disinfection over time and may be further optimized depending on the specific application. For example, water disinfection studies showed activity against protozoan cysts (*Giardia* and *Acanthamoeba*) that generally show higher resistance to chemical microbicides [168]. Cysticidal activity was observed against *Giardia* cysts but not *Acanthamoeba* over a 30 min illumination time, being overall less effective than control UV studies. Other investigations have shown little to no appreciable sporicidal activity in recent surface studies [169]. Further, microbicidal activity is significantly affected by the presence of interfering organic or inorganic materials [170]. However, many of these studies may be limited by the methods of preparation and illumination by UV light; for example nanometer films of titania may have some optimal benefits of bactericidal and cysticidal activity over conventional deposition methods [171, 172].

Conclusions

The use of physical techniques to inactivate microorganisms in some types of foods, pharmaceutical products and medical devices, without the application of heat, or with the use of less heat (or required time), is particularly attractive from the point of view of product quality. A wide range of methodologies such as high pressures, high-intensity light and sonication are potential alternatives for such applications. Three facts limit their widespread use and current usefulness for niche applications. First, bacterial endospores remain the organisms most tolerant to all the techniques, so that sterilization, as opposed to various levels of disinfection, is not yet possible. Further developments and specific applications (e.g. with supercritical fluids) may overcome this limitation with some of these technologies. Second, the kinetics of inactivation that result from some of the techniques are different from those resulting from heating. This means that a careful new approach, for example with respect to the potential for survival of low numbers of pathogens, and consequent

implications for product safety, will be needed if application of the techniques continues to be considered. Third, with the exception of hydrostatic pressure, which is now well established commercially, the efficacy of the other techniques is impaired by product structure and may, therefore, be limited to liquid products or products containing small particulates, or (for light pulses) transparent products and surfaces, etc. At the same time, combination techniques, in which newer technologies are only one component of the total disinfection/preservation system, have already been described. If these are further developed and proved to be effective, the opportunities for use of the new techniques are very likely to grow in the future.

Changes in alternative chemical and biological processes for disinfection and sterilization, with some exceptions, have evolutionary and not revolutionary characteristics. For instance, the use of hydrogen peroxide for disinfection and sterilization involves new versions of an existing technology. Despite this, there are some novel microbicidals that have been developed recently. Applications of microbicides with nitrous oxide are in the early developmental phase but show promise in various disinfection and terminal sterilization uses. However, significant research is required to materialize this development. The main factor limiting the use of new microbicidal compounds is the extreme cost of registration due to governmental regulation, which is retarding the consideration and development of new and innovative compounds. In the meantime, it is likely that further improvements will be made to the optimal use of microbicides in formulation and in synergistic mixtures.

References

1 McDonnell, G. (2007) *Antisepsis, Disinfection, and Sterilization: Types, Action and Resistance*, ASM Press, Washington DC.
2 Goddard, P.A. and McCue, K.A. (2001) Phenolic compounds, in *Disinfection, Sterilization and Preservation*, 5th edn (ed. S.S. Block), Lippincott Williams & Wilkins, New York, pp. 255–282.
3 Kostenbauder, H.K. (1991) Physical factors influencing the activity of antimicrobial agents, in *Disinfection, Sterilization and Preservation*, 4th edn (ed. S.S. Block), Lea & Febiger, Philadelphia, pp. 59–71.
4 Russell, A.D. *et al.* (1992) *Principles and Practices of Disinfection, Preservation, and Sterilization*, 2nd edn, Blackwell Scientific Publications, Oxford.
5 US Department of Health and Human Services, Food and Drug Administration and Center for Devices and Radiological Health (2000) *Guidance for Industry and FDA Reviewers: Content and Format of Premarket Notification (510(k)) Submissions for Liquid Chemical Sterilants/High Level Disinfectants*, US Department of Health and Human Services, Rockville, MD.
6 CEN (2006) *EN 14885. Chemical Disinfectants and Antiseptics. Application of European Standards for Chemical Disinfectants and Antiseptics*. European Committee for Standardization (CEN), Brussels.
7 Justi, C. *et al.* (2000) Demonstration of a sterility assurance level for a liquid chemical sterilisation process. *Zentral Sterilisation*, **9**, 170–181.
8 Amin, N.S. *et al.* (2010) *Enzyme for the Production of Long Chain Peracid*, United States Patent 7,754,460.
9 International Standards Organization (ISO) (2007) *ISO 11135-1. Sterilization of Health Care Products. Ethylene Oxide. Part 1: Requirements for development, validation and routine control of a sterilization process for medical devices*, ISO, Geneva.

10 International Standards Organization (ISO) (2009) *ISO 25424. Sterilization of Medical Devices. Low Temperature Steam Formaldehyde. Requirements for development, validation and routine control of a sterilization process for medical device*, ISO, Geneva.

11 Turcot, R. *et al.* (2009) *Method and Apparatus for Ozone Sterilization*, United States Patent 7,588,720.

12 Hijnen, W.A. *et al.* (2006) Inactivation credit of UV radiation for viruses, bacteria and protozoan (oo)cysts in water: a review. *Water Research*, **40**, 3–22.

13 Beekes, M. *et al.* (2010) Fast, broad-range disinfection of bacteria, fungi, viruses and prions. *Journal of General Virology*, **91** (2), 580–589.

14 McDonnell, G. *et al.* (2005) Cleaning investigations to reduce the risk of prion contamination on manufacturing surfaces and materials. *European Journal of Parenteral and Pharmaceutical Sciences*, **10** (3), 67–72.

15 Miner, N. (1999) *Glutaraldehyde plus Alcohol Product*, United States Patent 5,863,547.

16 Lambert, R.J. *et al.* (2003) Theory of antimicrobial combinations: biocide mixtures – synergy or addition? *Journal of Applied Microbiology*, **94** (4), 747–759.

17 Lehmann, R.H. (2001) Synergism in disinfectant formulation, in *Disinfection, Sterilization and Preservation*, 5th edn (ed. S.S. Block), Lippincott Williams & Wilkins, Philadelphia, pp. 459–472.

18 McDonnell, G. and Pretzer, D. (2001) New and developing chemical antimicrobials, in *Disinfection, Sterilization, and Preservation*, 5th edn (ed. S.S. Block), Lippincott Williams & Wilkins, Philadelphia, pp. 431–443.

19 Basset, J. and Machebouf, M.A. (1932) Étude sur les effets biologiques des ultrapressions: résistance de bactéries, de diastases et de toxines aux pressions très élévées. *Comptes Rendus Hebdomaire Science Academie Sciences*, **196**, 1431–1442.

20 Selman, J. (1992) New technologies for the food industry. *Food Science and Technology Today*, **6**, 205–209.

21 Knorr, D. (1995) Hydrostatic pressure treatment of food: microbiology, in *New Methods of Food Preservation* (ed. G.W. Gould), Blackie Academic & Professional, Glasgow, pp. 159–175.

22 Palaniappan, S. (1996) High isostatic presure processing of foods, in *New Processing Technologies Yearbook* (ed. P.I. Chandarana), National Food Processors Association, Washington, DC, pp. 51–66.

23 Heremans, K. (1995) High pressure effects on biomolecules, in *High Pressure Processing of Foods* (eds D.A. Ledward *et al.*), Nottingham University Press, Nottingham, pp. 81–97.

24 Isaacs, N.S. *et al.* (1995) Studies on the inactivation by high pressure of microorganisms, in *High Pressure Processing of Foods* (eds D.A. Ledward *et al.*), Nottingham University Press, Nottingham, pp. 65–79.

25 Hoover, D.G. *et al.* (1989) Biological effects of high hydrostatic pressure on food microorganisms. *Food Technology*, **43**, 99–107.

26 Smelt, J.P. *et al.* (2001) Effects of high pressure on vegetative microorganisms, in *Ultra High Pressure Treatments of Foods* (eds M.E.G. Hendrickx and D. Knorr), Kluwer Academic/Plenum Publishers, New York, pp. 55–76.

27 Ludwig, H. *et al.* (1992) Inactivation of microorganisms by hydrostatic pressure, in *High Pressure Biotechnology* (eds C. Balny *et al.*), Colloque INSERM/J, Libby Eurotext, Brussels, pp. 25–32.

28 Patterson, M.F. *et al.* (1995) Effects of high pressure on vegetative pathogens, in *High Pressure Processing of Foods* (eds D.A. Ledward *et al.*), Nottingham University Press, Nottingham, pp. 47–63.

29 Eze, M.O. (1990) Consequences of the lipid bilayer to membrane associated reactions. *Journal of Chemical Education*, **67**, 17–20.

30 Carlez, A. *et al.* (1992) Effects of high pressure and bacteriostatic agents on the destruction of *Citrobacter freundii* in minced beef muscle, in *High Pressure and Biotechnology* (eds C. Balny *et al.*), Colloque INSERM/J, Libby Eurotech, Brussels, pp. 365–368.

31 Palou, E. *et al.* (1997) High hydrostatic pressure as a hurdle for *Saccharomyces bailii* inactivation. *Journal of Food Science*, **62**, 855–857.

32 Metrick, C. *et al.* (1989) Effects of high hydrostatic pressure on heat-sensitive strains of *Salmonella*. *Journal of Food Science*, **54**, 1547–1564.

33 Dring, J.G. (1976) Some aspects of the effects of hydrostatic pressure on microorganisms, in *Inhibition and Inactivation of Microorganisms* (eds F.A. Skinner and W.B. Hugo), Academic Press, London, pp. 257–277.

34 Shigahisa, T. *et al.* (1991) Effects of high pressure on the characteristics of pork slurries and inactivation of microorganisms associated with meat and meat products. *International Journal of Food Microbiology*, **12**, 207–216.

35 Suárez-Jacobo, A. *et al.* (2010) Effect of UHPH on indigenous microbiota of apple juice: a preliminary study of microbial shelf-life. *International Journal of Food Microbiology*, **136** (3), 261–267.

36 Pereda, J. *et al.* (2007) Effects of ultra-high pressure homogenization on microbial and physicochemical shelf life of milk. *Journal of Dairy Science*, **90** (3), 1081–1093.

37 Sale, A.J.H. *et al.* (1970) Inactivation of bacterial spores by hydrostatic pressure. *Journal of General Microbiology*, **60**, 323–334.

38 Wills, P.A. (1974) Effects of hydrostatic pressure and ionizing radiation on bacterial spores. *Atomic Energy Australia*, **17**, 2–10.

39 Seyerderholm, I. and Knorr, D. (1992) Reduction of *Bacillus stearothermophilus* spores by combined high pressure and temperature treatments. *Journal of Food Industry*, **43** (4), 17–20.

40 Hayakawa, I. *et al.* (1994) Application of high pressure for spore inactivation and protein denaturation. *Journal of Food Science*, **59**, 159–163.

41 Heinz, V. and Knorr, D. (2001) Effects of high pressure on spores, in *Ultra High Pressure Treatments of Foods* (eds M.E.G. Hendrickx and D. Knorr), Kluwer Academic/Plenum Publishers, New York, pp. 77–113.

42 Spilimbergo, S. and Bertucco, A. (2003) Non-thermal bacterial inactivation with dense CO(2). *Biotechnology and Bioengineering*, **84** (6), 627–638.

43 Kim, S.R. *et al.* (2008) Analysis of survival rates and cellular fatty acid profiles of *Listeria monocytogenes* treated with supercritical carbon dioxide under the influence of cosolvents. *Journal of Microbiological Methods*, **75** (1), 47–54.

44 Hemmer, J.D. *et al.* (2007) Sterilization of bacterial spores by using supercritical carbon dioxide and hydrogen peroxide. *Journal of Biomedical Materials Research. Part B, Applied Biomaterials*, **80** (2), 511–518.

45 White, A. *et al.* (2009) Effective terminal sterilization using supercritical carbon dioxide. *Journal of Biomedical Materials Research. Part B, Applied Biomaterials*, **91** (2), 572–578.

46 Shieh, E. *et al.* (2009) Sterilization of *Bacillus pumilus* spores using supercritical fluid carbon dioxide containing various modifier solutions. *Journal of Microbiological Methods*, **76** (3), 247–252.

47 Castro, A.I. *et al.* (1993) Microbial inactivation in foods by pulsed electric fields. *Journal of Food Processing and Preservation*, **17**, 47–73.

48 Jayaram, S. *et al.* (1992) Kinetics of sterilization of *Lactobacillus brevis* by the application of high voltage pulses. *Biotechnology and Bioengineering*, **40**, 1412–1420.

49 Molina, J.F. *et al.* (2002) Inactivation by high intensity pulsed electric fields, in *Control of Foodborne Microoganisms* (eds V.K. Juneja and J.N. Sofos), Marcel Dekker, New York, pp. 383–397.

50 Tsong, T.Y. (1991) Minireview: electroporation of cell membranes. *Biophysical Journal*, **60**, 297–316.

51 Barbosa-Canovas, G.V. *et al.* (1995) State of the art technologies for the sterilization of foods by non-thermal processes: physical methods, in *Food Preservation by Moisture Control: Fundamentals and Applications* (eds G.V. Barbosa-Canovas and J. Welti-Chanes), Technomic Publishing, Lancaster, PA, pp. 493–532.

52 Hamilton, W.A. and Sale, A.J.H. (1967) Effects of high electric fields on microorganisms II. Mechanism of action of the lethal effect. *Biochimica et Biophysica Acta*, **148**, 789–795.

53 Mertens, B. and Knorr, D. (1992) Development of non-thermal processes for food preservation. *Food Technology*, **46** (5), 124–133.

54 Qin, B. *et al.* (1996) Nonthermal pasteurization of liquid foods using high-intensity pulsed electric fields. *Critical Reviews in Food Science and Nutrition*, **36**, 603–607.

55 Kalchayanand, N. *et al.* (1994) Hydrostatic pressure and electroporation have increased bactericidal efficiency in combination with bacteriocins. *Applied and Environmental Microbiology*, **60**, 4174–4177.

56 Uesugi, A.R. and Moraru, C.I. (2009) Reduction of *Listeria* on ready-to-eat sausages after exposure to a combination of pulsed light and nisin. *Journal of Food Protection*, **72**, 347–353.

57 Luksiene, Z. *et al.* (1999) Advanced high-power pulsed light device to decontaminate food from pathogens: effects on *Salmonella typhimurium* viability *in vitro*. *Applied and Environmental Microbiology*, **65** (3), 1312–1315.

58 Cobb, C.M. *et al.* (1992) A preliminary study on the effects of the Nd:YAG laser on root surfaces and subgingival microflora *in vivo*. *Journal of Periodontology*, **63**, 701–707.

59 Rooney, J. *et al.* (1994) A laboratory investigation of the bactericidal effect of a Nd: Yag laser. *British Dental Journal*, **176**, 61–64.

60 Degitz, K. (2007) Phototherapy, photodynamic therapy and lasers in the treatment of acne. *Journal of Applied Microbiology*, **103** (5), 1545–1552.

61 Dunn, J.E. *et al.* (1988) *Method and Apparatus for Preservation of Foodstuffs*, International Patent WO88/03369.

62 Rowan, N.J. *et al.* (2007) Pulsed-light inactivation of food-related microorganisms. *Letters in Applied Microbiology*, **45** (5), 564–567.

63 Lamont, Y. *et al.* (2007) Pulsed UV-light inactivation of poliovirus and adenovirus. *Applied and Environmental Microbiology*, **73** (17), 5663–5666.

64 Wainwright, K.E. *et al.* (1994) Physical inactivation of *Toxoplasma gondii* oocysts in water. *ASAIO Journal (American Society for Artificial Internal Organs)*, **40** (3), M371–M376.

65 Costa, J.L. and Hofmann, G.A. (1987) *Malignancy Treatment*, US Patent 4,665,898.

66 Hofmann, G.A. (1985) *Inactivation of Microorganisms by an Oscillating Magnetic Field*, US Patent 4,524,079 and International Patent WO85/02094.

67 Barbosa-Canovas, G.V. *et al.* (2002) Magnetic fields as a potential nonthermal technology for the inactivation of microorganisms, in *Control of Foodborne Microooganisms* (eds V.K. Juneja and J.N. Sofos), Marcel Dekker, New York, pp. 399–418.

68 Benson, D.E. *et al.* (1994) Magnetic field enhancement of antibiotic activity in biofilm forming *Pseudomonas aeruginosa*. *Water Environment Research: A Research Publication of the Water Environment Federation*, **81** (7), 695–701.

69 Scherba, G. *et al.* (1991) Quantitative assessment of the germicidal efficacy of ultrasonic energy. *Applied and Environmental Microbiology*, **57**, 2079–2084.

70 Alliger, H. (1975) Ultrasonic disruption. *American Laboratory*, **10**, 75–85.

71 Ahmed, F.I.K. and Russell, C. (1975) Synergism between ultrasonic waves and hydrogen peroxide in the killing of microorganisms. *Journal of Applied Bacteriology*, **39**, 31–40.

72 Sanz, B. *et al.* (1985) Effect of ultrasonic waves on the heat resistance of *Bacillus stearothermophilus* spores, in *Fundamental and Applied Aspects of Bacterial Spores* (eds G.J. Dring *et al.*), Academic Press, London, pp. 215–259.

73 Burgos, J. *et al.* (1972) Effect of ultrasonic waves on the heat resistance of *Bacillus cereus* and *Bacillus coagulans* spores. *Applied Microbiology*, **24**, 497–498.

74 Ordonez, J.A. *et al.* (1984) A note on the effect of combined ultrasonic and heat treatments on the survival of thermoduric streptococci. *Journal of Applied Bacteriology*, **56**, 175–177.

75 Ordonez, J.A. *et al.* (1987) Effects of combined ultrasonic and heat treatment (thermosonication) on the survival of a strain of *Staphylococcus aureus*. *Journal of Dairy Research*, **54**, 61–67.

76 Salleh-Mack, S.Z. and Roberts, J.S. (2007) Ultrasound pasteurization: the effects of temperature, soluble solids, organic acids and pH on the inactivation of *Escherichia coli* ATCC 25922. *Ultrason Sonochemistry*, **14** (3), 323–329.

77 Sala, F.J. *et al.* (1995) Effect of heat and ultrasound on microorganisms and enzymes, in *New Methods of Food Preservation* (ed. G.W. Gould), Blackie Academic & Professional, Glasgow, pp. 176–204.

78 Yong, H.N. *et al.* (2009) Effect of sonication on UV disinfectability of primary effluents. *Water Environment Research: A Research Publication of the Water Environment Federation*, **81** (7), 695–701.

79 Friedrich, E.G. Jr. and Phillips, L.E. (1988) Microwave sterilization of *Candida* on underwear fabric. A preliminary report. *Journal of Reproductive Medicine*, **33** (5), 421–422.

80 Xi, X. *et al.* (2000) An experiment on disinfection using high power microwave. *Sheng Wu Yi Xue Gong Cheng Xue Za Zhi*, **17** (2), 231–232.

81 Patel, S.S. *et al.* (2010) Microwave sterilization of bovine pericardium for heart valve applications. *Journal of Artificial Organs*, **13** (1), 24–30.

82 Fais, L.M. *et al.* (2009) Influence of microwave sterilization on the cutting capacity of carbide burs. *Journal of Applied Oral Science: Revista FOB*, **17** (6), 584–589.

83 Chan, J.L. *et al.* (2009) Adequacy of sanitization and storage of catheters for intermittent use after washing and microwave sterilization. *Journal of Urology*, **182** (4), 2085–2089.

84 Diaz, L.F. *et al.* (2005) Alternatives for the treatment and disposal of healthcare wastes in developing countries. *Waste Management (New York.)*, **25** (6), 626–637.

85 Kim, S.Y. *et al.* (2009) Destruction of *Bacillus licheniformis* spores by microwave irradiation. *Applied Microbiology*, **106** (3), 877–885.

86 Sakudo, A. and Shintani, H. (2010) *Sterilization and Disinfection by Plasma: Sterilization Mechanisms, Biological and Medical Applications*, Nova Science, Hauppauge, NY.

87 Jacobs, P.T. and Lin, S.-M. (1987) *Hydrogen Peroxide Plasma Sterilization System*, US Patent 4,643,876.

88 Caputo, R.A. *et al.* (1992) *Plasma Sterilizing Process with Pulsed Antimicrobial Agent*, US Patent 5,084,239.

89 McDonnell, G. (2010) Current and future perspectives of gas plasma for decontamination, in *Sterilization and Disinfection by Plasma: Sterilization Mechanisms, Biological and Medical Applications* (eds A. Sakudo and H. Shintani), Nova Science, Hauppauge, NY, pp. 99–109.

90 Perni, S. *et al.* (2008) Cold atmospheric plasma disinfection of cut fruit surfaces contaminated with migrating microorganisms. *Journal of Food Protection*, **71** (8), 1619–1625.

91 Rupf, S. *et al.* (2010) Killing of adherent oral microbes by a non-thermal atmospheric plasma jet. *Journal of Medical Microbiology*, **59** (2), 206–212.

92 Jacobs, P.T. and Lin, S.-M. (1988) *Hydrogen Peroxide Plasma Sterilization System*, US Patent 4,756,882.

93 Meszaros, J.E. *et al.* (2005) Area fumigation with hydrogen peroxide vapor. *Applied Biosafety*, **10** (2), 91–100.

94 Krebs, M.C. *et al.* (1998) Gas plasma sterilization: relative efficiency of the hydrogen peroxide phase as compared to that of the plasma phase. *International Journal of Pharmaceutics*, **160**, 75–81.

95 Schumb, W.C. (1955), *Hydrogen Peroxide*, American Chemical Society Monograph Series, Reinhold Publishing, New York.

96 Block, S.S. (1991) Peroxygen compounds, in *Disinfection, Sterilization and Preservation*, 4th edn (ed. S.S. Block), Lea & Febiger, Philadelphia, pp. 167–181.

97 Kokubo, M. *et al.* (1998) Resistance of common environmental spores of the genus *Bacillus* to vapor hydrogen peroxide vapor. *PDA Journal of Pharmaceutical Science and Technology*, **52**, 228–231.

98 McDonnell, G. and Burke, P. (2009) New low temperature sterilization processes. *International Journal of Infection Control*, **5** (2), 1–4.

99 Fichet, G.E. *et al.* (2004) Novel methods for disinfection of prion-contaminated medical devices. *Lancet*, **364**, 521–526.

100 Fichet, G. *et al.* (2007) Prion inactivation using a new gaseous hydrogen peroxide sterilisation process. *Journal of Hospital Infection*, **67**, 278–386.

101 Roberts, S. *et al.* (2006) Studies on the decontamination of surfaces exposed to cytotoxic drugs in chemotherapy workstations. *Journal of Oncology Pharmacy Practice*, **12** (2), 95–104.

102 Finnegan, M. *et al.* (2010) The mode of action of hydrogen peroxide and other oxidizing agents: differences between liquid and gas form. *Journal of Antimicrobial Chemotherapy*, **65**, 2108–2115.

103 Hultman, C. *et al.* (2007) The physical chemistry of decontamination with gaseous hydrogen peroxide. *Pharmaceutical Engineering*, **27** (1), 22–32.

104 McDonnell, G. (2005) Hydrogen peroxide fogging/fumigation. *Journal of Hospital Infection*, **62**, 385–386.

105 Gaspar, M.C. *et al.* (1995) Preliminary study on the efficacy of sterilization with AbTox system: comparison with ethylene oxide. *Medicina Preventiva*, **1**, 1–6.

106 Gates, D.J. (1998) *The Chlorine Dioxide Handbook*, Water Disinfection Series, AWWA Publishing, Denver, CO.

107 Morrissey, R.F. (1996) Changes in the science of sterilization and disinfection. *Biomedical Instrumentation and Technology*, **30**, 404–406.

108 Rosenblatt, A.A. and Knapp, J.E. (1989) *Chorine Dioxide Gas Sterilization. Sterilization in the 1990s*, HIMA Report 89-1, 75–80.

109 Knapp, D.L. and Battisti, D.L. (2001) Chlorine dioxide, in *Disinfection, Sterilization and Preservation*, 5th edn (ed. S.S. Block), Lippincott Williams & Wilkins, New York, pp. 215–228.

110 Han, Y. *et al.* (2004) Decontamination of strawberries using batch and continuous chlorine dioxide gas treatments. *Journal of Food Protection*, **67** (11), 2450–2455.

111 Aly, R. *et al.* (1998) Clinical efficacy of a chlorous acid preoperative skin antiseptic. *American Journal of Infection Control*, **26** (4), 406–412.

112 Boddie, R.L. *et al.* (1998) Germicidal activity of a chlorous acid-chlorine dioxide teat dip and a sodium chlorite teat dip during experimental challenge with *Staphylococcus aureus* and *Streptococcus agalactiae*. *Journal of Dairy Science*, **81** (8), 2293–2298.

113 Bedard, C. *et al.* (2009) *Ozone Sterilization Method*, United States Patent 7,582,257.

114 Dessy, C. and Ferron, O. (2004) Pathophysiological roles of nitric oxide: in the heart and the coronary vasculature. Current medical chemistry – anti-inflammatory and anti-allergy. *Agents in Medicinal Chemistry*, **3** (3), 207–216.

115 Shami, P.J. *et al.* (1995) Nitric oxide modulation of the growth and differentiation of freshly isolated acute non-lymphocytic leukemia cells. *Leukemia Research*, **19** (8), 527–533.

116 Nguyen, T. *et al.* (1992) DNA damage and mutation in human cells exposed to nitric oxide *in vitro*. *Proceedings of the National Academy of Sciences of the United States of America*, **89** (7), 3030–3034.

117 Arnold, E.V. *et al.* (2007) *Sterilization System and Device*, United States Patent Application 20070014686.

118 Green, S.J. and Keefer, L.K. (1998) *Encapsulated and Non-encapsulated Nitric Oxide Generators used as Antimicrobial Agents*, World Patent 9509612 A1 950413.

119 Cornforth, D. (1996) Nitric oxide, in *Role of Nitric Acid in the Treatment of Foods* (ed.J. Lancaster), Academic Press, San Diego, pp. 259–287.

120 Stanford, K. *et al.* (2010) Oral delivery systems for encapsulated bacteriophages targeted at *Escherichia coli* O157:H7 in feedlot cattle. *Journal of Food Protection*, **73** (7), 1304–1312.

121 Gupta, R. and Prasad, Y. (2011) Efficacy of polyvalent bacteriophage P-27/HP to control multidrug resistant *Staphylococcus aureus* associated with human infections. *Current Microbiology*, **62**, 255–260.

122 Kumari, S. *et al.* (2010) Evidence to support the therapeutic potential of bacteriophage Kpn5 in burn wound infection caused by *Klebsiella pneumoniae* in BALB/c mice. *Journal of Microbiology and Biotechnology*, **20** (5), 935–941.

123 McDonnell, G. and Pretzer, D. (2000) New and developing chemical antimicrobials, in *Disinfection, Sterilization and Preservation*, 5th edn (ed. S.S. Block), Lippincott Williams & Wilkins, Philadelphia, pp. 431–444.

124 Pathan, F.K. *et al.* (2010) Recent patents on antimicrobial peptides. *Recent Patents on DNA and Gene Sequence*, **4** (1), 10–16.

125 Gallo, R.L. and Huttner, K.M. (1998) Antimicrobial peptides: an emerging concept in cutaneous biology. *Journal of Investigative Dermatology*, **111**, 739–743.

126 Giuliani, A. *et al.* (2007) Antimicrobial peptides: an overview of a promising class of therapeutics. *Central European Journal of Biology*, **2**, 1–33.

127 Rathinakumar, R. *et al.* (2009) Broad-spectrum antimicrobial peptides by rational combinatorial design and high-throughput screening: the importance of interfacial activity. *Journal of the American Chemical Society*, **131** (22), 7609–7617.

128 Wang, G. *et al.* (2009) APD2: the updated antimicrobial peptide database and its application in peptide design. *Nucleic Acids Research*, **37**, D933–D937.

129 Bellomio, A. *et al.* (2007) J25 has dual and independent mechanisms of action in *Escherichia coli*: RNA polymerase inhibition and increased superoxide production. *Journal of Bacteriology*, **189** (11), 4180–4186.

130 Oyston, P. *et al.* (2009) Novel peptide therapeutics for treatment of infections. *Journal of Medical Microbiology*, **58**, 977–987.

131 Yeaman, M.R. and Yount, N.Y. (2003) Mechanisms of antimicrobial peptide action and resistance. *Pharmacological Reviews*, **55** (1), 27–55.

132 Hansen, J.N. (1994) Nisin as a model food preservative. *Critical Reviews in Food Science and Nutrition*, **34**, 69–93.

133 Hooven, H. *et al.* (1996) Three-dimensional structure of the antibiotic nisin in the presence of membrane-mimetic micelles of dodecylphosphocholine and of sodium dodecylsulphate. *FEBS Journal*, **235** (1–2), 382–393.

134 Bohlander, R. *et al.* (2001) *Method for Producing Glucoprotamines*, United States Patent 6,331,607.

135 Disch, K. (1994) Glucoprotamine – a new antimicrobial substance. *Zentralblatt fur Hygiene und Umweltmedizin*, **195** (5–6), 357–365.

136 Widmer, A.E. and Frei, R. (2003) Antimicrobial activity of glucoprotamin: a clinical study of a new disinfectant for instruments. *Infection Control and Hospital Epidemiology*, **24** (10), 762–764.

137 Meyer, B. and Kluin, C. (1999) Efficacy of glucoprotamin containing disinfectants against different species of atypical mycobacteria. *Journal of Hospital Infection*, **42** (2), 151–154.

138 Svetlíková, Z. *et al.* (2009) Role of porins in the susceptibility of *Mycobacterium smegmatis* and *Mycobacterium chelonae* to aldehyde-based disinfectants and drugs. *Antimicrobial Agents and Chemotherapy*, **53** (9), 4015–4018.

139 Tyski, S. *et al.* (2009) Antimicrobial activity of glucoprotamin-containing disinfectants. *Polish Journal of Microbiology*, **58** (4), 347–353.

140 Meakins, J.L. (2009) Silver and new technology: dressings and devices. *Surgical Infections*, **10** (3), 293–296.

141 Page, K. *et al.* (2009) Antimicrobial surfaces and their potential in reducing the role of the inanimate environment in the incidence of hospital-acquired infections. *Journal of Materials Chemistry*, **19**, 3819–3831.

142 Casey, A.L. *et al.* (2010) Role of copper in reducing hospital environment contamination. *Journal of Hospital Infection*, **74**, 72–77.

143 Mikolay, A. *et al.* (2010) Survival of bacteria on metallic copper surfaces in a hospital trial. *Applied Microbiology and Biotechnology*, **87**, 1875–1879.

144 Noyce, J.O. *et al.* (2006) Use of copper cast alloys to control *Escherichia coli* O157 cross-contamination during food processing. *Applied and Environmental Microbiology*, **72** (6), 4239–4244.

145 Zatcoff, R.C. *et al.* (2008) Treatment of tinea pedis with socks containing copper-oxide impregnated fibers. *Foot (Edinburgh, Scotland)*, **18** (3), 136–141.

146 Wheeldon, L.J. *et al.* (2008) Antimicrobial efficacy of copper surfaces against spores and vegetative cells of *Clostridium difficile*: the germination theory. *Journal of Antimicrobial Chemotherapy*, **62** (3), 522–525.

147 Weaver, L. *et al.* (2008) Survival of *Clostridium difficile* on copper and steel: futuristic options for hospital hygiene. *Journal of Hospital Infection*, **68** (2), 145–151.

148 Ren, G. *et al.* (2009) Characterisation of copper oxide nanoparticles for antimicrobial applications. *International Journal of Antimicrobial Agents*, **33** (6), 587–590.

149 Rai, M. *et al.* (2009) Silver nanoparticles as a new generation of antimicrobials. *Biotechnology Advances*, **27** (1), 76–83.

150 Gravante, G. *et al.* (2009) Nanocrystalline silver: a systematic review of randomized trials conducted on burned patients and an evidence-based assessment of potential advantages over older silver formulations. *Annals of Plastic Surgery*, **63** (2), 201–205.

151 Casey, A.L. and Elliott, T.S. (2010) Prevention of central venous catheter-related infection: update. *British Journal of Nursing*, **19** (2), 78, 80, 82 passim.

152 Monteiro, D.R. *et al.* (2009) The growing importance of materials that prevent microbial adhesion: antimicrobial effect of medical devices containing silver. *International Journal of Antimicrobial Agents*, **34** (2), 103–110.

153 Santo, C.E. *et al.* (2010) Isolation and characterization of bacteria resistant to metallic copper surfaces. *Applied and Environmental Microbiology*, **76** (5), 1341–1348.

154 Loh, J.V. *et al.* (2009) Silver resistance in MRSA isolated from wound and nasal sources in humans and animals. *International Wound Journal*, **6** (1), 32–38.

155 Barnela, S.B. *et al.* (1987) Syntheses and antibacterial activity of new N-halamine compounds. *Journal of Pharmaceutical Sciences*, **76** (3), 245–247.

156 Chen, Z. and Sun, Y. (2006) N-halamine-based antimicrobial additives for polymers: preparation, characterization and antimicrobial activity. *Industrial and Engineering Chemistry Research*, **45** (8), 2634–2640.

157 Worley, S.D. *et al.* (1999) *Surface Active N-halamine Compounds*, US Patent 5,902,818.

158 Sun, X. *et al.* (2010) Electrospun composite nanofiber fabrics containing uniformly dispersed antimicrobial agents as an innovative type of polymeric materials with superior antimicrobial efficacy. *ACS Applied Materials and Interfaces*, **2** (4), 952–956.

159 Eknoian, M.W. *et al.* (1998) Monomeric and polymeric N-halamine disinfectants. *Industrial and Engineering Chemistry Research*, **3**, 2873–2877.

160 Eknoian, M.W. and Worley, S.D. (1998) New N-halamine microbicidal polymers. *Journal of Bioactive and Compatible Polymers*, **13**, 303–314.

161 Worley, S.D. *et al.* (1996) *Polymeric Cyclic N-halamine Microbicidal Compounds*, US patent 5,490,983.

162 Coulliette, A.D. *et al.* (2010) Evaluation of a new disinfection approach: efficacy of chlorine and bromine halogenated contact disinfection for reduction of viruses and microcystin toxin. *American Journal of Tropical Medicine and Hygiene*, **82** (2), 279–288.

163 McLennan, S.D. *et al.* (2009) Comparison of point-of-use technologies for emergency disinfection of sewage-contaminated drinking water. *Applied and Environmental Microbiology*, **22**, 7283–7286.

164 Cao, Z. and Sun, Y. (2009) Polymeric N-halamine latex emulsions for use in antimicrobial paints. *ACS Applied Materials and Interfaces*, **1** (2), 494–504.

165 Sun, Y. and Chen, Z. (2009) *Method for Transformation of Conventional and Commercially Important Polymers into Durable and Rechargeable Antimicrobial Polymeric Materials*, US patent 7,541,398.

166 Sordo, C. *et al.* (2010) Solar photocatalytic disinfection with immobilised TiO(2) at pilot-plant scale. *Water Science and Technology: A Journal of the International Association on Water Pollution Research*, **61** (2), 507–512.

167 Zhao, Y.K. *et al.* (2010) Application of nanoscale silver-doped titanium dioxide as photocatalyst for indoor airborne bacteria control: a feasibility study in medical nursing institutions. *Journal of the Air and Waste Management Association*, **60** (3), 337–345.

168 Sökmen, M. *et al.* (2008) Photocatalytic disinfection of *Giardia intestinalis* and *Acanthamoeba castellani* cysts in water. *Experimental Parasitology*, **119** (1), 44–48.

169 Muranyi, P. *et al.* (2010) Antimicrobial efficiency of titanium dioxide-coated surfaces. *Journal of Applied Microbiology*, **108**, 1966–1973.

170 Block, S.S. *et al.* (1997) Chemically enhanced sunlight for killing bacteria. *Journal of Solar Energy Engineering*, **119**, 85–91.

171 Kambala, V.S. and Naidu, R. (2009) Disinfection studies on TiO2 thin films prepared by a sol-gel method. *Journal of Biomedical Nanotechnology*, **5** (1), 121–129.

172 Sunnotel, O. *et al.* (2010) Photocatalytic inactivation of *Cryptosporidium parvum* on nanostructured titanium dioxide films. *Journal of Water and Health*, **8** (1), 83–91.

17 Preservation of Medicines and Cosmetics

Sarah J. Hiom

Research and Development, St. Marys Pharmaceutical Unit, Cardiff and Vale University Health Board, Cardiff, Wales, UK

Nature of medicines and cosmetics

Medicines are formulated to assist in the administration of drugs to treat or prevent diseases or to alleviate symptoms in patients. Medicines can be delivered by a wide variety of routes, from relatively non-invasive topical applications to highly invasive injections. Cosmetics, however, are designed to deliver agents that enhance personal appearance, modify body odor or assist in body cleansing. Application is largely restricted to the skin, although such products as toothpaste or those for "feminine hygiene" may come into contact with mucous membranes. Eye-area cosmetics may also come into secondary contact with the cornea and conjunctiva.

Although the intended outcomes for medicines and cosmetics are fundamentally different, there are many similarities in the nature of the formulations created and the uses (and abuses) to which both can be subjected, including common microbiological problems. In order to create elegant products that are also efficacious, stable and safe to use throughout their intended shelf-life, it is often necessary to include several other ingredients in addition to the specific therapeutic agent or that producing the cosmetic effect. While a few formulations may be simple aqueous solutions or dry powders, many are extremely complex, both in the number of ingredients used and in their physicochemical complexity. Some indications of this variation and complexity of medicinal and cosmetic formulations can be obtained from the reviews of Frick [1] and Lund [2].

The possibility that microorganisms might contaminate medicines and cosmetics during manufacture, storage or use must be addressed to ensure the continued stability and safety of the product. The complex chemical and physicochemical nature of many formulations is often found to be conducive to the survival and even multiplication of such contaminants, unless specific precautions are taken to prevent it. Such survival, and even growth, may result in appreciable damage to the product as spoilage and/or the user as infection. Good manufacturing practices should provide adequate control of contamination from raw materials and processing activities [3–5]. This includes attention to the packaging, which should minimize the access of microorganisms, so that the quality of the product is maintained throughout the stresses of manufacturing, distribution, storage and use [6]. The ideal approach to reduce contamination risks would be to present the product as a sterile single-dose unit in robust packaging. However, this is only economically practical for high-risk dosage forms such as eye drops for hospital use or where preservatives cannot be used due to overriding toxicity concerns. One procedure adopted to limit the establishment of microbial contamination after manufacture is to include antimicrobial preservatives in the formulations. Preservatives, however, must never be added to mask contamination that arises from unsatisfactory manufacturing procedures or inadequate packaging.

The selection of a preservative system is a complex issue. It is essential to understand and fully evaluate the preservative needs and problems of individual products and be aware of how potential antimicrobial agents may behave in that formula.

The ideal properties of a preservative have been described [7–9] and include: being non-toxic and non-allergenic, having a broad spectrum of activity, being effective and stable over the range of pH values encountered in cosmetics and pharmaceuticals, be compatible with packaging and other ingredients in the formulation, be free from strong odor or color and not affect the physical properties of the product, be available at effective concentrations in the aqueous phase of the product, have an ability to meet regulatory requirements and be cost effective. Very few preservatives are able to meet all the required criteria and it is

often a case of "best choice under current circumstances". However, the selection process will include consideration of the properties of the formulation, preservative and likely challenge microbes, together with an evaluation of the intended use of the product and the associated contamination risks.

While there is little in the manner of official lists of recommended preservatives for medicines, there are bodies of unofficial regulatory beliefs which consider that certain preservatives would or would not be suitable for particular medicines. Thus, the use of bronopol and chloroform in new applications for oral medicines is most unlikely to be permitted, despite any data submitted to support its by-mouth usage. Since public disclosure of the preservative content of medicines is not generally mandatory, it is difficult to get a detailed pattern of usage. However, examination of partial disclosures in the *British National Forumulary* (*BNF*) [10] and by some manufacturers does provide an indication of UK usage. From anecdotal information and experience, it would appear that a limited range is suitable for use in medicines, and that parabens are by far the most commonly selected. Detailed monographs on the preservatives commonly used in medicines have

Table 17.1 Selected preservatives used in pharmaceutical formulations showing some typical in-use concentrations (%w/v) and optimal pH ranges.

Preservative	Formulation type				pH
	Parenteral	Ophthalmic	Topical	Oral	
Benzalkonium chloride	0.01	0.01–0.02	+		4–10
Benzethonium chloride	0.01–0.02	0.01–0.02	0.5		4–10
Benzoic acid	0.17		0.1–0.2	0.01–0.1	2–5
Benzyl alcohol	1.0		1.0	1.0	<5
Bronopol			0.02		5–7
Butylparabens			0.02–0.4	0.006–0.05	4–8
Cetrimide		0.005	+		4–10
Chlorhexidine		0.01	+		5–8
Chlorobutanol	≤0.5	≤0.5			4
Chlorocresol	0.1	0.05	0.075–0.2		<8.5
Chloroxylenol			0.1–0.8		4–10
Cresol	0.15–0.3		+		<7
Ethanol				≥10	<7
Imidurea			0.03–0.5		3–9
Methylparabens	(+)	(+)	0.02–0.3	0.015–0.2	4–8
Phenol	0.5		+		<7
Phenoxyethanol	+*		0.5–1.0		Broad
Phenylethanol		0.25–0.5	1.0		<7
Phenylmercuric acetate	(+)	(+)			>6
Phenylmercuric nitrate	(+)	(+)			>6
Potasssium sorbate			0.1–0.2	0.1–0.2	<6
Propionic acid (+salts)			+	+	<5
Propylene glycol			15–30	+	Broad
Propylparabens	(+)	(+)	0.01–0.6	0.01–0.02	4–8
Sodium benzoate	0.5		0.1–0.5	0.02–0.5	2–5
Sorbic acid			0.05–0.2	0.05–0.2	<6
Thiomersal	0.01	0.001–0.15	0.01		7–8

(+) now generally regarded as being unsuitable; +* generally for vaccines.

been produced [9–12]. A selection are presented in Table 17.1, showing the common types of formulations they are used in together with some in-use concentrations and optimal pH ranges.

Consequences of microbial contamination

Microorganisms possess diverse metabolic activities and are likely to present a variety of hazards (e.g. infection, toxicity, degradation of the formulation) both to the user and to the stability of the products, if allowed to persist. The European Pharmacopoeia Commission [13] sets limits for the presence of microorganisms in medicines, which vary depending on the product and its intended use. However, microbial contamination over and above these pharmacopoeial levels are still reported in distributed UK medicines [14, 15], although stricter regulatory controls have improved the situation compared with that of the pre-1970 period [16]. Other indications that the risk of microbial contamination is still a problem include reports that 13% of the UK drug alerts between January 2009 and January 2010 were due to an inability to provide microbial assurance to the required level [17] and that 4.9% of European Medicines Agency inspection deficiency reports (1995–2005) [18] were associated with the potential for microbial contamination. In-use contamination hazards also continue to be a problem, particularly for multidose eye drops [19] and multidose injections [20]. In the USA, concern currently centers on the microbial hazards that accumulate during the use of cosmetics [21, 22]. Few recent published data have been found for cosmetic contamination in the UK, although anecdotal evidence suggests a similar situation to that in the USA.

The most commonly reported microbial hazards found in liquid medicines and cosmetics are pseudomonads and their related Gram-negative rods, with spores (bacterial and fungal) predominating in dry tablets, capsules and cosmetic powders. Shared-use cosmetics accumulate human microflora, such as *Staphylococcus epidermidis*, *Staphylococcus aureus* and corynebacteria, as well as pathogenic fungi, yeasts and bacterial spores. Those that contain water or become wet during use reveal pseudomonads and related bacteria. The clinical and pharmaceutical significance of such contamination of medicines has been reviewed by Ringertz and Ringertz [23], Martone *et al.* [24] and Denyer [25] and for cosmetics by Sharpell and Manowitz [26]. The implications for product spoilage of both have been discussed by Spooner [27] and Beveridge [7].

The risk (likelihood of harm actually occurring) associated with delivery of contaminated products is less clearly determined. It will depend upon the type of microorganism present, the infective dose (dependent on the ability of the formulation to encourage microbial survival and the level of preservative protection built into it), the route of administration of the product and the host's resistance to infection (including immune status or degree of tissue damage at site of application). Prior to the 1960s, incidents of infection attributed to contaminated products seemed to be regarded as unfortunate but isolated occurrences, these

included severe eye infections from contaminated ophthalmic solutions [28] and tetanus infection of newborn children from contaminated talc dusting powders [29]. During the 1960s, a number of key investigations demonstrated the existence of a much wider problem. Ayliffe *et al.* [30] reported on an extensive UK outbreak of severe eye infections, traced to traditional but wholly inadequate official guidelines for the preservation and manufacture of ophthalmic solutions. The "Evans Medical disaster", in which contaminated infusion fluids caused serious injury and contributed to some deaths, precipitated public awareness and led to an official inquiry [31]. In Sweden, Kallings *et al.* [32] linked an outbreak of salmonellosis to contaminated thyroid tablets and eye and other infections to a range of contaminated pharmaceuticals. Bruch [33] in the USA similarly reported links between microbial contaminants in medicines and cosmetics and infections. Wilson [34] implicated contaminated eye-area cosmetics with severe eye infections. The more general role of opportunistic pathogens, such as the pseudomonads, and their implication in nosocomial infections was also becoming more recognized at this time. These reports stimulated an appreciable tightening of regulatory controls in many countries, and it is generally believed that the present situation is greatly improved. Comprehensive reviews of this topic can be found by Spooner [27], Beveridge [7], Fassihi [35] and Sharpell and Manowitz [26].

There are still difficulties in preventing the build-up of pathogenic contaminants in multidose eye drop containers during use [19]. The limited range of preservatives that are not damaging to the eye is also creating problems in controlling microbial proliferation, for example in contact lens maintenance [36, 37]. Additionally, there are currently small but serious outbreaks of protozoal infections by *Acanthamoeba*, for which effective and safe preservatives are difficult to find [38, 39].

Contaminated injections can result in the most serious infection outbreaks, as demonstrated by the administration of contaminated dextrose solution with the subsequent death of six UK hospital patients [40]. Despite major advances in the quality of large-volume parenteral infusions, high numbers of localized and systemic infections occur which are directly attributable to the administration devices themselves, such as catheters and cannulae [41]. Total parenteral nutrition infusions, compounded aseptically from sterile components, are conducive to microbial growth but cannot contain preservatives, due to their large volume [42]; they are therefore currently considered an area of great concern. Cases of fatal infections from contaminated units indicate a continuous need for improved systems for dispensing and protecting them from contamination [43–47].

Patients whose resistance has been weakened by trauma, chemotherapy, tissue damage or other disease often succumb to infection by opportunist contaminants that are unlikely to cause harm to "normal" patients [48]. The infection of haemophiliacs with human immunodeficiency virus (HIV) from human-derived factor VIII [49] and hepatitis C from blood-derived products [50] has stimulated action on possible virus contamination of other products derived from human or biotechnology-derived origin, as has the contraction of Creutzfeld–Jakob disease by patients treated with human growth hormone products from human origin [51]. More recently, a report links contamination from ultrasound gel to postoperative infections with *Burkholderia cepacia* [52].

Despite many well-publicised incidents, infection of patients with burned or otherwise damaged skin caused by using antiseptic cleaning solutions contaminated with *Pseudomonas* spp. continues [53–55], as does infection from contaminated nebulizer solutions [56, 57].The liberation of endotoxins by growth of Gram-negative contaminants in large-volume intravenous infusions and peritoneal dialysis fluids remains a problem [58, 59]. More recent are incidents of algal toxins, such as mycocystins, surviving in process water and causing damage and even death when used for the dilution of kidney dialysates [60]. The implications of aflatoxin contamination in cosmetics has become of interest [61], with the suggestion that these toxins could penetrate the epidermis [62].

With the link between infection and contaminated cosmetics long established [33, 34], current concerns center on the practice of in-store cosmetic multiuser testers. These have been shown to accumulate appreciable levels of contamination, including a variety of hazardous bacteria, yeasts and fungi, which are able to initiate severe eye infections and infections associated with the use of contaminated hand creams and lotions [21, 22].

The weight of published evidence, both past and present, on the implications of microbial contamination for medicines and cosmetics demands that a careful and specific microbiological risk assessment is made for each individual product at its design and validation stages, using conventional risk-assessment techniques [63–66]. These must take into account worst-case scenarios, such as the possibility that eye cosmetics may be applied while driving, where an applicator might scratch the cornea [67], or that multidose eye drop units may well receive varied and appreciable contamination during use by the lay public. Such assessments should take into account the highly critical expectations of the public concerning standards for medicines and other consumer products, which are usually far greater than those for their food.

Effect of formulation parameters on microbial contamination and spoilage

The formulation may have an effect on microbial contamination in one of two ways. Firstly, through modification of the physicochemical environment of any contaminant, which will challenge its ability to multiply and/or survive; and secondly, by having an effect on the efficacy of any preservative present.

Formulation effects on microbial growth

The nutritional requirements of most saprophytic, non-fastidious spoilage contaminants are likely to be well met in almost all pharmaceuticals and cosmetics, since many ingredients are easily biodegradable, and even the trace residues of non-specific chemical contaminants present in most commercial ingredients are likely to provide ample nutrients to permit growth. For example, even standard distilled and demineralized water contains sufficient trace nutrients to permit ample growth of pseudomonads and related species [68]. For microorganisms to multiply and/or survive there must also be appropriate physicochemical conditions that allow them to maintain adequate homeostasis. From the formulator's point of view the main conditions that can be modified include the amount of available water present and conducive temperatures and pH. Such manipulations form the basis for the preservation and protection of many foodstuffs, where the ability to add antimicrobial preservatives is strictly limited by law. A wealth of basic and applied food-protection research is available for those who wish to assess these principles for application to medicines and cosmetics, and the reviews of Chirife and Favetto [69], Dillon and Board [70], Gould [71] and Roberts [72] are recommended. Their application to pharmaceuticals and cosmetics has been considered briefly by Orth [73] and Beveridge [7].

Available water

Most microorganisms require over 70% water to grow [74], which necessitates that, if they are to replicate, they must successfully compete for ready access to water against the other ingredients of a formulation – which the microorganisms may interact with often in strong and complex ways [75]. The amount of water available to microorganisms in a product is given by:

$$A_w = \frac{\text{Vapor pressure of product}}{\text{Vapor pressure of water}}$$

Certain organisms will only grow at specific available water (A_w) levels (Table 17.2)

The manipulation of product water activity to a level below the minimum essential for growth offers a major potential for the protection of some products. It is possible to reduce the A_w of tablets, pastilles, capsules and powders sufficiently by drying to provide their major mode of spoilage protection, although some contaminants may continue to survive in a senescent state for a

Table 17.2 Available water (A_w) requirements of common microbial species.

Microorganism	A_w
Pseudomonas aeruginosa	0.97
Escherichia coli	0.95
Gram-negative rods	0.95
Staphylococcus aureus	0.90
Gram-positive rods	0.90
Molds and yeasts	0.85
Aspergillus niger	0.77
Osmotolerant yeasts	0.70
Aspergillus glaucus	0.61

considerable time [76]. Friedl [77] has proposed reducing the number of microbiological attribute tests carried out on pharmaceuticals based on information collated on the A_w content of different types of products and the ideal A_w growth requirements of the likely contaminating microorganisms [78]. These figures may also be used to assist decisions concerning the need to include preservatives in a product. For example, rectal ointments have an A_w of approximately 0.26 and as no organisms are expected to proliferate below an A_w of 0.6, preservatives are not recommended in these type of preparations. The proposed reduction in A_w must be maintained throughout the life of the product, possibly by using water vapor-resistant bottles or film-strip packing, otherwise protection will be lost. The use of vapor-repellent film coatings [79] has been suggested to assist in the control of spoilage of bulk tablets intended for distribution to humid climates [80]. The A_w of some aqueous systems can be lowered sufficiently to give useful protection by the addition of quite large amounts of water-binding low molecular weight solutes: sucrose (66% w/v, approximate $A_w = 0.86$) in, for example, reconstituted antibiotic syrups; sorbitol (c. >35% w/v) for dentifrice pastes [81]; glycerol (c. >40%) for cosmetic lotions and urea (10–20%) for some cosmetics [82]. Limtner [83] described the use of polyacrylamide hydrogels in cosmetic creams to enhance formulation robustness, presumably by very effectively lowering A_w. Ointments have a low A_w and it is not usual to add preservatives to these formulations. Strongly alcoholic formulations, such as perfumes, also have a low A_w, as well as being antimicrobial in their own right.

Condensed-moisture films can develop with sufficiently high A_w on the surfaces of waxy cosmetics, such as lipsticks, or highly viscous formulations, such as toothpastes, or on compressed cosmetic powders to permit localized fungal growth. This can happen when they are persistently exposed to humid environments, such as steamy bathrooms, or if moisture is regularly applied by mouth or applicator during use. Growth of contaminants has occurred in condensed films under the tops of containers formed when hot aqueous products have been packed into cold containers. This effect can also result in appreciable dilution and loss of localized efficiency of any preservative present [84]. Should sparse fungal growth be initiated on marginally dried products or those which have become damp during storage, such as tablets packed in bulk, water generated by respiration will create locally raised A_w levels and initiate a cycle of enhanced rates of growth, leading to appreciable levels of spoilage [75].

pH

The optimum pH for bacterial growth is normally between 7.4 and 7.8. However, fungi prefer more acidic conditions of 6.5 to 7.0. At extremes outside the range pH 3 to 11, growth of most species is inhibited. The food industry's wide use of pH reduction or gas environment modification of redox potentials to control spoilage is more limited in application to medicines and cosmetics due to physiological acceptability and formulation stability. However, the pH of a product will influence the type of spoilage

that might be initiated, although this itself may result in a pH change, allowing other contaminants to take over. Thus, the low pH of fruit juice-flavored medicines may aid fungal spoilage but suppress bacterial growth, while the slightly alkaline antacid mixtures would favor the growth of pseudomonads and related bacteria. It is unlikely that the redox potential of most pharmaceuticals or cosmetics is likely to be low enough to favor anaerobic spoilage, as is seen in some foodstuffs.

Temperature

Low temperatures will slow growth and rising temperatures will increase growth. Above optimum temperatures, growth is inhibited and microbes will eventually be killed, however most microorganisms can survive at low temperatures even if they do not grow. Most fungi considered to be contaminants to pharmaceuticals and cosmetics are recovered at 25°C and bacteria at 30°C.

Low-temperature storage (8–12°C) is used to improve the short-term stability of some unpreserved, or weakly preserved, medicines, such as unpreserved eye drops [85] and reconstituted antibiotic syrups. Where dispensed products are to be "stored in a cool place" during use, the growth-inhibitory effect of the reduced temperature needs to be balanced against the consequent, and often significant, reduction in efficacy of any preservative present (see below).

The response of contaminants to the physicochemically complex environment of many pharmaceutical and cosmetic formulations will differ significantly from that in simple laboratory media [7], being markedly influenced by their spatial arrangement [86] and the phase status of the systems [87]. There are many reports of modified behavior of microorganisms at solid–liquid and liquid–liquid interfaces, but the evidence for increased resistance or longevity compared with freely planktonic situations is far from clear [88]. An increasing understanding of the survival strategies of microorganisms in sparse ecosystems [89] may provide an insight into the longevity of vegetative contaminants in seemingly unlikely products. For example *Salmonella* spp. in chocolate [90] and thyroid tablets [91] or vegetative bacteria in "dry" powdered ingredients such as plant material, starch, hydroxymethyl cellulose and gels such as aluminum hydroxide [92, 93].

Formulation effects on preservative efficacy

The choice of a preservative depends on many factors, including the intrinsic properties of the agent (see Chapters 2 and 5), the extrinsic environment (product formulation) and the nature of product usage. The factors influencing the efficacy of antimicrobial preservatives has been dealt with in detail elsewhere in this book (see Chapter 3) and include consideration of the concentration, temperature coefficients and environmental pH. These areas will be briefly reviewed in relation to formulation effects, together with a more detailed discussion on additional areas such as water availability, chemical interaction and stability, adsorption, partitioning in multiphase formulations and inactivation.

Concentration

The exponential effect of change in preservative concentration on microbial death is given by the equation $Cnt = k$, where C is the preservative concentration, n is the concentration exponent, t is time to achieve a certain kill effect and k is a constant. The concentration exponent is a measure of the effect of change in concentration or dilution on microbial death and will depend on the type of preservative being used [94, 95]. The activity of a preservative depends on the free concentration of the active form of the molecule in the aqueous phase and will be affected by partitioning in complex multiphase formulations and pH effects.

Partitioning

When preservatives are incorporated into multiphase formulations, their efficacy is generally markedly attenuated by a variety of competing interactive possibilities, which have been reviewed by Attwood and Florence [96], van Doorne [97] and Dempsey [98]. The partitioning of preservatives between oil and water phases will occur, in line with their partition coefficients, which may be different for commercial-grade systems from those of simple laboratory-devised oil–water mixtures of purified ingredients. Appreciable migration into oil phases of lipophilic preservatives, such as the parabens and phenolic agents, is likely, with less effect on the more hydrophilic preservatives, such as imidazolidinyl urea or the isothiazolinones. The oil:water ratio will also significantly influence the extent of overall migration, and there is the probability that localized preservative concentration will occur at the oil–water interface. Since microbes also concentrate at interfaces, there are reasonable theoretical grounds for anticipating enhanced activity here [96]. Some evidence for this was provided by Bean et al. [99], but was discounted by Dempsey [98].

When preservatives are added to complex formulations, the above phenomena are likely to interact competitively and the eventual distribution of preservative molecules by the different phenomena between the different ingredients and phases will be determined by the relative affinities of each for the other and the relative proportions of each. In highly viscous and complex systems, full equilibration might never happen within the life of the product. As contaminant microorganisms will represent a minute mass in proportion to the vast amounts of the other components, their "share" could be expected to be dramatically restricted in many situations. It is generally believed that the proportion of total added preservative responsible ("available") for any inhibition of contaminants is principally that which remains "free" or unbound to other ingredients in the aqueous phase [96–98]. Preservative molecules in the oil or micellar phases, or bound to other ingredients, are considered not to contribute directly, except that slow back-migration should occur as preservative concentrations become depleted in the aqueous phase. Experimental evidence for this is limited and might be difficult to obtain. However, there is very good indirect physicochemical evidence to support this contention.

Attempts have been made to develop equations to calculate probable free, or unbound, preservative concentrations, based on partition coefficients, oil:water ratios, solubilization constants and polymer-binding constants, which have been reviewed by Attwood and Florence [96]. For example, Mitchell and Kamzi [100] proposed equations such as the following for estimating the free or available preservative in the aqueous phase of an emulsified system:

$$C = C_w[1 + nK(M)/(1 + KC_w) + K_w^o\phi](1 + \phi)$$

where C is the gross concentration of preservative in the system; C_w is the "unbound" preservative in the aqueous phase; n is the number of binding sites on the surfactant; K is the association constant for the preservative and surfactant; M is the preservative:surfactant ratio for a given surfactant concentration; K_w^o is the oil:water partition coefficient; and ϕ is the oil:water phase ratio.

Mitchell and Kamzi were able to produce some correlation of experimentally determined measurements of bactericidal activity for chlorocresol in cetomacrogol emulsified systems with estimates obtained using their equations [101]. While these equations have been of value in resolving theoretical concerns and in providing some limited practical information, in general there is difficulty in obtaining adequate values for commercially available ingredients for them to be of general practical application. Another approach has been to estimate the unbound preservative in the aqueous phase by dialysis and measurement of the agent in the dialysate [96, 102], with some formulators believing that useful practical information can be obtained. Kurup et al. [103] compared estimates of "unbound" preservative in the aqueous phases of emulsified systems as obtained by equilibrium dialysis with direct measurements of antimicrobial activity. They reported that the efficacy of the emulsified systems was greater than that of the corresponding simple aqueous solutions containing those concentration of preservatives estimated from the dialysis determinations to be "available" in the aqueous phase of these systems.

pH

Environmental pH has an effect on the efficacy of many preservatives (see Table 17.1), predominantly through ionic changes and the impact this has on preservative potency and/or direct interaction with cellular target sites. Depending on the preservative's mode of action (see Chapter 5) some are active in the non-ionized state (benzoic and sorbic acid) and will have greatest potency at or below their pK_a. It is possible to determine the extent of ionization using the equation below and figures for pK_a can be found in various monographs [12, 42]:

Undissociated fraction of weak acid preservative
$$= 1/1 + \text{antilog}(pH - pK_a)$$

Temperature

The effect of temperature on preservative efficacy may be described by the equation,

$Q_{10} = t_{(T)}/t_{(T+10)}$

where Q_{10} is the change in activity per 10°C change in temperature, $t_{(T)}$ is the death time at temperature T°C and $t_{(T+10)}$ is the death time at $(T + 10)$°C.

Preservatives respond differently to temperature changes and this must be taken into account when predicting activity and when recommended storage temperatures are different to those of preservative efficacy testing conditions.

Water availability

It is commonly believed that preservatives are usually far less effective at low A_w and virtually inactive at the very low A_w levels expected of powders, tablets or capsules, although there is only limited published work to support this. Low levels of various electrolytes have long been known to influence the activity of phenolic disinfectants, often with enhancement of effect [104]. Cooper [105, 106] and Anagnostopoulos and Kroll [107] generally found marked reductions in the efficacy of phenolic and other disinfectants and preservatives in solutions with the A_w appreciably lowered by addition of higher concentrations of sucrose, glycerol and similar glycols. There is good anecdotal evidence that manufacturers generally find the efficacy of preservatives in syrups and cosmetics such as toothpastes to be appreciably weaker than in simple aqueous solutions with high A_w. Bos *et al.* [108] found that the incorporation of parabens and sorbate into lactose-starch tablets contaminated with *Bacillus brevis* spores did not reduce subsequent spore viability while maintained at a suitably low A_w. Ethylene oxide [109] and high temperatures [110] are markedly less effective as sterilizing agents for powders and "dry" products with very low A_w, when compared with medicines with high A_w. It might be extremely difficult to devise an experiment to evaluate fully the *in situ* efficacy of preservatives under the very low A_w conditions of powders on vegetative microbial cells, since attempts to assess survivors would generally raise A_w and activate the preservatives during the recovery phase. When the A_w of the external environment is lowered below the osmoregulatory capacity of a microbial cell by non-permeant solutes, growth and other activities cease or are reduced to very low levels. This is due to the inability of the cell to accumulate sufficient intracellular water for the necessary metabolic reactions to occur [111]. It is possible that the apparent minimal efficacy of preservatives at very low A_w indicates a similar critical influence of intracellular water levels upon antimicrobial reactions.

Chemical interactions

Preservatives can react with polymeric suspending and thickening agents, such as tragacanth, alginates, starch mucilage and polyethylene glycols, by displacement of water of hydration, even to the extent of forming insoluble sticky complexes [102, 112]. Cyclodextrins have also been found to interact with a variety of preservatives [113]. However, there are also reports of enhancement of activity for some preservative/polymer combinations [114].

The aqueous solubility of some commonly used preservatives is low and some form salts or complexes with very low-solubility products, which precipitate from solution. Thus, the usefulness of chlorhexidine is restricted by its ability to form insoluble products with chloride, sulfate, phosphate or citrate ions and anionic surfactants. Quaternary ammonium preservatives form insoluble complexes with anionic surfactants and a range of anionic inorganic ions. Benzoates and parabens form insoluble and discoloring complexes with iron salts, chlorocresol precipitates with phosphates, and phenylmercuric nitrate precipitates with chloride ions. Bronopol has formed complexes with unprotected aluminum in flexible tubes.

Adsorption

Adsorption on to the surfaces of suspended drug and cosmetic ingredients can also significantly reduce preservative efficacy. Examples include adsorption of parabens on to magnesium trisilicate [115] and other natural hydrocolloids [116], loss of chlorhexidine on to mineral earths, such as kaolin and calamine [117], parabens on to cosmetic pigments [118] and benzoic acid on to sulphadimidine particles [119] and various other incidences of adsorption [102]. In some cases, adsorption is followed by absorption into the solids to form a "solid" solution. This is a particular problem with preservatives and plastic containers. For example, phenolics and parabens absorb appreciably into nylon and plasticized PVC [120] and chlorobutanol is absorbed appreciably into polyethylene bottles during autoclaving [121]. Kakemi *et al.* [122] examined the absorption of parabens and benzalkonium chloride into various container plastics. Aspinall *et al.* [123] found that the absorption of phenylmercuric acetate into low-density polythene eye drop bottles could be inhibited by the presence of phosphate ions. Methods for assessing possible preservative–plastic interactions are provided by Wang and Chien [124].

Inactivation

As preservative molecules inactivate microorganisms, they themselves become inactivated and are no longer available to inhibit subsequent additions of contaminants. For those preservatives with high-concentration exponents, such as the phenolic agents, this steady depletion of available agent can result in significant attenuation in preservative efficacy during repeated use and in the contamination of multidose formulations. The relative nonspecificity of preservative reactivity will mean that appreciable preservative depletion will also occur from interaction with a significant amount of non-microbial detritus ("dirt") also introduced during repeated and prolonged use. This must be allowed for when deciding upon the necessary preservative capacity of a formulation at the design stage.

It is clear that effective preservation of complex formulations is only likely to be successful if there is a good appreciation of these interactive problems. Even then, it may not be possible to provide highly effective preservation for many multiphase systems without recourse to more potent preservatives whose enhanced antimicrobial potency is matched by unacceptable levels of irritancy. Provided the problem of preservation is fully explored at the earliest stages of formulation development, it is sometimes possible to reduce the worst interactive effects by knowledgeable selection of ingredients and preservative(s) to maximize the levels of "free" agent in the aqueous phase.

Chemical stability

Finally, the chemical stability of the preservative must also be considered, for example with respect to the processing procedures of the product. Thus, isothiazolinones [125] and bronopol [102] deteriorate significantly if processing temperatures exceed 55°C. Chlorobutanol is unstable around neutral or alkaline pH and suffers appreciable destruction at autoclaving temperatures [121]. Unless light-proof containers are used, the photocatalyzed deterioration of preservatives such as the phenolics and quaternary ammonium and organomercurial agents may become significant. Paraben loss will occur by steam distillation at process temperatures approaching 100°C and has poor stability in slightly alkaline and above products [126]. Transesterification between parabens and polyols, such as sorbitol, may occur and result in significant loss of activity [127]. Alternatively, the formaldehyde-releasing agents depend on suitable conditions to provide a slow, steady decomposition and release of formaldehyde. This ensures preservative protection over the full life of the product, without too rapid a conversion early on in the product's life leaving little reservoir for the later stages of use; an example is pH 5–6.5 for bronopol [128]. It cannot be presumed that preservative degradation products will be inert. Thus, an excessive rate of formaldehyde release might create undue irritancy, and bronopol degradation releases nitrite ions, which might result in the formation of potentially toxic nitrosamines if ingredients such as amine soaps are present in the formulation or if it comes into contact with dietary amines [21, 128].

Use of preservatives in medicines and cosmetics

The preceding sections of this chapter have indicated not only that the survival of contaminant microorganisms in medicines and cosmetics may present serious risks for both users and the formulations themselves, but also that the use of antimicrobial agents to limit these risks will introduce additional problems. This is due to the relatively non-specific interactive nature of preservatives, readily combining as they do with formulation ingredients and users, as well as microbial contaminants.

There is general acceptance that preservatives should only be included in formulations to deal with possible contamination during storage or use of a product. Formulations that require a preservative generally fall into two categories: (i) those that are required to be sterile but are delivered in multidose containers (e.g. injections, eye drops/ointments, applications to wounds) where the preservative is necessary to ensure safety throughout its use; and (ii) those that are not required to be sterile but must

maintain organisms at an acceptable level to prevent spoilage and/or the delivery of high levels of microorganisms or specific pathogens to the recipient.

Concerns over preservative toxicity by medicine licensing authorities means that applicants for marketing authorizations must fully justify the inclusion or exclusion of any preservative in a formulation, and are expected to adopt alternative strategies for product protection where realistic. With cosmetics, regulatory attitudes often differ, placing the emphasis upon the use of preservatives with acceptable levels of toxicity at specified concentrations, and placing exclusions on others. There must therefore be a balance between the presence of microorganisms with their potential infective risks and the toxicity of the preservative.

It is essential that adequate precautions be taken in the manufacture and packaging of medicines and cosmetics to minimize the access of microorganisms. Awareness of the microbial quality of raw materials is essential, especially those of natural origin which may have a high initial microbial load. For UK medicines, the British Pharmacopoeia (BP) indicates microbial limits for raw materials both in terms of bioburden and absence of particular organisms (Table 17.3). Good manufacturing practice (GMP) also includes attention to atmospheric control, appropriate design of premises and equipment processes and training of staff [4, 5].

Sterile products must demonstrate, by the sterility test or validation of the sterilization process, that when released for use they contain no viable microorganisms. Sterile products being used for multidose purposes and non-sterile products containing a preservative must then demonstrate adequate preservation throughout their use by adherence to the efficacy of antimicrobial preservation test (see below). Non-sterile finished products

Table 17.3 Microbiological test requirements for selected raw materials (adapted from European Pharmacopoeia 2010 texts).

Raw material	TAMC	TYMC	Absence of
Acacia	10^4	10^2	*Escherichia coli, Salmonella*
Agar	10^3	10^2	*E. coli, Salmonella*
Alginic acid	10^2		*E. coli, Salmonella*
Aluminum hydroxide	10^3	10^2	*E. coli*, bile-tolerant Gram-negative bacteria
Bentonite	10^3		
Gelatin	10^3	10^2	*E. coli, Salmonella*
Kaolin	10^3	10^2	
Lactose	10^2		*E. coli*
Pancreatin			*E. coli, Salmonella*
Sterculia			*E. coli*
Talc, purified (cutaneous use)	10^2		
Talc, purified (oral use)	10^3	10^2	
Tragacanth	10^4	10^2	*E. coli, Salmonella*
Xanthan gum	10^3	10^2	

TAMC, total aerobic microbial count (cfu/g or cfu/ml); TYMC, total yeast/mold count (cfu/g or cfu/ml).

Table 17.4 Acceptance criteria for microbiological quality of non-sterile dosage forms (adapted from European Pharmacopoeia 2010 texts).

Route of administration	TAMC	TYMC	Specified microorganisms
Oral, non-aquous	10^3	10^2	Absence of *Escherichia coli*
Oral, aqueous	10^2	10^1	Absence of *E. coli*
Rectal	10^3	10^2	
Oromucosa, nasal, auricular	10^2	10^1	Absence of *Staphylococcus aureus*, *Pseudomonas aeruginosa*
Vaginal	10^2	10^1	Absence of *S. aureus*, *P. aeruginosa*, *Candida albicans*
Transdermal patches	10^2	10^1	Absence of *S. aureus*, *P. aeruginosa*
Inhalation	10^2	10^1	Absence of *S. aureus*, *P. aeruginosa*, bile-tolerant Gram-negative bacteria
Oral, natural raw materials[a]	10^4	10^2	Absence of *E. coli*, *Salmonella*, *S. aureus*, $\leq 10^2$ cfu bile-tolerant Gram-negative bacteria
Herbal medicines, boiling water added	10^7	10^5	$\leq 10^2$ cfu *E. coli*
Herbal medicines, no boiling water added	10^5	10^4	Absence of *E. coli*, *Salmonella*, $\leq 10^3$ cfu bile-tolerant Gram-negative bacteria

TAMC, total aerobic microbial count (cfu/g or cfu/ml); TYMC, total yeast/mold count (cfu/g or cfu/ml).

[a]Special EP provisions for oral dosage forms containing raw materials of natural origin where antimicrobial pretreatment is not feasible and where the TAMC of raw material exceeding 10^3 cfu is acceptable.

must also adhere to certain regulatory guidelines on total viable counts (TVC) and the absence of particular objectionable microbial species (Table 17.4). Total bioburden is an indication of the "cleanliness" of the material and objectional organisms are indicative of pathogenic or opportunistic pathogens. Unfortunately the requirements of various National Pharmacopoeias differ and limits applied "in-house" must often be based on a compilation of official critieria. The International Conference on Harmonization (ICH) was set up in the late 1990s to harmonize pharmacopoeial criteria between Europe (EP), USA (USP) and Japan (JP) and is currently still in progress. Within the UK, if a monograph is present in the EP it will take precedence over a BP monograph.

In general, the more potent antimicrobial agents are usually associated with problems of toxicity. There is only a limited range of materials with both reasonable preservative efficacy and acceptably low toxicity, and extremely few with sufficient potential to kill bacterial spores. In complex multiphase formulations, attenuating preservative interactions are so appreciable that it can be very difficult to achieve more than weak antimicrobial efficacy. This is reflected in the low efficacy criteria set for creams by the BP, and other pharmacopoeias, efficacy test protocols (see below). The difficulty of adequately balancing efficacy with toxicity considerations has led to an almost complete shift from preserved multidose units to sterile single-dosage forms for parenteral

medicines [10]. Occasionally, a higher risk of infection for a product justifies the use of preservatives considered too toxic for general application, such as the allowance by the US Food and Drug Administration (FDA) of organomercurial preservatives for cosmetics to be used around the eye, but not for other body-area products [21].

The longer a product is in use, the greater the opportunity for contamination to accumulate and the chance of growth and spoilage to ensue. Medicines prepared extemporaneously under Section 10 exemption of the Medicines Act (1968) are dispensed with short shelf-lives in an attempt to reduce the risk of growth and contamination. Oldham and Andrews [85] found that contamination could be held at reasonable levels in many types of unpreserved eye drops for up to 7 days, provided they were also stored in a refrigerator.

Medicines
Parenterals

Due to concerns over toxicity and the build-up of contamination in multidose vials [129], preserved multidose containers of injections have been largely replaced by sterile single-dose units without the need for preservatives, leaving only multidose units for parenterals such as campaign vaccines and insulin [130]. Organomercurial preservatives are rarely used in new formulations due to concerns of toxicity and have been replaced mainly with benzyl alcohol, phenol, phenoxyethanol and occasionally parabens [131]. Thiomersal has long been used in the preparation and preservation of vaccines and there is some suggestion that it has a positive effect on the efficacy of the antigen. Although no evidence of harm is presented it is discouraged for use in infant and toddler preparations and a general move towards its removal from formulations is supported, although the issues of reformulation and validation are acknowledged. However "the balance of risks and benefits of thiomersal-containing vaccines is considered positive" by current government guidelines [132]. Benzyl alcohol is still used, but not for injections that might be used in children. Preservatives are not permitted in solutions for direct injection into spinal, cranial or ophthalmic tissues, or in doses of greater than 15 ml, where the risks of toxic damage become greater [133, 134]. As a consequence, these must always be supplied as single-use vials or ampoules. Preservatives are no longer included in oily injections, as they are considered to be ineffective in non-aqueous systems (see Chapter 3).

Eye drops

Multidose containers of eye drops are still widely supplied for domestic use, due the perceived high cost of single-dose units. These require good preservative protection to minimize the appreciable risk of infections from organisms such as *Pseudomonas* and *Staphylococcus* [135], to which the damaged eye is particularly susceptible. Benzalkonium chloride, often in combination with ethylenediamine tetraacetic acid (EDTA), now appears to be the most commonly used preservative, with chlorhexidine and organomercurials occasionally reported [10].

However, concern at the appreciable damaging effect of quaternary ammonium antimicrobial agents on the cornea and their involvement in "dry eye" syndrome has resulted in the widespread use of unpreserved eye drops and artificial tears, usually in single-dosage units, for people suffering from this and related problems [136].

Creams

The complex distribution of preservatives in creams makes it difficult to obtain rapid inactivation of contamination. However, the major risk is seen as that of spoilage rather than of infection, and the poor levels of inactivation achieved with those preservatives considered to be sufficiently non-irritant for medicinal use, is accepted by licensing authorities as the best that is possible. Parabens are again by far the most commonly used preservative, with chlorocresol and benzyl alcohol lagging well behind [10]. Formaldehyde-releasing agents are used, but not widely, and the isothiazolinones are not considered suitable for potentially damaged skin. Most non-aqueous ointments are unpreserved, as the risk of accumulation and replication of contaminants is considered to be low. For high-risk areas, such as the eye, sterile ointments are used. Many UK medicinal creams and ointments which might be used on damaged skin are supplied to microbial specifications approaching those for sterile products.

Orals

Parabens are also the most commonly used preservative for oral aqueous medicines, probably due to their long usage with apparent safety [137] and the need to perform expensive oral toxicological evaluation if replacement systems are used. Weakly alkaline medicines, such as antacid suspensions, are difficult to preserve as parabens are relatively unstable at these pH levels [138]. Chloroform has been an excellent preservative for oral products supplied in well-sealed containers and with a short use life, but it is now banned in some countries over fears of toxicity. Although it may still be used as a preservative in UK medicines it is unlikely to pass regulatory approval as a new product constituent. Oral medicines supplied as a dry powder for reconstitution prior to use usually require a preservative to cope with possible in-use contamination once dispensed. Many contain parabens, although the presence of large amounts of sugar or other solutes to provide a low A_w solution for additional protection against spoilage, as well as for taste, often reduces their efficacy.

Tablets

There are suggestions that the inclusion of preservatives into tablets would give protection should they become damp during storage or use [80]. Bos *et al.* [108] suggested that this might be appropriate for tablets for use in tropical and humid environments. However, if tablets became damp, they would be inherently spoiled as the low A_w also offers protection against non-biological degradation, which is accelerated in the presence of water, as well as being physically damaged. Whiteman [79] has recommended the use of water vapor-resistant film coatings to reduce vapor uptake and assist in the maintenance of low A_w for bulk-packed tablets. The main protection must, however, remain adequate A_w reduction during manufacture and the use of water vapor-resistant packaging. It is understood that the UK licensing authorities will not condone the incorporation of preservatives into new tablet formulations.

Some medicinal ingredients have an intrinsic capability to inactivate likely microbial contamination, and no additional preservative is then necessary. Thus, lindane cream, some alkaloid solutions, furosemide (frusemide) injection, some local anesthetic injections and some broad-spectrum antibiotic creams are able to cope with contaminants adequately without the need for additional preservation. However, the mere presence of an antibiotic should not be presumed automatically to provide an adequate spectrum of preservative cover; there is still the need for a full efficacy-testing program.

Cosmetics

There is some difference of approach to the preservation of cosmetics compared with that for medicines. It is generally accepted that cosmetics are for use on a more restricted range of body sites involving healthy skin, and occasionally membranes, or around undamaged eyes, with lower risks of infection from contaminants than for some medicinal routes of administration. Contamination and spoilage possibilities for some cosmetics, however, may be high, due to their physicochemical complexity and the high potential for consumer abuse, such as regular fingering, repeated contact with saliva, repeated and communal application and possibilities for in-use dilution of remaining product, such as for shampoos or soap in the shower [139]. Although some manufacturers do not include preservatives in formulations such as dusting powders, block cosmetics, lipsticks, stick deodorants or alcohol-based perfumes with low A_w, many others do so for added reassurance and to cater for in-use abuse. Considerations of preservative toxicity, irritancy and sensitizing potential take into account the duration of contact and regularity of use on healthy skin for stay-on cosmetics, and the general levels of adverse reactions to other formulation ingredients. Higher levels of potentially more problematic preservatives may be used in rinse-off cosmetics, where the period of contact may be short and significant dilution will take place during application. Accordingly, many agents are used which would be considered too toxic for medicinal applications. Where the risk of infection by contaminants is deemed to be higher than for most situations, preservatives with greater efficiency may be used, despite their increased toxicity potential, such as the use of organomercurial agents in eye-area cosmetics.

Voluntary disclosure to the FDA revealed the use of over 100 preservatives for cosmetics in the USA [140, 141]. Parabens were by far the most commonly used preservatives, followed by imidazolidinyl urea, isothiazolinones, Quaternium 15, formaldehyde, phenoxyethanol and bronopol. The range of preservatives now in use in the EU is considerably less, but it is believed that those in most common usage are comparable to those in the USA, with parabens still topping the range. Sterile cosmetics are not in common use, except for eye conditioning, brightening and coloring drops, which should be supplied sterile, and preserved if in multidose containers. The range of preservatives and their applicability to cosmetic protection is indicated in the new Cosmetic Product Regulation (see below) and references [142, 143].

Other attempts to reduce in-use contamination include the replacement of wide-mouthed jars (with ready access for fingers) by flexible tubes for creams and ointments, the redesign of bottles to reduce the accumulation of liquid residues around the mouth and neck and the introduction of plastic "squeezy" eye drop bottles instead of the conventional glass-dropper bottles [144]. Brannan and Dille [145] also found that slit-top and pump-action closures provided greater protection for shampoo and skin lotion than a conventional screw-cap closure. Wet in-use bars of soap have also been recognized as a source of microbes and there has been a move towards liquid soap dispensers in an attempt to reduce hand contamination.

Potentiation and synergy

There have been numerous attempts to enhance preservative efficacy by using preservatives in combination with each other or together with various potentiators [146]. For this strategy to be successfully applied, there must be clear evidence of enhancement for any selected combination, rather than the creation of multi-component preservative systems on the basis of wishful thinking.

It is generally believed that, by using combinations of parabens, each approaching its aqueous solubility maximum, greater levels of unbound paraben will remain in the aqueous phase of multiphase systems, with some evidence that this offers enhanced preservative protection for such formulations [147]. It may also be possible to reduce the extent of such migration into the lipophilic regions by the addition of hydrophilic co-solvents to modify oil:water and micellar distribution coefficients more in favor of preservative retention in the aqueous phase. For example, Darwish and Bloomfield [148] were able to improve the efficacy of parabens in an emulsion by the incorporation of modest concentrations of ethanol, propylene glycol or glycerol as hydrophilic co-solvents.

Individual preservatives are sometimes less effective against certain microbial species than others, and the careful selection of preservative combinations can offer protection from a wider range of likely contaminants. Thus, it is believed that mixtures of methyl, propyl and butyl parabens have a wider combined antimicrobial spectrum than each individual ester alone [147]. Imidazolidinyl ureas have weak antifungal properties and parabens are less effective against pseudomonads, but combinations of both yield usefully improved protection against both contaminants [149]. Combinations of parabens with phenoxyethanol are also reported to provide a wider spectrum of activity than either alone [150].

The effectiveness of some preservatives can be enhanced by the presence of a variety of materials which in themselves are not strongly antimicrobial. Thus, the chelating agent EDTA usefully potentiates the activity of quaternary ammonium agents, ethanol, parabens, phenolics and sorbic acid among others [151], and is now used to a significant extent in cosmetic formulations. It is also used to potentiate various preservative systems towards pseudomonads and similar microorganisms in medicines, particularly those for use in and around the eyes [152]. Essential oils and fragrances [153] and humectants, such as glycerol and propylene glycol, in modest concentration can assist in overall protection. The gallate ester antioxidants, butylated hydroxyanisole (BHT) and butylated hydroxytoluene (BHA) also reveal modest antimicrobial activity, which can assist conventional antimicrobial preservatives [154].

Biochemical explanations for such enhancements of antimicrobial activity are not always clear. However, in a number of cases, there is good evidence to indicate that enhancement is related to the ability of chaotropic agents, such as EDTA, to disorganize lipopolysaccharides in the outer membranes of Gram-negative bacteria, a well-known barrier to the penetration of many agents [155]. Phenoxyethanol [156] and benzalkonium chloride [155] are known to disrupt the barrier properties of the cytoplasmic membrane. In both cases, this would then aid greater penetration of the main preservative to its site of lesion. In other cases, such as the synergy of chlorocresol with phenylethanol [157] and acetates with lactates or propionates [158], there are indications of more specific mechanistic interactions.

Synergy is the activity observed with combinations of agents greater than that anticipated from the sum of their activities when individually applied. It is often confused with cases where a widening of antimicrobial spectrum, or simple addition, has been observed. True synergism is often species-specific and most apparent at quite specific ratios of the agents involved. Practically useful examples of preservative synergy include mixtures of parabens [159], parabens with imidazolidinyl ureas [149], parabens with phenoxyethanol [150], chlorocresol with phenoxyethanol [157], parabens with acrylic acid homopolymers and copolymers [159], and others [142]. Laboratory techniques, such as those described by Pons *et al.* [160] and Gilliland *et al.* [159], often demonstrate synergy between combinations of antimicrobial agents, although only a few prove to be of effective value in practical situations. It is therefore essential to confirm any apparent indications of synergy by full testing in complete formulations before placing any commercial reliance upon them.

Antagonism between preservatives is uncommon [160], but there are reports of antagonism between sorbic acid and parabens [161] and between benzalkonium chloride and chlorocresol [160].

The limited list of currently authorized preservatives is likely to increase the use of combinations of preservatives and enhancers. This approach together with hurdle technology is also a likely way forward to exploit the use of low-level chemical preservation [162].

Regulatory aspects of the preservation of medicines and cosmetics

European Community Directives are legislative instruments and must be implemented into national legislation within a defined period of time. The EC Directive 65/65/EEC (1965) laid down original standards and procedures for the safe and effective use of medicines within the EU and was reflected in the UK Medicines Act 1968. A marketing authorization from the relevant licensing authority must be obtained before a company can market a product. Detailed scrutiny of the quality, safety and efficacy data for the product will be examined and this will include any data on excipients such as preservatives. In the UK the regulatory authority is the Medicines and Healthcare Products Regulatory Agency (MHRA), however European-wide approval may now also be obtained through relevant member state mutual recognition procedures or alternatively as a centralized submission to the Committee for Medicinal Products for Human Use (CHMP) Scientific Committee, overseen by the European Medicine Agency (EMEA). An analogous system operates in the USA for medicines via the Federal Food, Drug, and Cosmetic Act, as Amended (Title 21 USC, 350 *et seq.*), enforced through the FDA. Similar control of medicines in Japan is made under the Pharmaceutical Affairs Law (No. 96, 2002), administered through the Pharmaceutical and Food Safety Bureau.

Specific formal control of cosmetic safety across the EU commenced in 1976 with Council Directive 76/768/EEC, followed subsequently by the new Cosmetic Product Regulation 1223/2009, which aims to phase out animal testing by 2013. From January 1997, disclosure of cosmetic ingredients including preservatives had to be made on labels [163]. Cosmetics in the UK are controlled under the Cosmetic Products Regulation and are regulated via the Department of Industry. There are obligations for suitable qualified persons to carry out safety assessments for the manufacturer to maintain detailed product and processing information in a product information pack (PIP). However, regulatory action can only be taken once the product is offered for sale and believed to be defective. In the USA, cosmetics are regulated by the FDA through the Federal Food, Drug, and Cosmetic Act (2002); again action can only be taken once the product is offered for sale and is believed unsafe. There are only limited lists of banned substances and no formal ingredient recommendations are made.

Japanese control of cosmetics is made through the same laws as for medicine (Pharmaceutical Affairs Law, established in 1960) where prior approval by the Pharmaceutical and Food Safety Bureau is required before a cosmetic may be placed on the Japanese market.

The following publications provide a wider insight into the legislative arena: EU and UK medicines [164, 165], EU cosmetics (Cosmetics Products Regulation 2009), USA medicines and cosmetics (http://fda.gov; [166]) and Japanese regulations [167].

Regulatory bodies generally place the onus on applicants to fully justify the safety, effectiveness and stability of a proposed medicine, including the steps that have been taken to assess and minimize the risks of microbial contamination and spoilage by all relevant means. Where preservatives are deemed necessary, preservative efficacy tests must demonstrate adequate protection throughout the life of the product, and success in the appropriate national pharmacopoeial efficacy test is usually taken as a minimum requirement. Evidence of the safety of any preservatives used is also required, together with reasons for inclusion, details of labeling and methods of control in the finished product. Lists of approved preservatives are rarely issued, although some official compendia, such as pharmacopoeias, may give indications of possible preservatives for various purposes. Acceptance of the suitability of the proposals, including preservatives, usually depends on the panels of experts, who assess the choices in the light of the desirable balanced against the possible. When a preservative system is chosen which has been in common usage for similar medicines, the amount of toxicological data required by licensing authorities is usually considerably less than that for newer and less established preservatives. This tends to encourage applicants to go for the former, despite the possible advantages of the latter. The high cost of extensive toxicological testing for preservatives has minimized the likelihood of novel agents being brought into use. In both the EU and the UK, there is an obligation on producers of cosmetics to include microbiological risk assessments in the development process, to take steps to limit such risks and to record this in the PIP. The choice of preservatives is restricted by lists of banned, approved, provisionally approved and restricted-use preservatives. The FDA strongly recommends that preservative tests are carried out to prevent subsequent product failure and prosecution should defective products be offered for sale. Applications for cosmetic product licenses in Japan must include full risk assessments for microbiological problems, including details of preservative efficacy testing and a full toxicity evaluation. Restrictive lists of approved ingredients are published.

Various other regulations will have an impact on preservative usage, such as the banning of chloroform as a preservative, except for medicines in the UK (SI 1979 No. 382) and in all products in the USA, due to some reports of carcinogenicity in animals. Detailed environmental impact assessments will be required for preservatives (and other ingredients) under environmental protection legislation being brought into effect in most western countries, since cosmetic and medicinal components will eventually be disposed of into the biosphere. Increasingly strict direct product liability laws may offer a clearer route to compensation for users who believe they have suffered damage from a microbiologically inadequate medicine or cosmetic. International reviews of the legislation and impact relating to damage from contact dermatitis have been made by Frosch and Rycroft [168] and Hogan and Ledet [169].

Prediction of preservative efficacy

Due to the many interactive possibilities for both microorganisms and preservatives in complex formulations (see above), it is almost impossible to predict, with any reasonable degree of precision, the ultimate effectiveness of a preservative in all but the simplest solutions. It is therefore necessary to obtain some assurance of likely in-use and abuse performance, by conducting a direct microbiological preservative efficacy test on the complete formulation. Detailed reviews of such test procedures and the problems associated with them have been made by Baird [170] for medicines and by Brannan [171], Perry [172] and Leak et al. [173] for cosmetics, while Hopton and Hill [174] reviewed test methodology for a wider range of commercial materials.

Most conventional preservative efficacy testing protocols share common features and intentions, although the fine details and interpretation of the results vary significantly. Aliquots of complete formulations should be tested in their final containers, where possible, as these can influence overall efficacy [145, 175]. The testing of diluted cosmetic products should also be considered where dilution in use might occur, such as with shampoos in bottles or bars of soap taken into the shower or bath, as well as the addition of an organic load to simulate in-use soiling [143, 171, 176]. Formulations without preservative should be examined for possible inherent inhibitory activity. Samples should be tested within a general stability test program to determine whether preservative efficacy will remain throughout the intended life of the product. A limited range of test microorganisms, representative of likely contaminants, is usually selected from official culture collections, and often supplemented in individual companies with known problem strains such as osmophilic yeasts for sugary formulations, "wild" strains from the factory environment or those isolated from previously spoiled batches [177]. Usually, only elementary methods of cultivation and harvesting of inocula are used, despite much evidence that even minor variations here can dramatically influence the antimicrobial sensitivity of the resultant test suspension [178, 179]. In general, routine cultivation is well known to attenuate survival and spoilage potential appreciably, and numerous attempts have been made to develop maintenance systems that retain the aggressiveness of wild isolates, often with only limited success. Thus, Spooner and Croshaw [177] cultivated contaminant isolates in unpreserved product, and Flawn et al. [180] maintained the shampoo-degrading activity of tapwater isolates by routine cultivation in mineral salt media containing anionic surfactants. The ability of pseudomonads and related environmental isolates to degrade parabens, phenolic preservatives and a variety of surfactants could be retained over considerable periods by routine cultivation in minimal liquid media containing the agents as the primary carbon source.

Formulations are usually challenged by intimate mixing with the microbial suspensions and incubation at temperatures relevant to likely use conditions. Where solid formulations (e.g. powders or cakes), oily or waxy products (e.g. lipsticks), viscous creams or gels are to be examined, it may be necessary first to disperse them in an aqueous medium; this can be done either directly or with the aid of a dispersant such as a surfactant. For some solid products (e.g. soap bars), however, direct surface inoculation is a more realistic option [172, 181]. Single-species inocula are more commonly used than mixed challenges, although there might be potential advantages to multiple-species inoculation. The latter is not generally used for medicines [170] but is often used for cosmetic testing [173, 181, 182]. Inocula are commonly added as a single large challenge (single-challenge testing) and monitored for inhibition over a specified period. Multiple challenges (repeat-challenge testing), which repeat the inoculation at set intervals for a specified number of cycles or until the product fails, are also used, particularly for cosmetics [177, 183, 184].

Preservative efficacy is estimated by cultivating and counting survivors from small aliquots of the inoculated formulation added to culture media, either by conventional colony formation or via membrane filtration or by using most probable number schemes with liquid media [185]. This presumes an initial uniform distribution of inoculum and any subsequent growth in the product, both assumptions being unlikely to be correct [171]. Neutralization of residual preservative must be ensured before recovery is undertaken. Appropriate neutralizers have been documented [186], however work carried out by Johnston et al. [187] describes a rapid method to assist in the choice. Many of the standard laboratory media are somewhat stressful to damaged microorganisms [188]. Confirmation must be sought that the recovery procedures are capable of resuscitating viable but damaged microorganisms, and that they are not inhibitory.

For the purpose of preservative efficacy testing of medicines, products are divided into groups, each having their own compliance criteria (Table 17.5). The number of categories described in the BP [189], EP [190] and USP [191] monographs are now similar after changes to the USP (although the content of some groups vary), although compliance criteria are still less stringent in the USP. The basic test uses four stock cultures of *Aspergillus niger*, *Candida albicans*, *Pseudomonas aeruginosa* and *S. aureus*, which may be supplemented with other strains or species that may represent likely challenges for that product. Most monographs will detail the "preparation of inoculum" as variation in this can have a considerable effect on preservative sensitivity. Studies have been carried out to validate alternative preparative methods [192]. A single challenge of 10^5–10^6 microorganisms/g (or ml) of formulation is used; the product is incubated at 20–25°C and aliquots are tested for survivors at specified intervals by conventional plate count or membrane-filtration techniques. Two levels of criteria, A and B, are given for acceptable performance in the test – level A being the recommended level of efficiency, except where this is not possible for reasons such as toxicity, and then level B applies. The relatively weak compliance criteria for some formulations are indicative of the problems in achieving adequate preservative efficacy in complex products and potential toxicity issues.

Table 17.5 Compliance criteria for the efficacy of antimicrobial preservation, European Pharmacopoeia 2010.

Type of product	Type of inoculum	Level criteria	Required log$_{10}$ reduction of inoculum by time shown					
			6 h	1 day	2 days	7 days	14 days	28 days
Parenteral and ophthalmic preparations	Bacteria	A	2	3	–	–	–	NR
		B	–	1	–	3	–	NI
	Fungi	A	–	–	–	2	–	NI
		B	–	–	–	–	1	NI
Oral preparations	Bacteria		–	–	–	–	3	NI
	Fungi		–	–	–	–	1	NI
Topical preparations	Bacteria	A	–	–	2	3	–	NI
		B	–	–	–	–	3	NI
	Fungi	A	–	–	–	–	2	NI
		B	–	–	–	–	1	NI

NI, no increase in numbers over previous count; NR, no organisms to be recovered.

Although preservative efficacy evaluation with panels of volunteers, using test formulations under controlled conditions, is not generally realistic for medicines, this type of follow-up test is quite common for cosmetics [193, 194]. Thus, Farrington *et al.* [195] developed a panel test whereby volunteers applied the test products for a specified number of times to axillary areas, ensuring that the application fingers came into contact with residual product. Formulations were then examined for any accumulated contamination. There is some agreement that results obtained from in-use panel tests do show a reasonable correlation with estimates obtained from *in vitro* challenge testing and general in-use performance for cosmetics, including the ability to differentiate between products which subsequently perform well during use and those which do not [171, 194–196]. Spooner and Davison [197] compared the performance of an extensive array of medicines in the BP efficacy test with levels of contamination detected in used and returned medicines. They concluded that compliance in the official test generally indicated products that would perform adequately in the marketplace. Fels *et al.* [198] determined that a wide range of European preserved medicines found to be microbiologically reliable over many years gave predictive indications of failure when submitted retrospectively to the BP efficacy test. Applicants for marketing authorization in the UK for a new medicine must normally demonstrate that, if a preservative is necessary, the product at least satisfies the basic compliance criteria of the BP test, as the licensing authority believes that this gives a reasonable estimate of likely microbial stability in use. Orth has promoted an alternative to the conventional challenge test, in that, although the methodology is comparable, formal decimal reduction times (*D*-values) are determined for the inactivation of inocula, and predictions on the efficacy of formulations are obtained by extrapolation of data to estimate times of contact necessary to yield prescribed log levels of reduction [199]. Although there is some evidence to show that reliable information can be obtained for preliminary screening purposes, the short time of the test protocol necessitates additional testing to check for possible regrowth phenomena after long delays.

Conventional preservative challenge test procedures are time consuming and expensive, so attempts have been made to develop and assess alternatives [186, 200]. Impedance changes during the growth and death of microorganisms can be detected and used for rapid preservative efficacy screening [201, 202]. Other methods to estimate cell viability such as direct epifluorescence (DEF) and adenosine triphosphate (ATP) bioluminescence have been examined and considered unlikely alternatives to positron emission tomography (PET) [203]. However, more recent workers have included them together with flow cytometry, polymerase chain reaction (PCR) and immunoassays as rapid methods in use for the microbiological surveillance of pharmaceuticals, ultimately leading to real-time monitoring [204].

Adverse reactions of users to preservatives

The non-specific and reactive nature of preservatives not only results in interaction with many formulation ingredients (see above), but is also reflected by incidences of adverse reactions of users to preserved products. Significant incidences of senitization and dermatitis have been recorded to most of the commonly used preservatives at a frequency of approximately 0.5–1.0% of those tested. However, this needs to be seen in the context of overall levels of around 5% senitization to all cosmetic ingredients [205–208]. Regulatory activity exerts appreciable control to limit the risks of adverse reactions, by detailed specification of toxicity testing requirements, as well as attempting to allay public concerns over the use of animals for the purpose [209]. Screening studies of sensitivity are periodically carried out and highlight emerging allergens. For example, increased sensitivity to methyl-dibromoglutaronitrile was reported [210, 211], resulting in the

European Commission performing an expert review on its safety [212]. A more recent UK review of preservative sensitivity by patch testing identified formaldehyde and the isothiazolines as having the highest positive rates and chloroxylenol the lowest, with parabens having the highest irritancy rate [213]. The risk of preservative damage will be related to the frequency and duration of product contact, the route and site of administration as well as the concentration of preservative used. Thus, preservatives in rinse-off shampoos might be expected to present lower risks of senitization than those in prolonged-contact products, such as stay-on creams. Direct injection into the central nervous system or ophthalmic tissue is far more likely to be damaging than administration by the oral or topical routes.

This section can only illustrate the problems with selected examples, and interested readers are directed to the reviews of D'Arcy [214], de Groot and White [205] and Goon [215] for a more detailed treatment of the topic.

Injections preserved with chlorocresol, chlorobutanol, benzyl alcohol and organomercurials have all induced appreciable hypersensitivity and severe adverse reactions [216, 217]. Benzyl alcohol has been of particular concern with small children, who are unable to metabolize it effectively, and a number of neonatal deaths have been attributed to its use [218, 219]. A variety of eye-damaging reactions have been reported due to preservatives in multidose eye drops, and the particularly distressing condition of "dry eye" has been related to their use [220]. Benzalkonium chloride and other quaternary ammonium preservatives have been found to be particularly damaging to the cornea, by interfering with tear-film stability and direct toxic effects on the cells [221, 222]. Their use with local anesthetic eye drops (which reduce the blink reflex and therefore prolong contact time) is discouraged due to the risk of increased toxicity; single-use minims without preservatives are recommended instead. Nebulizers containing antimicrobials have also induced bronchoconstriction in asthmatic patients [57, 223, 224].

The parabens are by far the most commonly used preservatives in cosmetics and pharmaceuticals, reflecting their ability to meet many of the criteria associated with an ideal preservative, despite possessing only modest preservative efficacy [141, 208, 225]. Formaldehyde-releasing agents have been regarded as very effective preservatives for rinse-off cosmetics, but fears over carcinogenicity and sensitivity [211, 213] have limited their use. Topical medicines are implicated as the cause of 14–40% of all allergic contact dermatitis reports, the majority of these, however, being related to the therapeutic agents. There is a rather limited range of preservatives used in medicines, parabens paradoxically are the most commonly used but are reported as the most common irritant [213] and are generally well tolerated [137]. The majority of contact dermatitis reactions recede once the offending product is identified and use ceases. However, re-exposure to the preservative in another formulation will usually provoke further adverse effects [205].

Systemic damage from the topical application of preservatives is rare, but there are reports of serious to fatal reactions from skin absorption following the use of cord dusting powders containing hexachlorophene on neonates and its application to burned and damaged skin or mucous membranes [226]. More recently, reports relating to both parabens [227] and tricolsan [228] have been associated with antiandrogenic effects and the topical administration of parabens through underarm body care products with breast cancer [229].

References

1 Frick, E.W. (1992) *Cosmetic and Toiletry Formulations*, 2nd edn, Noyes Publications, Park Ridge, NJ.

2 Lund, W. (ed.) (1994) *The Pharmaceutical Codex*, 12th edn, Pharmaceutical Press, London.

3 Clegg, A. and Perry, B.F. (1996) Control of microbial contamination during manufacture, in *Microbial Quality Assurance in Cosmetics, Toiletries and Non-Sterile Pharmaceuticals*, 2nd edn (eds R.M. Baird and S.F. Bloomfield), Taylor & Francis, Basingstoke, pp. 49–66.

4 Medicines and Healthcare Products Regulatory Agency (2007) *Rules and Guidance for Pharmaceutical Manufacturers and Distributors*, The Stationary Office, London.

5 Beaney, A.M. (ed.) (2006) *Quality Assurance of Aseptic Preparation Services*, 4th edn, Pharmaceutical Press, London.

6 Kirsch, L.E. (2007) Package integrity testing, in *Guide to Microbiological Control in Pharmaceuticals and Medical Devices*, 2nd edn (eds S. Denyer and R. Baird), CRC Press, Boca Raton, FL, pp. 367–381.

7 Beveridge, E.G. (1998) Microbial spoilage and preservation of pharmaceutical products, in *Pharmaceutical Microbiology*, 6th edn (eds W.B. Hugo and A.D. Russell), Blackwell Scientific Publications, Oxford, pp. 355–374.

8 Lund, W. (ed.) (1994) Control of microbial contamination and growth, in *The Pharmaceutical Codex*, 12th edn, Pharmaceutical Press, London, p. 300.

9 English, D.J. (2006) Factors in selecting and testing preservatives in product formulations, in *Cosmetic and Drug Microbiology* (eds D.S. Orth *et al.*), Informa Healthcare, New York, pp. 57–108.

10 Royal Pharmaceutical Society of Great Britain and British Medical Association (2009) *British National Formulary, No.58*, BMJ Group and RPS Publishing, London.

11 Denyer, S.P. (2007) Antimicrobial preservatives and their properties, in *Guide to Microbiological Control in Pharmaceuticals and Medical Devices*, 2nd edn (eds S. Denyer and R. Baird), CRC Press, Boca Raton, FL, pp. 367–381.

12 Rowe, R.C. *et al.* (2009) *Handbook of Pharmaceutical Excipients*, 6th edn, Pharmaceutical Press, London and American Pharmaceutical Association, Washington, DC.

13 European Pharmacopoeia Commission (2010) *European Pharmacopoeia, 6th edn, 5.1.4 General text: Microbiology Quality of Non-Sterile Pharmaceutical Preparations and Substances for Pharmaceutical Use*, Council of Europe, Strasbourg.

14 Baird, R.M. (1988) Incidence of microbial contamination in medicines in hospitals, in *Biodeterioration 7* (eds D.R. Houghton *et al.*), Elsevier Applied Science. London, pp. 152–156.

15 Bloomfield, S.F. (1990) Microbial contamination: spoilage and hazard, in *Guide to Microbiological Control in Pharmaceuticals* (eds S.P. Denyer and R. Baird), Ellis-Horwood, Chichester, pp. 29–52.

16 Beveridge, E.G. (1975) The microbial spoilage of pharmaceutical products, in *Microbial Aspects of the Deterioration of Materials*, Society for Applied Bacteriology Technical Series No. 9 (eds D.W. Lovelock and R.J. Gilbert), Academic Press, London, pp. 213–235.

17 Medicines and Healthcare Products Regulatory Agency drug alerts, http://www.mhra.gov.uk/Safetyinformation/Safetywarningsalertsandrecalls/Drug alerts/index.html (accessed June 8, 2012).

18 European Medicines Agency (2007) *Good Manufacturing Practice: An Analysis of Regulatory Inspection Findings in the Centralised Procedure*, EMEA/INS/GMP/23022/2007, http://www.ema.europa.eu/Inspections/docs/2302207en.pdf (accessed June 8, 2012).

19 Tasli, H. and Cosar, G. (2001) Microbial contamination of eye drops. *Central European Journal of Public Health*, **9**, 162–164.

20 McHugh, G.J. and Roper, G.M. (1995) Propofol emulsion and bacterial contamination. *Canadian Journal of Anesthesia*, **42**, 801–804.

21 Anon. (1992) *Cosmetics Handbook*, Food and Drugs Administration, Washington, DC.

22 Tran, T.T. and Hitchins, A.D. (1994) Microbial survey of shared-use cosmetic test kits available to the public. *Journal of Industrial Microbiology*, **13**, 389–391.

23 Ringertz, O. and Ringertz, S. (1982) The clinical significance of microbial contamination in pharmaceutical and allied products, in *Advances in Pharmaceutical Sciences*, vol. 5 (eds H.S. Bean *et al.*), Academic Press, London, pp. 201–226.

24 Martone, W.J. *et al.* (1987) The epidemiology of nosocomial epidemic *Pseudomonas cepacia* infections. *European Journal of Epidemiology*, **3**, 222–232.

25 Denyer, S.P. (1988) Clinical consequences of microbial action on medicines, in *Biodeterioration 7* (eds D.R. Houghton *et al.*), Elsevier Applied Science, London, pp. 146–151.

26 Sharpell, F. and Manowitz, M. (1991) Preservation of cosmetics, in *Disinfection, Sterilisation and Preservation* (ed. S.E. Block), Lea & Febinger, Malvern, PA, pp. 887–900.

27 Spooner, D.F. (1996) Hazards associated with the microbiological contamination of cosmetics, toiletries, and non-sterile medicines, in *Microbial Quality Assurance in Cosmetics, Toiletries and Non-Sterile Pharmaceuticals*, 2nd edn (eds R.M. Baird and S.E. Bloomfield), Taylor & Francis, Basingstoke, pp. 9–27.

28 Theodore, F.H. and Feinstein, R.R. (1952) *Serratia* keratitis transmitted by contaminated eye droppers. *American Journal of Ophthalmology*, **93**, 723–726.

29 Tremewan, H.C. (1946) Tetanus neonatorum in New Zealand. *New Zealand Medical Journal*, **45**, 312–313.

30 Ayliffe, G.A.J. *et al.* (1966) Postoperative infection with *Pseudomonas aeruginosa*. *Lancet*, **i**, 1113–1117.

31 Clothier, C.M. (1972) *Report of the Committee Appointed to Look into the Circumstances, Including the Production, Which Led to the Use of Contaminated Infusion Fluids in the Devenport Section of Plymouth General Hospital*, HMSO, London.

32 Kallings, L.O. (1973) Contamination of therapeutic agents, in *Contamination in the Manufacture of Pharmaceutical products*, Secretariat of the Eurpoean Trade Association, Geneva, pp. 17–23.

33 Bruch, C.W. (1972) Objectionable micro-organisms in non-sterile drugs and cosmetics. *Drug and Cosmetic Industry*, **3**, 50–56.

34 Wilson, L.A. and Ahearn, D.G. (1977) *Pseudomonas*-induced corneal ulcers associated with contaminated eye mascaras. *American Journal of Ophthalmology*, **84**, 114–119.

35 Fassihi, R.A. (1991) Preservation of medicines against microbial contamination, in *Disinfection, Sterilisation and Preservation* (ed. S.E. Block), Lea & Febinger, Malvern, PA, pp. 871–886.

36 Hay, J. *et al.* (1996) Single-solution lens care systems. *Pharmaceutical Journal*, **256**, 824–825.

37 Sweeney, D.F. *et al.* (1999) Incidence of contamination of preserved saline solution during normal use. *CLAO Journal*, **25**, 167–175.

38 Seal, D.V. (1994) *Acanthamoeba* keratitis. *British Medical Journal*, **308**, 1116–1117.

39 Lim, L. *et al.* (2000) Antimicrobial susceptibility of 19 Australian corneal isolates of Acanthamoeba. *Clinical and Experimental Ophthalmology*, **28** (2), 119–124.

40 Meers, P.D. *et al.* (1973) Intravenous infusion of contaminated dextrose infusion: the Davenport incident. *Lancet*, **ii**, 1189–1198.

41 Tebbs, S.E. *et al.* (1996) Microbial contamination of intravenous and arterial catheters. *Intensive Care Medicine*, **22**, 272–273.

42 British Pharmacopoeia Commission (2009) *British Pharmacopoeia*, The Stationary Office, London.

43 Freund, H.R. and Rimon, B. (1990) Sepsis during total parenteral nutrition. *Journal of Parenteral and Enteral Nutrition*, **14**, 39–41.

44 Anon. (1995) Accidental death verdict on children infected by TPN at a Manchester hospital. *Pharmaceutical Journal*, **254**, 313.

45 Allwood, M.C. *et al.* (1997) Microbiological risks in parenteral nutrition compounding. *Nutrition*, **13** (1), 60–61.

46 Langford, S. (2000) Microbial survival in infusion fluids – the relevance to the management of aseptic facilities. *Hospital Pharmacist*, **7** (8), 228–236.

47 Bethune, K. *et al.* (2001) Use of filters during the preparation and administration of parenteral nutrition: position paper and guidelines prepared by a british pharmaceutical nutrition group working party. *Nutrition*, **17**, 403–408.

48 Millership, S.E. *et al.* (1986) The colonisation of patients in an intensive treatment unit with Gram-negative flora: the significnce of the oral route. *Journal of Hospital Infection*, **7**, 226–235.

49 Brown, L.K. *et al.* (1995) HIV-infected adolescents with hemophilia: adaptation and coping. *Pediatrics*, **96**, 459–463.

50 Anon. (1994) 111 cases of hepatitis C linked to Gamagard. *American Journal of Hospital Pharmacy*, **51**, 23–26.

51 Anon. (1996) A case of justice only half done. *New Scientist*, **151**, 3.

52 Hutchinson, J. *et al.* (2004) *Burkholderia cepacia* infections associated with intrinsically contaminated unltrasound gel: the role of microbial degradation of parabens. *Infection Control and Hospital Epidemiology*, **25** (4), 291–296.

53 Norman, P. *et al.* (1986) Pseudo-bacteraemia associated with contaminated skin cleaning agent. *Lancet*, **i**, 209.

54 Arjunwadkar, V.P. *et al.* (2001) Contaminated antiseptics – an unnecessary hospital hazard. *Indian Journal of Medical Sciences*, **55**, 393–398.

55 Bloomfield, S.F. (1988) Biodeterioration and disinfectants, in *Biodeterioration 7* (ed. D.R. Houghton), Elsevier Applied Science, London, pp. 135–145.

56 Hamil, R.J. *et al.* (1995) An outbreak of *Burkholderia* (formerly *Pseudomonas*) *cepacia* respiratory tract colonisation and infection associated with nebulised salbuterol therapy. *Annals of Internal Medicine*, **122**, 762–766.

57 Dautzenberg, B. (2001) Prevention of nosocomial infection during nebulization and spirometry. *Revue de Pneumologie Clinique*, **57** (2), 91–98.

58 Jarvis, W.R. and Highsmith, A.K. (1984) Bacterial growth and endotoxin production in lipid emulsion. *Journal of Clinical Medicine*, **19**, 17–20.

59 Mangram, A.J. *et al.* (1998) Outbreak of sterile peritonitis among continuous cycling peritoneal dialysis patients. *Kidney International*, **54** (4), 1367–1371.

60 Anon. (1996) Deadly blooms reach Britain's rivers. *New Scientist*, **151**, 5.

61 El-Dessouki, S. (1992) Aflatoxins in cosmetics containing substrates for aflatoxin-producing fungi. *Food and Chemical Toxicology*, **30**, 993–994.

62 Riley, R.T. *et al.* (1985) Penetration of aflatoxins through isolated human epidermis. *Journal of Toxicology and Environmental Health*, **15**, 769–777.

63 Smith, J.L. (1984) Evaluating your microbiology programme, in *The Cosmetic Industry: Scientific and Regulatory Foundations*, Cosmetic Science and Technology Series (ed. N.F. Estrin), Marcel Dekker, New York, pp. 301–320.

64 McIntosh, D.A. (1987) Risk assessment and protection against civil and criminal liability in the pharmaceutical industry, in *Proceedings of the 9th BIRA Annual Symposium*, pp. 18–29.

65 Begg, D.I.R. (1990) Risk assessment and microbiological auditing, in *Guide to Microbiological Control in Pharmaceuticals* (eds S. Denyer and R. Baird), Ellis Horwood, Chichester, pp. 366–379.

66 Rodford, R. (1996) Safety of preservatives, in *Microbial Contamination–Determination–Eradication. Proceedings, Society of Cosmetic Chemists Symposium, Daresbury*, Miller Freeman Publishers, London, pp. 1–23.

67 Anon. (1991) Cosmetic safety: more complex that at first blush. *FDA Consumer*, **November**, 2.

68 Favero, M.S. *et al.* (1971) *Pseudomonas aeruginosa*: growth in distilled water. *Science*, **173**, 836–838.

69 Chirife, J. and Favetto, G.J. (1992) Some physicochemical basis of food preservation by combined methods. *Food Research International (Ottawa, Ontario)*, **25**, 389–396.

70 Dillon, V.M. and Board, R.G. (1994) Ecological, concepts of food preservation, in *Natural Antimicrobial Systems and Food Preservation* (eds V.M. Dillon and R.G. Board), CAB International, Wallingford, pp. 1–13.

71 Gould, G.W. (1996) Methods for preservation and extension of shelf life. *International Journal of Food Microbiology*, **33**, 51–64.

72 Roberts, T.A. (1995) Microbial growth and survival: developments in predictive modelling. *International Biodeterioration and Biodegradation*, **36**, 297–309.

73 Orth, D.S. (1993) *Microbiological considerations in product development*, in *Handbook of Cosmetic Microbiology* (ed. D.S. Orth), Marcel Dekker, New York, pp. 103–118.

74 Wiggins, P.W. (1990) Role of water in some biological processes. *Microbiological Reviews*, **54**, 432–449.

75 Beveridge, E.G. and Bendall, D. (1988) Water relationships and microbial biodeterioration of some pharmaceutical tablets. *International Biodeterioration*, **24**, 197–203.

76 Flatau, T.C. *et al.* (1996) Preservation of solid oral dosage forms, in *Microbial Quality Assurance in Cosmetics, Toiletries and Non-Sterile Pharmaceuticals*, 2nd edn (eds R.M. Baird and S.E. Bloomfield), Taylor & Francis, Basingstoke, pp. 113–132.

77 Friedl, R.R. (1999) The application of water activity measurement to microbiological attributes testing of raw materials used in the manufacture of nonsterile pharmaceutical products. *Pharmacopeial Forum*, **25** (5), 8974–8981.

78 Cundell, A.M. (1998) *Reduced Testing in the Microbiology Laboratory*, PharMIG Annual Meeting, November 24–25.

79 Whiteman, M. (1995) Evaluating the performance of tablet coatings. *Manufacturing Chemist*, **66**, 24–27.

80 Fassihi, R.A. *et al.* (1978) The preservation of tablets against microbial spoilage. *Drug Development and Industrial Pharmacy*, **4**, 515–527.

81 Morris, C. and Leech, R. (1996) Natural and physical preservative systems, in *Microbial Quality Assurance in Cosmetics, Toiletries and Non-Sterile Pharmaceuticals*, 2nd edn (eds R.M. Baird and S.E. Bloomfield), Taylor & Francis, Basingstoke, pp. 69–97.

82 Jackson, E.M. (1993) The science of cosmetics. *American Journal of Contact Dermatitis: Official Journal of the American Contact Dermatitis Society*, **4**, 47–49.

83 Limtner, K. (1997) Physical methods of preservation. *Inside Cosmetics*, **March**, 23–29.

84 Bhadauria, R. and Ahearn, D.G. (1980) Loss of effectiveness of preservative systems of mascara with age. *Applied and Environmental Microbiology*, **39**, 665–667.

85 Oldham, G.B. and Andrews, V. (1996) Control of microbial contamination in unpreserved eyedrops. *British Journal of Ophthalmology*, **80**, 588–591.

86 Wimpenny, J.W.T. (1981) Spatial order in microbial ecosystems. *Biological Reviews*, **56**, 295–342.

87 Verrips, C.T. (1989) Growth of micro-organisms in compartmentalised producs, in *Mechanisms of Action of Food Preservation Procedures* (ed. G.W. Gould), Elsevier Applied Science, London, pp. 363–399.

88 van Loosdrecht, M.C.M. *et al.* (1990) Influence of interfaces on microbial activity. *Microbiological Reviews*, **54**, 75–87.

89 Roszac, D.B. and Colwell, R.R. (1987) Survival strategies of bacteria in the natural environment. *Microbiological Reviews*, **51**, 365–379.

90 Greenwood, M.H. and Hooper, W.L. (1983) Chocolate bars contaminated with *Salmonella napoli*: an infectivity study. *British Medical Journal*, **286**, 1394.

91 Kallings, L.O. *et al.* (1966) Microbiological contamination of medical preparations. *Acta Pharmaceutica Suecica*, **3**, 219–227.

92 Payne, D.N. (1990) Microbial ecology of the production process, in *Guide to Microbiological Control in Pharmaceuticals* (eds S. Denyer and R. Baird), Ellis Horwood, Chichester, pp. 53–67.

93 Kneifel, W. *et al.* (2002) Microbial contamination of medicinal plants – a review. *Planta Medica*, **68**, 5–15.

94 Hugo, W.B. and Denyer, S.P. (1987) The concentration exponent of disinfectants and preservatives, in *Preservatives in the Food, Pharmaceutical and Environmental Industries*, Society for Applied Bacteriology Technical Series No. 22

(eds R.G. Board *et al.*), Blackwell Scientific Publications, Oxford, pp. 281–291.

95 Russell, A.D. and McDonnell, G. (2000) Concentration: a major factor in studying biocidal action. *Journal of Hospital Infection*, **44**, 1–3.

96 Attwood, D. and Florence, A.T. (1983) *Surfactant Systems*, Chapman & Hall, London.

97 van Doorne, H. (1990) Interactions between preservatives and pharmaceutical components, in *Guide to Microbiological Control in Pharmaceuticals* (eds S. Denyer and R. Baird), Ellis Horwood, Chichester, pp. 274–291.

98 Dempsey, G. (1996) The effect of container materials and multiple-phase formulation components on the activity of antimicrobial agents, in *Microbial Quality Assurance in Cosmetics, Toiletries and Non-Sterile Pharmaceuticals*, 2nd edn (eds R.M. Baird and S.F. Bloomfield), Taylor & Francis, Basingstoke, pp. 87–97.

99 Bean, H.A. *et al.* (1962) The bactericidal activity against *Escherichia coli* of phenol in oil-in-water dispersions. *Bollettino Chimico Farmaceutico*, **101**, 339–346.

100 Mitchell, A.G. and Kamzi, J.A. (1975) Preservative availability in emulsified systems. *Canadian Journal of Pharmaceutical Sciences*, **10**, 67–68.

101 Kamzi, S.J.A. and Mitchell, A.G. (1978) Preservation of solubilised and emulsified systems II: theoretical development of capacity and its role in antimicrobial activity of chlorocresol in cetomacrogol-stabilised systems. *Journal of Pharmaceutical Sciences*, **67**, 1266–1271.

102 McCarthy, T.J. (1984) Formulated factors affecting the activity of preservatives, in *Cosmetic and Drug Preservation: Principles and Practice*, Cosmetic Science and Technology Series, vol. 1 (ed. J.J. Kabara), Marcel Dekker, New York, pp. 359–388.

103 Kurup, T.R.R. *et al.* (1991) Availability and activity of preservatives in emulsified systems. *Pharmaceutica Acta Helvetiae*, **66**, 76–83.

104 McCulloch, E.C. (1945) *Disinfection and Sterilisation*, 2nd edn, Henry Kimpton, London, p. 221.

105 Cooper, E.A. (1947) The influence of organic solvents on the bactericidal action of the phenols. Part II. *Journal of the Society of Chemical Industry (London)*, **66**, 48–50.

106 Cooper, E.A. (1948) The influence of ethylene glycol and glycerol on the germicidal power of aliphatic and aromatic compounds. *Journal of the Society of Chemical Industry (London)*, **67**, 69–70.

107 Anagnostopoulos, G.D. and Kroll, R.G. (1978) Water activity and solute effect on the bactericidal action of phenol. *Microbios Letters*, **7**, 69–74.

108 Bos, C.E. *et al.* (1989) Microbiological stability of tablets stored under tropical conditions. *International Journal of Pharmaceutics*, **55**, 175–183.

109 Burgess, D.J. and Reich, R.R. (1993) Industrial ethylene oxide sterilisation, in *Sterilization Technology: a Practical Guide for Manufacturers and Users of Health Care Products* (eds R.F. Morrissey and C.B. Phillips), Van Nostrand Reinhold, New York, pp. 152–195.

110 Wood, R.T. (1993) Sterilization with dry heat, in *Sterilization Technology: a Practical Guide for Manufacturers and Users of Health Care Products* (eds R.F. Morrissey and C.B. Phillips), Van Nostrand Reinhold, New York, pp. 81–119.

111 Gould, G.W. (1989) Drying, raised osmotic pressure and low water activity, in *Mechanisms of Action of Food Preservation Procedures* (ed. G.W. Gould), Elsevier Applied Science, London, pp. 97–117.

112 Wedderburn, D.L. (1964) Preservation of emulsions against microbial attack, in *Advances in Pharmaceutical Sciences*, vol. I (eds H.A. Bean *et al.*), Academic Press, London, pp. 195–268.

113 Loftsson, T. *et al.* (1992) Interactions between preservatives and 2-hydroxypropyl-β-cylcodextrin. *Drug Development and Industrial Pharmacy*, **18**, 1477–1484.

114 Yousef, R.T. *et al.* (1973) Effect of some pharmaceutical materials on the bactericidal activities of preservatives. *Canadian Journal of Pharmaceutical Sciences*, **18**, 54–56.

115 Allwood, M.C. (1982) The adsorption of esters of *p*-hydroxybenzoic acid by magnesium trisilicate. *International Journal of Pharmaceutics*, **11**, 101–107.

116 Kurup, T.R.R. *et al.* (1992) Interaction of preservatives with macromolecules: part 1. Natural hydrocolloids. *Pharmaceutica Acta Helvetiae*, **67**, 301–307.

117 Qawas, A. *et al.* The adsorption of bactericides by solids and the fitting of adsorption data to the Langmuir equation by a non-linear least-squares method. *Pharmaceutical Acta Helvetica*, 1986; **61**, 314–319.

118 Sakamoto, T. *et al.* (1987) Effects of some cosmetic pigments on the bactericidal activities of preservatives. *Journal of the Society of Cosmetic Chemists*, **38**, 83–98.

119 Beveridge, E.G. and Hope, I.A. (1967) Inactivation of benzoic acid in sulphadimidine mixture for infants BPC. *Pharmaceutical Journal*, **198**, 457–458.

120 Dean, D.A. (1992) *Packaging of Pharmaceuticals: Packages and Closures*, Practical Packaging Series, Institute of Packaging, Melton Mowbray.

121 Holdsworth, D.G. *et al.* (1984) Fate of chlorobutanol during storage in polyethylene dropper containers and simulated patient used. *Journal of Clinical and Hospital Pharmacy*, **9**, 29–39.

122 Kakemi, K.K. *et al.* (1971) Interaction of parabens and other pharmaceutical adjuvants with plastic containers. *Chemical and Pharmaceutical Bulletin of Japan*, **19**, 2523–2529.

123 Aspinall, J.E. *et al.* (1983) The effect of low density polyethylene containers on some hospital-manufactured eyedrop formulations II: inhibition of the sorption of phenylmercuric acetate. *Journal of Clinical and Hospital Pharmacy*, **8**, 233–240.

124 Wang, Y.J. and Chien, Y.W. (1984) *Sterile Pharmaceutical Packaging: Compatibility and Stability*, Parenteral Drug Association Technical Report No. 5, Parenteral Drug Association, Pennsylvania.

125 Anon. (n.d.) *Kathon CG Microbicide: Cosmetics and Toiletries*, Technical Bulletin, Rohm & Haas, Croydon.

126 Reiger, M.M. (1994) Methylparaben, in *Handbook of Pharmaceutical Excipients*, 2nd edn (eds A. Wade and P.J. Welter), Pharmaceutical Press, London and American Pharmaceutical Association, Washington, DC, pp. 310–313.

127 Runesson, B. and Gustavii, K. (1986) Stability of parabens in the presence of polyols. *Acta Pharmaceutica Suecica*, **23**, 151–162.

128 Allwood, M.C. *et al.* (1994) Bronopol, in *Handbook of Pharmaceutical Excipients*, 2nd edn (eds A. Wade and P.J. Welter), Pharmaceutical Press, London and American Pharmaceutical Association, Washington, DC, pp. 40–42.

129 Thompson, D.F. *et al.* (1989) Contamination risks of multidose medication vials: a review. *Journal of Pharmacy Technology*, **5**, 249–253.

130 Anon. (1996) Design and use of IV products. *Pharmaceutical Journal*, **257**, 772–773.

131 Meyer, B.K. *et al.* (2007) Antimicrobial preservative use in parenteral products: past and present. *Journal of Pharmaceutical Sciences*, **96** (12), 3155–3167.

132 Medicines and Healthcare Products Agency (2012) *Thiomersal (Ethylmercury) Containing Vaccines*, http://www.mhra.gov.uk/Safetyinformation/ (accessed June 8, 2012).

133 Hetherington, N.J. and Dooley, M.J. (2000) Potential for patient harm from intrathecal administration of preserved solutions. *Medical Journal of Australia*, **173** (3), 141–143.

134 British Pharmacopoeia Commission (2009) *British Pharmacopoeia*, The Stationary Office, London.

135 Rahman, M.Q. *et al.* (2006) Microbial contamination of preservative free eye drops in multiple application containers. *British Journal of Ophthalmology*, **90**, 139–141.

136 Anon. (1996) Seven day life of unpreserved eye-drops. *Pharmaceutical Journal*, **257**, 206.

137 Soni, M.G. *et al.* (2001) Safety assessment of propyl paraben: a review of the published literature. *Food and Chemical Toxicology: An International Journal Published for the British Industrial Biological Research Association*, **39** (6), 513–532.

138 Vanhaecke, E. *et al.* (1987) A comparative study of the effectiveness of preservatives in twelve antacid suspensions. *Drug Developments in Industrial Pharmacy*, **13**, 1429–1446.

139 Orth, D.S. *et al.* (1992) The required D-value: evaluating product preservation in relation to packaging and consumer use/abuse. *Cosmetics and Toiletries*, **107**, 39–43.

140 Anon. (1990) Frequency of preservative use in cosmetic formulas as disclosed to FDA – 1990. *Cosmetics and Toiletries*, **105**, 45–47.

141 Anon. (1993) Preservative frequency of use: FDA data, June 1993 update. *Cosmetics and Toiletries*, **108**, 47–48.

142 Anon. (1993) *CTPA Guidelines for Effective Preservation*, Cosmetic Toiletry and Perfumery Association, London, p. 1.

143 Orth, D.S. (1993) Preservation of cosmetic products, in *Handbook of Cosmetic Microbiology* (ed. D.S. Orth), Marcel Dekker, New York, pp. 75–102.

144 Allwood, M.C. (1990) Package design and product integrity, in *Guide to Microbiological Control in Pharmaceuticals* (eds S. Denyer and R. Baird), Ellis Horwood, Chichester, pp. 341–355.

145 Brannan, D.K. and Dille, J.C. (1990) Type of closure prevents microbial contamination of cosmetics during consumer use. *Applied and Environmental Microbiology*, **56**, 1476–1479.

146 Denyer, S.P. (1996) Development of preservative systems, in *Microbial Quality Assurance in Cosmetics, Toiletries and Non-Sterile Pharmaceuticals*, 2nd edn (eds R.M. Baird and S.E. Bloomfield), Taylor & Francis, Basingstoke, pp. 133–147.

147 Haag, T.E. and Loncrini, D.F. (1984) Esters of *para*-hydroxybenzoic acid, in *Cosmetic and Drug Preservation: Principles and Practice*, Cosmetic Science and Technology Series, vol. 1 (ed. J.J. Kabara), Marcel Dekker, New York, pp. 63–77.

148 Darwish, R.M. and Bloomfield, S.F. (1995) The effect of co-solvents on the antibacterial activity of paraben preservatives. *International Journal of Pharmaceutics*, **119**, 183–192.

149 Rosen, W.E. and Berke, P.A. (1984) German 115: a safe and effective preservative, in *Cosmetic and Drug Preservation: Principles and Practice*, Cosmetic Science and Technology Series, vol. 1 (ed. J.J. Kabara), Marcel Dekker, New York, pp. 191–205.

150 Hall, A.L. (1984) Cosmetically acceptable phenoxyethanol, in *Cosmetic and Drug Preservation: Principles and Practice*, Cosmetic Science and Technology Series, vol. 1 (ed. J.J. Kabara), Marcel Dekker, New York, pp. 79–110.

151 Hart, J.R. (1984) Chelating agents as preservative potentiators, in *Cosmetic and Drug Preservation: Principles and Practice*, Cosmetic Science and Technology Series, vol. 1 (ed. J.J. Kabara), Marcel Dekker, New York, pp. 323–337.

152 Cook, R.S. and Youssuf, N. (1994) Edetic acid, in *Handbook of Pharmaceutical Excipients*, 2nd edn (eds A. Wade and P.J. Welter), Pharmaceutical Press, London and American Pharmaceutical Association, Washington, DC, pp. 176–179.

153 Woodruff, J. (1995) Preservatives to fight the growth of mould. *Manufacturing Chemist*, **66**, 34–35.

154 Kabara, J.J. (1984) Food-grade chemicals in a systems approach to cosmetic preservation, in *Cosmetic and Drug Preservation: Principles and Practice*, Cosmetic Science and Technology Series, vol. 1 (ed. J.J. Kabara), Marcel Dekker, New York, pp. 339–356.

155 Vaara, M. (1992) Agents that increase the permeability of the outer membrane. *Microbiological Reviews*, **56**, 395–411.

156 Gilbert, P. *et al.* (1977) The lethal action of 2-phenoxyethanol and its analogues upon *Escherichia coli* NCTC 5933. *Microbios*, **19**, 125–141.

157 Denyer, S.P. *et al.* (1986) The biochemical basis of synergy between the antibacterial agents, chlorocresol and 2-phenylethanol. *International Journal of Pharmaceutics*, **29**, 29–36.

158 Moon, N.J. (1983) Inhibition of the growth of acid tolerant yeasts by acetate, lactate and propionate and their synergistic mixtures. *Journal of Applied Bacteriology*, **55**, 453–460.

159 Gilliland, D. *et al.* (1992) Kinetic evaluation of claimed synergistic paraben combinations using a factorial design. *Journal of Applied Bacteriology*, **72**, 258–261.

160 Pons, J.-L. *et al.* (1992) Evaluation of antimicrobial interactions between chlorhexidine quaternary ammonium compounds, preservatives and exipients. *Journal of Applied Bacteriology*, **73**, 395–400.

161 Rehm, H.-J. (1959) Untersuchung zur Wirkung von Konservierungsmittelkombinationen. Die Wirkung einfacher Konserviersmittelkombinationen auf *Escherichia coli*. *Zeitschrift fur Lebensmittel-Untersuchung und -Forschung*, **110**, 356–363.

162 Kabara, J.J. (2006) Hurdle technology for cosmetic and drug preservation, in *Cosmetic and Drug Microbiology* (eds D.S. Orth *et al.*), Informa Healthcare, New York, pp. 163–184.

163 Committee for Proprietary Medicinal Products (CPMP) (1997) *Inclusion of Antioxidants and Antimicrobial Preservatives in Medicinal Products (CPMP/QWP/115/95)*, European Agency for the Evaluation of Medicinal Products, London.

164 Applebe, G.E. and Wingfield, J. (1993) *Dale and Applebe's Pharmacy Law and Ethics*, 5th edn, Pharmaceutical Press, London.

165 Permanand, G. (2006) *EU Pharmaceutical Regulation, the Politics of Policy-Making*, Manchester University Press, Manchester.

166 Pisano, D.J. and Mantous, D. (2005) *FDA Regulatory Affairs: a Guide for Prescription Drugs, Medical Devices and Biologics.* Taylor & Francis E-Library, CRC Press, New York.

167 Japanese Pharmaceutical Manufacturers Association (n.d.) *Information in English on Japanese Regulatory Affairs*, http://www.jpma.or.jp/english/parj/1203.html (accessed June 13, 2012).

168 Frosch, P.J. and Rycroft, R.J.G. (1995) International legal aspects of contact dermatitis, in *Textbook of Contact Dermatology*, 2nd edn (eds R.J.G. Rycroft *et al.*), Springer-Verlag, Berlin, pp. 752–768.

169 Hogan, D. and Ledet, J.J. (2009) Impact of regulation on contact dermatitis. *Dermatologic Clinics*, **27** (3), 385–394.

170 Baird, R.M. (1995) Preservative efficacy testing in the pharmaceutical industries, in *Microbiological Quality Assurance: a Guide Towards Relevance and Reproducibility of Inocula* (eds M.R.W. Brown and P. Gilbert), CRC Press, New York, pp. 149–162.

171 Brannan, D.K. (1995) Cosmetic preservation. *Journal of the Society of Cosmetic Chemists*, **46**, 199–220.

172 Perry, B.F. (1995) Preservation efficacy testing in the cosmetics and toiletries industries, in *Microbiological Quality Assurance: a Guide Towards Relevance and Reproducibility of Inocula* (eds M.R.W. Brown and P. Gilbert), CRC Press, New York, pp. 163–187.

173 Leak, R.F. *et al.* (1996) Challenge tests and their predictive ability, in *Microbial Quality Assurance in Cosmetics, Toiletries and Non-Sterile Pharmaceuticals*, 2nd edn (eds R.M. Baird and S.F. Bloomfield), Taylor & Francis, Basingstoke, pp. 199–216.

174 Hopton, J.W. and Hill, E.C. (eds) (1987) *Industrial Microbiological Testing*, Society for Applied Bacteriology Technical Series No. 23, Blackwell Scientific Publications, Oxford.

175 Akers, M.J. and Taylor, C.J. (1990) Official methods of preservative evaluation and testing, in *Guide to Microbiological Control in Pharmaceuticals* (eds S. Denyer and R. Baird), Ellis Horwood, Chichester, pp. 292–303.

176 Chan, M. and Prince, H. (1981) Rapid screeing test for ranking preservative efficacy. *Drug and Cosmetic Industry*, **129**, 34–37, 80–81.

177 Spooner, D.F. and Croshaw, B. (1981) Challenge testing: the laboratory evaluation of the preservation of pharmaceutical preparations. *Antonie van Leeuwenboek Journal of Serology*, **47**, 168–169.

178 Brown, M.R.W. and Gilbert, P. (eds) (1995) *Microbiological Quality Assurance: a Guide to Relevance and Reproducibility of Inocula*, CRC Press, New York.

179 Gilbert, P. and Brown, M.R.W. (1995) Factors affecting the reproducibility and predictivity of performance tests, in *Microbiological Quality Assurance: a Guide to Relevance and Reproducibility of Inocula* (eds M.R.W. Brown and P. Gilbert), CRC Press, New York, pp. 135–147.

180 Flawn, P.C. *et al.* (1973) Assessment of the preservative capacity of shampoos. *Journal of the Society of Cosmetic Chemists*, **24**, 229–238.

181 Curry, A.S. *et al.* (1993) *CTFA Microbiology Guidelines*, Cosmetic, Toiletry and Fragrance Association, Washington, DC.

182 Muscatiello, M.J. (1993) CTFA's preservation guidelines: a historical perspective and review. *Cosmetics and Toiletries*, **108**, 53–59.

183 Shaqra, Q.M. and Husari, N. (1987) Preservation of some commercially available antacid suspensions against *Pseudomonas aeruginosa* (ATCC 9027). *International Biodeterioration*, **23**, 47–51.

184 Sabourin, J.R. (1990) Evaluation of preservatives for cosmetic products. *Drug and Cosmetic Industry*, **147**, 24–27, 64–65.

185 Fels, P. (1995) An automated personal computer-enhanced assay for antimicrobial preservative efficacy testing by the most probable number technique using microtiter plates. *Pharmazeutische Industrie*, **57**, 585–590.

186 Hugo, W.B. and Russell, A.D. (1998) Evaluation of non-antibiotic antimicrobial agents, in *Pharmaceutical Microbiology*, 6th edn (eds W.B. Hugo and A.D. Russell), Blackwell Scientific Publications, Oxford, pp. 229–254.

187 Johnston, M.D. *et al.* (2002) A rapid method for assessing the suitability of quenching agents for individual biocides as well as combinations. *Journal of Applied Microbiology*, **92** (4), 784–789.

188 Baird, R.M. and Bloomfield, S.F. (1996) *Microbial Quality Assurance in Cosmetics, Toiletries and Non-Sterile Pharmaceuticals*, 2nd edn, Taylor & Francis, Basingstoke.

189 British Pharmacopoeia Commission (2009) Efficacy of antimicrobial preservation, Appendix XVIC, in *British Pharmacopoeia*, The Stationary Office, London.

190 European Pharmacopoeia (2009) Efficacy of antimicrobial preservation, in *European Pharmacopoeia. Supplement*, 6th edn, EDQM, Strasbourg, pp. 528–529.

191 Unites States Pharmacopoeial Convention (2009) Antimicrobial effectiveness testing <51>, in *United States Pharmacopeia 32*, Webcom Ltd, Ontario, pp. 67–69.

192 Casey, W.M. and Muth, H. (2000) The effects of antimicrobial preservatives on organisms derived from fresh versus frozen cultures. *Pharmacopeial Forum*, **26**, 519–533.

193 Lindstrom, S.M. (1986) Consumer use testing: assurance of microbiological product safety. *Cosmetics and Toiletries*, **101**, 71–73.

194 Anon. (1990) CTFA survey: test methods companies use. *Cosmetics and Toiletries*, **105**, 79–82.

195 Farrington, J.K. *et al.* (1994) Ability of laboratory methods to predict in-use efficacy of antimicrobial preservatives in an experimental cosmetic. *Applied and Environmental Microbiology*, **60**, 4553–4558.

196 Tran, T.T. *et al.* (1994) Adequacy of cosmetic preservation: chemical analysis, microbiological challenge and in-use testing. *International Journal of Cosmetic Science*, **16**, 61–76.

197 Spooner, D.F. and Davison, A.L. (1993) The validity of the criteria for pharmacopoeial antimicrobial preservative efficacy tests. *Pharmaceutical Journal*, **251**, 602–605.

198 Fels, P. *et al.* (1987) Antimicrobial preservation. *Pharmazeutische Industrie*, **49**, 631–637.

199 Orth, D.S. (2007) Preservation evaluation and testing: the linear regression method, in *Guide to Microbiological Control in Pharmaceuticals and Medical Devices* (eds S.P. Denyer and R.M. Baird), Taylor & Francis Group, Boca Raton, FL, pp. 383–396.

200 Denyer, S.P. (1990) Monitoring microbiological quality: application of rapid microbiological methods to pharmaceuticals, in *Guide to Microbiological Control in Pharmaceuticals* (eds S.P. Denyer and R.M. Baird), Ellis Horwood, Chichester, pp. 146–156.

201 Connolly, P. *et al.* (1994) The use of impedance for preservative efficacy testing of pharmaceuticals and cosmetic products. *Journal of Applied Bacteriology*, **76**, 66–74.

202 Zhou, X. and King, V.M. (1995) An impedimetric method for rapid screening of cosmetic preservatives. *Journal of Industrial Microbiology*, **15** (2), 103–107.

203 Connolly, P. *et al.* (1993) A study of the use of rapid methods for preservative efficacy testing of pharmaceuticals and cosmetics. *Journal of Applied Bacteriology*, **75**, 456–462.

204 Jimenez, L. (2001) Rapid methods for the microbiological surveillance of pharmaceuticals. *PDA Journal of Pharmaceutical Science and Technology*, **55** (5), 278–285.

205 de Groot, A.C. and White, I.R. (1995) Cosmetics and skin care products, in *Textbook of Contact Dermatology*, 2nd edn (eds R.J.G. Rycroft *et al.*), Springer-Verlag, Berlin, pp. 461–476.

206 Jacobs, M.C. *et al.* (1995) Patch testing with preservatives at St John's from 1982 to 1993. *Contact Dermatitis*, **33**, 247–254.

207 Berne, B. *et al.* (1996) Adverse effects of cosmetics and toiletries reported to the Swedish Medical Products Agency. *Contact Dermatitis*, **34**, 359–362.

208 Schnuch, A. *et al.* (1998) Patch testing with preservatives, antimicrobials and industrial biocides. Results from a multicentre study. *British Journal of Dermatology*, **138**, 467–476.

209 Pauwels, M. and Rogiers, V. (2009) Human health safety evaluation of cosmetics in the EU: a legally imposed challenge to science. *Toxicology and Applied Pharmacology*, **243**, 260–274

210 Geier, J. *et al.* (2000) Patch testing with methyldibromoglutaronitrile. *American Journal of Contact Dermatitis: Official Journal of the American Contact Dermatitis Society*, **11** (4), 207–212.

211 Wilkinson, J.D. *et al.* (2002) Monitoring levels of preservative sensitivity in Europe. A 10-year overview (1991–2000). *Contact Dermatitis*, **46**, 207–210.

212 Scientific Committee on Cosmetic Products and Non-food Products (SCCNFP) (2002) *Opinion of the Scientific Committee on Cosmetic Products and Non-food Products Intended for Comsumers Concerning Methyldibromo Glutaronitrile (SCCNFP/0585/02)*, European Commission, Brussels.

213 Jong, C.T. *et al.* (2007) Contact sensitivity to prservatives in the UK, 2004–5: results of a multicentre study. *Contact Dermatitis.*, **57** (3), 165–168.

214 D'Arcy, P.F. (1990) Adverse reactions to excipients in pharmaceutical formulations, in *Formulation Factors in Adverse Reactions* (eds A.T. Florence and E.G. Salole), Wright, Butterworth Science, London, pp. 1–22.

215 Goon, A. *et al.* (2006) Safety and toxicological properties of preservatives, in *Cosmetic and Drug Microbiology* (eds D.S. Orth *et al.*), Informa Healthcare, New York, pp. 153–162.

216 Allwood, M.C. (1990) Adverse reactions in parenterals, in *Formulation Factors in Adverse Reactions* (eds A.T. Florence and E.G. Salole), Wright, Butterworth Science, London, pp. 56–74.

217 Audicana, M.T. *et al.* (2002) Allergic contact dermatitis from mercury antiseptics and derivatives: study protocol of tolerance to intramuscular injections of thiomersal. *American Journal of Contact Dermatitis*, **13**, 3–9.

218 Anon. (1983) Benzyl alcohol: toxic agent in neonatal units. *Pediatrics*, **72**, 356–358.

219 LeBel, M. *et al.* (1988) Benzyl alcohol metabolism and elimination in neonates. *Developmental Pharmacology and Therapeutics*, **11** (6), 347–356.

220 Burstein, N.L. (1985) The effects of topical drugs and preservatives on the tears and corneal epithelium in dry eye. *Transactions of the Ophthalmological Societies of the United Kingdom*, **104**, 402–409.

221 Olson, R.J. and White, G.L. (1990) Preservatives in ophthalmic topical medications: a significant cause of disease. *Cornea*, **9**, 362–364.

222 Sasaki, H. *et al.* (1995) Ophthalmic preservatives as absorption promoters for ocular drug delivery. *Journal of Pharmacy and Pharmacology*, **47**, 703–707.

223 Beasley, R. *et al.* (1998) Preservatives in nebulizer solutions: risks without benefit. *Pharmacotherapy*, **18**, 130–139.

224 Beasley, R. *et al.* (1988) Adverse reactions to the non-drug constituents of nebuliser solutions. *British Journal of Clinical Pharmacology*, **25**, 283–287.

225 Soni, M.G. *et al.* (2005) Safety assessment of esters of *p*-hydroxybenzoic acid (parabens). *Food and Chemical Toxicology*, **43**, 985–1015.

226 Anon. (1996) *Martindale: the Extra Pharmacopoeia*, 31st edn, Pharmaceutical Press, London.

227 Chen, J. *et al.* (2007) Antiandrogenic properties of parabens and other phenolic containing small molecules in personal care products. *Toxicology and Applied Pharmacology*, **221**, 278–284.

228 Kumar, V. *et al.* (2009) Alteration of testicular steroidogenesis and histopathology of reproductive system in male rats treated with triclosan. *Reproductive Toxicology*, **27**, 177–185.

229 Harvey, P.W. and Darbe, P. (2004) Endocrine disrupters and human health: could oestrogenic chemicals in body care cosmetics adversely affect breast cancer incidence in women? *Journal of Applied Toxicology*, **24** (3), 167–176.

18 Sterility Assurance: Concepts, Methods and Problems

Richard Bancroft

Albert Browne Ltd, Leicester, UK

Introduction

Preceding chapters have described in some detail the processes used in both healthcare and industry of rendering a product sterile. This chapter considers the factors necessary to achieve the state of "sterile" and how this may be assessed.

Sterile, sterilized

The definition of the term sterile is an absolute term meaning free from (all) viable (living) microorganisms. It is not possible, therefore, to have degrees of sterility – a device or product must be either sterile or non-sterile. In practice sterility is defined in terms of a probability of a surviving organism being present [1, 2]. The process by which this state is created is known as sterilization, which generally infers the destruction, or removal, of all viable microorganisms, which include vegetative cells, bacterial spores, fungi (yeasts and molds), protozoa and viruses. Sterilization processes are based on exposure of a device or product to a sterilizing agent in order to destroy, or inactivate, these viable microorganisms. It is also possible to sterilize some liquids or gases by passing them through a retentive filter, although this does raise other issues, which are referred to later. Sterilization processes typically utilize heat (either dry or moist), biocidal chemicals (in vapor or liquid form) or ionizing radiation.

One of the greatest issues with sterilization is that demonstrating complete freedom from a viable microorganism on a device or in a product is virtually impossible to show in practice. In order to detect the presence of a microorganism, an understanding of the nature of that microorganism is a prerequisite; certain microorganisms grow only at a particular temperature or have a requirement for specific growth conditions. So, in order to detect an unspecified microorganism, a large range of potentially destructive (to the device or the product) tests must be conducted.

We then must consider that loss of viability of the microorganism (viability being the only practical way of determining the presence of the cell) may be temporary due to the sterilant causing sublethal injury. This can be characterized by a loss of selective permeability of the cell membrane, leakage of intracellular components into the surrounding medium, degradation of ribosomes and ribonucleic acid, and decreased enzyme activity. Such damaged cells may require specialized recovery conditions for the repair of these injuries; failure to provide these may result in failure to detect these stressed cells [3]. However, should their specialized metabolic requirements be met in the future, these cells may repair the damage and subsequently grow.

Russell, Hugo & Ayliffe's: Principles and Practice of Disinfection, Preservation and Sterilization, Fifth Edition. Edited by Adam P. Fraise, Jean-Yves Maillard, and Syed A. Sattar.
© 2013 Blackwell Publishing Ltd. Published 2013 by Blackwell Publishing Ltd.

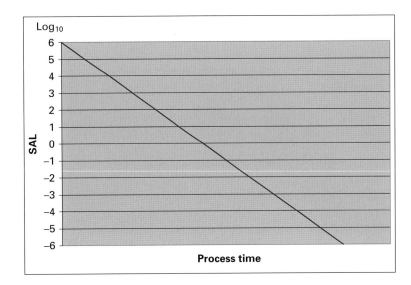

Figure 18.1 The 12-log cycle, showing sterility assurance level (SAL) against time needed to reach lethality.

Sterility and sterility assurance

The number of microorganisms will decrease exponentially during exposure to a sterilization process. Only by infinite exposure to the sterilizing agent can absence of all viable organisms be assured with certainty. At the same time, it is acknowledged that indefinite exposure to the lethal agent is impractical and may have deleterious effects on the device or product being processed. A compromise must be struck between assuring the sterility of the final device or product and also ensuring that the device or product remains fit for purpose. Hence the required sterility assurance level (SAL) is derived from what is considered to constitute the maximum acceptable risk, based on the intended use of the product.

The European standard EN556-1 describes the requirements for terminally sterilized devices to be designated sterile [2]; EN556-2 describes the requirements for aseptically produced devices [4]. The theoretical probability of there being a viable microorganism present should be equal to or less than 1×10^{-6} if the device or product is to be labeled sterile (that is a probability of less than 1 in 1,000,000 of having a viable microorganism present). In the USA, the Association for the Advancement of Medical Instrumentation (AAMI) has been instrumental in defining the term sterility assurance level [5]. The SAL is normally expressed as 10^{-x}; a SAL of 10^{-6} is hence identical in meaning to the European standard requirement, that a theoretical probability of there being a viable microorganism present should be equal to or less than 1×10^{-6}.

Figure 18.1 shows how a population of 1,000,000 (1×10^6) microorganisms will be destroyed exponentially during exposure

to a given sterilization process. It can be seen that at the halfway position, 6 logs (1 million) of microorganisms have been destroyed, however at 10^0 there is still a finite possibility of a surviving microorganism remaining. At a SAL of 10^{-1} there will be a probability of one survivor in 10. In order to achieve the level of assurance specified by regulatory authorities (a probability of a surviving viable microorganism to be equal to or less than 1×10^{-6} or a SAL of 10^{-6}), then the process will have to deliver lethality to a point at the end of the graphic line. It can be seen that depending upon the initial bioburden, the exposure time will be commensurately less as the process will be starting further down the extrapolated line. For the overkill approach, it is usual to assume that the initial bioburden is 1×10^6; hence the cycle is sometimes referred to as a 12D or 12-log cycle.

A less stringent SAL of 10^{-3} may, however, be acceptable in certain circumstances, owing to the nature of the product or the way in which it is to be used. This may be the case for aseptically made preparations, where a heat sterilization process is inappropriate owing to the nature of the material. In the USA, for certain medical devices which only come into contact with intact skin or mucous membranes, this less rigorous standard may be acceptable, although in Europe this level would be more likely to be described as "disinfected" rather than sterilized.

Factors affecting sterility assurance

A population of organisms exposed to a sterilizing agent will not die simultaneously. It will exhibit varying resistance to the sterilizing agent. As can be seen from Figure 18.2, there are significantly different mechanisms for the destruction of microorganisms. Some microorganisms are known to be more susceptible to sterilization processes than others, in general progressing from the more susceptible large viruses, to vegetative forms of bacteria and fungi, to fungal spores and small viruses, and finally to bacterial spores used as reference organisms to determine the efficacy of sterilization processes.

The concept of being sterile is, therefore, quite straightforward. However, just because a device or product has been sterilized does not mean that it will be sterile at the point of use; this is more a question of sterility maintenance than it is of inadequacy of the sterilization process (see below).

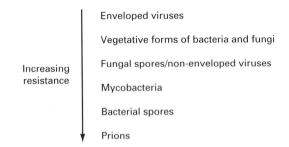

Increasing resistance

Enveloped viruses

Vegetative forms of bacteria and fungi

Fungal spores/non-enveloped viruses

Mycobacteria

Bacterial spores

Prions

Figure 18.2 Relative susceptibilities of microorganisms to sterilization processes.

The bioburden of any pharmaceutical product or medical device undergoing sterilization is likely to be composed of a mixed microbial flora, with varying levels of intrinsic resistance to the sterilization process. This may well contrast with laboratory sterilization studies involving the determination of resistance, which are more likely to use stock microbial cultures with well-characterized resistance patterns.

A given sterilization process can be considered as delivering a specific inactivation of microorganisms. Hence the initial bioburden of the device or product prior to sterilization will have a profound effect on the resulting SAL. Clearly, the higher the bioburden, the greater the challenge to the sterilizing process and, by the same token, the greater the probability of finding microbial survivors. Longer or more efficacious sterilization processes may need to be specified to ensure that a given SAL is achieved.

One factor common to all sterilization processes is contact with the sterilant; microorganisms that are occluded or protected from the sterilant will have significantly different inactivation kinetics than those that are readily presented to the sterilant. The most obvious example is the penetration of steam in a moist-heat process. Many different types of load can entrain air and hence prevent steam penetration. Thermometric mapping may only indicate temperature differences of several degrees cooler in these locations, but the fact that there is air present at these temperatures, and not steam, as the sterilant, will effectively render devices or products non-sterile. Device cleanliness is another similar factor, which is significant in the healthcare reprocessing of medical devices. Soiling from inadequate cleaning, hydrophobic instrument lubricants and even device design can significantly affect the sterilization outcome.

When considering pharmaceutical products, the chemical nature of such products may alter the resistance of the microorganisms to that expected in laboratory studies.

Sterility assurance in practice

There are two routes that can be utilized in order to be able to demonstrate achievement of the correct SAL. The traditional approach to sterility assurance has been based on the sterility test, whereby a direct assessment is made of the microbiological status of the article or product in question. A representative sample of the batch purporting to be sterile is selected and either inoculated into a suitable culture medium or passed through a membrane filter and then inoculated into an appropriate culture medium. Following incubation, the culture media are examined for evidence of microbial growth and, based on the absence or presence of this visual inspection, the sample passes or fails the test, respectively. The other route, parametric release, involves not only a detailed monitoring of the sterilization process itself but also using this information to make indirect inferences about the microbiological status of the product, based upon the treatment to which it has been exposed.

Due to the severe limitations of the sterility test, emphasis has been placed on parametric release whenever possible. However, both methods continue to be used today for both terminally-sterilized and aseptically-made products, there being no alternative test in the case of the latter. However, in terms of status, it must be emphasized that nowadays the sterility test, as applied to the finished product, should only be regarded as the last in a series of control measures by which sterility is assured. Thus, compliance with the test for sterility alone does not constitute absolute assurance of freedom from microbial contamination. Reliable manufacturing procedures provide a greater assurance of sterility.

Sterility testing

While the concept of performing a sterility test is simple and straightforward, both in practice and in theory it is fraught with difficulty; furthermore, it presents not only a technical but also a mathematical challenge. From a technical point of view, the test must be performed under suitable conditions, designed to minimize the risk of accidental microbial contamination. In practice, this involves a suitably qualified, carefully trained and appropriately-clad operator (i.e. wearing sterile, clean-room clothing) carrying out the test in a properly maintained laminar flow cabinet.

Clearly, staff involved in this testing should have a high level of proficiency in aseptic technique. This should be regularly monitored and recorded, using sterile broth-filling trials. The US Pharmacopeia (USP) Committee of Revision [6] suggested that a false positive rate not exceeding 0.5% was desirable. Records of routine failure rates for each operator should also be kept and, if warranted, an individual's requalification in sterility testing may be required.

While samples taken for sterility testing should be representative of the entire batch, it is accepted that the sampling should take particular account of those parts of the batch considered to be most at risk from contamination. Thus, for aseptically filled products, samples should include not only those containers filled at the beginning, middle and end of the batch, but also those filled after any significant interruption in the filling environment. Likewise, for heat-sterilized products in their final container, the sampling scheme should be skewed to account for those samples taken from the coolest part of the load, as determined during commissioning studies.

Detailed sampling instructions and testing procedures are given in the current pharmacopoeias. These form the basis of legal referee data in the event of litigation, legal validation or regulatory requirements. The test may be applied not only to parenteral and non-parenteral sterile products, but also to other articles that are required to be sterile.

As alluded to above, the mathematics of sampling pose a number of problems for those involved in sterility testing. As explained in detail below, the results are determined by both the number of samples taken and the incidence of contamination. In mathematical terms, if n is the number of containers tested, p the proportion of contaminated containers and q the proportion of non-infected containers in a batch, then:

$$p + q = 1$$

From this it can be deduced that:

the probability of rejection $= 1 - (1 - p)^n$

The implications of this are shown in Table 18.1, where it can be seen that, with a constant sample size of 20 containers and with varying proportions of the batch contaminated, the probability of drawing 20 consecutive sterile items is given. It can be seen that, with random sampling of the batch, very low levels of contamination cannot be detected with certainty by the test. Hence, if 10 items remained contaminated in a batch of 1000 units (i.e. $p = 0.01$), the probability of accepting the entire batch as sterile, based on a 20 unit sample size, would be $(1 - 0.01)^{20} = 0.99^{20} = 0.82$. Thus, in 82 instances out of 100, all 20 random samples would give negative results and the entire batch would be passed as sterile, although the batch actually contained 10 unsterilized units.

Table 18.1 Sampling in sterility testing.

	Contaminated items in batch (%)					
	0.1	1	5	10	20	50
p	0.001	0.01	0.05	0.1	0.2	0.5
q	0.999	0.99	0.95	0.9	0.8	0.5
Probability, P, of drawing 20 consecutive sterile items:						
First sterility test[a]	0.98	0.82	0.36	0.12	0.012	<0.00001
First retest[b]	0.99	0.99	0.84	0.58	0.11	0.002

[a]Calculated from $P = (1 - p)20 = q20$.
[b]Calculated from $P = (1 - p)20 [2 - (1 - p)20]$.
p, proportion of contaminated containers in batch; q, proportion of non-contaminated containers in batch.

Clearly, the chance of detecting an individual contaminated unit in a batch increases both as the batch contamination rate rises and as the number of samples increases. All pharmacopoeias provide guidance on the number of samples to be tested, depending on the type of product, its intended use and the size of the batch. During its performance, the sterility test is prone to accidental contamination (through faulty aseptic technique or materials), and, again, all current pharmacopoeias make allowance for this by permitting a retest if the first test is shown to be invalid. In this case, the probability of passing a defective batch on the basis of testing a further 20 samples actually increases, as can be seen from the same table, since a proportion of the contaminated samples have already been removed in the first test. In mathematical terms, the probability of passing a defective batch at the first retest is:

$$(1 - p)^n [2 - (1 - p)^n]$$

In recent years, there has been considerable progress in terms of harmonizing the individual pharmacopoeial sterility test methods. Current editions of the European Pharmacopoeia (EP) and USP bear a close resemblance to one another in terms of their test requirements. Pharmacopoeial products are nowadays tested for sterility using a membrane-filtration technique (0.45 μm filter pore size), any contaminating organisms being retained on the surface of the filter. If, however, this proves to be unsuitable, a direct inoculation technique may be used. Similarly, suitable test media are described for the growth of aerobic, anaerobic and fungal organisms. Before use, these must be tested not only for their sterility but also for their ability to support microbial growth, using specified test organisms. In addition, it must be shown that any microbicidal activity inherent in the preparation under test has been neutralized sufficiently for it to support the growth of a small inoculum of named test organisms (approximately 100 colony-forming units (cfu)).

Process monitoring and parametric release

Owing to the severe limitations of the sterility test, an alternative method of assuring sterility of sterilized products is utilized whenever possible. The parametric release concept has been widely accepted by the medical device, pharmaceutical and European healthcare areas, while healthcare settings in North America place heavy emphasis on the use of biological indicators (BIs). Sterility is assured by adopting an approach based upon process monitoring. In essence, this proposition rests upon the assumptions that if the sterilizing equipment is in proper working order, if the product has been subjected to a validated sterilizing treatment and if good manufacturing practices (GMPs) prevail, then the batch or load will be sterile and can be released for use.

It follows, therefore, that this approach is based upon three related components, discussed in detail below:

• *Equipment function tests*, proving proper mechanical operation of the sterilizer.

• *Performance verification tests*, showing product exposure for the correct sterilization cycle.

• *Process validation practices* which indicate bioburden levels, verify the kinetics of microbial inactivation, justify the design of sterilizing treatments and ensure correct pre- and post-handling of the product.

This method of assuring sterility by monitoring only the physical conditions of the sterilization process is termed "parametric release". It has been defined as the release of sterile products based on process compliance to physical specification [7]. Parametric release is currently used for product release from steam, ethylene oxide, vapor phase hydrogen peroxide, dry heat and ionizing radiation sterilization processes, where the physical conditions are understood and can be monitored directly.

Parametric release is inappropriate for filtration sterilization processes. There is always a probability, albeit remote, that a microorganism can pass through one of the few pores at the larger pore size extreme of the pore size distribution of the filter. Additionally, the absorption process in filtration involves a degree of probability of retention. Thus, sterile filtration must be regarded as a probability function and not as absolute. Moreover, filtration is a unit operation, wherein process validation is not practicable, unlike other sterilization methods. Thus, full aseptic precautions must be observed during processing, and a high SAL is dependent upon GMP and an initial low bioburden in the product. Stringent tests for sterility are also required. The parametric release of product in practice is discussed in further detail below.

Equipment function tests

Regardless of the method of sterilization, proper design, construction, installation and operation of the sterilizer are fundamental to sterility assurance. Validation is an intrinsic part of this process; validation is generally recognized to consist of a planned sequence of installation qualification (IQ), operational qualification (OQ) and performance qualification (PQ). Before being taken into routine use, correct functioning of the equipment must be shown, first by a process of IQ, then OQ and finally by PQ. The responsibility for these tasks is usually by the equipment manufacturer, the installer and the legal user of the equipment. Installation qualification involves the demonstration and certification that all parts of the sterilizer have been correctly installed, all measuring instruments have been correctly calibrated and all items of equipment comply with their performance specifications. During OQ, it must be demonstrated that, for any given load, the sterilizer performs reliably under automatic control, and that sterilization conditions are attained within every part of the load. Test and surrogate loads are often used at this stage to show that sterilization conditions are capable of being delivered to defined loads. The European standard for steam sterilizers, EN285, for example, gives type and performance test requirements that could be used as part of the OQ stage [8]. ISO 17665-1, *Sterilization of Health Care Products – Moist Heat – Part 1*

– *Requirements for the development, validation and routine control of a sterilization process for medical devices* [9], gives specific information for moist-heat sterilization validation, with guidance on Part 1 given in Part 2 [10]. Permanent records, in the form of chart recordings, computer printouts or electronic data archives, will provide evidence that sterilization conditions have been generated in the load.

Tests carried out during OQ and PQ studies will vary according to the method of sterilization used. In the case of heat sterilizers, heat distribution and penetration studies are undertaken, using thermocouples positioned at strategically determined places within the chamber and load. Such tests would normally need to be reviewed and if necessary repeated if there is any change in such variables as product type, shape or size of load. In the case of irradiation sterilization, the penetration of the ionizing radiation within the load is best monitored by the use of an adequate number of dosimeters, again strategically distributed. Where gas sterilizers are used, temperature, relative humidity and gas concentration are measured by physical sensors within the chamber and/or load. BIs may also be used during validation to demonstrate attainment of the critical parameters necessary for sterilization, although use of a BI in full cycle conditions may not solely be capable of demonstrating a SAL of 10^{-6}.

OQ of sterilizing filters is focused upon filter-integrity testing, pressure differentials and flow rate measurements. Additionally, environmental control and its validation during the filtration process itself must be considered an integral part of the sterile filtration process [11].

Performance verification tests

Equipment function tests, as discussed above, prove that the sterilizer and its process are performing to specification. However, it must then be shown that these conditions within the chamber are simultaneously provided within the microenvironments throughout the load, and sometimes irrespective of the packaging materials used. Chemical indicators (CIs) and biological indicators (BIs) are widely used to verify this.

Chemical indicators

Chemical indicators may be described as a test system that reveals change in one or more predefined process variables based on a chemical or physical change resulting from exposure to a process. This chemical or physical change usually presents in the form of a color change that is then interpreted by the user according to the instructions provided by the CI manufacturer. The point of the color change is defined as the end-point. CIs are available for many types of sterilization process. The performance of CIs is specified in ISO 11140-1, where they are identified according to the sterilization process they are designed to be used in, and the class of indicator in terms of their intended application and function (see classification below). Their reliability, stability and safety must also be considered when choosing which type and class of CI is best suited to the particular application. As is the case for any sterilization process monitor, CIs should be viewed as one of several complementary indicators of sterilization conditions that include both biological and physical parameter indicators (such as thermocouples). It should be noted that while CIs have either a qualitative or semiquantitative response (they cannot necessarily give a quantification of the variables they have been exposed to), they can discriminate between different media such as air and steam in a steam sterilizer, whereas a thermocouple can give a quantitative response but cannot discriminate between these two media. CIs are typically marked with their lot number and the expiry date, together with storage criteria. In all cases, the instructions given by the manufacturer must be followed if the CIs are to function as specified.

ISO 11140-1 defines six classes of CI that have different functions and these must be considered when choosing which CI to use:

1. *Class 1 indicators*, sometimes referred to as process indicators, are intended for use with individual packs or load components to show that the load component has been exposed to a sterilization process (i.e. to show that a load item has been processed, for example autoclave tape or adhesive labels with an indicator printed onto it).

2. *Class 2 indicators* are designed for use in specific test procedures, such as the Bowie–Dick test [12]. ISO 17665-1 requires that a Bowie–Dick test is performed at the commencement of each day (after a warm-up cycle) in all pre-vacuum steam sterilizers to assess the ability of the sterilizer to penetrate steam into a load of defined resistance. A Bowie–Dick indicator should be placed into an otherwise empty chamber as this is the worst case scenario for steam penetration.

3. *Class 3 indicators* will respond only to a single sterilization variable, such as time or temperature. As such, Class 3 indicators are not usually considered useful in processes that have two or more critical variables.

4. *Class 4 indicators* are multivariable indicators that will respond to two or more of the variables for the sterilization process for which they are intended. These indicators are designed to be placed within the load to monitor attainment of sterilization critical variables.

5. *Class 5 indicators* are designed to integrate all sterilization variables and to be equivalent to, or exceed, the performance of BIs that are specified in the ISO 11138 series for BIs. These indicators are designed to be placed within the load to monitor attainment of sterilization critical variables.

6. *Class 6 indicators*, sometimes termed cycle verification indicators, are designed to integrate all sterilization variables with their performance correlated to the actual settings of the sterilization cycle. These indicators are designed to be placed within the load to monitor attainment of sterilization critical variables.

Class 3, 4, 5 and 6 indicators are defined by the CI manufacturer in terms of their performance by stated values (SVs). These SVs should be carefully considered by the user to ensure that the performance of the indicator is suitable for their intended application. For example, a class 6 indicator may have SVs of 134°C and 3.5 min. This means that the indicator will reach its end-point (point of color change) after 3.5 min at 134°C. It therefore stands to reason that this indicator is suited to monitoring a 134°C, 3.5 min sterilization process. If the same indicator were to be used in a 134°C, 18 min process, the indicator would be giving much less information about the total process; in this latter case, an indicator with SVs of 134°C and 18 min would be more appropriate.

Biological indicators

Biological indicators are used extensively in sterilization cycle validation. They integrate all the sterilization variables such as time, temperature, gas concentration, humidity, etc. In common with CIs, since BIs are placed directly in the container or load, they will reflect the actual sterilizing conditions in the product or load itself, rather than just in the sterilizer environment in which the container or load has been placed. BIs generally utilize a bacterial strain that has been specially selected for its high resistance to the given sterilization process. Moreover, since the microbial load on the BI is likely to present considerably more of a challenge – in terms of numbers and resistance to the sterilization process – than the expected bioburden of the product, then considerable confidence can be placed in the expected level of sterility assurance associated with the process.

Biological indicators are commercially available preparations containing known numbers of microorganisms deposited on a carrier, often in the form of either metal foil or paper strips or disks. BIs are also available in a "self-contained" format with both the inoculated carrier and recovery medium in a sealed container. After processing, the recovery medium is released and the BI can be incubated as a whole unit. This significantly minimizes the chances of inadvertent contamination of the BI during aseptic transfer to the recovery medium. In some instances, BIs consist of inoculated units of the actual device or product. The microbial challenge usually comprises aerobic bacterial endospore formers (*Bacillus* and *Geobacillus* spp.), although occasionally *Clostridium* spp. may be used, selected on the basis of their resistance to a given sterilization process. BIs are, therefore, characterized by the strain of test organism, the number of colony-forming units per test piece, the *D*-value (decimal reduction value) determined under defined (and specified) conditions and the *z*-value (relating the heat resistance of a microorganism to changes in temperature). BIs are typically labeled with the above information, together with the lot and expiry date. *D*- and *z*-values are presented in Chapters 15.1 and 15.2.

Following exposure to the sterilization process, BIs are cultured in suitable media and under appropriate recovery conditions, as specified by the manufacturer. This latter point is of significance as small changes in the formulation of the recovery medium can have great consequences for the growth of the organism. If no growth occurs, the level of lethality can be calculated to be greater than the log of the population of the BI; in the event of growth occurring, it is normal to establish whether the growth is derived from the original inoculum or whether it represents accidental contamination during handling or culturing.

A number of factors are known to affect the reliability of BIs. These include the basis of the genotypically determined resistance, environmental influences during growth and sporulation, the environment during storage, the influence of the environment during sterilization, and finally the influence of recovery media and conditions. A discussion of these factors is outside the scope of this chapter, but the reader is referred to Quesnel [13]. Thus, as with all biological systems, because of their inherent variability BIs must be considered as less precise indicators of events than physical parameters. Hence, in the event of failure to comply with a physical specification, a sterilization cycle will be regarded as unsatisfactory in spite of contrary evidence from the BI supporting the lethality of the sterilizing process.

The performance of BIs is specified in the ISO 11138 series of standards. As well as specifying standardized labeling requirements, the performance of BIs using specified methods is given. Recommended reference strains of the organisms are also listed, but typically the following organisms are used:

• Steam and other moist-heat processes: *Geobacillus stearothermophilus*.
• Dry-heat processes: *Bacillus atrophaeus*.
• Ethylene oxide sterilization: *B. atrophaeus*.

Note that BIs are not commonly used for ionizing radiation processes, but if they are, *Bacillus pumilus* has been used as the organism.

Further information on the use of BIs in sterilizers employed in the manufacture of sterile medical devices can be obtained from the biological indicator guidance document ISO 14161. Specific requirements for BIs are given in ISO 11138-1 (general requirements), ISO 11138-2 (ethylene oxide sterilization), ISO 11138-3 (moist-heat sterilization), ISO 11138-4 (dry-heat sterilization) and ISO 11138-5 (low-temperature steam and formaldehyde (LTSF)).

BIs may be used for three main purposes: cycle development, validation and routine monitoring of sterilization processes. During cycle development, the ability of a given sterilization process to destroy a challenge from resistant organisms must be assessed. These contaminants can originate from a number of sources, including raw materials, operators or the production environment itself. Once their resistance has been characterized, they can then be used as resistant microbiological reference standards. In effect, such reference organisms in turn become BIs and can be used to evaluate the required cycle to achieve the desired SAL. The term "validation" describes tests on a sterilizer and a given product to determine that the sterilization process operates efficiently and performs repeatedly as expected. Any validation exercise must therefore assess not only the physical performance of the sterilizer but also the sterilization performance of the process on the product. The term "monitoring", on the other hand, implies the routine control of a process.

The use of BIs in practice depends not only upon the regulatory requirements of the country or region in question but also on the efficacy of alternative methods. In some instances, they represent the only practical method of monitoring sterilization cycles, whereas in other situations physical and chemical indicator methods offer a much more reliable and efficient alternative.

On an industrial scale, routine monitoring of ethylene oxide sterilization is largely based on physical parameter measurement (parametric release); however, the use of BIs in routine monitoring is prevalent, largely as this is a regulatory requirement in some parts of the world. Smaller-scale or hospital utilization of ethylene oxide sterilization, for example, would not necessarily have the expensive gas concentration monitoring equipment, and so would place increased reliance on BIs, in combination with other methods, namely physical parameter and CI monitoring. In some circumstances BIs may be used as part of the validation program for moist- or dry-heat sterilization cycles. However, they have little use in routine monitoring cycles since the required SAL can be defined in terms of easily and reliably measured physical parameters. Occasionally, their use may be justified in performance qualification, when difficulties arise in ensuring adequate contact and penetration of steam in a particular product.

With regard to sterilization by irradiation, BIs are regarded to be of little value since the process is defined in terms of a minimum absorbed dose of radiation, best and most reliably measured by dosimeters. In some countries, such as France, their use is obligatory for routine monitoring of irradiation sterilization in each batch. During validation work, they may, however, be used for initial characterization of inactivation rates within a given product.

Process validation practices

As discussed previously, sterilization practices nowadays place much greater emphasis upon the concept of sterility assurance, rather than reliance on end-product testing. By understanding the kinetics of microbial inactivation, individual sterilization protocols can be designed to destroy a known and previously determined bioburden with a desired level of confidence in the procedure in question. In other words, by introducing the notion of required margin of safety, the probability of detecting a viable survivor of the sterilizing process can be assessed on a mathematical scale, known as the SAL. As a result, by investing confidence in process validation practices, a system of parametric release can be used for approval of products, as discussed in detail later.

A specific microbial population exposed to a given sterilization cycle has a characteristic response, and the death curve follows a logarithmic pattern. This will depend upon the resistance of the organism concerned, the physicochemical environment where the treatment takes place and the lethality of the process itself. However, if these do not vary, the number of survivors in a known population can be computed after a given period of exposure to the lethal process. Microbial death can be measured in terms of the D-value, which is the time in minutes to reduce the microbial population by 90% or 1-log cycle at a certain temperature (or the dose in kGy when ionizing radiation is used).

As can be seen from Figure 18.3 (line A), if the original population is 10^2 spores and if the D-value is 1 min at 121°C, then after 1 min at 121°C the population will have been reduced to 10^1

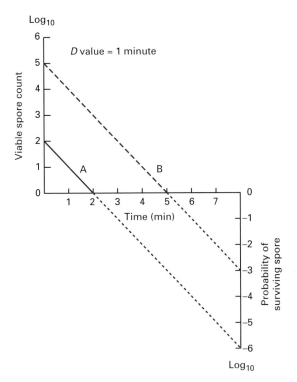

Figure 18.3 Relationship between D-value, initial contamination level and level of sterility assurance.

the method of sterilization. Ionizing radiation will be able to penetrate aluminum packaging that steam would clearly not be able to penetrate.

The maximum likely bioburden, the D-value of the most resistant spore-former in the load and the required SAL will affect the nature of the cycle when the sterilization method has been chosen. With regard to the pre-sterilization bioburden, this requires quantitative evaluation over a period of time. Spore-formers isolated from the bioburden must then be cultured and D-values determined for the resulting spore suspensions under the proposed sterilizing conditions.

In the healthcare setting, many hospitals adopt the "overkill" approach where sterilization cycles are designed in theory to inactivate considerably larger populations than are likely to be present in actual situations. A conservatively high bioburden of 1×10^6 resistant spores per load is usually assumed. When considering that loads reprocessed in a hospital would have been processed in a washer–disinfector prior to packaging under controlled conditions, it is highly unlikely that both the number and the resistant nature of the reference organism would ever be realized.

In accordance with GMP, the processor must document all aspects of the sterilization process. If the load has unusual characteristics that may pose a problem for sterilization, it would be normal to conduct pilot sterilization studies, using actual and surrogate products, with identical packaging to the ultimate process. These packs will previously have been artificially inoculated with either resistant spores from the natural bioburden or BI, outnumbering the normal spore flora both in terms of inoculum size and D-values. Having successfully completed pilot studies, the processor may reasonably assume that the required SAL will be achieved, so long as the process parameters remain unchanged. In this way, the sterilization cycle is literally designed for the product concerned, balancing the likely bioburden challenge and the required SAL against any deleterious effect of the sterilization process on the product or device itself.

Monitoring the sterilization cycle

Reproducibility of sterilization conditions is essential if sterility is to be assured with the required margin of safety. In practice this means that all monitoring equipment, as well as CIs and BIs, must show that the correct sterilizing conditions are being achieved within the microenvironment of the product or device itself. Additionally, microbiological monitoring of the bioburden challenge and its resistance should be shown not to differ significantly from those of the validation studies. Moreover, the packaging and loading of containers should remain unchanged.

Control of the complete process

Regardless of the sterilization method involved, no sterilization process can be considered in isolation, but must be viewed in the context of GMP or a quality system such as that detailed in ISO 13485 or the US Food and Drug Administration (FDA) Quality System Requirement. A discussion of these requirements is outside the scope of this chapter, but essentially it

spores. For each additional minute of exposure to the sterilizing cycle, a further reduction of 1-log cycle in the population will ensue. Thus, after an 8 min cycle at 121°C, the population will have been reduced by a total of 8-log cycles, i.e. from 10^2 to 10^{-6}. In other words, there is a one in a million chance that a viable spore exists per product. Clearly, this probability of contamination cannot be demonstrated in practice using end-product testing in the form of a sterility test. The effect that the bioburden level has on the ensuing SAL of a given process can also be clearly seen from Figure 18.3 (line B). If the original population is 10^5 spores, then the same 8 min cycle will result in a SAL of 10^{-3}. The importance of minimizing bioburden levels in any article ready for sterilization is therefore immediately obvious.

In essence, there are three components to process validation: selection and validation of the sterilizing cycle; monitoring of the cycle; and control of the complete process.

Selection and validation of the sterilization process

In selecting an appropriate sterilization process account must be taken of the nature of the load to be processed. Some load materials or configurations would eliminate some sterilization methods. In all cases, the sterilizing agent must be able to penetrate all parts of the load to be sterilized. Sealed areas of the load where the sterilizing agent cannot access will not be sterilized, but as long as this is well understood and those parts of the load will remain sealed at point of use then this may not ultimately present a problem. The method and nature of the packaging may dictate is based on a well-developed system of documentation and record-keeping. Thus, all records associated with the sterilization process itself must be retained for reference purposes, including sterilizer planned preventive maintenance (PPM) and breakdown records, physical parameter monitoring records, chemical and biological indicator results and experimental data on bioburden and *D*-values, as well as protocols and their validation. Regulatory agencies and notified bodies would expect to scrutinize all such data, along with the records of any ancillary processes such as cleaning and microbiological monitoring of associated controlled environmental areas; equipment maintenance and calibration; personnel training and qualification; and control over the packaging, labeling, wrapping, handling and storage of sterile items.

Bioburden estimation

The bioburden of the pre-sterilized product will be determined not only by the microbial flora of incoming raw materials and components and how they are stored, but also by the microbiological control applied to the environment where the product is manufactured, assembled and packed. Reliable, accurate and reproducible bioburden data must be collected. Any underestimation of the bioburden population would result in a miscalculation of the sterilization requirements for a given product and possible validation failures. Conversely, an overestimation of the bioburden would result in excessive exposure to the sterilizing agent, which in turn could affect the stability or functioning of the product or device. When using the overkill method, a basic understanding of the product bioburden is good practice.

As a group, medical devices present a challenge in terms of bioburden testing. They comprise a large, diverse collection of product types and there is no single, universally applicable technique which is appropriate to all devices. Considerable differences in bioburden levels have been reported [14]. In one study of a diverse group of medical devices, these ranged from less than 1 cfu/device in the case of a syringe to 10^7–10^9 cfu in the case of a biological tissue patch of raw material. The microbiologist must therefore use his/her knowledge and judgment to select the most appropriate technique. Ideally, bioburden estimates should be carried out for each product on a regular basis, although this may not always be practicable. In the latter case, selected testing of groups of products with a common raw material or perhaps a common manufacturing process may be acceptable, provided that the rationale behind such decisions is documented and it is shown that the data are representative of all product groups.

Detailed guidance on the estimation of bioburden in medical devices has been published [15, 16]. Five distinct stages are involved: sample selection; removal of microorganisms from the device, involving one or a combination of suggested techniques; transfer of microorganisms to recovery conditions; enumeration of microorganisms with specific characteristics; and

interpretation of data, involving the application of correction factors determined during validation studies. In addition, where the medical device is shown or known to release inhibitory substances (which may in turn affect bioburden recovery), the method should incorporate a validated neutralization or filtration step.

Parametric release of product in practice

As discussed previously, parametric release is accepted as the preferential method for routine sterility testing for the batch release of finished sterile products. Products or devices exposed in their final packaging to predetermined, fully validated terminal sterilizing conditions using steam, ethylene oxide, dry heat or ionizing radiation may be released batch by batch on the basis of accumulated process data, subject to the approval of the relevant regulatory agencies. Through parametric release, the manufacturer can provide assurance that the product or device is of the stipulated quality, thus meeting its specification, based on evidence of successful validation of the manufacturing process and review of the documentation on process monitoring carried out during manufacturing.

Parametric release is common practice in the sterile medical device industry for the release of batches sterilized by ethylene oxide processes, providing that the requirements of ISO 11135 [17] are met. If alternative methods of sterilization are used, sterility testing may be required depending on the type of device, company practice or the intended destination of the product.

When using parametric release, the manufacturer must demonstrate not only sufficient experience and control of the general manufacturing process through GMP compliance (based on both historical and current batch data) but also that the sterilization process is adequately validated and reliably controlled, and meets the requirements of the relevant pharmacopoeia. In particular, standard operating procedures (SOPs) of significance for sterility should be in place to ensure control of the quality of starting and packaging materials, process water and the manufacturing environment. SOPs should also detail the reporting and course of action to be taken for both approval and rejection of devices or product. With regard to sterilization issues, the choice of a particular sterilization method must be well founded, based on either device manufacturers' reprocessing instructions, or knowledge of product stability and information gained during development studies. As discussed earlier in this chapter, qualification of sterilization equipment and validation of the process (including heat distribution and penetration studies for a given load), accompanied by biological validation, are expected to be demonstrated in accordance with GMP guidelines [18]. Once defined the sterilization process should be shown to be reproducible and appropriate for a bioburden of known magnitude and heat resistance. Moreover, specific GMP requirements for parametric release must be met, for example segregation of sterilized from non-sterile products.

In the case of ionizing radiation sterilization, parametric release can be applied to those products exposed to a minimum absorbed dose of 25 kGy. However, lower doses may be acceptable if justified by low, routinely checked bioburden levels and adequate validation data.

Once parametric release has been approved as the releasing mechanism, release or rejection decisions of a batch must then be based on the approved specification. Such decisions cannot be subsequently over-ruled by use of sterility tests.

In summary, the introduction of parametric release for terminally-sterilized devices or products removes or reduces the requirement for sterility testing of the final device or product. However, it clearly requires increased technical understanding and awareness of the complete process from design, through manufacture, until final batch release.

Sterile barrier systems

The purpose of packaging is principally to enable a sterilized device or product to be presented in a sterile state at point of use. Hence sterilization packaging is increasingly referred to as a sterile barrier system (SBS). The maintenance of sterility during storage is dependent on SBS integrity. Provided this is not compromised in any way, sterility will be maintained, irrespective of the time for which it is stored. Klapes *et al.* [19] showed that the probability of contamination in freshly sterilized packs did not differ statistically from that in packs which had been stored for up to a year. It is good practice, however, to ensure that sterile goods are stored in controlled and clean areas and that a shelf-life (expiration date) is used to help in good practice stock rotation to ensure that older products are used first.

It is for sterility maintenance reasons that wet loads from steam sterilizers are rejected; the presence of water will allow microorganisms to grow through SBS materials that would normally, in the dry state, serve as an efficient barrier.

References

1 International Standards Organization (ISO) (2005) *ISO/TS 11139. Sterilization of Health Care Products – Vocabulary*, ISO, Geneva.

2 European Committee for Standardization (CEN) (2001) *European Standard EN556-1. Sterilization of Medical Devices. Requirements for a Terminally Sterilized Device to be Labelled "Sterile"*, CEN, Brussels.

3 Busta, F.F. (1978) Introduction to injury and repair of microbial cells. *Advances in Applied Microbiology*, **23**, 195–201.

4 European Committee for Standardization (CEN) (2003) *European Standard EN556-2. Sterilization of Medical Devices. Requirements for medical devices to be designated "STERILE". Requirements for aseptically processed medical devices*, CEN, Brussels

5 Association for the Advancement of Medical Instrumentation (AAMI) (2010) *ST79 Comprehensive Guide to Steam Sterilization and Sterility Assurance in Health Care Facilities*, AAMI, Arlington, VA.

6 (1995) *USP Open Conference: Microbiological Compendial Issues.*

7 Hoxey, E.V. (1989) The case for parametric release, in *Proceedings of the Eucomed Conference on Ethylene Oxide Sterilization, 21–22 April, 1989, Paris*, Eucomed, London, pp. 25–32.

8 European Committee for Standardization (CEN) (2010) *European Standard EN285. Sterilization – Steam Sterilizers – Large Sterilizers*, CEN, Brussels

9 International Standards Organization (ISO) (2006) ISO 17665-1. *Sterilization of Health Care Products – Moist Heat – Part 1 – Requirements for the development, validation and routine control of a sterilization process for medical devices*, ISO, Geneva.

10 International Standards Organization (ISO)/TS (2009) *17665-2:2009 Sterilization of Health Care Products. Moist Heat. Guidance on the Application of ISO 17665-1*, ISO, Geneva.

11 Wallhaeusser, K.-H. (1988) *In Praxis Der Sterilisation–Desinfektion–Konservierung*, 4th edn, Thieme, Stuttgart.

12 Bowie, J.H. *et al.* (1963) The Bowie and Dick autoclave tape test. *Lancet*, **i**, 586.

13 Quesnel, L.B. (1984) Biological indicators and sterilization processes, in *Revival of Injured Microbes*, Society for Applied Bacteriology Symposium Series No. 12 (eds M.H.E. Andrew and A.D. Russell), Academic Press, London, pp. 257–291.

14 Hoxey, E. (1993) Validation of methods for bioburden estimation, in *Sterilization of Medical Products*, vol. VI (ed. R.F. Morrissey), PolyScience, Morin Heights, Canada, pp. 176–180.

15 International Standards Organization (ISO) (2006) EN ISO 11737-1:2006. *Sterilization of Medical Devices. Microbiological Methods. Determination of a Population of Microorganisms on Products*, ISO, Geneva

16 International Standards Organization (ISO) (2009) EN ISO 11737-2:2009. *Sterilization of Medical Devices. Microbiological Methods. Tests of Sterility Performed in the Definition, Validation and Maintenance of a Sterilization Process*, ISO, Geneva.

17 International Standards Organization (ISO) (2007) *ISO 11135-1. Sterilization of Health Care Products. Ethylene Oxide, Requirements for Development, Validation and Routine Control of a Sterilization Process for Medical Devices*, ISO, Geneva.

18 Anon. (1997) *The Rules Governing Medicinal Products in the European Community*, vol. IV, Office for Official Publications of the EC, Luxembourg.

19 Klapes, N.A. *et al.* (1987) Effect of long term storage on sterile status of devices in surgical packs. *Infection Control*, **8**, 289–293.

19.1   Hand Hygiene

Benedetta Allegranzi[1] and Didier Pittet[2]

[1] World Health Organization Patient Safety, World Health Organization, Geneva, Switzerland
[2] Infection Control Program and WHO Collaborating Centre on Patient Safety, University of Geneva Hospitals and Faculty of Medicine, Geneva, Switzerland

Transmission of healthcare-associated pathogens through hands

Healthcare-associated infections (HAIs) are spread in different ways, but contaminated hands of healthcare-workers (HCWs) are the most common vehicle. By evaluating available evidence, Pittet and colleagues identified a five-step sequence leading to microbial transmission through hands during healthcare delivery [1]:

1. Pathogens shed by an infected or colonized patient can contaminate the immediate surroundings.

2. The hands of the HCW can become contaminated by contact with the patient's skin or environmental surfaces.

3. The pathogen must remain viable on the HCW's hands for at least several minutes.

4. The HCW may omit hand decontamination entirely or use an inappropriate product/procedure.

5. The HCW's contaminated hands can then either transfer the pathogen directly to another patient or indirectly by depositing the pathogen on a medical device or an environmental surface in the patient's immediate vicinity.

Healthcare-associated pathogens can be recovered not only from infected or draining wounds, but also from frequently colonized areas of normal, intact patient skin [2–15]. The perineal or inguinal areas tend to be most heavily colonized, but the axillae, trunk and upper extremities (including the hands) are also frequently colonized [2–15]. The number of organisms present on intact areas of some patient's skin, such as *Staphylococcus aureus*, *Proteus mirabilis*, *Klebsiella* spp. and *Acinetobacter* spp., can vary from 100 to 10^6 colony-forming units (CFU)/cm^2 [6, 8, 12, 16].

Russell, Hugo & Ayliffe's: Principles and Practice of Disinfection, Preservation and Sterilization, Fifth Edition. Edited by Adam P. Fraise, Jean-Yves Maillard, and Syed A. Sattar.
© 2013 Blackwell Publishing Ltd. Published 2013 by Blackwell Publishing Ltd.

As almost 10^6 skin squamae containing viable microorganisms are shed daily from normal skin [17], it is not surprising that patient gowns, bed linen, bedside furniture and other objects in the immediate environment of the patient become contaminated with patient flora [13–15, 18–26]. Through repeated hand contact, frequently touched surfaces even not placed in the immediate patient surroundings, such as computer keyboards and mobile phones, have been found to be contaminated with nosocomial pathogens and probably play a role in transmission dynamics [27–29]. Surface contamination is most likely to be due to staphylococci, enterococci or *Clostridium difficile*, which are more resistant to desiccation. Certain Gram-negative rods, such as *Acinetobacter baumannii*, can also play an important role in environmental contamination due to their long-time survival capacities [30–34].

Many studies have documented that HCWs can contaminate their hands or gloves with pathogens such as Gram-negative bacilli, *S. aureus*, enterococci or *C. difficile* by performing "clean procedures" or touching hospitalized patients' intact areas of skin [8, 9, 15, 21, 22, 34–38]. Following contact with patients and/or a contaminated environment, microorganisms can survive on hands for differing durations of time (2 to 60 min). HCWs' hands become progressively colonized with commensal flora, as well as with potential pathogens during patient care [35, 36]. In the absence of hand hygiene, the longer the duration of care, the higher the degree of hand contamination (Figure 19.1.1) [35].

Defective hand cleansing (e.g. use of an insufficient amount of product and/or insufficient duration of hand hygiene) leads to

poor hand decontamination. Obviously, when HCWs fail to clean their hands during the sequence of care of a single patient and/or between patient contacts, microbial transfer is likely to occur. Contaminated HCWs' hands have been associated with endemic HAIs [39, 40] and several HAI outbreaks [41–49].

Products and methods for hand antisepsis and infrastructures required for optimal hand hygiene

Hand hygiene can be performed either by washing with soap and water or by rubbing with an alcohol-based formulation. Many hand hygiene products are commercially available and differ in formulation, method of application and length of contact needed for hand decontamination.

Soaps are available in various forms including bar, tissue, leaf and liquid preparations. Plain soap can be used for routine handwashing, despite the fact that it has minimal, if any microbicidal activity [50, 51]. Through its detergent properties, lipids and adhering dirt, soil and various organic substances, as well as loosely adherent transient flora, can be removed from the hands.

Various microbicidal agents are suitable for hand antisepsis and are included in hand hygiene products. The most common agents are alcohols, chlorhexidine, chloroxylenol, hexachlorophene, iodine and iodophors, quaternary ammonium compounds (QACs) and triclosan. These are all effective against Gram-positive and Gram-negative bacteria with maximum efficacy demonstrated by alcohols [52–60] and iodophors, with low activity against Gram-negative bacteria by chloroxylenol, hexachlorophene and QACs [50]. Mycobacteria and fungi are most effectively eliminated by alcohols, and less effectively by chlorhexidine, chloroxylenol and hexachlorophene. Most enveloped (lipophilic) viruses, such as herpesvirus, human immunodeficiency virus, influenza viruses, respiratory syncytial virus and vaccinia virus, are susceptible to alcohols, chlorhexidine and iodophors [52, 61–69]. A recent *in vivo* study demonstrated that both handwashing with plain soap and handrubbing with alcohol-based products (containing either 61.5% or 70% ethanol or 70% isopropyl alcohol) are effective to significantly reduce hand contamination by H1N1 virus [70]. Other enveloped viruses (hepatitis B and probably hepatitis C) are less susceptible to alcohols, but are killed by higher concentrations (70–80% v/v) [71, 72]; alcohols also showed some *in vivo* activity against a number of non-enveloped viruses (rotavirus, adenovirus, rhinovirus, hepatitis A virus, enteroviruses) [71–75]. *In vitro* virucidal activity against surrogate strains of norovirus was demonstrated by 70% alcohol-based formulations, particularly ethanol [76, 77], and by the World Health Organization (WHO) recommended formulation [78] based on 80% ethanol [79]. Furthermore, several norovirus outbreaks were controlled with various preventive measures, including handrubbing with alcohol-based solutions [80, 81]. In general, ethanol has a greater activity against viruses than isopropanol [82]. Iodophors, and to a minor extent chlorhexidine, are

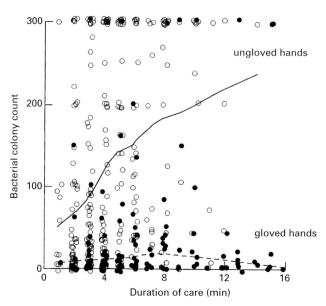

Figure 19.1.1 Relationship between duration of patient care and bacterial contamination of hands of hospital staff who wore gloves (solid circles and dashed line) and those who did not wear gloves (open circles and solid line) in 417 observations conducted at the University Hospitals of Geneva in 1996. Lines represent the average trend in each group, obtained using non-parametric regression (locally weighted scatterplot smoothing) (Reproduced with permission from [35].)

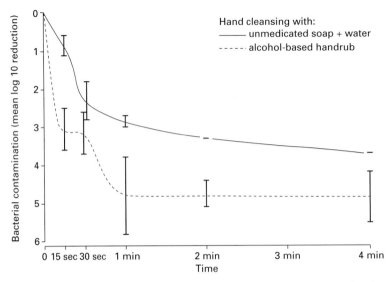

Figure 19.1.2 Time course of efficacy of unmedicated soap and water and alcohol-based handrub in reducing the release of test bacteria from artificially contaminated hands (reproduced with permission from Pittet D, Boyce JM (2001) Hand hygiene and patient care: pursuing the Semmelweis legacy. *Lancet Infect Dis* 1, 9–20).

also active against enveloped and some non-enveloped viruses. None of the listed antiseptic agents has activity against bacterial spores or protozoan oocysts. Only iodophors are slightly sporicidal, but at potentially toxic concentrations higher than the ones used in antiseptics [83]. However, the mechanical effect of hand-washing with soap and water can allow partial removal of bacterial spores or protozoan oocysts. For this reason, handwashing with a non-microbicidal or microbicidal soap and water following glove removal after caring for patients with diarrhea is recommended during *C. difficile*-associated outbreaks, in addition to strict adherence to contact precautions and environmental control measures [50, 51, 84].

According to the Centers for Disease Control and Prevention (CDC) [51] and WHO recommendations [50] (see Appendix 19.1), when an alcohol-based handrub is available it should be used as the preferred means for routine hand hygiene in health-care. The main reasons for the preferential use of these products for routine hand hygiene are the following: (i) alcohols have the broadest microbicidal spectrum compared to other agents; (ii) the handrubbing technique requires a shorter time (20–30 s) for effective microbial decontamination (Figure 19.1.2); (iii) alcohol-based handrub dispensers are more easily available at the point of care (i.e. where and when care is provided); (iv) alcohol-based handrubs have better skin tolerability; and (v) there is no need for any particular infrastructure, such as access to a clean water supply, washbasin, soap or handtowel [50, 78]. Situations (indications) where handwashing with either plain or microbicidal soap and water should be preferred are when hands are visibly dirty or soiled with blood or other body fluids, when exposure to potential spore-forming organisms is strongly suspected or proven, or after using the lavatory [50, 51].

Although comparing the results of laboratory studies investigating the *in vivo* efficacy of plain soap, microbicidal soaps and alcohol-based handrubs may be problematic for various reasons [50], it has been shown that alcohol-based rubs are more efficacious than antiseptic detergents and the latter are usually more efficacious than plain soap. However, various studies conducted in the community setting indicate that medicated and plain soaps are roughly equal in preventing the spread of microorganisms and reducing childhood gastrointestinal, upper respiratory tract infections, impetigo and other infections [85–87] and/or absenteeism due to these diseases [88–91]. In healthcare settings where alcohol-based handrubs are available, plain soap should be provided to perform handwashing when indicated [50]. Advantages and feasibility of alcohol-based handrub use in the community have also been recently demonstrated, with consequent significant reduction of absenteeism due to gastrointestinal and upper respiratory tract infections [92, 93].

The efficacy of the alcohol-based handrub depends on the quality of the product, the amount used, the time spent rubbing and a complete coverage of the hands' surface, which is achieved by performing specific movements in a defined sequence (Figure 19.1.3). These parameters for efficacy also apply to handwashing with soap and water. Alcohol-based handrub formulations containing 60–80% alcohol are usually considered to have adequate microbicidal activity (with concentrations higher than 90% being less potent), provided that they meet the recommended laboratory testing standards (i.e. European Norm (EN) or American Society for Testing and Materials (ASTM) International; see also Chapter 13) [71, 72]. Alcohol-based handrubs with optimal microbicidal efficacy usually contain 75–85% ethanol, isopropanol or *n*-propanol, or a combination of these products. The WHO recommended formulations contain either 75% v/v isopropanol or 80% v/v ethanol [50, 78].

Alcohol-based handrubs are available in different formulations as liquids (with low viscosity), gels and foams. Impregnated wipes

How to Handrub?

RUB HANDS FOR HAND HYGIENE! WASH HANDS WHEN VISIBLY SOILED

🕐 **Duration of the entire procedure: 20-30 seconds**

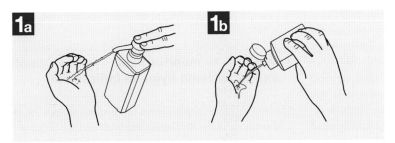

Apply a palmful of the product in a cupped hand, covering all surfaces;

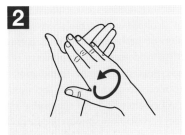

Rub hands palm to palm;

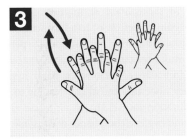

Right palm over left dorsum with interlaced fingers and vice versa;

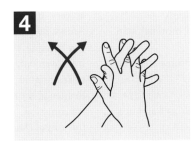

Palm to palm with fingers interlaced;

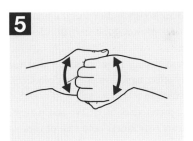

Backs of fingers to opposing palms with fingers interlocked;

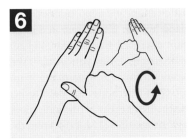

Rotational rubbing of left thumb clasped in right palm and vice versa;

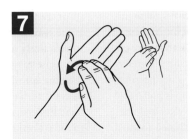

Rotational rubbing, backwards and forwards with clasped fingers of right hand in left palm and vice versa;

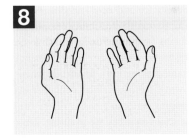

Once dry, your hands are safe.

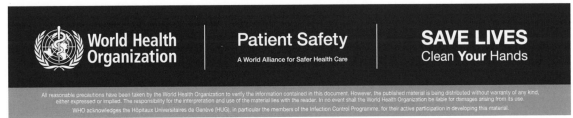

Figure 19.1.3 Hand hygiene technique with an alcohol-based formulation (reproduced with permission from [50]).

also exist, but are not as effective at reducing bacterial counts on HCWs' hands as alcohol-based handrubs or washing hands with microbicidal soap and water. Therefore, they cannot be considered a substitute for the use of an alcohol-based handrub or microbicidal soap.

Until recently, gels were generally considered to have a lower microbicidal efficacy than other formulations [94–96], but new generations of gel formulations with higher microbicidal efficacy than previous products have since been proposed [70, 82]. However, further studies are warranted to determine the relative efficacy of alcohol-based formulations and gels in reducing the transmission of healthcare-associated pathogens. Furthermore, it is worth considering that compliance is probably of higher importance; thus, if a specific formulation with lower *in vitro* activity is more frequently used, the overall outcome is still expected to be better [97]. No substantial evidence on microbicidal efficacy is available to support the use of alcohol-impregnated wipes and alcohol-based foams for hand hygiene [98].

Important aspects need to be evaluated when selecting commercially-produced hand hygiene products [50, 78]:
• Proven efficacy according to ASTM or EN standards for hygienic hand antisepsis and/or surgical hand preparation.
• Tested and proven good dermal tolerance and minimal skin reactions.
• Minimum drying time (products that require longer drying times may affect hand hygiene best practice).
• Cost issues.
• Esthetic preferences of HCWs and patients such as fragrance, color, texture, "stickiness" and ease of use.
• Availability, convenience and functioning of dispensers.
• Ability to prevent contamination.

Rational location of facilities for hand hygiene (i.e. sinks and alcohol-based handrub dispensers) at the point of care, as well as good maintenance and user-friendliness, are essential prerequisites for improving the feasibility of optimal hand hygiene compliance during healthcare delivery. While not all settings have a continuous water supply, tap water (ideally, drinkable) is preferable for handwashing [50]. In settings where this is not possible, water "flowing" from a prefilled container with a tap is preferable to still-standing water in a basin. Where running water and adequate financial resources are available, sensor-activated manual or elbow- or foot-activated taps could be considered the optimal standard within healthcare settings. Each sink should be always equipped with soap (preferably liquid rather than bars) and disposable towels, and located as close as possible to the point of care with an overall sink to patient bed ratio of 1:10 as the minimum requirement [50, 99].

When feasible, the different forms of alcohol-based handrub dispensers, for example wall-mounted or those for use at the point of care, should be used in combination to achieve maximum compliance. Wall-mounted handrub dispensers should be positioned in locations that facilitate hand hygiene at the point of care. Containers with a pump can also be placed easily on any horizontal surface, such as a cart/trolley or nightstand/bedside

table, or affixed to the bed rail. Individual, portable dispensers (e.g. pocket bottles) are ideal, especially if combined with wall-mounted dispensing systems, to increase point of care access and enable use in units where wall-mounted dispensers should be avoided or cannot be installed. Recent designs of both wall-mounted dispensers and pocket bottles have the added asset of including a monitoring device that allows detection of dispensing events and use of alcohol-based handrubs [100–102]. As many types of dispensers are used as disposable items, environmental considerations should also be taken into account.

Methods to monitor hand hygiene compliance and other hand hygiene indicators

Hand hygiene performance in healthcare can be monitored directly or indirectly. Direct methods include direct observation, patient assessment or HCW self-reporting. Indirect methods include monitoring product consumption, such as soap or alcohol-based handrub, and automated monitoring of the use of sinks and handrub dispensers. Monitoring hand hygiene practices is very important in the context of improvement strategies. Among others, the main objectives of hand hygiene monitoring are baseline evaluation, incentive for continuous performance improvement, outbreak investigation, staffing management and infrastructure design [103–113]. However, hand hygiene performance is only one node in a causal tree leading to pathogen transmission, colonization and HAI. As a process element in this causal chain, hand hygiene compliance itself is influenced by many factors, not least the structural aspects related to the quality and availability of products (e.g. soap, handrubs) and facilities (e.g. sinks) at the point of care.

A crucial point specific to hand hygiene monitoring is the distinction between indications and opportunities. The *indication* is the reason why hand hygiene is necessary at a given moment to effectively interrupt microbial transmission and corresponds to precise moments occurring during patient care. Very close to the concept of indication, the term *opportunity* is much more relevant to the observer. It determines the need to perform the hand hygiene action, whether the reason (the indication that leads to the action) be single or multiple [114, 115]. From the observer point of view, the opportunity exists whenever one of the indications for hand hygiene occurs and is observed. Several indications may arise simultaneously and create a single opportunity. Most importantly, the opportunity constitutes the denominator for calculating compliance, that is the number of times that HCWs perform hand hygiene actions when required at all observed moments.

With these concepts in mind, measurement technologies and methods can be divided into two main categories: those with a measured denominator and those without. The hand hygiene action can be performed either by handrubbing with an alcohol-based formulation or by handwashing with soap and water and constitutes the numerator for calculating compliance.

Monitoring hand hygiene by direct observation methods

Detection of hand hygiene compliance by a validated observer (direct observation) is currently considered the gold standard in hand hygiene compliance monitoring [50, 51]. It is the only method that allows following the entire sequence of care and thus identifies all hand hygiene opportunities occurring and actions performed at the appropriate time. Observations are usually performed by trained and validated observers who observe care activity directly, count the number of hand hygiene opportunities, and determine the proportion met by hand hygiene actions. It is essential that hand hygiene opportunities, indications and actions are clearly defined. The validation of observers is essential for the quality of observation data.

Opportunities for hand hygiene action using alcohol-based handrubs can be distinguished from those requiring handwashing with soap and water. Whereas routine monitoring needs to be kept simple and straightforward, observations for research purposes can be more detailed. This can comprise glove use, handrubbing technique, application time and other quality parameters that affect hand hygiene efficacy, such as the wearing of jewelry and fingernail status. A major drawback of direct observation is the major effort required (trained and validated staff and many working hours).

The most important causes of potential bias arising from hand hygiene direct observation are observation, observer and selection bias. Observation bias is generated by an observer whose overt presence influences the behavior of the observed HCWs towards a higher compliance (the so-called "Hawthorne effect") or by increased attention to the topic under study. It can also induce increased recourse to hand hygiene action at inappropriate times not associated with a true improvement in compliance during the sequence of care. If observational surveys are conducted periodically, this bias would be equally distributed among all observations [116]. Observation bias might be eliminated by covert observation, but this method is not recommended when implementing promotional interventions as it can create a climate of mistrust among observed HCWs. This bias can also be attenuated by desensitizing HCWs through the frequent presence of observers or unobtrusive conduct during observation sessions. On the other hand, the Hawthorne effect can be used deliberately to stimulate hand hygiene compliance with a promotional intention, rather than to obtain objective quantitative results [117–119]. Obtaining a sustained and never-ending Hawthorne effect associated with improved compliance with hand hygiene and decreased infection and cross-transmission rates could certainly represent an ideal perspective [117].

Observer bias refers to the systematic error introduced by inter-observer variation in the observation method. To reduce this bias, observers must be validated. Of note, even the same observer can unconsciously change his/her method over time. If hand hygiene compliance is monitored to assess the impact of a hand hygiene promotion intervention, observers could introduce another bias through knowledge of the intervention. As recently documented by Fuller and colleagues [120], blinding observers would be particularly important when conducting randomized control trials of this type.

Selection bias results from systematically selecting HCWs, care settings, observation times or healthcare sectors with a specific hand hygiene behavior. In practical terms, this bias can be minimized by randomly choosing locations, times of day and HCWs.

Another threat to meaningful hand hygiene compliance results is the inclusion of a small sample size. In a comparative quantitative analysis of hand hygiene performance during two different periods, a sufficiently large sample is needed to exclude the influence of chance. If hand hygiene monitoring is used to compare healthcare sectors or periods, confounding factors should be included in the dataset and corrected for by stratification, adjustment or by keeping them unchanged between monitoring sets. Typical confounders in this field are professional category, time of day and healthcare setting. Critical reviews of observation methods have been published on this topic [121–123].

Direct observation of hand hygiene practices is an essential component of the WHO Hand Hygiene Improvement Strategy. WHO has proposed a standardized hand hygiene observation method [50] based on the concept of "My five moments for hand hygiene" [50, 124] and a method validated by several studies (Figure 19.1.4) [103, 109, 125, 126]. All relevant theoretical concepts that form the basis of this method have been described by Sax and colleagues [115] and the practical aspects of observation are detailed in the *Hand Hygiene Technical Reference Manual* included in the WHO Implementation Toolkit [114]. The latter includes also an observation form for data collection and a compliance calculation form to facilitate immediate performance feedback consistent with the proposed method. For a more

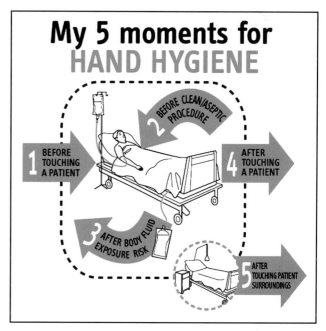

Figure 19.1.4 "My five moments for hand hygiene" (reproduced with permission from [124]).

comprehensive analysis of observation data from multiple sessions, Epi Info data entry and analysis tools are available [127].

Patients could also be observers of HCWs' hand hygiene compliance [128]. Some studies recently reported data on HCWs' practices collected by patients [129–131], but this is a novel approach to hand hygiene monitoring that has never been objectively evaluated [132] and requires further research [133, 134]. Patients may not feel comfortable in a formal role as observers and are not always physically or mentally able to execute this task [135–137].

Although self-assessment by HCWs can be carried out, it has been demonstrated that self-reports do not correlate well with compliance measured by direct observation and markedly overestimate hand hygiene compliance [106, 108, 138–141]. Observers must be aware of the multiple potential biases introduced by the observation process and they can help to minimize these by gaining a full understanding of the methodology. A stringent adherence to the same methodology over space and time is required.

Indirect monitoring of hand hygiene

Monitoring hand hygiene product consumption, such as alcohol-based handrubs or liquid soap, has been identified as a surrogate method of evaluating hand hygiene practices and, in some studies, to estimate the number of hand hygiene actions [103, 104, 118, 142–151]. To make these monitoring techniques more meaningful, the quantity of handrub was translated into a number of hand hygiene actions by using the average amount per action as a divider.

Methods based on product consumption cannot determine if hand hygiene actions are performed at the right moment during care or if the technique is correct. However, the advantages are that they are simple and less demanding in terms of time, human resources and expertise. In addition, they can provide continuous information and a global picture that remains unaffected by selection or observer bias and, most likely, observation bias. The amount of alcohol-based handrub used in healthcare settings has been selected as one of the indicators. Nevertheless, it has to be considered that this measure may not exactly reflect product consumption by HCWs and could include amounts used by visitors or patients, especially if dispensers are also located in public areas and are wall-mounted.

Some studies [103, 118, 142] have shown that the consumption of products used for hand hygiene correlated with observed hand hygiene compliance, whereas others have not [151, 152]. An increasing number of studies have investigated the relation between hand hygiene product consumption and HAI over the past decade, in particular methicillin-resistant *S. aureus* (MRSA) bacteremia, mostly through time series analysis [103, 148–150, 153–161]. By pooling the results of several studies, Sroka and colleagues demonstrated that an increase in alcohol-based handrub consumption significantly correlated with a reduction of MRSA bacteremia or the incidence of MRSA clinical isolates [162]. Although this approach provides new, encouraging

perspectives, some interventions were probably not limited to hand hygiene, and the reliability of these correlations and the best statistical methods to describe these still need to be fully ascertained.

Thus, the use of this measure as a surrogate for monitoring hand hygiene practices deserves further validation. Other studies found that feedback based on measured soap and paper towel consumption did not have an impact on hand hygiene [163, 164].

Automated monitoring of hand hygiene

The use of sinks and handrub dispensers can be monitored electronically [100, 101, 145, 165–170]. These methods are based on the use of liquid soap or hand sanitizer (dispensing events) and/or patient room entries as surrogate markers for hand hygiene compliance. Quantitative estimates of hand hygiene activity can be obtained with the only costs being installation and system maintenance. Changes over time can be assessed. Some studies have attempted to measure the need for hand hygiene by monitoring patient room entries and linking each entry to the use of a sink or a handrub dispenser. These systems can include further sophisticated technology, such as prompting messages [168] and sensors able to identify HCWs when using a sink or a handrub dispenser through their badges (under development), but no comparative studies exist so far to validate the appropriateness of the electronic detection of hand hygiene opportunities.

Wireless devices placed inside handrub or soap dispensers can provide useful information regarding patterns of hand hygiene frequency. A recent study evaluated wireless devices that were placed inside handrub dispensers on a general medical ward and in a surgical intensive care unit. During a 6-month trial period, 105,462 hand hygiene events using handrub were recorded on the surgical intensive care unit at a rate of 48.7 events/patient-day; on the medical ward, detected events were 44,845 with a rate of 12.2 hand hygiene events/patient-day [100]. By mapping the location of each device, it was observed that dispensers located in patient rooms were used significantly less often in medical wards than in the surgical intensive care unit ($P < 0.001$).

Hand hygiene practices among healthcare workers

Caregivers' hands are known to be the most common vehicle of healthcare-associated pathogens [1]. As a consequence, hand hygiene is considered the primary measure to prevent HAI and the spread of microbicidal resistance. However, dynamics during healthcare delivery and the behavior of HCWs significantly influence actual compliance with best hand hygiene practices. Despite a very high perception of their own adherence to hand hygiene recommendations [171–177], HCWs' compliance is usually very low. Through evaluation of the available evidence, the *WHO Guidelines on Hand Hygiene in Health Care* reported mean baseline compliance rates ranging from 5% to 89% with an overall average of 38.7% [50]. Similar data resulted from a recent review on this topic [178]. Some studies document that hand hygiene compliance is particularly low in settings with limited resources in the absence of any promotional activity [179–182]. In these settings, a careful assessment of resources and equipment available for hand hygiene (e.g. soap, alcohol-based handrub) is particularly important because performance of good practices may be actually prevented mainly by lack of resources.

Hand hygiene performance varies according to work intensity, type of ward, professional category, time of day/week and several other factors [50, 178]. In observational studies conducted in hospitals, HCWs cleaned their hands on average from five to as many as 42 times per shift and 1.7 to 15.2 times per hour. The duration of hand-cleansing episodes ranged on average from as short as 6.6 s to 30 s. Compliance is usually higher among nurses than medical doctors [103, 112, 118, 125, 135, 183–186], even if several studies documented that the latter group performs significantly better than the former in developing countries [50, 180, 181]. A recent review including 96 published studies reported that unadjusted compliance rates were lower in intensive care units (30%–40%) than in other settings (50%–60%), lower among physicians (32%) than among nurses (48%), and lower before (21%) rather than after (47%) patient contact [178]. Furthermore, according to many studies, HCWs tend to comply more frequently with indications that protect themselves from being contaminated or infected (e.g. after potential exposure to body fluids, after glove use, after contact with the patient or the patient environment) [50, 181, 187]. Many studies assessed risk factors for non-adherence, reported reasons for the lack of adherence to recommendations, and additional factors perceived as important to facilitate appropriate HCW behavior. Multiple factors determining poor hand hygiene have been identified and/or reported by HCWs (Table 19.1.1) [50].

Strategies to improve hand hygiene compliance

Understanding the factors determining barriers to optimal hand hygiene and reasons for non-compliance by HCWs has been crucial identifing the best strategies to improve practices in healthcare. Most, if not all, identified factors can be addressed through specific interventions that lead to best effects when combined together in a multimodal and multidisciplinary approach.

The interest in the topic of hand hygiene promotion has grown tremendously over the past 30 years as evidenced by the scientific literature published especially in the field of infection control, but also in other specialty areas [218]. A huge number of studies have investigated the effect of specific strategies either as single components or in combination, although the intervention type and duration, the method of hand hygiene compliance assessment, selected indicators and the duration of follow-up varied significantly. Despite different methodologies, most interventions have been associated with an increase in hand hygiene compliance and improvement of other structure, process and outcome indicators.

While listing the main risk factors associated with poor hand hygiene compliance and those reported by HCWs, Table 19.1.1 also shows strategic actions potentially targeting these factors with the ultimate aim of improving hand hygiene performance. Indeed, interventions aimed at hand hygiene improvement can include one or more strategy components: system change; HCW education; monitoring of hand hygiene compliance and other indicators; performance feedback; use of reminders in the workplace; improvement of the institutional safety climate; and patient participation. Most successful strategies include multiple components [103, 104, 106, 109, 111, 112, 144, 153, 169, 179, 182, 194, 204, 216, 219–232] and have been implemented both at facility level and national or subnational level in some countries [50, 153, 225, 232–239]. Although all these elements are important, the selection of the most appropriate strategy components at facility level should be based on a careful preliminary evaluation of the local situation and needs regarding hand hygiene performance and promotion [180, 240–243].

System change represents a number of actions aimed at ensuring that the necessary equipment and facilities for hand hygiene are in place, for example the introduction and continuous provision of alcohol-based handrubs and the installation of an adequate number of sinks as close as possible to the point of care, the continuous provision of water, soap and disposable towels, and the use of automated sinks [99, 103, 109, 110, 112, 113, 118, 142, 144, 145, 147, 154, 155, 165, 166, 219–221, 244–257]. This strategic element is intended to make hand hygiene possible and easier and to overcome barriers such as lack of time, lack of facilities, high workload or the inconvenient location of sinks and dispensers (Table 19.1.1).

Education is of paramount importance in a hand hygiene promotion program [50, 153, 157, 179, 182, 194, 220–223, 225, 249, 258–269]. Many factors or beliefs associated with lack of hand hygiene compliance can be targeted through staff education (Table 19.1.1) by providing solid evidence on hand transmission, the need for improvement of hand hygiene practices, the burden and impact of HAI, and by explaining basic infection control principles and key hand hygiene indications and methods in a simple, user-friendly manner. Negative behavior detected in specific healthcare professional categories can be targeted by training sessions selectively dedicated to these professionals while referring to their particular tasks and role in healthcare delivery. HCW education can be achieved using regular presentations, e-learning modules, posters, focus groups, reflective discussion, videos, self-learning modules, practical demonstrations, feedback from assessment, buddy systems or combinations of different methods. Assessment of the impact of training on HCW understanding and knowledge is recommended to identify remaining gaps and areas for continuous education [180, 258, 270].

Monitoring of hand hygiene compliance and other indicators together with the feedback of results to HCWs and/or senior managers are key elements to plan, successfully implement and evaluate hand hygiene promotion programs. The value,

Table 19.1.1 Observed risk factors and obstacles reported by healthcare workers for poor hand hygiene compliance and components of hand hygiene improvement strategies potentially addressing theses issues.

Risk factors for poor compliance with recommended hand hygiene practices (with study references)	Strategy component
Observed factors[a]	
Doctor status (rather than a nurse)	Education
[103, 112, 118, 125, 135, 183–186]	Monitoring and feedback
	Institutional safety climate
Nursing assistant status (rather than a nurse)	Education
[112, 118, 125, 135, 183, 185, 188, 189]	Monitoring and feedback
	Institutional safety climate
Working in an intensive care unit	System change
[112, 118, 125, 135, 171, 190]	Education
	Monitoring and feedback
Working in a surgical care unit	System change
[171, 183, 184]	Education
	Monitoring and feedback
Wearing gown/gloves	Education
[125, 181, 192–194]	Monitoring and feedback
	Reminders
Activities with high risk of cross-transmission	Education
[103, 118, 125, 135, 185]	Monitoring and feedback
	Reminders
Understaffing or overcrowding	Institutional safety climate
[103, 125, 135, 190, 195, 196, 197]	
High number of opportunities for hand hygiene per hour of patient care	System change
[103, 118, 125, 126, 135, 185, 190, 194, 197]	
Self-reported factors	
Handwashing agents cause irritation and dryness	System change
[103, 125, 173, 198–207]	Education
Sinks are inconveniently located or shortage of sinks	System change
[103, 125, 198, 200, 201, 203–205, 208]	Monitoring and feedback
	Institutional safety climate
Lack of soap, paper, towel or handwashing agents	System change
[103, 125, 173, 201, 205, 209, 210]	Monitoring and feedback
	Institutional safety climate
Often too busy or insufficient time	Education
[103, 125, 135, 142, 173, 198, 200, 201, 203, 204, 207, 209, 211–215]	Institutional safety climate
Patient needs take priority	Education
[125, 204, 206]	
Hand hygiene interferes with healthcare worker–patient relationship	Education
[125, 203, 204]	
Wearing gloves or belief that glove use obviates the need for hand hygiene	Education
[103, 125, 135, 173, 207]	Reminders
Lack of institutional guidelines/lack of knowledge of guidelines and protocols	Education
[49, 198, 200, 203, 204, 209, 216]	Institutional safety climate
Lack of knowledge, experience and education	Monitoring and feedback
[198, 200, 207, 209]	Education
Lack of rewards/encouragement	Monitoring and feedback
[198, 200, 209]	Institutional safety climate
Lack of role model from colleagues or superiors	Institutional safety climate
[103, 125, 198, 200, 209, 217]	
Not thinking about it, forgetfulness	Education
[103, 125, 173, 203, 204, 206]	Reminders
	Institutional safety climate
Skepticism about the value of hand hygiene	Education
[51, 103, 125, 173]	Institutional safety climate
Lack of scientific information about definitive impact of improved hand hygiene on healthcare-associated infection rates	Education
[103, 125, 214]	Monitoring and feedback
	Institutional safety climate

[a]Only factors identified in at least three studies published in the literature are cited.

objectives and methods for evaluating hand hygiene practices have been discussed above. Evaluation of the infrastructure available for hand hygiene and HCWs' perception and knowledge about hand transmission of infection and the importance of hand hygiene also bring invaluable data to inform the planning of the most appropriate strategy locally [243, 257, 269–271]. Many studies aimed at hand hygiene improvement included the monitoring component within the implemented strategy [50, 103–109, 111, 112, 118, 140, 142, 153, 169, 179, 182, 184, 194, 216, 217, 219, 221–225, 245, 255, 272–274]. The selected indicators should be assessed before starting a hand hygiene campaign and then periodically (at least annually, but ideally more frequently) during and after the implementation period. Feedback of monitored indicators is essential to keep HCWs and managers involved in the campaign and contribute to establish an institutional safety climate where HCWs become more accountable due to an increased awareness of their hand hygiene practices.

In association with other strategy components, reminders in the workplace are key tools to prompt and remind HCWs about the importance of hand hygiene and the appropriate indications and procedures for its performance [103, 105, 106, 109, 112, 118, 140, 144, 153, 154, 179, 182, 217, 219–223, 225, 232, 244, 245, 248, 251, 272, 275, 276]. They are also means of informing patients and their visitors of the standard of care that they should expect from their HCWs with respect to hand hygiene. Posters are the most common type of reminder and these should be placed as close as possible to the point of care. Good maintenance and a regular renewal of posters are very important aspects to achieve maximum impact with these tools. Other types of reminders are pocket leaflets that individual HCWs can carry in their pockets, stickers posted at the point of care, special labels including prompting slogans stuck on alcohol-based handrub dispensers, and gadgets such as badges with the hand hygiene logo.

To be successful, especially in the long term, a hand hygiene campaign must be embedded in a deeply-rooted institutional safety climate where individual HCWs, managers and the institution as a whole show clear commitment, reliability and accountability about patient safety issues while guaranteeing consideration of hand hygiene improvement as a high priority at all levels [103, 112, 125, 153, 154, 184, 204, 269, 277]. The creation and maintenance of this climate is not easy and requires leadership, together with high motivation and human and financial resources, to tackle patient safety from different angles and disseminate safety principles and spirit. Continuous progress in the development of stable systems for adverse event detection and quality assessment is also required, hand hygiene being one of the key indicators. Strategies to achieve this goal can be actions at the group level (e.g. the unit or the ward) and may include education and performance feedback on hand hygiene compliance, efforts to prevent high workloads (e.g. downsizing and understaffing) and encouragement and role modeling from senior staff and key HCWs on the ward. At the institutional level,

targets for improvement include a lack of written guidelines, available or suitable hand hygiene agents, skin care promotion/agents or hand hygiene facilities, lack of culture or tradition of adherence, and a lack of administrative leadership, sanctions, rewards or support.

Patient participation is another interesting strategic element that could contribute to the creation of an institutional safety climate [50, 133, 134, 137]. Several studies have investigated if patients' awareness and understanding of hand hygiene and their positive encouragement to HCWs could motivate the latter to implement optimal hand hygiene [50, 128, 133, 134, 179, 223, 278, 279]. In this way, patients may feel more involved in their own process of care and in the efforts to make it safer. Furthermore, the performance of correct hand hygiene in full view of the patient can promote patient confidence and partnership between patients and HCWs. Based on the available evidence from most of these investigations it appears that patient participation is indeed an important aspect to be considered in a multimodal hand hygiene improvement program. Ideally, this component should not be implemented in a setting where the culture of hand hygiene promotion has not yet been created, but rather at a more advanced stage and after considering local beliefs, the social level of development and the cultural features of the local environment.

Effectiveness of hand hygiene programs to reduce healthcare-associated infections, including cost-saving issues

As described in steps 4 and 5 of the hand transmission model by Pittet and colleagues [1], failure to perform appropriate hand hygiene leads to the transmission of healthcare-associated microorganisms, the spread of microbicidal resistance and ultimately to the occurrence of HAI, including outbreak situations. The evaluation of studies aimed at assessing the effectiveness of hand hygiene to reduce pathogen transmission and HAI rates is challenged by differences in study design, surveillance definitions and the coexistence of the implementation of various infection control measures among others. However, according to studies based on multimodal strategies for hand hygiene improvement, there is convincing evidence that improved hand hygiene can reduce HAI [50]. In addition, although not reporting infection rates, several studies showed a sustained decrease of the incidence of multidrug-resistant bacterial isolates and patient colonization following the implementation of hand hygiene improvement strategies [219, 220, 280–282].

Among about 30 hospital-based studies investigating the impact of hand hygiene interventions on HAI occurrence and published between January 1977 and February 2011 (Table 19.1.2), only three [140, 182, 221] failed to demonstrate that improved hand hygiene significantly reduces HAI. Most of the reports showed a temporal relation between improved hand hygiene practices and reduced infection and cross-transmission

Table 19.1.2 Most relevant studies assessing the impact of hand hygiene promotion on HAI (January 1977–February 2011).

Year	Authors	Country	Hospital setting	Intervention	Impact on hand hygiene compliance	Impact on HAI	Follow-up duration	Reference
1977	Casewell and Phillips	UK	Adult ICU	Promotion of HW with a chlorhexidine hand cleanser	NA	Significant reduction in the percentage of patients colonized or infected by *Klebsiella* spp.	2 years	[283]
1989	Conly *et al.*	Canada	Adult ICU	Education, observation, performance feedback	HH compliance increase from 14% to 73% (before patient contact) and from 28% to 81% (after patient contact)	Significant reduction in HAI rates after HW promotion (from 33% to 12% and from 33% to 10%, respectively, after two intervention periods 4 years apart)	6 years	[105]
1990	Simmons *et al.*	USA	Adult ICU	HW promotion	HH compliance increase from 22% to 29.9%	No impact on HAI rates (no statistically significant improvement of HH adherence)	11 months	[140]
1992	Doebbeling *et al.*	USA	Adult ICUs	Prospective multiple cross-over trial on HH with either chlorhexidine soap or HR with 60% isopropyl alcohol with optional HW with plain soap	NA	Significant reduction of HAI rates using HW with chlorhexidine soap	8 months	[247]
1994	Webster *et al.*	Australia	NICU	Introduction of HW with triclosan 1% w/v	NA	Elimination of MRSA when combined with multiple other infection control measures. Reduction of vancomycin use. Significant reduction of nosocomial bacteremia (from 2.6% to 1.1%) using triclosan compared with chlorhexidine for HW	9 months	[284]
1995	Zafar *et al.*	USA	Newborn nursery	Introduction of HCW HW and neonate bathing with triclosan 0.3% w/v	NA	Control of a MRSA outbreak	3.5 years	[285]
2000	Larson *et al.*	USA	MICU/NICU	Organizational climate intervention	NA	Significant (85%) relative reduction of the vancomycin-resistant enterococci rate at the intervention hospital; statistically insignificant (44%) reduction at the control hospital; no significant change in MRSA	8 months	[6, 104]
2000	Pittet *et al.*	Switzerland	Hospital-wide	Introduction of alcohol-based HR, HH observation, training, performance feedback, posters	Significant increase of HH compliance from 48% to 66%	Significant reduction in annual overall prevalence of HAI (42%) and MRSA[a] cross-transmission rates (87%). A follow-up study showed continuous increase in HR use, stable HAI rates and cost savings derived from the strategy	8 years	[103]

Year	Author	Country	Intervention	HH compliance	Outcome	Duration	Reference
2003	Hilburn et al.	USA	Orthopedic surgical unit	Introduction of alcohol-based HR, posters, feedback on HAI rates, patient education and involvement	NA	36% reduction of UTI and SSI rates (from 8.2% to 5.3%)	10 months	[286]
2004	MacDonald et al.	UK	Hospital-wide	Introduction of alcohol-based HR, HH observation, posters, performance feedback, informal discussions	No statistically significant increase of HH compliance before and after patient contact	Significant reduction in hospital-acquired MRSA cases (from 1.9% to 0.9%)	1 year	[146]
2004	Swoboda et al.	USA	Adult intermediate care unit	HH electronic monitoring at exit from patient rooms, direct observation, voice prompts	No statistically significant increase of compliance by electronic monitoring (from 19.1% to 27.3%)	Reduction in HAI rates (not statistically significant)	2.5 months	[145]
2004	Lam et al.	Hong Kong SAR (China)	NICU	Introduction of alcohol-based HR, HH observation, training, HH protocols, posters	HH compliance increase from 40% to 53% (before patient contact) and from 39% to 59% (after patient contact)	Reduction (not statistically significant) in HAI rates (from 11.3/1000 patient-days to 6.2/1000 patient-days)	6 months	[110]
2004	Won et al.	China (Taiwan)	NICU	Education, written instructions, HH observation, posters, performance feedback, financial incentives	HH compliance increase from 43% to 80%	Significant reduction in HAI rates (from 15.1/1000 patient-days to 10.7/1000 patient-days), in particular of respiratory infections	2 years	[113]
2005	Zerr et al.	USA	Hospital-wide	Introduction of alcohol-based HR, HH observation, training, posters	HH compliance increase from 62% to 81%	Significant reduction in hospital-associated rotavirus infections	4 years	[184]
2005	Rosenthal et al.	Argentina	Adult ICUs	HW observation, training, guideline dissemination, posters, performance feedback	HH compliance increase from 23.1% to 64.5%	Significant reduction in HAI rates (from 47.5/1000 patient-days to 27.9/1000 patient-days)	21 months	[216]
2005	Johnson et al.	Australia	Hospital-wide	Introduction of alcohol-based HR, HH observation, training, posters, promotional gadgets	HH compliance increase from 21% to 42%	Significant reduction (57%) in MRSA bacteremia	36 months	[154]
2007	Le et al.	Vietnam	Neurosurgery	Introduction of alcohol-based HR, training, posters, case–control study	NA	Reduction (54%, NS) of overall incidence of SSI. Significant reduction (100%) of superficial SSI; significantly lower SSI incidence in intervention ward compared with control ward	2 years	[251]
2007	Pessoa-Silva et al.	Switzerland	Neonatal unit	Posters, focus groups, HH observation, HCWs' perception assessment, feedback on performance, perception and HAI rates	HH compliance increase from 42% to 55%	Reduction of overall HAI rates (from 11 to 8.2 infections/1000 patient-days) and 60% decrease of HAI risk in very low birth weight neonates (from 15.5 to 8.8 episodes/1000 patient-days)	27 months	[194]

(Continued)

429

Table 19.1.2 (Continued)

Year	Authors	Country	Hospital setting	Intervention	Impact on hand hygiene compliance	Impact on HAI	Follow-up duration	Reference
2008	Rupp et al.	USA	ICU	Introduction of alcohol-based HR, education, and posters, prospective controlled cross-over trial in two units	HH compliance increase from 38–37% to 68–69%	No impact on device-associated infection and infections due to multidrug-resistant pathogen	2 years	[221]
2008	Grayson et al.	Australia	(i) Six pilot hospitals (ii) All public hospitals in Victoria (Australia)	Introduction of alcohol-based HR, HH observation, training, posters, promotional gadgets	(i) Compliance increase from 21% to 48% (ii) Compliance increase from 20% to 53%	(i) Significant reduction of MRSA bacteremia (from 0.05/100 patient-discharges to 0.02/100 patient-discharges per month) and of clinical MRSA isolates (ii) Significant reduction of MRSA bacteremia (from 0.03/100 patient-discharges to 0.01/100 patient-discharges per month) and of clinical MRSA isolates	(i) 2 years (ii) 1 year	[153]
2008	Capretti et al.	Italy	NICU	Introduction of alcohol-based HR, training, posters	NA	Significant reduction of HAI incidence (4.1/1000 patient-days vs 1.2/1000 patient-days)	18 months	[222]
2008	Picheansathian et al.	Thailand	NICU	Introduction of alcohol-based HR, HH observation, training, posters, performance feedback, focus groups	HH compliance increase from 6.3% to 81.2%	No impact on HAI rates (9.7/1000 patient-days vs 13.5/1000 patient-days)	7 months	[182]
2009	Lederer et al.	USA	Hospital-wide, seven acute care facilities	Education, HH observation, performance feedback, posters, memos and poster-board communications, visitor education program, internal marketing campaign	Compliance increase from 49% to 98% with sustained rates greater than 90%	Significant reduction of MRSA rates from 0.52 episodes/1000 patient-days to 0.24/1000 patient-days	3 years	[223]
2008	Cromer et al.	USA	Hospital-wide	Direct HH observation, including technique and feedback, in a setting where HH promotion had been implemented during previous years	HH compliance increase from 72.5% to 90.3%	Significant reduction in facility-acquired MRSA from 0.85 to 0.52/1000 patient-days	10 months	[224]
2008	Nguyen KM et al.	Vietnam	Urology ward	Education of staff and patient relatives, posters, introduction of bed-mounted bottles of alcohol-based HR, direct HH observation	Baseline HH compliance assumed to be close to 0%. Overall compliance after intervention not reported. Highest HH compliance after wound care (67.9%) and lowest for breaks in intravenous lines (9.3%)	Significant reduction in HAI incidence from 13.1% to 2.1%	6 months	[179]

2008	Marra et al.	Brazil	Two adult step-down units	Electronic monitoring of alcohol-based HR use and feedback, prospective controlled study	No significant difference in HH episodes recorded by electronic monitoring	No significant difference in BSI, UTI and pneumonia infection episodes/1000 device-days	6 months	[169]
2009	McLaws et al.	Australia	Hospital-wide in 208 public hospitals (state-wide)	Introduction of alcohol-based HR, HH observation, training, performance feedback, posters	Significant HH compliance increase from 47% to 61%	Significant reduction of 6% of overall MRSA infections/10 000 patient-days. Reductions of 16% in MRSA infection in non-sterile sites in ICU and of 25% in sterile sites in non-ICU wards	18 months	[225, 287]
2010	Helder et al	The Netherlands	NICO	A HH education program, encouragement of role models, and culture change in favour of better HH	Significant increase in HH compliance before patient contact from 68.8% to 86.9% and after patient contact from 68.9% to 83.9%	Significant reduction in the incidence of BSI and (from 44.5% to 36.1%) and of overall HAI (from 17.3 to 13.5/1000 patients-days)	18 months	[269]
2010	Cheng et al	Hong Kong SAR (China)	Adult ICU	Phase 1: baseline; Phase 2: ICU renovation with introduction of single room isolation; Phase 3: HH campaign with alcohol-based HR introduction, briefing and discussion sessions, posters, HH observation	HH compliance increase* from 29% at baseline (2nd quarter of 2006) to 46% (4th quarter of 2006), 54% (4th quarter of 2007), and 64% (3rd quarter of 2008)	Significant reduction of incidence density of ICU onset bacteraemic and non bacteraemic MRSA infection in the intervention units between Phase 3 and Phase 2.	3 yrs (follow up from Phase 2)	[274]
2011	Yeung et al	Hong Kong SAR (China)	7 LTCFs	Alcohol-based HR introduction in pocket bottles, education, reminders (intervention LCTFs) vs basic life support education (control LTCFs)	Significant HH compliance increase from 25.8% to 33.3% in the intervention LTCFs	In the intervention LTCFs, significant reduction of incidence of serious infections (from 1.42 cases/1000 resident-days to 0.65 cases/1000 resident-days) and significant reduction of mortality due to infection. In the control LTCFs, significant increase of infection incidence and no change in mortality	7 months	[227]

BSI, bloodstream infection; HAI, healthcare-associated infection; ICU, intensive care unit; HH, hand hygiene; HR, handrub; HW, handwashing; MICU, medical intensive care unit; MRSA, methicillin-resistant *Staphylococcus aureus*; NA, not available; NS, not significant; NICU, neonatal intensive care unit; SSI, surgical site infection; UTI, urinary tract infection.
[a]MRSA active surveillance cultures and contact precautions were implemented during same time period.

rates. In most, if not all the studies, the hand hygiene improvement strategy was multimodal and included the strategy components described in above. Among these, staff education and the introduction of an alcohol-based handrub were included in the vast majority of studies. The settings were adult and neonatal intensive care units [104, 105, 110, 182, 216, 221, 222, 247, 269, 274, 283, 284, 287] in most cases, but in some the scope was much broader with hospital-wide extension [103, 146, 153, 154, 184, 191] and coverage of an entire region, state or country [225]. Most of these studies showed that hand hygiene improvement, demonstrated by a significant increase of compliance with best practices, has an impact on the incidence rates of overall HAI and specific sites of infection [103, 105, 110, 113, 145, 179, 191, 194, 216, 222, 227, 247, 251, 269, 274, 284, 286, 288] In addition, many showed a reduction in MRSA infections, bacteremia and clinical isolates, and an effectiveness to control MRSA outbreaks [103, 146, 153, 154, 191, 223–225, 274, 284, 285]. Some studies also demonstrated an impact on other specific microorganisms, such as vancomycin-resistant enterococci, *Klebsiella* spp. and rotavirus [104, 184, 283]. Although this effect was shown at follow-up of less than one year in most cases, several studies demonstrated sustained effects for longer periods of time [103, 105, 113, 153, 154, 184, 191, 194, 216, 222, 223, 225, 251, 274, 283, 285]. In addition, hand hygiene programs were at the core of many studies implementing broader infection control interventions and showing an impact on HAI rates.

Furthermore, the incidence of MRSA bacteremia and MRSA isolates dramatically decreased at national level in countries such as England and France following implementation of targeted prevention programs with a very strong hand hygiene component [153, 154, 289–291].

However, while evaluating this substantial evidence on hand hygiene promotion effectiveness, it is important to consider the limitations in that most studies used an observational before/after design. For this reason, cluster-randomized, controlled and/or stepped-wedge studies and/or solid mathematical models should be strongly encouraged to better explore the relationship between hand hygiene compliance and the ultimate outcomes of HAI and the spread of microbicidal resistance. This should include an assessment of the impact of specific strategy components on short-term and sustained improvement.

Reinforcement of hand hygiene practices also helps control epidemics in healthcare facilities [283, 285]. Outbreak investigations have suggested an association between infection and understaffing or overcrowding that was consistently linked with poor adherence to hand hygiene [292–294]. Although the above-mentioned studies used hand hygiene compliance as the gold standard for assessing hand hygiene improvement, an increasing number of studies over the past decade have investigated the correlation between the consumption of hand hygiene products and HAI rates following a hand hygiene promotion intervention [103, 148, 153, 154, 157, 159, 160, 265, 295]. In particular, increased consumption of alcohol-based handrub was accompanied by a reduction of MRSA bacteremia or clinical isolates in some studies, although statistical correlation between the two parameters was not assessed in all [103, 148–150, 153–155, 157, 159, 295]. By pooling the results of several studies using the Spearman correlation coefficient, Sroka and colleagues were able to demonstrate that an increase in the provision of alcohol-based handrubs significantly correlated with a reduction of MRSA bacteremia or the incidence of clinical isolates [162]. This approach and related evidence provide new, encouraging perspectives, but the reliability of this correlation and the best methods to demonstrate it still need to be established with more accuracy.

The costs of hand hygiene promotion programs include the costs of hand hygiene installations and products plus the costs associated with HCW time and the educational and promotional materials required by the program. To assess the cost savings of hand hygiene promotion programs, it is necessary to consider the potential savings that can be achieved by reducing the incidence of HAIs. Several studies provided some quantitative estimates of the cost savings from hand hygiene promotion programs [103, 193, 284].

In a study conducted in a Russian neonatal intensive care unit, the authors estimated that the added cost of one healthcare-associated bloodstream infection (US$1100) would cover 3265 patient-days of hand antiseptic use ($0.34/patient-day) [219]. In another study, it was estimated that cost savings achieved by reducing the incidence of *C. difficile*-associated disease and MRSA infections far exceeded the additional cost of using an alcohol-based handrub [144]. Similarly, MacDonald and colleagues reported that the use of an alcohol-based hand gel combined with education sessions and HCW performance feedback reduced the incidence of MRSA infections and expenditures for teicoplanin (used to treat such infections) [146]. For every UK£1 spent on alcohol-based gel, £9–20 were saved on teicoplanin expenditure.

Pittet and colleagues [103] estimated direct and indirect costs associated with a hand hygiene program to be less than US$57,000 per year for a 2600-bed hospital, an average of $1.42 per patient admitted. The authors concluded that the hand hygiene program was cost-saving if less than 1% of the reduction in HAIs observed was attributable to improved hand hygiene practices. An effective hand hygiene program implemented in a neonatal intensive care unit in Italy could allow the avoidance of approximately 10 HAI episodes/year at a cost of $10,000 per episode [222]. Using a different methodology, with two models simulating sequential patient contacts by a hand hygiene non-compliant HCW, a study recently conducted in North Carolina, USA, estimated that a 200-bed hospital incurs $1,779,283 in annual MRSA infection-related expenses attributable to hand hygiene non-compliance. A 1% increase in hand hygiene compliance resulted in annual savings of $39,650 for this hospital [296].

An economic analysis of the "clean*your*hands" hand hygiene promotion campaign conducted in England and Wales concluded that the program would be cost beneficial if HAI rates decreased by as little as 0.1% [297].

The World Health Organization multimodal hand hygiene improvement strategy and toolkit

The *WHO Guidelines on Hand Hygiene in Health Care* [50], issued by WHO Patient Safety in 2009, are considered the most recently updated and comprehensive document currently available on this topic. Their recommendations have been adopted by more than 150 countries and healthcare settings worldwide as the gold standard for hand hygiene. To translate the evidence-based recommendations into practice and help healthcare settings to succeed in hand hygiene improvement, the WHO Multimodal Hand Hygiene Improvement Strategy and a wide range of implementation tools were developed and made available in parallel to the WHO guidelines [298]. The concepts underpinning the strategy are supported by the literature on implementation science, behavioral change, spread methodology, diffusion of innovation and impact evaluation. Implementation of the guidelines' recommendations, together with the strategy and tools, was proven to be feasible, effective and sustainable according to the results of pilot testing in a large variety of sites worldwide [50]. The WHO Multimodal Hand Hygiene Improvement Strategy includes essential elements of proven efficacy to improve hand hygiene performance (see Part 5 of the strategy), such as system change, training and education, evaluation and feedback, reminders in the workplace, and the creation of an institutional safety climate [298]. Following the implementation of the strategy in pilot sites, a significant increase in hand hygiene compliance was observed across all sites [50]. In addition, an improvement in HCWs' perception of the importance of HAI and its prevention, as well as their knowledge about hand transmission and hand hygiene practices, was observed. Furthermore, a substantial system change was achieved with an improvement in the facilities and equipment available for hand hygiene, including the local production of the WHO recommended alcohol-based formulations [78] in settings where these products were not available commercially [180].

The innovative approach of the "My five moments for hand hygiene" is central to the implementation of the recommendations at the point of care (see Figure 19.1.4) [50, 114, 124, 299]. Considering the scientific evidence, this concept merges the hand hygiene indications recommended by the *WHO Guidelines on Hand Hygiene in Health Care* (see Part II) into five moments when hand hygiene is required. This approach proposes a unified vision for HCWs, trainers and observers to minimize interindividual variation and enable a global increase in adherence to effective hand hygiene practices. According to this concept, HCWs are requested to clean their hands: (i) before touching a patient; (ii) before clean/aseptic procedures; (iii) after body fluid exposure/risk; (iv) after touching a patient; and (v) after touching patient surroundings. This concept has been integrated into the various WHO tools to educate, monitor, summarize, feedback and promote hand hygiene in healthcare settings.

The WHO Multimodal Hand Hygiene Improvement Strategy is accompanied by a toolkit, including a range of tools corresponding to each strategy component to facilitate its practical implementation. A guide was developed to assist healthcare facilities to implement hand hygiene programs [298]. It illustrates the strategy components in detail, including the objectives and utility of each tool, indicates the resources necessary for implementation, provides a template action plan, and proposes a stepwise approach for practical implementation at the healthcare setting level. The following are essential steps, particularly in facilities where a hand hygiene improvement program has to be initiated from the very beginning.

- Step 1: Facility preparedness – readiness for action.
- Step 2: Baseline evaluation – establishing the current situation.
- Step 3: Implementation – introducing the improvement activities.
- Step 4: Follow-up evaluation – evaluating the implementation impact.
- Step 5: Action planning and review cycle – developing a plan for the next 5 years (minimum).

Adverse events related to hand hygiene and in particular to the use of alcohol-based handrubs

Repeated performance of hand hygiene actions and the alcohol-based nature of handrubs may lead to some adverse events that may affect the HCW, patients and healthcare setting. These events are mostly rare and specific measures have been identified for their prevention.

Skin reactions may appear on the hands of HCWs because of the necessity for frequent hand hygiene during patient care. There are two major types of skin reactions associated with hand hygiene. The first and most common is irritant contact dermatitis, and includes symptoms such as dryness, irritation, itching and, in some cases, even cracking and bleeding. The second type of skin reaction, allergic contact dermatitis, is rare and represents an allergy to some ingredients in a hand hygiene product. Symptoms can range from mild and localized to severe and generalized. In its most serious form, allergic contact dermatitis may be associated with respiratory distress and other symptoms of anaphylaxis. HCWs with skin reactions or complaints related to hand hygiene should have access to an appropriate referral service. In general, irritant contact dermatitis is more commonly reported with iodophors [139], but other antiseptic agents that may cause irritation include chlorhexidine, chloroxylenol, triclosan and alcohol-based products, in order of decreasing frequency. However, numerous reports confirm that alcohol-based formulations are well tolerated and associated with better acceptability and tolerance than other hand hygiene products [50, 300–309].

Allergic reactions to antiseptic agents including QACs, iodine or iodophors, chlorhexidine, triclosan, chloroxylenol and alcohols [310–320] have been reported, as well as possible toxicity in relation to dermal absorption of products [321, 322]. Allergic contact dermatitis attributable to alcohol-based handrubs is very uncommon. Damaged, irritated skin is undesirable, not only because it causes discomfort and even lost workdays for the professional, but also because hands with damaged skin may in fact increase the risk of transmission of infections to patients.

The use of clear parameters for the selection of products that are both efficacious and as safe as possible for the skin is of the utmost importance. Several studies have demonstrated that alcohol-based handrubs containing humectants are tolerated better by HCWs and are associated with a better skin condition when compared with either plain or microbicidal soap [103, 142, 323–329]. With rubs, a shorter time required for hand antisepsis may increase acceptability and compliance [212]. Despite this strong evidence, HCWs (particularly nurses) often perceive that the use of these products leads to more skin-damaging effects [330] and this may become a major cause of poor acceptance of alcohol-based handrubs in hospitals [331, 332]. Although many hospitals have provided HCWs with plain soaps in the hope of minimizing dermatitis, frequent use of such products has been associated with even greater skin damage, dryness and irritation than some antiseptic preparations [139, 325, 326].

Ways to minimize the possible adverse effects of hand hygiene include selecting less irritating products, using skin moisturizers and modifying certain hand hygiene behaviors such as unnecessary washing [50, 333]. Certain practices can increase the risk of skin irritation and should be avoided. For example, washing hands regularly with soap and water immediately before or after using an alcohol-based product is not only unnecessary, but may lead to dermatitis [334]. The use of very hot water for handwashing should be avoided as it increases the likelihood of skin damage. When clean or disposable towels are used, it is important to pat the skin rather than to rub it to avoid cracking. Additionally, donning gloves while hands are still wet from either washing or applying alcohol increases the risk of skin irritation.

Other relevant safety issues related to the use of alcohol-based handrubs are risk of fire, accidents with ingestion by psychiatric or pediatric patients, potential alcohol inhalation and skin absorption. Alcohols are flammable and alcohol-based handrubs should be stored away from high temperatures or flames in accordance with national and local regulations [50]. However, the risk of fires associated with such products is very low. For example, none of 798 healthcare facilities surveyed in the USA in 2003 reported a fire related to an alcohol-based handrub dispenser [335]. In Europe, where alcohol-based handrubs have been used extensively for many years, the incidence of fires related to such products has been extremely low [336]. A study conducted in German hospitals found that with an overall usage of 35 million liters for all settings, only seven non-severe fire incidents were reported (0.9% of hospitals), thus corresponding to an annual incidence per hospital of 0.0000475% [337]. Most reported incidents were associated with deliberate exposure to a naked flame, for example lighting a cigarette. A summary of incidents related to the use of alcohol-based handrubs from the start of the "clean*your*hands" campaign from February 2003 to July 2008 recorded

only two fire events out of 692 incidents reported in 187 acute trusts in England and Wales [338].

Accidental and intentional ingestion of alcohol-based preparations used for hand hygiene have been reported and may lead to acute, and in some cases severe, alcohol intoxication [339–343]. In the "clean*your*hands" campaign incidents summary [338], 189 cases of ingestion were recorded in healthcare settings. However, the vast majority was graded as of no or low harm, 12 as moderate, two as severe, and one death was reported (but the patient had been admitted already the previous day for severe alcohol intoxication). It is clear that security measures are needed, especially in pediatric and psychiatric wards. These may involve placing the preparation in secure wall dispensers, labeling dispensers to make the alcohol content less clear at a casual glance and adding a warning against consumption, and the inclusion of an additive in the product formula to reduce its palatability. In the meantime, medical and nursing staff should be aware of this potential risk.

Alcohols can be absorbed by inhalation and through intact skin, although the latter route (dermal uptake) is very low. Several studies have evaluated alcohol dermal absorption and inhalation following its application or spraying on skin [322, 344–347]. In all cases, either no or very low (much less than levels achieved with mild intoxication, i.e. 50 mg/dl) blood concentrations of alcohols were detected and no symptoms were noticed. Indeed, while there are no data showing that the use of alcohol-based handrub may be harmful because of alcohol absorption, it is well-established that reduced compliance with hand hygiene will lead to preventable HAIs.

Appendix 19.1 World Health Organization recommendations on hand hygiene in health care

Consensus recommendations*

Recommendations were formulated based on evidence described in the various sections of the WHO guidelines and expert consensus. Evidence and recommendations were graded using a system adapted from the one developed by the Healthcare Infection Control Practices Advisory Committee (HICPAC) of the CDC, Atlanta, GA (Table 19.1.A1).

1. Indications for hand hygiene

A. Wash hands with soap and water when visibly dirty or visibly soiled with blood or other body fluids (IB) or after using the toilet (II).

B. If exposure to potential spore-forming pathogens is strongly suspected or proven, including outbreaks of *C. difficile*, handwashing with soap and water is the preferred means (IB).

C. Use an alcohol-based handrub as the preferred means for routine hand antisepsis in all other clinical situations described in items D(a) to D(f) listed below if hands are not visibly soiled

---

*Adapted with permission from reference [50].

Table 19.1.A1 Ranking system used to grade the guidelines' recommendations.

Category	Criteria
IA	Strongly recommended for implementation and strongly supported by well-designed experimental, clinical or epidemiological studies
IB	Strongly recommended for implementation and supported by some experimental, clinical or epidemiological studies and a strong theoretical rationale
IC	Required for implementation as mandated by federal and/or state regulation or standard
II	Suggested for implementation and supported by suggestive clinical or epidemiological studies or a theoretical rationale or the consensus of a panel of experts

(IA). If alcohol-based handrub is not obtainable, wash hands with soap and water (IB).

D. Perform hand hygiene:

    a. before and after touching the patient (IB);

    b. before handling an invasive device for patient care, regardless of whether or not gloves are used (IB);

    c. after contact with body fluids or excretions, mucous membranes, non-intact skin or wound dressings (IA);

    d. if moving from a contaminated body site to another body site during care of the same patient (IB);

    e. after contact with inanimate surfaces and objects (including medical equipment) in the immediate vicinity of the patient (IB);

    f. after removing sterile (II) or non-sterile gloves (IB).

E. Before handling medication or preparing food, perform hand hygiene using an alcohol-based handrub or wash hands with either plain or microbicidal soap and water (IB).

F. Soap and alcohol-based handrub should not be used concomitantly (II).

2. Hand hygiene technique

A. Apply a palmful of alcohol-based handrub and cover all surfaces of the hands. Rub hands until dry (IB) (see Figure 19.1.3).

B. When washing hands with soap and water, wet hands with water and apply the amount of product necessary to cover all surfaces. Rinse hands with water and dry thoroughly with a single-use towel. Use clean, running water whenever possible. Avoid using hot water, as repeated exposure to hot water may increase the risk of dermatitis (IB). Use a towel to turn off the tap/faucet (IB). Dry hands thoroughly using a method that does not recontaminate the hands. Make sure towels are not used multiple times or by multiple people (IB).

C. Liquid, bar, leaf or powdered forms of soap are acceptable. When bar soap is used, small bars of soap in racks that facilitate drainage should be used to allow the bars to dry (II).

3. Recommendations for surgical hand preparation

A. Remove rings, wrist watch and bracelets before beginning surgical hand preparation (II). Artificial nails are prohibited (IB).

B. Sinks should be designed to reduce the risk of splashes (II).

C. If hands are visibly soiled, wash hands with plain soap before surgical hand preparation (II). Remove debris from underneath fingernails using a nail cleaner, preferably under running water (II).

D. Brushes are not recommended for surgical hand preparation (IB).

E. Surgical hand antisepsis should be performed using either a suitable microbicidal soap or suitable alcohol-based handrub, preferably with a product ensuring sustained activity, before donning sterile gloves (IB).

F. If quality of water is not assured in the operating theater, surgical hand antisepsis using an alcohol-based handrub is recommended before donning sterile gloves when performing surgical procedures (II).

G. When performing surgical hand antisepsis using a microbicidal soap, scrub hands and forearms for the length of time recommended by the manufacturer, typically 2–5 min. Long scrub times (e.g. 10 min) are not necessary (IB).

H. When using an alcohol-based surgical handrub product with sustained activity, follow the manufacturer's instructions for application times. Apply the product to dry hands only (IB). Do not combine surgical handscrub and surgical handrub with alcohol-based products sequentially (II).

I. When using an alcohol-based handrub, use sufficient product to keep hands and forearms wet with the handrub throughout the surgical hand preparation procedure (IB).

J. After application of the alcohol-based handrub as recommended, allow hands and forearms to dry thoroughly before donning sterile gloves (IB).

4. Selection and handling of hand hygiene agents

A. Provide HCWs with efficacious hand hygiene products that have low irritancy potential (IB).

B. To maximize acceptance of hand hygiene products by HCWs, solicit their input regarding the skin tolerance, feel and fragrance of any products under consideration (IB). Comparative evaluations may greatly help in this process.

C. When selecting hand hygiene products:

    a. determine any known interaction between products used to clean hands, skin care products and the types of glove used in the institution (II);

    b. solicit information from manufacturers about the risk of product contamination (IB);

    c. ensure that dispensers are accessible at the point of care (see Part I.1 of the guidelines for the definition) (IB);

    d. ensure that dispensers function adequately and reliably and deliver an appropriate volume of the product (II);

    e. ensure that the dispenser system for alcohol-based handrubs is approved for flammable materials (IC);

    f. solicit and evaluate information from manufacturers regarding any effect that hand lotions, creams or alcohol-based handrubs may have on the effects of microbicidal soaps being used in the institution (IB);

g. cost comparisons should only be made for products that meet requirements for efficacy, skin tolerance and acceptability (II).

D. Do not add soap (IA) or alcohol-based formulations (II) to a partially empty soap dispenser. If soap dispensers are reused, follow recommended procedures for cleansing.

5. Skin care

A. Include information regarding hand-care practices designed to reduce the risk of irritant contact dermatitis and other skin damage in education programs for HCWs (IB).

B. Provide alternative hand hygiene products for HCWs with confirmed allergies or adverse reactions to standard products used in the healthcare setting (II).

C. Provide HCWs with hand lotions or creams to minimize the occurrence of irritant contact dermatitis associated with hand antisepsis or handwashing (IA).

D. When alcohol-based handrub is available in the healthcare facility for hygienic hand antisepsis, the use of microbicidal soap is not recommended (II).

E. Soap and alcohol-based handrub should not be used concomitantly (II).

6. Use of gloves

A. The use of gloves does not replace the need for hand hygiene by either handrubbing or handwashing (IB).

B. Wear gloves when it can be reasonably anticipated that contact with blood or other potentially infectious materials, mucous membranes or non-intact skin will occur (IC).

C. Remove gloves after caring for a patient. Do not wear the same pair of gloves for the care of more than one patient (IB).

D. When wearing gloves, change or remove gloves during patient care if moving from a contaminated body site to either another body site (including non-intact skin, mucous membrane or medical device) on the same patient or the environment (II).

E. The reuse of gloves is not recommended (IB). In the case of glove reuse, implement the safest reprocessing method (II).

7. Other aspects of hand hygiene

A. Do not wear artificial fingernails or extenders when having direct contact with patients (IA).

B. Keep natural nails short (tips less than 0.5 cm long or approximately 1/4 inch) (II).

8. Educational and motivational programs for healthcare workers

A. In hand hygiene promotion programs for HCWs, focus specifically on factors currently found to have a significant influence on behavior and not solely on the type of hand hygiene products. The strategy should be multifaceted and multimodal and include education and senior executive support for implementation (IA).

B. Educate HCWs about the type of patient care activities that can result in hand contamination and about the advantages and disadvantages of various methods used to clean their hands (II).

C. Monitor HCWs' adherence to recommended hand hygiene practices and provide them with performance feedback (IA).

D. Encourage partnerships between patients, their families and HCWs to promote hand hygiene in healthcare settings (II).

9. Governmental and institutional responsibilities
9.1 For healthcare administrators

A. It is essential that administrators ensure that conditions are conducive to the promotion of a multifaceted, multimodal hand hygiene strategy and an approach that promotes a patient safety culture by implementation of points B to I below.

B. Provide HCWs with access to a safe, continuous water supply at all outlets and access to the necessary facilities to perform handwashing (IB).

C. Provide HCWs with a readily accessible alcohol-based handrub at the point of patient care (IA).

D. Make improved hand hygiene adherence (compliance) an institutional priority and provide appropriate leadership, administrative support, financial resources and support for hand hygiene and other infection prevention and control activities (IB).

E. Ensure that HCWs have dedicated time for infection control training, including sessions on hand hygiene (II).

F. Implement a multidisciplinary, multifaceted and multimodal program designed to improve adherence of HCWs to recommended hand hygiene practices (IB).

G. With regard to hand hygiene, ensure that the water supply is physically separated from drainage and sewerage within the healthcare setting and provide routine system monitoring and management (IB).

H. Provide strong leadership and support for hand hygiene and other infection prevention and control activities (II).

I. Alcohol-based handrub production and storage must adhere to the national safety guidelines and local legal requirements (II).

9.2 For national governments

A. Make improved hand hygiene adherence a national priority and consider provision of a funded, coordinated implementation program while ensuring monitoring and long-term sustainability (II).

B. Support strengthening of infection control capacities within healthcare settings (II).

C. Promote hand hygiene at the community level to strengthen both self-protection and the protection of others (II).

D. Encourage healthcare settings to use hand hygiene as a quality indicator (II).

Disclaimer

WHO takes no responsibility for the information provided or the views expressed in this chapter.

References

1 Pittet, D. *et al.* (2006) Evidence-based model for hand transmission during patient care and the role of improved practices. *Lancet Infectious Diseases*, **6**, 641–652.

2 Lowbury, E.J.L. (1969) Gram-negative bacilli on the skin. *British Journal of Dermatology*, **81**, 55–61.

3 Noble, W.C. (1969) Distribution of the *Micrococcaceae*. *British Journal of Dermatology*, **81** (Suppl. 1), 27–32.

4 McBride, M.E. *et al.* (1976) Microbial skin flora of selected cancer patients and hospital personnel. *Journal of Clinical Microbiology*, **3**, 14–20.

5 Casewell, M.W. (1981) The role of hands in nosocomial gram-negative infection, in *Skin Microbiology Relevance to Clinical Infection* (eds H.I. Maibach and R. Aly), Springer-Verlag, New York, pp. 192–202.

6 Larson, E.L. *et al.* (2000) Differences in skin flora between inpatients and chronically ill patients. *Heart and Lung: Journal of Critical Care*, **29**, 298–305.

7 Larson, E.L. *et al.* (1986) Composition and antimicrobic resistance of skin flora in hospitalized and healthy adults. *Journal of Clinical Microbiology*, **23**, 604–608.

8 Ehrenkranz, N.J. and Alfonso, B.C. (1991) Failure of bland soap handwash to prevent hand transfer of patient bacteria to urethral catheters. *Infection Control and Hospital Epidemiology*, **12**, 654–662.

9 Sanderson, P.J. and Weissler, S. (1992) Recovery of coliforms from the hands of nurses and patients: activities leading to contamination. *Journal of Hospital Infection*, **21**, 85–93.

10 Coello, R. *et al.* (1994) Prospective study of infection, colonization and carriage of methicillin-resistant *Staphylococcus aureus* in an outbreak affecting 990 patients. *European Journal of Clinical Microbiology and Infectious Diseases: Official Publication of the European Society of Clinical Microbiology*, **13**, 74–81.

11 Sanford, M.D. *et al.* (1994) Efficient detection and long-term persistence of the carriage of methicillin-resistant *Staphylococcus aureus*. *Clinical Infectious Diseases*, **19**, 1123–1128.

12 Bertone, S.A. *et al.* (1994) Quantitative skin cultures at potential catheter sites in neonates. *Infection Control and Hospital Epidemiology*, **15**, 315–318.

13 Bonten, M.J.M. *et al.* (1996) Epidemiology of colonisation of patients and environment with vancomycin-resistant *Enterococci*. *Lancet*, **348**, 1615–1619.

14 Vernon, M.O. *et al.* (2006) Chlorhexidine gluconate to cleanse patients in a medical intensive care unit: the effectiveness of source control to reduce the bioburden of vancomycin-resistant enterococci. *Archives of Internal Medicine*, **166**, 306–312.

15 Riggs, M.M. *et al.* (2007) Asymptomatic carriers are a potential source for transmission of epidemic and nonepidemic *Clostridium difficile* strains among long-term care facility residents. *Clinical Infectious Diseases*, **45**, 992–998.

16 Leyden, J.J. *et al.* (1987) Skin microflora. *Journal of Investigative Dermatology*, **88**, 65s–72s.

17 Noble, W.C. (1975) Dispersal of skin microorganisms. *British Journal of Dermatology*, **93**, 477–485.

18 Bhalla, A. *et al.* (2007) *Staphylococcus aureus* intestinal colonization is associated with increased frequency of *S. aureus* on skin of hospitalized patients. *BMC Infectious Diseases*, **7**, 105–111.

19 Walter, C.W. *et al.* (1959) The spread of *Staphylococci* to the environment. *Antibiotics Annual*, **6**, 952–957.

20 Boyce, J.M. *et al.* (1994) Outbreak of multidrug-resistant *Enterococcus faecium* with transferable *vanB* class vancomycin resistance. *Journal of Clinical Microbiology*, **32**, 1148–1153.

21 McFarland, L.V. *et al.* (1989) Nosocomial acquisition of *Clostridium difficile* infection. *New England Journal of Medicine*, **320**, 204–210.

22 Samore, M.H. *et al.* (1996) Clinical and molecular epidemiology of sporadic and clustered cases of nosocomial *Clostridium difficile* diarrhea. *American Journal of Medicine*, **100**, 32–40.

23 Boyce, J.M. *et al.* (1997) Environmental contamination due to methicillin-resistant *Staphylococcus aureus*: possible infection control implications. *Infection Control and Hospital Epidemiology*, **18**, 622–627.

24 Grabsch, E.A. *et al.* (2006) Risk of environmental and healthcare worker contamination with vancomycin-resistant enterococci during outpatient procedures and hemodialysis. *Infection Control and Hospital Epidemiology*, **27**, 287–293.

25 Hayden, M.K. *et al.* (2008) Risk of hand or glove contamination after contact with patients colonized with vancomycin-resistant enterococcus or the colonized patients' environment. *Infection Control and Hospital Epidemiology*, **29**, 149–154.

26 Dancer, S.J. (2008) Importance of the environment in meticillin-resistant *Staphylococcus aureus* acquisition: the case for hospital cleaning. *Lancet Infectious Diseases*, **8**, 101–113.

27 Brady, R.R. *et al.* (2009) Review of mobile communication devices as potential reservoirs of nosocomial pathogens. *Journal of Hospital Infection*, **71**, 295–300.

28 Lu, P.L. *et al.* (2009) Methicillin-resistant *Staphylococcus aureus* and *Acinetobacter baumannii* on computer interface surfaces of hospital wards and association with clinical isolates. *BMC Infectious Diseases*, **9**, 164–170.

29 Jeske, H.C. *et al.* (2007) Bacterial contamination of anaesthetists' hands by personal mobile phone and fixed phone use in the operating theatre. *Anaesthesia*, **62**, 904–906.

30 Levin, A.S. *et al.* (2001) Environmental contamination by multidrug-resistant *Acinetobacter baumannii* in an intensive care unit. *Infection Control and Hospital Epidemiology*, **22**, 717–720.

31 Aygun, G. *et al.* (2002) Environmental contamination during a carbapenem-resistant *Acinetobacter baumannii* outbreak in an intensive care unit. *Journal of Hospital Infection*, **52**, 259–262.

32 Denton, M. *et al.* (2004) Role of environmental cleaning in controlling an outbreak of *Acinetobacter baumannii* on a neurosurgical intensive care unit. *Journal of Hospital Infection*, **56**, 106–110.

33 Zanetti, G. *et al.* (2007) Importation of *Acinetobacter baumannii* into a burn unit: a recurrent outbreak of infection associated with widespread environmental contamination. *Infection Control and Hospital Epidemiology*, **28**, 723–725.

34 Morgan, D.J. *et al.* (2010) Frequent multidrug-resistant *Acinetobacter baumannii* contamination of gloves, gowns, and hands of healthcare workers. *Infection Control and Hospital Epidemiology*, **31**, 716–721.

35 Pittet, D. *et al.* (1999) Bacterial contamination of the hands of hospital staff during routine patient care. *Archives of Internal Medicine*, **159**, 821–826.

36 Pessoa-Silva, C.L. *et al.* (2004) Dynamics of bacterial hand contamination during routine neonatal care. *Infection Control and Hospital Epidemiology*, **25**, 192–197.

37 Ojajarvi, J. (1980) Effectiveness of hand washing and disinfection methods in removing transient bacteria after patient nursing. *Journal of Hygiene*, **85**, 193–203.

38 Duckro, A.N. *et al.* (2005) Transfer of vancomycin-resistant *Enterococci* via health care worker hands. *Archives of Internal Medicine*, **165**, 302–307.

39 Foca, M. *et al.* (2000) Endemic *Pseudomonas aeruginosa* infection in a neonatal intensive care unit. *New England Journal of Medicine*, **343**, 695–700.

40 Sartor, C. *et al.* (2000) Nosocomial *Serratia marcescens* infections associated with extrinsic contamination of a liquid nonmedicated soap. *Infection Control and Hospital Epidemiology*, **21**, 196–199.

41 Boyce, J.M. *et al.* (1990) A common-source outbreak of *Staphylococcus epidermidis* infections among patients undergoing cardiac surgery. *Journal of Infectious Diseases*, **161**, 493–499.

42 Zawacki, A. *et al.* (2004) An outbreak of *Pseudomonas aeruginosa* pneumonia and bloodstream infection associated with intermittent otitis externa in a healthcare worker. *Infection Control and Hospital Epidemiology*, **25**, 1083–1089.

43 El Shafie, S.S. *et al.* (2004) Investigation of an outbreak of multidrug-resistant *Acinetobacter baumannii* in trauma intensive care unit. *Journal of Hospital Infection*, **56**, 101–105.

44 Hernandez-Castro, R. *et al.* (2010) Outbreak of *Candida parapsilosis* in a neonatal intensive care unit: a health care workers source. *European Journal of Pediatrics*, **169**, 783–787.

45 Mayank, D. *et al.* (2009) Nosocomial cross-transmission of *Pseudomonas aeruginosa* between patients in a tertiary intensive care unit. *Indian Journal of Pathology and Microbiology*, **52**, 509–513.

46 Girou, E. *et al.* (2008) Determinant roles of environmental contamination and noncompliance with standard precautions in the risk of hepatitis C virus transmission in a hemodialysis unit. *Clinical Infectious Diseases*, **47**, 627–633.

47 Laporte, F. *et al.* (2009) Mathematical modeling of hepatitis C virus transmission in hemodialysis. *American Journal of Infection Control*, **37**, 403–407.

48 Ivanova, D. *et al.* (2008) Extended-spectrum beta-lactamase-producing *Serratia marcescens* outbreak in a Bulgarian hospital. *Journal of Hospital Infection*, **70**, 60–65.

49 Rushton, S.P. *et al.* (2010) The transmission of nosocomial pathogens in an intensive care unit: a space-time clustering and structural equation modelling approach. *Epidemiology and Infection*, **138**, 915–926.

50 World Health Organization (WHO) (2009) *WHO Guidelines on Hand Hygiene in Health Care*, WHO, Geneva, http://whqlibdoc.who.int/publications/2009/9789241597906_eng.pdf (accessed September 21, 2012).

51 Boyce, J.M. and Pittet, D. (2002) Guideline for hand hygiene in health-care settings. Recommendations of the Healthcare Infection Control Practices Advisory Committee and the HICPAC/SHEA/APIC/IDSA Hand Hygiene Task Force. Society for Healthcare Epidemiology of America/Association for Professionals in Infection Control/Infectious Diseases Society of America. *MMWR. Morbidity and Mortality Weekly Report*, **51**, 1–45.

52 Larson, E.L. and Morton, H.E. (1991) Alcohols, in *Disinfection, Sterilization and Reservation*, 4th edn (ed. S.S. Block), Lea & Febiger, Philadelphia, pp. 191–203.

53 Price, P.B. (1939) Ethyl alcohol as a germicide. *Archives of Surgery*, **38**, 528–542.

54 Harrington, C. and Walker, H. (1903) The germicidal action of alcohol. *Boston Medical and Surgical Journal*, **148**, 548–552.

55 Coulthard, C.E. and Sykes, G. (1936) The germicidal effect of alcohol with special reference to its action on bacterial spores. *Pharmaceutical Journal*, **137**, 79–81.

56 Pohle, W.D. and Stuart, L.S. (1940) The germicidal action of cleaning agents – a study of a modification of price's procedure. *Journal of Infectious Diseases*, **67**, 275–281.

57 Gardner, A.D. (1948) Rapid disinfection of clean unwashed skin. *Lancet*, **2**, 760–763.

58 Sakuragi, T. *et al.* (1995) Bactericidal activity of skin disinfectants on methicillin-resistant *Staphylococcus aureus*. *Anesthesia and Analgesia*, **81**, 555–558.

59 Kampf, G. *et al.* (1998) Limited effectiveness of chlorhexidine-based hand disinfectants against methicillin-resistant *Staphylococcus aureus* (MRSA). *Journal of Hospital Infection*, **38**, 297–303.

60 Kampf, G. *et al.* (1999) Efficacy of hand disinfectants against vancomycin-resistant *Enterococci* in vitro. *Journal of Hospital Infection*, **42**, 143–150.

61 Platt, J. and Bucknall, R.A. (1985) The disinfection of respiratory syncytial virusby isopropanol and a chlorhexidine-detergent handwash. *Journal of Hospital Infection*, **6**, 89–94.

62 Krilov, L.R. and Hella Harkness, S. (1993) Inactivation of respiratory syncytial virus by detergents and disinfectants. *Pediatric Infectious Disease Journal*, **12**, 582–584.

63 Narang, H.K. and Codd, A.A. (1983) Action of commonly used disinfectants against *Enteroviruses*. *Journal of Hospital Infection*, **4**, 209–212.

64 Larson, E.L. (1995) APIC guideline for handwashing and hand antisepsis in health care settings. *American Journal of Infection Control*, **23**, 251–269.

65 Gottardi, W. (1991) Iodine and iodine compounds, in *Disinfection, Sterilization and Preservation* (ed. S.S. Block), Lea & Febiger, Philadelphia, pp. 152–166.

66 Goldenheim, P.D. (1993) In vitro efficacy of povidone-iodine solution and cream against methicillin-resistant *Staphylococcus aureus*. *Postgraduate Medical Journal*, **69** (Suppl. 3), S62–S65.

67 Traore, O. *et al.* (1996) An in-vitro evaluation of the activity of povidone-iodine against nosocomial bacterial strains. *Journal of Hospital Infection*, **34**, 217–222.

68 McLure, A.R. and Gordon, J. (1992) In-vitro evaluation of povidone-iodine and chlorhexidine against methicillin-resistant *Staphylococcus aureus*. *Journal of Hospital Infection*, **21**, 291–299.

69 Davies, J.G. *et al.* (1993) Preliminary study of test methods to assess the virucidal activity of skin disinfectants using poliovirus and bacteriophages. *Journal of Hospital Infection*, **25**, 125–131.

70 Grayson, M.L. *et al.* (2009) Efficacy of soap and water and alcohol-based hand-rub preparations against live H1N1 influenza virus on the hands of human volunteers. *Clinical Infectious Diseases*, **48**, 285–291.

71 Wolff, M.H. (2001) Hepatitis A virus: a test method for virucidal activity. *Journal of Hospital Infection*, **48** (Suppl. A), S18–S22.

72 Steinmann, J. *et al.* (1995) Two in-vivo protocols for testing virucidal efficacy of handwashing and hand disinfection. *Zentralblatt fur Hygiene Und Umweltmedizin*, **196**, 425–436.

73 Ansari, S.A. *et al.* (1991) Comparison of cloth, paper, and warm air drying in eliminating viruses and bacteria from washed hands. *American Journal of Infection Control*, **19**, 243–249.

74 Ansari, S.A. *et al.* (1989) In vivo protocol for testing efficacy of hand-washing agents against viruses and bacteria: experiments with *Rotavirus* and *Escherichia coli*. *Applied and Environmental Microbiology*, **55**, 3113–3118.

75 Sattar, S.A. *et al.* (2000) Activity of an alcohol-based hand gel against human adeno-, rhino-, and rotaviruses using the fingerpad method. *Infection Control and Hospital Epidemiology*, **21**, 516–519.

76 Gehrke, C. *et al.* (2004) Inactivation of feline Calicivirus, a surrogate of Norovirus (formerly Norwalk-like viruses), by different types of alcohol in vitro and in vivo. *Journal of Hospital Infection*, **56**, 49–55.

77 Steinmann, J. (2004) Surrogate viruses for testing virucidal efficacy of chemical disinfectants. *Journal of Hospital Infection*, **56** (Suppl. 2), S49–S54.

78 World Health Organization (WHO) (2010) *Guide to Local Production: WHO-Recommended Handrub Formulations*, WHO, Geneva, http://www.who.int/gpsc/5may/tools/system_change/en/index.html (accessed August 23, 2011).

79 Steinmann, J. *et al.* (2010) Virucidal activity of 2 alcohol-based formulations proposed as hand rubs by the World Health Organization. *American Journal of Infection Control*, **38**, 66–68.

80 Centers for Disease Control and Prevention (2009) Norovirus outbreaks on three college campuses – California, Michigan, and Wisconsin, 2008. *MMWR. Morbidity and Mortality Weekly Report*, **58**, 1095–1100.

81 Cheng, V.C. *et al.* (2009) Successful control of norovirus outbreak in an infirmary with the use of alcohol-based hand rub. *Journal of Hospital Infection*, **72**, 370–371.

82 Kampf, G. and Kramer, A. (2004) Epidemiologic background of hand hygiene and evaluation of the most important agents for scrubs and rubs. *Clinical Microbiology Reviews*, **17**, 863–893.

83 Rotter, M.L. (1996) Hand washing and hand disinfection, in *Hospital Epidemiology and Infection Control* (ed. G. Mayhall), Williams & Wilkins, Baltimore, pp. 1052–1068.

84 Oughton, M.T. *et al.* (2009) Hand hygiene with soap and water is superior to alcohol rub and antiseptic wipes for removal of *Clostridium difficile*. *Infection Control and Hospital Epidemiology*, **30**, 939–944.

85 Luby, S.P. *et al.* (2005) Effect of handwashing on child health: a randomized controlled trial. *Lancet*, **366**, 225–233.

86 Luby, S.P. *et al.* (2004) Effect of intensive handwashing promotion on childhood diarrhea in high-risk communities in Pakistan: a randomized controlled trial. *Journal of the American Medical Association*, **291**, 2547–2554.

87 Larson, E.L. *et al.* (2004) Effect of antibacterial home cleaning and handwashing products on infectious disease symptoms: a randomized, double-blind trial. *Annals of Internal Medicine*, **140**, 321–329.

88 Nandrup-Bus, I. (2011) Comparative studies of hand disinfection and handwashing procedures as tested by pupils in intervention programs. *American Journal of Infection Control*, **39**, 450–455.

89 Talaat, M. *et al.* (2011) Effects of hand hygiene campaigns on incidence of laboratory-confirmed influenza and absenteeism in schoolchildren, Cairo, Egypt. *Emerging Infectious Diseases*, **17**, 619–625.

90 Nandrup-Bus, I. (2009) Mandatory handwashing in elementary schools reduces absenteeism due to infectious illness among pupils: a pilot intervention study. *American Journal of Infection Control*, **37**, 820–826.

91 Aiello, A.E. *et al.* (2008) Effect of hand hygiene on infectious disease risk in the community setting: a meta-analysis. *American Journal of Public Health*, **98**, 1372–1381.

92 Sandora, T.J. *et al.* (2008) Reducing absenteeism from gastrointestinal and respiratory illness in elementary school students: a randomized, controlled trial of an infection-control intervention. *Pediatrics*, **121**, e1555–e1562.

93 Hubner, N.O. *et al.* (2010) Effectiveness of alcohol-based hand disinfectants in a public administration: impact on health and work performance related to acute respiratory symptoms and diarrhoea. *BMC Infectious Diseases*, **10**, 250.

94 Ojajarvi, J. (1991) Handwashing in Finland. *Journal of Hospital Infection*, **18**, 35–40.

95 Kramer, A. *et al.* (2002) Limited efficacy of alcohol-based hand gels. *Lancet*, **359**, 1489–1490.

96 Dharan, S. *et al.* (2003) Comparison of waterless hand antisepsis agents at short application times: raising the flag of concern. *Infection Control and Hospital Epidemiology*, **24**, 160–164.

97 Traore, O. *et al.* (2007) Liquid versus gel handrub formulation: a prospective intervention study. *Critical Care*, **11**, 52.

98 Kampf, G. *et al.* (2010) Efficacy of ethanol-based hand foams using clinically relevant amounts: a cross-over controlled study among healthy volunteers. *BMC Infectious Diseases*, **10**, 78–82.

99 World Health Organization (WHO) (2008) *Essential Environmental Health Standards in Health Care* (eds J.B. Adams and Y. Chartier) WHO, Geneva.

100 Boyce, J.M. *et al.* (2009) Evaluation of an electronic device for real-time measurement of alcohol-based hand rub use. *Infection Control and Hospital Epidemiology*, **30**, 1090–1095.

101 Sahud, A.G. and Bhanot, N. (2009) Measuring hand hygiene compliance: a new frontier for improving hand hygiene. *Infection Control and Hospital Epidemiology*, **30**, 1132.

102 Marra, A.R. *et al.* (2010) Measuring rates of hand hygiene adherence in the intensive care setting: a comparative study of direct observation, product usage, and electronic counting devices. *Infection Control and Hospital Epidemiology*, **31**, 796–801.

103 Pittet, D. *et al.* (2000) Effectiveness of a hospital-wide programme to improve compliance with hand hygiene. *Lancet*, **356**, 1307–1312.

104 Larson, E.L. *et al.* (2000) An organizational climate intervention associated with increased handwashing and decreased nosocomial infections. *Behavioral Medicine (Washington, DC)*, **26**, 14–22.

105 Conly, J.M. *et al.* (1989) Handwashing practices in an intensive care unit: the effects of an educational program and its relationship to infection rates. *American Journal of Infection Control*, **17**, 330–339.

106 Dubbert, P.M. *et al.* (1990) Increasing ICU staff handwashing: effects of education and group feedback. *Infection Control and Hospital Epidemiology*, **11**, 191–193.

107 Raju, T.N. and Kobler, C. (1991) Improving handwashing habits in the newborn nurseries. *American Journal of the Medical Sciences*, **302**, 355–358.

108 Tibballs, J. (1996) Teaching hospital medical staff to handwash. *Medical Journal of Australia*, **164**, 395–398.

109 Harbarth, S. *et al.* (2002) Interventional study to evaluate the impact of an alcohol-based hand gel in improving hand hygiene compliance. *Pediatric Infectious Disease Journal*, **21**, 489–495.

110 Lam, B.C. *et al.* (2004) Hand hygiene practices in a neonatal intensive care unit: a multimodal intervention and impact on nosocomial infection. *Pediatrics*, **114**, e565–e571.

111 Larson, E.L. *et al.* (1997) A multifaceted approach to changing handwashing behavior. *American Journal of Infection Control*, **25**, 3–10.

112 Rosenthal, V.D. *et al.* (2003) Effect of education and performance feedback on handwashing: the benefit of administrative support in Argentinean hospitals. *American Journal of Infection Control*, **31**, 85–92.

113 Won, S.P. *et al.* (2004) Handwashing program for the prevention of nosocomial infections in a neonatal intensive care unit. *Infection Control and Hospital Epidemiology*, **25**, 742–746.

114 World Health Organization (WHO) (2010) *Hand Hygiene Technical Reference Manual*, WHO, Geneva, http://www.who.int/gpsc/5may/tools/training_education/en/index.html (accessed September 29, 2010).

115 Sax, H. *et al.* (2009) The World Health Organization hand hygiene observation method. *American Journal of Infection Control*, **37**, 827–834.

116 Pittet, D. and Boyce, J.M. (2003) Revolutionising hand hygiene in health-care settings: guidelines revisited. *Lancet Infectious Diseases*, **3**, 269–270.

117 Pittet, D. (2002) Promotion of hand hygiene: magic, hype, or scientific challenge? *Infection Control and Hospital Epidemiology*, **23**, 118–119.

118 Hugonnet, S. *et al.* (2002) Alcohol-based handrub improves compliance with hand hygiene in intensive care units. *Archives of Internal Medicine*, **162**, 1037–1043.

119 Bittner, M.J. and Rich, E.C. (1998) Surveillance of handwashing episodes in adult intensive care units by measuring an index of soap and paper towel consumption. *Clinical Performance and Quality Health Care*, **4**, 179–182.

120 Fuller, C. *et al.* (2010) Technical note: assessment of blinding of hand hygiene observers in randomized controlled trials of hand hygiene interventions. *American Journal of Infection Control*, **38**, 332–334.

121 Haas, J.P. and Larson, E.L. (2007) Measurement of compliance with hand hygiene. *Journal of Hospital Infection*, **66**, 6–14.

122 Gould, D.J. *et al.* (2007) Measuring handwashing performance in health service audits and research studies. *Journal of Hospital Infection*, **66**, 109–115.

123 Gould, D.J. *et al.* (2007) Interventions to improve hand hygiene compliance in patient care. *Cochrane Database of Systematic Reviews*, Art. No. CD005186.

124 Sax, H. *et al.* (2007) "My five moments for hand hygiene": a user-centred design approach to understand, train, monitor and report hand hygiene. *Journal of Hospital Infection*, **67**, 9–21.

125 Pittet, D. (2000) Improving compliance with hand hygiene in hospitals. *Infection Control and Hospital Epidemiology*, **21**, 381–386.

126 Pittet, D. *et al.* (2003) Hand-cleansing during postanesthesia care. *Anesthesiology*, **99**, 530–535.

127 World Health Organization (WHO) (2010) *Instructions for Data-Entry and Data-Analysis*, WHO, Geneva, http://www.who.int/gpsc/5may/tools/training_education/en/index.html (accessed September 29, 2010).

128 Longtin, Y. *et al.* (2009) Patients' beliefs and perceptions of their participation to increase healthcare worker compliance with hand hygiene. *Infection Control and Hospital Epidemiology*, **30**, 830–839.

129 McGuckin, M. *et al.* (2001) Evaluation of a patient-empowering hand hygiene programme in the UK. *Journal of Hospital Infection*, **48**, 222–227.

130 McGuckin, M. *et al.* (2004) Evaluation of a patient education model for increasing hand hygiene compliance in an inpatient rehabilitation unit. *American Journal of Infection Control*, **32**, 235–238.

131 Bittle, M.J. and LaMarche, S. (2009) Engaging the patient as observer to promote hand hygiene compliance in ambulatory care. *Joint Commission Journal on Quality and Patient Safety*, **35**, 519–525.

132 Williams, T. (2002) Patient empowerment and ethical decision making: the patient/partner and the right to act. *Dimensions of Critical Care Nursing*, **21**, 100–104.

133 McGuckin, M. *et al.* (2011) Patient empowerment and multimodal hand hygiene promotion: a win-win strategy. *American Journal of Medical Quality*, **26**, 10–17.

134 Longtin, Y. *et al.* (2010) Patient participation: current knowledge and applicability to patient safety. *Mayo Clinic Proceedings*, **85**, 53–62.

135 Pittet, D. *et al.* (1999) Compliance with handwashing in a teaching hospital. *Annals of Internal Medicine*, **130**, 126–130.

136 Wade, S. (1995) Partnership in care: a critical review. *Nursing Standard*, **9**, 29–32.

137 Pittet, D. *et al.* (2011) Involving the patient to ask about hospital hand hygiene: a National Patient Safety Agency feasibility study. *Journal of Hospital Infection*, **77**, 299–303.

138 Broughall, J.M. (1984) An automatic monitoring system for measuring handwashing frequency. *Journal of Hospital Infection*, **5**, 447–453.

139 Larson, E. *et al.* (1986) Physiologic and microbiologic changes in skin related to frequent handwashing. *Infection Control*, **7**, 59–63.

140 Simmons, B. *et al.* (1990) The role of handwashing in prevention of endemic intensive care unit infections. *Infection Control and Hospital Epidemiology*, **11**, 589–594.

141 McLane, C. *et al.* (1983) A nursing practice problem: failure to observe aseptic technique. *American Journal of Infection Control*, **11**, 178–182.

142 Bischoff, W.E. *et al.* (2000) Handwashing compliance by health care workers: the impact of introducing an accessible, alcohol-based hand antiseptic. *Archives of Internal Medicine*, **160**, 1017–1021.

143 McGuckin, M. *et al.* (1999) Patient education model for increasing handwashing compliance. *American Journal of Infection Control*, **27**, 309–314.

144 Gopal Rao, G. *et al.* (2002) Marketing hand hygiene in hospitals – a case study. *Journal of Hospital Infection*, **50**, 42–47.

145 Swoboda, S.M. *et al.* (2004) Electronic monitoring and voice prompts improve hand hygiene and decrease nosocomial infections in an intermediate care unit. *Critical Care Medicine*, **32**, 358–363.

146 MacDonald, A. *et al.* (2004) Performance feedback of hand hygiene, using alcohol gel as the skin decontaminant, reduces the number of inpatients newly affected by MRSA and antibiotic costs. *Journal of Hospital Infection*, **56**, 56–63.

147 Colombo, C. *et al.* (2002) Impact of teaching interventions on nurse compliance with hand disinfection. *Journal of Hospital Infection*, **51**, 69–72.

148 Kaier, K. *et al.* (2009) The impact of antimicrobial drug consumption and alcohol-based hand rub use on the emergence and spread of extended-spectrum beta-lactamase-producing strains: a time-series analysis. *Journal of Antimicrobial Chemotherapy*, **63**, 609–614.

149 Vernaz, N. *et al.* (2008) Temporal effects of antibiotic use and hand rub consumption on the incidence of MRSA and *Clostridium difficile*. *Journal of Antimicrobial Chemotherapy*, **62**, 601–607.

150 Kappstein, I. *et al.* (2009) [Prevention of transmission of methicillin-resistant *Staphylococcus aureus* (MRSA) infection: standard precautions instead of isolation: a 6-year surveillance in a university hospital.] *Chirurgia (Bucharest, Romania: 1990)*, **80**, 49–61.

151 Scheithauer, S. *et al.* (2009) Compliance with hand hygiene on surgical, medical, and neurologic intensive care units: direct observation versus calculated disinfectant usage. *American Journal of Infection Control*, **37**, 835–841.

152 van de Mortel, T. and Murgo, M. (2006) An examination of covert observation and solution audit as tools to measure the success of hand hygiene interventions. *American Journal of Infection Control*, **34**, 95–99.

153 Grayson, M.L. *et al.* (2008) Significant reductions in methicillin-resistant *Staphylococcus aureus* bacteraemia and clinical isolates associated with a multisite, hand hygiene culture-change program and subsequent successful statewide roll-out. *Medical Journal of Australia*, **188**, 633–640.

154 Johnson, P.D. *et al.* (2005) Efficacy of an alcohol/chlorhexidine hand hygiene program in a hospital with high rates of nosocomial methicillin-resistant *Staphylococcus aureus* (MRSA) infection. *Medical Journal of Australia*, **183**, 509–514.

155 Harrington, G. *et al.* (2007) Reduction in hospitalwide incidence of infection or colonization with methicillin-resistant *Staphylococcus aureus* with use of antimicrobial hand-hygiene gel and statistical process control charts. *Infection Control and Hospital Epidemiology*, **28**, 837–844.

156 Laustsen, S. *et al.* (2009) Amount of alcohol-based hand rub used and incidence of hospital-acquired bloodstream infection in a Danish hospital. *Infection Control and Hospital Epidemiology*, **30**, 1012–1014.

157 Sakamoto, F. *et al.* (2010) Increased use of alcohol-based hand sanitizers and successful eradication of methicillin-resistant *Staphylococcus aureus* from a neonatal intensive care unit: a multivariate time series analysis. *American Journal of Infection Control*, **38**, 529–534.

158 Eveillard, M. *et al.* (2006) Impact of the reinforcement of a methicillin-resistant *Staphylococcus aureus* control programme: a 3-year evaluation by several indicators in a French university hospital. *European Journal of Epidemiology*, **21**, 551–558.

159 Christiaens, G. *et al.* (2006) [Hand hygiene: first measure to control nosocomial infection.] *Revue Medicale de Liege*, **61**, 31–36.

160 Herud, T. *et al.* (2009) Association between use of hand hygiene products and rates of health care-associated infections in a large university hospital in Norway. *American Journal of Infection Control*, **37**, 311–317.

161 Kaier, K. *et al.* (2009) Two time-series analyses of the impact of antibiotic consumption and alcohol-based hand disinfection on the incidences of nosocomial methicillin-resistant *Staphylococcus aureus* infection and *Clostridium difficile* infection. *Infection Control and Hospital Epidemiology*, **30**, 346–353.

162 Sroka, S. *et al.* (2010) Impact of alcohol hand-rub use on meticillin-resistant *Staphylococcus aureus:* an analysis of the literature. *Journal of Hospital Infection*, **74**, 204–211.

163 Lankford, M.G. *et al.* (2003) Influence of role models and hospital design on hand hygiene of healthcare workers. *Emerging Infectious Diseases*, **9**, 217–223.

164 Bittner, M.J. *et al.* (2002) Limited impact of sustained simple feedback based on soap and paper towel consumption on the frequency of hand washing in an adult intensive care unit. *Infection Control and Hospital Epidemiology*, **23**, 120–126.

165 Swoboda, S.M. *et al.* (2007) Isolation status and voice prompts improve hand hygiene. *American Journal of Infection Control*, **35**, 470–476.

166 Venkatesh, A.K. *et al.* (2008) Use of electronic alerts to enhance hand hygiene compliance and decrease transmission of vancomycin-resistant Enterococcus in a hematology unit. *American Journal of Infection Control*, **36**, 199–205.

167 Kinsella, G. *et al.* (2007) Electronic surveillance of wall-mounted soap and alcohol gel dispensers in an intensive care unit. *Journal of Hospital Infection*, **66**, 34–39.

168 Boscart, V.M. *et al.* (2008) Acceptability of a wearable hand hygiene device with monitoring capabilities. *Journal of Hospital Infection*, **70**, 216–222.

169 Marra, A.R. *et al.* (2008) Controlled trial measuring the effect of a feedback intervention on hand hygiene compliance in a step-down unit. *Infection Control and Hospital Epidemiology*, **29**, 730–735.

170 Boscart, V.M. *et al.* (2010) Defining the configuration of a hand hygiene monitoring system. *American Journal of Infection Control*, **38**, 518–522.

171 Pittet, D. *et al.* (2004) Hand hygiene among physicians: performance, beliefs, and perceptions. *Annals of Internal Medicine*, **141**, 1–8.

172 Pessoa-Silva, C.L. *et al.* (2005) Attitudes and perceptions toward hand hygiene among healthcare workers caring for critically ill neonates. *Infection Control and Hospital Epidemiology*, **26**, 305–311.

173 Malekmakan, L. *et al.* (2008) Hand hygiene in Iranian health care workers. *American Journal of Infection Control*, **36**, 602–603.

174 Allegranzi, B. *et al.* (2009) Successful implementation of the WHO multimodal hand hygiene improvement strategy and tools: a survey of 230 hospitals worldwide. Poster presented at 19th European Congress of Clinical Microbiology and Infectious Diseases, Helsinki, Finland, 16–19 May 2009.

175 Burnett, E. (2009) Perceptions, attitudes, and behavior towards patient hand hygiene. *American Journal of Infection Control*, **37**, 638–642.

176 Tai, J.W. *et al.* (2009) Nurses and physicians' perceptions of the importance and impact of healthcare-associated infections and hand hygiene: a multicenter exploratory study in Hong Kong. *Infection*, **37**, 320–333.

177 De Wandel, D. *et al.* (2010) Behavioral determinants of hand hygiene compliance in intensive care units. *American Journal of Critical Care*, **19**, 230–239.

178 Erasmus, V. *et al.* (2010) Systematic review of studies on compliance with hand hygiene guidelines in hospital care. *Infection Control and Hospital Epidemiology*, **31**, 283–294.

179 Nguyen, K.V. *et al.* (2008) Effectiveness of an alcohol-based hand hygiene programme in reducing nosocomial infections in the urology ward of Binh Dan Hospital, Vietnam. *Tropical Medicine and International Health*, **13**, 1297–1302.

180 Allegranzi, B. *et al.* (2010) Successful implementation of the World Health Organization hand hygiene improvement strategy in a referral hospital in Mali, Africa. *Infection Control and Hospital Epidemiology*, **31**, 133–141.

181 Asare, A. *et al.* (2009) Hand hygiene practices in a neonatal intensive care unit in Ghana. *Journal of Infectious Diseases*, **3**, 352–356.

182 Picheansathian, W. *et al.* (2008) The effectiveness of a promotion programme on hand hygiene compliance and nosocomial infections in a neonatal intensive care unit. *International Journal of Nursing Practice*, **14**, 315–321.

183 Lipsett, P.A. and Swoboda, S.M. (2001) Handwashing compliance depends on professional status. *Surgical Infections*, **2**, 241–245.

184 Zerr, D.M. *et al.* (2005) Decreasing hospital-associated rotavirus infection: a multidisciplinary hand hygiene campaign in a children's hospital. *Pediatric Infectious Disease Journal*, **24**, 397–403.

185 Pan, A. *et al.* (2007) Hand hygiene and glove use behavior in an Italian hospital. *Infection Control and Hospital Epidemiology*, **28**, 1099–1102.

186 Saint, S. *et al.* (2009) Marked variability in adherence to hand hygiene: a 5-unit observational study in Tuscany. *American Journal of Infection Control*, **37**, 306–310.

187 Borg, M.A. *et al.* (2009) Self-protection as a driver for hand hygiene among healthcare workers. *Infection Control and Hospital Epidemiology*, **30**, 578–580.

188 Arenas, M.D. *et al.* (2005) A multicentric survey of the practice of hand hygiene in haemodialysis units: factors affecting compliance. *Nephrology, Dialysis, Transplantation: Official Publication of the European Dialysis and Transplant Association – European Renal Association*, **20**, 1164–1171.

189 Novoa, A.M. *et al.* (2007) Evaluation of hand hygiene adherence in a tertiary hospital. *American Journal of Infection Control*, **35**, 676–683.

190 O'Boyle, C.A. *et al.* (2001) Understanding adherence to hand hygiene recommendations: the theory of planned behavior. *American Journal of Infection Control*, **29**, 352–360.

191 Pittet, D. *et al.* (2004) Cost implications of successful hand hygiene promotion. *Infection Control and Hospital Epidemiology*, **25**, 264–266.

192 Thompson, B.L. *et al.* (1997) Handwashing and glove use in a long-term-care facility. *Infection Control and Hospital Epidemiology*, **18**, 97–103.

193 Khatib, M. *et al.* (1999) Hand washing and use of gloves while managing patients receiving mechanical ventilation in the ICU. *Chest*, **116**, 172–175.

194 Pessoa-Silva, C.L. *et al.* (2007) Reduction of health care associated infection risk in neonates by successful hand hygiene promotion. *Pediatrics*, **120**, e382–e390.

195 Haley, R.W. and Bregman, D. (1982) The role of understaffing and overcrowding in recurrent outbreaks of staphylococcal infection in a neonatal special-care unit. *Journal of Infectious Diseases*, **145**, 875–885.

196 Harbarth, S. *et al.* (1999) Outbreak of *Enterobacter cloacae* related to understaffing, overcrowding, and poor hygiene practices. *Infection Control and Hospital Epidemiology*, **20**, 598–603.

197 Kuzu, N. *et al.* (2005) Compliance with hand hygiene and glove use in a university-affiliated hospital. *Infection Control and Hospital Epidemiology*, **26**, 312–315.

198 Larson, E. and Killien, M. (1982) Factors influencing handwashing behavior of patient care personnel. *American Journal of Infection Control*, **10**, 93–99.

199 Larson, E. (1985) Handwashing and skin physiologic and bacteriologic aspects. *Infection Control*, **6**, 14–23.

200 Pettinger, A. and Nettleman, M.D. (1991) Epidemiology of isolation precautions. *Infection Control and Hospital Epidemiology*, **12**, 303–307.

201 Heenan, A. (1992) Handwashing practices. *Nursing Times*, **88**, 70.

202 Zimakoff, J. *et al.* (1992) A multicenter questionnaire investigation of attitudes toward hand hygiene, assessed by the staff in fifteen hospitals in Denmark and Norway. *American Journal of Infection Control*, **20**, 58–64.

203 Larson, E. and Kretzer, E.K. (1995) Compliance with handwashing and barrier precautions. *Journal of Hospital Infection*, **30** (Suppl.), 88–106.

204 Kretzer, E.K. and Larson, E.L. (1998) Behavioral interventions to improve infection control practices. *American Journal of Infection Control*, **26**, 245–253.

205 Huskins, W.C. *et al.* (1999) Infection control in countries with limited resources, in *Hospital Epidemiology and Infection Control*, 2nd edn (ed. C.G. Mayhall), Williams & Wilkins, Baltimore, pp. 1489–1513.

206 Patarakul, K. *et al.* (2005) Cross-sectional survey of hand-hygiene compliance and attitudes of health care workers and visitors in the intensive care units at King Chulalongkorn Memorial Hospital. *Journal of the Medical Association of Thailand*, **88** (Suppl. 4), S287–S293.

207 Barrett, R. and Randle, J. (2008) Hand hygiene practices: nursing students' perceptions. *Journal of Clinical Nursing*, **17**, 1851–1857.

208 Kaplan, L.M. and McGuckin, M. (1986) Increasing handwashing compliance with more accessible sinks. *Infection Control*, **7**, 408–410.

209 Suchitra, J.B. and Lakshmi Devi, N. (2007) Impact of education on knowledge, attitudes and practices among various categories of health care workers on nosocomial infections. *Indian Journal of Medical Microbiology*, **25**, 181–187.

210 Yuan, C.T. *et al.* (2009) Perceptions of hand hygiene practices in China. *Journal of Hospital Infection*, **71**, 157–162.

211 Williams, C.O. *et al.* (1994) Variables influencing worker compliance with universal precautions in the emergency department. *American Journal of Infection Control*, **22**, 138–148.

212 Voss, A. and Widmer, A.F. (1997) No time for handwashing!? Handwashing versus alcoholic rub: can we afford 100% compliance? *Infection Control and Hospital Epidemiology*, **18**, 205–208.

213 Boyce, J.M. (1999) It is time for action: improving hand hygiene in hospitals. *Annals of Internal Medicine*, **130**, 153–155.

214 Weeks, A. (1999) Why I don't wash my hands between each patient contact. *British Medical Journal (Clinical Research Ed.)*, **319**, 518–518.

215 Dedrick, R.E. *et al.* (2007) Hand hygiene practices after brief encounters with patients: an important opportunity for prevention. *Infection Control and Hospital Epidemiology*, **28**, 341–345.

216 Rosenthal, V.D. *et al.* (2005) Reduction in nosocomial infection with improved hand hygiene in intensive care units of a tertiary care hospital in Argentina. *American Journal of Infection Control*, **33**, 392–397.

217 Muto, C.A. *et al.* (2000) Hand hygiene rates unaffected by installation of dispensers of a rapidly acting hand antiseptic. *American Journal of Infection Control*, **28**, 273–276.

218 Graafmans, W. *et al.* (2010) Trends in scientific publications as an indicator for hand hygiene awareness, in *50th Interscience Conference on Antimicrobial Agents and Chemotherapy. Boston, USA, 12–15 September 2010*, American Society for Microbiology, Abstract P1775.

219 Brown, S.M. *et al.* (2003) Use of an alcohol-based hand rub and quality improvement interventions to improve hand hygiene in a Russian neonatal intensive care unit. *Infection Control and Hospital Epidemiology*, **24**, 172–179.

220 Trick, W.E. *et al.* (2007) Multicenter intervention program to increase adherence to hand hygiene recommendations and glove use and to reduce the incidence of antimicrobial resistance. *Infection Control and Hospital Epidemiology*, **28**, 42–49.

221 Rupp, M.E. *et al.* (2008) Prospective, controlled, cross-over trial of alcohol-based hand gel in critical care units. *Infection Control and Hospital Epidemiology*, **29**, 8–15.

222 Capretti, M.G. *et al.* (2008) Impact of a standardized hand hygiene program on the incidence of nosocomial infection in very low birth weight infants. *American Journal of Infection Control*, **36**, 430–435.

223 Lederer, J.W. *et al.* (2009) A comprehensive hand hygiene approach to reducing MRSA health care-associated infections. *Joint Commission Journal on Quality and Patient Safety*, **35**, 180–185.

224 Cromer, A.L. *et al.* (2008) Monitoring and feedback of hand hygiene compliance and the impact on facility-acquired methicillin-resistant *Staphylococcus aureus*. *American Journal of Infection Control*, **36**, 672–677.

225 McLaws, M.L. *et al.* (2009) Improvements in hand hygiene across New South Wales public hospitals: clean hands save lives, part III. *Medical Journal of Australia*, **191**, S18–S24.

226 Helms, B. *et al.* (2010) Improving hand hygiene compliance: a multidisciplinary approach. *American Journal of Infection Control*, **38**, 572–574.

227 Yeung, W.K. *et al.* (2011) Clustered randomized controlled trial of a hand hygiene intervention involving pocket-sized containers of alcohol-based hand rub for the control of infections in long-term care facilities. *Infection Control and Hospital Epidemiology*, **32**, 67–76.

228 Doron, S.I. *et al.* (2011) A multifaceted approach to education, observation, and feedback in a successful hand hygiene campaign. *Joint Commission Journal on Quality and Patient Safety*, **37**, 3–10.

229 van den Hoogen, A. *et al.* (2010) Improvement of adherence to hand hygiene practice using a multimodal intervention program in a neonatal intensive care unit. *Journal of Nursing Care Quality*, June 26 (epub ahead of print).

230 Chou, T. *et al.* (2010) Changing the culture of hand hygiene compliance using a bundle that includes a violation letter. *American Journal of Infection Control*, **38**, 575–578.

231 Mayer, J. *et al.* (2011) Dissemination and sustainability of a hospital-wide hand hygiene program emphasizing positive reinforcement. *Infection Control and Hospital Epidemiology*, **32**, 59–66.

232 Forrester, L.A. *et al.* (2010) Clean hands for life: results of a large, multicentre, multifaceted, social marketing hand-hygiene campaign. *Journal of Hospital Infection*, **74**, 225–231.

233 Allegranzi, B. *et al.* (2007) The 1st Global Patient Safety Challenge: catalyzing hand hygiene national campaigns worldwide, in *47th Interscience Conference on Antimicrobial Agents and Chemotherapy, Chicago, USA, 13–20 September 2007*, American Society for Microbiology, Abstract K1376.

234 Mathai, E. *et al.* (2010) A survey examining promotion of hand hygiene in healthcare through campaigns and programmes coordinated at a national/sub-national level. *Clinical Microbiology and Infection*, **16** (Suppl. 2), S100.

235 Magiorakos, A.P. *et al.* (2009) National hand hygiene campaigns in Europe, 2000–2009. *Euro Surveillance*, **14**, 1–7.

236 Magiorakos, A.P. *et al.* (2010) Pathways to clean hands: highlights of successful hand hygiene implementation strategies in Europe. *Euro Surveillance*, **15**, 1–5.

237 Storr, J. (2005) The effectiveness of the national cleanyourhands campaign. *Nursing Times*, **101**, 50–51.

238 Allegranzi, B. *et al.* (2010) Successful implementation of the WHO hand hygiene improvement strategy in 41 Italian intensive care units, in *50th Interscience Conference on Antimicrobial Agents and Chemotherapy, Boston, USA, 12–15 September 2010*, American Society for Microbiology, Abstract K506.

239 Mathai, E. *et al.* (2011) Promoting hand hygiene in healthcare through national/subnational campaigns. *Journal of Hospital Infection*, **77**, 294–298.

240 Pantle, A.C. *et al.* (2009) A statewide approach to systematising hand hygiene behaviour in hospitals: clean hands save lives, part I. *Medical Journal of Australia*, **191**, S8–S12.

241 Fitzpatrick, K.R. *et al.* (2009) Culture change for hand hygiene: clean hands save lives, part II. *Medical Journal of Australia*, **191**, S13–S17.

242 World Health Organization (WHO) (2010) *Hand Hygiene Self-Assessment Framework*, WHO, Geneva, http://www.who.int/gpsc/country_work/hhsa_framework/en/index.html (accessed September 29, 2010).

243 Ahmed, K. (2010) Audit of hand hygiene at Broadmoor, a high secure psychiatric hospital. *Journal of Hospital Infection*, **75**, 128–131.

244 Hayden, M.K. *et al.* (2006) Reduction in acquisition of vancomycin-resistant enterococcus after enforcement of routine environmental cleaning measures. *Clinical Infectious Diseases*, **42**, 1552–1560.

245 Maury, E. *et al.* (2000) Availability of an alcohol solution can improve hand disinfection compliance in an intensive care unit. *American Journal of Respiratory and Critical Care Medicine*, **162**, 324–327.

246 Mayer, J.A. *et al.* (1986) Increasing handwashing in an intensive care unit. *Infection Control*, **7**, 259–262.

247 Doebbeling, B.N. *et al.* (1992) Comparative efficacy of alternative handwashing agents in reducing nosocomial infections in intensive care units. *New England Journal of Medicine*, **327**, 88–93.

248 Santana, S.L. *et al.* (2007) Assessment of healthcare professionals' adherence to hand hygiene after alcohol-based hand rub introduction at an intensive care unit in Sao Paulo, Brazil. *Infection Control and Hospital Epidemiology*, **28**, 365–367.

249 Raskind, C.H. *et al.* (2007) Hand hygiene compliance rates after an educational intervention in a neonatal intensive care unit. *Infection Control and Hospital Epidemiology*, **28**, 1096–1098.

250 Haas, J.P. and Larson, E.L. (2008) Impact of wearable alcohol gel dispensers on hand hygiene in an emergency department. *Academic Emergency Medicine*, **15**, 393–396.

251 Le, T.A. *et al.* (2007) Reduction in surgical site infections in neurosurgical patients associated with a bedside hand hygiene program in Vietnam. *Infection Control and Hospital Epidemiology*, **28**, 583–588.

252 McGuckin, M. *et al.* (2006) The effect of random voice hand hygiene messages delivered by medical, nursing, and infection control staff on hand hygiene compliance in intensive care. *American Journal of Infection Control*, **34**, 673–675.

253 Girou, E. and Oppein, F. (2001) Hand washing compliance in a French university hospital: new perspective with the introduction of hand rubbing with a waterless alcohol-based solution. *Journal of Hospital Infection*, **48** (Suppl. A), 55–57.

254 Gordin, F.M. *et al.* (2007) A cluster of hemodialysis-related bacteremia linked to artificial fingernails. *Infection Control and Hospital Epidemiology*, **28**, 743–744.

255 Aspock, C. and Koller, W. (1999) A simple hand hygiene exercise. *American Journal of Infection Control*, **27**, 370–372.

256 Giannitsioti, E. *et al.* (2009) Does a bed rail system of alcohol-based handrub antiseptic improve compliance of health care workers with hand hygiene? Results from a pilot study. *American Journal of Infection Control*, **37**, 160–163.

257 Caniza, M.A. *et al.* (2009) A practical guide to alcohol-based hand hygiene infrastructure in a resource-poor pediatric hospital. *American Journal of Infection Control*, **37**, 851–854.

258 Mathai, E. *et al.* (2010) Educating healthcare workers to optimal hand hygiene practices: addressing the need. *Infection*, **38**, 349–356.

259 Widmer, A.F. *et al.* (2007) Introducing alcohol-based hand rub for hand hygiene: the critical need for training. *Infection Control and Hospital Epidemiology*, **28**, 50–54.

260 Lee, T.C. *et al.* (2009) Impact of a mandatory infection control education program on nosocomial acquisition of methicillin-resistant *Staphylococcus aureus*. *Infection Control and Hospital Epidemiology*, **30**, 249–256.

261 Wisniewski, M.F. *et al.* (2007) Effect of education on hand hygiene beliefs and practices: a 5-year program. *Infection Control and Hospital Epidemiology*, **28**, 88–91.

262 Caniza, M.A. *et al.* (2007) Effective hand hygiene education with the use of flipcharts in a hospital in El Salvador. *Journal of Hospital Infection*, **65**, 58–64.

263 Benton, C. (2007) Hand hygiene-meeting the JCAHO safety goal: can compliance with CDC hand hygiene guidelines be improved by a surveillance and educational program? *Plastic Surgical Nursing*, **27**, 40–44.

264 Howard, D.P. *et al.* (2009) A simple effective clean practice protocol significantly improves hand decontamination and infection control measures in the acute surgical setting. *Infection*, **37**, 34–38.

265 Laustsen, S. *et al.* (2009) E-learning may improve adherence to alcohol-based hand rubbing: a cohort study. *American Journal of Infection Control*, **37**, 565–568.

266 Dierssen-Sotos, T. *et al.* (2010) Evaluating the impact of a hand hygiene campaign on improving adherence. *American Journal of Infection Control*, **38**, 240–243.

267 Conrad, A. *et al.* (2010) Are short training sessions on hand hygiene effective in preventing hospital-acquired MRSA? A time-series analysis. *American Journal of Infection Control*, **38**, 559–561.

268 Jang, J.H. *et al.* (2010) Focus group study of hand hygiene practice among healthcare workers in a teaching hospital in Toronto, Canada. *Infection Control and Hospital Epidemiology*, **31**, 144–150.

269 Helder, O.K. *et al.* (2010) The impact of an education program on hand hygiene compliance and nosocomial infection incidence in an urban neonatal intensive care unit: an intervention study with before and after comparison. *International Journal of Nursing Studies*, **47**, 1245–1252.

270 van de Mortel, T.F. *et al.* (2010) A comparison of the hand hygiene knowledge, beliefs, and practices of Greek nursing and medical students. *American Journal of Infection Control*, **38**, 75–77.

271 Lockhart, D.E. and Smith, A.J. (2009) An evaluation of a pilot study of a web-based educational initiative for educating and training undergraduate dental students in infection prevention. *British Dental Journal*, **207**, 223–226.

272 Avila-Aguero, M.L. *et al.* (1998) Handwashing practices in a tertiary-care, pediatric hospital and the effect on an educational program. *Clinical Performance and Quality Health Care*, **6**, 70–72.

273 McAteer, J. *et al.* (2007) Use of performance feedback to increase healthcare worker hand-hygiene behaviour. *Journal of Hospital Infection*, **66**, 291–292; author reply 292–293.

274 Cheng, V.C. *et al.* (2010) Sequential introduction of single room isolation and hand hygiene campaign in the control of methicillin-resistant *Staphylococcus aureus* in intensive care unit. *BMC Infectious Diseases*, **10**, 263.

275 McKinley, T. *et al.* (2005) Focus group data as a tool in assessing effectiveness of a hand hygiene campaign. *American Journal of Infection Control*, **33**, 368–373.

276 das Neves, Z.C. *et al.* (2006) Hand hygiene: the impact of incentive strategies on adherence among healthcare workers from a newborn intensive care unit. *Revista Latino-Americana de Enfermagem*, **14**, 546–552.

277 Pittet, D. (2004) The Lowbury lecture: behaviour in infection control. *Journal of Hospital Infection*, **58**, 1–13.

278 Fletcher, M. (2009) Hand hygiene and infection in hospitals: what do the public know; what should the public know? *Journal of Hospital Infection*, **73**, 397–399.

279 Lent, V. *et al.* (2009) Evaluation of patient participation in a patient empowerment initiative to improve hand hygiene practices in a Veterans Affairs medical center. *American Journal of Infection Control*, **37**, 117–120.

280 Allegranzi, B. and Pittet, D. (2009) Role of hand hygiene in healthcare-associated infection prevention. *Journal of Hospital Infection*, **73**, 305–315.

281 Gordin, F.M. *et al.* (2005) Reduction in nosocomial transmission of drug-resistant bacteria after introduction of an alcohol-based handrub. *Infection Control and Hospital Epidemiology*, **26**, 650–653.

282 Girou, E. *et al.* (2006) Association between hand hygiene compliance and methicillin-resistant *Staphylococcus aureus* prevalence in a French rehabilitation hospital. *Infection Control and Hospital Epidemiology*, **27**, 1128–1130.

283 Casewell, M. and Phillips, I. (1977) Hands as route of transmission for *Klebsiella* species. *British Medical Journal (Clinical Research Ed.)*, **2**, 1315–1317.

284 Webster, J. *et al.* (1994) Elimination of methicillin-resistant *Staphylococcus aureus* from a neonatal intensive care unit after hand washing with triclosan. *Journal of Paediatrics and Child Health*, **30**, 59–64.

285 Zafar, A.B. *et al.* (1995) Use of 0.3% triclosan (Bacti-Stat) to eradicate an outbreak of methicillin-resistant *Staphylococcus aureus* in a neonatal nursery. *American Journal of Infection Control*, **23**, 200–208.

286 Hilburn, J. *et al.* (2003) Use of alcohol hand sanitizer as an infection control strategy in an acute care facility. *American Journal of Infection Control*, **31**, 109–116.

287 McLaws, M.L. *et al.* (2009) More than hand hygiene is needed to affect methicillin-resistant *Staphylococcus aureus* clinical indicator rates: clean hands save lives, part IV. *Medical Journal of Australia*, **191**, S26–S31.

288 Nguyen, D.M. *et al.* (2007) Risk factors for neonatal methicillin-resistant *Staphylococcus aureus* infection in a well-infant nursery. *Infection Control and Hospital Epidemiology*, **28**, 406–411.

289 Health Protection Agency Centre for Infections (2009) *Healthcare-associated Infections in England: 2008–2009 Report*. Health Protection Agency, London.

290 Jarlier, V. *et al.* (2010) Curbing methicillin-resistant *Staphylococcus aureus* in 38 French hospitals through a 15-year institutional control program. *Archives of Internal Medicine*, **170**, 552–559.

291 Struelens, M.J. and Monnet, D.L. (2010) Prevention of methicillin-resistant *Staphylococcus aureus* infection: is Europe winning the fight? *Infection Control and Hospital Epidemiology*, **31** (Suppl. 1), S42–S44.

292 Fridkin, S. *et al.* (1996) The role of understaffing in central venous catheter-associated bloodstream infections. *Infection Control and Hospital Epidemiology*, **17**, 150–158.

293 Vicca, A.F. (1999) Nursing staff workload as a determinant of methicillin-resistant *Staphylococcus aureus* spread in an adult intensive therapy unit. *Journal of Hospital Infection*, **43**, 109–113.

294 Robert, J. *et al.* (2000) The influence of the composition of the nursing staff on primary bloodstream infection rates in a surgical intensive care unit. *Infection Control and Hospital Epidemiology*, **21**, 12–17.

295 Eveillard, M. *et al.* (2006) Evaluation of a strategy of screening multiple anatomical sites for methicillin-resistant *Staphylococcus aureus* at admission to a teaching hospital. *Infection Control and Hospital Epidemiology*, **27**, 181–184.

296 Cummings, K.L. *et al.* (2010) Hand hygiene noncompliance and the cost of hospital-acquired methicillin-resistant *Staphylococcus aureus* infection. *Infection Control and Hospital Epidemiology*, **31**, 357–364.

297 Cleanyourhands campaign (2004) *The Economic Case: Implementing Near-patient Alcohol Handrub in your Trust*, National Patient Safety Agency, London.

298 World Health Organization (WHO) (2009) *A Guide to the Implementation of the WHO Multimodal Hand Hygiene Improvement Strategy*, WHO, Geneva, http://www.who.int/gpsc/5may/Guide_to_Implementation.pdf (accessed September 29, 2010).

299 World Health Organization (WHO) (2009) *Tools for Training and Education*, WHO, Geneva, http://www.who.int/gpsc/5may/tools/training_education/en/index.html (accessed September 29, 2010).

300 Picheansathian, W. (2004) A systematic review on the effectiveness of alcohol-based solutions for hand hygiene. *International Journal of Nursing Studies*, **10**, 3–9.

301 Graham, M. *et al.* (2005) Low rates of cutaneous adverse reactions to alcohol-based hand hygiene solution during prolonged use in a large teaching hospital. *Antimicrobial Agents and Chemotherapy*, **49**, 4404–4405.

302 Pittet, D. *et al.* (2007) Double-blind, randomized, crossover trial of 3 hand rub formulations: fast-track evaluation of tolerability and acceptability. *Infection Control and Hospital Epidemiology*, **28**, 1344–1351.

303 Girard, R. *et al.* (2006) Tolerance and acceptability of 14 surgical and hygienic alcohol-based hand rubs. *Journal of Hospital Infection*, **63**, 281–288.

304 Houben, E. *et al.* (2006) Skin condition associated with intensive use of alcoholic gels for hand disinfection: a combination of biophysical and sensorial data. *Contact Dermatitis*, **54**, 261–267.

305 Pedersen, L.K. *et al.* (2005) Less skin irritation from alcohol-based disinfectant than from detergent used for hand disinfection. *British Journal of Dermatology*, **153**, 1142–1146.

306 Kampf, G. *et al.* (2006) Do atopics tolerate alcohol-based hand rubs? A prospective randomized double-blind clinical trial. *Acta Dermato-Venereologica*, **157**, 140–143.

307 Loffler, H. *et al.* (2007) How irritant is alcohol? *British Journal of Dermatology*, **157**, 74–81.

308 Slotosch, C.M. *et al.* (2007) Effects of disinfectants and detergents on skin irritation. *Contact Dermatitis*, **57**, 235–241.

309 Souweine, B. *et al.* (2009) Comparison of acceptability, skin tolerance, and compliance between handwashing and alcohol-based handrub in ICUs: results of a multicentric study. *Intensive Care Medicine*, **35**, 1216–1224.

310 Denton, G.W. (1991) Chlorhexidine, in *Disinfection, Sterilization and Preservation*, 4th edn (ed. S.S. Block), Lea & Febiger, Philadelphia, pp. 274–289.

311 Rosenberg, A. *et al.* (1976) Safety and efficacy of the antiseptic chlorhexidine gluconate. *Surgery, Gynecology and Obstetrics*, **143**, 789–792.

312 Ophaswongse, S. and Maibach, H.I. (1994) Alcohol dermatitis: allergic contact dermatitis and contact urticaria syndrome. A review. *Contact Dermatitis*, **30**, 1–6.

313 De Groot, A.C. (1987) Contact allergy to cosmetics: causative ingredients. *Contact Dermatitis*, **17**, 26–34.

314 Perrenoud, D. *et al.* (1994) Frequency of sensitization to 13 common preservatives in switzerland. Swiss contact dermatitis research group. *Contact Dermatitis*, **30**, 276–279.

315 Kiec-Swierczynska, M. and Krecisz, B. (2000) Occupational skin diseases among the nurses in the region of Lodz. *International Journal of Occupational Medicine and Environmental Health*, **13**, 179–184.

316 Garvey, L.H. *et al.* (2001) Anaphylactic reactions in anaesthetised patients – four cases of chlorhexidine allergy. *Acta Anaesthesiologica Scandinavica*, **45**, 1290–1294.

317 Pham, N.H. *et al.* (2000) Anaphylaxis to chlorhexidine. Case report. Implication of immunoglobulin e antibodies and identification of an allergenic determinant. *Clinical and Experimental Allergy: Journal of the British Society for Allergy and Clinical Immunology*, **30**, 1001–1007.

318 Nishioka, K. *et al.* (2000) The results of ingredient patch testing in contact dermatitis elicited by povidone-iodine preparations. *Contact Dermatitis*, **42**, 90–94.

319 Wong, C.S.M. and Beck, M.H. (2001) Allergic contact dermatitis from triclosan in antibacterial handwashes. *Contact Dermatitis*, **45**, 307–307.

320 Cimiotti, J. *et al.* (2003) Adverse reactions associated with an alcohol-based hand antiseptic among nurses in a neonatal intensive care unit. *American Journal of Infection Control*, **31**, 43–48.

321 Scott, D. *et al.* (1991) An evaluation of the user acceptability of chlorhexidine handwash formulations. *Journal of Hospital Infection*, **18**, 51–55.

322 Turner, P. *et al.* (2004) Dermal absorption of isopropyl alcohol from a commercial hand rub: implications for its use in hand decontamination. *Journal of Hospital Infection*, **56**, 287–290.

323 Girard, R. *et al.* (2001) Better compliance and better tolerance in relation to a well-conducted introduction to rub-in hand disinfection. *Journal of Hospital Infection*, **47**, 131–137.

324 Larson, E.L. *et al.* (2001) Assessment of two hand hygiene regimens for intensive care unit personnel. *Critical Care Medicine*, **29**, 944–951.

325 Boyce, J.M. *et al.* (2000) Skin irritation and dryness associated with two hand-hygiene regimens: soap-and-water hand washing versus hand antisepsis with an alcoholic hand gel. *Infection Control and Hospital Epidemiology*, **21**, 442–448.

326 Winnefeld, M. *et al.* (2000) Skin tolerance and effectiveness of two hand decontamination procedures in everyday hospital use. *British Journal of Dermatology*, **143**, 546–550.

327 Newman, J.L. and Seitz, J.C. (1990) Intermittent use of an antimicrobial hand gel for reducing soap-induced irritation of health care personnel. *American Journal of Infection Control*, **18**, 194–200.

328 Kownatzki, E. (2003) Hand hygiene and skin health. *Journal of Hospital Infection*, **55**, 239–245.

329 Jungbauer, F.H. *et al.* (2004) Skin protection in nursing work: promoting the use of gloves and hand alcohol. *Contact Dermatitis*, **51**, 135–140.

330 Stutz, N. *et al.* (2009) Nurses' perceptions of the benefits and adverse effects of hand disinfection: alcohol-based hand rubs vs. hygienic handwashing: a multi-centre questionnaire study with additional patch testing by the German Contact Dermatitis Research Group. *British Journal of Dermatology*, **160**, 565–572.

331 Steere, A.C. and Mallison, G.F. (1975) Handwashing practices for the prevention of nosocomial infections. *Annals of Internal Medicine*, **83**, 683–690.

332 Dineen, P. and Hildick-Smith, G. (1965) Antiseptic care of the hands, in *Skin Bacteria and their Role in Infection* (eds H.I. Maibach and G. Hildick-Smith), McGraw-Hill, New York, pp. 291–309.

333 Kampf, G. and Löffler, H. (2007) Prevention of irritant contact dermatitis among health care workers by using evidence-based hand hygiene practices: a review. *Industrial Health*, **45**, 645–652.

334 Kampf, G. and Loffler, H. (2003) Dermatological aspects of a successful introduction and continuation of alcohol-based hand rubs for hygienic hand disinfection. *Journal of Hospital Infection*, **55**, 1–7.

335 Boyce, J.M. and Pearson, M.L. (2003) Low frequency of fires from alcohol-based hand rub dispensers in healthcare facilities. *Infection Control and Hospital Epidemiology*, **24**, 618–619.

336 Widmer, A.F. (2000) Replace hand washing with use of a waterless alcohol hand rub? *Clinical Infectious Diseases*, **31**, 136–143.

337 Kramer, A. and Kampf, G. (2007) Hand rub-associated fire incidents during 25 038 hospital-years in Germany. *Infection Control and Hospital Epidemiology*, **28**, 745–746.

338 National Patient Safety Agency (2009) *Organization Patient Safety Reports: Quarterly Data Summaries*, The Stationery Office, London.

339 Roberts, H.S. *et al.* (2005) An unusual complication of hand hygiene. *Anaesthesia*, **60**, 100–101.

340 Fahlen, M. and Duarte, A.G. (2001) Gait disturbance, confusion, and coma in a 93-year-old blind woman. *Chest*, **120**, 295–297.

341 Archer, J.R. *et al.* (2007) Alcohol hand rubs: hygiene and hazard. *British Medical Journal (Clinical Research Ed.)*, **335**, 1154–1155.

342 May, C. (2009) The risks to children of alcohol-based hand gels. *Paediatric Nursing*, **21**, 36–37.

343 Henry-Lagarrigue, M. *et al.* (2010) Severe alcohol hand rub overdose inducing coma, watch after H1N1 pandemic. *Neurocritical Care*, **12**, 400–402.

344 Pendlington, R.U. et al. (2001) Fate of ethanol topically applied to skin. *Food and Chemical Toxicology: an International Journal Published for the British Industrial Biological Research Association*, **39**, 169–174.

345 Miller, M.A. *et al.* (2006) Does the clinical use of ethanol-based hand sanitizer elevate blood alcohol levels? A prospective study. *American Journal of Emergency Medicine*, **24**, 815–817.

346 Brown, T.L. *et al.* (2007) Can alcohol-based hand-rub solutions cause you to lose your driver's license? Comparative cutaneous absorption of various alcohols. *Antimicrobial Agents and Chemotherapy*, **51**, 1107–1108.

347 Kinnula, S. *et al.* (2009) Safety of alcohol hand gel use among children and personnel at a child day care center. *American Journal of Infection Control*, **37**, 318–321.

19.2 Decontamination of the Environment and Medical Equipment in Hospitals

Adam P. Fraise

Microbiology Department, Queen Elizabeth Medical Centre, Pathology – University Hospitals Birmingham NHS Foundation Trust, Birmingham, UK

Introduction

Infection has always been a problem in hospitals and, before the introduction of antiseptic techniques by Lister [1], mortality following surgery was often high. John Bell [2] wrote about the "hospital sore", describing it as an epidemic ulcer occurring in all hospitals, but particularly in the larger ones. He described how difficult it was for young surgeons in the Hotel Dieu in Paris when they saw many of their patients dying of hospital "gangrene". Following Lister's use of antiseptics in surgery (see Chapter 1), a gradual evolution has occurred in aseptic, sterilization and disinfection techniques. Hospitals now have access to sterile service departments for instruments, dressings and many other items, and operating theaters have mechanical ventilation systems providing filtered air. Nevertheless, although mortality has been considerably reduced, morbidity remains and approximately 10% of patients in hospital at any one time have acquired a nosocomial infection [3–6].

The main hospital-acquired infections are of the urinary tract, surgical operation or traumatic wounds and the respiratory tract. Most of the infections are endogenous in origin (acquired from a patient's own bacterial flora) and may be difficult to prevent [7]. The elderly, newborn and the seriously ill are particularly likely to acquire a hospital infection, as are patients with diabetes, leukemia or undergoing radiotherapy or receiving treatment with steroids or immunosuppressive drugs. Infection is also commonly associated with invasive procedures, such as intravenous and urinary tract catheterization and mechanical ventilation of the respiratory tract. Patients are often crowded together in the same environment and some are admitted for the treatment of an existing infection. Hospital staff provide many opportunities for transfer of infection by successive close contact with infected and susceptible patients.

The use of antibiotics has been associated not only with more effective treatment of infection, but also with the emergence of antibiotic-resistant organisms and their transmission. In recent years, methicillin-resistant *Staphylococcus aureus* (MRSA) has spread to hospitals in most countries of the world [8, 9] and at least 17 epidemic strains have been described in England and Wales [10]. These epidemic strains have been difficult to control [11–13]. Furthermore, there have been reports of strains of MRSA demonstrating intermediate [14] and even high-level resistance to vancomycin [15]. Although usually highly resistant to antibiotics, MRSA does not show significantly increased resistance to the disinfectants commonly used in hospitals for environmental and equipment disinfection. Infections caused by coagulase-negative staphylococci have also increased, particularly following intravascular catheterization and implant surgery and in immunocompromised patients. Vancomycin-resistant

Russell, Hugo & Ayliffe's: Principles and Practice of Disinfection, Preservation and Sterilization, Fifth Edition. Edited by Adam P. Fraise, Jean-Yves Maillard, and Syed A. Sattar.

enterococci (VRE) are also causing treatment problems in some hospitals [16]. Although some strains of enterococci show an increased resistance to heat, they remain sensitive to environmental disinfectants at in-use concentrations [17, 18]. Outbreaks of diarrhea in geriatric units caused by *Clostridium difficile* are also being increasingly reported [19–21]. Antibiotic-resistant strains of Gram-negative bacilli, such as *Pseudomonas aeruginosa*, *Klebsiella* and *Enterobacter* spp., *Serratia marcescens* and *Acinetobacter* spp., continue to cause infection problems, particularly in high-risk units, such as intensive care and burns. Although they have been exposed to disinfectants for many years, there is little evidence of increased resistance to disinfectants commonly used in US hospitals [22]. The nature of the hospital population and host susceptibility are more important contributory factors to infection than the inanimate environment, but despite this disinfection still has a role in the prevention of the spread of infection.

Disinfectants tend to be used indiscriminately, and the Public Health Laboratory Service Committee [23] described a wide range of disinfectants in use in hospitals at that time. Although recommendations were made by the committee, the situation had shown little improvement by 1969 [24]. Disinfectants were often used unnecessarily, and not used at all in situations where they could have been of value. Many of the products were unsuitable for hospital use, but were usually acceptable if they possessed a characteristic "disinfectant" or "antiseptic" smell. Dilutions of disinfectants were rarely measured and concentrations were often inadequate and associated with bacterial contamination [25, 26]. Failure to appreciate the effects of concentration and dilution on biocidal activity [27] is common (see Chapter 3). Although disinfectant policies have been introduced in most hospitals, implementation is still often unsatisfactory [28] and inappropriate disinfectants are still used, particularly in countries where infection-control services are not well developed (e.g. [29]). The hospital staff responsible for buying and using disinfectants are often not well trained and have little knowledge of microbiology. They are frequently advised by representatives of disinfectant manufacturers and the advice is usually based on the results of laboratory tests, which do not necessarily mimic hospital conditions [30]. Considerable sums of money are wasted in the unnecessary disinfection of floors and the inanimate environment [31, 32].

The increasing use of complex medical equipment, often heat labile, and the presence of potentially hazardous bloodborne infections, such as hepatitis B virus (HBV), hepatitis C virus (HCV) and human immunodeficiency virus (HIV), have increased the need for effective and well-defined decontamination procedures [33]. Defining adequate procedures is particularly important in the context of the transmissible spongiform encephalopathies (TSEs) as the agents causing these diseases are resistant to most of the commonly used disinfection procedures [34]. Medical equipment and the hospital environment must be rendered safe to use by a decontamination process, which consists of cleaning and disinfection or sterilization [35, 36].

1. *Cleaning* is a process that removes contaminants, including dust, soil, chemical residues, pyrogens, large numbers of microorganisms and the organic matter protecting them. Cleaning is usually a prerequisite to disinfection or sterilization.
2. *Disinfection* is a process that reduces the number of organisms, but not necessarily spores; it does not kill or remove all organisms but reduces their number to a level that is not harmful to health. High-level disinfection includes the killing or removal of *Mycobacterium tuberculosis* and enteroviruses, but not necessarily all mycobacteria, spores or prions.
3. *Sterilization* is a process used to render an object free from all microorganisms, but in practice usually excludes prions.

The decontamination processes vary in their microbiological effect, ranging from cleaning, which is the least effective, to sterilization, which is the most effective. They are not mutually exclusive. Cleaning could remove all organisms. It might be better to redefine these terms on the basis of making an item safe for a specified purpose.

A rational approach to disinfection: a disinfectant policy

Every hospital should have a disinfectant policy. The principles of preparing such a policy were described by Kelsey and Maurer [37] and, more recently, by Ayliffe *et al.* [35], Coates and Hutchinson [38], Fraise [39] and Hoffman *et al.* [36].

Policies essentially consist of: listing the purposes for which disinfectants are used; eliminating their use when sterilization rather than disinfection is the object; deciding where heat can be used and where single-use equipment can be economically used; and selecting a limited number of disinfectants for most of the remaining uses. In order to produce a realistic policy, the reason for disinfection should be considered in detail. Risks of infection from equipment or the environment should be categorized, priorities allocated and resources made available on the basis of this assessment.

Objective

When deciding whether or not disinfection is necessary, it is important to consider the reason for the procedure. The objective is to prevent infection but, in more practical terms, may be defined as the "reduction of microbiological contamination to such a level that an infective dose is unlikely to reach a susceptible site on a patient". However, an infective dose cannot easily be determined, due to the variability in virulence of organisms and resistance of the host. In some instances, one virus-containing particle or a single tubercle bacillus will initiate an infection, but for most organisms a much larger number is necessary in a healthy person [40]. In experiments with *S. aureus* in humans, over 10^6 organisms are required to cause a local infection following intradermal injection, but in the presence of a suture only 10^2 organisms are required [41]. An assessment of the value of disinfection in terms of a reduction in clinical infection would be very useful but is rarely possible. Trials would need to be large and the results could still be inconclusive because of the large number of interrelating factors, although occasional studies have failed to show differences in infection rates between wards using environmental disinfectants and those using detergents only [31]. Nevertheless, a rational decision can be made in most situations. For instance, chemical disinfection of an operating room floor is probably unnecessary, because the bacteria-carrying particles already on the floor are unlikely to reach an open wound in sufficient numbers to cause an infection [42, 43]. Cleaning alone, followed by drying, will considerably reduce the bacterial population.

The standards of hygiene expected by patients and staff must also be considered. Even when these standards are illogical, failure to meet them may erode confidence and could cause unnecessary anxiety.

Categories of risk to patients and treatment of equipment and environment

The objective must be considered carefully in any situation, categories of risk determined [44, 45] and the appropriate treatment applied [46, 47]. Four categories of risk may be considered: high, intermediate, low and minimal [48].

High risk

High-risk items of equipment are those in close contact with a break in the skin or mucous membrane or introduced into a sterile body cavity or into the vascular system. Items in this category should be sterilized by heat, if possible, or, if heat labile, may be treated with ethylene oxide (EO), low-temperature steam and formaldehyde, gas plasma or commercially by irradiation. In some instances, for example a heat-labile cystoscope, high-level disinfection with a chemical agent may be acceptable. The high-risk category includes surgical instruments, implants, surgical dressings, operative endoscopes, urinary and other catheters, parenteral fluids, syringes and needles and other equipment used in surgical operations or aseptic techniques.

Intermediate risk

This category includes items of equipment in close contact with intact mucous membranes or body fluids or contaminated with particularly virulent or highly transmissible organisms. These items will usually require disinfection. They include respiratory and anesthetic equipment, flexible endoscopes (e.g. gastroscopes and colonoscopies), vaginal speculae, tonometers and thermometers.

Low risk

These are items of equipment in contact with intact skin. Cleaning and drying will usually be sufficient, although some items are usually disinfected, such as stethoscopes, dressing-trolley tops, bedding, mattresses and baths.

Minimal risk

This category includes items not in close contact with the patient or his/her immediate surroundings. These items are unlikely either to be contaminated with significant numbers of potential pathogens or to transfer potential pathogens from them to a susceptible site on the patient. Cleaning and drying are usually adequate. Items in this category include floors, walls, ceilings, furniture and sinks. Disinfection may be required for removing contaminated spillage and occasionally for terminal disinfection or surface decontamination during outbreaks caused by organisms that survive well in the inanimate environment, such as MRSA, *C. difficile* or enterococci. Pouring disinfectants into sinks and drains is wasteful and of little value in the prevention of hospital infection [30].

Requirements of chemical disinfectants

All the requirements or desirable properties of disinfectants are not attainable by any single agent and a choice must be made depending on the particular use, for example equipment, environmental surfaces or skin. Requirements are described in more detail in European publications [49–51].

1. The disinfectant should preferably be bactericidal and its spectrum of activity should include all the common non-sporing pathogens, including tubercle bacilli. There is now a greater awareness of the risks of acquiring bloodborne infections, such as HBV, HCV and HIV. Virucidal activity is therefore a requirement for routine disinfection. Narrow-spectrum agents, such as some quaternary ammonium compounds (QACs) or pine fluids, may select *Pseudomonas* spp. or other resistant Gram-negative bacilli, which are potentially hazardous to highly susceptible patients.

2. Disinfectants used on surfaces should be rapid in action, since the microbicidal activity ceases when the surface is dry.

3. The disinfectant should not be readily neutralized by organic matter, soaps, hard water or plastics.

4. Toxic effects should be minimal, and in-use dilutions of disinfectants should, if possible, be relatively non-corrosive. Confused or mentally defective patients may accidentally swallow a disinfectant solution. Many of the environmental disinfectants in routine use are both toxic and corrosive, and care is required in their use and storage. Employers in the UK are now responsible for assessing health risks and measures to protect the health of workers from infection and toxic hazards [52].

5. The disinfectant should not damage surfaces or articles treated. This requirement may vary with the particular situation; for example the criteria for selecting a disinfectant for a toilet are obviously different from those for selecting one for an expensive endoscope.

6. Costs should be acceptable and supplies assured.

Choice of a disinfection method
Heat

Heat is the preferred method of disinfection for all medical equipment (Table 19.2.1). Heat penetrates well, is predictably effective and is readily controlled. Steam at high pressure (e.g. 121°C for

Table 19.2.1 Decontamination of equipment.

Method	Temperature (°C)	Time of exposure (min)	Level of decontamination
Heat			
Autoclave	134	3	Sterilization
	121	15	Sterilization
Low-temperature steam	73	10	Disinfection
Low-temperature steam and formaldehyde	73	180	Sterilization
Boilers	100	5–10	Disinfection
Pasteurizers	70–100	Variable	Disinfection
Washer disinfectors			
Bedpans	80	1	Cleaning and disinfection
Linen	65	10	Cleaning and disinfection
	71	3	Cleaning and disinfection
Medical devices	65–100	Variable	Cleaning and disinfection
Chemical[a]			
Ethylene oxide	55	60–360	Sterilization
Gas plasma	45	50–70[b]	Sterilization
Peracetic acid (0.2–0.35%)	RT	5	Disinfection
Chlorine dioxide (1000–1500 parts/10^6 available ClO_2)	RT	5	Disinfection
2% Glutaraldehyde	RT	10–60	Disinfection
Ortho-phthalaldehyde (0.55%)	RT	5	Disinfection
Superoxidized saline	RT	5	Disinfection
70% alcohol	RT	5–10	Disinfection

RT, room temperature.

[a]Some chemicals will kill bacterial spores and have been termed "sterilants"; however, rinsing is required to remove chemical residues. This introduces a risk of recontamination during the final rinse.

[b]Total cycle times.

15 min, 134°C for 3 min) will sterilize, and, although a sporicidal effect may not necessarily be required, steam is the most reliable method of microbial decontamination. Heat-labile equipment, such as ventilator and anesthetic tubing and used surgical instruments, may be decontaminated in a washer disinfector that reaches an appropriate temperature for disinfection, for example 71°C for 3 min, 80°C for 1 min or 90°C for 1 s [53, 54]. However, it must be borne in mind that the current European Standard (EN15883) uses the Ao concept which allows different time/ temperature combinations to be used with the important parameter being the amount of energy expended. (Using this concept, A is the time equivalent, in seconds at 80°C, needed to achieve a

specific level of disinfection.) The effect of using the Ao concept is that an increase in the contact time at the temperatures noted above may be required. This should be referred to when commissioning new washer disinfectors.

Low-temperature steam (73°C for 10 min) or immersion in water at 70–100°C for 5–10 min is effective in killing vegetative organisms and should inactivate most viruses, including HIV.

Chemical

A clear soluble phenolic and a chlorine-releasing agent (see Chapter 2) should be sufficient for most environmental disinfection. Clear soluble phenolics are comparatively cheap, are not readily neutralized and are active against a wide range or organisms, although not usually against non-enveloped viruses. They are suitable for environmental disinfection, but not for skin or for equipment likely to come into contact with skin or mucous membranes, or in food-preparation or storage areas. Their potential toxicity and the poor effect against some viruses have reduced their use in hospitals in recent years. Furthermore, since the introduction of the Biocides Directive (1998) they have been withdrawn and are no longer available in Europe. They are, however, still used in other countries.

Chlorine-releasing agents are very inexpensive, are active against a wide range of organisms, including viruses and bacterial spores (e.g., *C. difficile*), but are readily neutralized and tend to damage some metals and materials. They are relatively non-toxic when diluted and are useful in food-preparation areas. Powder or tablets containing sodium dichloroisocyanurate (NaDCC) are stable when dry and are useful for environmental decontamination [55, 56]. Chlorine-releasing agents at 1000–10,000 ppm of available Cl are increasingly used for routine disinfection and for removal of spillages, but at these concentrations can cause rapid deterioration of materials. Peroxygen compounds may be useful for the disinfection of some materials, for example carpets, which may be damaged by chlorine-releasing compounds [57], but some are deficient in activity against mycobacteria [58, 59]. Activated alkaline glutaraldehyde 2% is still widely used for decontaminating flexible endoscopes, but it is rapidly becoming obsolete for health and safety reasons (see below). It is relatively noncorrosive and will kill spores with prolonged exposure (3–10 h) [60], but is toxic and irritant. Possible alternatives to glutaraldehyde are *ortho*-phthalaldehyde (OPA), peracetic acid, chlorine dioxide (ClO_2) products and superoxidized water. These agents are rapidly sporicidal, mycobactericidal and virucidal, and some commercial preparations appear to be less irritant to staff than glutaraldehyde [61]. However, some are more corrosive, less stable and more expensive. None is clearly superior to the others and a thorough assessment needs to be performed before an alternative agent is chosen.

Ethyl or isopropyl alcohol 60–70% is a rapid and effective method for disinfecting skin, trolleys and the surfaces of medical equipment. Compounds of low toxicity, such as chlorhexidine or povidone-iodine (both of which were considered in Chapter 2), may be required for disinfecting skin or mucous membranes and occasionally for inanimate items likely to be in contact with skin or mucous membranes.

Implementation of the disinfectant policy

Although most hospitals have a policy, implementation is often inefficient. All hospital staff should be aware of the policy and of problems likely to arise if there are any major departures from that policy. Audits of the policy should be carried out at regular intervals in acute wards and special units. Audit tools, such as those developed by the Infection Prevention Society in the UK, are now available to assist staff in carrying out these audits.

Organization

The infection control committee and team have the responsibility of preparing a safe and effective policy and ensuring that the correct disinfectants and methods of application are used. The infection control committee and team will need to liaise closely with microbiologists, pharmacists, decontamination experts and sterile services managers. A microbiologist and an infection control nurse should be members of the committee. The nursing and domestic staff, who are mainly responsible for the actual practice of disinfection, are also advised through their own organizations, but responsibilities and priorities are often poorly defined. Information is not always passed to those who use the disinfectants [48].

Training

A logical, safe and effective approach to disinfection requires trained staff. They should have some knowledge of microbiology, mechanisms of transfer of infection, health and safety issues and properties of disinfectants. Alternatively, operatives should follow defined schedules and be supervised by trained staff. Decisions are still made too often by staff without adequate training. It is important that external contract cleaners are aware of the policy and are similarly trained to in-house staff. The infection control team should regularly update the policy.

Distribution and dilution of disinfectants

Since inaccurate dilution is one of the main causes of failure of disinfection, this aspect requires careful consideration. It is preferable to deliver disinfectants to departments at the use dilution, but this is not always possible or convenient. If not possible, suitable dispensers are required and the staff must be trained in their use. As pointed out earlier, the effect of dilution on disinfectant activity should always be borne in mind ([27]; see also Chapter 3).

Testing of disinfectants

Official tests have existed in some countries for several years now (e.g. Germany, France, the USA). However, national tests in Europe are gradually being replaced by agreed standard European suspension, surface and practical tests. These tests include virucidal, fungicidal, mycobactericidal and sporicidal activity, as well as tests using a range of bacteria (see Chapters 4 and 6). These tests are termed phase 1 tests (basic bactericidal activity in suspension), phase 2, step 1 tests (suspension tests using a wider range of organisms) and phase 2, step 2 tests (surface tests). It is eventually intended that phase 3 tests, which simulate practical conditions closely, will eventually be developed but, at the time of writing, such tests have not yet been drafted.

Tests of disinfectants should preferably be carried out by a reliable independent organization and results supplied to hospitals by the manufacturers. The manufacturer should also provide evidence of other properties of the disinfectant, such as the range of susceptible organisms, toxicity, stability and corrosiveness. Manufacturers of reusable medical devices in Europe are required to provide details of acceptable reprocessing methods, including decontamination [33].

Costs

Excessive costs may be due to unnecessary use, incorrect concentrations or inappropriate disinfectants being used. The cost of the disinfection procedure as well as that of the agent should be considered.

Problems with certain microorganisms

Bacterial spores

A process that kills spores is usually required for articles in the high-risk category (see above). Liquid preparations, such as glutaraldehyde, peracetic acid, ClO_2 and other chlorine-releasing agents may be used but are generally less reliable than heat: penetration is often poor, thorough rinsing is required before use of the treated item, items cannot be packed, and recontamination with microorganisms can occur during the rinsing process. Activated alkaline glutaraldehyde 2% requires a minimum exposure time of 3 h for an adequate sporicidal action [60] or up to 10 h on the basis of AOAC International's test [43]. However, some spores (e.g. *C. difficile*) appear to be killed by glutaraldehyde in a much shorter time [62, 63]. A number of glutaraldehyde preparations are now available and these show some variation in activity, stability and corrosiveness. Furthermore, glutaraldehyde is not used in many countries (such as the UK) due to its fixative properties and health and safety concerns. Repeated use of a glutaraldehyde solution is common practice, mainly due to its inexpense. The length of time a solution is repeatedly used should depend on the extent of contamination with organic matter or dilution during use and not on stability alone [64]. Peracetic acid (0.2–0.35%) and ClO_2 (1000–10 000 ppm available Cl) are sporicidal in less than 10 min [61]. Superoxidized water is also rapidly sporicidal [65]. Other chlorine-releasing agents are rapidly sporicidal in high concentrations [66] but have the disadvantage of corroding instruments.

Bloodborne viruses, hepatitis A virus and prions

Hepatitis B virus, HCV and other hepatitis non-A, non-B viruses are difficult or impossible to grow *in vitro*, and laboratory tests for inactivation are complex, often relying on animal models or molecular technology [67]. Limited studies in chimpanzees have indicated that HBV is inactivated by a temperature of 98°C for 2 min, but lower temperatures were not investigated. Glutaraldehyde, 70% ethanol, hypochlorite solutions and iodophors also inactivate the virus, for example different authors quote 0.1% glutaraldehyde (24°C) in 5 min, 2% glutaraldehyde in 10 min, 70% isopropanol in 10 min and 80% ethanol in 2 min [68, 69]. A product containing 3.2% glutaraldehyde reduced HBV surface antigen (HBsAg) activity to low levels in 30 s ([70]). Studies with the duck HBV model showed that the virus was inactivated by 2% glutaraldehyde preparations in 5 min [71, 72]. The resistance of HCV to disinfectants is unknown, but it can be predicted from its structure that it is not more resistant than HBV. Hepatitis A virus (HAV) spreads by the fecal–oral route and is one of the most resistant viruses to disinfectants. However, it is rapidly inactivated by 2% glutaraldehyde and high concentrations of chlorine-releasing agents [73].

HIV is an enveloped virus and is readily inactivated by heat and commonly used virucidal disinfectants [74, 75]. It is inactivated by 2% glutaraldehyde in 1 min, but 70% ethanol has shown variable results in surface tests [76, 77]. The inconsistent results were probably due to variability of penetration of dried organic material, and it is likely that 70% ethanol is rapidly effective against HIV on pre-cleaned surfaces.

HBV particles are usually present in larger numbers than HIV in blood, and infection is more readily transmissible, but thorough washing of equipment with a detergent to remove blood and body secretions will minimize the risk of infection from these viruses. However, the use of a chorine-releasing solution or powder should be effective in rapidly decontaminating blood spillage before cleaning, and is recommended particularly if the spillage is from an infected or high-risk patient [38, 48, 56, 78]. The agents causing viral hemorrhagic fevers (e.g. Lassa, Ebola, Marburg) are transmitted in blood or body fluids. They are inactivated by the same disinfectants as the other bloodborne viruses, for example chlorine-releasing agents and 2% glutaraldehyde [79].

The agents causing Creutzfeld–Jakob disease, kuru, scrapie and bovine spongiform encephalopathy (BSE) are termed prions. They have been transmitted via instruments used for neurosurgical procedures, from corneal implants and from pituitary growth hormone. The infectious agents are probably small protein particles (see Chapter 10), which are highly resistant to heat, EO, glutaraldehyde and formaldehyde. High concentrations of sodium hypochlorite (20,000 ppm available Cl) for 60 min are effective but are corrosive to most instruments. Moist heat at 134°C for 18 min is recommended but may not be effective against all strains. Thorough cleaning is of great importance because of the doubts on the effectiveness of decontamination methods and the probable variation in the resistance of different prions to heat and disinfectants ([80]).

Mycobacteria

Mycobacterium tuberculosis continues to be a major problem throughout the world, and resistance to useful systemic chemo-

therapeutic agents is increasing. This and other mycobacteria are often the cause of infections in patients with acquired immune deficiency syndrome (AIDS). Atypical mycobacteria, such as *Mycobacterium chelonae,* have been isolated from the rinsing tank of washer disinfectors and from washings from bronchoscopes. These have been responsible for pseudo-outbreaks and rarely for actual infections of the respiratory tract.

M. tuberculosis and some other mycobacteria are more resistant to chemical disinfectants than other non-sporing organisms. Heat is the preferred method of decontamination, but EO is appropriate for heat-labile items. Glutaraldehyde 2% is a less satisfactory alternative, but is still widely used for heat-labile endoscopes. A high-level disinfection process, for example immersion for at least 20 min, is required for *M. tuberculosis. Mycobacterium avium-intracellulare* is even more resistant to glutaraldehyde and requires immersion for 60–90 min [59, 81–84]. Strains of *M. chelonae* resistant to 2% glutaraldehyde have been isolated from washer disinfectors [85, 86]. Peracetic acid (0.2–0.35%) and chlorine dioxide (1100 ppm available Cl) are effective against most strains of mycobacteria, including *M. avium-intracellulare,* in 5 min. Ethanol 70% and chlorine-releasing compounds in high concentrations (5000–10,000 ppm available Cl) are effective against *M. tuberculosis, M. avium-intracellulare* and *M. chelonae* in less than 5 min [86]. The clear soluble phenolics are active against *M. tuberculosis* and are suitable for disinfection of rooms occupied by patients with open tuberculosis. Quaternary ammonium and peroxygen compounds and chlorhexidine usually show poor activity against tubercle bacilli, although one QAC, Sactimed Sinald, shows useful *in vitro* activity [59]. The resistance of mycobacteria to disinfectants is also considered in Chapter 6.3.

Prions

Prions are the causative agent of TSE. These degenerative diseases include include sporadic Creutzfeld–Jakob disease (sCJD) and variant Creutzfeld–Jakob disease (vCJD) as well as less well-known diseases such as Gerstmann–Sträussler–Scheinker syndrome (GSS), fatal familial insomnia (FFI) and kuru. The infective agents of these diseases are generally thought to be proteinaceous in nature and are resistant to most commonly used decontamination processes including sterilization by heat. Chemical agents that are active against these agents tend to be very aggressive compounds such as 1 M NaOH and chlorine-releasing agents providing 20,000 ppm of available Cl, although several newer technologies have been studied and have the ability to inactivate prions. For a more detailed discussion of prion decontamination see Chapter 10.

Contaminated disinfectant solutions

Solutions contaminated with Gram-negative bacilli are a particular hazard in hospitals, and infections originating from them have been reported [87–89]. Contamination is usually due to inappropriate use of disinfectants [90, 91], weak solutions [26], where there is poor appreciation of the concentration exponent of a particular agent [27] or "topping up" of containers. The last problem can usually be avoided by thorough cleaning and drying of the container before refilling, but an additional microbicide is sometimes necessary [92]. It is also important to prepare solutions as required rather than preparing in bulk and storing them.

Treatment of the environment and equipment

In many instances it is still difficult to decide on the appropriate method of decontamination, even after taking into consideration the nature and risk category of the item concerned. Cleaning alone may be adequate for most routine purposes, but disinfection may be required for the same item during outbreaks of infection. However, it is useful to remember that the risk of transmitting infection on an article that has been thoroughly washed and dried is very small [61, 93, 94]. Thorough cleaning also removes potential bacterial nutrients, as well as bacteria themselves. Methods of decontamination of equipment are summarized in Table 19.2.1. The variable temperatures and exposure times are due to procedural differences and often to practical requirements. Infection risks from equipment have been reviewed by Ayliffe [95].

Some of the problem areas in hospital are described in this section, but for more information see references [30, 45, 48, 96–102].

Walls, ceilings and floors
Walls and ceilings are rarely heavily contaminated, provided the surface remains intact and dry [56, 103]. In our own studies, using contact plates, bacterial counts on walls were in the range of 2–5 per 25 cm^2 and counts of 10 were unusually high (Table 19.2.2). The organisms were mainly Gram-positive, coagulase-negative cocci, with occasional aerobic, spore-bearing organisms and, rarely, S. aureus. The number of bacteria does not appear to increase even if walls are not cleaned, and frequent cleaning has

little influence on bacterial counts. Table 19.2.2 shows bacterial counts from an unwashed operating-theater wall over a 12-week period [42]. No increase in contamination occurred over this period. Additional studies showed no further increase over 6 months. Routine disinfection is therefore unnecessary, but walls should be cleaned when dirty.

Floors are more heavily contaminated than walls and a mean count of 380 organisms/25 cm^2 was obtained from ward floors in a study by the authors. As on the walls and other surfaces, most of the bacteria are from the skin flora of the occupants of the room. A small proportion – usually less than 1% – are potential pathogens, such as S. aureus. The number of bacteria in the room environment tends to be related to the number of people in the ward and their activity [104, 105]. Provided these factors remain relatively unchanged, the bacterial population on a surface will usually reach a plateau in a few hours. At this stage, the rates of deposition and death of organisms remain constant (Figure 19.2.1); cleaning the floor with a detergent reduces the number of organisms by about 80% and the addition of a disinfectant may increase the reduction to over 95%. In a busy hospital ward, recontamination is rapid and bacterial counts may reach the pre-cleaning or pre-disinfection level in 1–2 h [106, 107]. The transient reduction obtained does not appear to justify the routine use of a disinfectant. There is also evidence that skin organisms on the floor are not readily resuspended in the air [42, 43], provided a suitable method of cleaning is used (e.g. a dust-attracting mop, a vacuum cleaner with a filtered exhaust, wet-cleaning techniques).

Disinfection may still be required in areas of high risk or if the number of potential pathogens is thought to be high – for instance, in a room after the discharge of an infected patient – but, even in these circumstances, disinfection of walls and ceilings is rarely necessarily. Carpets are now often found in hospitals and may be exposed to heavy contamination from spillage of food, blood or feces. The carpets must be able to withstand regular cleaning and should have waterproof backing and the fibers

Table 19.2.2 Bacterial contamination of walls in an operating theater (data from [42]).

Time of sampling after washing	Mean counts from 10 contact plates (25 cm^2)	
	Total	*Staphylococcus aureus*
1 day	2.8	0
1 week	5.0	0
3 week	3.4	0.2
5 week	4.6	0.2
12 weeks	1.2	0

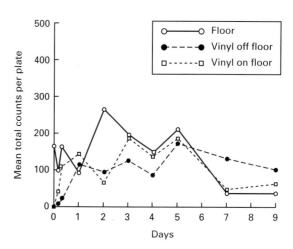

Figure 19.2.1 Mean total counts taken on impression plates at intervals after cleaning the floor in a female surgical ward during the course of 9 days.

should preferably not absorb water [108, 109]. Although there is no good evidence that carpets increase the risk of infection in clinical areas [110], infectious agents have been shown to survive in carpets for prolonged periods [111, 112] . Regular routine maintenance is required and many of the failures in the use of carpets have been due to an unpleasant smell associated with inadequate cleaning. This particularly applies to certain wards, for example the psychogeriatric ward, where spillage is excessive but carpets are preferred for esthetic reasons. Although the risk of infection is small, careful thought should be given before carpets are fitted in clinical areas or where spillage is likely to be considerable [109].

Air

Airborne spread of infection in hospitals is less important than previously thought [113, 114], but more recent evidence has demonstrated that airborne spread plays a major role in prosthetic surgery (e.g. [115]).

Outbreaks of *Aspergillus* infection have been reported in immunosuppressed patients, probably acquired by the airborne route, mainly during building demolition or structural renovation. This risk may be reduced by nursing susceptible patients in rooms supplied with high-efficiency particulate air (HEPA) filtered air [116–118]. Legionnaires' disease is caused by the spread of *Legionella* from cooling towers, showers and water supplies or other aerosol-producing systems [119, 120]. It does not spread from person to person. Prevention is possible by regular maintenance of systems, use of microbicides and improved design to avoid static water [121]. In the event of an outbreak, chlorination or heating of the hot-water supply to an appropriate temperature for preventing the growth of *Legionella* may be introduced. However, chlorination may corrode the water-storage and supply systems, and excessive heating of water may cause scalding, particularly in children and the elderly.

Disinfection of the air has been reviewed elsewhere [122] but is now rarely considered necessary in hospital. Good ventilation with filtered air is considered adequate for operating theaters, isolation rooms and safety cabinets [123]. Thorough cleaning of surfaces and disinfection are thought to be more reliable than "fogging", which is the production of a disinfectant aerosol or vapor, usually formaldehyde [124]. Systems that provide a mist of chemical (e.g. H_2O_2) or ozone are now being introduced. These may have a role in decontaminating the environment [125, 126] Methods of air disinfection and air sterilization are considered in Chapters 2 and 11.

Baths, washbowls and toilets

Bathwater contains large numbers of bacteria, including potential pathogens [127]. Many bacteria remain on the surface of the bath after emptying and may be transferred to the next patient. Thorough cleaning with a detergent after each use is usually sufficient, but disinfection is necessary in maternity or surgical units when bathing carriers of communicable multiresistant bacteria, such as MRSA, or where patients with open wounds use the same bath.

Chlorine-releasing solutions or powders are commonly recommended for disinfection [48, 128, 129]. Abrasive powders may damage certain bath surfaces and non-abrasive chlorine-releasing powders should be used. Washbowls are often stacked so that a small amount of residual water remains in each after emptying, and Gram-negative bacilli may grow to large numbers overnight [130]. Routine disinfection is usually unnecessary, but thorough cleaning and drying is always required. Toilets are an obvious infection risk during outbreaks of gastrointestinal infection. Disinfection of the seat of the toilet is probably of some value in these circumstances, but, for routine purposes, cleaning is usually sufficient. Risks of infection from aerosols after flushing are usually small [131].

Bedpans and urinals

These are required for patients confined to bed, but are used less often than formerly because of early mobilization of patients after surgical operations. After use, the contents require disposal and the container must be decontaminated, particularly if the patient is suffering from a gastrointestinal or urinary tract infection. Although bedpan washers without a disinfecting heat cycle are still used without evidence of cross-infection, a thermal disinfection cycle stage is now recommended on all machines [53, 54, 132]. This is the preferred method of decontamination, although the machines must be well maintained and comply with relevant standards (e.g. EN15883 parts 1 and 3). One report suggested that leaking bedpan washers were implicated in the transmission of vancomycin-resistant enterococci in a hematology unit [133]. Chemical methods should be avoided if possible as immersion of bedpans or urinals in tanks of disinfectant has been associated with the selection and growth of Gram-negative bacilli in the solution [134]. Macerators are a popular alternative to heat disinfection of metal or polypropylene pans and are satisfactory, if well maintained, but possible disadvantages, particularly drainage requirements, should be considered before installation [135, 136]. They have the advantage of saving nursing time by disposing of several pans in one cycle and avoiding the necessity of handling pans after disinfection. Bedpan supports are, however, reusable and require separate processing.

Crockery and cutlery

Handwashed crockery and cutlery are frequently heavily contaminated after processing, but bacterial counts decrease considerably on drying. The addition of a disinfectant to the wash water is unreliable as a disinfection process [137]. Washing in a machine at a minimum temperature of 50–60°C, with a final rinse at 80°C for 1 min or more, followed by a drying cycle, is a satisfactory disinfection process [30]. Table 19.2.3 shows the difference in contamination of plates after hand and machine washing. If a suitable dishwasher is not available, disposable crockery and cutlery may be used for patients with open tuberculosis enteric infections and some other communicable infections, although the risks from washed and dried crockery and cutlery are minimal.

Table 19.2.3 Bacterial contamination of crockery (plates) after washing.

Method of washing	No. of plates	No. of plates in contamination range		
		0–10 bacteria/ 25 cm²	11–1000 bacteria/ 25 cm²	>1000 bacteria/ 25 cm²
Machine	72	67 (93%)	2	3
Hand	108	40 (37%)	46	22

Cleaning equipment

Floor mops are often heavily contaminated with Gram-negative bacilli. Although the opportunities for these organisms to reach a susceptible site on a patient are small, the presence of a large reservoir of potentially pathogenic Gram-negative bacilli is undesirable. Mops should be periodically disinfected, preferably by heat. Mopheads washed by a machine will usually be adequately disinfected, but soaking overnight in disinfectant is not recommended. Some phenolics may be partially inactivated by plastic floor mops [30, 138]. Moisture retained in mop buckets, trapped in the tanks of scrubbing machines or retained in the reservoir of spray cleaners can also encourage the growth of Gram-negative bacilli [139]. If the fluid used is capable of supporting bacterial growth, the equipment should be dried, cleaned and stored dry. Poorly maintained or badly designed scrubbing machines, carpet cleaners or spray-cleaning equipment can produce contaminated aerosols. Staff should understand the need to decontaminate equipment for use in a certain area, but especially where there is a specific risk of infection.

Babies' incubators

Surfaces of incubators are rarely heavily contaminated, but there is always a risk of transfer of infection from one baby to the next. Thorough cleaning and drying of surfaces, seals and humidifier are important and are usually sufficient for routine treatment. If disinfection is considered necessary in an addition to cleaning, wiping over with 70% alcohol or a chlorine-releasing solution (125 ppm available Cl) is adequate [140].

Respiratory ventilators and associated equipment

The accumulation of moisture and the warm conditions in ventilators and associated equipment are often associated with the growth of Gram-negative bacilli, particularly *P. aeruginosa* and *Klebsiella* spp. There is some experimental evidence that organisms are able to reach the patient from contaminated ventilator tubing [141] and that infection can subsequently occur [142]. Nebulization of contaminated droplets has caused lung infections [143]. Apart from a contaminated nebulizer, the greatest infection risk is from the part of the circuit nearest to the patient. Changing the reservoir bag, tubing and connectors every 48 h is an important measure in the prevention of infection [144]. Respiratory circuits are preferably decontaminated by heat (see below).

Disposable circuits are expensive. Ventilators are difficult to clean and disinfect, and most available methods are not entirely satisfactory [48, 145].

The use of filters or heat–moisture exchangers (HMEs) for microbiologically isolating the machine from the patient is a better method of preventing contamination of the machine and subsequent cross-infection. It is important to recognize that HMEs are primarily designed to retain humidity in the circuit and are not as effective at preventing the passage of bacteria as purpose-designed bacterial filters. Similarly bacterial filters are less effective at maintaining humidity. The importance of protecting a circuit with filters is most crucial when the tubing is used on more than one patient, and there is some debate about whether filters are necessary to protect circuits used on one patient only (e.g. in the intensive care unit) [146]. The amount of condensate associated with water humidification is minimal if a HME is used, and the circuitry can be changed less frequently, for example between patients or weekly. Less condensate is also produced with most neonatal ventilating systems, and a change of circuitry every 7 days would often appear to be adequate [147]. Nevertheless, careful surveillance and monitoring of infection rates are necessary if a reversion to less frequent changing of circuits is introduced. Many ventilators now have reusable circuits, which may be cleaned and disinfected thermally in a dedicated washer disinfector. Nebulizers should preferably be capable of withstanding disinfection by heat, but, if not, should be chemically disinfected or cleaned and dried every day [148].

Anesthetic equipment

Patients are usually connected to anesthetic machines for a shorter period of time than to respiratory ventilators in intensive care units, and machines are rarely heavily contaminated, providing that the associated tubing is regularly changed [149]. It is obviously preferable to provide each patient with a decontaminated circuit, but this could be expensive. Since contamination is usually not great, sessional replacement may be an acceptable compromise, provided decontaminated facemasks, endotracheal tubes and airways are available for each patient during a session of about 9–10 operations [150]. The corrugated tubing should be disinfected with low-temperature steam or in a washing machine that reaches temperatures of 70–80°C [53, 54]. Chemical disinfection is less reliable and should be avoided if possible [151]. A single-use circuit may be preferred if a patient with known tuberculosis is anaesthetized. The possible transmission of HCV by anesthetic equipment has been reported [152], but this is an unlikely route of spread for a bloodborne virus. Based on this uncertain evidence, it has been suggested that filters should be used and replaced after each patient. Filters can prevent the transfer of bacteria and viruses [153], but there is little evidence from earlier studies that they reduce clinical infection [154, 155]. The cost-effectiveness of using a new filter for each patient requires careful consideration [156, 157].

Endoscopes

Endoscopes are extremely complex medical devices which are now used for a wide range of diagnostic and therapeutic procedures. Those used for minimal-access surgery (e.g. laparoscopes and arthroscopes) are usually rigid and can be steam sterilized, whereas the flexible instruments for gastrointestinal endoscopy and bronchoscopy are not. These are often grossly contaminated and difficult to clean and they require chemical sterilization or disinfection processes, which have several disadvantages. For a full discussion on the various aspects of decontamination of endoscopes see Chapter 19.3.

Miscellaneous items of medical equipment
Vaginal specula and other vaginal devices

There is little reported evidence of spread of infection from these devices, but there is a potential risk of acquiring HIV, hepatitis viruses, herpesvirus, papillomavirus or other organisms causing sexually transmitted infections. Single-use items are preferred whenever possible, but, if not available or if too expensive, decontamination by thorough cleaning and heat (autoclaving, immersion in boiling water for 5–10 min or processing in a washer disinfector at 70–100°C) should be effective [48, 158]. There are no data on the susceptibility of human papillomavirus to disinfectants, but there is no evidence that it is particularly resistant to the usual decontamination processes. If the item is heat labile, chemical methods after thorough cleaning should be effective, such as immersion in 70% alcohol or a chlorine-releasing agent (1000 parts/10^6 available Cl for 5–10 min), but these have the disadvantages already described.

Tonometers

Viruses, such as adenovirus 8, herpesvirus and HIV, may be transferred from eye to eye by these items if not properly decontaminated after each use. There is also a theoretical risk that prion diseases such CJD can be transmitted via these items although the risk is thought to be low. Tonometer heads are usually heat labile and chemical disinfection is required ([159]). Thorough rinsing and immersion in a chlorine-releasing agent (500 parts/10^6 available Cl), 3–6% stabilized hydrogen peroxide or 70% alcohol for 5–10 min is commonly recommended although this would not be effective against prions. If transmissible spongiform encephalopathy is a possibility, disposable tonometer heads are available. The manufacturer should state whether these processes would damage the tonometer. Thorough rinsing after disinfection (or allowing alcohol to evaporate) is important to prevent damage to the conjunctiva.

Stethoscopes and sphygmomanometer cuffs

Although these are only in contact with intact skin, transfer of staphylococci can occur [160, 161]. Thorough cleaning of the stethoscope head with 70% alcohol at regular intervals and after use on patients colonized or infected with MRSA or other organisms transferred by this route should reduce the risks of spread.

Alternatively, a dedicated stethoscope could be made available for each patient but the stethoscope must be decontaminated between patients. A sphygmomanometer cuff should be kept for each infected or colonized patient and terminally decontaminated by thorough washing and drying.

Other items

Dressing trolleys, mattress covers, supports, hoists, etc. may require decontamination and similar principles apply. Thorough cleaning is always necessary. Decontamination by heat is preferable to chemical disinfection. Immersion in a chlorine-releasing agent may be used if appropriate for the instrument. Wiping with 70% alcohol is less effective than immersion (e.g. for 5–10 min) but may be necessary for large items. Glutaraldehyde 2% should be avoided but, if used, appropriate environmental precautions should be taken to contain or extract the irritant vapor.

Conclusions

The increased use of invasive techniques in a hospital population consisting of both infected and highly susceptible patients has increased the risk of spread of infection. Disinfection has a role in reducing these risks, but, in the past, too great a reliance has been placed on chemical methods, which are often used in an indiscriminate, illogical and inefficient manner. Heat is the preferred method of microbial decontamination, but the continued use of complex, heat-sensitive equipment means that less satisfactory alternatives are still required. In recent years, there has also been an increase in the use of medical devices labeled "single use" (see Chapter 24 for a critical and comprehensive account of the reuse of disposable items). These may be expensive although it is important to include the cost of reprocessing when comparing the cost of reusable versus single-use equipment. Often the extra cost of a single-use item is minimal although their use should be discouraged if clearly not cost-effective. Manufacturers should be encouraged to produce equipment that can be readily cleaned and will withstand heat at least to 70–80°C or, preferably, autoclaving at high temperature. A limited range of chemical disinfectants should be available and techniques of application should be standardized according to a well-defined policy. Allocation of resources for disinfection should be related to risks of infection and priorities decided according to the principles already described. Some of the chemical disinfectants, such as glutaraldehyde, are potentially toxic, irritant and allergenic to staff and require special handling and controlled environmental conditions. Alternative agents are needed, but prolonged testing under in-use conditions should be undertaken before they are accepted for routine use. All grades of staff should be trained in methods of disinfection and other control of infection techniques to an agreed level, depending on their role in the hospital. Decontamination methods should be routinely audited.

Acknowledgment

We thank the Editor of the *Journal of Hygiene* for permission to publish Figure 19.2.1.

References

1 Lister, J. (1868) An address on the antiseptic system of treatment in surgery. *British Medical Journal*, **ii**, 53–56, 101–102.

2 Bell, J. (1801) *The Principles of Surgery*, Edinburgh. Printed for T. Cadell, Jun. & W. Davies (Strand); T.N. Longman & O. Rees (Paternoster Row); W Creech, P. Hill and Manners & Miller.

3 Meers, P.D. *et al.* (1981) Report on the national survey of infection in hospitals, 1980. *Journal of Hospital Infection*, **2** (Suppl.), 1–53.

4 Mayon-White, R.T. *et al.* (1988) An international survey of the prevalence of hospital-acquired infection. *Journal of Hospital Infection*, **11** (Suppl. A), 43–48.

5 Emmerson, A.M. *et al.* (1996) The Second National Prevalence Survey of Infection in Hospitals – overview of the results. *Journal of Hospital Infection*, **32**, 175–190.

6 Smyth, E.T.M. *et al.* (2008) Four Country Healthcare Associated Infection Prevalence Survey 2006: overview of the results. *Journal of Hospital Infection*, **69**, 230–248.

7 Ayliffe, G.A.J. (1986) Nosocomial infection and the irreducible minimum. *Infection Control*, **7**, 92–95.

8 Wenzel, R.P. *et al.* (1991) Methicillin-resistant *Staphylococcus aureus*: implications for the 1990s and control measures. *American Journal of Medicine*, **91** (Suppl. 3B), 221S–227S.

9 Ayliffe, G.A.J. (1997) The progressive intercontinental spread of methicillin-resistant *Staphylococcus aureus*. *Clinical Infectious Diseases*, **24** (Suppl. 1), S74–S79.

10 Report of a Combined Working Party of the British Society of Antimicrobial Chemotherapy and the Hospital Infection Society, prepared by G. Duckworth and R. Heathcock (1995) Guidelines on the control of methicillin-resistant *Staphylococcus aureus* in the community. *Journal of Hospital Infection*, **35**, 1–12.

11 Report of a Combined Working Party of the Hospital Infection Society and the British Society for Antimicrobial Chemotherapy (1990) Revised guidelines for the control of epidemic methicillin-resistant *Staphylococcus aureus*. *Journal of Hospital Infection*, **16**, 351–377.

12 Duckworth, G.J. (1993) Diagnosis and management of methicillin-resistant *Staphylococcus aureus* infection. *British Medical Journal*, **307**, 1049–1052.

13 Cox, R.A. *et al.* (1995) A major outbreak of methicillin-resistant *Staphylococcus aureus* caused by a new phage type (EMRSA 16). *Journal of Hospital Infection*, **29**, 87–106.

14 Hiramatsu, K. *et al.* (1997) Methicillin-resistant *Staphylococcus aureus* clinical strain with reduced vancomycin susceptibility. *Journal of Antimicrobial Chemotherapy*, **40**, 135–136.

15 Centers for Disease Control and Prevention (2002) *Staphylococcus aureus* reistant to vancomycin – United States, 2002. *MMWR. Morbidity and Mortality Weekly Report*, **51**, 565–567.

16 Wade, J.J. (1995) Emergence of *Enterococcus faecium* resistant to glycopeptides and other standard agents – a preliminary report. *Journal of Hospital Infection*, **30** (Suppl.), 483–493.

17 Kearns, A.M. *et al.* (1995) Nosocomial enterococci: resistance to heat and sodium hypochlorite. *Journal of Hospital Infection*, **30**, 193–199.

18 Bradley, C.R. and Fraise, A.P. (1996) Heat and chemical resistance of enterococci. *Journal of Hospital Infection*, **34**, 191–196.

19 Cartmill, T.D. *et al.* (1994) Management and control of a large outbreak of diarrhoea due to *Clostridium difficile*. *Journal of Hospital Infection*, **27**, 1–15.

20 Bartlett, J.G. (2006) Narrative review: the new epidemic of *clostridium difficile*–associated enteric disease. *Annals of Internal Medicine*, **145**, 758–764.

21 Kelly, C.P. and LaMont, J.T. (2008) *Clostridium difficile* – more difficult than ever. *New England Journal of Medicine*, **359**, 1932–1940.

22 Rutala, W.A. *et al.* (1997) Susceptibility of antibiotic-susceptible and antibiotic-resistant hospital bacteria to disinfectants. *Infection Control and Hospital Epidemiology*, **18**, 417–421.

23 Public Health Laboratory Service (1965) Committee on the testing and evaluation of disinfectants. *British Medical Journal*, **i**, 408–413.

24 Ayliffe, G.A.J. *et al.* (1969) Varieties of aseptic practice in hospital wards. *Lancet*, **ii**, 1117–1120.

25 Kelsey, J.C. and Maurer, I.M. (1966) An in-use test for hospital disinfectants. *Monthly Bulletin of the Ministry of Health and the Public Health Laboratory Service*, **25**, 180–184.

26 Prince, J. and Ayliffe, G.A.J. (1972) In-use testing of disinfectants in hospitals. *Journal of Clinical Pathology*, **25**, 586–589.

27 Hugo, W.B. and Denyer, S.P. (1987) The concentration exponent of disinfectants and preservatives (biocides), in *Preservatives in the Food, Pharmaceutical and Environmental Industries*, Society for Applied Bacteriology Technical Series No. 22 (eds R.G. Board *et al.*), Blackwell Scientific Publications, Oxford, pp. 281–291.

28 Cadwallader, H. (1989) Setting the seal on standards. *Nursing Times*, **85**, 71–72.

29 Zaidi, M. *et al.* (1995) Disinfection and sterilization practices in Mexico. *Journal of Hospital Infection*, **31**, 25–32.

30 Maurer, I. (1985) *Hospital Hygiene*, 3rd edn, Edward Arnold, London.

31 Danforth, D. *et al.* (1987) Nosocomial infections on nursing units with floors cleaned with a disinfectant compared with detergent. *Journal of Hospital Infection*, **10**, 229–235.

32 Daschner, E. (1991) Unnecessary and ecological cost of hospital infection. *Journal of Hospital Infection*, **18** (Suppl. A), 73–78.

33 Department of Health Medical Devices Directorate (1993, 1996) *Sterilization, Disinfection and Cleaning of Medical Devices and Equipment: Guidance on Decontamination from the Microbiological Advisory Committee to Department of Health*, Parts 1 and 2, HMSO, London.

34 Taylor, D.M. (2000) Inactivation of transmissible degenerative encephalopathy agents: a review. *Veterinary Journal (London, England: 1997)*, **159**, 10–17.

35 Ayliffe, G.A.J. *et al.* (1993) *Chemical Disinfection in Hospitals*, Public Health Laboratory Service, London.

36 Hoffman, P. *et al.* (2008) *Disinfection in Healthcare*, 3rd edn, John Wiley & Sons, Hoboken, NJ.

37 Kelsey, J.C. and Maurer, I.M. (1972) *The Use of Chemical Disinfectants in Hospitals*, Public Health Laboratory Service Monograph No. 2, HMSO, London.

38 Coates, D. and Hutchinson, D.N. (1994) How to produce a hospital disinfection policy. *Journal of Hospital Infection*, **26**, 57–68.

39 Fraise, A.P. (1999) Choosing disinfectants. *Journal of Hospital Infection*, **43**, 255–264.

40 McKinney, R.W. *et al.* (2001) The hazard of infectious agents in microbiological laboratories, in *Disinfection, Sterilization and Preservation*, 5th edn (ed. S. Block), Lea & Febiger, Philadelphia, pp. 1115–1122.

41 Elek, S.D. and Conen, P.E. (1957) The virulence of *Staphylococcus pyogenes* for man. *British Journal of Experimental Pathology*, **38**, 573–586.

42 Ayliffe, G.A.J. *et al.* (1967) Ward floors and other surfaces as reservoirs of hospital infection. *Journal of Hygiene*, **65**, 515–536.

43 Hambraeus, A. *et al.* (1978) Bacterial contamination in a modern operating suite 3. Importance of floor contamination as a source of airborne contamination. *Journal of Hygiene*, **80**, 169–174.

44 Favero, M.S. and Bond, W.W. (2001) Chemical disinfection of medical and surgical materials, in *Disinfection, Sterilization and Preservation*, 5th edn (ed. S. Block), Lea & Febiger, Philadelphia, pp. 881–917.

45 Rutala, W.A. (1996) APIC guidelines for selection and use of disinfectant. *American Journal of Infection Control*, **24**, 313–342.

46 Ayliffe, G.A.J. and Gibson, G.L. (1975) Antimicrobial treatment of equipment in the hospital. *Health and Social Services Journal*, **85**, 598–599.

47 Ayliffe, G.A.J. *et al.* (1976) Environment hazards – real and imaginary. *Health and Social Services Journal*, **86** (Suppl. 3), 3–4.

48 Ayliffe, G.A.J. *et al.* (1992) *The Control of Hospital Infection: a Practical Handbook*, 3rd edn, Chapman & Hall, London.

49 Reber, H. *et al.* (1972) *Bewertung Und Prüfung Von Disinfektionsmitteln Und Verfahren*, Auftrag der schweizerischen Mikrobiologischen Gesellschaft, Basel.

50 Schmidt, B. (1973) Das 2. Internationale Colloquium uber die Wertbestimmung von Disinfektionsmitteln in Europa. *Zentralblatt für Bakteriologie, Parasitenkunde, Infections-krankheiten und Hygiene 1. Abteilung Originale Reihe B*, **157**, 411–420.

51 Babb, J.R. (1996) Application of disinfectants in hospitals and other health-care establishments. *Infection Control Journal of Southern Africa*, **1**, 4–12.

52 Department of Health (1988) *Control of Substances Hazardous to Health Regulations*, HMSO, London.

53 Collins, B.J. and Phelps, M. (1985) Heat disinfection and disinfector machines. *Journal of Sterile Services Management*, **3**, 7–8.

54 British Standard Institution (1993) *BS 2745. Washer Disinfectors for Medical Purposes*, Parts 1–3, British Standards Institution, London.

55 Bloomfield, S.F. and Uso, E.E. (1985) The antibacterial properties of sodium hypochlorite and sodium dichloroisocyanurate as hospital disinfectants. *Journal of Hospital Infection*, **6**, 20–30.

56 Coates, D. (1988) Comparison of sodium hypochlorite and sodium dichloroisocyanurate disinfectants: neutralization by serum. *Journal of Hospital Infection*, **11**, 60. 67.

57 Coates, D. and Wilson, M. (1992) Powders, composed of chlorine-releasing agent acrylic resin mixtures or based on peroxygen compounds, for spills of body fluids. *Journal of Hospital Infection*, **21**, 241–252.

58 Broadley, S.J. *et al.* (1993) Antimicrobial activity of "Virkon". *Journal of Hospital Infection*, **23**, 189–197.

59 Holton, J. *et al.* (1994) Efficacy of selected disinfectants against mycobacteria and cryptosporidia. *Journal of Hospital Infection*, **27**, 105–115.

60 Babb, J.R. *et al.* (1980) Sporicidal activity of glutaraldehydes and hypochlorites and other factors influencing their selection for the treatment of medical equipment. *Journal of Hospital Infection*, **1**, 63–75.

61 Babb, J.R. and Bradley, C.R. (1995) Endoscope decontamination, where do we go from here. *Journal of Hospital Infection*, **30** (Suppl.), 543–551.

62 Dyas, A. and Das, B.C. (1985) The activity of glutaraldehyde against *Clostridium difficile*. *Journal of Hospital Infection*, **6**, 41–45.

63 Rutala, W.A. *et al.* (1993) Inactivation of *Clostridium difficile* spores by disinfectants. *Infection Control and Hospital Epidemiology*, **14**, 36–39.

64 Babb, J.R., Bradley, C.R. and Barnes, A.R. (1992) Question and Answer. *Journal of Hospital Infection*, **20**, 51–54.

65 Selkon, J.B. *et al.* (1999) Evaluation of the antimicrobial activity of a new super-oxidized water, Sterilox, for the disinfection of endoscopes. *Journal of Hospital Infection*, **41**, 59–70.

66 Coates, D. (1996) Sporicidal activity of sodium dichloroisocyanurate, peroxygen and glutaraldehyde disinfectants against *Bacillus subtilis*. *Journal of Hospital Infection*, **32**, 283–294.

67 Wang, C. *et al.* (2002) Development of viral disinfectant assays for duck hepatitis B virus using cell culture/PCR. *Journal of Virological Methods*, **106**, 39.

68 Bond, W.W. *et al.* (1983) Inactivation of hepatitis B virus by intermediate to high level disinfectant chemicals. *Journal of Clinical Microbiology*, **18**, 535–538.

69 Kobayashi, H. *et al.* (1984) Susceptibility of hepatitis B virus to disinfectants or heat. *Journal of Clinical Microbiology*, **20**, 214–216.

70 Akamatsu, T. *et al.* (1997) Evaluation of the efficacy of a 3.2% glutaraldehyde product for disinfection of fibreoptic endoscopes with an automatic machine. *Journal of Hospital Infection*, **35**, 47–57.

71 Murray, S.M. *et al.* (1991) Duck hepatitis B virus: a model to assess efficacy of disinfectants against hepadnavirus activity. *Epidemiology and Infection*, **106**, 435–443.

72 Deva, A.K. *et al.* (1996) Establishment of an in-use method for evaluating disinfection of surgical instruments using the duck hepatitis B model. *Journal of Hospital Infection*, **33**, 119–130.

73 Mbithi, J.N. *et al.* (1990) Chemical disinfection of hepatitis A virus on environmental surfaces. *Applied and Environmental Microbiology*, **56**, 3601–3604.

74 Kurth, R. *et al.* (1986) Stability and inactivation of the human immunodeficiency virus. *Aids-Forschung*, **ii**, 601–607.

75 Resnick, L. *et al.* (1986) Stability and inactivation of HTLV/LAV under clinical and laboratory environments. *Journal of the American Medical Association*, **255**, 1887–1891.

76 Hanson, P.J.V. *et al.* (1989) Chemical inactivation of HIV on surfaces. *British Medical Journal*, **298**, 862–864.

77 Van Bueren, J. *et al.* (1989) Inactivation of HIV on surfaces by alcohol. *British Medical Journal*, **299**, 459.

78 Bloomfield, S.F. *et al.* (1990) Evaluation of hypochlorite-releasing disinfectants against the human immunodeficiency virus. *Journal of Hospital Infection*, **15**, 273–278.

79 Advisory Committee on Dangerous Pathogens, Department of Health (1996) *Management and Control of Viral Haemorrhagic Fevers*, HMSO, London.

80 Advisory Committee on Dangerous Pathogens/Spongiform Enchepholopathy Advisory Committee (1998) Guidance – *Transmissible Spongiform Encephalopathy Agents: Safe Working and the Prevention of Infection*, HMSO, London.

81 Collins, F.M. (1986) Bactericidal activity of alkaline glutaraldehyde solution against a number of atypical mycobacterial species. *Journal of Applied Bacteriology*, **61**, 247–251.

82 Best, M. *et al.* (1990) Efficacies of selected disinfectants against *Mycobacterium tuberculosis*. *Journal of Clinical Microbiology*, **28**, 2234–2239.

83 Lynam, P.A. *et al.* (1995) Comparison of the mycobactericidal activity of 2% alkaline glutaraldehyde and NuCidex (0.35% peracetic acid). *Journal of Hospital Infection*, **30**, 237–239.

84 Russell, A.D. (1996) Activity of biocides against mycobacteria. *Journal of Applied Bacteriology*, **81** (Symposium Suppl.), 67S–101S.

85 Van Klingeren, B. and Pullen, W. (1993) Glutaraldehyde resistant mycobacteria from endoscope washers. *Journal of Hospital Infection*, **25**, 147–149.

86 Griffiths, P.A. *et al.* (1998) *Mycobacterium terrae*: a potential surrogate for *Mycobacterium tuberculosis* in a standard disinfectant test. *Journal of Hospital Infection*, **38**, 183–192.

87 Lee, J.C. and Fialkow, P.J. (1961) Benzalkonium chloridesource of hospital infection with Gram-negative bacteria. *Journal of the American Medical Association*, **177**, 708–710.

88 Bassett, D.C.J. *et al.* (1970) Wound infection with *Pseudomonas multivorans*. *Lancet*, **i**, 1188–1191.

89 Speller, D.C.E. *et al.* (1971) Hospital infection by *Pseudomonas capacia*. *Lancet*, **i**, 798–799.

90 Sanford, J.P. (1970) Disinfectants that don't. *Annals of Internal Medicine*, **72**, 282–283.

91 Centers for Disease Control (CDC) (1974) Disinfectant or infectant: the label doesn't always say, *National Nosocomial Infections Study, Fourth Quarter 1973*, CDC, Altanta, GA, pp. 18–23.

92 Burdon, D.W. and Whitby, J.L. (1967) Contamination of hospital disinfectants with *Pseudomonas* species. *British Medical Journal*, **ii**, 153–155.

93 Nÿstrom, B. (1981) Disinfection of surgical instruments. *Journal of Hospital Infection*, **2**, 363–368.

94 Hanson, P.J. *et al.* (1990) Elimination of high titre HIV from fibreoptic endoscopes. *Gut*, **31**, 657–659.

95 Ayliffe, G.A.J. (1988) Equipment-related infection risks. *Journal of Hospital Infection*, **11** (Suppl. A), 279–284.

96 Block, S. (ed.) (1991) *Disinfection, Sterilization and Preservation*, 4th edn, Lea & Febiger, Philadelphia.

97 Gardner, J.F. and Peel, M.M. (1998) *Introduction to Sterilization, Disinfection and Infection Control*, 3rd edn, Harcourt Brace, London.

98 Bennett, J.V. and Brachman, P.S. (eds) (1992) *Hospital Infections*, 3rd edn, Little Brown, Boston.

99 Taylor, E.W. (ed.) (1992) *Infection and Surgical Practice*, Oxford Medical Publications, Oxford.

100 Rutala, W.A. (1997) Disinfection sterilization and waste disposal, in *Prevention and Control of Nosocomial Infections*, 3rd edn (ed. R.P. Wenzel), Williams & Wilkins, Baltimore.

101 Philpott-Howard, J. and Casewell, M. (1994) *Hospital Infection Control: Policies and Practical Procedures*, Saunders, London.

102 Mayhall, C.G. (ed.) (1996) *Hospital Epidemiology and Infection Control*, Williams & Wilkins, Baltimore.

103 Wypkema, W. and Alder, V.G. (1962) Hospital cross-infection and dirty walls. *Lancet*, **ii**, 1066–1068.

104 Williams, R.E.O. *et al.* (1966) *Hospital Infection – Causes and Prevention*, Lloyd-Luke, London.

105 Noble, W.C. and Somerville, D.A. (1974) *Microbiology of Human Skin*, Saunders, London.

106 Vesley, D. and Michaelsen, G.S. (1964) Application of a surface sampling method technique to the evaluation of the bacteriological effectiveness of certain hospital house-keeping procedures. *Health Laboratory Science*, **1**, 107.

107 Ayliffe, G.A.J. *et al.* (1966) Cleaning and disinfection of hospital floors. *British Medical Journal*, **ii**, 442–445.

108 Ayliffe, G.A.J. *et al.* (1974) Carpets in hospital wards. *Health and Social Services Journal*, **84** (Suppl.), 12–13.

109 Collins, B.J. (1979) How to have carpeted luxury. *Health and Social Services Journal*, **September** (Suppl.).

110 Anderson, R.L. *et al.* (1982) Carpeting in hospital: an epidemiologic evaluation. *Journal of Clinical Microbiology*, **15**, 408–415.

111 Skoutelis, A.T. *et al.* (1994) Hospital carpeting and epidemiology of *Clostridium difficile*. *American Journal of Infection Control*, **22**, 212–217.

112 Cheesbrough, J.S. *et al.* (2000) Widespread environmental contamination with Norwalk-like viruses (NLV) detected in a prolonged hotel outbreak of gastroenteritis. *Epidemiology and Infection*, **125**, 93–98.

113 Brachman, P.S. (1971) *Proceedings of the International Conference on Nosocomial Infections 1970*, American Hospital Association, Chicago, pp. 189–192.

114 Ayliffe, G.A.J. and Lowbury, E.J.L. (1982) Airborne infection in hospital. *Journal of Hospital Infection*, **3**, 217–240.

115 Lidwell, O.M. *et al.* (1983) Airborne contamination of wounds in joint replacement operations: the relationship to sepsis rates. *Journal of Hospital Infection*, **4**, 111–131.

116 Rogers, T.R. and Barnes, R.A. (1988) Prevention of airborne fungal infection in immunocompromised patients. *Journal of Hospital Infection*, **11** (Suppl. A), 15–20.

117 Walsh, T.J. and Dixon, G.M. (1989) Nosocomial aspergillus: environmental microbiology, hospital epidemiology, diagnosis and treatment. *European Journal of Epidemiology*, **5**, 131–142.

118 Rhame, F.S. (1991) Prevention of nosocomial aspergillosis. *Journal of Hospital Infection*, **18** (Suppl. A), 466–472.

119 Bartlett, C.L.R. *et al.* (1986) *Legionella Infections*, Arnold, London.

120 Department of Health (1994) *The Control of Legionellae in Healthcare Premises – a Code of Practice*, HTM 2040, HMSO, London.

121 Health and Safety Commission (2000) *Legionnaires' Disease. The Control of Legionella Bacteria in Water Systems; Approved code of practice and guidance*, Health & Safety Executive, Sheffield.

122 Sykes, G. (1965) *Disinfection and Sterilization*, 2nd edn, E. & F.N. Spon, London.

123 Department of Health (1994) *Ventilation in Healthcare Premises*, HTM 2025, HMSO, London.

124 Centers for Disease Control (CDC) (1972) Fogging, an ineffective measure, *National Nosocomial Infections Study, Third Quarter 1972*, CDC, Atlanta, GA, pp. 19–22.

125 French, G.L. *et al.* (2004) Tackling contamination of the hospital environment by methicillin-resistant *Staphylococcus aureus* (MRSA): a comparison between conventional terminal cleaning and hydrogen peroxide vapour decontamination. *Journal of Hospital Infection*, 57, 31–37.

126 Shapey, S. *et al.* (2008) Activity of a dry mist hydrogen peroxide system against environmental *Clostridium difficile* contamination in elderly care wards. *Journal of Hospital Infection*, **70**, 136–141

127 Ayliffe, G.A.J. *et al.* (1975) Disinfection of baths and bathwater. *Nursing Times*, **11 September**, 22–23.

128 Boycott, J.A. (1956) A note on the disinfection of baths and basins. *Lancet*, **ii**, 678–679.

129 Alder, V.G. *et al.* (1966) Disinfection and cleaning of baths in hospital. *Monthly Bulletin of the Ministry of Health and the Public Health Laboratory Service*, 25, 18–20.

130 Joynson, D.H.M. (1978) Bowls and bacteria. *Journal of Hygiene*, **80**, 423–425.

131 Newsom, S.W.B. (1972) Microbiology of hospital toilets. *Lancet*, **ii**, 700–703.

132 Ayliffe, G.A.J. *et al.* (1974) Tests of disinfection by heat in a bedpan washing machine. *Journal of Clinical Pathology*, **27**, 760–763.

133 Chadwick, P.R. and Oppenheim, B.A. (1994) Vancomycin-resistant enterococci and bedpan washer machines. *Lancet*, **344**, 685.

134 Curie, K. *et al.* (1978) A hospital epidemic caused by a gentamicin-resistant *Klebsiella* aerogenes. *Journal of Hygiene*, **80**, 115–123.

135 Gibson, G.L. (1973) Bacteriological hazards of disposable bed-pan systems. *Journal of Clinical Pathology*, **26**, 146–153.

136 Gibson, G.L. (1973) A disposable bed-pan system using an improved disposal unit and self-supporting bedpans. *Journal of Clinical Pathology*, **26**, 925–928.

137 Department of Health and Social Security (1986) *Health Service Catering Manual: Hygiene*, HMSO, London.

138 Leigh, D.A. and Whittaker, C. (1967) Disinfectants and plastic mop-heads. *British Medical Journal*, **iii**, 435.

139 Medcraft, J.W. *et al.* (1987) Potential hazard from spray cleaning of floors in hospital wards. *Journal of Hospital Infection*, **9**, 151–157.

140 Ayliffe, G.A.J. *et al.* (1975) Hygiene of babies' incubators. *Lancet*, **i**, 923.

141 Babington, P.C.B. *et al.* (1971) Retrograde spread of organisms from ventilator to patient via the expiratory limb. *Lancet*, **i**, 61–62.

142 Phillips, I. and Spencer, G. (1965) *Pseudomonas aeruginosa* cross-infection due to contaminated respirators. *Lancet*, **ii**, 1325–1327.

143 Sanford, J.P. and Pierce, A.K. (1979) Lower respiratory tract infections, in *Hospital Infections* (eds J.V. Bennett and P.S. Brachman), Little Brown, Boston, pp. 255–286.

144 Craven, D.I. *et al.* (1982) Contamination of mechanical ventilators with tubing changes every 24 or 48 hours. *New England Journal of Medicine*, **306**, 1505–1509.

145 Phillips, I. *et al.* (1974) Control of respirator-associated infection due to *Pseudomonas aeruginosa*. *Lancet*, **ii**, 871–873.

146 Das, I. and Fraise, A.P. (1998) How useful are microbial filters in respiratory apparatus. *Journal of Hospital Infection*, 4, 263–272.

147 Cadwallader, H.L. *et al.* (1990) Bacterial contamination and frequency of changing ventilator circuitry. *Journal of Hospital Infection*, **15**, 65–72.

148 La Force, F.M. (1992) Lower respiratory tract infections, in *Hospital Infections*, 3rd edn (eds J.V. Bennett and P.S. Brachman), Little Brown, Boston, pp. 611–639.

149 du Moulin, G.C. and Saubermann, A.J. (1977) The anaesthesia machine and circle system are not likely to be sources of bacterial contamination. *Anaesthesiology*, **47**, 353–358.

150 Deverill, C.E.A. and Dutt, K.K. (1980) Methods of decontamination of anaesthetic equipment: daily sessional exchange of circuits. *Journal of Hospital Infection*, **1**, 165–170.

151 George, R.H. (1975) A critical look at chemical disinfection of anaesthetic apparatus. *British Journal of Anaesthesia*, **47**, 719–721.

152 Ragg, M. (1994) Transmission of hepatitis C via anaesthetic tubings. *Lancet*, **343**, 1419.

153 Vandenbroucke-Grauls, C.M.J.E. *et al.* (1995) Bacterial and viral removal efficiency, heat and moisture exchange properties of four filtration devices. *Journal of Hospital Infection*, **29**, 45–56.

154 Feeley, T.W. *et al.* (1981) Sterile anesthesia breathing circuits do not prevent post operative pulmonary infection. *Anesthesiology*, **54**, 369–372.

155 Garibaldi, R.A. *et al.* (1981) Sterile anesthesia breathing circuits do not prevent pulmonary infection. *Anesthesiology*, **54**, 364–368.

156 Snowden, S.L. (1994) Hygiene standards for breathing systems. *British Journal of Anaesthesia*, **72**, 143–144.

157 Das, I. and Fraise, A.P. (1997) How useful are microbial filters in respiratory apparatus? *Journal of Hospital Infection*, **37**, 263–272.

158 Working Party Report (1997) *HIV Infection in Maternity Care and Gynaecology*, Royal College of Obstetricians and Gynaecologists Press, London.

159 Centers for Disease Control (1985) Recommendations for preventing possible transmission of human T lymphotrophic virus type 111/lymphadenopathyassociated virus from tears. *MMWR. Morbidity and Mortality Weekly Report*, **34**, 533–534.

160 Breathnach, A.S. *et al.* (1992) Stethoscopes as possible vectors of infection by staphylococci. *British Medical Journal*, **305**, 1573–1574.

161 Wright, I.M.R. *et al.* (1995) Stethoscope contamination in the neonatal intensive care unit. *Journal of Hospital Infection*, **29**, 65–68.

19.3 Decontamination of Endoscopes

Michelle J. Alfa[1] and Christina Bradley[2]

[1] Diagnostic Services of Manitoba, St. Boniface General Hospital, Winnipeg, Manitoba, Canada
[2] Hospital Infection Research Laboratory, Queen Elizabeth Hospital, Birmingham, UK

Introduction

Since the introduction of rigid endoscopes and subsequently that of flexible endoscopes, there has been an astounding expansion in the routine use of these minimally invasive devices [1–5]. Endoscopes in general are used throughout the world for both diagnosis and treatment of a wide range of disorders. Laparoscopic surgical procedures often utilize rigid endoscopes with fiberoptics that allow visualization of the site of interest either directly through an eye-piece or by digitizing and transmitting the image onto a monitor. Both the rigid endoscope and the minimally invasive surgical (MIS) devices such as graspers, clamps and scissors are introduced through small incisions. MIS procedures facilitate tissue collection to help with diagnosis, and the range of surgical procedures using minimally invasive surgery has greatly expanded [6]. For flexible endoscopy, the mouth provides access to the stomach and upper gastrointestinal (GI) tract while the lungs, urethra, rectum and genital tract allow entry into other body cavities. Like MIS procedures, the diagnostic and treatment approaches utilizing flexible endoscopes have greatly expanded. Colonoscopies in particular have increased significantly in number due to recent recommendations that all persons over 50 undergo screening for bowel cancer. This rapid increase in endoscopies entails a corresponding increase in the risk from infections if improperly designed or incorrectly reprocessed devices are used [7–11].

The patient population is also changing worldwide with an on-going increase in the relative numbers of the elderly and the immunocompromised. The population in general is at a higher risk not just from infections acquired during endoscopy but also from adverse reactions due to inflammatory responses to foreign organic material as well as exposure to microbicidal chemicals.

Generally, it is the manual cleaning phase in endoscope reprocessing that is most often suboptimal, thus raising the risk of spreading infections [1, 5, 12–18]. In flexible endoscopy of the GI tract, the risk of infection from residual organisms in or on the device is low because the GI tract is already colonized with normal microbiota [5, 18]. As such, the introduction of exogenous microorganisms frequently goes undetected [19, 20] unless a primary pathogen such as *Salmonella* or *Helicobacter* is involved. This likely explains why most published reports of serious infections are related to bronchoscopies (especially when there are design flaws) and not GI endoscopies [7–11, 21]. Any exogenous microorganisms introduced into the lower and normally sterile portion of the lungs pose a much higher risk of infection, especially if the alveoli are damaged during endoscopy. Since rigid endoscopes are normally used for surgery in sterile parts of the body, any exogenous microorganisms introduced have a much high risk of causing an infection. However, despite the high risk, the use of

Russell, Hugo & Ayliffe's: Principles and Practice of Disinfection, Preservation and Sterilization, Fifth Edition. Edited by Adam P. Fraise, Jean-Yves Maillard, and Syed A. Sattar.
© 2013 Blackwell Publishing Ltd. Published 2013 by Blackwell Publishing Ltd.

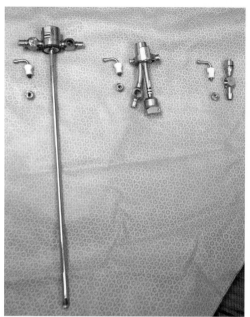
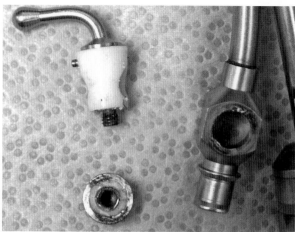

Figure 19.3.1 Accumulated "crud" build-up in a cystoureteroscope insertion trochar and attachments. Staff who were responsible for reprocessing these instruments were not aware that the "stopcock" portion was to be removed to facilitate cleaning. In other models these components look exactly the same and the manufacturer stipulated that they are not to be removed for cleaning. These instruments were taken from a cleaned, steam-sterilized tray that was ready to use on the next patient.

high-level disinfection (HLD) for MIS endoscopes and accessories is common in the USA and reports of infection from such procedures are rare [5, 6].

The primary objective of this chapter is to review the issues pertaining to decontamination (including cleaning and disinfection/sterilization) of both rigid and flexible endoscopes as well as providing recommendations regarding how to minimize these risks.

Rigid endoscopes

Infections can arise after surgical procedures involving rigid endoscopes and the associated MIS accessory devices [22]. These infections may be from endogenous microorganisms (patient's own microbes) or exogenous ones (microbes on the surgical instruments that were acquired from the previous patient or during reprocessing). Because most rigid scopes do not have channels or lumens and are heat tolerant, they are thus easier to reprocess and the risk of infection from them is quite remote [6]. However, accessory devices such as the trochars used to puncture the skin as well as the MIS accessory instruments themselves have many complex moving parts and channels. These MIS instruments are "critical" devices based on the Spaulding classification [23] and are "high risk" in terms of causing infections if residual viable microorganisms are present after reprocessing. Fortunately, these MIS instruments (including the rigid endoscope) are steam sterilizable so infections associated with such instruments are not common.

What is common is the accumulation of organic material over repeated uses as a result of lapses in reprocessing. Figure 19.3.1 shows one such MIS device where the accumulated material is readily visible. This problem occurred because the reprocessing staff were unaware that the device was to be disassembled for cleaning. Since fluid is frequently flushed through the channel of this device during the patient procedure (to clear the lens of the rigid endoscope or flush the surgical site to improve visualization of the tissues), it is very likely that some of the accumulated debris could have been introduced into the abdominal cavity and/or the surgical site. Because steam sterilization was used to reprocess these instruments, the accumulated debris was likely sterile, but it could still elicit an adverse inflammatory reaction at the surgical site. Also, any foreign material introduced into a sterile body site can act as a nidus that can protect endogenous microorganisms introduced from host defenses, thereby increasing the risk of infection.

The use of "loaner" instrument sets (i.e. sets of MIS instruments including rigid endoscopes shared between different healthcare facilities) requires special attention to ensure proper reprocessing by the sending site and also adequate packing and proper transportation to maintain sterility. Most guidelines recommend that healthcare facilities require the "loaner" set to be completely cleaned and resterilized prior to patient use [24, 25]. However, such on-site reprocessing may not be feasible if there is delayed arrival of the set at a site with surgery already scheduled. In addition, there is need for traceability of any reprocessed device in case it is suspected as the source of an infection.

The key issues include the following:

1. Insist that the manufacturer provide device-specific instructions that clearly show how to disassemble an instrument for the cleaning protocol validated for that instrument and how to reassemble and package it for the validated sterilization process.

2. Ensure that reprocessing personnel are properly trained in cleaning of such instruments, conduct on-going audits to ensure compliance and are retrained in case of lack of compliance.

3. Implement labeling and tracking of instruments (or minimally the MIS instrument set) as part of the quality process for MIS instruments.

Flexible endoscopes

Infections associated with flexible endoscopy

There is little published evidence of the true infection rate in relation to the number of procedures carried out. In proportion to the number of flexible endoscopies performed the risk of infection is low, but such infections continue to occur [26, 27]. It was estimated in an American Society of Gastroenterology report in 1996 [28] that the incidence of infection following GI endoscopy was 1 in 1.8 million [29]. In the 28 reported cases, infection resulted from a breach in the recommended decontamination procedure or contamination of the automated endoscope reprocessor (AER) [29].

In a review, Nelson [21] examined 120 reports from 1974 to 2001. Publications related to gastroscopy have identified numerous causative organisms including *Pseudomonas aeruginosa*, *Salmonella* spp. and *Helicobacter pylori* [21]. The number of patients involved ranged from 1 to 126 [21].. The reasons for failure were identified as selection of an unsuitable disinfectant (e.g. cetrimide/chlorhexidine, cetrimide, benzethonium chloride), inadequate cleaning, failure to use sterile water, failure to irrigate channels, failure to dry with 70% alcohol, failure to sterilize the waterbottle, and failure to access all channels of the endoscope. Similarly, publications [30] related to endoscopic retrograde pancreatography (ERCP) identified numerous causative organisms including *P. aeruginosa*, *Serratia marcescens*, *Enterococcus cloacae*, *Klebsiella pneumoniae* and *Salmonella* spp. Nelson [21] examined 16 publications from 1975 to 1993. The number of patients involved ranged from 1 to 17 and similar reasons were cited for failures in the decontamination procedure. Infections from bronchoscopy have also been reported [31]. Failures in the decontamination procedure were associated with "out-of-hours" use of bronchoscopes without immediate reprocessing. A systematic literature review published in 2006 [31] identified 31 publications related to flexible endoscopy, but no articles related to possible transmission of HIV were identified [32]. A recent report by Aumeran *et al.* [33] indicated that manual cleaning and drying stages before storage of ERCP scopes were inadequate and had led to an outbreak of multidrug-resistant *K. pneumoniae* infections.

Risk assessment

Most flexible endoscopes are considered semicritical items as they are not intentionally invasive but are in contact with intact mucous membranes (e.g. gastroscope, colonoscope, sigmoidoscope), so high-level disinfection is acceptable to reprocess them [23]. Those endoscopes that are invasive (e.g. angioscope, choledochoscope) should be subjected to a sterilization procedure.

Problems associated with flexible endoscopes

Although there are some bronchoscopes that are autoclavable, most currently used flexible endoscopes are heat sensitive and will not withstand temperatures in excess of 60°C. Therefore, only low-temperature decontamination methods are recommended. It is important that the manufacturer's recommendations are adhered to at all times. Flexible endoscopes are complex devices, some with numerous long and narrow channels [5, 23]. It is imperative that all personnel responsible for reprocessing are familiar with the structure of the endoscopes they handle so that all critical parts of the devices are thoroughly cleaned and decontaminated [12, 33–35]. In particular, all staff must be trained to check prior to disinfection that no channels are blocked. Flexible endoscopes are comparatively expensive and most endoscopy units only have a limited number of them on hand. As a result, reprocessing staff in busy endoscopy units are under considerable pressure for rapid turnaround of devices. The recent observation study by Ofstead *et al.* [36] confirmed that only 1.4% of endoscopes reprocessed using manual cleaning (in conjunction with HLD in an AER) complied with guidelines, whereas 75.4% of endoscopes reprocessed using a validated AER cleaning cycle (in conjunction with HLD in an AER) complied with reprocessing guidelines.

Decontamination procedure

It is preferable to use a well-designed and maintained AER, following manufacturer's instructions, to ensure perfusion of all channels and adequate exposure of devices to the disinfectant. Use of an AER ensures reproducibility in the decontamination procedure and protects staff from exposure to potentially harmful chemicals. Many countries have published national guidelines and these should be taken into account when local policies and procedures are prepared.

Decontamination of flexible endoscopes consists of precleaning, leak testing, manual cleaning, high-level disinfection and a final rinse.

Steps in the decontamination procedure
Pre-cleaning or bedside cleaning
Immediately after use of the endoscope, while the scope is still attached to the light source, all channels should be flushed with water or detergent solution and external surfaces wiped with a non-linting cloth. Such immediate bedside pre-cleaning will

remove easily detachable patient-derived organic material, which may be more difficult to remove once dry. During this part of the process, users can make initial checks for channel blockages. Adaptors are available for easy flushing of the air and water channels. The scope is then securely transferred to a dedicated reprocessing room.

Leak testing

Prior to commencing the manual cleaning, it is recommended that a leak test is carried out to ensure the integrity of the instrument. An undetected leak in the endoscope can lead to damage and ingress of contaminated material into the internal workings.

Manual cleaning

This stage is required irrespective of whether disinfection is carried out manually or within an AER. However, manual cleaning must be performed thoroughly at all times by all staff [4, 15, 34] using written standard operating procedures (SOPs) to be provided to all staff following their initial training [1, 4, 5, 20, 36–39]. All SOPs should be based on the recommendations of the endoscope and disinfectant manufacturers. They should include all aspects of the process including dismantling of valves, etc., endoscope channel configuration and instructions for access to all channels, any safety warnings associated with the chemicals used and recommendations on the use of personal protective equipment (PPE).

Manual cleaning should include wiping all external surfaces, brushing (or use of an equivalent device) of all accessible channels (if recommended by the endoscope manufacturer) and flushing of all channels, whether they have been used or not, with freshly prepared detergent solution. The detergent solution should be accurately prepared at the correct concentration and temperature. The valves should also be manually cleaned using suitable brushes. Endoscope manufacturers provide accessories such as tubing connectors to ensure access to all channels and the instructions for use should be followed at all times. It is important that the correct diameter and length of channel brush or other channel cleaning device is used for each endoscope (note that not all channels can be brushed so ensure manufacturer instructions are followed). The brush or device itself will collect debris as it passes through the channels. This should be removed by cleaning the brush until no visible debris remains before withdrawing it back through the channel. The brush should be repeatedly passed through the channel until there is no more visible debris on the cleaning brush (a minimum of three passes through the channel should be performed). All brushing procedures should take place while the endoscope is submerged in cleaning fluid and the brush inserted into the channel below the level of the cleaning fluid to reduce the risk of aerosol production. Decontamination of the cleaning brush is required after use on each endoscope. These are not easy to clean and in some countries (e.g. the UK) single-use brushes are now recommended. These have the advantage of ensuring a

standard quality of brush every time a channel is cleaned and eliminates the risk of protein residues remaining on the brush being transferred to the next endoscope that is cleaned. The quality of the bristles on reusable brushes can deteriorate over time, the cable can become distorted and kinks may develop which may damage the endoscope. Staff should wear appropriate PPE including gloves, waterproof apron and a full facial visor. There is risk of aerosol production, particularly while brushing the channels. This can be minimized by ensuring the brush is immersed under the cleaning fluid as it emerges from the channel. Staff should be immunized against relevant infectious agents (e.g. hepatitis B) in line with hospital policy and their immune status established.

The detergent solution should be freshly prepared for each endoscope and should be accurately measured to ensure the correct concentration is used. The detergent manufacturer's instructions should be followed (i.e. concentration, contact time, temperature). Some cleaning chemicals may be damaging to endoscopes and advice should be obtained from the endoscope manufacturer on the selection of a suitable cleaning agent. A detergent with a neutral pH is usually selected, which may or may not be enzyme-based. Detergent action is dependent on contact time and temperature. The temperature should not exceed 35°C as higher temperatures may cause protein coagulation. Cleansing efficacy is mainly achieved by friction (i.e. brushing and flushing). There are some enzymatic detergents (e.g. subtilisin-based enzymatics) that can lead to respiratory sensitization, so appropriate PPE should be used by reprocessing staff [4, 5, 40].

After cleaning with detergent the endoscope should be rinsed to remove detergent residues. Fresh rinsewater should be used for each endoscope. Freshly drawn tapwater is considered suitable at this stage. A separate sink for rinsing is advised. If this is not possible then the sink should be thoroughly rinsed to remove detergent residues before rinsing the endoscope. All channels of the endoscope and all external surfaces should be thoroughly rinsed during this part of the procedure. After rinsing, the channels should be flushed with air to expel excess fluid before the endoscope is processed in an AER.

Automated cleaning

Recently, AERs with validated cleaning cycles have become commercially available [41]. The value of replacing the manual cleaning with an automated cycle was reported by Ofstead *et al.* [36]. Their observational study confirmed that lack of compliance with manual cleaning guidelines was a major shortcoming.

High-level disinfection

After the cleaning procedure, all internal channels and external surfaces of the endoscope should be exposed to an approved (the approval process varies in different countries), effective, compatible disinfectant at the correct temperature and contact time to provide HLD. The HLD process should preferably take place in an AER as this ensures standardized, controlled exposure. However, in some countries these are not widely available and manual disinfection using immersion is carried out. Whichever method is used it is important to ensure that all internal and external surfaces are exposed to the disinfectant at the correct concentration and temperature (in accordance with the manufacturer's recommendations) for the correct contact time. There may be health and safety issues with some chemicals (e.g. vapors from glutaraldehyde) and reprocessing staff should wear appropriate PPE to ensure protection from skin contact and respiratory exposure.

The disinfectant should be effective against bacteria, including *Mycobacterium tuberculosis* and viruses. Sporicidal activity may be required for invasive endoscopes that cannot be processed by any other method. Test data should be made available by the disinfectant manufacturer to support the efficacy claims of the disinfectant at the concentration, temperature and contact time recommended. Numerous liquid disinfectants are available (e.g. aldehydes, peracetic acid, chlorine dioxide, superoxidized water, etc.). Further information on the properties of disinfectants can be found in Chapter 2. In the UK, France and Australia, the use of aldehyde-based disinfectants is no longer recommended due to their fixative properties and/or workplace safety concerns related to fumes [33].

Final rinse to removal of disinfectant residues

Rinsing with freshwater is required to remove the disinfectant residues after HLD [42]. The water should be of a quality that will not recontaminate the endoscope. For the higher-risk procedures with a potential for infection or misdiagnosis of infection (e.g. ERCP, bronchoscopy, cystoscopy) bacteria-free water is recommended. This may be achieved by submicron filtration of potable water, reverse osmosis or the addition of a microbicide that has been proven to be biocompatible. In North America the guidelines recommend that all scopes should be rinsed with bacteria-free water or preferably sterile water [5, 20, 28, 40] after HLD. If tapwater is used for the final rinse (e.g. manual HLD) then the channels should have an alcohol flush followed by forced air drying [3, 5, 43].

Drying of all channels and external surfaces

After the decontamination procedure, excess fluid should be expelled from the channels. This can be achieved using forced air or alcohol followed by forced air. In the UK, the use of alcohol is no longer recommended for GI endoscopes due to its fixative properties and the potential risk of prion transmission [32]. Alcohol facilitates the drying process so if it is not used it is important that the duration of forced air drying is thorough enough to ensure no moisture remains in the channels [44]. Drying between patient use is not necessary but drying thoroughly before flexible endoscopes are placed in storage is critical [20, 44, 45]. Recently, storage cabinets have been developed that facilitate the drying process by flushing HEPA filtered air through the channels for a defined length of time [46].

Selection of a chemical disinfectant for HLD

The chemical disinfectant chosen must have the following characteristics:
• It should have a spectrum of activity suitable for the devices being processed – bactericidal, virucidal, mycobactericidal and, if required, sporicidal [48].
• It should be compatible with the instrument and the washer disinfector.
• It should be used in such a manner that the user and patient are not put at risk.

In the UK, washer disinfectors have to comply with the recommendations in HTM 2030 *Washer Disinfectors* [48] for operational management, design and validation. Other countries may have adopted the ISO guidance documents 15883 parts 1 to 5 [49] or use their own national guidelines. HTM 2030 [48] design considerations state that ideally the disinfectant solution should be used once and discarded. If, however, the disinfectant is reused a means should be incorporated to ensure that the disinfectant remains active and contains the minimum effective concentration (MEC). Similar MEC testing recommendations are made in a range of other guidance documents [3–5, 40, 43].

When purchasing an AER, the facility has to decide whether to reuse the disinfectant or not (i.e. single use). One of the deciding factors for use of a reusable versus single-use disinfectant is often cost. Costing should take into account the cost of disinfectant per cycle and not just the cost per liter of the high-level disinfectant. This cost must be balanced against infection risk, health and safety issues to staff from exposure to chemicals, the risk to patients of potential exposure to process residues, and the risk of inactivation/dilution of the disinfectant when reused. Where GI scopes are processed from patients in a risk category for vCJD, single-use disinfectants are advised as the potential risk of carry-over of high-risk tissue is removed by discarding the disinfectant each time it is used.

However, whether a single-use or reusable disinfectant is used, tests must take place to ensure that the disinfectant concentration does not fall below the MEC. The disinfectant manufacturer should specify the MEC and how to test the MEC as well as the use-life of the disinfectant. The machine manufacturer should indicate the number of cycles that can be run before the MEC is reached. This information should be programmed into the machine to ensure the disinfectant is not overused or used beyond the specified use-life. However, this must also be validated with daily MEC testing. This could be achieved by using a monitoring system within the AER or a test kit supplied by the disinfectant manufacturer to be employed by the user.

If a single-use disinfectant is used, tests must be carried out to ensure that the disinfectant concentration when prepared for use within the washer disinfector is reproducible. Tests are described in HTM 2030 [48] (under Validation and verification 9.279 to 9.289) for establishing the reproducibility of the chemical dosing system and for ensuring the AER can detect low levels in the dispensing containers. It is recommended that these tests be carried out yearly.

A test is also described in HTM 2030 [48] (under Validation and verification 9.343 to 9.352) for establishing that process chemical residues in the final rinsewater are below those recommended by the disinfectant manufacturer.

Automated endoscope reprocessors

Typical AER cycle including a validated cleaning cycle

A cycle as described in HTM 2030 and EN ISO 15883 part 4 [50] consists of the following stages:

- Leak test to verify that the endoscope is undamaged.
- Flushing with water not exceeding 35°C.
- Flow test to verify that all channels are free of blockages for effective cleaning, disinfection and rinsing to take place.
- Washing with detergent solution at an appropriate temperature not exceeding 60°C and an appropriate contact time.
- Rinsing to remove detergent residues.
- Drying to remove excess fluid which may dilute the disinfectant.
- Disinfection with a suitable agent that is microbiologically effective and compatible with the endoscope and washer disinfector. Contact time, temperature and concentration should be controlled by the washer disinfector.
- Rinsing to remove disinfectant residues.
- Drying to remove excess fluid so the endoscope is available for immediate patient use.

Endoscope washer disinfectors: issues

It is important for the user to appreciate and understand the range of issues associated with the use of endoscope washer disinfectors and how to avoid these problems (Table 19.3.1).

Contamination of the washer disinfector

The AER should be designed so as to discourage the proliferation of microorganisms within the AER. Pipework should be free-draining and there should be no water storage tanks. In the UK, the Medicines and Healthcare Products Regulatory Agency (MHRA) [51] recommend that the AER should be subjected to a daily self-disinfect process, preferably at the start of the day. This may be carried out thermally or chemically. HTM 2030 [48] states that the chemical used to disinfect the AER should be different to that used for disinfection of the endoscope. This is to avoid the selection of disinfectant-resistant strains, which has been reported when glutaraldehyde was used [51, 52]. Ideally, the machine should have the facility to be programmed to perform the self-disinfect cycle at the start of the day so the AER is ready for use when the staff arrive for duty. Proof of the self-disinfection cycle having taken place should be available.

Treatment of the incoming water supply

It is recommended that the final rinsewater used for cystoscopes, bronchoscopes and ERCP procedures be bacteria-free to reduce the risk of infection and/or misdiagnosis of infection. Different

countries have guidelines on the recommended levels of bacteria permissible in the final rinsewater. In Europe this level is <10 cfu/100 ml of water provided these are not *P. aeruginosa*, atypical mycobacteria or legionellae [53]. In the UK HTM 2030 [48] recommends that 100 ml samples of rinsewater taken on a weekly basis should contain no bacteria. Incoming water will contain bacteria and are to be removed using physical methods (e.g. submicron filtration, reverse osmosis). The water-treatment system itself may become a source of contamination and like the washer disinfector should also be subjected to a regular disinfection regime. The AAMI TIR34 [50] recommends that high-purity water (e.g. reverse osmosis, deionized or distilled water) should have <10 cfu /ml and that tapwater used for medical device reprocessing should have <200 cfu/ml. Although many guidance documents suggest that the water quality of the final rinsewater used by the AER be monitored, in North America this is not widely implemented as manufacturers have not provided recommended methods for this type of testing.

Suitability of endoscope connection systems for the endoscopes being processed

The AER should be capable of processing all makes and models of endoscopes used within the department. Suitable channel connectors should be available to ensure access to all channels including the elevator bridge (forceps raiser) channel (may also be referred to as the elevator wire channel). The pump capacity of the AER should be sufficient to ensure adequate flow within all of the channels to achieve the required disinfectant contact time. It is important for users to ensure that the AER can process the elevator wire channel otherwise they must ensure it is fully reprocessed using manual cleaning and manual HLD. Reprocessing personnel should never modify the manufacturer-supplied connectors as there would be no validation to confirm the efficacy of the modified connector.

Verification of all-channel irrigation

It is important to ensure that all channels are accessed during the decontamination process and that no channel blockages are present. These are often detected during the manual cleaning procedure. However, the AER should ideally have a means to detect individual channel blockages and/or disconnections of the channel connectors. This will ensure that all internal surfaces are perfused properly, ensuring adequate exposure to the chemical disinfectant.

Traceability

It is important to ensure that all stages of the endoscope decontamination process are documented and linked to the patient on whom the endoscope has been used. In the event of an infection occurring that is thought to be linked to an endoscopic procedure, a "look back" exercise may be undertaken. Investigators will need proof of which endoscope was used on the index patient and any subsequent patients. They will also require evidence of a satisfactory decontamination process. The documentation may

Table 19.3.1 Flexible endoscope reprocessing: summary of potential problems and how to avoid them.

Problem	Basis for problem	How can this be detected?	How can this be avoided?
Improper cleaning: • not cleaning all channels present in flexible endoscope (e.g. elevator wire channel, auxiliary water channel), • not cleaning accessories • not cleaning adequately; using short-cuts like not immersing scope for cleaning	Staff not properly trained and unaware of new channels on new model of endoscope. Short-cuts to manual cleaning due to staff being pressured to rush	If periodic competency audits are made of staff it will be detected. Otherwise hard to detect unless a staff member points it out or the channel becomes blocked	Require that vendor provide on-site training of physicians, nurses and reprocessing personnel and they must sign a record sheet documenting training and date. On-going yearly competency assessments of all staff who reprocess endoscopes
No manual brushing and cleaning; scope placed in an AER that has no cleaning cycle or has no validated cleaning cycle	Staff in a rush, rely blindly on the AER to do cleaning. Staff do not understand the implications of problems this can create in the AER (e.g. biofilm)	Unless staff identify this as a problem or unless there are infections that are traced back to the endoscopy procedure it is hard to detect	Implement yearly audit of staff competency (observe process of reprocessing and use checklist of expected competencies)
Scope incorrectly connected to the AER leading to suboptimal or no flow through channels	Staff inadequately trained or unaware of correct connectors to use	If AER has channel flow detectors the cycle would be aborted. If AER does not have channel flow detectors it may be hard to detect	Implement yearly audit of staff competency (observe process of reprocessing and use checklist of expected competencies)
Wrong chemical delivered during cycle, e.g. swapped connectors for detergent and alcohol	Reservoirs that do not have unique connectors or refillable reservoirs that had wrong chemical introduced	May go unnoticed if staff do not recognize the error. Some AER manufacturers are building units with unique tubing connectors that prevent this issue	Have co-signature when bottles are replaced to verify correct chemical has been attached with the correct connector. Ensure each bottle or reservoir has unique connector so mistakes cannot happen
Liquid chemical provides inadequate HLD	Reused high-level disinfectant may have become diluted or inactivated with organic material	May go undetected if staff do not notice	Use daily MEC test strips to ensure appropriate active concentration of high-level disinfectant. Ensure the results are documented (e.g. on a record sheet or electronically by the AER)
Tracking: unable to determine what scope was used on which patient and unable to determine which AER was used for that scope	No tracking system implemented as part of the quality system	Often will be undetected until patient problem occurs and infection control system needs to track problematic scope	Master record (or other method) of tracking each scope each time it is used so patient and AER can all be linked each time the scope is used. Need to have after-hours protocol for tracking scopes used for emergency procedures
Non-disinfected scope used by accident for patient procedure (e.g. damaged scope waiting for repair, or scope waiting for HLD)	Inadequate labeling of damaged or contaminated scopes in reprocessing area. After-hours staff who are not knowledgeable about endoscope storage area taking incorrect endoscope	May not be detected until staff notice that scope was used (e.g. day staff return and note that damaged non-disinfected scope was used by after-hours staff)	Ensure policy developed to prohibit after-hours access to endoscopy area for untrained personnel. Ensure labeling of scope that warns scope is not disinfected and should not be used on patients

AER, automated endoscope reprocessor; HLD, high-level disinfection; MEC, minimum effective concentration.

be recorded in an electronic format by means of a computer-based tracking and traceability package or manually using paper records.

Accessories

Any accessories used during the endoscopic procedure or the decontamination procedure should be single-use or decontaminated after each use if reusable. This includes biopsy forceps, guide wires, cleaning brushes, etc. Many of the reusable accessories are heat tolerant and can be processed in a steam sterilizer; alternatively they can be decontaminated by the same process used for the endoscope.

Documentation

Manual cleaning is most commonly done prior to the HLD process in an AER (even if the AER includes a "wash" stage prior to the HLD stage). As such, records should ideally be kept of all manual processes undertaken. This should include the result of the leak test and that visual inspection of endoscopes after cleaning was undertaken by the operator carrying out the procedure. Those AERs with validated cleaning and HLD cycles have print-outs that document the entire process (i.e. cleaning and HLD). All print-outs from the AER, including evidence of machine self-disinfection, should be retained and linked to the patient records. Documentation of initial staff training and on-going competency is required by most guidance documents [4, 5, 33, 40].

Facilities

A dedicated decontamination room with a clear pathway from a "dirty" decontamination area to a "clean" storage area should be available. Separate appropriately-sized sinks should be used for manual cleaning and rinsing. Dedicated handwashing facilities should be available. Ventilation and air handling should be adequate for the tasks performed and chemicals used for endoscope reprocessing. The endoscope reprocessing room should be a restricted-access area where eating and drinking are prohibited.

Storage of endoscopes

After the decontamination procedure, the endoscopes should be stored in such a way that allows free draining of any residual fluid from the channels and protects them from any possible damage or theft. This could be in a cupboard with dedicated cradles to accommodate the control box of the endoscope or in dedicated storage cupboards [47] which allows filtered air to pass down all channels. If this type of cabinet is not used then it is recommended in some countries [49] that the endoscope should be used within a 3 h period after HLD. This is based on the potential for any residual contamination to multiply to significant numbers if left for periods longer than 3 h [54]. The use of dying cabinets allows the endoscopes to be stored for periods in excess of 72 h without the need for reprocessing of the endoscope before patient use. In North America the alternative to the drying cabinets is the use of an alcohol rinse combined with forced air drying to ensure the scope channels are thoroughly dried prior to storage [4, 40].

Current data suggest that properly dried and stored flexible GI endoscopes may be kept for 5–7 days without needing to reprocess them prior to patient use [55–57].

Cleaning verification of reprocessed endoscopes

There is increasing evidence that reprocessing of rigid and flexible endoscopes should incorporate a quality process that includes some way to ensure verification of the cleaning stage. A wide range of products to assess cleaning efficacy are now commercially available in many countries (Table 19.3.2). In addition, there is a wide range of test soils and cleaning verification approaches outlined in national guidance documents from various countries [48, 53, 64]. However, there remains a lot of controversy regarding what defines "adequately clean" for the surface and/or lumen of any medical instrument or device. Currently, visual inspection is most widely used – that is does the instrument look clean when visually inspected. The "visual" audit tool is very crude and cannot assess reliably serrated, hinged or lumen components. Other approaches have been to take samples from the instrument using swabs or elution methods [19, 61, 62, 65] and then test these instrument samples to assess if the level of residuals is considered excessive or not. The efficiency of the sampling method will greatly affect any direct testing of medical devices but this is the only approach that will determine if that specific device has unacceptable levels of residuals after manual cleaning. Another generally accepted approach is to assess the automated washer itself and try to ensure that the washer is providing adequate cleaning. It can then be assumed that the instruments processed have been adequately cleaned (process monitoring rather than direct medical instrument monitoring). It would seem there is merit in both approaches for ensuring on-going assurance of cleaning efficacy.

Despite the merit in either approach it has been hard to reach consensus regarding what marker to target and for this marker, what level of residuals on the exterior or lumen surface of a medical device is unacceptable. Some argue that protein is the most appropriate target and that it should take into consideration concerns regarding prion residuals on surgical instruments. The protein "cut-offs" that have been suggested include 0.1 µg/device [66], 5.5 µg/cm^2 [67] and 6.4 µg/cm^2 [59]. Other studies have suggested targeting bioburden, hemoglobin or carbohydrate as markers of cleaning adequacy [59]. The other aspect that is yet to be agreed upon is how difficult it should be to remove the test soil. Should cleaning efficacy of an automated washer be defined based on whether or not it can remove a test soil formulated to be strongly adherent or should the test soil mimic clinically relevant soiling conditions?

Despite the controversies and lack of consensus there is one thing that seems evident – any of the test methods or approaches currently published or commercially available provide a better assessment of manual cleaning efficacy compared with simply visually inspecting instruments that have been cleaned either

Table 19.3.2 Summary of some types of currently commercially available tests to assess cleaning adequacy.[a]

Cleaning test (manufacturer)	Application	Parameter assessed	Cut-off for adequate cleaning
Automated washers			
TOSI (Healthmark Industries Co. Inc.)	Automated washers – assess cleaning provided by washer	Removal of blood–protein marker soil	Visual assessment that blood–protein has been completely removed [58] Website: http://hmark.com
Lumchek (Healthmark Industries Co. Inc.)	Automated washers – assess cleaning provided by lumen flushing ports	Removal of blood–protein marker soil on carrier inserted into lumen holder	Visual assessment that blood–protein has been completely removed [58] Website: http://hmark.com
Washer monitors based on dye removal Flexicheck and lumen check (Healthmark Co. Inc.) Wash checks (SteriTec Products Inc.)	Automated washers – assess cleaning provided by washer	Removal of colored dye from carrier strip (may have protective cover or lumen to provide difficulty in removing marker)	Visual assessment that colored marker has been completely removed Websites: http://hmark.com, http://steritecproducts.com
Test soil Browne soil (STERIS Corp), ATS (Healthmark Industries Co. Inc.), etc. as well as use-prepared test soils outlined in ISO and AAMI	Automated washers – assess cleaning provided by washer	Removal of test soil from carrier or inside wall of washer	Visual assessment that test soil have been completely removed [48] Quantitative assessment of residuals: <6.4 μg/cm² protein, <4-log₁₀ cfu/cm² [59, 60]
Devices			
ATP (various including 3M, Scil Diagnostics)	Device – assess cleaning of surfaces or lumens of endoscopes or other instruments	Detection of ATP residuals remaining on instruments after cleaning. ATP reflects living microbes or human cellular components	Currently suggested cut-off of 500 relative light units for site sampled. Cut-off varies for different ATP kits and validation studies are lacking. [60, 61, 68]
ChannelCheck™ (Healthmark Industries Co. Inc.)	Device, endoscopes – cleaned manually Sample collected from channel (sample collected by flushing 10 ml sterile deionized water through channel)	Residual protein, carbohydrate and hemoglobin	Color change on test pads confirming protein <6.4 μg/cm², carbohydrate <1.8 μg/cm² and hemoglobin <2.2 μg/cm² (check manufacturer's website for details) Website: http://hmark.com
ProCheckII™ (Healthmark Industries Co. Inc.)	Device, instrument surfaces – collect surface sample using a swab	Residual protein	Color change occurs if 1 μg of protein is on swab Website: http://steritecproducts.com
EndoCheck™ (Healthmark Industries Co. Inc.)	Device, flexible endoscope – sample from biopsy channel collected using a swab	Residual protein or blood	Color change indicates blood or protein residuals Limit of detection not specified Website: http://hmark.com

AAMI, Association for the Advancement of Medical Instrumentation; ATP, adenosine tri-phosphate; ATS, Artificial Test Soil; ISO, International Standards Organization; TOSI, this is the actual name it is not an abbreviation.
[a]The list of devices and manufacturers is not exhaustive and is meant to reflect the range of tests available.

manually or through an automated washer. At a minimum it would be useful for healthcare facilities to adopt methods to assess washer efficacy as well as to provide on-going cleaning competency assessment of reprocessing personnel. This is particularly true for countries such as the USA, Canada and Australia where installation qualification testing and on-going performance qualification testing for automated instrument washers used for rigid and flexible endoscopes is not currently required.

Another aspect of reprocessing rigid and flexible endoscopes is the need to ensure the water used for the final rinse is appropriate. For rigid endoscopes this final rinsewater should be free of organic residuals such as protein and endotoxins. As reported by Alfa *et al.* [58], surgical instruments processed through automated washers may have high levels of endotoxins after the final rinse. This is unacceptable as steam sterilization does not completely inactivate endotoxins, so any endotoxin residuals on surgical instruments could lead to adverse reactions in patients. Checking the water quality as part of an on-going quality program is essential for rigid endoscopes and the accessory devices used with them. For flexible endoscopes the final rinsewater should as a minimum be "bacteria-free". For automated washers this is most commonly achieved using submicron filtration of the water. This is generally effective providing the filters are monitored for breaks and changed as per the manufacturer's recommendations.

The key issues are:

1. Ensure automated washers used for endoscope cleaning are periodically tested on an on-going basis to ensure they are still providing adequate cleaning.

2. Ensure the water used (high-purity feedwater and/or final rinsewater) is monitored to ensure adequacy. The heterotrophic plate count is generally used to ensure unacceptable microorganism counts are not present [56].

3. Testing the flexible endoscopes to assess cleaning adequacy may be a valuable addition to the on-going quality process in endoscopy and is a key component during training of new personnel and for on-going compliance assessment.

4. No internationally accepted cut-offs are available to guide users in cleaning adequacy of rigid or flexible endoscopes, so users are recommended to ask manufacturers of endoscope cleaning tests for their validation data to help determine which tests best suit their needs.

Staff training

Written procedures

One of the main problems with any decontamination procedure, particularly when manual stages are involved, is ensuring that the correct procedure is followed at all times by all staff [36]. Therefore, written SOPs should be available which will provide a standard method for all staff to follow. These should be based on the recommendations of the manufacturers of the endoscope, AER and detergent/disinfectant. They should include all aspects of the process, including dismantling of valves, etc., endoscope channel configuration and instructions for access to all channels, any safety warnings associated with the chemicals used and recommendations on the use of protective clothing [3–5, 14]. These written procedures should form the basis of the staff training.

Training

Training programs should be in place for new staff and there should also be on-going training programs held on a regular basis (e.g. yearly) for all staff. Training should be available for the users of the endoscopes (nurses and doctors) and for staff carrying out the decontamination procedure. Staff should familiarize themselves with the instructions provided with each endoscope. They should have a full understanding of the anatomy of each instrument used within the department to ensure all surfaces and channels are accessed during the complete decontamination process, which should include the manual cleaning. In some countries there are AERs that have validated cleaning cycles that have been approved to replace the manual cleaning. The SOPs should form the framework of the training program. It is recommended that the department manager retains documentation of the training records for each member of staff. Topics for inclusion in the training program should include disassembly and assembly of the endoscopes, manual processing, use of automated systems, the importance of traceability and how to use the system in that healthcare facility, maintenance of the decontamination equipment etc.

Acknowledgment

Figure 19.3.1 was kindly provided by Louise Buelow-Smith, Winnipeg, MB.

References

1 Mehta, A.C. *et al.* (2005) [Corrected] consensus statement: prevention of flexible bronchoscopy-associated infection. *Chest*, **128**, 1742–1755.

2 Alvarado, C.J. and Reichelderfer, M. (2000) APIC guideline for infection prevention and control in flexible endoscopy. Association for Professionals in Infection Control. *American Journal of Infection Control*, **28**, 138–155.

3 (2003) Multi-society guideline for reprocessing flexible gastrointestinal endoscopes. *Gastrointestinal Endoscopy*, **58** (1), 1–8.

4 Canadian Standard Association ISBN 978-1-55436-652-1 (CSA) (2008) *CSA Z314.8-08. Decontamination of Reusable Medical Devices*, Canadian Standard Association.

5 Rutala, W.A. and Weber, D.J. (2004) Reprocessing endoscopes: United States perspective. *Journal of Hospital Infection*, **56** (Suppl. 2), S27–S39.

6 Ayliffe, G. (2000) Decontamination of minimally invasive surgical endoscopes and accessories. *Journal of Hospital Infection*, **45** (4), 263–277.

7 Cetre, J.C. *et al.* (2005) Outbreaks of contaminated broncho-alveolar lavage related to intrinsically defective bronchoscopes. *Journal of Hospital Infection*, **61** (1), 39–45.

8 Srinivasan, A. *et al.* (2003) An outbreak of *Pseudomonas aeruginosa* infections associated with flexible bronchoscopes. *New England Journal of Medicine*, **348** (3), 221–227.

9 Kirschke, D.L. *et al.* (2003) *Pseudomonas aeruginosa* and *Serratia marcescens* contamination associated with a manufacturing defect in bronchoscopes. *New England Journal of Medicine*, **348** (3), 214–220.

10 Cetre, J.C. *et al.* (2003) Outbreaks of infection associated with bronchoscopes. *New England Journal of Medicine*, **348** (20), 2039–2040; author reply, 40.

11 MMWR. (2002) *Morbidity and Mortality Weekly Report*, March 8, **51** (9), 190. http://www.cdc.gov/mmwr/preview/mmwrhtml/mm5109a5.htm.

12 Moses, F.M. and Lee, J.S. (2004) Current GI endoscope disinfection and QA practices. *Digestive Diseases and Sciences*, **49** (11–12), 1791–1797.

13 Mean, M. *et al.* (2006) Gastrointestinal endoscopes cleaned without detergent substance following an automated endoscope washer/disinfector dysfunction. *Gastroenterologie Clinique et Biologique*, **30** (5), 665–668.

14 Alfa, M. (1999) Flexible endoscope reprocessing: staff training verification to ensure reproducibility. *Infection Control Today*, May 1999, 9–20.

15 Kaczmarek, R.G. *et al.* (1992) Multi-state investigation of the actual disinfection/sterilization of endoscopes in health care facilities. *American Journal of Medicine*, **92** (3), 257–261.

16 Heeg, P. (2004) Reprocessing endoscopes: national recommendations with a special emphasis on cleaning – the German perspective. *Journal of Hospital Infection*, **56** (Suppl. 2), S23–S26.

17 Wood-Baker, R. *et al.* (2001) Fibre-optic bronchoscopy in adults: a position paper of The Thoracic Society of Australia and New Zealand. *Internal Medicine Journal*, **31** (8), 479–487.

18 Vesley, D. *et al.* (1999) Microbial bioburden in endoscope reprocessing and an in-use evaluation of the high-level disinfection capabilities of Cidex PA. *Gastroenterology Nursing*, **22** (2), 63–68.

19 Buss, A.J. *et al.* (2008) Endoscope disinfection and its pitfalls – requirement for retrograde surveillance cultures. *Endoscopy*, **40** (4), 327–332.

20 Beilenhoff, U. *et al.* (2008) ESGE-ESGENA guideline: cleaning and disinfection in gastrointestinal endoscopy. *Endoscopy*, **40** (11), 939–957.

21 Nelson, D.B. (2003) Infectious disease complications of GI endoscopy: part II, exogenous infections. *Gastrointestinal Endoscopy*, **57** (6), 695–711.

22 Furuya, E.Y. *et al.* (2008) Outbreak of *Mycobacterium abscessus* wound infections among "lipotourists" from the United States who underwent abdominoplasty in the Dominican Republic. *Clinical Infectious Diseases*, **46** (8), 1181–1188.

23 Spaulding, E. (1970) The role of chemical disinfection in the prevention of nosocomial infections, in *Proceeedings of International Conference on Nosocomial Infections* (eds P.S. Brachman and T.C. Eickof), American Hospital Association, Chicago, pp. 254–274.

24 American Society for Healthcare Central Service Personnel/International Association of Healthcare Central Service Materiel Management (ASHCSP/IAHCSMM) (2004) *Position Paper on Loaner Instrumentation*, http://www.iahcsmm.org.

25 CSA-Z314.22-04 (CSA) (2004) *Management of Loaned, Shared, and Leased Medical Devices*, Canadian Standards Association.

26 Bisset, L. *et al.* (2006) A prospective study of the efficacy of routine decontamination for gastrointestinal endoscopes and the risk factors for failure. *American Journal of Infection Control*, **34** (5), 274–280.

27 Spach, D.H. *et al.* (1993) Transmission of infection by gastrointestinal endoscopy and bronchoscopy. *Annals of Internal Medicine*, **118** (2), 117–128.

28 American Society for Gastrointestinal Endoscopy (1996) Reprocessing of flexible gastrointestinal endoscopes. *Gastrointestinal Endoscopy*, **43** (5), 540–545.

29 Leung, J.W. (2000) Reprocessing of flexible endoscopes. *Journal of Gastroenterology and Hepatology*, **15** (Suppl.), G73–G77.

30 Anderson, D.J. *et al.* (2008) Infectious complications following endoscopic retrograde cholangiopancreatography: an automated surveillance system for detecting postprocedure bacteremia. *American Journal of Infection Control*, **36** (8), 592–594.

31 Bou, R. *et al.* (2006) Nosocomial outbreak of *Pseudomonas aeruginosa* infections related to a flexible bronchoscope. *Journal of Hospital Infection*, **64** (2), 129–135.

32 Morris, J. *et al.* (2006) Gastrointestinal endoscopy decontamination failure and the risk of transmission of blood-borne viruses: a review. *Journal of Hospital Infection*, **63** (1), 1–13.

33 Aumeran, C. *et al.* (2010) Multidrug-resistant *Klebsiella pneumoniae* outbreak fater endoscopic retrograde cholangiopancreatography. *Endosopy*, **42** (11), 957–959.

34 (BSG) BSoG (1998) *BSG Guidelines for the Decontamination of Equipment for Gastrointestinal Endoscopy*.

35 Alfa, M. (2000) Medical Device Reprocessing, Infection Control and Hospital Epidemiology, **21**, 496–498.

36 Ofstead, C. *et al.* (2010) Endoscope reprocessing methods. *Society of Gastroenterology Nurses and Associates*, **33** (4), 304–311.

37 Vickery, K. *et al.* (2009) The effect of multiple cycles of contamination, detergent washing, and disinfection on the development of biofilm in endoscope tubing. *American Journal of Infection Control*, **37** (6), 470–475.

38 HealthCanada (1998) *Infection Control Guidelines – Hand Washing, Cleaning, Disinfection and Sterilization in Health Care*, Canada Communicabale Disease Report 24S8, HealthCanada, Ottawa.

39 Association of periOperative Registered Nurses (AORN) (2002) Recommended practices for cleaning and caring for surgical instruments and powered equipment. *AORN Journal*, **75** (3), 627–630, 633–636, 638 passim.

40 Society of Gastrointestinal Nursing Association (SGNA) (2007) *Guideline for Use of High Level Disinfectants and Sterilants for Reprocessing Flexible Gastrointestinal Endoscopes*, SGNA. http://www.sgna.org/Portals/0/Education/Practice%20Guidelines/HLDGuideline.pdf.

41 Ontario Public Health Division MoH, Provincial Infectious Diseases Advisory Committee (PIDAC) (2006) *Best Practices for Cleaning, Disinfection and Sterilization: In all Healthcare Settings*, Ottawa, ON, Canada. http://www.health.gov.on.ca/english/providers/program/infectious/diseases/ic_cds.html.

42 Ahishali, E. *et al.* (2008) Chemical colitis due to glutaraldehyde: case series and review of the literature. *Digestive Diseases and Sciences*, **54** (12), 2541–2545.

43 Alfa, M. *et al.* (2010) Evotech® endoscope cleaner and reprocessor (ECR) simulated-use and clinical-use evaluation of cleaning efficacy. *BMC Infectious Diseases (Electronic Resource)*, **10**, 200.

44 Martin, M.A. and Reichelderfer, M. (1994) APIC guidelines for infection prevention and control in flexible endoscopy. Association for Professionals in Infection Control and Epidemiology, Inc. 1991, 1992, and 1993 APIC Guidelines Committee. *American Journal of Infection Control*, **22** (1), 19–38.

45 Alfa, M.J. and Sitter, D.L. (1991) In-hospital evaluation of contamination of duodenoscopes: a quantitative assessment of the effect of drying. *Journal of Hospital Infection*, **19** (2), 89–98.

46 Pineau, L. *et al.* (2008) Endoscope drying/storage cabinet: interest and efficacy. *Journal of Hospital Infection*, **68** (1), 59–65.

47 Miner, N. *et al.* (2007) Sporicidal activity of disinfectants as one possible cause for bacteria in patient-ready endoscopes. *Gastroenterology Nursing*, **30** (4), 285–290.

48 NHS Estates (1997) *Health Management Memorandum HTM 2030. Washer Disinfectors, Operational Management, Design Consideratinos, Validation and Verificatino*, HMSO, London.

49 International Standards Organization (ISO) (2006) *ISO 15883. Washer Disinfectors – Part 1 and Part 5*, ISO, Geneva.

50 British Standards Institution (BSI) (2006) BS EN ISO 15883. Washer Disinfectors (Parts 1–4), BSI, Milton Keynes.

51 Medicines and Healthcare Products Regulatory Agency (MHRA, MaHPRA) (2002) *MDS DB 2002(05). Device Bulletin, Decontamination of Endoscopes*, Medical Devices Agency, London.

52 Griffiths, P.A. *et al.* (1997) Glutaraldehyde-resistant *Mycobacterium chelonae* from endoscope washer disinfectors. *Journal of Applied Microbiology*, **82** (4), 519–526.

53 Martin, D.J. *et al.* (2008) Resistance and cross-resistance to oxidising agents of bacterial isolates from endoscope washer disinfectors. *Journal of Hospital Infection*, **69** (4), 377–383.

54 Association for the Advancement of Medical Instrumentation (AAMI) (2008) *AAMI TIR34:2007. Water for the Reprocessing of Medical Devices*. AAMI, Arlington, VA, USA. www.aami.org.

55 Gillespie, E.E. *et al.* (2008) Microbiological monitoring of endoscopes: 5-year review. *Journal of Gastroenterology and Hepatology*, **23** (7 Pt 1): 1069–1074.

56 Riley, R. *et al.* (2002) Establishing the shelf life of flexible colonoscopes. *Gastroenterology Nursing*, **25** (3), 114–119.

57 Rejchrt, S. *et al.* (2004) Bacteriologic testing of endoscopes after high-level disinfection. *Gastrointestinal Endoscopy*, **60** (1), 76–78.

58 Alfa, M.J. *et al.* (1999) Worst-case soiling levels for patient-used flexible endoscopes before and after cleaning. *American Journal of Infection Control*, **27** (5), 392–401.

59 Kruger, S. (1997) Testing the cleaning efficacy in decontamination equipment. Part 1. *Zentr Steril (Central Service)*, **5**, 333–334.

60 Alfa, M.J. *et al.* (2009) Cleaning efficacy of medical device washers in North American healthcare facilities. *Journal of Hospital Infection*, **74** (2), 168–177.

61 Beilenhoff, U. *et al.* (2007) ESGE-ESGENA guideline for quality assurance in reprocessing: microbiological surveillance testing in endoscopy. *Endoscopy*, **39** (2), 175–181.

62 Obee, P.C. *et al.* (2005) Real-time monitoring in managing the decontamination of flexible gastrointestinal endoscopes. *American Journal of Infection Control*, **33** (4), 202–206.

63 Hansen, D. *et al.* (2004) ATP measurement as method to monitor the quality of reprocessing flexible endoscopes. *German Medical Science*, **2**, 1612–3174.

64 Osborne, S. *et al.* (2007) Challenging endoscopy reprocessing guidelines: a prospective study investigating the safe shelf life of flexible endoscopes in a tertiary gastroenterology unit. *Endoscopy*, **39** (9), 825–830.

65 (AAMI) (2003) *AAMI TIR30:2003. A Compendium of Processes, Materials, Test Methods, and Acceptance Criteria for Cleaning Reusable Medical Devices.*

66 Lewis, T. *et al.* (2008) A modified ATP benchmark for evaluating the cleaning of some hospital environmental surfaces. *Journal of Hospital Infection*, **69** (2), 156–163.

67 Verjat, D. *et al.* (1999) Fluorescence-assay on traces of protein on re-usable medical devices: cleaning efficiency. *International Journal of Pharmaceutics*, **179** (2), 267–271.

68 Alfa, M. *et al.* (2005) Validation of ATS as an appropriate test soil. *Zentr Steril (Central Service)*, **13**, 387–402.

19.4 Issues Associated with the Decontamination of Laundry and Clinical Waste

Peter Hoffman

Laboratory of Healthcare-associated Infection, Health Protection Agency, London, UK

Introduction

This chapter deals with two areas with contrasting legislative coverage in the UK. The first section, healthcare laundry, has no specific legislative basis and is covered by more general legislation, primarily the Health and Safety at Work etc. Act (HSAWA) and the Control of Substances Hazardous to Health Regulations (COSHH). The second, the clinical waste component of healthcare waste, has a specific, substantial and varied legislative basis within the component nations of the UK covering the classification, transport and disposal of trades waste and hazardous substances, with healthcare waste being only one of many waste categories covered, as well as the HSAWA and COSHH. The UK approach is based on interpretations of regulations that apply throughout the European Union. This contrasts with the USA, where there are generally no federal regulations on medical waste generation, transport and disposal, and individual state regulations apply but there is a federal requirement for "cradle-to-grave" tracking of medical waste.

Healthcare laundry

The washing of fabrics is probably the largest, by weight, decontamination task in the healthcare sector, yet it remains the one with the least clinical input or appreciation of its components. As with many other preventative interventions, it is not possible to gauge precisely the value of effective healthcare laundry decontamination, but bacteria causing infections in patients have been found on their bedsheets [1]. Contact between patients and their bedding is close and prolonged, and should bedding not be decontaminated between successive uses, there is a clear and significant potential for such fabrics to act as a vector of infection. In the UK, healthcare linens tend to be supplied by laundries that serve several hospitals rather than being owned by an individual hospital. This increases the potential for interhospital transmission of microbial strains causing healthcare-associated infections should laundry decontamination fail. Such transmission is most significant if it is with microbes that are already adapted to spreading and causing problematic infections in healthcare, such as those involving bacteria resistant to multiple antibiotics.

Routine healthcare laundry

The laundering of fabrics can combine two factors that reduce microbial contamination: there is always dilution (inherent in the washing process) and there can also be additional disinfection (thermal and/or chemical). Ironically, commercial laundries use as little water, and thus dilution, as possible. It represents a major cost in buying it and disposing of it to a public sewer (both charged by volume); the more water is used, the more it costs to heat it to the right temperature and the more it costs in process chemicals (detergents, etc.) to attain the correct concentrations. So large-scale commercial laundries favor automated

Russell, Hugo & Ayliffe's: Principles and Practice of Disinfection, Preservation and Sterilization, Fifth Edition. Edited by Adam P. Fraise, Jean-Yves Maillard, and Syed A. Sattar.
© 2013 Blackwell Publishing Ltd. Published 2013 by Blackwell Publishing Ltd.

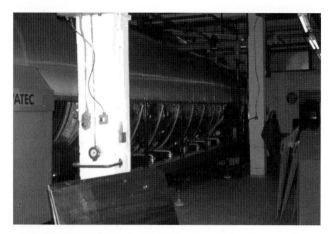

Figure 19.4.1 Example of a tunnel washer.

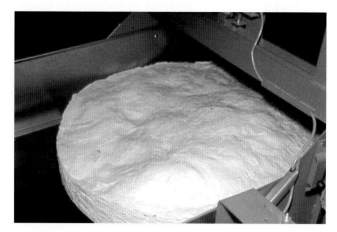

Figure 19.4.3 Linen processed by a tunnel washer.

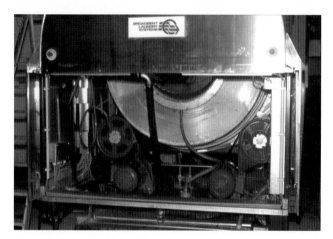

Figure 19.4.2 Detail of metal cylinder in a tunnel washer.

washing processes that have a high throughput and use low water volumes; this is exemplified in continuous tunnel washing machines.

Continuous tunnel washing machines

Continuous tunnel washing machines (CTWMs), also known as batch continuous washing machines or, more usually, tunnel washers, process the vast majority of healthcare laundry (Figure 19.4.1). A CTWM comprises a large metal cylinder (Figure 19.4.2), about 2 m in diameter and 15 m in length with an internal Archimedean screw that effectively divides it into a number of compartments, each of which contains one load of linen. This cylinder is on rollers, and rocks back and forth, agitating the linen in each compartment then, about every 2 min, the cylinder rotates 360°, moving each load of linen on to the next compartment. At the same time, another load of soiled laundry is added to the first compartment and a load of clean linen is ejected from the last compartment. Clean water is added to the last compartment and flows, either by gravity through small holes in the Archimedean screw or via pumps, backwards through the cylinder so, in essence, clean water and dirty linen flow countercurrent

to each other. Heat and wash chemicals can be added to individual compartments.

After clean linen is ejected from the last compartment (Figure 19.4.3), in the majority of laundries it proceeds automatically via a conveyer belt to a tumble drier set at a temperature and time appropriate to a particular linen type, for example sheets requiring less drying than towels. This dividing of linens into separate drying types for each load, essential for the economics of the process, requires laundry to be sorted before it is loaded into the CTWM. Such sorting is by hand, and the industrial conditions and high linen volumes mean that personal protective equipment used by staff is unlikely to be as effective as it would be when used by healthcare staff in clinical situations. Thus, safety requirements normally necessitate that linens contaminated with highly infectious microbes should not be processed by CTWMs.

Washer extractors

These are similar to large domestic or launderette washing machines where successive volumes of water and wash chemicals are added to linen in the wash compartment (Figure 19.4.4). These use high volumes of water and take about 40–50 min to process a single load (as opposed to a CTWM producing a load of clean linen every 2 min), making them highly uneconomic for processing anything but a very small proportion of laundry. They do have the advantage that a load of linen can be added with minimal staff contact, making them a much safer option for loads contaminated with highly infectious microbes.

Categorization of healthcare laundry

For the safety of laundry workers, linens contaminated with highly infectious microbes need to be clearly identifiable so that they can be loaded with minimal handling into washer extractors, rather than be hand-sorted for processing via a CTWM. The concept of "universal precautions" (treating all linens as infectious and processing them with minimal handling via washer extractors) has no place in healthcare laundries as there is too little washer-extractor capacity and it would be vastly uneconomic to process all linens this way. Microbiological safety in

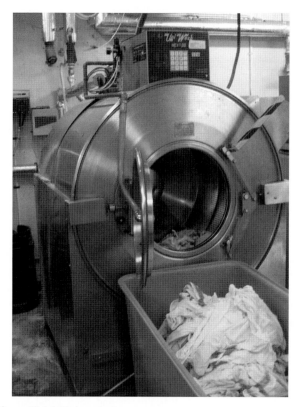

Figure 19.4.4 Washer extractor.

laundries is achieved by standard precautions (such as personal protective equipment, handwashing before eating or drinking, etc.) by those sorting linen for CTWM processing and additional precautions (minimal contact) by those loading linen contaminated with highly infectious microbes into washer extractors. This requires categorization of laundry into the two main types ("used" and "infectious" – see below) at the point of production by those aware of an individual patient's status.

• *Used linen.* This is the vast majority of healthcare linens. It can be soiled or contaminated with blood, feces or other body fluids ("fouled"). It can be from patients with infections that are not readily transmitted to laundry workers (e.g. the presence of methicillin-resistant *Staphylococcus aureus* (MRSA) or *Clostridium difficile* is acceptable on used linen).

• *Infectious linen.* This is linen contaminated with microbes that are an infectious hazard to those who may come into contact with it. These should be defined locally but could include microbes readily transmitted by the fecal–oral route (*Salmonella, Shigella*, norovirus, etc.) and linens bloodstained from known or suspected bloodborne virus carriers. This type of linen is sometimes misleadingly referred to as "infected", a term that encourages clinical staff to use this classification for linen from a patient with any infection, the vast majority of which pose a minimal hazard to those coming into contact with it.

• *Thermolabile linen.* This is linen that would be damaged by heat disinfection. It should form a very small proportion of

laundry from acute healthcare and is predominantly patients' own clothing in long-stay facilities.

Decontamination of laundry

Both "used" and "infectious" linen should be heat disinfected using a minimum of either 65°C for 10 min or 71°C for 3 min [2]. These holding times apply only from when the linen has equilibrated to the disinfection temperature. There is no difference in the decontamination parameters between these two categories, only in the handling before decontamination. Used linen is usually sorted into different drying types and is processed in a CTWM; infectious linen is usually loaded directly into a washer extractor with minimal handling.

Thermolabile linen is processed in a washer extractor at sub-disinfection temperatures and chemically disinfected with sodium hypochlorite at 150 ppm available chlorine and a contact time of at least 5 min in the penultimate rinse. This disinfection must be in a rinse phase as any organic matter present before washing could inactivate the low hypochlorite concentration needed to keep bleaching to a minimum. It is in the penultimate rinse, so that the last rinse can remove the odor of chlorine from the fabric. Some other chemical disinfection processes, such as the dosing of wash and rinsewater with ozone, may also be suitable for use in washer extractors if continuously monitored.

Chemical disinfection of used and infectious laundry

This remains largely unexplored on an industrial scale but the energy savings that could be made by using chemical disinfection at more modestly elevated temperatures are attractive. If this is to be used, disinfectants need to be shown to have sufficient activity at the concentration, exposure time and temperature that are achieved in practice. Laboratory data showing activity outside these parameters offers no indication of practical efficacy. Following laboratory tests, there would need to be verification that, with specified cycle parameters, effective disinfection can occur in the actual wash process used. That these parameters are being achieved in every wash should also be part of the quality assurance of the routine process and these parameters should be observable in real time rather than in retrospect.

Staff uniforms

The laundering of healthcare staff uniforms is a controversial and sometimes emotive area. This was examined in a review of available evidence and informed opinion [3], and guidance based on this was issued by the English Department of Health [4] which suggests that there is little hygienic difference between domestic and commercial washing of uniforms, even at lower wash temperatures. The uniforms of clinical staff can be washed in their own domestic washing machines as part of a mixed load at temperatures appropriate for that fabric type. If uniforms are heavily soiled, they should be washed domestically separately from other items or can be sent for commercial healthcare laundering.

Dry cleaning

There should be minimal need for dry cleaning of healthcare fabrics but it may occasionally be needed for patients' personal clothing or particularly treasured soft toys. While there is a little evidence that the process gives some reduction in enveloped viruses and some bacteria [5], for those microbes not killed by the solvent used there can be poor reduction produced by the dilution of the wash process alone. Where steam pressing can be used to finish garments, this will add a heat disinfection element. Dry cleaning should not be an infection control measure of first choice.

Washing machines in acute clinical areas

These should be generally discouraged, but there may be a few areas where their use is difficult to avoid. For example, some neonatal units may have small woolen items such as babies' socks that are unsuitable for industrial washing. If such units are forbidden washing machines, these items may only be rinsed out and dried on radiators between uses. If this is the case, the installation of washing machines and driers on a planned preventative maintenance schedule and agreements about what they can process, may represent acceptable risk control. There should also be an understanding that, in case of infection outbreaks, special measures in agreement with the local infection control team, such as treating delicate clothing items as single use, may be necessary.

Laundry quality assurance systems

The most common quality assurance system for laundries is based on the standard EN14065 *Textiles. Laundry Processed Textiles. Biocontamination Control System* [6]. This is similar to other hazard analysis critical control point (HACCP) systems but in this context is known as a risk analysis biocontamination control (RABC) system. In this system, representatives of the laundry and invited advisors decide what local parameters are important to the production of microbiologically acceptable textiles, how to measure them, what values are acceptable, the tolerances on those values and corrective actions when those values are exceeded. In practice, this system is reliable only if the team devising and implementing it are knowledgeable about what the critical parameters really are. It is possible to have RABC systems where irrelevant surfaces are sampled (the hoppers that contain fabrics pre-decontamination, for example) and pointless corrective actions taken. If appraising an RABC system, the most important steps are the decontamination parameters (usually monitoring of the temperature of disinfection and the duration it is maintained) and prevention of recontamination with healthcare-associated contamination (i.e. directly or indirectly from undecontaminated linen), both at the laundry and during transport (the same vehicle is usually used for collection of dirty linen and the delivery of clean linen).

Clinical waste

The classification, transport and disposal of clinical waste are governed by a stronger legislative base than most other areas of healthcare that involve decontamination and infection prevention. Essentially, waste from healthcare is classified as a category of industrial waste, different components of which may contain a wide variety of hazards, for example harmful, toxic, mutagenic, flammable and infectious. Wastes may also contain more than one hazard. Although this section will only cover those wastes classified under the Hazardous Waste Regulations as category H9 "infectious", healthcare establishments have an overall duty to meet legislative requirements for all types of waste that they produce, both for safety and environmental reasons. For example, the Health and Social Care Act 2008 Code of Practice on the prevention and control of infections and related guidance [7] requires that "The risks from waste disposal should be properly controlled" and "Systems should be in place to ensure that the risks to service users from exposure to infections caused by waste present in the environment are properly managed, and that duties under environmental law are discharged". Guidance on how to achieve this is given in the Department of Health's document *Safe Management of Healthcare Waste* [8]. The Code of Practice covers "registered providers of all healthcare and adult social care in England" – that is not just hospitals, but general medical practitioners, dentists, podiatrists, opticians, pharmacies, private and independent healthcare organizations, ambulance trusts, complementary and alternative treatments, residential homes and similar establishments.

Healthcare waste is defined as being waste specifically associated with the activity of healthcare. Wastes incidental to the activity of healthcare (examples would be waste oil from an ambulance or food waste from a hospital kitchen) are not healthcare waste.

Segregation of clinical waste

It is a legal requirement that items of healthcare waste be classified according to the risk or risks they possess such they can be transported and disposed of appropriately. With regard to infectious waste, it can be either category A or B:
• Category A infectious waste is: "an infectious substance which is transported in a form that, when exposure to it occurs, is capable of causing permanent disability, life-threatening or fatal disease to humans or animals".
• Category B infectious waste is: "an infectious substance which does not meet the criteria for inclusion in Category A".
The interpretation of category A waste is that from patients with viral hemorrhagic fevers, monkeypox virus and variola, and cultures of containment level 3 microorganisms. This means that all routine infectious clinical waste is category B.

In addition to the attribute "infectious", other hazards must be considered in the classification of infectious waste for transport and disposal. The main additional hazard classifications are:

sharp, cytotoxic or cytostatic, medicinal but not cytotoxic/cytostatic, radioactive, mercury amalgam and anatomical (this last category is not of itself a hazard but does carry additional legislative requirements). Infectious waste could have one or more of these additional attributes. Each attribute or group of attributes will require segregation from others.

Color coding of clinical waste containers

The color coding of clinical waste containers is vital in the early stages of the journey of clinical waste and communicates the pathway which that particular container should follow to final disposal.

Yellow is indicative of bagged waste that must be incinerated as its final disposal. Category A infectious waste and medicinal (not cytotoxic/cytostatic) will be put into yellow containers. Other colors may be used in addition to a predominantly yellow container to indicate additional hazards: red indicates anatomical waste; purple indicates cytotoxic/cytostatic-containing waste. These must all be incinerated.

If bagged clinical waste can be rendered safe by alternative treatments to incineration, essentially category B infectious waste with no additional hazards, it is placed in orange containers.

Sharps containers have a yellow body with different color lids denoting more specific risks and appropriate disposal methods: with orange lids for category B infectious sharps, with purple lids for sharps with cytotoxic/cytostatic contamination, with yellow lids for sharps with medicinal (not cytotoxic/cytostatic) contamination. The volume of medicinal waste retained in a discharged syringe is judged sufficiently small that it can be disposed of as non-medicinal waste. Syringes with more medicinal remnants than this must not be discharged just so they can be disposed of as non-medicinal waste. Syringes contaminated with even residual volumes of cytotoxic/cytostatic fluids must be disposed of as contaminated with these.

Infectious waste

The definition of infectious waste is waste that "may cause infection to any person (or animal) coming into contact with it". This is not particularly helpful to clinicians who will appreciate the highly subjective nature of such a definition. It is a legal definition that waste from an individual who has an infection is categorized as infectious when the waste is connected with that infection. For example, the urine of a patient with an ear infection is not considered infectious; the urine of a patient with a urinary tract infection is considered infectious. That the microorganisms infecting a highly susceptible patient in hospital may be of low pathogenicity and very unlikely to give rise to infections in those who come into contact with the waste is not to be considered in this legal definition. Some body fluids may also be generically classified as infectious, blood for example would normally be classified as infectious unless it had specifically been screened; empty blood transfusion bags could, for example, be considered as offensive waste (see below) rather than infectious.

Offensive waste

This is healthcare waste that does not have the hazardous properties of clinical waste but may cause offense. Examples being incontinence pads, nappies and sanitary waste from healthcare. Offensive waste should be collected in yellow bags with prominent black stripes ("tiger stripe" bags). This waste can go to landfill sites licensed for this type of waste or be incinerated at municipal (i.e. not clinical waste) incinerators such as energy-from-waste facilities; such final disposal is significantly less expensive than either clinical waste incineration or alternative treatments. This is a substantially underused healthcare waste category and if a higher proportion of offensive waste were classified as such, it would represent a substantial cost and energy saving in healthcare waste disposal.

The risk assessment for waste being offensive rather than infectious can be done on a generic basis, for example incontinence pads from units where these are in routine use and are not associated with infectious conditions could generically be considered as offensive waste. This would change if there were clinical suspicion of the presence of infection, for example if there were a norovirus outbreak.

Storage of clinical waste

Bulk waste should be stored before collection in an enclosed, secure, cleanable area that can be locked when access in not required. There should be segregation of different waste types within this area. It should have washing facilities for staff.

Transfer documentation

Bulk wastes must have documentation that accurately describes the waste and its origins. This documentation (a "waste transfer note") must follow the waste from its origin to the point of final disposal. Small amounts of waste, for example that carried in an individual ambulance or produced by a GP practice, do not require such documentation, but when that waste is collected into a bulk quantity, documentation is required.

Accidents and incidents

Within any waste management policy should be actions to be taken in case of spillage. Staff should be trained in how to deal with spills of infectious waste, including sharps. Suitable spill kits and disinfectants should be provided.

Final disposal method

Final disposal by incineration was traditionally the fate of all infectious clinical waste. A variety of constraints, principally stringent pollution controls, make this an expensive option and likely to become more so. It is accepted that a variety of alternative treatments to incineration can render certain categories of infectious waste safe, and can be less expensive and less damaging to the environment. These are generically known as "alternative treatments" and may involve heating by microwaves, steam under pressure or other technologies.

All infectious waste must be rendered safe as part of its disposal. The accepted definition of rendering clinical waste safe (excluding laboratory cultures) is a process that has been demonstrated to achieve at least a million-fold (6-$\log_{10}$) reduction in vegetative bacteria and a 10,000-fold (4-$\log_{10}$) reduction in bacterial spores. In addition to any microbicidal action, for patient confidentiality any patient identifiable data (such as names on specimen containers) should be rendered unrecognizable.

Types of disposal

Incineration

Clinical waste incinerators are becoming increasingly sophisticated and costly, not to ensure adequate microbial kill (any burning method would produce sufficient reductions), but to reduce the output of pollutant combustion products. Incinerators have two chambers; the first where the load is broken down into gaseous molecules at 800–1000°C and which feeds in to a second chamber with a temperature of at least 1100°C and a dwell time of at least 2 s, where large gaseous molecules are broken down even further. Gas scrubbing before emission will remove the majority of toxic pollutants such as sulfur dioxide and hydrogen chloride.

Variations on incineration are pyrolysis and gasification, where waste is heated in the absence (pyrolysis) or minimal amounts (gasification) of air in a primary chamber, and the resultant gases fed into a secondary chamber at 1100°C.

Alternative technologies

Alternatives to incineration tend to be less costly and, as they require less extensive plant, can be on or close to the site of waste production.

Microwave-based treatments generally shred the waste, add water (usually as steam) to the load and then use microwaves to produce atmospheric pressure steam in the waste to thermally disinfect it. This can be done on a continuous basis with an auger moving shredded waste past the microwave sources. Similar systems inject steam directly into the auger and use the energy from that to disinfect without extra energy from microwaves.

Clinical waste autoclaves use steam under pressure to treat batches of clinical waste. There also exist chemical disinfection systems where the disinfectant is added to shredded waste. If these are used, it should be ensured that one hazard in the waste (microbial) is not replaced with another hazard (chemical) and, while the disinfectant is effective, that it does not leave toxic substances in the treated waste.

Conclusions

Healthcare laundry currently faces a number of issues that need to be resolved. For large-scale laundries, a crucial issue is that of energy efficiency, with the requirement for thermal disinfection being one of the more substantial uses of energy. If safe and effective chemical disinfection could achieve acceptable results at lower temperatures, this would save considerable energy but needs to be within a reliably high-quality assurance process. Suitable processes and means of monitoring them on a real-time basis are needed. Another issue is that of the laundering requirements of a variety of establishments outside the acute healthcare sector. To what extent do the laundering requirements of, for example, a care home need to be the same as those for providers of linen for high-dependency healthcare? If different requirements are applicable to less acute healthcare, what should these be and how should they be graded across the spectrum this sector offers? As the non-acute care sectors generate a high proportion of laundry that cannot be thermally disinfected, mostly personal clothing, do they need to be chemically disinfected or is the dilution in a washing process sufficient, as has been judged adequate for staff uniforms?

For clinical waste, a significant future issue is the development of more alternatives to incineration. The vast majority of infectious clinical waste can be made safe by comparatively simple treatments before it progresses to a less environmentally damaging final disposal, which is also considerably less costly than the more traditional incineration. The category of "offensive waste" is currently very underused, probably caused by difficulties in practical classification of waste into this category. Use of this classification would allow less rigorous transport and disposal at significantly reduced cost. A survey by the UK Royal College of Nursing (RCN) [9] estimated a national saving of over £5 million if 20% of what is currently infectious waste were to be reclassified as offensive waste. A similar logic applies to the overall reduction in the generation of infectious waste. Repeated surveys show that hospital staff are poor at distinguishing in practice between what should go in the domestic (black bag) waste stream and the infectious (orange bag) waste stream. The same RCN survey estimated that if 20% of infectious waste were reclassified as domestic waste, the savings would be nearly £9 million [9].

References

1 Sanderson, P.J. and Alshafi, K.M. (1995) Environmental contamination by organisms causing urinary tract infection. *Journal of Hospital Infection*, **29**, 301–303.

2 Department of Health (2012) Choice Framework for local Policy and Procedures 01-04 – Decontamination of linen for health and social care: Engineering, equipment and validation manual. Department of Health, London.

3 Wilson, J.A. *et al.* (2007) Uniform: an evidence review of the microbiological significance of uniforms and uniform policy in the prevention and control of healthcare-associated infections. *Journal of Hospital Infection*, **66**, 301–307.

4 Department of Health (2010) *Uniforms and Workwear: Guidance on Uniform and Workwear Policies for NHS Employers*, Department of Health, London.

5 Bates, C.J. *et al.* (1993) The efficacy of hospital dry cleaning in disinfecting material contaminated with bacteria and viruses. *Journal of Hospital Infection*, **23**, 255–262.

6 British Standards Institution (2002) *BS EN 14065. Textiles. Laundry Processed Textiles. Biocontamination Control System*, BSI, London.

7 Department of Health (2010) *The Health and Social Care Act 2008 Code of Practice on the Prevention and Control of Infections and Related Guidance*, Department of Health, London.

8 Department of Health (2012) *Safe Management of Healthcare Waste, version 2.0*, Department of Health, London.

9 Royal College of Nursing (2011) *Freedom of Information Report on Waste Management*, RCN Publication Code 004 108, Royal College of Nursing, London.

Further reading

1 Department of Health (2006) *Standards for Better Health*, http://www.dh.gov.uk/en/Publicationsandstatistics/Publications/PublicationsPolicyAndGuidance/DH_4086665 (accessed June 12, 2012).

19.5 Treated Recreational Water Venues

Darla M. Goeres[1], Philippe Hartemann[2] and John V. Dadswell[3]

[1] Center for Biofilm Engineering, Montana State University, Bozeman, MT, USA
[2] Department of Environment and Public Health, Nancy School of Medicine, Lorraine University, Vandoeuvre-Nancy, France
[3] Reading, UK

Introduction

Swimming is an activity enjoyed by people of all ages and abilities in all parts of the world. Swimming promotes known health benefits. The water provides support for the body, making it an ideal activity for people with joint pain or who are recovering from an injury. In addition to exercise, soaking in hot tubs or hot springs promotes relaxation and soothes sore muscles. With the notable health benefits and enjoyment associated with swimming, it is important that the water and facility do not become a source of disease and/or injury. Swimming may be thought of as communal bathing. Bathers introduce varying amounts of organics into the water including sweat, urine, dead skin, hair, oils, lotions and microorganisms every time they enter. The type and concentration of organics introduced by the bather is a function of the individual and the facility they are using. A small child in swim diapers in a splash pool is very different to an adult competitive swimmer practicing in a lap pool. Regardless, it is the responsibility of the facility operator to maintain healthy water quality.

Four factors contribute to maintaining a healthy water quality in a recreational water facility: engineering design, water chemistry, disinfection and facility management. All factors must be operating properly for a facility to maintain a healthy bathing environment. For instance, if a facility operator does not adhere to their policies in remediating a fecal accident in the pool water, then even if the facility has a disinfectant residual when the event occurred, they have still placed the other bathers at risk. This chapter will present a holistic approach for the maintenance of recreational water. This includes a discussion on the engineering aspects that define the different facilities, a general discussion on maintaining balanced water chemistry, the use and evaluation of disinfectants and a general discussion at the end on the importance of well-trained facility managers. An overview of the various illnesses that are associated with recreational water which is not maintained correctly are presented as a cautionary note. Finally, like any industry, recreational water is subject to trends, which will be addressed in the appropriate sections.

Engineering design considerations

People have enjoyed built communal swimming pools for centuries. The original design for these pools was simple. Hot water, typically from a spring, was piped into an enclosed structure and the spent water flowed out. Over time, this simple design evolved to include recycle, filtration and heat exchangers so that a cold source water could be used. At some point, disinfectants were added and the water chemistry was balanced. In recent history, recreational water facilities have evolved well beyond a simple swimming pool to include complex water parks with specialized pools. The engineer who designs the facility must balance fundamental concepts, such as filtration, recycle rates, material choices and safety with energy costs, ease of maintenance and, of course, bather enjoyment. A poorly designed facility is virtually impossible to maintain, whether it is new or old. An old facility, though, poses special engineering challenges including high maintenance costs and the challenge of retrofitting new technology in an old system. This section will discuss a selection of recreational water facilities and the engineering design parameters that set them apart from each other.

Swimming pools and water parks

Historically, swimming pools were simple geometric shapes constructed out of concrete, tile or vinyl. The swimming pool was filled with water that was continuously recycled through skimmers to remove gross contamination, a filter to remove smaller particles and a heat exchanger to warm the water before going back into the pool. Although the water is recycled, a small percent of freshwater is routinely added to public pools. The turnover rate, also known as recycle rate, is the time required for the entire volume of water in the swimming pool to make it through the entire process. A typical turnover rate for swimming pools is 6 h, which means that the entire pool volume passes through the filter four times every day. The actual turnover rate is set by the design guidelines under which the pool is operating. A well-designed pool has no dead spaces, where water is allowed to stagnate and avoid going through the filter. Dead spaces occur when the placement of the inlets from the filter and outlets to the filter create a flow channel. In addition to preventing channeling, inlets and outlets are designed with swimmer safety in mind. It is important that the inlets and outlets are designed to prevent reasonably small items from entering the filter, "trapping" swimmers under water or causing injury from exposed rusty or sharp edges.

One of the most important engineering parameters in swimming pool design is the filter. Swimming pool filters are generally constructed from diatomaceous earth, sand or compressed synthetic fibers housed inside a cartridge. The goal of filtration is to remove very small particles, on the order of magnitude of 20–100 μm. The filter loading rate is defined as volume per time per area. Filter loading rates are specified in swimming pool design guidelines. Filters are sized based upon the requirements for the filter loading and turnover rates and the volume of water in the pool. The actual surface area available in a swimming pool filter is much greater than the calculated cross-sectional surface area. This large surface area provides an ideal location for bacteria and other charged particles to attach, which means over time the filter will start to foul. Fouling is indicated by an increase in the pressure drop across the filter. In practical terms, more power is required to push water through a plugged filter at the same rate as an unplugged filter. As a filter becomes plugged, the water will begin to find a preferred path or channel through which to flow. Once this happens, the

filter is no longer operating according to design specifications. To keep the filters operating properly, it is important that they are cleaned regularly using a backwashing procedure, and replaced when backwashing does not decrease the pressure drop to an acceptable level.

A more recent trend in swimming pool filtration technology is the use of coagulants and flocculants to reduce turbidity and improve water quality by the removal of particles smaller than 20 μm. For instance, researchers are investigating the use of flocculation for the improved removal of *Cryptosporidium* oocysts [1]. Another research area is the use of filters filled with granular activated carbon (GAC) which would filter out both microbial contaminants and organics, thereby reducing the formation of disinfection by-products [2].

Swimming pools are found both indoors and outdoors. Both locations pose their own set of challenges. For outdoor swimming pools, increased exposure to the elements will lead to increased levels of contamination from dust, dirt, pollen, leaves, insects, etc. that find their way into the pool water from the environment. An intense rainfall will impact the water's chemistry and sunlight will cause both evaporation and chlorine degradation. Air quality is a concern for swimming pools located indoors, including the accumulation of disinfection by-products and increased humidity, which can lead to higher microbial contamination rates of items located next to the swimming pool, such as carpets and painted walls.

In recent years, the complexity of swimming pools has grown dramatically with the popularity of water theme-parks that include features to encourage play and a fun swimming experience. These may include slides, wave pools, features that spray water, collect and dump water or toys anchored in water, all of which may pose a challenge for maintaining healthy water quality [3]. Many of these features are designed specifically for small children that are not yet potty trained. It is not uncommon to find these water parks inside, especially in colder climates. This enables the water park to operate year-round to maximize profits. The new designs, although fun, have resulted in new challenges for maintaining the water quality. The aerosolized water may spread contaminants [4], increase the rate of chlorine degradation and make it more challenging to maintain balanced water chemistry. Features such as slides have a large surface area and intimate contact with people yet little treated water flowing over them. Often all the water from the various features will be piped to one filter system. Therefore, in case of a fecal accident, the quick spread of the contaminate to the other features could put the health of many bathers at risk.

As energy becomes more expensive, the costs associated with operating a swimming pool will also increase. The energy required to heat a pool is significant, but the costs of pumping water through the system cannot be overlooked. There are multiple avenues that may be pursued for a more environmentally-friendly and affordable means of energy (e.g. the use of solar power is a viable option given that many pools and water parks are located in warmer climates [5]), better insulation, wind breaks and the use of pool blankets. It is important to consider the impact an engineering cost-saving design "improvement" has on the entire system, though. For instance, even though fewer turnovers per day would save money, the impact on the sanitary condition of the water and therefore increased risk of infection would not balance the cost savings.

Hot tubs and spas

Hot tubs (also known as spas) are smaller tubs of water that are used recreationally for relaxation or for therapy. Hot tubs contain a separate circulation system with air blowers and hydrotherapy jets, which help soothe sore muscles, increase blood flow to the central organs, provide respiratory exercise and provide a relaxing effect [6]. As with the increase in popularity of water parks, hot tubs have also become more common. Like swimming pools, the water quality in a hot tub is maintained through the use of filtration and addition of chemicals. These common features resulted in hot tubs being regulated and maintained as small swimming pools, although there are numerous design and operational parameters that distinguish them from swimming pools, including high operational temperatures, heavy bather loads, aeration, large surface area to volume ratios and different water turnover rates. These particular features elucidate the difficulty in maintaining balanced water quality in a hot tub, which may allow for the formation of biofilm within the piping and filter [7], resulting in an increased risk of exposure to microorganisms.

Hot springs and natural pools

Hot springs or natural pools are filled with water from thermal features that usually contain geochemical properties that bathers enjoy. The water most often flows through the pool and is not recycled through a filter, and there is no need to heat the water. Typically these pools are drained and cleaned every day. Disinfectants are often not added to hot springs and natural pools, which place bathers at risk of exposure to microorganisms shed by the bather next to them.

Whirlpool baths and birthing pools designed for a single user

Hydrotherapy pools, birthing pools and drain-and-fill whirlpool bath tubs are fundamentally different from the previously described features in that they are designed for a single user and are drained and cleaned between each use. These features are included in this chapter because most of them contain jets that are used to soothe sore muscles and promote relaxation. Typically, the jets are not readily accessible for cleaning, and if the water does not completely drain from the tubing or housing, then bacterial biofilms may start to form. This poses a problem if the biofilm detaches while the jets are operating, exposing the bather to aerosolized bacteria [4, 8]. Maintenance of these systems requires adding a liquid disinfectant to the water once the bather has exited the bath and running the jets for a specified contact time.

Water chemistry

Balanced water chemistry is the second of the four factors that contribute to maintaining healthy water quality in a recreational water facility. The term "balanced" refers to the water's saturation or Langelier index. The five parameters that are used to calculate the saturation index are: temperature, pH, total alkalinity, calcium hardness and total dissolved solids. The first four parameters are easily measured and adjusted. If the total dissolved solids measurement becomes too high, then either some of the pool water must be drained and make-up water added, or a flocculent added and the solids filtered out of the water. A discussion on how to calculate the Langelier index is beyond the scope of this chapter, and may be found in water chemistry texts [9, 10].

Unsaturated water is corrosive and attacks the equipment and pool surfaces; conversely, overly saturated water results in scale deposits and cloudy water. In addition to the negative impacts unbalanced water has upon the facility's equipment, it may also result in bather discomfort by irritating the skin or eyes. Finally, many disinfectants, particularly the halogens, depend upon balanced water chemistry to achieve the desired levels of water decontamination.

Disinfection

The need for proper disinfection of swimming pool water has been known for a long time [11]. The primary function of a disinfectant is to make the water microbiologically safe for swimmers, and this is accomplished by bringing to an acceptable level the number of viable organisms found both in the pool water and as biofilms on all the exposed surfaces. While an "acceptable level" remains difficult to define, the goal is to minimize the risk of illness to those using the recreational facility.

Chorine is the most common chemical used to disinfect water in recreational facilities. Although chlorine is used in various forms and under different trade names, the mechanism of its microbicidal action remains the same. In water, chlorine forms hypochlorous acid and hypochlorite ions, and the total concentration of these two compounds is known as the free available chlorine (FAC) level in the treated water. The relative proportions of the hypochlorous acid and hypochlorite depend upon the pH of the water. Under acidic conditions the proportion of hypochlorous acid is higher but under alkaline conditions hypochlorite ions predominate. Whether the pH of treated water increases or decreases depends upon the chemical formulation of the product used. The pH of the water is, therefore, critical because hypochlorous acid is a stronger microbicide than hypochlorite ions. Another challenge with chlorine disinfection in swimming pools is that inorganic chlorine compounds are degraded by direct sunlight. Cyanuric acid is combined with chlorine to form a more stabilized compound; two examples of stabilized chlorine are sodium dichloro-*s*-triazinetrione and trichloro-*s*-triazinetrione.

The strong oxidizing potential of chlorine also helps reduce the levels of organics in recreational waters, thus improving its overall quality. Incomplete oxidation results in the formation of combined chlorine compounds. The difference between the total chlorine concentration and FAC concentration is the combined chlorine concentration. If the combined chlorine concentration becomes too high (>0.2–0.3 mg/l), then the water should be subjected to breakpoint chlorination. The reaction of chlorine with organics in water may lead to the formation of potentially harmful disinfection by-products (DBPs), as discussed below. This also requires maintaining a fine balance between the necessary level of disinfectant residual while minimizing the generation of toxic DBPs. Improved water filtration is among the approaches used to reduce the risk of DBP generation in recreational waters [2, 12].

Numerous other options exist for disinfecting waters in recreational facilities. Products based on other halogens such as bromine and iodine face many of the same challenges as described for chlorine. Ozone and UV light are also used to disinfect swimming pool water in many facilities. The use of ozone or UV does not impact the pH, odor or taste of water. However, neither ozone nor UV leaves a disinfectant residual and this may promote the formation of biofilms in the system. Therefore, ozone and UV should be used in conjunction with another disinfectant that is capable of maintaining a disinfectant residual. Additional options for recreational water disinfection include biguanides, silver and copper ions. These options require an additional chemical to oxidize the water. In addition to products formulated to sanitize and/or oxidize the water, many companies sell additives such as algaecides, scale removers, chelating agents, degreasers, defoamers, flocculants or enzymes to improve the overall quality of the water.

The rapid and continuing evolution of the disinfection of recreational waters market would quickly outdate any listing of current strategies. Nor is it likely that a "perfect" product or technique will soon be found for this purpose. Thus, the selection from what is available must be based on the specific needs of the site, the age of the system under consideration and its user profile, while remembering that even the best system will likely fail without proper training of the operators and routine maintenance and monitoring of the facility.

Efficacy testing disinfectants
Much has been published on the testing of various swimming pool disinfectants [13–16] and the laboratory tests available for this purpose [17, 18]. Nevertheless, proper and routine testing under field conditions is vital for bather safety as well as longevity of the infrastructure. The list of parameters to monitor may include:
• Dose (concentration and quantity) of disinfectant added.
• Disinfectant residual maintained.
• Daily record of the water chemistry parameters previously described.

• Bulk water and surface (biofilm) samples to quantify numbers of viable organisms.
• Engineering parameters that define the system such as number of turnovers per day; filtration type and rate, facility location, number of pools, etc.
• Addition of other chemicals such as flocculants, algaecides, sequestering agents, degreasers, defoamers and stabilizing agents.
• Hours of operation and number of users per hour.
• Duration of the field test.
• Description of the area around swimming pool, for instance is the pool surrounded by cement, grass, tile, carpet or sand?
• Training received by facility operators.

A field test will not gauge a disinfectant's "true" efficacy if biofilm samples are not collected alongside those from the bulk water [15, 17, 19–21]; this is particularly crucial for hot tubs [7] as pathogens in biofilms may be better protected from disinfectants [22–25]. Although information on the importance of biofilms in recreational waters dates back to the late 1980s, regulators, public health officials and facility managers have been slow to appreciate this.

Health effects

Swimming in public pools and sharing hot tubs is tantamount to communal bathing. While such activities may spread infections [26], there is a recent upsurge of interest in the potential of chemically-disinfected recreational waters to cause respiratory disorders, especially in young swimmers [27]. This section will address health issues from both infectious agents and chemicals in recreational waters.

Skin, ear and eye irritation and infection
Disinfectant chemicals frequently cause skin irritation in pool users, chlorine sensitivity being less common than the "bromine rash" which may be associated with dimethylhydantoin [28, 29]. Such skin sensitivity is related to the degree of exposure, and physiotherapists who may spend a lot of time in a hydrotherapy pool are particularly at risk. Initially, the rash may appear about 12 h after exposure but, once sensitized, it may do so almost immediately after contact with the water.

In contrast, the itchy rash from *Pseudomonas aeruginosa* infection may take 12–24 h to manifest [28]. This condition, which is an infection of the hair follicles, resolves itself in about a week in otherwise healthy persons. It is more often associated with spa pools, where the raised temperature and agitation of the waters render the skin more susceptible. The introduction of *P. aeruginosa* in the follicles is also facilitated by the pressure during water-massage.

Otitis externa may also be caused by chemical irritation or by infection with *P. aeruginosa*, especially when the uncovered head is submerged during swimming. The condition is more common in competitive swimmers and divers.

Swimming bath granuloma, caused by *Mycobacterium marinum*, can be acquired in pools with cracked and roughened surfaces wherein the organism can proliferate. Infections with *Mycobacterium avium* and *Mycobacterium abscessus* have also been reported [30, 31]. Fungal infections of the feet and viral warts are often associated with pool use but are more likely to be spread from contact with contaminated surfaces surrounding the pool rather than the pool water itself. The sharing of towels and bath sponges was the likely cause of an outbreak of molluscum contagiosum, a viral infection of the skin [32].

Conjunctivitis is not an uncommon complaint among swimmers but is usually the result of chemical irritation, such as with a low pH value or high combined chlorine levels. Infective conjunctivitis is more likely to be spread directly from person to person by shared towels than by the water, but outbreaks of eye infections due to adenoviruses can occur from swimming in pools with inadequate levels of disinfectant residuals.

Gastrointestinal infections

Outbreaks of infections due to *Giardia* [33], *Cryptosporidium* [34], *Escherichia coli* O157:H7 [35], norovirus [36] and hepatitis A virus [37] have been reported in swimming pool users. Such outbreaks are now rare due to better maintenance and monitoring of disinfectant levels in public pools.

Respiratory irritation and infections

Some bathers, asthmatics in particular, may experience wheezing from exposure to the chemicals in the pool atmosphere. This is now well established to be due to disinfection by-products [27].

Every swimmer contributes about 2.3–2.6 billion potentially pathogenic microorganisms in a swimming pool [38]. The microbicidal properties of several agents, especially chlorine, are used to avoid cross-transmission of such pathogens and eventual infections [39]. But the reaction of chlorine with organic matter generates some DBPs. Even though this topic is still controversial, in epidemiological studies the exposure to DPBs through drinking water consumption is linked with the development of bladder cancers [40] and less often colorectal cancers [41]. Recent works have discussed hazards for the workers and users of indoor swimming pools [42, 43] that come from acute respiratory exposure to trichloramine (or nitrogen trichloride).

The most common DBP is the family of trihalomethanes (THMs), which contains chloroform, bromodichloromethane (BDCM), dibromochloromethane (DBCM) and bromoform. The trihalomethanes were chosen as the markers of DBP contamination because information about their toxicity and effects are known. Chloroform is classified as 2B (possible human carcinogen) by the International Agency for Research on Cancer (IARC) and B2 (probable human carcinogen) by the US Environmental Protection Agency (EPA). The situation is identical for BDCM, which is classified as 3 by the IARC (not classifiable for human carcinogenicity) and C by the EPA (possible human carcinogen). Bromoform is classified as 3 by the IARC but 2B by the EPA.

Much research has been carried out in many countries to determine the exposure and doses of DBPs through domestic uses of drinking water [41, 44, 45]. Others European studies have tried to determine the exposure during swimming activities [38, 46–49]. THMs in pool water may reach much higher concentrations than those normally found and regulated in drinking water [48, 50]. Chloroform is the dominant and most abundant species in pools treated with chlorine and ozone, but brominated THMs levels are higher in pools treated with electrochemically generated mixed oxidants [51].

Outdoor pools are usually disinfected with chlorinated isocyanurates (stabilized forms of chlorine more resistant to UV degradation). Thus potent irritants as chloramines, haloacetic acids or acetonitriles may be also found in such pools [52].

Given their volatility, THMs can be found in the airspace above the water and in the air in indoor swimming pools. Thus they may be taken up by swimmers through the skin, but also through ingestion and by inhalation. Studies on elite swimmers were among the first to suggest that the chlorinated atmosphere of indoor pools could be detrimental to the lungs by increasing the risk of asthma, bronchial hyperreactivity and airways inflammation [53–55]. Other studies performed on recreational swimmers have provided further evidence that exposure to indoor chlorinated pools might contribute to the development of allergic diseases [56–58]. Life guards and others who work near a swimming pool are also at risk through the inhalation of DBPs, therefore this is also a problem of occupational health [43, 59, 60].

Studies on children attending indoor chlorinated swimming pools have shown that trichloramine, together with presumably aerosolized hypochlorous acid and chloramines, can damage the lung epithelium and promote the development of asthma, particularly among children with higher concentrations of total serum immunoglobulin IgE [27, 42, 61, 62]. A recent paper of Schöefer *et al.* [63], demonstrated during a 6-year follow-up of a prospective birth cohort study, some relationships between swimming pool attendance and health problems for swimming babies. Babies who did not participate in baby swimming programs had lower rates of infection in the first year of life (diarrhea: OR 0.68; otitis media: OR 0.81, airways infections: OR 0.85). No clear association could be found between late or non-swimmers and atopic dermatitis or hay fever until the age of 6 years, while higher rates of asthma were found (OR 2.15).

Another recent paper of Bernard *et al.* [52] illustrated a significant increase of ever and current asthma with the lifetime number of hours spent in outdoor pools by up to four and eight times, respectively, among adolescents with the highest attendance (>500 h) and a low exposure to indoor pools (<250 h). Use of residential outdoor pools was also associated with higher risks of elevated exhaled nitric oxide and sensitization to cat or house dust mite allergens. Thus even outdoor chlorinated swimming pool attendance is associated, according to this study, with higher risks of asthma, airways inflammation and some respiratory allergies.

Taking into account the increased prevalence of asthma or atopic dermatitis among children and adolescents in Europe, even though this increase is certainly due to multiple factors, questions arises about the mandatory participation in swimming pool activities for school-age children. The debate continues, with some associations considering it to be a public health problem. Thus research is needed to confirm both the efficacy and toxicology of any new disinfectants.

In contrast with the frequency of these pulmonary irritation syndromes, other reported infections including legionnaires' disease and Pontiac fever in users of spa pools, where water agitation can produce aerosols [64], are rare. A Pontiac fever-like illness was associated with a pool contaminated with *Legionella micdadei* [65]. *Mycobacterium chelonae* infection has been also reported in children with cystic fibrosis who used a poorly maintained hydrotherapy pool [66], and this leads to the more general question of immune-suppressed patients frequenting pools.

Other infectious diseases

Urinary tract infection with *P. aeruginosa* in a spa pool user is possible and primary amoebic meningoencephalitis in users of warm-water pools has been described in some countries [67]. Bloodborne infections, such as hepatitis B and human immunodeficiency virus infection, have not been associated with pool use.

Management and reporting

Ultimately, of the four factors that contribute to maintaining healthy water quality in a recreational water facility, facility management is the most important [68]. Good management includes staff involved in the safe operation of the system according to the guidelines specified by the country in which the facility is located. All equipment will eventually fail, as will all disinfectants. Swimming pools will become contaminated with a variety of organisms and organic and inorganic compounds. When this happens, the staff must know how to immediately respond to minimize the risk to the bathers. A reporting system should be in place to alert public health officials of outbreaks so that they are immediately available to help document and contain the impact on human health. Facility operators should be in constant contact with the engineers who designed the system and the chemical suppliers.

Access to recreational water facilities is a great way for people to maintain a healthy lifestyle. The health benefits associated with recreational water will be negated if a bather's health is put at risk due to an unsafe facility with poor water and/or air quality. A safe and healthy bathing experience will occur when the engineering design, water chemistry and disinfection are functioning optimally, and the entire system is being monitored by a highly trained facility manager.

References

1 Croll, B.T. *et al.* (2007) Simulated *Cryptosporidium* removal under swimming pool filtration conditions. *Water and Environment Journal*, **21**, 149–156.

2 Uhl, W. and Hartmann, C. (2005) Disinfection by-products and microbial contamination in the treatment of pool water with granular activated carbon. *Water Science and Technology*, **52**, 71–76.

3 Davis, T.L. *et al.* (2009) Bacteriological analysis of indoor and outdoor water parks in Wisconsin. *Journal of Water and Health*, **7**, 452–463.

4 Schafter, M.P. *et al.* (2003) Rapid detection and determination of the aerodynamic size range of airborne *Mycobacteria* associated with whirlpools. *Applied Occupational and Environmental Hygiene*, **18**, 41–50.

5 Michels, A. *et al.* (2008) Fossil fuel saving through a direct solar energy water heating system. *Clean-Soil Air Water*, **36**, 743–747.

6 Becker, B.E. (1997) Biophysiologic aspects of hydrotherapy, in *Comprehensive Aquatic Therapy* (eds B.E. Becker and A.J. Cole), Butterworth-Heinemann, Boston, pp. 17–48.

7 Goeres, D.M. (2010) Understanding the importance of biofilm growth in hot tubs, in *Applied Biomedical Microbiology: a Biofilms Approach* (ed. D.S. Paulson), CRC Press, Boca Raton, FL, pp. 133–148.

8 Hanak, V. *et al.* (2006) Hot tub lung: presenting features and clinical course of 21 patients. *Respiratory Medicine*, **100**, 610–615.

9 Snoeyink, V.L. and Jenkins, D. (1980) *Water Chemistry*, John Wiley & Sons, New York.

10 Pontius, F.W. (1990) *Water Quality and Treatment: a Handbook of Community Water Supplies*, 4th edn, McGraw-Hill, New York.

11 Mallmann, W.L. (1928) Streptococcus as an indicator of swimming pool pollution. *American Journal of Public Health*, **18**, 771–776.

12 Barbot, E. and Moulin, P. (2008) Swimming pool water treatment by ultrafiltration-adsorption process. *Journal of Membrane Science*, **314**, 50–57.

13 Anipsitakis, G.P. *et al.* (2008) Chemical and microbial decontamination of pool water using activated potassium peroxymonosulfate. *Water Research*, **42**, 2899–2910.

14 Black, A.P. *et al.* (1970) The disinfection of swimming pool waters: part 1 – comparison of iodine and chlorine as swimming pool disinfectants. *American Journal of Public Health*, **60**, 535–345.

15 Goeres, D.M. *et al.* (2004) Evaluation of disinfectant efficacy against biofilm and suspended bacteria in a laboratory swimming pool model. *Water Research*, **38**, 3103–3109.

16 Mood, E.W. (1950) Effect of free and combined available residual chlorine upon bacteria in swimming pools. *American Journal of Public Health*, **40**, 459–466.

17 Goeres, D.M. *et al.* (2007) A laboratory hot tub model for disinfectant efficacy evaluation. *Journal of Microbiological Methods*, **68**, 184–192.

18 Ortenzio, L.F. and Stuart, L.S. (1964) A standard test for efficacy of germicides and acceptability of residual disinfecting activity in swimming pool water. *Journal of AOAC International*, **47**, 540–547.

19 Price, D. and Ahearn, D.G. (1988) Incidence and persistence of *Pseudomonas aeruginosa* in whirlpools. *Journal of Clinical Microbiology*, **26**, 1650–1654.

20 Seyfried, P.L. and Fraser, D.J. (1980) Persistence of *Pseudomonas aeruginosa* in chlorinated swimming pools. *Canadian Journal of Microbiology*, **26**, 350–355.

21 Storey, A. (1989) Microbiological problems of swimming pools. *Environmental Health*, **97**, 260–262.

22 De Groote, M.A. and Huitt, G. (2006) Infections due to rapidly growing mycobacteria. *Emerging Infections*, **42**, 1756–1763.

23 Hall-Stoodley, L. and Lappin-Scott, H. (1998) Biofilm formation by the rapidly growing mycobacterial species *Mycobacterium fortuitum*. *FEMS Microbiology Letters*, **168**, 77–84.

24 Hall-Stoodley, L. and Stoodley, P. (2005) Biofilm formation and dispersal and the transmission of human pathogens. *Trends in Microbiology*, **13**, 7–10.

25 Murga, R. *et al.* (2001) Role of biofilms in the survival of *Legionella pneumophila* in a model potable-water system. *Microbiology*, **147**, 3121–3125.

26 Jones, F. and Bartlett, C.L.R. (1985) Infections associated with whirlpools and spas. *Journal of Applied Bacteriology*, **59** (Suppl.), 61–66.

27 Bernard, A. *et al.* (2006) Chlorinated pool attendance, atopy and the risk of asthma during childhood. *Environmental Health Perspectives*, **114**, 1567–1573.

28 Penny, P.T. (1991) Hydrotherapy pools of the future – the avoidance of health problems. *Journal of Hospital Infection*, **18** (Suppl. A), 535–542.

29 Pool Water Treatment Advisory Group (1999) *Swimming Pool Water: Treatment and Quality Standards*, Pool Water Treatment Advisory Group, Diss.

30 Lee, W.J. *et al.* (2000) Sporotrichoid dermatosis caused by *Mycobacterium abscessus* from a public bath. *Journal of Dermatology*, **27**, 264–268.

31 Sugita, Y. *et al.* (2000) Familial cluster of cutaneous *Mycobacterium avium* infection resulting from use of a circulating, constantly heated bath water system. *British Journal of Dermatology*, **142**, 789–793.

32 Choong, K.Y. and Roberts, L.J. (1999) Molluscum contagiosum, swimming and bathing: a clinical analysis. *Australian Journal of Dermatology*, **40**, 89–92.

33 Porter, J.D. *et al.* (1988) *Giardia* transmission in a swimming pool. *American Journal of Public Health*, **78**, 659–662.

34 Craun, G.F. *et al.* (2005) Outbreaks associated with recreational waters in the US. *Journal of Environmental Health Research*, **15**, 243–262.

35 Friedman, M.S. *et al.* (1999) *Escherichia coli* O157:H7 outbreak associated with an improperly chlorinated swimming pool. *Clinical Infectious Diseases*, **29**, 298–303.

36 Kappus, K.D. *et al.* (1989) An outbreak of Norwalk gastroenteritidis associated with swimming in a pool and secondary person-to-person transmission. *American Journal of Epidemiology*, **116**, 834–839.

37 Mahoney, F.J. *et al.* (1992) An outbreak of hepatitis A associated with swimming in a public school. *Journal Infection Diseases*, **165**, 613–618.

38 Gabrio, T. *et al.* (2005) Untersuchung der Belastung von Taucher mit Trihalogenmethanen zur Abklärung ihres Aufnahmepfades. *A.B. Archives des Badewesen*, **58**, 160–164.

39 World Health Organization (WHO) (2000) *Guidelines for Safe Recreational-water Environments Vol.2: Swimming Pools, Spas and Similar Recreational-water Environments*, WHO, Geneva.

40 Villanueva, C.M. *et al.* (2007) Bladder cancer and exposure to water disinfection by-products through ingestion, bathing, showering, and swimming in pools. *American Journal of Epidemiology*, **165**, 148–156.

41 Vandentorren, S. et al. (2004) *Evaluation des risques sanitaires des sous-produits de chloration de l'eau potable: partie 1. Caractérisation des dangers: effets sanitaires et valeurs toxicologiques de référence*, Institut de Veille Sanitaire, Saint-Maurice, p. 44.

42 Bernard, A. *et al.* (2003) Lung hyperpermeability and asthma prevalence in schoolchildren: inexpected associations with the attendance of indoor chlorinated pools. *Occupational and Environmental Medicine*, **60**, 385–394.

43 Massin, N. *et al.* (1998) Respiratory symptoms and bronchial responsiveness in lifeguards exposed to nitrogen trichloride in indoor swimming pools. *Occupational and Environmental Medicine*, **55**, 258–263.

44 Williams, D.T. *et al.* (Health Canada) (1997) Disinfection by-products in Canadian drinking water. *Chemosphere*, **34**, 299–316.

45 US Environmental Protection Agency (EPA) (2006) *Exposure and International Doses of Trihalomethanes in Humans: Multi-Route Contributions from Drinking Water*, EPA, Office of Research and Development, National Center for Environmental Assessment, Washington, DC.

46 Agazotti, G. *et al.* (1998) Blood and breath analyses as biological indicators of exposure to trihalomethanes in indoor swimming pools. *Science of the Total Environment*, **30**, 155–163.

47 Caro, J. and Gallego, M. (2007) Assessment of exposure of workers and swimmers to trihalomethane in an indoor swimming pool. *Environmental Science and Technology*, **41**, 4793–4798.

48 Erdinger, L. *et al.* (2004) Pathways of trihalomethane uptake in swimming pools. *International Journal of Hygiene and Environmental Health*, **207**, 571–575.

49 Gagnaire, F. *et al.* (1994) Comparison of the sensory irritation response in mice to chlorine and nitrogen chloride. *Journal of Applied Toxicology*, **14**, 405–409.

50 Chu, H. and Nieuwenhuijsen, M.J. (2002) Distribution and determinants of trihalomethane concentrations in indoor swimming pools. *Occupational and Environmental Medicine*, **59**, 243–247.

51 Lee, J. *et al.* (2009) Characteristics of trihalomethane (THM) production and associated health risk assessment in swimming pool waters treated with different disinfection methods. *Science of the Total Environment*, **407**, 1990–1997.

52 Bernard, A. *et al.* (2008) Outdoor swimming pools and the risk of asthma and allergies during adolescence. *European Respiratory Journal*, **32**, 979–988.

53 Bernard, A. (2007) Chlorination products: emerging links with allergic diseases. *Current Medicinal Chemistry*, **14**, 1771–1782.

54 Helenius, I.J. *et al.* (1998) Asthma and increased bronchial responsiveness in elite athletes: atopy and sport event as risk factors. *Journal of Allergy and Clinical Immunology*, **101**, 646–652.

55 Helenius, I.J. *et al.* (2002) Effect of continuing or finishing high-level sports on airway inflammation, bronchial hyper responsiveness, and asthma: a 5-year prospective follow-up study of 42 highly trained swimmers. *Journal of Allergy and Clinical Immunology*, **109**, 962–968.

56 Lagerkvist, B. *et al.* (2004) Pulmonary epithelial integrity in children – relationship to ambient ozone exposure and swimming pool attendance. *Environmental Health Perspectives*, **112**, 1767–1772.

57 Stav, D. and Stav, M. (2005) Asthma and whirlpool baths. *New England Journal of Medicine*, **353**, 1635–1636.

58 Kohlhammer, Y. *et al.* (2006) Swimming pool attendance and hay fever rates later in life. *Allergy*, **61**, 1305–1309.

59 Thickett, K.M. *et al.* (2002) Occupational asthma caused by chloramines in indoor swimming-pool air. *European Respiratory Journal*, **19**, 827–832.

60 Jacobs, J.H. *et al.* (2007) Exposure to trichloramine and respiratory symptoms in indoor swimming pool workers. *European Respiratory Journal: Official Journal of the European Society for Clinical Respiratory Physiology*, **29**, 690–698.

61 Carbonelle, S. *et al.* (2002) Changes in serum pneumoproteins caused by short-term exposures to nitrogen trichloride in indoor chlorinated swimming pools. *Biomarkers*, **7**, 464–478.

62 Bernard, A. *et al.* (2007) Infant swimming, pulmonary epithelium integrity and the risk of allergic and respiratory diseases later in childhood. *Pediatrics*, **119**, 1095–1103.

63 Schöefer, Y. *et al.* (2008) Health risk of early swimming pool attendance. *International Journal of Hygiene and Environmental Health*, **211**, 367–373.

64 Bartlett, C.L.R. *et al.* (1986) Legionella Infections, Edward Arnold, London.

65 Godberg, D.J. *et al.* (1989) Lochgoilhead fever: outbreak of non-pneumonic legionellosis due to *Legionella micdadeï*. *Lancet*, **i**, 316–318.

66 Basavaraj, D.S. *et al.* (1985) *Mycobacterium chelonei* associated with a hydrotherapy poll. *PHLS Disease Report*, **41**, 3–4.

67 Bard, D. and Siclet, F. (1995) *Amibes Libres et Santé Publique*, Co-édition Ecole Nationale de Santé Publique/EDF, Rennes.

68 Buss, B.E. *et al.* (2009) Association between swimming pool operator certification and reduced pool chemistry violations – Nebraska, 2005–2006. *Journal of Environmental Health*, **71**, 36–40.

20.1   Antimicrobial Surfaces

Gareth J. Williams

ECHA Microbiology Ltd, Willowbrook Technology Park, Cardiff, Wales, UK

Introduction

Bacteria have a marked preference to live as sessile cells on surfaces, rather than as planktonic cells in suspension [1]. Numerous studies have reported on the ability of organisms such as methicillin-resistant *Staphylococcus aureus* (MRSA) to contaminate surfaces and persist in the healthcare environment [2]. These pathogens can be readily cross-transmitted from hospital surfaces [3, 4] and there is evidence suggesting that surfaces in the healthcare environment have been the direct source of outbreaks [5]. There are similar concerns about surface hygiene in the food industry. Microorganisms in this context have the potential to contaminate food and impact on the quality of the product and of course cause disease in the consumer [6].

Cleaning regimes alone might be ineffective at eliminating microbial contamination from surfaces [7–9]. The use of disinfectants is therefore of prime importance, and there is considerable emphasis placed on ensuring disinfection regimes are fit for purpose [10–12]. It is therefore justified that antimicrobial surface materials are evaluated for their ability to provide an extra level of protection as part of the overall strategy to prevent the survival of microorganisms in the healthcare and food-processing environments.

There has long been a tendency to regard all microorganisms as entities that need to be destroyed. It is possible that fears over microbial contamination have been magnified by the regular and sometimes sensationalist media coverage of hospital "superbugs".

This may explain why there is currently such an emphasis on the control of microbes in the home environment. At present, there is a high likelihood that any plastic or fabric products used in the home have been manufactured to have antimicrobial properties.

If conditions are favorable for microbial growth, microorganisms colonizing surfaces will divide and produce biofilms, often embedded in a gel-like polysaccharide matrix [1]. Bacteria growing in biofilms in natural and industrial environments are resistant to diverse microbicides and bacteriophages used to combat biofouling in industrial processes [1]. In medical terms, biofilms can survive host immune responses and they are much less susceptible to chemotherapeutic antibiotics than their planktonic counterparts [13]. Biofilms are particularly problematic in the context of medical device-associated infection. The traditional materials used in the manufacture of implanted medical devices, such as silicone and latex, impair local host defenses and do not resist microbial attachment and the formation of biofilm. Biofilms are central to the failure of medical devices such as central venous catheters, urinary catheters, prosthetic joints and pacemakers to name but few [14, 15]. These devices have been coated or impregnated with antimicrobial agents in attempts to reduce the incidence of medical device-associated infections (see Chapter 20.2).

This chapter will review and evaluate the state of the art with regards to current and emerging antimicrobial technologies, focusing on the development of passive and reactive surface technologies for environmental surfaces and indwelling medical devices, particularly urinary catheters.

Russell, Hugo & Ayliffe's: Principles and Practice of Disinfection, Preservation and Sterilization, Fifth Edition. Edited by Adam P. Fraise, Jean-Yves Maillard, and Syed A. Sattar.

© 2013 Blackwell Publishing Ltd. Published 2013 by Blackwell Publishing Ltd.

Passive surfaces

Microorganisms are ubiquitous in the environment and thus surfaces can become contaminated following contact with soil, air, water, animals and plants. Microorganisms may be brought into close proximity to an implanted medical device, for example by a stream of fluid flowing over the surface or in a directed fashion via chemotaxis and motility [16, 17]. The initial step in colonization and subsequent biofilm formation is bacterial attachment to a surface. Microbial attachment is dependent on attractive or repulsive forces generated between the organism and the surface. When a bacterium reaches a critical proximity to a surface (<1 nm), short-range chemical interactions (ionic, hydrogen, covalent bonding) may influence bacterial attachment [17, 18]. Flagellar-mediated motility and/or pili-mediated motility may help to overcome repulsive forces between the bacterium and a surface and contribute to the early stages of biofilm development [19].

Some surface materials have been developed which possess physical properties that can attenuate the attractive forces and inhibit the binding of microorganisms. These include, for example, diamond-like carbon (DLC) coating, polyethylene oxide (PEO) brush coatings and polymers coated with "benign" cultures of microorganisms – a strategy defined as bacterial interference. These "passive" surfaces, which do not kill microorganisms, are being developed as potential surfaces for medical devices, particularly urinary catheters.

Diamond-like carbon

It was shown that strongly electron-donating polymers, such as polyvinyl alcohols and agarose, were less vulnerable to colonization by the important catheter-associated urinary tract pathogen *Proteus mirabilis* than more hydrophobic polymers [20]. Once this organism gains access into the catheterized bladder, however, it generates the enzyme urease, which hydrolyzes urea to ammonia and carbon dioxide, increasing the pH of urine. This generates conditions under which crystals of calcium and magnesium precipitate from solution. It has been shown *in vitro* that once the urinary pH rises to the level at which crystals form, *P. mirabilis* biofilms can be initiated on surfaces that inhibit bacterial cell attachment. Indeed the crystals bind to surfaces and allow microorganisms to bind to it [21].

Diamond-like carbon has emerged as a material with which to coat medical devices. Polymers coated with DLC have been found to reduce the adherence of pathogens such as *Pseudomonas aeruginosa*, *S. aureus* and *Escherichia coli* [22–26]. In addition, it has been reported that DLC coating can reduce the deposition of calcium and magnesium crystals, thus marking it to be a potential coating for urinary catheters and stents which commonly become colonized with crystalline bacterial biofilms [22, 27]. It appears the effectiveness of this approach can be further enhanced by the incorporation of silicon and nitrogen, making DLC even more resistant to microbial attachment [23–25].

Polyethylene oxide brush coatings

It is important to remember that implanted medical devices are likely to become coated in a conditioning film comprising of host proteins [18, 28, 29]. This has the potential to compromise the "non-stick" nature of surfaces thus enabling microorganisms to gain a foothold and proliferate. PEO brush coatings are an exciting prospect for medical implant development since it has been reported that they can be manufactured to repel proteins and microorganisms [30–34]. PEO brushes are chains of PEO that are grafted onto a surface and stretch into the surrounding medium. PEO is also known as polyethylene glycol (PEG). The process of attaching PEG or PEO chains to a surface is commonly referred to as PEGylation.

Studies *in vitro* have shown that when applied to surfaces, PEO brush coatings can reduce the adherence of *Staphylococcus epidermidis*, *S. aureus*, *Streptococcus salivarius*, *E. coli* and yeasts and that adhesion is influenced by PEO chain length [31, 32]. It is thought that as a microorganism penetrates the PEO brush it compresses the polymer chains. The compressed chains therefore create a physical barrier between the surface and the approaching organism and thus inhibit attachment [34]. It has been noted that the surfaces are unable to resist the attachment of certain strains of *P. aeruginosa* [34]. This has been attributed to their more hydrophobic nature and the secretion of extracellular substances which may have attractive interactions with PEO chains. It has been shown, however, that the microorganisms that do adhere to PEO brush coatings are weakly associated and are more easily removed by shear forces compared with organisms on uncoated surfaces [32–34].

Bacterial interference

Instead of trying to prevent microbial attachment other researchers are adopting the opposite strategy – producing surfaces coated with live cultures of "benign" microorganisms [35–38]. Here, urinary catheters are simply placed into a broth which is inoculated with a non-pathogenic strain of *E. coli* and incubated for 2 days at 37°C. The catheters become coated with a bacterial biofilm. *In vitro* studies have shown that these surfaces can resist colonization by a range of uropathogens, including *Enterococcus faecalis*, pathogenic strains of *E. coli*, *Providencia stuartii* and *Candida albicans* [35, 36]. Pilot studies examining the approach revealed that the rates of urinary tract infection were reduced in patients whose bladders subsequently became colonized by the non-pathogenic strain following the insertion of the catheters [37, 38].

The strategy is defined as bacterial interference, but the mechanisms by which these surfaces prevent bacterial binding are unclear. It has been postulated that the benign colonizers: (i) impose spatial constraints and block further microbial attachment on the surface; (ii) may outcompete pathogens for available nutrients; or (iii) may even secrete inhibitory agents [35]. This promising approach does have some limitations. The use of such catheters coated with live cultures of microorganisms may be precluded in immunocompromised individuals [37]. In addition, the pilot studies found that the benign culture of *E. coli* could be eliminated from both the bladder and the surface of the catheter by the bacterium *Proteus* [37, 38]. This is an unfortunate development in view of the complications to catheter care caused by this organism [39].

Reactive surfaces

Reactive surfaces can be defined as those that possess an antimicrobial activity. Many such surfaces have been developed. The challenges associated with the development of effective reactive surfaces in the context of urinary catheters will be explored further. Current and emerging reactive technologies will be reviewed for other applications. For instance, reactive surfaces that continuously release antimicrobial agents and those which kill microorganisms upon contact will be discussed. The controlled release of antimicrobial agents from "smart" reactive polymers will also be considered. This is a more ingenious approach whereby antimicrobials are released from surfaces "on command" through the application of an external stimulus or "on demand" in response to the presence of microorganisms.

Challenges associated with the development of reactive surfaces: Urinary catheters

What are the desirable properties of a reactive antimicrobial surface? Ideally, the "gold standard" should possess a broad spectrum of antimicrobial activity and resist microbial colonization and subsequent biofilm formation [40]. This activity needs to endure for the lifetime of the surface and should not select for antimicrobial resistance. Has the gold standard been achieved in the case of urinary catheters? They are the most frequently used prosthetic devices in modern medicine, with more than 30 million inserted into patients every year in the USA alone [41]. While catheters provide a convenient way to drain urine from the dysfunctional bladder, they also provide access for bacteria from a contaminated external environment into a vulnerable body cavity. The presence of the catheter also undermines the basic defenses of the urinary tract against infection. These factors induce a vulnerability to infection enabling contaminating organisms to gain a foothold and proliferate.

It has been proposed that catheters impregnated with an effective antimicrobial agent may offer great potential for reducing the rates of catheter-associated urinary tract infection [42]. Other researchers, however, have expressed concerns over the use of antimicrobial-containing catheters. For example, it is thought that the constant efflux of antimicrobial agents from catheters could result in subinhibitory concentrations in urine which could encourage resistance in the colonizing microbes [43]. Others have warned that the mixed microbial flora that commonly colonizes the urinary tract of catheterized patients would be extremely challenging for antimicrobial-impregnated catheters [40]. Despite these concerns, urinary catheters impregnated with antimicrobial agents continue to be developed.

It is unlikely that antimicrobials fixed in the catheter polymer will solve the problem. Conditioning films comprised of fibronectin, fibrinogen, collagen and other host proteins immediately coat prosthesis *in vivo* [18, 28, 29] and will likely shield subsequent colonizers from the bound agent. In addition any primary colonizers that might be killed on adherence will protect subsequent colonizers from the bound agent [44]. In theory, a better strategy would be to ensure that the active agents elute from the catheter [45–47]. In this way, planktonic bacteria in the vicinity of the device can be attacked before they colonize the surface and adopt the biofilm's resistant phenotype.

Studies evaluating the release from catheters impregnated with microbicides, such as chlorhexidine, and frontline antibiotics, such as gentamicin and norfloxacin, have shown that the agents were generally released in an uncontrolled manner with an initial burst at day 1 followed by a negligible release thereafter [48–51]. In attempts to control the release of antimicrobial agents improved technologies have been developed. Kwok *et al.* [52], for example, showed that a more controlled release could be achieved by depositing a thin polymer film of poly(butylmethacrylate) or p(BMA) around polyurethane that had been impregnated with the antibiotic ciprofloxacin. The antibiofilm properties of this polymer, however, have only been evaluated over 24 h [53]. An alternative approach was developed by DiTizio *et al.* [54]. The authors showed that catheters coated with hydrogel containing ciprofloxacin lost their entire antibiotic content *in vitro* within 4 h. The release of the antibiotic could be extended over 7 days when they coated the catheters with a ciprofloxacin liposome-containing hydrogel.

Silver has a broad antimicrobial spectrum [55] and catheters have been manufactured coated with silver oxide or silver alloy. Latex-based catheters with a silver alloy/hydrogel coating are currently on the market and it is claimed they exert their antibacterial activity by releasing silver ions over prolonged periods. Their use has been recommended to reduce the incidence of infection in patients undergoing short-term catheterization [56]. It must be remembered that catheters are used to manage chronic urinary incontinence in the elderly and in patients whose bladder function has been impaired by trauma or neuropathies such as multiple sclerosis. There is evidence to suggest catheters coated with silver alloy do not resist microbial attachment and biofilm formation in patients requiring catheterization long term [57].

Catheters have been impregnated with combinations of agents in order to broaden their spectrum of antimicrobial activity and decrease the risk of emergence of resistant microorganisms [42, 58]. For example, catheters impregnated with minocycline and rifampicin have been tested in a clinical study [42]. The performance of the impregnated catheters was compared with standard unmedicated silicone catheters in a group of 124 patients. It was observed that it took significantly longer for patients who were fitted with the antimicrobial catheters to develop urinary tract infections. There were also significantly lower rates of infection associated with the use of the antimicrobial catheters after 7 and 14 days [42]. The antimicrobial catheters significantly reduced the rates of infection with Gram-positive bacteria. Interestingly, similar rates of infection with Gram-negative bacteria and yeasts were observed in the control and test groups [42]. This demonstrated how challenging the polymicrobial flora of the catheterized urinary tract can be for an antimicrobial catheter.

Overall, the antimicrobial-containing catheters developed so far may have a role in patients who require short-term catheterization. No approach, however, has achieved a sustained release of active concentrations of antimicrobial agents over the period of time equivalent to the normal lifespan of a long-term indwelling catheter, which can be up to 12 weeks. The main obstacle appears to be loading catheters with sufficient antimicrobial agent and then controlling its release. A promising approach is using the catheter's bladder retention balloon as a large reservoir for the delivery of antimicrobial agents. Subsequent experiments using a laboratory model have shown that the microbicide triclosan can diffuse through the balloons of catheters and inhibit the formation of catheter-blocking biofilms generated by the important pathogen *P. mirabilis* [46, 47]. In these experiments catheters inflated with water blocked within 48 h, whereas triclosan-inflated catheters reduced the viability of *P. mirabilis* and prevented the formation of crystalline biofilm for the duration of 7-day experiments. The approach has yet to be tested in a clinical study.

In the context of urinary catheterization it could be argued that the gold standard has not been achieved yet [40]. It is doubtful, on this evidence, that simply incorporating an antimicrobial agent into a polymer will frustrate the colonization mechanisms of microorganisms.

Other reactive surfaces that continuously release antimicrobial agents

The majority of the reactive technologies developed in the context of urinary catheters rely on the continuous release of antimicrobial agents in order to reduce microbial colonization and subsequent biofilm formation (see above). The active agents are therefore constantly available to exert their antimicrobial activity. Antimicrobial metals, particularly copper and silver, are being evaluated for a number of other applications. Antimicrobial delivery systems, zeolites and carbide-derived carbons (CDCs), have been developed to have "nanopores" that release metal ions or gases. An emergent approach is the development of surfaces that can mitigate biofilm formation through the release of quorum-sensing antagonists or dispersin B.

Antimicrobial metals

Silver has been used for many centuries as an antimicrobial agent and has been shown to have activity against viruses, bacteria and fungi [55]. Despite its long use, the mechanisms by which it exerts these effects are not fully understood [59]. It is known that the ionic form of silver interacts with thiol (sulfhydryl) groups located within structural proteins and enzymes resulting in a loss

of function and can also bind to nucleic acid and inhibit replication [55, 60, 61]. It has also been proposed that silver ions released from the metal catalyze the production of antimicrobial reactive oxygen species within the microorganism, which contribute to cellular damage and the death of the organism [62]. A desirable property of an antimicrobial surface is that the agent used should possess a broad spectrum of antimicrobial activity. Silver has such a broad antimicrobial spectrum and therefore it is not surprising that silver and its compounds have been widely used, for example as coatings for catheters, wound dressings and dental implants [56, 59, 63–66].

Copper and its alloys have antimicrobial properties, also due to the release of toxic metal ions and the generation of reactive oxygen species, and are being evaluated as an alternative to stainless steel in food-processing environments [67–69]. A common mode of transmission of microorganisms in the healthcare environment is via the hands of healthcare workers [70, 71]. Therefore, surfaces commonly touched by staff and patients may act as sources of cross-contamination [72–74]. Copper surfaces are being assessed to reduce the survival of microorganisms in the healthcare environment, for example on door handles, door push plates, tap handles and toilet seats [75, 76].

In a laboratory analysis, copper surfaces brought about a >7-$\log_{10}$ reduction in MRSA numbers after 90 min of contact [77]. Activity has also been reported against vegetative cells of *Clostridium difficile*, *Listeria monocytogenes*, *P. aeruginosa* and *E. coli* O157 [67–69, 78, 79]. Trials of copper-containing items in the healthcare environment have revealed that they become colonized by lower levels of bioburden than those that do not contain the metal [75, 76]. Casey *et al.* [75], for example, reported a crossover study comparing the efficacy of copper-containing items with the equivalent standards in an acute medical ward over 10 weeks. Copper-containing items were colonized by 90–100% lower numbers of viable microorganisms than the control equivalents. Important pathogens associated with development of healthcare-associated infections (methicillin-susceptible *S. aureus* (MSSA), vancomycin-resistant *Enterococcus faecium* (VRE) and *E. coli*) were isolated from the control surfaces over the course of the study. None of these microorganisms, however, were isolated from the copper-containing surfaces. A laboratory study by Airey and Verran [80] suggested that soiling materials may bind more strongly to copper than stainless steel, possibly due to the more reactive nature of copper. Therefore, if copper surfaces are introduced into the clinical or industrial environment it would be important to rigorously evaluate cleaning procedures since the generation of a conditioning film could compromise their antimicrobial properties.

Antimicrobial delivery systems

Metal ions with antimicrobial properties, for example silver ions, can be incorporated into inorganic ceramic matrices known as zeolites. Zeolites are synthesized to have a three-dimensional grid-like structure with a network of nanopores that harbor the metal ions. When a microorganism makes contact with the zeolite, silver ions are transferred to the organism whereupon they exert their antimicrobial activity [62]. Zeolites have been investigated as potential "self-disinfecting" coatings for indwelling catheters [81], dental implants [82–85], air ventilation systems [86] and hospital surfaces [87]. They have also been tested for efficacy against common food-spoilage organisms, respiratory pathogens and agents of bioterrorism [86, 88–90].

A zeolite consisting of an aluminum silicate ceramic loaded with silver (2.5% w/w) and zinc ions (14% w/w) has been developed as a commercial product called AgION® by AK Steel Corporation (Ohio, USA). In laboratory analyses, the coating achieved >99.99% reductions in *S. aureus*, *E. coli*, *P. aeruginosa* and *L. monocytogenes* after 24 h [90]. Similar activity was achieved against *Legionella pneumophila* [86]. While these results appear promising, the activity of AgION against bacterial spores was disappointing. While the zeolite coating produced approximately 3-$\log_{10}$ inactivation of vegetative *Bacillus anthracis*, *Bacillus cereus* and *Bacillus subtilis* within a 5–24 h period, it had no effect on the viability of the endospores formed by these organisms [89].

In addition to trapping antimicrobial silver ions inside a matrix it is also feasible to trap chlorine. A class of porous carbons known as CDCs can also be manufactured to have nanopores, in the range of 2 nm and below, which can retain gas molecules effectively [91, 92]. When tested as a suspension it was shown that CDCs loaded with chlorine achieved considerable reductions of spores and vegetative forms of *B. anthracis* following 2 h exposures [92]. Based on these results it was proposed that CDCs, which can be manufactured as a powder, coating or membrane, could have applications in a range of settings.

Release of factors that can disrupt biofilm formation
Quorum-sensing antagonists

In recent years evidence has been presented suggesting that regulatory mechanisms are important in controlling the development of biofilms. Acylated homoserine lactones (AHLs) have been shown to be produced by a range of bacteria to regulate cell density-dependent gene expression by a mechanism known as quorum sensing [93]. Evidence to suggest that this signaling system is important in biofilm formation was reported in a study by Davies *et al.* [94]. In this work, *P. aeruginosa* mutants unable to produce the signaling molecules formed poorly developed biofilms that, unlike the wild-type biofilms, were susceptible to the microbicide sodium dodecyl sulfate.

A number of research efforts have identified compounds that can interfere with the signaling systems of specific microorganisms [93]. One class of compounds receiving considerable attention is the furanones. Furanones are produced by the red algae *Delisea pulchra* and are able to antagonize quorum sensing in a number of organisms including *P. aeruginosa*, *Salmonella enterica* serovar Typhimurium and *E. coli* [95–97]. It was recently shown that a synthetic furanone could potentiate the activity of microbicides against *Salmonella* in biofilms [97]. One can conceive of applications in which the synergistic combinations of antimicrobial agents and quorum-sensing inhibitors are incorporated into

polymers in order to mitigate biofilm formation. An exciting prospect is the development of a polymer that can actively sequester quorum-sensing signaling molecules [98].

Dispersin B

There are multiple mechanisms of biofilm resistance to antimicrobials, which may vary with the bacteria present in the biofilm and the agent being applied [15, 99, 100]. For example, studies have reported an apparent failure of certain antimicrobial agents to penetrate biofilms [101, 102]. At present there is much interest in β-*N*-acetylglucosaminidase secreted by the Gram-negative pathogen *Aggregatibacter actinomycetemcomitans*. This enzyme, known as dispersin B, has been found to hydrolyze the exopolysaccharide matrix that envelopes microbial biofilms and enable the penetration of antimicrobial agents [103, 104].

A study by Donelli *et al.* [103] showed that *S. aureus* and *S. epidermidis* biofilms that coated dispersin B-impregnated surfaces were more susceptible to treatment with an antibiotic solution than the biofilms that coated control surfaces. The synergy between dispersin B and antimicrobial agents was also noted in a study by Darouiche *et al.* [104]. Here vascular catheters impregnated with both dispersin B and the microbicide triclosan significantly reduced colonization by *S. aureus*, *S. epidermidis*, *E. coli* and *C. albicans* over a 24 h period and exhibited a prolonged superior antimicrobial activity in comparison with catheters coated with chlorhexidine and silver sulfadiazine. Both types of catheter had a similar efficacy when challenged with *S. aureus* in an animal model but were more efficacious than standard unmedicated catheters [104].

Reactive surfaces that kill microorganisms on contact

A number of reactive surface technologies have been developed that require direct contact with the contaminating microorganism in order for them to exert their antimicrobial activity. Surfaces impregnated with microbicides are finding increasing application in the home. By the early 2000s, such surfaces were commonly impregnated with triclosan. More recently, surfaces coated with silver nanoparticles have become de rigueur. Concerns over antibiotic and microbicide cross-resistance are driving interest in natural antimicrobial agents. Surfaces have been coated with natural antimicrobial agents such as honey, bacteriophages and antimicrobial peptides. Surfaces which are manufactured to have a strong positive charge are also being investigated for their ability to kill microorganisms upon contact.

Surfaces impregnated with microbicides
Triclosan

By the early 2000s, the microbicide triclosan had almost become a staple ingredient of personal care products and was being incorporated into the surfaces of a range of household goods. Several authors warned that triclosan was being overused and that this could not only result in the selection of bacteria resistant to it, but also cross-resistance to other antimicrobial agents [105–108]. This is because there are similarities in the way in which bacteria resist the action of triclosan and antibiotics – target mutations, degradative enzymes, increased target expression and efflux pumps [106, 107]. Surveys and laboratory studies have failed to establish a link between triclosan use and antibacterial resistance [108–111]. It has been emphasized, however, that important microbicides like triclosan should not be used indiscriminately, but should be limited to clinically useful situations [105, 108, 112]. Some European countries are taking note of these concerns and have banned the use of triclosan in a number of applications.

There is a real potential for using triclosan in the clinic to control the formation of crystalline biofilms formed by *P. mirabilis*, which block urinary catheters (discussed above). Triclosan-impregnated sutures are also being evaluated to reduce infection and promote wound healing following surgery. Studies, *in vitro* and *in vivo*, have shown that the sutures are active against a range of pathogenic microorganisms and can reduce the number of adherent bacteria compared with standard unmedicated sutures [113, 114]. Triclosan-impregnated sutures have been evaluated in a clinical trial. A retrospective analysis revealed that the rate of wound infection following abdominal surgery in the year triclosan-impregnated sutures were introduced was significantly lower than the rate in the preceding year [115].

Metal nanoparticles

Elemental silver in the form of nanoparticles also directly possesses antimicrobial activity in addition to any silver ions that they may release into solution. Products coated with "nanosilver" technology are already widely available. Applications include coatings for laundry machines, dishwashers, computer keyboards, toilet seats and clothing [56]. Silver nanoparticles, in the size range 1–10 nm, have been shown to bind to GP120 glycoprotein knobs on the surface of HIV and prevent the virus from attaching to and infecting susceptible cells [116]. Slightly larger nanoparticles with mean size <50 nm are directly toxic for *E. coli*, causing disruption of the cell membrane which results in the loss of cellular constituents and allows nanoparticles to gain access to the interior of the cell where they are thought to interact with other cellular components [60, 117]. A recent study showed that the antibacterial activity of silver nanoparticles was linked to their shape, with triangular nanoparticles showing the most activity against *E. coli* compared with spherical and rod-shaped nanoparticles [60]. One could hypothesize that triangular particles are more efficient at interacting with cellular constituents and generating antibacterial radicals. Thus by optimizing the shape of silver nanoparticles immobilized on surfaces it should be possible to enhance the antimicrobial potential of silver-coated surfaces.

Other nanoparticle metals are being developed and investigated for their antibacterial properties. Jones *et al.* [118] recently investigated the antibacterial activity of zinc oxide particles, while other groups are interested in the development of copper nanoparticles for application in disinfectant and coating formulations [119–122]. In addition, nanocrystalline metal oxides such as magnesium oxide and calcium oxide can be produced to retain halogen gases such as chlorine and bromine. On contact with bacteria the particles are taken up, whereupon they adhere to proteins and DNA and release the halogen. They have been shown to be extremely effective against vegetative cells of *E. coli*, *B. cereus* or *Bacillus globigii*, achieving >90% kill within a few minutes. They are less effective against the endospores of *Bacillus* species, with decontamination taking several hours [123].

Surfaces impregnated with natural antimicrobial agents
Honey

In terms of infection and disease, alternative natural therapies have the potential to reduce antibiotic and microbicide usage, and thus preserve their efficacy. Traditionally, honey has been used for the treatment of various disorders. The antimicrobial properties of Manuka honey have been revisited and it has been shown to have activity against common opportunistic pathogens such as *P. aeruginosa*, *S. aureus* and coagulase-negative staphylococci [124–127]. Some types of honey also possess antioxidant activity. This is a property that may aid the demonstrated ability of honey to help resolve the chronic inflammation associated with wounds [128]. Wound dressings impregnated with Manuka honey are now available on the drug tariff in the UK due to its broad spectrum of activity and its ability to promote wound healing.

Bacteriophages

One strategy that is attracting increasing attention is bacteriophage (phage) therapy, which has been used for almost a century to treat various infections, particularly in eastern Europe [129]. Bacteriophages are naturally occurring bacterial viruses that selectively recognize and kill vegetative bacteria. Recently, the Listex™ P100 bacteriophage has been approved for the treatment of ready-to-eat meat and poultry products in the USA and cheese in the European Union to protect consumers from the life-threatening pathogen *L. monocytogenes*.

Urinary catheters coated with phages have been produced in attempts to mitigate biofilm development. It was reported, for example, that biofilm formation by *S. epidermidis*, *P. mirabilis* or *E. coli* was significantly reduced after 24 h on catheter segments pretreated with bacteriophages which specifically infected these microorganisms [130, 131]. An advantage to the approach is that bacteriophage replication will be triggered when the virus infects the pathogen and the levels will continue to rise until host cells have been destroyed [129]. However, a drawback is that a few cells within a heterogeneous population may be intrinsically resistant to the bacteriophage and therefore could be responsible for biofilm regrowth [132]. A solution to this problem could be the exploitation of cultures comprising of several bacteriophage strains, a phage "cocktail", to reduce the likelihood of resistance emerging and to ensure that the majority of isolates of a particular organism can be killed. It has been shown *in vitro* that pretreating catheters with a five-phage cocktail reduced biofilm formation by *P. aeruginosa* by 99.9% over 48 h and limited biofilm regrowth [132]. Other researchers are investigating ways of immobilizing bacteriophages on surfaces, which could enhance this approach further [133]. The specificity of bacteriophages could complicate their use in urinary catheterization. While single-species biofilms are found on catheters in patients, urine biofilms are commonly contaminated by polymicrobial communities of uropathogens [47]. In addition, the production of phage-neutralizing antibodies in the body could reduce the efficacy of the approach [134].

Antimicrobial peptides

Antimicrobial peptides are generally short peptides between 8 and 30 amino acids in length and constitute a significant component of the innate immune response of a number of eukaryotes including plants, insects, amphibians and mammals [135]. There has been considerable interest in this area in recent years and, as a consequence, a wide range of peptides have been described. Probably the best characterized is nisin, a heat-stable bacteriocin produced by certain strains of the bacterium *Lactococcus lactis*. When incorporated into antimicrobial food packaging as a polymer film, nisin has been shown to have an antibacterial effect against a range of foodborne bacterial pathogens [136–138].

The human immune system has proved to be a useful source of antimicrobial peptides that demonstrate activity against a range of microorganisms [139–142]. Antimicrobial peptides of human origin (histatins, defensins) were recently evaluated *in vitro* as potential antifungal coatings for dentures and other oral prostheses [142]. It was shown that the surfaces had a limited efficacy, producing less than 1-$\log_{10}$ reductions of *C. albicans* over 72 h. Etienne *et al.* [143] described a strategy whereby a mosquito-derived peptide was inserted into multilayer films consisting of alternate layers of polyanions and polycations. In an adherence assay, the efficacy of the approach increased with the number of peptide layers incorporated into the films, with 10 layers, the highest number tested, reducing the viability of adhered *E. coli* by 98.75% after 30 min contact. Based on these results the authors proposed that this technology could have biomedical applications.

Synthetic antimicrobial peptides can be manufactured. For example, flexible sequence-random polymers containing cationic and lipophilic subunits that act as functional mimics of host-defense peptides have been reported [144]. One such polymer, with an average length of 21 residues, was able to disrupt bacterial cell membranes [145]. Reactive Surfaces, Ltd, a US-based company, claim to have developed polymers of amino acid peptides with activity against algae, fungi, bacteria (including the spore form of such microorganisms) and certain viruses, which they have incorporated into their ProteCoat® product line of coatings. They also claim the system can be used alone or synergistically in combination with existing microbicides (http://reactivesurfaces.com/).

Cationic surfaces

Several research groups have investigated the potential of cationic or positively charged surfaces to inactivate microorganisms that have adhered to a surface. Abel *et al.* [146] developed surfaces bearing carbohydrate units modified in a two-step process to incorporate lipophilic and polycationic functionalities. The rationale for the use of a lipophilic and cationic surfactant is that the cationic site of the agent is able to bind to anionic sites of the bacterial cell wall surface. With a significant lipophilic component present, it is then able to diffuse through the cell wall and bind to the membrane. The surfactant is then able to disrupt the membrane and permit the release of cellular constituents leading to cell death. The group produced eight carbohydrate materials with various surface structures and showed that several could inhibit the growth of *E. coli*, *Enterobacter aerogenes*, *Enterobacter cloacae*, *Proteus vulgaris*, *B. cereus*, *Micrococcus luteus* and *S. aureus*. The surfaces continued to inhibit growth when repeatedly challenged with the bacteria.

Bouloussa *et al.* [147] described a technique for fabricating highly positively charged nanometric thin films on materials bearing hydroxylated groups on their outermost surface, conferring on them the ability to kill bacteria on contact. This approach uses a bifunctional copolymer bearing simultaneously trimethoxysilane, which anchors the polymer to a surface, and quaternary ammonium groups, which provide the cationic charges for the biocidal behavior. The surfaces showed activity against *E. coli*, *B. subtilis* (vegetative cells), *S. epidermidis* and *Streptococcus mutans* and a 98–100% kill was cited. The authors also stated that the surfaces can be reused after the inactivated bacteria have been removed by washing.

Terada *et al.* [148] performed a study whereby they introduced positively charged ethylamino and diethylamino groups into polymer sheets and examined the adhesion and viability of *E. coli* and vegetative *B. subtilis*. The density of the amino groups was proportional to the membrane potential and high membrane potentials were associated with increased bacterial adhesion (more than −7.8 mV for *E. coli* and more than −8.3 mV for *B. subtilis*). However, as the membrane potential increased there were reductions in the viability of adhered bacteria. For example, 80% of *E. coli* cells adhering to sheets with high membrane potential were inactivated after 8 h and 60% of adhered *B. subtilis* cells were inactivated. *E. coli* viability appeared to be affected significantly when membrane potentials were higher than −8 mV, whereas *B. subtilis* viability decreased gradually as membrane potential increased.

Reactive surfaces that release antimicrobial agents on command

The properties of reactive surfaces that continuously release their antimicrobial agents have been discussed (see above). The constant efflux of agents means that the concentration of available agents will continuously decline. There are concerns that this could result in subinhibitory concentrations being released, which could encourage resistance [43]. A better approach would be to trap the active agent within a polymer and only make it available when it is needed. Reactive surfaces have been developed to be responsive to light (UV), electricity, ultrasound, magnetic

Table 20.1.1 The efficacy of titanium dioxide coatings irradiated with UVA.

Agent	Microorganism tested	Efficacy		Reference
		Reduction	Time	
TiO$_2$-coated glass	Escherichia coli	>6.3-log$_{10}$	1 h	Kuhn et al. [150]
	Pseudomonas aeruginosa	>5.4-log$_{10}$	1 h	
	Staphylococcus aureus	>3.9-log$_{10}$	1 h	
	Enterococcus faecium	3.1-log$_{10}$	1 h	
	Candida albicans	1.2-log$_{10}$	1 h	
TiO$_2$-coated glass	Bacteriophage T4	c. 6-log$_{10}$	3 h	Ditta et al. [149]
	E. coli	c. 6-log$_{10}$	3 h	
TiO$_2$/CuO hybrid	Bacteriophage T4	c. 9-log$_{10}$	80 min	
TiO$_2$-coated glass	Kocuria rhizophilus	3.3-log$_{10}$	4 h	Muranyi et al. [151]
	Bacillus atrophaeus (vegetative cells)	3.5-log$_{10}$	4 h	
	B. atrophaeus (spores)	No reduction	4 h	
	Aspergillus niger (spores)	No reduction	4 h	

fields, temperature and pH. Another approach is the development of polymers which can be "programmed" to release active agents at predetermined time points.

Surfaces with photocatalytic activity

The irradiation of some metal oxides with UV light generates reactive oxygen species which can react together to form hydrogen peroxide [149]. There is considerable interest in this technology as a means of generating surfaces that can "self-clean". In the following summarized studies (Table 20.1.1), titanium dioxide (TiO$_2$) coatings were inoculated with various microorganisms and irradiated with UVA light (320–400 nm). It is apparent that the TiO$_2$ coatings can considerably reduce the viability of microorganisms. The study by Ditta et al. [149] reported that an enhanced kill was achieved when the surface was manufactured to contain TiO$_2$ and copper oxide (CuO) and attributed this to the additional release of toxic copper ions. TiO$_2$ coatings, however, appear to have little or no activity against fungal and bacterial spores [151]. Chen et al. [152] have adopted a slightly different approach. They developed magnetic nanoparticles comprised of iron oxide coated with TiO$_2$ with pathogen-specific antibodies immobilized on its surface. These nanoparticles were shown to capture high numbers of pathogenic bacteria and inactivate them following exposure to UV light.

Photosensitive dyes such as Rose Bengal also generate oxygen radicals upon exposure to light. The dye achieves this by transferring energy provided in the form of light to molecular oxygen before returning to its electronic ground state whereupon it is able to absorb another photon and repeat the cycle. Recent studies have shown that the activity of the dye can be enhanced when it is incorporated into films comprising of silver nanoparticles [153, 154]. This raises the possibility of developing a decontamination system based on a combination of silver nanoparticles and a photosensitizer.

Anthraquinone is a naturally-occurring aromatic organic compound used in the manufacture of dyes. Bilyk et al. [155] developed a novel polymeric surface consisting of modified poly(ethylene imine) (PEI) polymers containing anthraquinone moieties attached covalently to the PEI chains. These polymers were applied from solution to the surface of polyethylene films. Exposure to low-energy UV light resulted in the production of hydrogen peroxide from the coated film on exposure to air. No work has been conducted to see if the amounts of hydrogen peroxide produced at the surface are sufficient to inactivate microorganisms.

Surfaces responsive to electricity

As previously described, the ionic forms of silver, zinc and copper possess intrinsic antimicrobial activity. A relatively simple way of generating ions is to pass an electric current through a wire composed of the metal of choice. Researchers have examined this "iontophoretic" approach in vitro where a low-current power source was used to drive the release of antimicrobial silver ions from silver wires attached to catheters [156, 157]. Raad et al. [156], for example, showed that the electrified catheters could prevent the migration of S. epidermidis from the highly contaminated hub to the sterile tip for 40 days, whereas silver-impregnated catheters could only delay this migration for 3 days. Chakravarti et al. [157] used a model of the catheterized bladder to examine the iontophoretic approach. This group reported that control catheters became blocked with crystalline P. mirabilis biofilm within 48 h. It took up to 156 h, however, for the catheter-blocking biofilms to develop on the electrified catheters. A recent refinement of this approach has been the development of a washing machine that releases 0.2 ppm silver ions into the laundry [61, 158]. Laboratory studies confirmed that this concentration of silver ions was able to achieve a 5-log$_{10}$ reduction against S. aureus and E. coli after 90 min contact [61]. Gelatin-containing microemulsion-based organogels (MBGs) are electrically conducting and have been employed for the iontophoretic delivery of a model drug through excised pig skin. Iontophoresis using MBGs gave substantially higher release rates for sodium salicylate compared with passive diffusion, and fluxes were proportional to the drug loading and the current density [159, 160].

Ultrasound activated release of antimicrobial agents

Ultrasound has been developed as an "off–on" switch to regulate the release of drugs. Kwok and colleagues initially developed an impermeable layer based on self-assembled methylene chains, which changed shape in response to exposure to ultrasound [161]. Using this ultrasound responsive layer they were able to regulate the release of a polymer carrier containing insulin. In a further adaptation of this approach, researchers have developed a novel drug delivery polymer matrix consisting of a poly(2-hydroxyethyl methacrylate) hydrogel coated with ordered methylene chains to form an ultrasound-responsive coating [162]. This system retained the antibiotic ciprofloxacin within the polymer and was subsequently released on exposure to low-intensity ultrasound. It was reported that daily 20 min 43 kHz treatments reduced biofilm formation by *P. aeruginosa* over a 72 h period.

Shchukin and colleagues [163] investigated the effect of ultrasonic treatments of different intensity and duration on the integrity and permeability of polyelectrolyte capsules comprising of poly(allylamine)/poly(styrene sulfonate) and Fe_3O_4 (magnetite)/poly(allylamine)/poly(styrene sulfonate). They reported that ultrasonic treatment of the capsules induced the destruction of the polyelectrolyte shell and the subsequent release of the encapsulated material following a 5 s ultrasonic burst. The presence of magnetite nanoparticles significantly improved the efficiency of the ultrasonically-stimulated release. These "microcontainers" are being developed for the potential delivery of toxic drugs in the treatment of diseases like cancer or tuberculosis [163]. In theory, they offer the potential to magnetically control drug delivery to the desired site before ultrasonic treatment triggers drug release. One can envisage applications whereby the microcontainers are loaded with microbicides and incorporated into surface coatings that release their load when exposed to ultrasound.

Magnetically controlled drug delivery

As well as being evaluated for the targeted delivery of drugs in medicine, magnetic particles are also being considered for surface applications. Lee *et al.* [164], for example, produced magnetic microspheres coated with silver nanoparticles which could be directed to a specific location on a surface to achieve a localized antimicrobial action. A different approach is the manufacture of small spheres comprising of magnetic particles that release their load when exposed to an oscillating magnetic field [165–167]. This technology may facilitate the future development of reactive surfaces capable of treating or preventing microbial colonization via "on command" microbicide release.

Hsu and Su [168] have developed magnetic lipid nanoparticles with the potential to serve as controlled delivery vehicles for the release of encapsulated drugs and microbicides. The nanoparticles can consist of multiple drugs enveloped within lipid matrices, which melt at around 45–55°C. In addition, super-paramagnetic γ-Fe_2O_3 particles, with sizes ranging from 5 to 25 nm, are dispersed uniformly in the lipid nanoparticles. When exposed to an alternating magnetic field, a solution of the nanoparticles (approximately 150 nm in diameter) showed a temperature increase from 37 to 50°C in 20 min. The dissipated heat melted the surrounding lipid matrices and resulted in an accelerated release of the encapsulated drugs. Release rates could be elevated further by decreasing the size of the lipid nanoparticles.

An alternative approach has been investigated by Liu and colleagues [169] where active agents can be released from a polymer on command when the magnetic field is switched off. A magnetic-sensitive hydrogel (ferrogel) has been developed consisting of a cross-linked polymer network containing magnetic particles. The theory is that when the magnetic field is switched on, the attraction of the magnetic particles interspersed throughout will reduce the pore size of the polymer. When the field is switched off, the pores in the polymer will reopen. Therefore, ferrogels can be developed with a precise opening and closure of pores, allowing a burst release or no release of an active agent which can be controlled externally and magnetically.

Surfaces responsive to temperature and pH

A number of polymers and hydrogels have been developed that can expel entrapped drug molecules in response to changes in pH and temperature [170]. For instance, when a critical pH or temperature is reached some polymers can undergo a reversible phase transition that results in the collapse of the structure and the release of the drug. This technology has mostly been evaluated for the controlled delivery of therapeutic drugs within the body [170]. In theory, environmental applications could be explored.

An interesting approach is the development of surfaces which can slough off accumulated material in response to external stimuli. For example, a thermally responsive polymer, poly(*N*-isopropyl acrylamide) (PNIPAM), has been developed which has a lower critical solubility temperature (LCST) of 32°C, making it insoluble in water above this temperature. In a laboratory study examining surfaces coated with this polymer it was demonstrated that >90% of microorganisms attached to the surfaces were immediately removed when they were washed with cold (4°C) water [171]. Systems based on this technology could be explored for their ability to detach biofilms from surfaces in the environment.

Double-responsive systems are also being developed which respond to both temperature and pH [170]. For example, Gupta and colleagues [172] described a drug delivery system based on a smart polymer gel composed of a random terpolymer of *N*-isopropyl acrylamide, butyl methacrylate and acrylic acid. The system was engineered to coat vaginal tissue with a stable gel layer and to potentially release entrapped antiviral agents in response to the presence of semen, which increases the pH of the vagina. It is thought that the thermoresponsive properties of the gel will promote its retention within the body.

Programmable release of active agents from implants

Another approach is the rational selection of polymer constituents that have defined stabilities over time. In this way the polymer can be "programmed" to release active agents as its constituents gradually degrade. Vogelhuber *et al.* [173] developed matrices consisting of various polymers (polyanhydrides, poly(D,L-lactic acid) or poly(D,L-lactic acid co-glycolic acid)). These polymers exhibited different stabilities and began to degrade and release an associated drug at different time points. This offered the possibility of combining these matrices in the development of a system that can be programmed to release drugs at several predetermined time points. Guse *et al.* [174] investigated the development of programmable implants by using triglycerides as core materials. The core materials were loaded with the model drug (pyranine) and used to produce the implant matrices. The matrices produced release periods from 2 to 16 weeks depending on the core material used. Overall, therefore, it could be possible to program drug release from a polymer so there is a delayed onset of release followed by several weeks of controlled release.

Reactive surfaces that release antimicrobial agents on demand

An emergent approach to the exploitation of antibacterial agents in the protection of surfaces is the "on demand" release of antimicrobial agents in response to the presence of contaminating microorganisms. Several studies have investigated the possibility of attaching drugs to polymers via a linker which operates as an infection sensor at the site of infection [175, 176]. Tanihara *et al.* [175] for instance noted that the exudate from wounds infected with *S. aureus* had thrombin-like activity, an enzyme involved in the formation of blood clots. A polymer–drug conjugate was subsequently synthesized where the antibiotic gentamicin was bound to a hydrogel polymer through a thrombin-sensitive linker. In subsequent experiments gentamicin was released from the polymer in the presence of infected exudate but, importantly, was not released in the presence of sterile wound exudate. Another approach targeted the macrophage-derived enzyme cholesterol esterase which is secreted during infection [176]. It may be possible to develop a system whereby a broad-spectrum antimicrobial is attached to a polymer via a linker which can be degraded by an enzyme secreted by a range of microorganisms.

A more general approach has been proposed by Loher and colleagues [177] in a report on the potential of a microorganism-triggered silver nanoparticle release system. This coating system consists of 1–2 nm silver particles decorating the surface of 20–50 nm biodegradable, phosphate-based carrier particles. As the organisms grow they take up nutrients and minerals from the coating, which dissolves the matrix and thus triggers the release of silver nanoparticles. In laboratory experiments it was demonstrated that the surface reduced the viability of *E. coli*, *P. aeruginosa* and *C. albicans* by 5–6-$\log_{10}$, 6-$\log_{10}$ and 4-$\log_{10}$ after 24 h, respectively. The surface, however, had little effect on *S. aureus* or fungal spores (*Aspergillus niger*). Encouraging pathogens to actively grow on contaminated surfaces under some circumstances, for example in the healthcare environment, may be considered to be unwise.

Conclusions

Considerable research effort has focused on the development of indwelling medical devices, such as urinary catheters, which can resist microbial colonization and biofilm formation. This is warranted since urinary catheters are the leading cause of infections acquired by patients in healthcare facilities [178–180]. In theory, the efficacy of many antimicrobial surface technologies can be examined in medical and environmental settings. This has been the case for antimicrobial delivery systems such as zeolites.

Passive surfaces that inhibit microbial attachment have been developed as potential coatings for implanted medical devices. The principal challenge associated with the development of an effective passive surface is controlling the formation of protein conditioning films which have the potential to compromise their "non-stick" nature. However, passive coatings comprising of diamond-like carbon (DLC) and polyethylene oxide (PEO) polymer brushes have been noted for their ability to reduce both the adherence of microorganisms and other debris. The interest in these coatings for the development of medical devices appears to be justified. These passive technologies have not been evaluated for use on environmental surfaces. In theory, a coating based on the PEO polymer brushes could be investigated since it has been reported that the microbes that attach to polymer brushes are weakly associated and more easily removed by physical shear than uncoated surfaces. This may offer the potential to develop a surface which can be easily cleaned.

A logical approach to combat the formation of biofilms on medical devices or to kill microorganisms attached to environmental surfaces has been to incorporate microbicides or antibiotics into the surface. A range of reactive surfaces that possess antimicrobial activity have been described for various applications. A review of the reactive technologies developed for urinary catheters helped to identify the challenges involved in the development of effective reactive surfaces. The challenges can be summarized as follows:

1. Surfaces in the environment and those used for implanted medical devices come into contact with a range of microorganisms with different susceptibilities to antimicrobial agents.

2. If conditions are favorable for microbial growth, subsequent biofilm development will further decrease the susceptibility of the colonizing microorganisms to antimicrobial agents.

3. Whatever the application, reactive surfaces could become compromised by extraneous factors. The presence of soiling materials, for example, could prevent the active agent from accessing the microorganism.

4. The antimicrobial activity should provide protection over the long term.

5. The delivery of subinhibitory concentrations of antimicrobial agents could induce resistance in colonizing microbes.

Traditionally, reactive surfaces have been developed where the antimicrobial agents are continuously released or they are fixed into the surface. In this way, the active agents are constantly available to exert their antimicrobial activity. Coating surfaces with live microorganisms, bacteria or bacteriophages, are promising approaches which deserve further examination. A major difficulty in the development of effective reactive surfaces appears to be loading materials with sufficient active agent and then controlling its release. The concentration of available agents will constantly decline. With the exploitation of live cultures, however, the organisms are capable of replication and thus renewing themselves [37, 129].

For environmental and medical applications, the ability to activate antimicrobial activity "on command" or "on demand" could result in the development of an extremely effective coating system. In this way, the antimicrobial agents are not being used prophylactically and it would reduce the risk of selecting resistant species since they are not being exploited indiscriminately. In addition, the ability to activate antimicrobial activity when needed would increase the lifespan of the systems. With the exception of TiO_2 surfaces developed to have photocatalytic activity, the majority of these technologies are at an early stage in their development.

The development of combinational or synergistic approaches should continue. It is well known that microbes growing in biofilms are more resistant to antimicrobial agents than their planktonic counterparts. The ability to make cells growing in biofilms more susceptible to antimicrobial agents would be an attractive capability. The development of surfaces that release dispersin B is one approach which is showing promise. The incorporation of quorum-sensing inhibitors should also be explored. In theory it may be possible to combine passive and reactive technologies or exploit several reactive properties. Li *et al.* [181], for example, constructed thin film coatings comprising two distinct layered functional regions. The bottom layer acted as a reservoir for the loading of silver nanoparticles, which released antimicrobial ions. This layer was capped by another layer bearing quaternary ammonium salts. Therefore, this technology is able to release antimicrobial agents into the surrounding medium but also kill microorganisms upon contact.

Several of the researchers investigating the efficacy of reactive polymers have noted an inability to inactivate endospores [79, 89, 151, 177]. The spore form of bacteria is designed to allow the organism to survive many physical insults that the environment might expose them to until conditions change for the better. As a consequence, spores are considerably more resistant to microbicides than their vegetative counterparts. There is particular interest in the identification of approaches capable of inactivating bacterial spore-formers such as *Clostridium difficile* [79]. *C. difficile* is a major contaminant of the hospital environment and

significant cause of morbidity and mortality as a consequence of environmental spread between patients [182].

In theory, a strategy which could induce the organism to convert from a microbicide-resistant spore to its more susceptible vegetative form, a process called germination, would therefore increase the susceptibility of the organism to antimicrobial agents. A study by Wheeldon *et al.* [79] showed that copper surfaces were rapidly active against the vegetative form of *C. difficile*, but had no activity against the spore form of this organism. However, when *C. difficile* spores were premixed with a solution of sodium taurocholate, a bile salt known to induce the germination of this organism, copper surfaces achieved close to 3-$\log_{10}$ reductions after 3 h. Other applications should be explored where germinants are simply mixed with disinfectant solutions or incorporated into reactive polymers, which trick the spores into germinating so they can be attacked by antimicrobial agents.

It is important to realize that no single antimicrobial surface is likely to provide a panacea for the prevention of microbial contamination since these rapidly evolving organisms are likely to overcome any intervention. However, the utilization of such surfaces is justified, particularly in the healthcare and food processing environments, since they have the potential to reduce the level of bioburden on surfaces and prevent the survival of potential pathogens. The research evidence suggests that a strategy to replace high-contact surfaces in these settings with copper and its alloys could be beneficial. Microbicides, particularly triclosan and silver nanoparticles, have been incorporated into a plethora of household appliances. It is understandable that consumers want to protect themselves from harmful "germs" that can colonize surfaces and fabrics. Reactive surfaces in this context may help to provide peace of mind to those who might be particularly susceptible to infection. Others, however, subscribe to the view that these technologies should be reserved for more clinically useful situations [105, 108, 112].

It could be argued that the introduction of antimicrobial surfaces into the environment could create complacency with regards to hygiene. There is no evidence to suggest that antimicrobial surfaces can replace cleaning and disinfection. In fact, one could argue that reactive technologies in the environment would not be effective unless they are regularly cleaned to prevent conditioning film development, which could mask the antimicrobial activities of any surface. There is ample evidence showing that these surfaces could have a positive impact as an adjunct to cleaning and disinfection strategies. The introduction of these surfaces, however, has to be evidence-based and it would be prudent to closely monitor the adhered flora for signs of the emergence of less susceptible strains or the selection of intrinsically resistant species.

References

1 Costerton, J.W. *et al.* (1987) Bacterial biofilms in nature and disease. *Annual Review of Microbiology*, **41**, 435–464.

2 Kramer, A. *et al.* (2006) How long do nosocomial pathogens persist on inanimate surfaces? A systematic review. *BMC Infectious Diseases*, **6**, 130.

3 Boyce, J.M. *et al.* (1997) Environmental contamination due to methicillin-resistant *Staphylococcus aureus*: possible infection control implications. *Infection Control and Hospital Epidemiology*, **18**, 622–627.

4 Boyce, J.M. (2007) Environmental contamination makes an important contribution to hospital infection. *Journal of Hospital Infection*, **65** (Suppl. 2), 50–54.

5 Hardy, K.J. *et al.* (2006) A study of the relationship between environmental contamination with methicillin-resistant *Staphylococcus aureus* (MRSA) and patients' acquisition of MRSA. *Infection Control and Hospital Epidemiology*, **27**, 127–132.

6 Kumar, C.G. and Anand, S.K. (1998) Significance of microbial biofilms in food industry: a review. *International Journal of Food Microbiology*, **42**, 9–27.

7 Werry, C. *et al.* (1988) Contamination of detergent cleaning solutions during hospital cleaning. *Journal of Hospital Infection*, **11**, 44–49.

8 Dharan, S. *et al.* (1999) Routine disinfection of patients' environmental surfaces. Myth or reality? *Journal of Hospital Infection*, **42**, 113–117.

9 Barker, J. *et al.* (2004) Effects of cleaning and disinfection in reducing the spread of Norovirus contamination via environmental surfaces. *Journal of Hospital Infection*, **58**, 42–49.

10 Coia, J.E. *et al.* (2006) Guidelines for the control and prevention of meticillin-resistant *Staphylococcus aureus* (MRSA) in healthcare facilities. *Journal of Hospital Infection*, **63** (Suppl. 1), 1–44.

11 Williams, G.J. *et al.* (2007) The development of a new three-step protocol to determine the efficacy of disinfectant wipes on surfaces contaminated with *Staphylococcus aureus*. *Journal of Hospital Infection*, **67**, 329–335.

12 Williams, G.J. *et al.* (2009) Limitations of the efficacy of surface disinfection in the healthcare setting. *Infection Control and Hospital Epidemiology*, **30**, 570–573.

13 Costerton, J.W. *et al.* (1999) Bacterial biofilms: a common cause of persistent infections. *Science*, **284**, 1318–1322.

14 Donlan, R.M. (2001) Biofilms and device-associated infections. *Emerging Infectious Diseases*, **7**, 277–281.

15 Donlan, R.M. and Costerton, J.W. (2002) Biofilms: survival mechanisms of clinically relevant microorganisms. *Clinical Microbiology Reviews*, **15**, 167–193.

16 Lappin-Scott, H.M. and Bass, C. (2001) Biofilm formation: attachment, growth, and detachment of microbes from surfaces. *American Journal of Infection Control*, **29**, 250–251.

17 Dunne, W.M. Jr. (2002) Bacterial adhesion: seen any good biofilms lately? *Clinical Microbiology Reviews*, **15**, 155–166.

18 Gristina, A.G. (1987) Biomaterial-centered infection: microbial adhesion versus tissue integration. *Science*, **25**, 1588–1595.

19 O'Toole, G.A. and Kolter, R. (1998) Flagellar and twitching motility are necessary for *Pseudomonas aeruginosa* biofilm development. *Molecular Microbiology*, **30**, 295–304.

20 Downer, A. *et al.* (2003) Polymer surface properties and their effect on the adhesion of *Proteus mirabilis*. *Proceedings of the Institution of Mechanical Engineers. Part H, Journal of Engineering in Medicine*, **217**, 279–289.

21 Stickler, D.J. *et al.* (2006) Observations on the adherence of *Proteus mirabilis* onto polymer surfaces. *Journal of Applied Microbiology*, **100**, 1028–1033.

22 Jones, D.S. *et al.* (2006) Examination of surface properties and *in vitro* biological performance of amorphous diamond-like carbon-coated polyurethane. *Journal of Biomedical Materials Research. Part B, Applied Biomaterials*, **78**, 230–236.

23 Liu, C. *et al.* (2008) Reduction of bacterial adhesion on modified DLC coatings. *Colloids and Surfaces. B, Biointerfaces*, **61**, 182–187.

24 Zhao, Q. *et al.* (2009) Bacterial attachment and removal properties of silicon- and nitrogen-doped diamond-like carbon coatings. *Biofouling*, **25**, 377–385.

25 Shao, W. *et al.* (2010) Influence of interaction energy between Si-doped diamond-like carbon films and bacteria on bacterial adhesion under flow conditions. *Journal of Biomedical Materials Research. Part A*, **93**, 133–139.

26 Levon, J. *et al.* (2010) Patterned macroarray plates in comparison of bacterial adhesion inhibition of tantalum, titanium, and chromium compared with diamond-like carbon. *Journal of Biomedical Materials Research. Part A*, **92**, 1606–1613.

27 Laube, N. *et al.* (2007) Diamond-like carbon coatings on ureteral stents – a new strategy for decreasing the formation of crystalline bacterial biofilms? *Journal of Urology*, **177**, 1923–1927.

28 Ohkawa, M. *et al.* (1990) Bacterial and crystal adherence to the surfaces of indwelling urethral catheters. *Journal of Urology*, **143**, 717–721.

29 Tieszer, C. *et al.* (1998) Conditioning film deposition on ureteral stents after implantation. *Journal of Urology*, **160**, 876–881.

30 Currie, E.P. *et al.* (2003) Tethered polymer chains: surface chemistry and their impact on colloidal and surface properties. *Advances in Colloid and Interface Science*, **100–102**, 205–265.

31 Roosjen, A. *et al.* (2003) Inhibition of adhesion of yeasts and bacteria by poly(ethylene oxide)-brushes on glass in a parallel plate flow chamber. *Microbiology*, **149**, 3239–3246.

32 Roosjen, A. *et al.* (2004) Microbial adhesion to poly(ethylene oxide) brushes: influence of polymer chain length and temperature. *Langmuir*, **20**, 10949–10955.

33 Roosjen, A. *et al.* (2005) Stability and effectiveness against bacterial adhesion of poly(ethylene oxide) coatings in biological fluids. *Journal of Biomedical Materials Research. Part B, Applied Biomaterials*, **73**, 347–354.

34 Roosjen, A. *et al.* (2006) Bacterial factors influencing adhesion of *Pseudomonas aeruginosa* strains to a poly(ethylene oxide) brush. *Microbiology*, **152**, 2673–2682.

35 Trautner, B.W. *et al.* (2002) Pre-inoculation of urinary catheters with *Escherichia coli* 83972 inhibits catheter colonization by *Enterococcus faecalis*. *Journal of Urology*, **167**, 375–379.

36 Trautner, B.W. *et al.* (2003) *Escherichia coli* 83972 inhibits catheter adherence by a broad spectrum of uropathogens. *Urology*, **61**, 1059–1062.

37 Trautner, B.W. *et al.* (2007) Coating urinary catheters with an avirulent strain of *Escherichia coli* as a means to establish asymptomatic colonization. *Infection Control and Hospital Epidemiology*, **28**, 92–94.

38 Prasad, A. *et al.* (2009) A bacterial interference strategy for prevention of UTI in persons practicing intermittent catheterization. *Spinal Cord*, **47**, 565–569.

39 Stickler, D.J. and Feneley, R.C. (2010) The encrustation and blockage of long-term indwelling bladder catheters: a way forward in prevention and control. *Spinal Cord*, **48**, 784–790.

40 Stickler, D.J. (2000) Biomaterials to prevent nosocomial infections: is silver the gold standard? *Current Opinion in Infectious Diseases*, **13**, 389–393.

41 Darouiche, R.O. (2001) Device-associated infections: a macroproblem that starts with microadherence. *Clinical Infectious Diseases*, **33**, 1567–1572.

42 Darouiche, R.O. *et al.* (1999) Efficacy of antimicrobial-impregnated bladder catheters in reducing catheter-associated bacteriuria: a prospective, randomized, multicenter clinical trial. *Urology*, **54**, 976–981.

43 Rosch, W. and Lugauer, S. (1999) Catheter-associated infections in urology: possible use of silver-impregnated catheters and the Erlanger silver catheter. *Infection*, **27** (Suppl. 1), 74–77.

44 Stickler, D.J. *et al.* (1994) Bacterial biofilm growth on ciprofloxacin treated urethral catheters. *Cells and Materials*, **4**, 387–398.

45 Danese, P.N. (2002) Antibiofilm approaches: prevention of catheter colonization. *Chemistry and Biology*, **9**, 873–880.

46 Williams, G.J. and Stickler, D.J. (2007) Some observations on the diffusion of antimicrobial agents through the retention balloons of Foley catheters. *Journal of Urology*, **178**, 697–701.

47 Williams, G.J. and Stickler, D.J. (2008) Effect of triclosan on the formation of crystalline biofilms by mixed communities of urinary tract pathogens on urinary catheters. *Journal of Medical Microbiology*, **57**, 1135–1140.

48 Whalen, R.L. *et al.* (1997) An infection inhibiting urinary catheter material. *ASAIO Journal (American Society for Artificial Internal Organs: 1992)*, **43**, M842–M847.

49 Cho, Y.H. *et al.* (2001) Prophylactic efficacy of a new gentamicin-releasing urethral catheter in short-term catheterized rabbits. *BJU International*, **87**, 104–109.

50 Park, J.H. *et al.* (2003) Norfloxacin-releasing urethral catheter for long-term catheterization. *Journal of Biomaterials Science. Polymer Edition*, **14**, 951–962.

51 Richards, C.L. *et al.* (2003) Development and characterization of an infection inhibiting urinary catheter. *ASAIO Journal (American Society for Artificial Internal Organs: 1992)*, **49**, 449–453.

52 Kwok, C.S. *et al.* (1999) Design of infection-resistant antibiotic-releasing polymers. II. Controlled release of antibiotics through a plasma-deposited thin film barrier. *Journal of Controlled Release*, **62**, 301–311.

53 Hendricks, S.K. *et al.* (2000) Plasma-deposited membranes for controlled release of antibiotic to prevent bacterial adhesion and biofilm formation. *Journal of Biomedical Materials Research*, **50**, 160–170.

54 DiTizio, V. *et al.* (1998) A liposomal hydrogel for the prevention of bacterial adhesion to catheters. *Biomaterials*, **19**, 1877–1884.

55 Russell, A.D. and Hugo, W.B. (1994) Antimicrobial activity and action of silver. *Progress in Medicinal Chemistry*, **31**, 351–370.

56 Edwards-Jones, V. (2009) The benefits of silver in hygiene, personal care and healthcare. *Letters in Applied Microbiology*, **49**, 147–152.

57 Morgan, S.D. *et al.* (2009) A study of the structure of the crystalline bacterial biofilms that can encrust and block silver Foley catheters. *Urological Research*, **37**, 89–93.

58 Gaonkar, T.A. *et al.* (2007) Efficacy of a silicone urinary catheter impregnated with chlorhexidine and triclosan against colonization with *Proteus mirabilis* and other uropathogens. *Infection Control and Hospital Epidemiology*, **28**, 596–598.

59 Maillard, J.Y. and Denyer, S.P. (2006) Focus on silver. *EWMA Journal*, **6**, 5–7.

60 Pal, S. *et al.* (2007) Does the antibacterial activity of silver nanoparticles depend on the shape of the nanoparticle? A study of the Gram-negative bacterium *Escherichia coli*. *Applied and Environmental Microbiology*, **73**, 1712–1720.

61 Jung, W.K. *et al.* (2008) Antibacterial activity and mechanism of action of the silver ion in *Staphylococcus aureus* and *Escherichia coli*. *Applied and Environmental Microbiology*, **74**, 2171–2178.

62 Matsumura, Y. *et al.* (2003) Mode of bactericidal action of silver zeolite and its comparison with that of silver nitrate. *Applied and Environmental Microbiology*, **69**, 4278–4281.

63 Davenport, K. and Keeley, F.X. (2005) Evidence for the use of silver-alloy-coated urethral catheters. *Journal of Hospital Infection*, **60**, 298–303.

64 Maillard, J.Y. and Denyer, S.P. (2006) Demystifying Silver. European Wound Management Association, Position Document: Management of Wound Infection, MEP Ltd, London.

65 Chopra, I. (2007) The increasing use of silver-based products as antimicrobial agents: a useful development or a cause for concern? *Journal of Antimicrobial Chemotherapy*, **59**, 587–590.

66 Das, K. *et al.* (2008) Surface coatings for improvement of bone cell materials and antimicrobial activities of Ti implants. *Journal of Biomedical Materials Research. Part B, Applied Biomaterials*, **87**, 455–460.

67 Wilks, S.A. *et al.* (2005) The survival of *Escherichia coli* O157 on a range of metal surfaces. *International Journal of Food Microbiology*, **105**, 445–454.

68 Noyce, J.O. *et al.* (2006) Use of copper cast alloys to control *Escherichia coli* O157 cross-contamination during food processing. *Applied and Environmental Microbiology*, **72**, 4239–4244.

69 Wilks, S.A. *et al.* (2006) Survival of *Listeria monocytogenes* Scott A on metal surfaces: implications for cross-contamination. *International Journal of Food Microbiology*, **111**, 93–98.

70 Conly, J.M. *et al.* (1989) Handwashing practices in an intensive care unit: the effects of an educational program and its relationship to infection rates. *American Journal of Infection Control*, **17**, 330–339.

71 Bauer, T.M. *et al.* (1990) An epidemiological study assessing the relative importance of airborne and direct contact transmission of microorganisms in a medical intensive care unit. *Journal of Hospital Infection*, **15**, 301–309.

72 Blythe, D. *et al.* (1998) Environmental contamination due to methicillin-resistant *Staphylococcus aureus* (MRSA). *Journal of Hospital Infection*, **38**, 67–69.

73 Griffith, C.J. *et al.* (2003) Environmental surface cleanliness and the potential for contamination during handwashing. *American Journal of Infection Control*, **31**, 93–96.

74 Bhalla, A. *et al.* (2004) Acquisition of nosocomial pathogens on hands after contact with environmental surfaces near hospitalized patients. *Infection Control and Hospital Epidemiology*, **25**, 164–167.

75 Casey, A.L. *et al.* (2010) Role of copper in reducing hospital environment contamination. *Journal of Hospital Infection*, **74**, 72–77.

76 Mikolay, A. *et al.* (2010) Survival of bacteria on metallic copper surfaces in a hospital trial. *Applied Microbiology and Biotechnology*, **87**, 1875–1879.

77 Noyce, J.O. *et al.* (2006) Potential use of copper surfaces to reduce survival of epidemic meticillin-resistant *Staphylococcus aureus* in the healthcare environment. *Journal of Hospital Infection*, **63**, 289–297.

78 Mehtar, S. *et al.* (2008) The antimicrobial activity of copper and copper alloys against nosocomial pathogens and *Mycobacterium tuberculosis* isolated from healthcare facilities in the Western Cape: an *in-vitro* study. *Journal of Hospital Infection*, **68**, 45–51.

79 Wheeldon, L.J. *et al.* (2008) Antimicrobial efficacy of copper surfaces against spores and vegetative cells of *Clostridium difficile*: the germination theory. *Journal of Antimicrobial Chemotherapy*, **62**, 522–525.

80 Airey, P. and Verran, J. (2007) Potential use of copper as a hygienic surface; problems associated with cumulative soiling and cleaning. *Journal of Hospital Infection*, **67**, 271–277.

81 Khare, M.D. *et al.* (2007) Reduction of catheter-related colonisation by the use of a silver zeolite-impregnated central vascular catheter in adult critical care. *Journal of Infection*, **54**, 146–150.

82 Matsuura, T. *et al.* (1997) Prolonged antimicrobial effect of tissue conditioners containing silver-zeolite. *Journal of Dentistry*, **25**, 373–377.

83 Hotta, M. *et al.* (1998) Antibacterial temporary filling materials: the effect of adding various ratios of Ag-Zn-Zeolite. *Journal of Oral Rehabilitation*, **25**, 485–489.

84 Padachey, N. *et al.* (2000) Resistance of a novel root canal sealer to bacterial ingress *in vitro*. *Journal of Endodontics*, **26**, 656–659.

85 Abe, Y. *et al.* (2004) Effect of saliva on an antimicrobial tissue conditioner containing silver-zeolite. *Journal of Oral Rehabilitation*, **31**, 568–573.

86 Rusin, P. *et al.* (2003) Rapid reduction of *Legionella pneumophila* on stainless steel with zeolite coatings containing silver and zinc ions. *Letters in Applied Microbiology*, **36**, 69–72.

87 Bright, K.R. *et al.* (2002) Rapid reduction of *Staphylococcus aureus* populations on stainless steel surfaces by zeolite ceramic coatings containing silver and zinc ions. *Journal of Hospital Infection*, **52**, 307–309.

88 Inoue, Y. *et al.* (2002) Bactericidal activity of Ag-zeolite mediated by reactive oxygen species under aerated conditions. *Journal of Inorganic Biochemistry*, **92**, 37–42.

89 Galeano, B. *et al.* (2003) Inactivation of vegetative cells, but not spores, of *Bacillus anthracis*, *B. cereus*, and *B. subtilis* on stainless steel surfaces coated with an antimicrobial silver- and zinc-containing zeolite formulation. *Applied and Environmental Microbiology*, **69**, 4329–4331.

90 Cowan, M.M. *et al.* (2003) Antimicrobial efficacy of a silver-zeolite matrix coating on stainless steel. *Journal of Industrial Microbiology and Biotechnology*, **30**, 102–106.

91 Gogotsi, Y. *et al.* (2003) Nanoporous carbide-derived carbon with tunable pore size. *Nature Materials*, **2**, 591–594.

92 Gogotsi, Y. *et al.* (2008) Bactericidal activity of chlorine-loaded carbide-derived carbon against *Escherichia coli* and *Bacillus anthracis*. *Journal of Biomedical Materials Research. Part A*, **84**, 607–613.

93 Njoroge, J. and Sperandio, V. (2009) Jamming bacterial communication: new approaches for the treatment of infectious diseases. *EMBO Molecular Medicine*, **1**, 201–210.

94 Davies, D.G. *et al.* (1998) The involvement of cell-to-cell signals in the development of a bacterial biofilm. *Science*, **280**, 295–298.

95 Han, Y. *et al.* (2008) Identifying the important structural elements of brominated furanones for inhibiting biofilm formation by *Escherichia coli*. *Bioorganic and Medicinal Chemistry Letters*, **18**, 1006–1010.

96 Liu, H.B. *et al.* (2010) Inhibitors of the *Pseudomonas aeruginosa* quorum-sensing regulator, QscR. *Biotechnology and Bioengineering*, **106**, 119–126.

97 Vestby, L.K. *et al.* (2010) A synthetic furanone potentiates the effect of disinfectants on *Salmonella* in biofilm. *Journal of Applied Microbiology*, **108**, 771–778.

98 Piletska, E.V. *et al.* (2010) Attenuation of *Vibrio fischeri* quorum sensing using rationally designed polymers. *Biomacromolecules*, **11**, 975–980.

99 Mah, T.F. and O'Toole, G.A. (2001) Mechanisms of biofilm resistance to antimicrobial agents. *Trends in Microbiology*, **9**, 34–39.

100 Stewart, P.S. and Costerton, J.W. (2001) Antibiotic resistance of bacteria in biofilms. *Lancet*, **358**, 135–138.

101 De Beer, D. *et al.* (1994) Direct measurement of chlorine penetration into biofilms during disinfection. *Applied and Environmental Microbiology*, **60**, 4339–4344.

102 Hoyle, B.D. *et al.* (1992) *Pseudomonas aeruginosa* biofilm as a diffusion barrier to piperacillin. *Antimicrobial Agents and Chemotherapy*, **36**, 2054–2056.

103 Donelli, G. *et al.* (2007) Synergistic activity of dispersin B and cefamandole nafate in inhibition of staphylococcal biofilm growth on polyurethanes. *Antimicrobial Agents and Chemotherapy*, **51**, 2733–2740.

104 Darouiche, R.O. *et al.* (2009) Antimicrobial and antibiofilm efficacy of triclosan and DispersinB combination. *Journal of Antimicrobial Chemotherapy*, **64**, 88–93.

105 Levy, S.B. (2001) Antibacterial household products: cause for concern. *Emerging Infectious Diseases*, **7** (Suppl. 3), 512–515.

106 Schweizer, H.P. (2001) Triclosan: a widely used biocide and its link to antibiotics. *FEMS Microbiology Letters*, **202**, 1–7.

107 White, D.G. and McDermott, P.F. (2001) Biocides, drug resistance and microbial evolution. *Current Opinion in Microbiology*, **4**, 313–317.

108 SCCS (Scientific Committee on Consumer Safety) (2010) Preliminary opinion on triclosan (antimicrobial resistance), http://ec.europa.eu/health/scientific_committees/consumer_safety/docs/sccs_o_013.pdf (assessed 23 March, 2010).

109 Cole, E.C. *et al.* (2003) Investigation of antibiotic and antibacterial agent cross-resistance in target bacteria from homes of antibacterial product users and nonusers. *Journal of Applied Microbiology*, **95**, 664–676.

110 McBain, A.J. *et al.* (2003) Exposure of sink drain microcosms to triclosan: population dynamics and antimicrobial susceptibility. *Applied and Environmental Microbiology*, **69**, 5433–5442.

111 McBain, A.J. *et al.* (2004) Selection for high-level resistance by chronic triclosan exposure is not universal. *Journal of Antimicrobial Chemotherapy*, **53**, 772–777.

112 Russell, A.D. (2004) Whither triclosan? *Journal of Antimicrobial Chemotherapy*, **53**, 693–695.

113 Edmiston, C.E. *et al.* (2006) Bacterial adherence to surgical sutures: can antibacterial-coated sutures reduce the risk of microbial contamination? *Journal of the American College of Surgeons*, **203**, 481–489.

114 Ming, X. *et al.* (2008) *In vivo* and *in vitro* antibacterial efficacy of PDS plus (polidioxanone with triclosan) suture. *Surgical Infections*, **9**, 451–457.

115 Justinger, C. *et al.* (2009) Antibacterial coating of abdominal closure sutures and wound infection. *Surgery*, **145**, 330–334.

116 Elechiguerra, J.L. *et al.* (2005) Interaction of silver nanoparticles with HIV-1. *Journal of Nanobiotechnology*, **3**, 6.

117 Raffi, M. *et al.* (2008) Antibacterial characterization of silver nanoparticles against ATCC-15224. *Journal of Materials Science and Technology*, **24**, 192–196.

118 Jones, N. *et al.* (2008) Antibacterial activity of ZnO nanoparticle suspensions on a broad spectrum of microorganisms. *FEMS Microbiology Letters*, **279**, 71–76.

119 Cioffi, N. *et al.* (2005) Synthesis, analytical characterization and bioactivity of Ag and Cu nanoparticles embedded in poly-vinyl-methyl-ketone films. *Analytical and Bioanalytical Chemistry*, **382**, 1912–1918.

120 Yoon, K.Y. *et al.* (2007) Susceptibility constants of *Escherichia coli* and *Bacillus subtilis* to silver and copper nanoparticles. *Science of the Total Environment*, **373**, 572–575.

121 Ruparelia, J.P. *et al.* (2008) Strain specificity in antimicrobial activity of silver and copper nanoparticles. *Acta Biomaterialia*, **4**, 707–716.

122 Ren, G. *et al.* (2009) Characterisation of copper oxide nanoparticles for antimicrobial applications. *International Journal of Antimicrobial Agents*, **33**, 587–590.

123 Koper, O.B. *et al.* (2002) Nanoscale powders and formulations with biocidal activity toward spores and vegetative cells of *Bacillus* species, viruses, and toxins. *Current Microbiology*, **44**, 49–55.

124 Cooper, R.A. *et al.* (1999) Antibacterial activity of honey against strains of *Staphylococcus aureus* from infected wounds. *Journal of the Royal Society of Medicine*, **92**, 283–285.

125 Cooper, R.A. *et al.* (2002) The efficacy of honey in inhibiting strains of *Pseudomonas aeruginosa* from infected burns. *Journal of Burn Care and Rehabilitation*, **23**, 366–370.

126 French, V.M. *et al.* (2005) The antibacterial activity of honey against coagulase-negative staphylococci. *Journal of Antimicrobial Chemotherapy*, **56**, 228–231.

127 Henriques, A.F. *et al.* (2010) The intracellular effects of manuka honey on *Staphylococcus aureus*. *European Journal of Clinical Microbiology and Infectious Diseases*, **29**, 45–50.

128 Henriques, A. *et al.* (2006) Free radical production and quenching in honeys with wound healing potential. *Journal of Antimicrobial Chemotherapy*, **58**, 773–777.

129 Hanlon, G.W. (2007) Bacteriophages: an appraisal of their role in the treatment of bacterial infections. *International Journal of Antimicrobial Agents*, **30**, 118–128.

130 Curtin, J.J. and Donlan, R.M. (2006) Using bacteriophages to reduce formation of catheter-associated biofilms by *Staphylococcus epidermidis*. *Antimicrobial Agents and Chemotherapy*, **50**, 1268–1275.

131 Carson, L. *et al.* (2010) The use of lytic bacteriophages in the prevention and eradication of biofilms of *Proteus mirabilis* and *Escherichia coli*. *FEMS Immunology and Medical Microbiology*, **59**, 447–455.

132 Fu, W. *et al.* (2010) Bacteriophage cocktail for the prevention of biofilm formation by *Pseudomonas aeruginosa* on catheters in an *in vitro* model system. *Antimicrobial Agents and Chemotherapy*, **54**, 397–404.

133 Cademartiri, R. *et al.* (2010) Immobilization of bacteriophages on modified silica particles. *Biomaterials*, **31**, 1904–1910.

134 Smith, H.W. *et al.* (1987) Factors influencing the survival of bacteriophages in calves and in their environment. *Journal of General Microbiology*, **133**, 1127–1135.

135 Guani-Guerra, E. *et al.* (2010) Antimicrobial peptides: general overview and clinical implications in human health and disease. *Clinical Immunology (Orlando, Fla.)*, **135**, 1–11.

136 Jin, T. and Zhang, H. (2008) Biodegradable polylactic acid polymer with nisin for use in antimicrobial food packaging. *Journal of Food Science*, **73**, M127–M134.

137 Nguyen, V.T. *et al.* (2008) Potential of a nisin-containing bacterial cellulose film to inhibit *Listeria monocytogenes* on processed meats. *Food microbiology*, **25**, 471–478.

138 Ye, M. *et al.* (2008) Effectiveness of chitosan-coated plastic films incorporating antimicrobials in inhibition of *Listeria monocytogenes* on cold-smoked salmon. *International Journal of Food Microbiology*, **127**, 235–240.

139 Ericksen, B. *et al.* (2005) Antibacterial activity and specificity of the six human {alpha}-defensins. *Antimicrobial Agents and Chemotherapy*, **49**, 269–275.

140 Yadava, P. *et al.* (2006) Antimicrobial activities of human beta-defensins against *Bacillus* species. *International Journal of Antimicrobial Agents*, **28**, 132–137.

141 Sass, V. *et al.* (2010) Human beta-defensin 3 inhibits cell wall biosynthesis in staphylococci. *Infection and Immunity*, **78**, 2793–2800.

142 Pusateri, C.R. *et al.* (2009) Sensitivity of *Candida albicans* biofilm cells grown on denture acrylic to antifungal proteins and chlorhexidine. *Archives of Oral Biology*, **54**, 588–594.

143 Etienne, O. *et al.* (2004) Multilayer polyelectrolyte films functionalized by insertion of defensin: a new approach to protection of implants from bacterial colonization. *Antimicrobial Agents and Chemotherapy*, **48**, 3662–3669.

144 Mowery, B.P. *et al.* (2007) Mimicry of antimicrobial host-defense peptides by random copolymers. *Journal of the American Chemical Society*, **129**, 15474–15476.

145 Epand, R.F. *et al.* (2008) Dual mechanism of bacterial lethality for a cationic sequence-random copolymer that mimics host-defense antimicrobial peptides. *Journal of Molecular Biology*, **379**, 38–50.

146 Abel, T. *et al.* (2002) Preparation and investigation of antibacterial carbohydrate-based surfaces. *Carbohydrate Research*, **337**, 2495–2499.

147 Bouloussa, O. *et al.* (2008) A new, simple approach to confer permanent antimicrobial properties to hydroxylated surfaces by surface functionalization. *Chemical Communications (Cambridge, England)*, **28**, 951–953.

148 Terada, A. *et al.* (2006) Bacterial adhesion to and viability on positively charged polymer surfaces. *Microbiology*, **152**, 3575–3583.

149 Ditta, I.B. *et al.* (2008) Photocatalytic antimicrobial activity of thin surface films of TiO$_2$, CuO and TiO$_2$/CuO dual layers on *Escherichia coli* and bacteriophage T4. *Applied Microbiology and Biotechnology*, **79**, 127–133.

150 Kuhn, K.P. *et al.* (2003) Disinfection of surfaces by photocatalytic oxidation with titanium dioxide and UVA light. *Chemosphere*, **53**, 71–77.

151 Muranyi, P. *et al.* (2010) Antimicrobial efficiency of titanium dioxide-coated surfaces. *Journal of Applied Microbiology*, **108**, 1966–1973.

152 Chen, W.J. *et al.* (2008) Functional Fe$_3$O$_4$/TiO$_2$ core/shell magnetic nanoparticles as photokilling agents for pathogenic bacteria. *Small (Weinheim an der Bergstrasse, Germany)*, **4**, 485–491.

153 Zhang, Y. *et al.* (2007) Metal-enhanced singlet oxygen generation: a consequence of plasmon enhanced triplet yields. *Journal of Fluorescence*, **17**, 345–349.

154 Zhang, Y. *et al.* (2008) Plasmonic engineering of singlet oxygen generation. *Proceedings of the National Academy of Sciences of the United States of America*, **105**, 1798–1802.

155 Bilyk, A. *et al.* (2008) Photoactive nanocoating for controlling microbial proliferation on polymeric surfaces. *Progress in Organic Coatings*, **62**, 40–48.

156 Raad, I. *et al.* (1996) *In vitro* antimicrobial efficacy of silver iontophoretic catheter. *Biomaterials*, **17**, 1055–1059.

157 Chakravarti, A. *et al.* (2005) An electrified catheter to resist encrustation by *Proteus mirabilis* biofilm. *Journal of Urology*, **174**, 1129–1132.

158 Jung, W.K. *et al.* (2007) Antifungal activity of the silver ion against contaminated fabric. *Mycoses*, **50**, 265–269.

159 Kantaria, S. *et al.* (1999) Gelatin-stabilised microemulsion-based organogels: rheology and application in iontophoretic transdermal drug delivery. *Journal of Controlled Release*, **60**, 355–365.

160 Kantaria, S. *et al.* (2003) Formulation of electrically conducting microemulsion-based organogels. *International Journal of Pharmaceutics*, **250**, 65–83.

161 Kwok, C.S. *et al.* (2001) Self-assembled molecular structures as ultrasonically-responsive barrier membranes for pulsatile drug delivery. *Journal of Biomedical Materials Research*, **57**, 151–164.

162 Norris, P. *et al.* (2005) Ultrasonically controlled release of ciprofloxacin from self-assembled coatings on poly(2-hydroxyethyl methacrylate) hydrogels for *Pseudomonas aeruginosa* biofilm prevention. *Antimicrobial Agents and Chemotherapy*, **49**, 4272–4279.

163 Shchukin, D.G. *et al.* (2006) Ultrasonically induced opening of polyelectrolyte microcontainers. *Langmuir*, **22**, 7400–7404.

164 Lee, D. *et al.* (2005) Antibacterial properties of Ag nanoparticle loaded multilayers and formation of magnetically directed antibacterial microparticles. *Langmuir*, **21**, 9651–9659.

165 Edelman, E.R. *et al.* (1985) Regulation of drug release from polymer matrices by oscillating magnetic fields. *Journal of Biomedical Materials Research*, **19**, 67–83.

166 Saslawski, O. *et al.* (1988) Magnetically responsive microspheres for the pulsed delivery of insulin. *Life Sciences*, **42**, 1521–1528.

167 Zhang, Y. *et al.* (2006) Controlled drug delivery system based on magnetic hollow spheres/polyelectrolyte multilayer core-shell structure. *Journal of Nanoscience and Nanotechnology*, **6**, 3210–3214.

168 Hsu, M.H. and Su, Y.C. (2008) Iron-oxide embedded solid lipid nanoparticles for magnetically controlled heating and drug delivery. *Biomedical Microdevices*, **10**, 785–793.

169 Liu, T.Y. *et al.* (2008) Study on controlled drug permeation of magnetic-sensitive ferrogels: effect of Fe$_3$O$_4$ and PVA. *Journal of Controlled Release*, **126**, 228–236.

170 Schmaljohann, D. (2006) Thermo- and pH-responsive polymers in drug delivery. *Advanced Drug Delivery Reviews*, **58**, 1655–1670.

171 Ista, L.K. *et al.* (1999) Surface-grafted, environmentally sensitive polymers for biofilm release. *Applied and Environmental Microbiology*, **65**, 1603–1609.

172 Gupta, K.M. *et al.* (2007) Temperature and pH sensitive hydrogels: an approach towards smart semen-triggered vaginal microbicidal vehicles. *Journal of Pharmaceutical Sciences*, **96**, 670–681.

173 Vogelhuber, W. *et al.* (2001) Programmable biodegradable implants. *Journal of Controlled Release*, **73**, 75–88.

174 Guse, C. *et al.* (2006) Programmable implants – from pulsatile to controlled release. *International Journal of Pharmaceutics*, **314**, 161–169.

175 Tanihara, M. *et al.* (1999) A novel microbial infection-responsive drug release system. *Journal of Pharmaceutical Sciences*, **88**, 510–514.

176 Woo, G.L. *et al.* (2002) Biological characterization of a novel biodegradable antimicrobial polymer synthesized with fluoroquinolones. *Journal of Biomedical Materials Research*, **59**, 35–45.

177 Loher, S. *et al.* (2008) Micro-organism-triggered release of silver nanoparticles from biodegradable oxide carriers allows preparation of self-sterilizing polymer surfaces. *Small (Weinheim an der Bergstrasse, Germany)*, **4**, 824–832.

178 Warren, J.W. *et al.* (1989) The prevalence of urethral catheterization in Maryland nursing homes. *Archives of Internal Medicine*, **149**, 1535–1537.

179 Stamm, W.E. (1991) Catheter-associated urinary tract infections: epidemiology, pathogenesis, and prevention. *American Journal of Medicine*, **91**, 65S–71S.

180 Kunin, C.M. (1997) Care of the urinary catheter, in *Urinary Tract Infections: Detection, Prevention and Management*, 5th edn, Williams & Wilkins, Baltimore, pp. 227–279.

181 Li, Z. (2006) Two-level antibacterial coating with both release-killing and contact-killing capabilities. *Langmuir*, **22**, 9820–9823.

182 Cohen, S.H. *et al.* (2010) Clinical practice guidelines for *Clostridium difficile* infection in adults: 2010 update by the society for healthcare epidemiology of America (SHEA) and the infectious diseases society of America (IDSA). *Infection Control and Hospital Epidemiology*, **31**, 431–455.

20.2 Antimicrobial Devices

Brendan F. Gilmore and Sean P. Gorman

Faculty of Medicine, Health and Life Sciences, Queen's University Belfast, Belfast, Northern Ireland, UK

Introduction

The use of indwelling medical devices such as catheters, stents and artificial prostheses has become a cornerstone of modern surgical and clinical practice. In fact, it is estimated that each person will host an indwelling medical device at least once in their lifetime, and that tens of millions of devices are used in patients each year. The general trend in industrialized nations towards a steadily aging population has driven increasing reliance upon, and unprecedented demand for, medical devices that support the normal physiological functioning of the body, and improve pre- and post-operative care, diagnosis and patient quality of life. Such devices provide solutions for a diverse range of acute and chronic medical conditions and surgical procedures (Table 20.2.1). However, despite the technological advances made in the fields of biomaterials and medical device manufacture, a number of fundamental issues still plague their use *in vivo*. While complications may be specific to the type and placement of a given device, every type of indwelling medical device in current use is susceptible to microbial colonization and

biofilm formation, which remains the primary complication inherent to their use. The development of medical device-associated infections generally necessitates complete device removal which, depending on the type and site of the device, can either be relatively simple (i.e. a urological catheter) or require complete surgical removal.

In attempts to resolve the infectious complications associated with the use of indwelling medical devices, significant research has been directed towards the development of devices which are inherently antimicrobial or anti-infective, by either direct incorporation of antimicrobial agents or chemical/physical modification of the biomaterial surface. In addition to increased demand for indwelling medical devices, an unprecedented growth in high-value combination products (drug–device combinations) such as drug-eluting arterial stents and antimicrobial devices (primarily urological and central venous catheters) is fueling an average annual growth rate of *c.* 12.4% in the global medical device coatings market. By 2010, annual worldwide sales (medical device coatings) are forecast to reach US$5.31 billion. Clearly, there is an urgent need to develop devices that prevent or retard microbial colonization and biofilm formation, to

---

Russell, Hugo & Ayliffe's: Principles and Practice of Disinfection, Preservation and Sterilization, Fifth Edition. Edited by Adam P. Fraise, Jean-Yves Maillard, and Syed A. Sattar.
© 2013 Blackwell Publishing Ltd. Published 2013 by Blackwell Publishing Ltd.

Table 20.2.1 Number of medical implants used in the USA (adapted from [5]).

Device	Number/year
Intraocular lens	2,700,000
Contact lens	30,000,000
Vascular graft	250,000
Hip and knee prostheses	500,000
Catheter	200,000,000
Heart valve	80,000
Stent (cardiovascular)	>1,000,000
Breast implant	192,000
Dental implant	300,000
Pacemaker	130,000
Renal dialyzer	16,000,000

address the ubiquitous problem of device-associated infection and to alleviate not only the unacceptably high levels of patient morbidity and mortality associated with their use, but also to reduce the significant financial implications to healthcare providers associated with increased patient morbidity and extended care costs. Currently, healthcare-associated infections (HAIs) are estimated to cost the UK National Health Service £1 billion per year [1].

Definition of medical device

According to the Medicines and Healthcare Products Regulatory Agency (MHRA), the regulator of medical devices in the UK, a medical device may be defined as:

. . . any instrument, apparatus, appliance, material or other article, whether used alone or in combination, including the software necessary for its proper application intended by the manufacturer to be used for human beings for the purpose of:
• diagnosis, prevention, monitoring, treatment or alleviation of disease,
• diagnosis, monitoring, treatment, alleviation of or compensation for an injury or handicap,
• investigation, replacement or modification of the anatomy or of a physiological process,
• control of conception,
and which does not achieve its principal intended action in or on the human body by pharmacological, immunological or metabolic means, but which may be assisted in its functions by such means. [2]

Medical devices typically fulfill their intended functions by physical means (e.g. mechanical action, physical barrier, support/replace organs, normal physiological functioning), but may contain a medicinal substance that acts on the body in a manner auxiliary to the device.

Biomaterials

The term biomaterial has been defined as any substance (other than a drug) or combination of substances, natural or synthetic, which can be used for any time as a whole or part of a system that treats, augments or replaces any tissue, organ or function of the body [3]. By definition, therefore, all materials employed in the manufacture of indwelling medical devices are described as biomaterials. The design of biomaterials will ultimately be dictated by their intended applications and the functional lifetime of the device, which can be temporary use (urinary catheters, sutures, central venous catheters, etc.) or permanent implant (orthopedic/dental implants, prosthetic heart valves, etc.). Importantly, biomaterials are characterized not only by their intended function, but also by their continuous or intermittent contact with bodily fluids and/or tissues. Therefore, biomaterials must be also be designed to reduce adverse events associated with intimate (direct or indirect) contact between the body and the material/medical device and must therefore exhibit biocompatibility.

Such is the extent of utilization of biomaterials that almost every human in technologically advanced societies will host a biomaterial at some point [4]. The high incidence of adverse side effects associated with biomaterials and implanted medical device usage has stimulated significant research into the design and production of materials to minimize the complications inherent in the clinical use of these devices.

Medical device applications of biomaterials

The medical device-related applications of biomaterials are contained within three broad categories: (i) extracorporeal applications, such as catheters, tubing and fluid lines, dialysis devices, ocular devices, wound dressings, etc.; (ii) permanently implanted devices such as orthopedic, dental or cardiovascular devices; and (iii) temporary implants, such as temporary vascular grafts, arterial stents, scaffolds for tissue growth or organ replacement, degradable sutures, implantable drug delivery systems, etc.

Biomaterials in medical device manufacture

Throughout the history of indwelling or implantable medical devices a wide range of materials have been employed in their manufacture, from natural materials to metals. Today, a diverse range of materials are employed in device manufacture including natural macromolecules (biopolymers), synthetic polymers, biodegradable polymers, metals, carbons and ceramics. Polymeric materials remain the most popular medical device material, thanks to their ease of processing, favorable mechanical and physical attributes and ease of modification post manufacture (e.g. coating) to increase biocompatibility. The development of vulcanized rubber in 1839 may be regarded as the pioneering step towards more patient-acceptable devices. The most common biomaterials employed in the manufacture of indwelling medical devices are discussed below.

Latex

Natural rubber latex (polyisoprene) had been utilized in the Americas for thousands of years but was first brought to Europe by Columbus in the late 1500s. It was the material employed for the manufacture of the first Foley urinary catheters and to this day is still widely employed, primarily as a base for "coated" devices. The material exhibits many properties desirable for use in medical devices, for example high tensile strength and superb elastic recovery. Latex is inexpensive, easily processed and hence production costs are low. Unfortunately, latex is neither especially biocompatible nor resistant to the development of biofilm formation. Additionally, latex may absorb up to 40% of its own weight in water, potentially increasing the external diameter of devices and reducing the lumen size. For this reason the useable lifespan of all-latex devices is generally only 14 days.

Silicone

Silicone was first developed by the chemist Kipping in the early 1900s and was thus named due to its similarity in structure with ketones. The resinous, polymeric material was first isolated as an impurity [5] and largely ignored until a commercially viable production process was developed in the 1940s. Its application in medical device manufacture followed shortly thereafter. Poly-dimethylsiloxane (PDMS) is the most widely utilized silicone polymer in modern medicine due to its stability and ease of manufacture. Silicone is widely used as a biomaterial of choice for catheter production. Exhibiting the mechanical benefits of latex rubber, silicone's inherent strength allows for the design of a large lumen within the device since the walls remain thin. However, although it appears that there is a slight reduction in the susceptibility for encrusted deposits to form on urological catheters, silicone is still highly susceptible to biofilm formation and, in the case of urological devices where it is widely used, development of encrustation [6, 7].

The primary disadvantage with all-silicone devices is the greater level of discomfort experienced by patients. Such discomfort is associated with the higher levels of rigidity when compared with all-latex or other coated devices and silicone's relatively low lubricity, particularly during insertion and removal of devices. For these reasons manufacturers favor the application of lubricious coatings on silicone and latex devices. Silicone may also be applied as a coating over latex devices, resulting in a device with improved mechanical characteristics while the propensity for stricture formation is reduced due to the latex base being "masked" beneath the more biocompatible polymer.

Polyvinyl chloride

Polyvinyl chloride (PVC) is widely employed in the manufacture of intermittent catheters since it is mechanically strong, inexpensive and has a relatively smooth, lubricious surface. The rigidity of the material is overcome in practice through the addition of plasticizers to yield a sufficiently flexible product that may be employed clinically. When compared with latex, the devices can have thinner walls and hence a larger lumen; however, even when a plasticizer is present the material is not sufficiently elastic to enable it to be comfortably utilized in the manufacture of indwelling devices.

Polytetrafluoroethylene

Polytetrafluoroethylene (PTFE, Teflon), has been employed since the mid 1960s as a catheter coating thanks to its low coefficient of friction and hydrophobic nature, thought to increase patient comfort and reduce device degradation *in situ*. Despite initial claims of reduced biofilm/encrustation formation, little evidence has emerged of any benefit of these devices over other materials. The characteristic paved texture of this material has been proposed to act as a nidus for bacterial attachment, promoting microbial adhesion and biofilm formation and facilitating the swarming of *Proteus* spp. [8], leading to encrustation deposition in urological applications [9]. PTFE is generally applied over a latex core, by dipping the latex device into a solution of PTFE particles in a binder (usually polyurethane). For this reason an even application is not always possible and, as the binder cures, tiny cracks may become evident. A PTFE coating may decrease water absorbency of the latex core of devices and allow for a potential 28-day indwelling duration.

Polyurethane

Polyurethanes are polymers containing the urethane linkage –OC(O)NH–. The term "polyurethane" refers to a broad variety of elastomers that are usually formed by the addition of a polyg-lycol to an isocyanate. They can be readily tailored for many applications by changing the chemicals used and thus a high degree of versatility in physical, chemical and biological/biocompatible characteristics is possible. Polyurethanes have good mechanical properties and are commonly used in permanent or semipermanent implanted medical devices (e.g. pacemakers, ureteral stents). This class of polymer also benefits from being relatively inexpensive.

Hydrogels

Hydrogels possess a number of physical characteristics such as biocompatibility, which make them attractive for medical device applications, and hydrophilicity, which can impart desirable release characteristics especially in combination devices (such as antimicrobial devices) where controlled drug release from a polymeric system is required. Hydrogels represent a relatively recent development in the manufacture of indwelling medical devices and are commonly employed as coatings over latex or silicone devices. At equilibrium, hydrogels swell to hold from 10% to 98% of water within their polymeric matrix. As such, they have at a minimum a moderately hydrophilic character and the extent of polymeric swelling is governed by both the polymer cross-link density and the degree of hydrophilicity of the polymer itself.

The trapping of water reduces the coefficient of friction, helping reduce patient discomfort since frictional irritation is reduced along with cell adhesion at the biomaterial–tissue interface. Various studies related to patient comfort and acceptability, for example that of Bull and colleagues [10], indicate that when contrasted with previous devices fitted, high proportions of patients indicated a preference for hydrogel-coated devices. A range of hydrogel materials have been employed including, hydroxyethyl methacrylate, *n*-vinyl pyrollidone and polyvinyl alcohol.

Although many benefits of hydrogel-coated devices have been proposed, evidence from trials has returned inconsistent results. A randomized controlled trial of device materials with a sufficiently large number of patients enrolled would be desirable to resolve the question of comparative benefits of materials. Gorman and co-workers [11] noted lower levels of encrustation compared with standard latex devices although there was increased adherence of hydrophilic bacterial strains. Sabbuba and colleagues [12] found that hydrogel coatings aid migration of pathogenic bacteria over samples. In contrast, Denyer and co-workers [13] noted significant reductions in the adherence of staphylococci to polyvinylpyrrolidine (PVP) and pHEMA. Coatings based upon polyethylene oxide (PEO) based multiblock copolymer/segmented polyurethane (SPU) blends have also demonstrated promise in the reduction of bacterial adherence and encrustation formation.

Complications associated with indwelling medical devices

Despite significant advances in the field of biomaterials over the past 50 years, the same complications associated with the earliest use of materials in human medicine remain a feature of modern devices. These include mechanical complications, adverse biological responses to implanted biomaterials and biomaterial- and device-related infections. In the case of mechanical failure, and biological adverse effects, many of these have been circumvented by the design of new polymeric materials, biologically inspired materials and materials capable of modulation of biological response either by virtue of drug release or surface modification. While much industry has been directed towards what is potentially the most serious and problematic of these complications – that is microbial colonization, biofilm formation and device infection – and while there has undoubtedly been progress in reducing the incidences of infections short term, there has been little in the way of real progress towards a biomaterial capable of ultimately resisting infection, especially in long-term use in patients.

Mechanical complications

As demand continues to grow for biomaterials that mimic as closely as possible the host tissue and environment with respect to biological, chemical, functional and mechanical attribute, significant advances in material design continue to deliver improved medical devices. The greatest potential diversity of properties, which can be tailored to a particular functional niche, exists within polymeric materials, driving the massive popularity of synthetic polymers in biomedical applications. As with any material, the functional demands placed on a device *in situ* (depending

mainly on placement within the body and intended function, i.e. load-bearing or non-load-bearing devices), can contribute to mechanical failure. This includes environmental stress cracking, material degradation, time-dependent deformation (creep), brittle fracture or fatigue. Mechanically-induced biological failure occurs when the functional demands on the medical device result in degradation of the device or liberation of particles of material, which results in the establishment of an inflammatory response *in vivo*, necessitating device removal.

Biocompatibility

Biomaterials by definition are designed to be in contact with host tissue or bodily fluids, a feature which distinguishes them from other materials commonly encountered in daily life, commerce or technology. A widely cited definition of biocompatibility is "the ability of a material to perform with an appropriate host response in a specific application" [14]. The interactions of a material within the host are undoubtedly complex and in many cases poorly elucidated; however, the concept of achieving an appropriate biocompatibility is a central tenet in the development of medical devices. The tests for assessment of biocompatibility of medical devices and the materials from which they are manufactured are described in the international standard ISO 10993, which covers the evaluation of genotoxicity, teratogenicity, antigenicity, thrombogenicity and carcinogenicity, basic *in vitro* screens for cytotoxicity, *in vivo* evaluation of biological response following implantation, toxicity of leachable or degradation by-products of medical devices, systemic toxicity, irritation and hypersensitivity. Furthermore, since the sterile device itself, not simply the material from which it was manufactured, must pass biocompatibility testing protocols, ISO 10993 also evaluates potential toxicities resulting from sterilization processes (e.g. ethylene oxide sterilization residuals). The specific potential biocompatibility complications (in common with all potential complications) will be dictated by the functional requirements of the device, as well as the site and duration of placement *in vivo*, and indeed may be related to mechanical and infectious complications resulting in degradation of the device and the resulting biological response.

Infectious complications

All implanted medical devices are susceptible to device-related infections, where microorganisms colonize the indwelling device and rapidly establish sessile, or surfaced-adhered, populations on the device surface. The development of microbial biofilms, surface-adhered microbial populations encased in a matrix of extracellular polymeric material (or "glycocalyx") under the control of a population density-dependent gene regulation mechanism (known as "quorum sensing"), is a ubiquitous survival strategy among microorganisms. It represents the predominant mode of growth of microorganisms in both the natural environment and in chronic infectious disease.

Critically, at least half of all cases of HAIs are associated with the use of implanted medical devices [15], with medical device use the greatest external predictor of HAIs. Indeed, many

Table 20.2.2 Rate of infection and attributable mortality of device-associated infections (adapted from [16]).

Medical device	Rate of infection (%)	Attributable mortality
Urinary catheters	10–30	Low
Central venous catheters	3–8	Moderate
Fracture fixation devices	5–10	Low
Dental implants	5–10	Low
Joint prostheses	1–3	Low
Vascular grafts	1–5	Moderate
Cardiac pacemakers	1–7	Moderate
Mammary implants, in pairs	1–2	Low
Mechanical heart valves	1–3	High
Penile implants	1–3	Low
Heart assist devices	25–50	High

biomaterials in current use exhibit surface characteristics that favor microbial surface colonization, such as poorly controlled, dynamic interfacial responses in physiological milieu, surface charge, hydrophobicity and microrugosity. While it is difficult to establish the exact magnitude and cost (in terms of patient morbidity, mortality and financial impact) of medical device-associated infections, Table 20.2.2 gives estimated rates of infection and attributable mortality for commonly implanted medical devices.

Factors that further increase the risk of implanted device infections include prolonged hospitalization, multiple surgical procedures at the time of implant, remote infections in other body parts, surgery duration and the amount of tissue devitalization [17]. The increased use of implanted medical devices and the growing number of immunocompromised and critically ill patients requiring interventions involving medical devices have also contributed to the rising number of medical device-related infections.

Healthcare-associated infections

Healthcare-associated infections are localized or systemic conditions resulting from an adverse reaction to the presence of an infectious agent(s) or its toxin(s). There must be no evidence that the infection was either present or incubating at the time of admission to the acute care setting. The causative organisms of HAIs may be from exogenous sources (e.g. patient carers, visitors, equipment, medical devices, healthcare environment) or endogenous sources (e.g. migration of organisms from normally colonized body sites: skin, mouth, nose, gastrointestinal tract, genitourinary tract).

The vast majority of nosocomial or HAIs occur at four major body sites, leading to their designation by the US Centers for Disease Control and Prevention (CDC) as the "Big Four" HAIs, namely surgical site infections (SSIs), pneumonia (PNEU), bloodstream infections (BSIs) and urinary tract infections (UTIs).

The incidences of three of these HAIs (pneumonia, urinary tract infections and bloodstream infections) are commonly associated with the use of medical devices, since each of these sites is amenable to instrumentation.

The urinary tract is the most common site for nosocomial infections, accounting for 23.2% of such infections in the UK, and greater than 30% of infections reported by acute care hospitals in the USA. The majority of these (up to 95%) follow instrumentation of the urinary tract, mainly urinary catheterization. In the USA alone, up to 13,000 deaths are associated with UTIs. This is followed closely by infections of the respiratory tract (22.9% of incidences), again commonly related to the use of implanted devices (more than 85% of cases) such as endotracheal tubes; the infection exhibiting the highest incidence is ventilator-associated pneumonia (VAP) [15]. SSIs account for 15% and 17% of all HAIs in the UK and US, respectively, and are associated with considerable morbidity, leading to an estimated doubling in the length of hospital stay. SSIs are also a significant cause of mortality among hospitalized patients, with one study estimating annual mortality rates associated with SSIs as high as 8% of all deaths attributable to HAIs (8000 in 100,000 HAI cases) [18]. However, significant reductions in SSI incidence can be achieved by improvements in pre- and postoperative care. In the UK, the highest incidences of SSIs are, perhaps unsurprisingly, recorded for small and large bowel surgery; however, the rate of SSI following orthopedic surgery has decreased significantly since 2004. Finally, it is estimated that approximately 248,000 bloodstream infections occur in US hospitals each year, with a large proportion of these associated with central venous catheters. In the UK, catheter-related blood stream infections (CRBSIs) represent between 10% and 20% of all HAIs. In general, of all device-associated infections, CRBSIs carry the highest rate of mortality.

Microorganisms typically encounter the implanted medical device either by gaining direct access to the device during placement or as systemically circulating opportunistic pathogens which colonize the device postimplantation (a latent infection). Therefore, the main causative organisms of medical device-related nosocomial infections are frequently normal skin biota including *Staphylococcus aureus* and coagulase-negative staphylococci, predominantly *Staphylococcus epidermidis*. The latter has been shown to be the most common cause of infections related to intravascular catheters and other implanted medical devices. A number of other key microorganisms have been shown to be significant causative organisms of medical device-related nosocomial infections, including *Pseudomonas aeruginosa* (VAP), enterococci, *Escherichia coli* (UTI, septicemia) and *Proteus* species, for example *Proteus mirabilis* (UTI, device encrustation).

Device-associated infections: Events following device implantation

The specter of medical device-related infection is one common to all types of implanted, indwelling medical devices. While

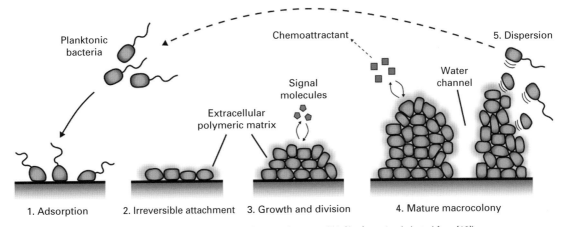

Figure 20.2.1 Medical device colonization by microorganisms showing surface attachment and biofilm formation (adapted from [19]).

causative organism may vary according to site or device, the process of biofilm formation on the biomaterial/device surface follows a series of discrete, well-characterized sequence of events, as shown in Figure 20.2.1 and described in detail in Chapter 21.2.

Deposition of conditioning film, colonization and biofilm formation

It is now well established that immediately after implantation the native medical device surface becomes rapidly modified, depending on the site, by adsorption of host-derived proteins, extracellular matrix proteins and coagulation products [20]. This is followed by rapid primary attachment of microorganism to the material surface and biofilm formation. Subsequent to the attachment of bacterial cells to the surface of a material, a number of phenotypic changes occur within the cells which lead to the formation of a microenvironment, conferring significant survival advantages over planktonic growth [21]. A biofilm can be defined as a microbially-derived sessile community of cells irreversibly attached to a substratum (biotic or abiotic), embedded within a matrix of extracellular polymeric substances that they have produced, and exhibiting an altered phenotype with respect to growth rate and gene transcription [22]

After the initial adherence of bacterial cells, the production of capsular exopolysaccharides is increased and coats the surface of the material and, for the majority of species, acts as an anchor to bind the bacterial colonies to the surface. The bacteria continue to divide within this protective matrix, with the rate of growth dependent upon the nutrient composition of the medium, its flow rate and whether there are any antimicrobial agents present [23]. The population of cells within a biofilm is heterogeneous with respect to metabolic activity, which contributes to their lack of sensitivity to standard antibiotic agents. Even so, the cells within the biofilm matrix reproduce, spreading over the surface of the material to form a more confluent coating. Cells are continually shed that may in turn form new colonies, the rate of which is determined by various factors including shear forces in the medium [24]. As a result, biofilms forming on indwelling medical devices may be considered a reservoir of infection.

Bacterial colonization of the surface and the production of extensive exopolysaccharide glycocalyxes provides a confluent-protected biofilm on medical devices. The biofilm provides and maintains an advantageous, protected microenvironment where organic nutrients and ions may be sequestered from the environment, antimicrobial penetration is retarded and cooperative activities such as genetic exchange, resistance transfer and cross-feeding are facilitated. Indeed, in some respects, biofilm communities may be regarded as a form of primitive tissue with channels present for the mass transit of both waste substances and nutrients, and a sophisticated quorum-sensing, population-dependent gene regulation system. The formation of a biofilm on a device–host tissue interface confers significant advantages to the bacteria within, in terms of tolerance/resistance to host defense mechanisms and antimicrobial agents [21]. The privileged microenvironment of the biofilm also facilitates, for example: (i) modulation of the physiological environment through maintenance of pH and electrochemical gradients; (ii) increased protection from phagocytosis and antimicrobial agents; (iii) improved ability to avoid recognition by natural defense mechanisms as capsular proteins of certain bacterial strains can mimic host structures; (iv) improved sustainability of growth through localization and concentration of nutrients and extracellular components within the interfaces of microcolonies with the exclusion of oxygen; and (v) increased access of extracellular enzymes, facilitating the absorption of molecules, may also occur, resulting in synergy within mixed cultures. The polysaccharide matrix also acts as an ion-exchange resin sequestering iron from host transferrin and lactoferrin. Irregular biofilm surfaces may increase turbulence at the interface between its surface and the surrounding medium, increasing the transfer of substrates from the medium up to three-fold [25].

Clinical management of device-related infections

The traditional management of device-associated infections involves the use of conventional antibiotic therapy directed against the identified or suspected causative organism, with the final choice of antibiotic ideally depending on microbiological susceptibility assay, as well as consideration of the pharmacological and toxicological properties of the antibacterial agent. At the biomaterial–device surface, antibiotics may induce direct kill or inhibit bacterial growth and can negatively affect the adhesion of microorganisms to the surface by interfering with bacterial adhesions, resulting in prevention of binding of planktonic bacteria [21]. Accepted clinical practice often includes combination therapy in which two or more antimicrobials are used to treat biofilm-associated infections. This approach introduces a broader spectrum of activity compared with single-agent treatment. Lower concentrations of the antimicrobials are required, resulting in more effective therapy and a decreased likelihood of resistance development [26]. Such approaches may also eradicate microorganisms, which despite being important mediators in mixed species biofilms, are not identified by standard culture techniques. Administration of prophylactic antibiotic therapy to prevent colonization is also common practice during surgical insertion of most devices. However, even in the presence of antibiotics, adherence, colonization and the establishment of infection can occur at medical device surfaces.

As discussed, a general characteristic of medical device-associated infections (and biofilm-mediated infections generally) is their recalcitrance to typical antimicrobial therapy and host defenses; such infections prove extremely difficult to eradicate and relapses occur frequently. Numerous factors contribute to the high antimicrobial tolerance of biofilm-mediated, medical device-associated infections including the distinct mode of growth displayed by biofilm populations and multidrug antimicrobial resistance.

Furthermore, standard susceptibility assays which often dictate antimicrobial choice may not be good predictors of the appropriate antimicrobial or concentration for biofilm eradication. This is because there may be no correlation between planktonic susceptibility to antimicrobial challenge (as assessed by the minimum inhibitory concentration (MIC)) and biofilm susceptibility of the same strain [27], thus contributing to the clinical failure rate of treating chronic biofilm-associated infections [17].

Development of antimicrobial biomaterials

The high incidences of device-associated infections and the significant limitations of conventional antimicrobial chemotherapy in their effective management, has prompted the development of device-based approaches. These are aimed at preventing the establishment of microbial biofilms rather than attempting to eradicate the infection once established as a sessile population. These approaches are focused on the development of bioactive, anti-infective or antimicrobial devices, which inhibit microbial adherence (by surface modification or irreversible tethering of antimicrobial to the surface) or microbial growth (by elution of the active agent).

In an effort to combat microbial adherence and biofilm formation on the surfaces of indwelling medical devices, a number of methods have been employed to modify polymer surfaces and/or load antimicrobial agents into medical device polymers, with the aim of producing bacteria-inhibitory and bactericidal surfaces (Figure 20.2.2). Bacteria-inhibitory surfaces prevent/discourage both bacterial colonization and proliferation, whereas bactericidal surfaces elute bactericides with the intent of killing planktonic and early colonizing microorganisms. Both systems aim to prevent microbial contamination from occurring on the surface of the medical device in the first instance and to inhibit bacterial colonization and subsequent biofilm formation. Such materials benefit from relatively low manufacturing costs, long shelf-lives and ease of processing (manufacturing/sterilization), and the overall function of a device is not compromised by the presence of the active agent [29]. Examples of methods employed in the loading of polymeric matrices with antimicrobial agents include immersion, coating, matrix loading and drug polymer conjugates [26].

Although straightforward, a major limitation of direct antimicrobial loading into a polymeric biomaterial matrix by coating or immersion is the optimization of drug release. Since release of standard antibacterial agents from the surface of the medical device is not coordinated with the presence of infecting organisms, the release of antimicrobial from a drug-loaded polymer matrix generally follows (according to Fick's law) a "burst" release

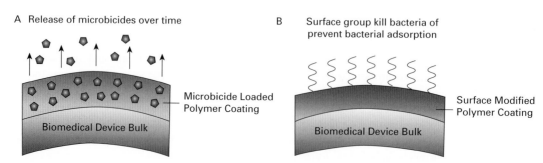

Figure 20.2.2 Antibacterial coating of medical devices. (a) Impregnation/loading of device coating with a polymeric layer (e.g. hydrogel) containing biocidal agents. (b) Permanent surface modification of a device with conjugates with either cidal or antiadherent activity. (Adapted from [28].)

profile (a major proportion of the drug is released at an early stage following implantation). This is followed by a slow leaching of potentially subinhibitory levels of the antimicrobial, which may be insufficient to prevent infection but may facilitate the selection of antimicrobial-resistant strains. The concentration of the polymer reservoir is then depleted and the "exhausted" device becomes susceptible to colonization by bacteria or fungi encountering the device surface at any time following the "burst" of antimicrobial release. Concerns have been raised that prophylaxis of device-associated infections using antibiotic-coated or loaded medical devices may lead to the proliferation of antimicrobial resistance, though further, long-term studies are necessary to confirm this.

Clinical experience with antimicrobial devices clearly indicates that due consideration must be given to mechanisms for achieving appropriate drug-release kinetics. Drug release which is uncontrolled and rapid, from a few hours to a few days, will in most clinical scenarios be inappropriate for preventing device-related infections [29]. Additionally, the mass of drug that can be incorporated is often insufficient for maintenance of prolonged bactericidal or bacteriostatic concentrations.

The formation of drug–polymer conjugates involves the covalent linkage of an agent to a monomer, prior to polymerization, resulting in the production of an extremely resilient drug–polymer material. Drug–polymer conjugates have been shown to significantly reduce bacterial adherence and encrustation in urinary catheters indicating the therapeutic potential of this approach for urinary catheter use in a site-specific manner. However, this approach is not without limitations, including increased cost of manufacture and limited antimicrobial choice (according to chemical compatibility of therapeutic agents with the synthetic reaction scheme) [26]. Furthermore, deposition of conditioning film or cellular material on the device surface may be sufficient to "mask" the antimicrobial activity of the biomaterial surface and to permit the establishment of a sessile microbial population.

Antiseptics

Antimicrobial impregnation/loading is not limited exclusively to conventional antibiotics. Coatings that release metals, namely silver and copper ions, and nonspecific antiseptic coatings (triclosan, hexetidine chlorhexidine, benzalkonium chloride) have been used effectively against device-associated infections. *Proteus mirabilis* is highly sensitive to triclosan with MICs of strains cultured from devices being reported as $0.5\,\mu g/ml$ [30], with other key pathogens also exhibiting high sensitivity to the compound. Triclosan has also been shown to inhibit *in vitro* biofilm growth of *E. coli*, *Klebsiella pneumoniae*, *S. aureus* and *P. mirabilis*, thus reducing encrustation formation. However, biofilm formation by some key pathogens such as *Serratia marcescens*, *Morganella morganii* and *P. aeruginosa* was not inhibited.

Silver

The use of silver in active medical devices has been the subject of much debate, with conflicting results from many studies since the first investigation indicating the potential for reduction in catheter-associated urinary tract infection (CAUTI) [31]. While much research has focused on the reduction of CAUTI by using silver-impregnated, silver-eluting or silver-coated urological catheters, silver (in various presentations and usually in combination with a broad-spectrum biocidal agent such as chlorhexidine) has been employed in commercially available endotracheal tubes, central venous catheters and wound dressings.

Silver ions have often been less effective than expected *in vivo* in relation to antimicrobial effects, although this may be related to their high reactivity with electron-donating groups such as sulfur, oxygen and nitrogen which are present in biological molecules. A sufficiently high concentration of free silver ions must be present since the rate of bacterial killing is directly proportional to concentration and, in the presence of albumin and/or Cl⁻ ions, activity may be reduced [31].

Due to the divergent views on the subject, Saint and co-workers [32] conducted a meta-analysis of eight clinical trials, the results indicating that there was a statistically significant benefit in the reduction of CAUTI in all patients where silver-coated catheters were used. However, their analysis indicated a significant benefit in silver alloy-coated catheters over silver oxide-coated catheters. The lack of evidence for benefit of these latter devices was a key factor in their withdrawal from the market. A more recent review [33] of antimicrobial catheters notes that more recent (post 1995) studies involving silver-coated devices demonstrate less significant advantages over control devices in reducing CAUTI. The authors argue that a combination of factors may be involved – the use of silicone devices rather than all-latex catheters as controls, better clinical practice and reduced background rates of bacteriuria due to improved clinical practice.

The Cochrane review of catheter trials [34] also criticizes the quality of most clinical trials involving the use of silver alloy- and silver oxide-containing urological catheters. The study did conclude, however, that silver alloy-containing catheters appeared to reduce levels of asymptomatic bacteriuria in patients catheterized for less than 7 days. Silver oxide-containing devices were not associated with significantly reduced risks of bacteriuria.

While debate continues to rage regarding the clinical effectiveness of silver-coated/impregnated devices, Niël-Weise and co-workers [35] concluded that, at present, there is insufficient evidence to justify recommendation of urological devices incorporating silver for routine use, based on current clinical trial data.

Antibiotics

Several antibiotics have been investigated as actives, either alone or in combination with a non-antibiotic, antimicrobial agent. The potential of nitrofurazone-impregnated devices against urinary pathogens was discussed as long ago as 1993 by Johnson and colleagues, with the growth of 75% of clinical isolates being inhibited [36] by cross-sections of catheter material placed on growth media. *In vivo* results, however, have been less conclusive, with several studies finding no significant benefit of this type of "active" device over standard silicone catheters in the reduction of CAUTI, except in patients catheterized for 5–7 days or in elderly patients. Al-Habdan and co-workers [37] did, however, suggest the potential for these devices to reduce the occurrence of nosocomial CAUTI in postoperative orthopedic and trauma patients catheterized short term. A randomized controlled trial by Maki and colleagues [38] indicated a significant risk reduction for CAUTI. However, this study involved a small number of patients and concerns over selection of antimicrobial drug-resistant uropathogens were not satisfactorily resolved.

Norfloxacin release from catheters coated with poly(ethylene covinyl) acetate (EVA) and an amphiphilic multiblock copolymer composed of PEO and PDMS has also been examined for periods of up to 30 days. Significant inhibition of *E. coli*, *Klebsiella pneumoniae* and *Proteus vulgaris* growth was only demonstrated for 10 days [39]. Cho and colleagues [40] demonstrated that a gentamicin sulfate-coated catheter reduced both biofilm formation and bacteriuria in a rabbit model at 3- and 5-day intervals. However, the sample size used in the investigation was small and the issues of efficacy and resistance in the longer term remain unanswered. The widespread use of an important broad-spectrum antimicrobial such as gentamicin in this manner may, however, be irresponsible since it may well encourage resistance. This issue is especially important s this antimicrobial is one of the most useful in the armamentarium of the urologist when treating potentially life-threatening septicemias which may result as a complication of CAUTIs. The use of rifampicin and minocycline in central venous catheters and urological catheters has been associated with significant reductions in CRBSIs and bacteriuria, respectively. The use of a range of active devices employing standard antibiotics will be discussed later in the chapter under specific devices.

Antimicrobial combinations

It has been demonstrated that synergistic combinations of a number of antimicrobials may result in increased efficacy and a broader spectrum of activity. Gaonkar and colleagues [41] demonstrated that latex and silicone catheters containing silver sulfadiazine, triclosan and chlorhexidine showed greater efficacy and broader spectrum than nitrofurazone-containing devices or any of the individual compounds or pairs, in terms of inhibition of bacterial colonization to the outer wall of devices. In addition, the benefits proposed for silver-containing devices must be weighed against the slightly increased costs associated with them.

Hydrogel coatings for catheters have significant advantages over other materials in modifying the "active" properties of the device. By tailoring the cross-linking agents employed, the rate of release of active agent may be easily altered according to the desired properties. This strategy has been elegantly employed to alter the release of chlorhexidine and fusidic acid from potential catheter coatings with the rate of drug release being directly proportional to the concentration of the cross-linking agent utilized in the manufacture of the polymers [42].

Soaking devices in solutions of antimicrobials has been demonstrated as a simple technique to reduce bacterial adherence. Devices soaked in gendine, a novel antiseptic containing Gentian violet and chlorhexidine, have exhibited promise, reducing the counts of

viable adhered methicillin-resistant *S. aureus* (MRSA), *E. coli* or *Candida parapsilosis* when compared with silver/hydrogel-coated urinary catheters or control uncoated catheters [43].

Darouiche and co-workers [44] demonstrated a significant reduction in Gram-positive bacteriuria in patients when contrasted with silicone control devices at both 7 days (15.2% versus 39.7%) and 14 days (58.5% versus 83.5%) using a silicone catheter impregnated with minocycline and rifampicin. The study did not demonstrate any increased efficacy with respect to Gram-negative organisms or *Candida*. This study also involved a small number of patients and concern has been expressed over selection of resistant strains.

The use of biomaterials combined with standard antimicrobial agents is a simple and straightforward strategy to reduce the chances of bacterial colonization and subsequent biofilm formation. In spite of significant limitations, the use of antimicrobial medical devices is now a common feature of clinical practice, with differing opinions regarding their long-term effectiveness in the prevention of medical device-associated infections.

Antimicrobial devices

Antimicrobial urological devices

Urethral catheters are widely used with approximately 96 million devices being sold worldwide annually, 25% of these sales being within the USA alone [45]. Studies estimate that somewhere in the region of 11% of hospitalized patients within Europe are catheterized at some point during their hospitalization and it is estimated that some 5 million patients in acute care hospitals are catheterized annually [46]. Levels of catheterization are generally higher in the USA, with estimates ranging from 15% to 25% of hospitalized patients. Within the secondary care setting, nosocomial infections are one of the key contributors to patient morbidity and mortality, with the urinary tract being the most common site of infection. Infection of the urinary tract is dependent on the duration of device insertion, with the incidence of bacteriuria being approximately 5–8% per day and, as such, 90% of patients undergoing long-term catheterization will develop bacteriuria within 4 weeks [47]. Approximately 10–25% of patients with bacteriuria progress to develop a UTI and around 3% to develop potentially life-threatening bacteriuria. Urinary tract infections account for 40% of all nosocomial infections, with 80% of these being CAUTIs [33]. Gram-negative organisms tend to be implicated most commonly with *E. coli*, *Proteus mirabilis*, *P. aeruginosa* and *Klebsiella pneumoniae* being the primary pathogenic species, although Gram-positive strains such as *S. epidermidis* and *Enterococcus faecalis* may also be implicated.

The potential of nitrofurazone- and nitrofuroxone-impregnated devices to prevent bacteraemia has been investigated and they have been shown to demonstrate efficacy in the reduction of nosocomial CAUTIs in postoperative orthopedic and trauma patients. The incorporation of synergistic combinations of antimicrobials may offer greater promise, however, with synergistic combinations of chlorhexidine, silver sulfadiazine and triclosan exhibiting a broader spectrum of activity and longer-term inhibition of bacterial colonization to the outer wall of devices when compared with nitrofurazone- or silver-containing devices in an *in vitro* model. The use of silver as a coating for urological catheters has also been investigated and the interpretation of clinical data has provoked much debate.

Urease-producing bacteria, primarily *Proteus mirabilis*, are implicated in the formation of encrusted deposits on urological devices (catheters and stents); these may damage the uroepithelium or block the device lumen, leading to device failure requiring removal. Colonization of the biomaterial surface with urease-producing bacteria causes alkalinization of the urine and the biofilm matrix (urease hydrolyzes urea, forming ammonia and carbon dioxide, and the ammonia becomes protonated, causing alkalinization of the urine). This lowers the solubility and initiates the precipitation of poorly soluble Mg^{2+} and Ca^{2+} salts in the form of struvite and hydroxyapatite, resulting in surface deposition and crystal formation. Encrustations associated with an infectious origin are primarily composed of magnesium ammonium phosphate (struvite) $[MgNH_4PO_46H_2O]$ or calcium phosphate (hydroxyapatite) $[Ca_{10}(PO_4)_6(OH)_2]$. In attempts to prevent biofilm formation and encrustation of ureteral stents, several biocidal agents have been evaluated for use in antimicrobial eluting stents. Currently, a number of triclosan eluting ureteral stents are commercially available (e.g. Triumph stent, Boston Scientific) for this application and have shown promise in reducing bacteriuria and biofilm formation, with clinical trials currently underway.

Antimicrobial central venous access devices/catheters

In common with other types of catheter and access devices, infection and biofilm formation leading to patient morbidity and mortality remain the most common and perplexing complications associated with central venous catheters (CVCs). CVCs are used in a vast array of primary and secondary care applications, often in critical care situations. In the USA, 5 million CVCs are used in patients annually [48] and are a major cause of nosocomial infections. Between 100,000 and 500,000 CRBSIs occur in the USA every year, contributing to increased patient morbidity, increased care costs (estimated between US$3700 and 28,000 per patient) and mortality – more than 25,000 patients die annually of CRBSIs [49]. Furthermore, CVCs are responsible for the highest proportion of nosocomial bacteremias and are the most common cause of nosocomial endocarditis [50]. Perhaps unsurprisingly, the most common causative organisms of catheter-related infections are derived from the patient's own skin microflora. The predominant causative organisms are the Gram-positive cocci, coagulase-negative staphylococci (e.g. *S. epidermidis*), followed by *S. aureus* and Gram-negative bacilli (Enterobacteriaceae). *Candida* species are also emerging as important pathogens in catheter-related infections. The range of microorganisms causing CVC-related infections is shown in Table 20.2.3.

Systemic or oral administration of antibiotic agents is not generally the preferred treatment option, therefore a number of

Table 20.2.3 Microorganisms causing central venous catheter-related infections (adapted from [51]]).

Organism	Approximate percentage
Coagulase-negative staphylococci, e.g. *S. epidermidis*	60–70
Staphylococcus aureus	15
Methicillin-resistant *Staphylococcus aureus* (MRSA)	<5
Candida species	<5
Enterococci	2–4
Enterobacteriaceae (coliforms)	5–10

antimicrobial CVCs have been developed and are commercially available in the UK and USA. Fundamentally, these devices rely on either non-antibiotic agents such as silver sulfadiazine and chlorhexidine or antibiotic agents such as rifampicin and minocycline. A summary of currently available antimicrobial CVCs is given in Table 20.2.4.

Data on the use of these devices are not currently available for the USA; however, data from National Health Service Logistics (UK) for the period 2003–2004 indicate that only 4.2% of all CVCs issued in this period were antimicrobial. Recent meta-analysis data suggest that, with respect to reduction in device colonization and CRBSI, antimicrobial CVCs performed better than standard devices. However, benzalkonium chloride-impregnated, silver alloy-coated, silver iontophoretic or silver-impregnated devices did not reduce colonization or CRBSI. First-generation chlorhexidine-silver sulfadiazine CVCs did, however, significantly reduce catheter colonization and CRBSI. Superior activity was recorded with rifampicin-minocycline catheters, which were shown to reduce the risk of both colonization and CRBSI. Rifampicin-miconazole catheters also significantly reduced catheter colonization, although a reduction in CRBSI was not demonstrated by limited clinical assessment [52].

Antimicrobial endotracheal tubes

The first *in vitro* study of an antimicrobial, silver-coated endotracheal tube (ETT) was published by Hartmann and co-workers [53]. These devices significantly reduced colonization by *P. aeruginosa*. Hexetidine-impregnated PVC ETTs were also shown to significantly reduce adherence of both *S. aureus* and *P. aeruginosa* [54]. Combinations of antiseptic and silver salts have also been examined, and in the case of chlorhexidine/silver carbonate-coated ETTs, significant reduction or total prevention of colonization of a range of pathogens was observed over 5 days. Animal models of ETT-associated infections have yielded positive data supporting the use of antimicrobial ETTs. Olson and co-workers [55] demonstrated the benefits of a silver/hydrogel-coated ETT *in vivo*, which resulted in a decreased bacterial burden in the lungs of mechanically ventilated dogs. Silver sulfadiazine and chlorhexidine have also shown significant promise for the prevention of bacterial colonization in a recent *in vitro* study [56]. A silver-coated ETT utilizing the patented Bacti-Guard® silver alloy

Table 20.2.4 Commercially available adult antimicrobial central venous catheters (USA and UK) (adapted from [52]).

Active	Activity	Name (manufacturer)	USA	UK
Silver with platinum and carbon (iontophoretic)	External and internal	Vantex CVC kits (Edwards Life Sciences)	✓	✓
Silver in ceramic zeolite matrix (impregnated)	External and internal	Multicath Expert range (Vygon Ltd)	✗	✓
1st generation chlorhexidine and silver sulfadiazine	External	ARROWg + ard Blue (Arrow International, Inc.)	✓	✓
2nd generation chlorhexidine and silver sulfadiazine	External (internal chlorhexidinde coating)	ARROWg + ard Blue Plus (Arrow International, Inc.)	✓	✓
Benzalkonium chloride	External and internal	Hydrocath Assure (BD Ltd)	✓	✓
Benzalkonium chloride-heparin bonded	External and internal	AMC Thrombosure (Edwards Life Sciences)	✓	✓
Minocycline and rifampicin	External and linternal	Cook Spectrum (Cook Medical, Inc.)	✓	✓
Miconazole and rifampicin	External and internal	Multistar (Vygon Ltd)	✗	✓

system is commercially available (Agento I.C., C.R. Bard Inc., USA) and marketed for prevention of VAP in patients at risk of intubation for 24 hours or longer.

Antimicrobial orthopedic devices

Given the nature and placement of orthopedic medical devices, the consequences of device-associated infections can be particularly acute, giving rise to increased morbidity and mortality in patients. Often the development of infection will require a further operation to remove and replace the infected device. To avoid the risks of device-associated infection a number of approaches have been adopted, including improvements to pre- and postoperative care and the use of antimicrobial devices such as antibiotic-loaded bone cements, fillers and implant coatings. Antibiotic-impregnated acrylic bone cements have been commercially available in Europe for more than 20 years, with gentamicin the most commonly employed antibiotic agent. Tobramycin-containing bone cements (e.g. Simplex P, Stryker Orthopedics) are also commercially available. It is common in practice for surgeons to mix a range of antibiotic agents directly into commercially available bone cements, depending on the infecting organism. Gentamicin-loaded polyurethane sheaths designed for external fixator pins to prevent pin-track infections are also commercially available (OrthoGuard AB, Smith & Nephew, USA). For a comprehensive review, see [57].

Antimicrobial peritoneal catheters

A number of complications are inherent to the use of peritoneal catheters. Catheter-related problems cause significant morbidity and often necessitate catheter removal. Indeed, up to 20% of patient transfers from peritoneal dialysis to hemodialysis are directly related to catheter complications. While a significant number of mechanical complications have been reported for peritoneal access devices – such as occlusion, infusion pain, peri-catheter leaks and cuff extrusion from the abdominal wall – these problems have been largely resolved either by improved design of the device/appropriate device selection, improved biomaterial design or by improvements to clinical practice [58].

However, in common with all types of implantable medical device, infectious complications (exit-site infection, tunnel infections, peritonitis) are common and problematic. Since the introduction of continuous ambulatory peritoneal dialysis (CAPD) in the 1970s, around 150,000 worldwide are on the treatment, some 15% of the global dialysis population [58]. Two prominent studies have placed the combined overall incidence of peritonitis and exit-site tunnel infections at between 11% and 13% [59, 60]. Both studies are in agreement that peritonitis rates are approximately 1 incidence per 16.7 patient-months. In common with other types of catheter infections (especially CVC-related infections), the most common causative organism of such infections is *S. epidermidis*. Recent studies (in this case the Network Nine Study) indicated that the most common causative organism of peritoneal catheter-associated infection and peritonitis was *S. epidermidis*, which accounted for 43% of Gram-positive organisms isolated, *S. aureus* (26%), enterococci (5%) and other Gram-positives (26%). *Pseudomonas* spp. accounted for 11% of all Gram-negative peritonitis cases recorded. Currently, there are no commercially available antimicrobial peritoneal catheters, although an antimicrobial modified silicone peritoneal catheter impregnated with rifampicin, triclosan and trimethoprim has been reported recently, which exhibits long-term activity against a range of clinically relevant pathogens in *in vitro* and *in vivo* animal studies [61].

Antimicrobial catheters for neurosurgery

Catheters are employed for a variety of indications in neurosurgery, primarily in the management of intracranial pressure in hydrocephalus by direct drainage of cerebrospinal fluid (CSF). Catheters, depending on placement, are referred to as either shunts (permanent) or external (short-term) ventricular drainage devices (EVDs). Around 4000 shunts are inserted annually in the UK; EVD data are not available but the numbers are likely to be significantly higher [62]. Infections remain serious complications and are associated with poor outcome, and generally require removal and replacement of the device. In shunt infections, the primary causative agents of catheter infection are the coagulase-negative staphylococci and *S. aureus*. Infections of EVDs are also caused by these organisms, though a greater proportion of Gram-negative organisms are implicated. The use of prophylaxis antibiotic cover during catheter insertion is an almost universal practice, most commonly using gentamicin, cephalosporins or vancomycin. While some studies appear to show improved clinical outcome with respect to device infection, others demonstrate no benefit [62]. Antimicrobial CSF shunt or EVD catheters have been the subject of considerable research and development and a number of commercially available examples are discussed below.

Silver has been widely employed in the design of antimicrobial catheters for neurosurgery, with a polyurethane-silver-impregnated EVD catheter (Silverline, Spiegelberg (GmbH & Co.)) commercially available. As with other devices using silver as an antimicrobial agent, there is significant debate surrounding the preclinical or clinical efficacy, with few data as yet available on patient outcomes. The impregnation of catheters with antibiotics has been examined, with both rifampicin and minocycline (Ventriclear) and rifampicin and clindamycin (Bactiseal) combinations commercially available.

Antimicrobial sutures

The development of wound or surgical site infections is common and the use of antimicrobial sutures or other closure devices has been the subject of debate for many years. In fact, it is known that suture-associated polymicrobial biofilms are responsible for chronic SSIs, and that contaminated sutures may act as a vector for the introduction of microorganisms to soft tissues. A number of recent studies have demonstrated the benefits of antimicrobial sutures in reducing SSIs. Triclosan is the antiseptic of choice, due to its broad spectrum of activity and a history of use in topical applications. The commercially available Vicryl Plus (triclosan-coated polyglactin) have been extensively studied and has demonstrated efficacy against a broad range of microorganisms as well as prevention of colonization and improved wound healing *in vivo* [63].

The future: Emerging strategies for anti-infective biomaterials

Elucidation of the molecular mechanisms of biofilm formation, and the production and regulation of virulence factors in microorganisms implicated in medical device-associated infections, has facilitated the development of a number of strategies. These strategies target functional molecules, gene systems and regulatory pathways, which maintain and control the overall development and maturation of the biofilm and, subsequently, the etiology of medical device-associated infection. Table 20.2.5 summarizes

Table 20.2.5 Novel approaches for biofilm dispersal and eradication (adapted from [64]).

Approach	Mechanism of action	Target
Quorum-sensing (QS) inhibitors	QS interruption Reducing adhesion and colonization	Population density-dependent gene regulation (adhesion, glycocalyx production)
Impairing adhesion Biosurfactants including RC14 biosurfactant "surlactin"	Anti-adhesive activity; interference with initial bacterial attachment	Microbial adhesion
Diterpenoids (salvipisone and aethiopinone)	Destabilizing biofilm matrix allowing detachment and altering bacterial cell surface hydrophobicity	Biofilm matrix and bacterial cell surface
Targetting slime formation N-acetyl-D-glucosamine-1-phosphate acetyltransferase (GlmU) inhibitors; N-substituted maleimides	Inhibiting bacterial cell wall synthesis and polysaccharide intercellular adhesion (PIA) formation	PIA biosynthetic enzymes; GlmU enzyme
N-acetylcysteine (NAC)	Reducing production of extracellular polysaccharide matrix and promoting disruption of mature biofilm	Extracellular polymeric matrix
Bacteriophage therapy	Lytic activity on biofilm cells	Biofilm glycocalyx (lysins) and biofilm cells
Immunotherapy Fibronectin (FN)-binding receptor monoclonal antibodies (MAbs)	Blocking adhesion	FN-binding receptor
Anti-PIA antibodies	Inhibition of PIA formation	PIA
Surface-binding protein/Fbe antibodies	Blocking adhesion	Fibronectin/fibrinogen binding protein (Fbe)
Anti-Aap domain B antiserum Aap antibodies	Inhibiting accumulation and intercellular adhesion	Aap
Enzymatic removal Oxidoreductases and polysaccharide-hydrolyzing enzymes	Enzymatic removal and disinfection of biofilm	Biofilm matrix
Lysostaphin (staphylolytic endopeptidase)	Disruption of biofilm matrix and killing of released bacteria	Peptidoglycan pentaglycine interpeptide bridges of staphylococcal cell wall
Dispersin B (DspB)	Enzymatic degradation of cell-bound exopolysaccharide adhesin, an essential component of the biofilm polymeric matrix	B-1, N-acetyl-D-glucosamine
Serratiopeptidase	Induces biofilm degradation via proteolytic activity, also enhances antibiotic activity	Biofilm slime matrix
Immunomodulation Interferon γ	Reversal of macrophage deactivation in the vicinity of implanted biomaterial	Macrophages

novel targets and the mode of action of a number of approaches that have been developed recently for the treatment and prevention of device-related infections, particularly with respect to *S. epidermidis*. These approaches have not, as yet, replaced the widely employed, standard antimicrobial combination devices since their evaluation has been, for the greater part, small-scale *in vitro* laboratory trials. Therapeutic strategies are aimed at the disintegration of established biofilms and include quorum sensing perturbation, which leads to the downregulation of molecules stabilizing the biofilm architecture, or the use of enzymes to dissolve the biofilm matrix.

Conclusions

Much progress has been made in the development of antimicrobial medical devices for the control and prevention of the ubiquitous specter of medical device-associated infections. The susceptibility of all implanted or indwelling medical devices to succumb to microbial infection remains the major disadvantage and complication associated with their use in patients. The changing global demographics towards a steadily aging population will impose even greater demands on healthcare providers and for the provision of improved devices that can resist infection and thus reduce patient morbidity and mortality. Improving the useful lifetime of a device also reduces the necessity for its removal and replacement and the attendant costs associated with increased hospitalization and care costs.

References

1 Plowman, R. *et al.* (2001) The rate and cost of hospital-acquired infections in patients admitted to selected specialties of a district general hospital in England and the national burden imposed. *Journal of Hospital Infection*, **47**, 198–209.

2 Medicines and Healthcare Products Regulatory Agency (MHRA) (2009) Bulletin No.17, Medical Devices and Medicinal Products, MHRA, London.

3 Boretos, J.W. and Eden, M. (eds) (1984) *Contemporary Biomaterials: Material and Host Response, Clinical Application, New Technology and Legal Aspects*, Noyes Publications, Park Ridge, NJ, pp. 27–88.

4 Gristina, A.G. *et al.* (1988) Infections from biomaterials and implants: a race for the surface. *Medical Progress Through Technology*, **14**, 205–224.

5 Castner, D.G. and Ratner, B.D. (2002) Biomedical surface science: foundations to frontiers. *Surface Science*, **500**, 28–60.

6 Denstedt, J.D. *et al.* (1998) Biomaterials used in urology: current issues of biocompatibility, infection and encrustation. *Journal of Endourology*, **12**, 493–500.

7 Morris, N.S. *et al.* (1997) Which indwelling urethral catheters resist encrustation by *Proteus mirabilis* biofilms? *British Journal of Urology*, **80**, 58–63.

8 Roberts, J.A. *et al.* (1990) Bacterial adherence to urethral catheters. *Journal of Urology*, **144**, 264–269.

9 Cormio, L. *et al.* (2001) Bacterial adhesion to urethral catheters: role of coating materials coating materials and immersion in antibiotic solution. *European Urology*, **40**, 354–358.

10 Bull, E. *et al.* (1991) Single-blind, randomised, parallel group study of the Bard Biocath catheter and a silicone elastomer coated catheter. *British Journal of Urology*, **68**, 394–399.

11 Gorman, S.P. *et al.* (1991) Microbial adherence and biofilm formation on latex and polymer-coated urinary catheters; role of hydrophobicity, in *Proceedings of 10th Pharmaceutical Conference, Bologna, Italy*, vol. 2, pp. 661–663.

12 Sabbuba, N. *et al.* (2002) The migration of *Proteus mirabilis* and other urinary tract pathogens over Foley catheters. *British Journal of Urology International*, **89**, 55–60.

13 Denyer, S.P. *et al.* (1993) Antimicrobial and other methods for controlling microbial adhesion in infection, in *Microbial Biofilms: Formation and Control* (eds. S.P. Denyer *et al.*), Blackwell Scientific Publications, Oxford, pp. 147–165.

14 Williams, D.F. (1987) Definitions in biomaterials, in *Proceedings of a Consensus Conference of the European Society for Biomaterials, Chester, England, 1986*, vol. 4, Elsevier, New York.

15 Richards, M.J. *et al.* (1999) Nosocomial infections in medical intensive care units in the United States. National Nosocomial Infections Surveillance System. *Critical Care Medicine*, **27**, 887–892.

16 Darouiche, R.O. (2001) Device-associated infections: a macroproblem that starts with microadherence. *Clinical Infectious Diseases*, **33** (9), 1567–1572.

17 Choong, S.K. and Whitfield, H.N. (2000) Urinary encrustation of alloplastic materials. *Journal of Endourology*, **14**, 19–23.

18 Condon, R.E. *et al.* (1983) Effectiveness of a surgical wound surveillance program. *Archives of Surgery*, **118**, 303–307.

19 Harrison, J.J. *et al.* (2005) Biofilms: a new understanding of these microbial communities is driving a revolution that may transform the science of microbiology. *American Scientist*, **93**, 508–515.

20 Fuller, R.A. and Rosen, J.J. (1986) Materials for Medicine. *Scientific American*, **255**, 118–125.

21 Habash, M. and Reid, G. (1999) Microbial biofilms: their development and significance for medical device-related infections. *Journal of Clinical Pharmacology*, **39**, 887–898.

22 Donlon, R.M. and Costerton, J.W. (2002) Biofilms: survival mechanisms of clinically relevant microorganisms. *Clinical Microbiology Reviews*, **15**, 167–193.

23 Donlan, R.M. (2001) Biofilms and device-associated infections. *Emerging Infectious Diseases*, **7**, 277–281.

24 Gristina, A.G. (1987) Biomaterial-centered infection: microbial adhesion versus tissue integration. *Science*, **237**, 1588–1595.

25 Fletcher, M. (1991) The physiological activity of bacteria attached to solid surfaces. *Advances in Microbial Physiology*, **32**, 53–85.

26 Gorman, S.P. and Jones, D.S. (2002) Antimicrobial Biomaterials for Medical Devices, World Markets Business Briefing: Medical Device Manufacturing and Technology, pp. 97–101.

27 Smith, A.L. *et al.* (2003) Susceptibility testing of *Pseudomonas aeruginosa* isolates and clinical response to parenteral antibiotic administration: lack of association in cystic fibrosis. *Chest*, **123**, 1495–1502.

28 Vasilev, K. *et al.* (2009) Antibacterial surfaces for biomedical devices. *Expert Review of Medical Devices*, **6**, 553–567.

29 Lin, T.L. *et al.* (2001) Antimicrobial coatings: a remedy for medical device-related infections. *Medical Device Technology*, **12**, 26–30.

30 Stickler, D. *et al.* (2003) Why are Foley catheters so vulnerable to encrustation and blockage by crystalline bacterial biofilm? *Urological Research*, **31**, 306–311.

31 Brehmer, B. and Marsden, P.O. (1972) Route and prophylaxis of ascending bladder infection in male patients with indwelling catheters. *Journal of Urology*, **108**, 719–721.

32 Saint, S. *et al.* (1998) The efficacy of silver coated urinary catheters in preventing urinary infection: a meta-analysis. *American Journal of Medicine*, **105**, 236–241.

33 Johnson, J.R. *et al.* (2006) Systematic review: antimicrobial urinary catheters to prevent catheter-associated urinary tract infection in hospitalized patients. *Annals of Internal Medicine*, **144**, 116–126.

34 Brosnahan, J. *et al.* (2004) Types of urethral catheters for management of short-term voiding problems in hospitalised adults. *Cochrane Database of Systematic Reviews* 1, Art. No. CD004013.

35 Niël-Weise, B.S. *et al.* (2002) Is there evidence for recommending silver-coated urinary catheters in guidelines? *Journal of Hospital Infection*, **52**, 81–87.

36 Johnson, J.R. *et al.* (1993) Activity of a nitrofurazone matrix urinary catheter against catheter-associated uropathogens. *Antimicrobial Agents and Chemotherapy*, **37**, 2033–2036.

37 Al-Habdan, I. *et al.* (2003) Assessment of nosocomial urinary tract infections in orthopaedic patients: a prospective and comparative study using two different catheters. *International Surgery*, **88**, 152–154.

38 Maki, D.G. *et al.* (1997) A prospective, randomized, investigator-blinded trial of a novel nitrofurazone-impregnated urinary catheter. *Infection Control and Hospital Epidemiology*, **18** (Suppl.), 50.

39 Park, J.H. *et al.* (2003) Norfloxacin-releasing urethral catheter for long-term catheterization. *Journal of Biomaterials Science, Polymer Edition*, **14**, 951–962.

40 Cho, Y.W. *et al.* (2003) Gentamicin-releasing urethral catheter for short-term catheterization. *Journal of Biomaterials Science – Polymer Edition*, **14** (9), 963–972.

41 Gaonkar, T.A. *et al.* (2003) Evaluation of the antimicrobial efficacy of urinary catheters impregnated with antiseptics in an *in vitro* urinary tract model. *Infection Control and Hospital Epidemiology*, **24**, 506–513.

42 Jones, D.S. *et al.* (2005) Characterization of crosslinking effects on the physicochemical and drug diffusional properties of cationic hydrogels designed as bioactive urological biomaterials. *Journal of Pharmacy and Pharmacology*, **57**, 1251–1259.

43 Chaiban, G. *et al.* (2005) A rapid method of impregnating endotracheal tubes and urinary catheters with gendine: a novel antiseptic agent. *Journal of Antimicrobial Chemotherapy*, **55**, 51–56.

44 Darouiche, R.O. *et al.* (1999) Efficacy of antimicrobial-impregnated ladder catheters in reducing catheter-associated bacteriuria: a prospective randomized, multicenter clinical trial. *Urology*, **54**, 976–981.

45 Saint, S. *et al.* (2002) Indwelling urinary catheters: a one-point restraint? *Annals of Internal Medicine*, **137**, 125–127.

46 Maki, D.G. and Tambyah, P.A. (2001) Engineering out the risk of infection with urinary catheters. *Emerging Infectious Diseases*, **7**, 1–6.

47 Leone, M. *et al.* (2004) Catheter-associated urinary tract infections in intensive care units. *Microbes and Infection*, **6**, 1026–1032.

48 Wu, P. and Grainger, D.W. (2006) Drug/device combinations for local drug therapies and infection prophylaxis. *Biomaterials*, **27**, 2450–2467.

49 Dimick, J.B. *et al.* (2001) Increased resource use associated with catheter-related bloodstream infection in the surgical intensive care unit. *Archives of Surgery*, **136**, 229–234.

50 Gouello, J.P. *et al.* (2000) Nosocomial endocarditis in the intensive care unit: an analysis of 22 cases. *Critical Care Medicine*, **28**, 377–382.

51 Elliott, T.S.J. (2009) The pathogenesis and prevention of intravascular catheter-related infections, in *Central Venous Catheters* (eds H. Hamilton and A.R. Bodenham), Wiley-Blackwell, Oxford, pp. 206–215.

52 Casey, A.L. *et al.* (2008) Antimicrobial central venous catheters in adults: a systematic review and meta-analysis. *Lancet Infectious Diseases*, **8**, 763–776.

53 Hartmann, M. *et al.* (1999) Reduction of the biomaterial load by the silver-coated endotracheal tube (SCET), a laboratory investigation. *Technology and Health Care*, **7**, 359–370.

54 Jones, D.S. *et al.* (2003) Characterisation and evaluation of novel surfactant bacterial anti-adherent coatings for endotracheal tubes designed for the prevention of ventilator-associated pneumonia. *Journal of Pharmacy and Pharmacology*, **55**, 43–52.

55 Olson, M.E., Harmon, B.G. and Kollef, M.H. (2002) Silver-coated endotracheal tubes associated with reduced bacterial burden in the lungs of mechanically ventilated dogs. *Chest*, **121** (3), 863–870.

56 Berra, L. *et al.* (2008) Antimicrobial coated endotracheal tubes: an experimental study. *Intensive Care Medicine*, **34**, 1020–1029.

57 Zilberman, M. and Elsner, J.J. (2008) Antibiotic-eluting medical devices for various applications. *Journal of Controlled Release*, **130**, 202–215.

58 Gilmore, B.F. *et al.* (2010) Catheter-based drug-device combination products: an overview, in *Drug-Device Combination Products; Delivery Technologies and Applications* (ed. A. Lewis), Woodhead Publishing, Cambridge, pp. 61–86.

59 Golper, T.A. *et al.* (1996) Risk factors for peritonitis in long-term dialysis: the Network 9 Peritonitis and Catheter Survival Studies. *American Journal of Kidney Diseases*, **38**, 428–436.

60 Lupo, A. *et al.* (1994) Long-term outcome in CAPD: a 10-year survey by the Italian Cooperative Peritoneal Dialysis study group. *American Journal of Kidney Diseases*, **24**, 826–837.

61 Bayston, R. *et al.* (2009) An antimicrobial modified silicone peritoneal catheter with activity against both Gram positive and gram negative bacteria. *Biomaterials*, **30**, 3167–3173.

62 Bayston, R. *et al.* (2007) Prevention of infection in neurosurgery: role of "antimicrobial" catheters. *Journal of Hospital Infection*, **65**, 39–42.

63 Gomez-Alonso, A. *et al.* (2007) Study of the efficacy of coated VICRYL Plus antibacterial suture (coated polyglactin 910 suture with triclosan) in two animal models of general surgery. *Journal of Infection*, **54**, 82–88.

64 McCann, M.T. *et al.* (2008) *Staphylococcus epidermidis* device-related infections: pathogenesis and clinical management. *Journal of Pharmacy and Pharmacology*, **60**, 1551–1571.

20.3 Antimicrobial Dressings

Valerie Edwards-Jones

School of Research, Enterprise and Innovation, Faculty of Science and Engineering, Manchester Metropolitan University, Manchester, UK

Introduction

Modern wound dressings are designed to protect and prepare the wound bed and create an optimal environment suitable to facilitate moist wound healing [1]. Effective tissue perfusion and oxygenation is required for the regenerating cells, with removal of excess exudate and toxins and protection against infection. No single dressing is suitable for the management of all wound types and each phase of wound healing may require a different dressing (Table 20.3.1). The wound healing process is well described and is divided into four, often indistinguishable, overlapping phases: hemostasis, inflammatory, proliferative and maturation. At each phase, the cascades of growth factors, enzymes and cells work in concert to ultimately lead to wound closure by regeneration and repair by epithelialization, wound contraction and laying down of connective tissue collagenous scar. Many of the biomolecules involved in the various phases have been identified and categorized with their interactions.

Healing through primary intention involves the wound edges being brought together using sutures or adhesive strips, usually after injury or surgical operation. Wound healing by secondary intention usually involves some loss of tissue, or following infection. These wounds are left open to allow the free drainage of exudate and pus and to form granulation tissue to fill the cavity left by dead or purulent material or excised tissue [2].

Wound healing to full closure usually occurs within 2–4 weeks but can take longer depending on the clinical status of the patient and any underlying pathological processes. Unfortunately, wounds that have delayed healing can result in the development of chronic wounds that can cause loss of function and increased pain, with the resultant complications of odor and exudate. A chronic wound can be defined as one that has not healed in 6 weeks despite optimal conditions.

If the orderly sequence of wound healing becomes disrupted by arterial or venous disorders, diabetes, unrelieved pressure or other pathology, the wound may remain chronic and unhealed for months or even years. The inflammatory response often becomes excessive, out of phase and inappropriate. This is a major challenge for the individual patient, their carer and wound care practitioner and successful closure of chronic wounds can change the quality of life for the patient.

Effective wound management depends on an understanding of all the factors needed for healing such as the type of wound being treated (i.e. acute or chronic), the phase of healing, a good knowledge of wound management and underlying pathologies, and to an extent the physical/chemical properties of the dressings. Depending upon the wound type (especially in the burned patient), skin substitutes may be used to provide a suitable wound bed for the epithelialization process to proceed optimally. Once the wound bed is prepared by a combination of debridement and attention to underlying disorders, then wound

Table 20.3.1 Desired properties of modern wound dressings [4].

Property	Function
Fluid control	Ability to absorb wound exudate and to donate water to a dry wound
Low adherence	Trauma free dressing removal
Physical barrier	Prevents bacterial contamination from the atmosphere and further damage to the tissue
Odor control	Prevents or minimizes wound odor
Microbial control	Bacteria need to be contained or removed
Debridement	Some dressings can accelerate the debridement process (i.e. removal of necrotic tissue) by providing the appropriate moisture, pH and temperature
Hemostatic effect	Prevention of bleeding to prevent excessive blood loss (important in surgical or traumatic wounds)
Reduced scarring	Any dressing that can reduce scar formation is of great benefit
Metal ion metabolism	Some metal ions are important in cellular activity, e.g. inhibition or activation of enzymes

dressings (including those with antimicrobial properties) are applied to accelerate the healing process or to increase the effectiveness of advanced therapies. Infected or critically colonized wounds with a high microbial load tend to generate larger amounts of purulent exudate with further tissue damage and often increasing odor. The choice of appropriate dressings by the wound care practitioner is based on its ability to absorb exudate and aid with debridement, contain odor and control microbial colonization [3] with a maximum wear-time and fewer dressing changes.

Following the increase in resistance with over- or misuse of antibiotics (predominantly methicillin-resistant *Staphylococcus aureus* or MRSA) and bacterial emergence (e.g. *Acinetobacter baumannii*), a number of wound dressings now contain antiseptics or topical antimicrobial agents that help to reduce bioburden and prevent infection while simultaneously facilitating wound healing. Antibiotics act selectively on a specific target site, whereas antiseptics have multiple targets with a broad spectrum of activity and associated toxicity; for this reason resistance following their use is rare. The choice of antiseptic used in wound care should be one that provides sustained antimicrobial activity, does not impede healing and has the least potential for local or systemic toxicity to the patient's tissues. In addition, there should be limited accumulation of any antimicrobial agent in tissues, which may lead to later complications.

Choosing an appropriate antimicrobial agent for incorporation into a dressing must not compromise the physical properties of the dressing and wherever possible must release the antimicrobial agent slowly or effect a targeted, sustained release. It must also show activity against microorganisms that are typically isolated from wounds as causative agents of wound infection, namely *S. aureus* (including MRSA), *Pseudomonas aeruginosa*, *Streptococcus pyogenes* and other hemolytic streptococci, Enterobacteriaceae

including *Escherichia coli*, *Klebsiella* spp. and other Gram-negative bacteria such as *Acinetobacter* spp., anaerobic bacteria and yeasts including *Candida albicans*. In addition, the topical antimicrobial agents should not be inactivated readily by the protein-rich matter in exudates, body fluids, necrotic tissue or any associated blood and pus.

Dressings that can control all these factors are therefore increasing in number, as is the popularity of their use. They are available with incorporated antimicrobials such as silver compounds, iodine, chlorhexidine, polyhexamethylene biguanide (PHMB) or honey.

Silver dressings

Further understanding of the physical chemistry, the mode of action, the importance of ionic state and concentration of silver compounds in the wound bed has led to the development of a plethora of sophisticated dressings. Examples of these are listed in Table 20.3.2. Some of these dressings release the silver into the wound bed, while others release silver ions into the dressing following activation by the exudate.

Silver nitrate ($AgNO_3$) soaks were introduced into modern burn wound management to prevent infection and were shown to be effective against typical wound pathogens such as *S. aureus*, *P. aeruginosa* and hemolytic streptococci [6, 7]. Unfortunately, $AgNO_3$ dissociates quickly and the silver ions (Ag^+) are rapidly inactivated by proteinaceous materials in the wound, necessitating up to four dressing changes daily. Silver sulphadiazine (SSD), introduced into wound care by Fox in 1968, allows the slower release of Ag^+ from SSD over a 24 h period. This resulted in fewer dressing changes [8] and SSD is still in use today. There is also a topical antibiotic effect from the sulphadiazine.

Four different states of silver are known to exist: Ag^+, Ag^{2+}, Ag^{3+} and Ag^0. Singly charged silver, Ag^+, is the most biologically active and is dependent upon solubility [9]; Ag^{2+} and Ag^{3+} show some activity but are more likely to form insoluble complexes and thus become readily inactivated. These different forms are incorporated into a wide range of wound care products; ultimately the release of Ag^+ determines the longevity of antimicrobial activity. Ag^+ has a broad spectrum of activity and inhibits the growth of bacteria and yeasts at levels between and including 8 and 80 ppm [10]. Silver acts on multiple sites within the bacterial cell, including the cell membrane, respiratory enzymes and intracellular enzymes; it also interacts with DNA (possibly through binding with purine and pyrimidine groups) [11–17]. Intrinsic resistance to silver is effected through prevention of entry into the cell or through efflux mechanisms. Reported cases of genuine silver resistance are minimal [18] and resistance is currently unknown in human pathogens but there are concerns that resistance may develop, as it has with antibiotics, because of misuse and overuse.

Different silver formulations, including nanocrystalline silver, are incorporated into alginates, hydrogels, hydrocolloids and

Table 20.3.2 Examples of silver dressings [5].

Dressing	Description	Manufacturer
Acticoat, Acticoat 7, Acticoat Absorbent, Acticoat Flex 3, Acticoat Flex 7, Acticoat Moisture Control	Two or three layers of a nanocrystalline, silver-coated, high-density, polyethylene mesh, enclosing a single layer of an apertured non-woven rayon and polyester fabric. Also available coating: an alginate fiber; a flexible, low-adherent polyester layer; and a three-layer foam dressing	Smith and Nephew Healthcare
Allevyn Ag Non-adhesive, Allevyn Ag Adhesive, Allevyn Ag Gentle, Allevyn Ag Gentle Border, Allevyn Ag Heel	Advanced, triple-layered, construction foam dressing containing SSD available as an adhesive dressing containing a vapor-permeable film backing. The Gentle preparation uses a soft gel adhesive wound contact. The Gentle Border version has a highly permeable waterproof outer film extended to the border. The final dressing has the same properties but is shaped for use on the heel	Smith and Nephew Healthcare
Aquacel Ag	Fleece of sodium carboxymethylcellulose fibers containing 1.2% ionic silver	Convatec
Atrauman Ag	Non-adherent, polyamide mesh, wound contact layer impregnated with neutral triglycerides coated with metallic silver	Paul Hartmann
Mepilex Ag	Soft silicone-faced polyurethane foam dressing with silver	Molnlycke Health Care
Melgisorb Ag	Highly absorbent antimicrobial alginate dressing	Molnlycke Health Care
Urgotul SSD, Urgotul Silver, UrgoCell Silver, UrgoCell Duo Silver, UrgoSorb Silver	Polyester mesh impregnated with hydrocolloid, white soft paraffin and SSD. Also available as a non-adherent, non-occlusive, antibacterial foam dressing with a polyester mesh impregnated with hydrocolloid, white soft paraffin and silver particles, and as a non-adherent, antibacterial foam dressing with a polyester mesh impregnated with hydrocolloid, white soft paraffin and silver particles combined with an absorbent polyurethane foam pad and a protective semipermeable polyurethane backing. UrgoSorb Silver consists of G-type calcium alginate fibers and hydrocolloid particles impregnated with silver	Urgo
Contreet Hydrocolloid	Hydrocolloid technology, also contains a silver complex	Coloplast
BioTain Ag, BioTain Ag Adhesive	Soft and flexible foam with a vapor-permeable backing and hydroactivated silver. The adhesive dressing has an adhesive backing	Coloplast
Actisorb Silver 220	Silver-impregnated activated charcoal cloth	Johnson and Johnson
Silvercel	Sterile, non-woven pad composed of high tensile strength alginate, CMC and silver-coated nylon fibers	Systagenix Wound Management
Avance A	A hydropolymer dressing that has a silver compound bonded to it	Avance
Sorbsan Silver, Sorbsan Silver Packing, **Sorbsan Silver Plus NA, ***Sorbsan Silver Plus SA, Sorbsan Silver Ribbon, Sorbsan	Calcium alginate fiber pad containing silver. **Sorbsan Silver Plus NA contains 1.5% silver effective over 7 days. ***Sorbsan Silver Plus SA is bonded to an absorbent viscose pad with a vapor-permeable thin foam backing	Aspen Medical Europe Ltd
Suprasorb A, Suprasorb Ag	Non-woven calcium alginate dressing with silver	Activa Healthcare
Tegaderm Alginate Ag	Highly absorbent, non-woven pad with guluronic acid, calcium alginate, CMC and ionic silver	3M Healthcare

CMC, carboxymethylcellulose; SSD, silver sulfadiazine.

foams to provide the dual properties of a modern dressing with the advantageous antimicrobial properties of silver. Their efficacy is dependent upon the nature of silver used and the effective levels released [19]. Nanocrystalline silver is more active than many of the silver salts as it presents a larger, sustained supply of active silver to the wound, as well as in terms of its immunological and antimicrobial properties [20–22] and its positive effect on wound healing in murine, guinea pig and porcine models. The production of nanoparticles of silver varies and improved antibacterial activity is dependent on both the size and the shape of the nanoparticles [23]. Acticoat™, marketed by Smith and Nephew Healthcare, is produced by sputtering silver salts by vapor deposition onto a dressing surface, creating a larger surface area with more availability of silver ions (particle size typically 20–120 nm). Ag^+ nanoparticles allow continual sustained release of Ag^+ when exposed to water, with antimicrobial activity still observed over 3–7 days equilibrium between the Ag^0/Ag^+ complexes. The reported levels of Ag^+ remain at approximately 100 ppm, facilitating fewer dressing changes provided the dressing is kept moist and the exudate is managed effectively [24]. It is recommended that dressings are changed at 3–7 days depending upon the release mechanism and sustainability of the levels of silver released. Nanocrystalline dressings need the least frequent changes.

Silver dressings can be used as a topical prophylactic agent when there is a high risk of infection, for example in major trauma with exposed tissues or in large burns, in the early stages of wound healing. They are used to reduce bacterial bioburden in wounds that show signs of heavy colonization or local infection and may offer a barrier to transmission of organisms between patients in infection control.

Cases of silver toxicity have been reported but are minimal and are primarily manifested as argyria, a blue discoloration of the skin. Recently, concerns have been raised over high serum silver levels in children following long-term use of silver [19, 25, 26]. Sensitization and stinging on application of silver dressings have been reported.

Iodine dressings

Iodine has been used extensively as an antiseptic for over 150 years. It has a broad spectrum of antimicrobial activity, inhibiting bacteria, yeasts, molds, protozoa and viruses. Prolonged use of iodine in wound care was limited as elemental iodine is absorbed systemically and can irritate the skin. Iodine denatures proteins by interacting with thiol and sulphydryl groups in proteins and inactivates enzymes, phospholipids and membrane structures by blocking hydrogen and bonding with amino acids within the cell. This results in changes to the structure and function of proteins in cell walls, membranes and cytoplasm leading to rapid cell death [27].

Newer formulations of iodine and associated compounds, used in advanced wound dressings, give sustained delivery without marked tissue damage or toxicity, with a reduction in pain and irritation because of its slow release. The active iodine is carried in aggregates and is gradually released in aqueous solution. The newer formulations use iodine carriers: polyoxymer iodophores, cationic surfactant iodophores, non-ionic surfactant iodophores and, the most commonly used, polyvinyl-pyrrolidone iodophores (PVP-I or povidone-iodine) [28].

Iodine is available in modern wound care in two forms: povidone-iodine (PVP-I) and cadexomer iodine. PVP-I (Betadine™ 10%) is available as an alcoholic and aqueous solution, aerosol spray, ointment, cream and wound dressing at varying concentrations. Inadine™ PVP-I is a non-adherent, knitted viscose fabric dressing impregnated with a polyethylene glycol (PEG) base containing 10% povidone-iodine, which is equivalent to 1.0% available iodine. This is a very common dressing used in the community because of its ease of application and low cost.

Cadexomer iodine (Iodosorb™), iodine aggregated onto starch beads, is incorporated into ointment, powders and wound dressings. Upon application the starch beads are swollen by wound exudate and slowly release the incorporated active iodine [29]. It is generally used for treatment in heavily exudating, sloughy ulcers showing signs of critical colonization or infection.

The slow release of iodine from wound dressings prevents high levels being "dumped" or deposited into the wound bed with resultant iodine being absorbed into the bloodstream leading to potential thyroid dysfunction. There have been concerns over the possible absorption of iodine through dressings in patients with extensive burns, in children and in pregnant or lactating mothers and caution should probably be advised [2].

A new generation of products, Oxyzyme™ and Iodozyme™, are two new dressings and both comprise a two-component,

occlusive, hydrogel layer. The dressing absorbs wound fluid, while its gel structure intimately conforms to the wound surface. The dressings incorporate glucose oxidase that produces a low level of hydrogen peroxide, which in turn generates iodine from the iodide salt held within the dressing. The amount of oxygen and iodine generated are related to the thicknesses of the gel sheets. Iodozyme has been formulated to produce a higher level of iodine at the wound interface than Oxyzyme [28, 30]. Reports of iodine resistance are limited [28].

Chlorhexidine dressings

Chlorhexidine has been used worldwide since 1954, has an excellent safety record and is used in a diverse range of applications, including wound care. It is commonly used as water-soluble chlorhexidine gluconate (CHL-G), a cationic (positively charged) biguanide that binds to the negatively charged bacterial cell wall, altering the bacterial cell osmotic equilibrium. It is used at concentrations between 0.5% and 4%, with and without alcohol (especially when being used for skin preparation prior to surgery). At low concentrations, CHL-G affects membrane integrity, but at high concentrations cytoplasmic contents precipitate, resulting in cell death [31]. CHL-G at 0.05% is effective against a wide range of Gram-positive bacteria, including MRSA, has limited activity against Gram-negative bacteria, facultative anaerobes, yeasts and some lipid-enveloped viruses, and is inactive against spores [32].

CHL-G 2% in 70% isopropyl alcohol is currently recommended in the UK for skin preparation prior to central venous line (CVC) insertion [33]. A CHL-G-impregnated, hydrophilic polyurethane foam dressing that can be fitted around intravascular catheter exit sites was evaluated for efficacy through a meta-analysis of randomized controlled trials and shown to reduce the rate of catheter colonization [34]. Further work has shown significant reductions in the associated rate of catheter-related bloodstream infections [35]. Other antimicrobial agents are also being used in this type of dressing as the success of chlorhexidine has reduced the numbers of intravenous line-related infections [36].

Chlorhexidine-impregnated tulle dressings containing 0.5% chlorhexidine acetate (Bactigras™, Smith and Nephew Healthcare) have been used for many years in wound care. However, the poor release of chlorhexidine from the paraffin base, its tendency to adhere to the wound and the need for frequent dressing changes (at least daily) has lessened its popularity. It can also cause maceration of the wound bed.

Polyhexamethylene biguanide dressings

Polyhexamethylene biguanide (synonyms: PHMB, polihexanide, polyaminopropyl biguanide) is used as an antimicrobial agent in contact lens cleaning solutions, cleansing products, swimming pool cleaners, baby wipes for cleansing the skin and, most recently, wound care dressings [37]. Toxicity and hypersensitivity are rare but a case of anaphylactic shock has been described following treatment with PHMB wound care products [38]. PHMB is a cationic (positively charged) polymeric biguanide with a molecular weight of 3000 Da having antimicrobial action against Gram-positive and Gram-negative bacteria. It has limited virucidal activity and recent studies have shown that exposure to PHMB results in the formation of viral aggregates [39]. The positively charged PHMB ions interact with the negatively charged acidic phospholipids in the bacterial cell membrane, resulting in disruption of integrity and function of the membrane [40]. The neutral phospholipids in human cell membranes are only marginally affected [41]. An *in vitro* study using a porcine model showed that PHMB prevented infection by *P. aeruginosa* at 200 mg/l. In the same study common wound pathogens, including elastase expressing *P. aeruginosa*, were inhibited in the presence of human wound fluid and PHMB [42].

PHMB is rapidly bactericidal at high concentrations and causes disruption of bacterial cytoplasmic membranes with eventual leakage and precipitation of cell contents [40, 43]. PHMB is tissue compatible and does not have any apparent negative effects on wound healing when used as a solution. Recent *in vitro* studies have shown that PHMB can protect keratinocytes from bacterial damage and can re-establish normal host cell proliferation [44].

PHMB induces aggregation of acidic lipids in the vicinity of the adsorption site [45], changing membrane permeability and possibly altering the function of membrane-associated enzymes causing leakage of cytoplasmic compounds. Hence, it seems reasonable that the protective effect of PHMB is mediated by the preferential reduction of the number of viable bacteria cells in a dose-dependent manner [41, 45]. PHMB is currently incorporated into foams, gauze and biocellulose dressings and case studies have demonstrated positive results in terms of wound healing and wound closure.

Honey dressings

Another topical treatment for heavily colonized chronic wounds is honey. Its mode of action is probably principally related to the osmotic effect produced by the high sugar content, hydrogen peroxide and non-peroxide antibacterials including properdin [46]. Honey was shown to be antimicrobial against 150 species of bacteria, including clinical strains of MRSA and vancomycin-resistant enterococci (VRE) [47], and there is no reported microbial resistance. It has been proven clinically to reduce bacterial bioburden in chronic wounds and to facilitate wound healing [48], and rarely causes adverse reactions. Medical-grade Manuka honey contains terpenoids of *Leptospermum scoparium* (Manuka oil) and there are several different brands available [48, 49]. More information is available in Chapter 22.1.

Evaluation and safety of wound dressings

Evaluation of the safety and clinical efficacy of dressings is undertaken using internationally recognized standardized methods, such as ISO 10993, and European legislation ensures the safety of medical devices (90/385/EEC, 93/42/EEC). The 93/42/EEC amendment was made mandatory in 2010. The amendment is necessary due to continual advancements in technology and the development of international initiatives. The standards cover biological and chemical testing. The biological evaluation of medical devices includes tests for genotoxicity, carcinogenicity and reproductive toxicity, *in vitro* cytotoxicity, irritation and sensitization and systemic toxicity. A comprehensive evaluation strategy for a topical antimicrobial solution determines the antimitotic activity of the agent using monolayer cell cultures of each of the cell types that occur in the target tissue (human or mouse fibroblasts, keratinocytes, polymorphonuclear leukocytes). The effect of an agent on processes pertinent to wound healing is tested (cell migration, angiogenesis, synthesis of extracellular matrix components, wound closure) using three-dimensional models. Finally, *in vivo* studies on animal models are performed and clinical evidence collected from humans [28].

References

1 Winter, G.D. (1962) Formation of the scab and the rate of epithelization of superficial wounds in the skin of the young domestic pig. *Nature*, **193**, 293–294.

2 Leaper, D.J. and Durani, P. (2008) Topical antimicrobial therapy of chronic wounds healing by secondary intention using iodine products. *International Wound Journal*, **5**, 361–368.

3 Thomas, S. *et al.* (1998) Odour-absorbing dressings. *Journal of Wound Care*, **7**, 246–250.

4 Qin, Y. (2001) Advanced wound dressings. *Journal of the Textile Institute*, **92**, 127–138.

5 Anon. (2010–2011) *Wound Care Handbook*, Journal of Wound Care, MA Healthcare Ltd, London.

6 Moyer, C.A. (1965) A treatment of burns. *Transactions and Studies of the College of Physicians of Philadelphia*, **33**, 53–103.

7 Moyer, C.A. *et al.* (1965) Treatment of large human burns with 0.5% silver nitrate solution. *Archives of Surgery*, **90**, 812–867.

8 Fox, C.L. (1968) Silver sulfadiazine-a new topical therapy for *Pseudomonas* in burns. *Archives of Surgery*, **96**, 184–188.

9 Richards, R.M.E. *et al.* (1991) An evaluation of antibacterial activities of sulphonamides, trimethoprim, dibromopropamidine and silver nitrate compared with their uptakes in selected bacteria. *Journal of Pharmaceutical Sciences*, **80**, 861–867.

10 Hamilton-Miller, J.M. *et al.* (1993) Silver sulphadiazine; a comprehensive *in vitro* reassessment. *Chemotherapy*, **39**, 405–409.

11 Chappell, J.B. and Greville, G.D. (1954) Effect of silver ions on mitochondrial adenosine triphosphatase. *Nature*, **174**, 930–931.

12 Semeykina, A.L. and Skulachev, V.P. (1990) Submicromolar Ag^+ increases passive Na^+ permeability and inhibits respiration-supported formation of Na^+ gradient in *Bacillus* FTU vesicles. *FEBS Letters*, **269**, 69–72.

13 Schreurs, W.J. and Roseberg, H. (1982) Effect of silver ions on transport and retention of phosphate by *Escherichia coli*. *Journal of Bacteriology*, **152**, 7–13.

14 Dibrov, P. *et al.* (2002) Chemiosmotic mechanism of antimicrobial activity of Ag⁺ in *Vibrio cholera*. *Antimicrobial Agents and Chemotherapy*, **46**, 2668–2670.

15 Modak, S.M. and Fox, C.L. Jr. (1973) Binding of silver sulfadiazine to the cellular components of *Pseudomonas aeruginosa*. *Biochemistry and Pharmacology*, **22**, 2391–2404.

16 Rosenkranz, H.S. and Rosenkranz, S. (1972) Silver sulfadiazine: interaction with isolated deoxyribonucleic acid. *Antimicrobial Agents and Chemotherapy*, **2**, 373–383.

17 Teng, Q.L. *et al.* (2000) Mechanistic study of the antibacterial effect of silver ions on *Escherichia coli* and *Staphylococcus aureus*. *Journal of Biomedical Material Research*, **52**, 662–668.

18 Silver, S. *et al.* (2006) Silver as biocides in burn and wound dressings and bacterial resistance to silver compounds. *Journal of Industrial Microbiology and Biotechnology*, **33**, 627–634.

19 Lansdown, A.B. (2006) Silver in health care: antimicrobial effects and safety in use. *Current Problems in Dermatology*, **33**, 17–34.

20 Bhol, K.C. *et al.* (2004) Anti-inflammatory effect of topical nanocrystalline silver cream on allergic contact dermatitis in a guinea pig model. *Clinical and Experimental Dermatology*, **3**, 282–287.

21 Bhol, K.C. and Schechter, P.T. (2005) Topical nanocrystalline cream suppresses proinflammatory cytokines and induces apoptosis of inflammatory cells in murine model of allergic contact dermatitis. *British Journal of Dermatology*, **152**, 1235–1242.

22 Wright, J.B. *et al.* (2002) Early healing events in a porcine model of contaminated wounds: effects of nanocrystalline silver on matrix metalloproteinases, cell apoptosis, and healing. *Wound Repair and Regeneration*, **10**, 141–151.

23 Pal, S. *et al.* (2007) Does the antibacterial activity of the silver nanoparticles depend on the shape of the nanoparticles? A study of the gram-negative bacterium *Escherichia coli*. *Applied and Environmental Microbiology*, **73**, 1712–1720.

24 Dunn, K. and Edwards-Jones, V. (2004) The role of Acticoat™ with nanocrystalline silver in the management of burns. *Burns*, **30** (Suppl. 1), S1–S9.

25 Payne, C.M. *et al.* (1992) Argyria from excessive use of topical silver sulphadiazine. *Lancet*, **340**, 126.

26 Poon, V.K. and Burd, A. (2004) *In vitro* cytotoxity of silver: implication for clinical wound care. *Burns*, **30**, 140–147.

27 Gottardi, W. (1991) Iodine and iodine compounds, in *Disinfection, Sterilization and Preservatives*, 4th edn (ed. S. Block), Lea & Febinger, Philadelphia, pp. 152–165.

28 Cooper, R.A. (2007) Iodine revisited. *International Wound Journal*, **4**, 124–137.

29 Noda, Y. *et al.* (2009) Critical evaluation of cadexomer-iodine ointment and povidone-iodine sugar ointment. *International Journal of Pharmaceutics*, **372**, 85–90.

30 Thorn, R.M. *et al.* (2006) An *in vitro* study of antimicrobial activity and efficacy of iodine-generating hydrogel dressings. *Journal of Wound Care*, **15**, 305–310.

31 Milstone, A.M. *et al.* (2008) Chlorhexidine: expanding the armamentarium for infection control and prevention. *Clinical Infectious Diseases*, **46**, 274–281.

32 McDonnell, G. and Russell, A.D. (1999) Antiseptics and disinfectants: activity, action, and resistance. *Clinical Microbiology Reviews*, **12**, 147–179.

33 Pratt, R.J. *et al.* (2007) epic2: national evidence-based guidelines for preventing healthcareassociated infections in NHS hospitals in England. *Journal of Hospital Infection*, **65** (Suppl. 1), 61–64.

34 Ho, K.M. and Litton, E. (2006) Use of chlorhexidine-impregnated dressing to prevent vascular and epidural catheter colonization and infection: a meta-analysis. *Journal of Antimicrobial Chemotherapy*, **58**, 281–287.

35 Timsit, J.F. *et al.* (2009) Chlorhexidine-impregnated sponges and less frequent dressing changes for prevention of catheter-related infections in critically-ill adults: a randomized controlled trial. *Journal of the American Medical Association*, **301**, 1231–1241.

36 Casey, A.L. and Elliott, T.S.J. (2010) Prevention of central venous catheter-related infection: update. *British Journal of Nursing*, **19**, 78–87.

37 White, R.J. *et al.* (2006) Topical antimicrobials in the control of wound bioburden. *Ostomy/Wound Management*, **52**, 26–58.

38 Kautz, O. *et al.* (2010) Severe anaphylaxis to the antiseptic polyhexanide. *Allergy*, **65**, 1068–1070.

39 Pinto, F. *et al.* (2010) Polyhexamethylene biguanide exposure leads to viral aggregation. *Journal of Applied Microbiology*, **108**, 1080–1088.

40 Gilbert, P. and Moore, L.E. (2005) Cationic antiseptics: diversity of action under a common epithet. *Journal of Applied Microbiology*, **99**, 703–715.

41 Ikeda, T. *et al.* (1983) Interaction of biologically active molecules with phospholipid membranes. I. Fluorescence depolarization studies on the effect of polymeric biocide bearing biguanide groups in the main chain. *Biochimica et Biophysica Acta*, **735**, 380–386.

42 Werthen, M. *et al.* (2004) *Pseudomonas aeruginosa*-induced infection and degradation of human wound fluid and skin proteins *ex vivo* are eradicated by a synthetic cationic polymer. *Journal of Antimicrobial Chemotherapy*, **54**, 772–779.

43 Broxton, P. *et al.* (1983) A study of the antibacterial activity of some polyhexamethylene biguanides towards *Escherichia coli* ATCC 8739. *Journal of Applied Bacteriology*, **54**, 345–353.

44 Wiegand, C. *et al.* (2009) HaCaT keratinocytes in co-culture with *Staphylococcus aureus* can be protected from bacterial damage by polihexanide. *Wound Repair and Regeneration*, **17**, 730–738.

45 Ikeda, T. *et al.* (1984) Interaction of a polymeric biguanide biocide with phospholipids membranes. *Biochimica et Biophysica Acta*, **769**, 57–66.

46 Molan, P.C. (2001) Honey as a topical antibacterial agent for treatment of infected wounds, *World Wide Wounds*, November, http://www.worldwidewounds.com/2001/november/Molan/honey-as -topical-agent.html (accessed April 3, 2010).

47 Kwakman, P.H. *et al.* (2008) Medical-grade honey kills antibiotic-resistant bacteria in vitro and eradicates skin colonization. *Clinical Infectious Diseases*, **46**, 1677–1682.

48 Molan, P.C. and Cooper, R.A. (2000) Honey and sugar as a dressing for wounds and ulcers. *Tropical Doctor*, **30**, 249–250.

49 Cooper, R.A. *et al.* (2002) The sensitivity to honey of gram positive cocci of clinical significance isolated from wounds. *Journal of Applied Microbiology*, **93**, 857–863.

20.4   Antimicrobial Textiles and Testing Techniques

Robert A. Monticello[1] and Peter D. Askew[2]

[1] International Antimicrobial Council, Washington, DC, USA
[2] Industrial Microbiological Services Ltd, Hartley Wintney, UK

Introduction

Microbial contamination of textile products is recognized as a major problem in the hospital environment and in the everyday use and abuse of apparel and construction fabrics [1, 2]. Hospital staff try their utmost to control unwanted microbial growth and persistence with the use of strict sterilization and disinfection protocols. Athletes recognize the effect of unwanted bacterial growth in textiles not only in the unpleasant odor they produce but in the deterioration of highly technical performance fabrics. Controlling microbial growth on textiles to both reduce odor and to reduce bacterial cross-contamination and microbial deterioration has been performed for decades [3]. The versatile and varied end uses and composition of textiles provide conditions where a wide variety of microorganisms can take up residence and cause problems for both the substrates and the users. The type of microorganism associated with the fabric will, of course, determine the extent and speed of its deterioration and odor generated from it [4]. More importantly, the degree of pathogen survival on and release from a given type of fabric will determine its potential for disseminating infections [5].

Textiles are ideal substrates for antimicrobial treatments with expected benefits for a wide variety of consumer, commercial and industrial products. However, the antimicrobial agents available are as diverse as the products to which they are to be applied and the performance expectations they are to meet. In a developmental setting, one must choose the appropriate antimicrobial agent along with a suitable method to measure and predict its activity in the field. In general, an antimicrobial agent should be broad spectrum (i.e. activity at least against bacteria and fungi) and capable of performing in the intended end use, with limited exposure of the wearer and the environment. Thus, a tiered approach for such testing must be chosen to screen potential antimicrobials and to best predict their end-use performance [6].

This chapter describes the relative strengths and shortcomings for testing available antimicrobial agents on textiles. It will also discuss the role of microorganisms in our daily lives as they relate to textiles, the mode(s) of action of antimicrobials and how this affects the end-use performances, human and environmental toxicity, and the possible generation of microbial tolerance/resistance.

Benefits of antimicrobial agents on textiles

Ever since microorganisms were recognized as a major cause of problems in buildings and on textiles, people have struggled against such organisms in an effort to provide a clean, pleasant

Russell, Hugo & Ayliffe's: Principles and Practice of Disinfection, Preservation and Sterilization, Fifth Edition. Edited by Adam P. Fraise, Jean-Yves Maillard, and Syed A. Sattar.
© 2013 Blackwell Publishing Ltd. Published 2013 by Blackwell Publishing Ltd.

and safe environment [7]. There has been an unending array of products, cleaners, chemicals, devices, strategies and methods available to combat microbial problems caused by organisms as diverse as fungi, algae, viruses and pathogenic bacteria.

Microbiological growth on Textiles

Microbial attack of finished textiles is usually associated with fungi and bacteria. Major points of microbial contamination on textiles occur not only during manufacturing but also in the shipment and storage of these finished goods. Growth occurs on the finished goods when the material is exposed to either high humidity or free water. The resultant growth causes either marking/discoloration or physical damage. Such damage may range from small blemishes to severe staining and musty odors and even structural failures of articles stored damp. While damage of textiles by microbial growth can usually be prevented by ensuring that insufficient moisture is present, such goods can also be treated to further reduce the risk of spoilage from microbial growth [8]. This use of preservative technology is well understood and a number of standard test protocols exist that can be used to optimize performance and predict durability [7, 9]. However, in recent years a number of antimicrobial textile-based goods have been produced not only to prevent deterioration in service, but also to provide an antimicrobial function in use. These articles include items of clothing fortified with microbicides to prevent body odors as well as to reduce cross-infection in clinical environments. Test protocols for these are less well defined and often fail to predict the in-service performance of the treated goods.

Microbiological issues associated with manufacturing and raw materials

Microorganisms cause problems with textile raw materials and processing chemicals, wet processes in the mills, roll or bulk goods in storage, finished goods in storage and transport, and goods as the consumer uses them. Similarly, microbial action in textile manufacturing processes causes losses in productivity as well as function (e.g. blockage of applicators of spin finishes/weaving ancillaries by either microbial growth or detached microbial biofilms resulting in either yarn being produced without antistatic agents/lubricants or areas of localized damage due to overheating on the loom and consequent damage to the finished product). Despite the emergence of many synthetics materials, with various levels of inherent resistance to microbial growth, the biodeterioration of textiles remains a problem in use, with microorganisms causing either discoloration of, or odors in, finished goods and loss of functionality, for example loss of tensile strength in canvas [10]. Microbial contamination at any of these sites during production can be extremely critical to a clean-room operator, a medical facility or a food-processing facility. It can also be an annoyance and esthetic problem to an athlete or normal consumer. The economic impact of microbial contamination is significant and the consumer interests and demands for protection are at an all-time high.

Natural and synthetic materials

In addition to the microbial challenges associated with textiles, the textile raw materials, as well as their function, structure and design have changed and matured over the years. Textiles have been produced and used by humans for millennia but until relatively recently their composition has been dominated by natural materials, usually from fibers derived from either plants or animals. However, in the last 100 years, natural fibers have been mixed with synthetics created either from polyolefin such as nylon or modified natural materials such as viscose and rayon. In many cases, synthetic fibers have either replaced traditional, natural fibers in modern textiles or added properties which could not previously be obtained (e.g. a high degree of elasticity) and other additives are being used increasingly to add new functionality (e.g. hydrophobicity and stay-fresh properties). Additionally, in 2010, the global cotton industry was affected by several natural disasters that have greatly affected the overall price of cotton. As a result, some manufacturers are changing harvesting and processing conditions of cotton in order to compensate for the added cost. These processing changes in the cotton industry have greatly affected the microbial contamination and susceptibility of these natural substrates. With the expansion of fabric materials and construction types and changes in standard processing conditions, the need for specialized antimicrobial agents becomes ever greater. Antimicrobial agents will need to be functional on a variety of substrates and efficient in countless different end uses. Protecting these fabrics from microbial contamination and deterioration, or eliminating them as a potential source for microbial contamination, is the primary goal for the addition of these chemicals into textiles.

Benefits in the hospital and home

Infections, particularly those caused by bacteria resistant to antibiotics in clinical use, are a growing concern in hospitals worldwide. In general, hospital workers do their utmost to lower the risk of disease transmission by reducing the number of bacteria in the surrounding environment through established cleaning and disinfection practices. Infection control and housekeeping professionals regularly scrutinize building spaces and remove any visible microbial growth. Even with these cleaning strategies, microorganisms can survive on most hospital surfaces from door handles and handrails to bed sheets and uniforms [7]. Eventually, the surface or textile is once again exposed to microbial colonization/attack. Beyond the typical cleaning practices, which vary widely from hospital to hospital, antimicrobial agents applied directly to articles during their manufacturing have been added to the list of protective agents that are at the disposal of the healthcare system. Durable antimicrobial agents can be added directly to the non-porous floors, ceilings, drapes and walls of surgical wards to give added protection both during use and between cleanings [11]. With the use of durable antimicrobial agents, residual protection is created in which the antimicrobial agent is not consumed as the organism is destroyed nor does it volatilize over time. This leaves a protective surface that is inhospitable to microbial contamination, not just directly after cleaning but for weeks after [12, 13]. The degree of function that this adds will vary depending on the technology employed and the conditions that prevail and this is discussed further below.

Textiles used in the hospital environment can be a significant potential reservoir of bacteria and can even be a source of cross-contamination [5]. While sterility is the goal during surgical procedures, up to 60,000 organisms can be deposited on a 3 m² sterile field during every hour of major operations [14]. Microorganisms are constantly being isolated from virtually every surface in the hospital. Recent infections and hospital-wide outbreaks have been linked to surfaces such as stretchers, handheld showers, electronic ear-probe thermometers and even the neckties worn by doctors [1, 15, 16].

Among the critical factors in the person-to-person transmission of microbes is their ability to remain viable outside hosts. Under suitable condition, microbial biofilms on environmental surfaces may become chronic sources of contamination with nuisance organisms as well as pathogens [17, 18]. The inhibition of biofilm formation is, therefore, crucial to the protection of textiles as well as the general protection of human health [19].

The protection of textiles in settings other than hospitals is generally viewed as an esthetic issue. Products available can enhance the freshness of many types of garments by interfering with the growth of body odor-causing bacteria [4]. High levels of humidity often extend the drying times of laundered fabrics and cause them to develop musty odors. Biofilm formation on textiles is responsible for both odor formation and deterioration of the product as well a degradation of tactile properties. Thus, preventing biofilm formation and/or removal of already formed biofilms on such materials can extend their use-life. Better protection of fabrics from microbial growth can also reduce the need for laundering, thereby cutting down on the risk of damage from the laundering process while reducing water and detergent consumption [20].

Antimicrobial agents

Here, the term "antimicrobial" refers to a broad range of technologies that can provide varying degrees of protection for textile products against microorganisms. Antimicrobial agents are very different in their chemical nature, mode of action and impact on people and the environment. Similarly they vary in their in-plant handling characteristics, durability on various substrates, costs and how they interact with microorganisms. Antimicrobials are used on textiles to control the growth of bacteria, fungi, mold and mildew, as well as algae. These organisms can also cause problems of deterioration, staining, odor, etc., in addition to the health concerns indicated above. Strategies to control the proliferation of disease-causing and nuisance organisms must ensure that beneficial and innocuous ones are not affected or become resistant to the active(s). For instance, an antimicrobial agent(s) applied

should ideally act against the undesirable microorganisms on the textile with minimal leaching into the environment and without affecting the natural skin microbiota. In addition, the antimicrobial agent used must remain effective over the life of the treated article.

Leaching and non-leaching agents

Antimicrobial agents can be classified into two main types: leaching and non-leaching. A leaching antimicrobial is one that must come off a treated substrate and enters microbial cells to exert its inhibitory action. Such substances include triclosan, silver, chitosan and soluble quaternary amine compounds; the degree to which they migrate out from the textile will depend on many factors including the type of proprietary technology used [21]. However, as it has proven difficult to fine-tune such leaching of chemicals to minimize risks to humans and the environment, many manufacturers have virtually eliminated their use on textiles. Non-leaching agents are fixed to the treated surface usually by covalent bonding and ionic associations [22, 23]. Examples of such antimicrobials include polyhexylmethylene biguanides or PHMBs (ionic association) and silane-functionalized quaternary compounds "silane-quat" (covalent association). Specific to the silane-quat technology, since these agents are covalently attached, there is generally no means for removal and therefore no means to diminish their overall strength [24, 25].

Mode of antimicrobial action

The vast majority of antimicrobials work by migrating from the surface on which they are applied to interact with the cells, probably eventually entering them to cause cell death. The actual mode of action varies from agent to agent but, in all cases, the gradual transfer of microbial agent from the textile to the environment will eventually determine the lifespan of the effect. Thus, the rate of release must be controlled to maximize durability and useful life, as well as to minimize any effects on the skin and its normal flora and to prevent crossing of the skin barrier and/or causing rashes and other irritations.

The bound antimicrobial, often presented as an organofunctional silane, kills microorganisms by direct surface contact [26]. Effective levels of such chemicals do not leach or lose effectiveness over time. When applied, the technology actually polymerizes with the substrate, making the surface antimicrobial [27, 28]. This type of antimicrobial technology is used in textiles that are likely to have human contact or where durability is of value.

Global regulatory compliance

Antimicrobial agents in general must have broad-spectrum antimicrobial activity (equally effective against bacteria, fungi and algae), present little risk to the product or to the people applying the product, and be compatible with current production systems. They must also be environmentally friendly, and be compliant with all global biocidal regulations. This is often a difficult task, and with today's regulatory environment, it is practically impossible.

Objectives and principles of antimicrobial testing

Several standardized test protocols have recently evolved to provide confidence in the interpolation from laboratory testing to real-world performance of treated fabric performance claims made by the manufacturer.

Tiered antimicrobial testing

Currently, the Organization for Economic Cooperation and Development (OECD), building on the experiences of standards organizations around the world, is defining protocols for studying the effectiveness of antimicrobial-treated textiles. These guidelines will provide a tiered approach of testing. Each tier will provide data vital in understanding the significance of, and for predicting end-use utility for, each antimicrobial agent tested. Tier 1 (proof of principle) involves the demonstration of antimicrobial activity using basic standardized laboratory techniques. These can include simple antimicrobial tests and chemical indicator tests. Tier 2 (simulation of claims) testing is intended to focus more on end-use applications but may involve the same microbiological principles established within tier 1 but with real-world and intended-use stresses applied to the test samples. Finally, tier 3 (demonstration of benefit) testing involves real-world-use studies such as wear trials and odor panel studies. This tiered approach [6] to testing allows for the correlation between simple laboratory tests and actual-use conditions. Such established correlation studies provide a solid base for further predictive laboratory studies. Based on test data from this kind of tiered approach, one can perform simple laboratory tests on antimicrobial treated fabrics and have strong evidence and confidence that these results will predict real-world activity that can support regulatory, sales and marketing claims.

Testing via zone of inhibition studies

As discussed above, antimicrobials primarily function in two different ways. The conventional leaching types of antimicrobials leave the textile and chemically enter or react with the microorganism to act as a poison. The non-leaching, bound antimicrobial agents stay affixed to the textile and, on a molecular scale, physically and ionically interact externally on the membrane of the microorganism on contact to kill it.

Some leaching antimicrobial technologies are incorporated into fibers or other binders that slow the release rate to extend the useful life of the antimicrobial. Even though these agents have a longer useful life due to the decreased release of the antimicrobial agent, the agent is not considered "bound" from a microbicidal standpoint. Whether leaching antimicrobials are extruded with the fiber, placed in a binder or simply added as a finish to fabrics or finished goods, they all function in the same manner. In all cases, leaching antimicrobial technologies produce a gradient of the active within any water that comes into contact with the textile. The concentration present will depend on several

factors, depending on the antimicrobial agent concerned, the technology used to control its release and the degree of demand from the environment. In some instances these gradients can be visualized in zone of inhibition bioassays such as AATCC 147; however, it should be noted that the lack of a zone of inhibition does not necessarily indicate a lack of activity. With some antimicrobial agents (such as silver ions) the interaction between the media used and the active substance is greater than with the microbial cells and the gradient cannot be visualized as a zone free of growth. With other technologies, the rate of release is controlled to such a degree that insufficient active substance seeps into the nutrient-rich medium to inhibit growth. Indeed, in many cases the presence of a wide zone of inhibition is an indicator that large amounts of the active are being lost readily from the textile, suggesting poor durability. In contrast, such methods can be useful indicators of performance where contact between the textile and a liquid/semiliquid environment is anticipated and where migration of the active substance is a desirable property, such as in dressings intended for suppurating wounds. As with all test strategies, the choice of method must be appropriate to the intended application.

Generation of resistant bacteria due to the antimicrobial agent

The killing or inhibitory action of a leaching antimicrobial agent is witnessed when zone of inhibition tests are performed. These tests are used to measure the zone of inhibition created by a leaching antimicrobial and clearly define the area of seepage of the antimicrobial. Repeated washing of fabrics treated with leaching antimicrobials will obviously lead to a gradual reduction in the amount of the active. Figure 20.4.1 shows inhibition of bacterial growth in a typical inhibition test. The zone is clearly seen surrounding the treated article. Smaller individual bacterial colonies can also be seen to be growing within the "kill" zone. These organisms have either gained an environmental advantage over the other organisms or represent a component of the population with higher tolerance to the antimicrobial agent. They may represent a fraction of the population that could eventually become completely resistant to the antimicrobial.

Figure 20.4.2 demonstrates these phenomena as seen on typical zone of inhibition test methods. The bright blue area represents a textile material treated with a leaching antimicrobial. The dark blue zone surrounding the substrate represents the zone of inhibition and the sublethal zone is shown in gray. The area at which the zones merge is presented as the zone of adaptation. As with any chemistry that migrates from the surface, a leaching antimicrobial agent is strongest in the reservoir or at the source and weakest the further it travels from the reservoir. The outermost edge of the zone of inhibition is where the sublethal dose can be found – the zone of adaptation. The presence of colonies within this zone is a clear indicator of the effect that articles treated with antimicrobial agents can have on the microbial populations they come in contact with, whether it is to provide a selective pressure for natural tolerance or a trigger to mutation. As with all

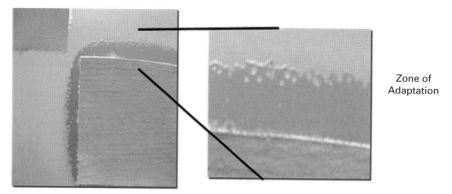

Zone of
Adaptation

Figure 20.4.1 Development of microbial resistance due to the presence of leaching antimicrobial agents.

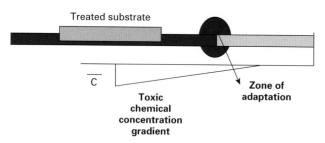

Treated substrate

C

Toxic
chemical
concentration
gradient

Zone of
adaptation

Figure 20.4.2 Graphic demonstration of zone of adaptation area created with the use of leaching microbicides on textiles.

applications employing antimicrobial agents the risk of tolerance/resistance is always present and needs to be considered when strategies for their deployment are being considered.

Antimicrobial test methods used to measure activity

The range of applications addressed by textiles designed to exhibit an antimicrobial/hygienic effect is extensive. As discussed above, products have been developed that are intended to enhance the freshness of garments through the prevention of odor resulting from unwanted microbial growth and metabolism. Other applications include antimicrobial wound dressings intended either to enhance wound healing or extend the intervals between the changing of dressings (see Chapter 20.3). Similarly, medical uniforms have been treated in an attempt to reduce the incidence of hospital-acquired infections, as have drapes used during surgical procedures and soft furnishings used in the hospital environment (e.g. curtains, seating fabric). Socks containing copper-based additives have been used to treat persistent ulcers in individuals with diabetes. The silane-quat technology has been used in socks for the prevention of athlete's foot and on silk to increase wound healing efficiency on burns patients. Antimicrobial pajamas that claim to eliminate methicillin-resistant *Staphylococcus aureus* (MRSA) from the skin are marketed for use prior to admission to hospital [18]. The range of claims is extensive; however,

relatively few standard test protocols exist to help substantiate them and fewer still provide useful models of end use.

Inherent "passive" microbial resistance and preservative testing

Microbial attack of finished textiles is heavily dependent on the presence of food, water and ideal environmental conditions optimal for fungal and bacterial growth. The resultant microbial growth causes obvious staining and discoloration of the material and also physical deterioration. Growth of microorganisms is usually prevented by ensuring that insufficient moisture is present but this is clearly not possible for all products with their variety of end uses. Many test methods have been developed over the decades to measure the inherent susceptibility of products to microbial contamination. With all of these tests, the objective is to produce an environment similar to the expected end use of the product tested while providing ideal conditions under which the organisms can grow. These "passive" test methods study the inherent resistance of materials to microbiological attack and often take months to complete. Many textiles, due to either the construction of the product or to the addition of auxiliary agents (hydrophobic chemicals), have inherent microbial resistance without the addition of antimicrobial agents.

Measuring "active" microbial properties on textiles

In recent years a number of textile-based goods have been produced that include antimicrobial properties intended to not merely prevent deterioration in service, but also to provide an antimicrobial function in use. These articles include items of clothing fortified with microbicides to prevent odors being formed from human sweat and bacterial colonization or to prevent cross-infection in clinical environments. The "active" antimicrobial agents have been directly applied to the textiles in order to achieve these functions. While passive tests measure the inherent resistance of a particular surface to microbial growth and may take months to complete, these active test methods measure the direct biocidal activity of the treated material against specific microorganisms and can be completed within days.

Table 20.4.1 Qualitative test methods used to measure the active antimicrobial activity of textiles.

Reference	Title	Description	Major principle
AATCC 147-2004	*Antibacterial Activity Assessment of Textile Materials: Parallel Streak Method*	Agar plates are inoculated with five parallel streaks (60 mm long) of either *Staphylococcus aureus* or *Klebsiella pneumoniae*. A textile sample is then placed over the streaks and in intimate contact with the surface of the agar and incubated. Activity is assessed based on either the mean zone of inhibition over the five streaks or the absence of growth behind the test specimen	Zone diffusion assay
JIS L 1902	*Testing Method for Antibacterial Activity of Textiles: Qualitative Test*	Three replicate samples of fabric, yarn or pile/wadding are placed in intimate contact with the surface of agar plates that have been inoculated with a cell suspension of either *S. aureus* or *K. pneumoniae* and incubated at 37°C for 24–48 h. The presence of and size of any zone of inhibition around the samples is then recorded	Zone diffusion assay
SN 195920	*Examination of the Antibacterial Effect of Impregnated Textiles by the Agar Diffusion Method*	Four replicate samples of fabric (25 ± 5 mm) are placed in intimate contact with a solid nutrient medium in a petri dish. The samples are then overlaid with semisolid nutrient media which have been inoculated with a cell suspension of either *S. aureus* or *Escherichia coli*. The plates are then incubated for between 18 and 24 h and then assessed as described in prEN ISO 20645	Zone diffusion assay
ISO 20645	*Textile Fabrics – Determination of the Antibacterial Activity – Agar Plate Test*	Four replicate samples of fabric (25 ± 5 mm) are placed in intimate contact with a solid nutrient medium in a petri dish. The samples are then overlaid with semisolid nutrient media which have been inoculated with a cell suspension of either *S. aureus*, *E. coli* or *K. pneumoniae*. The plates are then incubated for between 18 and 24 h and then assessed for growth based on either the presence of a zone of inhibition of >1 mm or the absence/strength of the growth in the media overlaying the test specimen	Zone diffusion assay
SN 195921	*Textile Fabrics – Determination of Antimycotic Activity: Agar Diffusion Plate Test*		Zone diffusion assay

Qualitative test methods

There are two major forms of tests for the microbiological effects of treated textiles: qualitative and quantitative. The first, typified by the qualitative component of JIS L1902 (AATCC147), are referred to as "zone of inhibition" or "zone diffusion" studies (Table 20.4.1). In these tests, samples of textile are placed onto agar plates which have been inoculated with bacteria and are then incubated. The intention is that intimate contact between the textile, the bacteria and the growth medium will result in the inhibition of growth either immediately adjacent to the textile or in an area around the textile should any antimicrobial agents that have been employed become dissolved in the growth medium. These zone of inhibition methods are generally acknowledged as being non-quantitative although they could potentially be employed as assays of certain antimicrobial products in the same manner that such techniques are used for some antibiotics. They can be useful as a screening tool and for investigating the effect of wash cycles on durability, for example.

Such methods are widely employed in the textile industry as they provide a highly graphic representation of antimicrobial activity. However, this can lead to a misunderstanding of the scale of effect seen (bigger zones of inhibition looking better) and the implications that active ingredient mobility has on service life (e.g. loss during laundering). For immobilized active

ingredients and for leaching active ingredients that interact with proteins, such as silver ion donors, these methods often have little utility. This is either because the active ingredient cannot migrate to form a zone (e.g. silane-quat) or the high concentration of proteins in the growth medium deactivates the antimicrobial agent (e.g. silver). Although these techniques are considered to be unsuitable for "quantifying" the effect of the antimicrobial effects of treated textiles, there are some disciplines in which they may provide data that are more relevant to the effect claimed than that delivered by a fully quantitative technique. For example, interactions with a microbial population on a semisolid, protein-rich medium can provide a useful model for wound dressings. These zone of inhibition test methods are presented in Table 20.4.1.

Quantitative test methods

In addition to the qualitative tests, there are at least four techniques that provide quantitative data on the effect of treated textiles on bacteria (Table 20.4.2). These are typified by the method described in ISO 20743 in which samples are inoculated with suspensions of bacteria and then incubated for a specified time before being examined for the size of population present. The methods differ in the form of the suspension medium, number of replicates examined, test species and, to a certain

Table 20.4.2 Quantitative methods used to measure the active antimicrobial activity of textiles.

Reference	Title	Description	Major principle
ASTM E2149-10	*Standard Test Method for Determining the Antimicrobial Activity of Immobilized Antimicrobial Agents Under Dynamic Contact Conditions*	Dynamic shake flask test. Test material is suspended in a buffer solution containing a known number of cells of *E. coli* and agitated for 1 h. Efficacy is determined by comparing the size of the population before and after a specified contact time	Relies on the interaction between the bacterial population and the surface of the material in suspension. Specific for non-leaching agents
AATCC 100-2004	*Antibacterial Finishes on Textile Materials: Assessment of*	Replicate samples of fabric are inoculated with individual bacterial species (*S. aureus* and *K. pneumoniae*) suspended in a nutrient or buffered medium. The samples are incubated under humid conditions at 37°C for a specified contact time. Activity is assessed by comparing the size of the initial population with that present following incubation. A neutralizer is employed during cell recovery	Cell suspension intimate contact test
XP G 39-010	*Propriétés des étoffes – Étoffes et surfaces polymériques à propriétés antibactériennes – Caractérisation et mesure de l activité antibactérienne*	Four replicate samples of test material are placed in contact with an agar plate that has been inoculated with a specified volume of a known cell suspension of either *S. aureus* or *K. pneumoniae* using a 200 g weight for 1 min. The samples are then removed. Duplicate samples are analyzed for the number of viable bacteria before and after incubation under humid conditions at 37°C for 24 h. A neutralizer is employed during cell recovery	Cell suspension intimate contact test
JIS L 1902	*Testing Method for Antibacterial Activity of Textiles: Quantitative Test*	Replicate samples of fabric (six of the control and three of the treated) are inoculated with individual bacterial species (*S. aureus* and *K. pneumoniae*) suspended in a heavily diluted nutrient medium. The samples are incubated under humid conditions at 37°C for a specified contact time. Activity is assessed by comparing the size of the initial population in the control with that present following incubation. No neutralizer is employed during cell recovery	Cell suspension intimate contact test.
SN 195924	*Textile Fabrics – Determination of the Antibacterial Activity: Germ Count Method*	Fifteen replicate samples (each replicate is comprised of sufficient specimens of 25 ± 5 mm to absorb 1 ml of test inoculum) are inoculated with cells of either *E. coli* or *S. aureus* suspended in a liquid nutrient medium and incubated in sealed bottles for up to 24 h at 27°C. After 0, 6 and 24 h, five replicate samples are analyzed for the size of the viable population present. A neutralizer is employed. An increase of 2 orders of magnitude of the population exposed to a control sample is required to validate the test. The method defines a textile as antibacterial if no more than a specified minimum level of growth is observed after 24 h in four of the five replicate groups of samples	Cell suspension intimate contact test.
ISO 20743	*Textiles – Determination of Antibacterial Activity of Antibacterial Finished Products*	1. Adsorption method: see JIS L 1902 – Quantitative Method 2. Transfer method: bacteria are transferred from a cell suspension to a sample of textile using the surface of an agar plate under defined conditions to simulate bacterial transfer from skin 3. Printing method: bacteria are transferred from a cell suspension to a sample of textile via a membrane filter under defined conditions to simulate the transfer of bacteria from dry environmental surfaces, etc.	Cell suspension intimate contact test

extent, conditions for incubation. The methods described in AATCC 100-2004 and JIS L 1902 appear to be the most commonly employed although the absorption method in ISO 20743 is cited more frequently. In addition, no fully quantitative methods yet exist for the examination of the effect of treated textiles against fungi (Tables 20.4.1 and 20.4.2). All of the fungal protocols described are zone diffusion assays of one form or another but, as with the antibacterial properties, these may be sufficient to substantiate certain claims. A fungal quantitative method is under development in Japan in the form of an early draft ISO standard, which employs the measurement of adenosing triphosphate (ATP) to predict/quantify the early stages of fungal spore germination and growth.

Test methods specific for claim validation
Understanding test methods for odor control
As discussed above, these methods are employed for a wide range of claims made by a number of antimicrobial treatments

and have emerged mainly from the need to determine the performance of textiles associated with healthcare applications (e.g. dressings, uniforms of medical staff) where relatively large or rapid antibacterial effects are required. However, the published methods are less well suited to exploring effects associated with either small bacterial populations or relatively low levels of metabolic activity, for example the transformation of sweat and sebum into odor compounds [29]. While the formation of body odor is attributed to a number of bacterial species associated with human skin, limited data are available for such transformations on textiles worn close to the skin [4]. Used sportswear often develops musty odors before being laundered and this is often associated with the presence of pseudomonads on the damp clothing. This odor does not usually develop when worn. The transformation of steroids, etc. to the main components of body odor appears to be attributed to a number of bacterial species, such as coryneform bacteria [30], probably functioning within consortia on the skin or in sebum glands. Some transformations may also occur on clothing. In contrast, a less diverse range of bacteria are associated with foot odor, with a number Gram-positive species including staphylococci being implicated [31, 32].

In contrast to a number of antibacterial effects (e.g. elimination of pathogens carried in splashes of contaminated body fluids on medical uniforms, prevention of growth of bacteria in dressings on suppurating wounds, etc. [33]), the control of odor in textiles caused by bacteria requires only a reduction in the rate of their metabolism to reduce the production of odor compounds. Thus, textiles that can inhibit their growth (rather than necessarily killing the populations) can affect the generation of odor within a garment. Ideally, any antimicrobial agent used for such purposes should not migrate to the skin. Textiles that control odor within the textile only may not require registration under the EU Biocidal Products Regulation. However, if the antimicrobial agents employed migrate to the skin registration is likely to be required [34]. It is important, therefore, that the choice of antimicrobial agent and the concentration of that agent are chosen with care. It is equally important that the method that is employed to measure activity is appropriate to the claim being made. As the control of odor requires relatively subtle antibacterial effects, the use of protocols that apply unrealistic demands on the system under test should be avoided, such that the textile is not "overtreated" resulting in migration of antimicrobial agent from the textile to the skin. For example, systems that employ silver ions to create antimicrobial effects are intended for relatively clean systems. The use of test protocols that employ a high concentration of nutrients, which might be suitable for healthcare scenarios, result in the deactivation of the silver ions released before they interact with microbial cells (they act as soiling agents as well as nutrients). For this reason a number of variants of the basic tests described above are under development that model better the end use of a textile and ensure that treatments are appropriate to the effect being targeted.

Claim validation test methods using a simulated microbial splash

Many of the methods described in Tables 20.4.1 and 20.4.2 were developed with medical applications in mind. Despite this, they provide a poor model for many end uses as they present a bacterial population as a cell suspension and maintain a wet system during the contact interval. Clearly, this is unrealistic for most end uses. The relevance of a test method to the intended application is critical to be of scientific value. For this reason a number of protocols have been developed that simulate certain exposure scenarios. One such scenario [33] is to examine the impact of a treatment on a textile on the survival of bacteria carried in small splashes of contaminated liquids when they alight on the surface; such as might occur and go unobserved during patient care in a hospital. The protocol is illustrated in Figure 20.4.3 and a model dataset is presented in Figure 20.4.4. This protocol is consistent with the basic principles of the initial antimicrobial tests (AATCC 100-2004/JIS L 1902) but creates an environment more similar to the end-use conditions. In this example the treatments have resulted in an increase in the rate of decline of a microbial population that has come into contact with the textile (simulating for example a splash of sputum on a medical uniform) compared with an untreated textile. Such effects could bring a benefit in reducing the risk of transfer of microbial contamination from patient to patient in a clinical setting.

Conclusions

Despite advances in modern materials technology and our ability to control the microenvironment surrounding textiles, many textiles are susceptible to spoilage by microbial growth when used in conditions that allow their growth. A wide range of tests exist that can be used to model such growth and determine the efficacy of preventative treatments. In addition to protecting textiles in service, a number of microbicidal treatments are now available that intend to introduce antimicrobial properties to textiles which bring hygienic or performance benefits.

Although a number of standard methods exist, in general these do not predict well the performance in service and fail to describe the benefit intended. Choosing the correct test method appropriate not only for the antimicrobial agent used but for the intended end use is critical. In most cases, such ideal industry-accepted test methods do not exist. It is, however, possible to design study protocols that allow performance to be measured under realistic simulations, support claims and illustrate benefits while keeping with the initial scientific principles associated with the industry-standard test methods. With the current regulatory climate and with justified concerns over the exposure of humans to microbicidal treatments (as well as the potential development of resistance by microorganisms to microbicidal treatments and clinical antimicrobial agents), the need to understand the functionality of antimicrobial treatments and any benefits they may bring is becoming increasingly important.

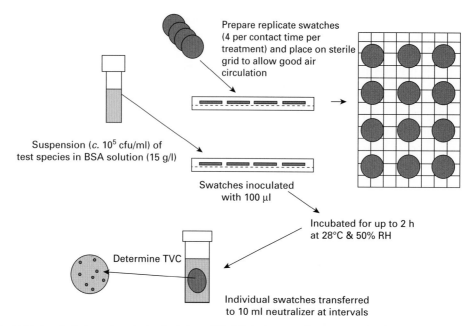

Figure 20.4.3 Antimicrobial test method scheme from simulated splash test [33]. BSA, bovin serum albumin; CFU, colony-forming units; RH, relative humidity; TVC, total viable count.

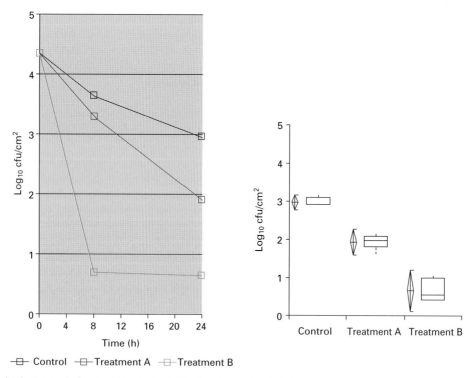

Figure 20.4.4 Bacterial reduction graphs from treated and untreated textiles using simulated splash test.

References

1 Knobben, B.A.S. *et al.* (2007) Transfer of bacteria between biomaterials surfaces in the operating room – an experimental study. *Journal of Biomedical Materials Research. Part A*, **80** (4), 790–799.

2 Neely, A.N. *et al.* (2000) Survival of enterococci and staphylococci on hospital fabrics and plastic. *Journal of Clinical Microbiology*, **38** (2), 724–726.

3 Abrams, E. (1948) Microbiological Deterioration of Organic Material: its prevention and Methods of Test, Miscellaneous Publication 188, Washington National Bureau of Standards, Washington, DC.

4 McQueen, R. *et al.* (2007) Odor intensity in apparel fabrics and the link with bacterial populations. *Textile Research Journal*, **77**, 449.

5 Neely, A. and Maley, M. (1999) Survival of Enterococci and Staphylococci on Hospital Fabrics and Plastic, Shriners Hospitals for Children, and Department of Surgery, University of Cincinnati College of Medicine, Cincinnati.

6 Organization for Economic Cooperation and Development (OECD) (2007) Analysis and Assessment of Current Protocols to Develop Harmonised Test Methods and Relevant Performance Standards for Efficacy Testing of Treated Articles/Treated Materials, ENV/JM/MONO(2007)4, OECD, Paris.

7 Maillard, J.-Y. (2005) Antimicrobial biocides in the healthcare environment: efficacy, usage, policies, and perceived problems. *Therapeutics and Clinical Risk Management*, **1** (4), 307–320.

8 Wypkema, A.W. (2005) Microbicides for the protection of textiles, in *Directory of Microbicides for the Protection of Materials – a Handbook* (ed. W. Paulus), Springer Verlag, Dordrecht, pp. 5.1.1–5.1.6.

9 La Brijn, J. and Kauffman, H.K. (1972) Fungal testing of textiles: a summary of the cooperative experiments carried out by the Working Group on Textiles of the International Biodeterioration Research Group (IBRG). *Biodeterioration of Materials*, **2**, 208–215.

10 Askew, P.D. (2006), Biogenic impact on materials – paper and textiles in *Springer Handbook of Materials Measurement Methods* (eds H. Czichos et al.), Springer Velag, Dordrecht, pp. 712–787.

11 Nikawa, H. et al. (2005) Immobilization of octadecyl ammonium chloride on the surface of titanium and its effect on microbial colonization *in vitro*. *Dental Materials Journal*, **24** (4), 570–582.

12 Gottenbos, B. et al. (2002) *In vitro* and *in vivo* antimicrobial activity of covalently coupled quaternary ammonium silane coatings on silicone rubber. *Biomaterials*, **23**, 1417–1423.

13 Kemper, R.A. et al. (1992) Improved control of microbial exposure hazards in hospitals: a 30-month field study, in *Annual Conference of the Association of Professionals in Infection Control and Epidemiology*.

14 Conn, J. et al. (1986) *In vivo* study of an antimicrobial surgical drape system. *Journal of Clinical Microbiology*, **24**, 803–808.

15 Wiener-Well, Y. et al. (2011) Nursing and physician attire as possible source of nosocomial infections. *American Journal of Infection Control*, **39** (7), 555–559.

16 Srinivasan, M. et al. (2007) The medical overcoat – is it a transmitting agent for bacterial pathogens? *Japanese Journal of Infectious Diseases*, **60**, 121–122.

17 Goeres, D.M. (2010) Understanding the importance of biofilm growth in hot tubs. *Applied Biomedical Microbiology: A Biofilms Approach*, **1** (4), 134–144.

18 Borkow, G. and Gabbay, J. (2008) Biocidal textiles can help fight nosocomial infections. *Medical Hypotheses*, **70**, 990–994.

19 Monticello, R.A. and White, C. (2010) Inhibition of foundation colonization of biofilm by surface modifications with organofunctional silanes. *Applied Biomedical Microbiology: A Biofilms Approach*, **1** (4), 45–58.

20 Monticello, R.A. (2011) Creating and Testing Innovative Textiles Containing Non-leaching Antimicrobial and Moisture Management Features, Techtextile North America, Las Vegas.

21 Gao, Y. and Cranston, R. (2008) Recent advances in antimicrobial treatments of textiles. *Textile Research Journal*, **78**, 60.

22 Murata, L. et al. (2007) Permanent, non-leaching antibacterial surfaces-2: how high density cationic surfaces kill bacterial cells. *Biomaterials*, **28**, 4870–4879.

23 Kenawy, E.R. et al. (2007) The chemistry and applications of antimicrobial polymers: a state-of-the-art review. *Biomacromolecules*, **8** (5), 1359–1384.

24 Andresen, M. et al. (2007) Nonleaching antimicrobial films prepared from surface-modified microfibrillated cellulose. *Biomacromolecules*, **8**, 2149–2155.

25 Huang, J.Y. et al. (2008) Nonleaching antibacterial glass surfaces via "grafting onto": the effect of the number of quaternary ammonium groups on biocidal activity. *Langmuir*, **24**, 6785–6795.

26 Kugler, R. et al. (2005) Evidence of a charge-density threshold for optimum efficiency of biocidal cationic surfaces. *Microbiology*, **151**, 1341–1348.

27 Bouloussa, O. et al. (2008) A new, simple approach to confer permanent antimicrobial properties to hydroxylated surfaces by surface functionalization. *Chemical Communications (Cambridge, England)*, 951–953.

28 Oosterhof, J.J. et al. (2006) Effects of quaternary ammonium silane coatings on mixed fungal and bacterial biofilms on tracheoesophageal shunt prostheses. *Applied and Environmental Microbiology*, **72**, 3673–3677.

29 James, A.G. et al. (2004) Generation of volatile fatty acids by axillary bacteria. *International Journal of Cosmetic Science*, **26** (3), 149–156.

30 Rennie, P.R. et al. (1990) The skin microflora and the formation of human axillary odour. *International Journal of Cosmetic Science*, **12** (5), 197–207.

31 Gettings, R.L. and Triplett, B.L. (1978) A new durable antimicrobial finish for textiles, in *Book of Papers, AATCC National Conference*, pp. 259–261.

32 Marshall, J. et al. (1988) A comparative study of the cutaneous microflora of normal feet with low and high levels of odour. *Journal of Applied Microbiology*, **65** (1), 61-68.

33 Askew, P.D. (2007) Exploring the functionality of antibacterial plastics and textiles, antimicrobials in plastic and textiles applications. Paper presented at the *PIRA Conference, Prague, Czech Republic, June*.

34 Anon. (2008) *Manual of Decisions for Implementation of Directive 98/8/EC concerning the Placing on the Market of Biocidal Products*, www.ec.europa,eu/environment/biocides/manual.htm.

21.1 Use of Microbicides in Disinfection of Contact Lenses

Patrick J. McCormick, Susan E. Norton and James J. Kaiser

Microbiology and Sterilization Sciences, Bausch and Lomb, Rochester, NY, USA

Introduction

Contact lenses have been used for decades to facilitate vision. Integral to the use of contact lenses is care of the lenses to ensure safe and comfortable wear, particularly from a microbiological perspective. This chapter provides an overview of contact lenses and the microbiological methods employed to evaluate the efficacy of lens care solutions.

Contact lenses are of two general types, rigid and soft contact lenses. Rigid lenses may be manufactured from materials such as polymethylmethacrylate (PMMA) or silicone acrylate and fluorosilicone acrylate. Those manufactured from the latter materials are known as rigid gas-permeable (RGP) lenses and provide for greater oxygen transmission to the eye as compared with lenses manufactured from PMMA. The use of rigid contact lenses requires a period of adaptation and they may not be well tolerated by all users. Soft contact lenses are manufactured from a variety of polymerized hydrophilic or hydrophobic monomers that allow oxygen to reach the eye. In contrast to rigid contact lenses, soft contact lenses require little or no adaptation and are generally well tolerated following initial fitting.

Soft contact lenses were developed in 1960 when Otto Wichterle, a Czechoslovakian chemist, successfully molded hydroxyethylmethacrylate (HEMA) lenses using a spin casting method. The rights to Wichterle's patents were acquired by Bausch and Lomb and the first commercial soft contact lens, Soflens® was introduced in 1971 [1]. Today, there is a wide range of soft contact lenses available for corrective, therapeutic and cosmetic applications. Due to their higher water content, soft contact lenses provide improved comfort on the eye but also exhibit a greater susceptibility to microbial colonization in comparison with rigid contact lenses. An important development in contact lens technology was the introduction of the silicone hydrogel soft contact lens. As with RGP lenses the use of silicone provides a high rate of oxygen transmission, allowing the lens to be worn for longer periods of time [2].

Contact lenses may be grouped into one of four categories depending on their water content and surface charge (Table 21.1.1). They may also be categorized based on their schedule of wear and replacement. Daily-wear lenses are removed from the eye on a daily basis for cleaning and disinfection. Extended-wear lenses may be worn overnight and remain in the eye for up to 1 week without being removed. Continuous-wear lenses may be worn for up to 30 days without being removed from the eye, while daily-disposable lenses are worn once and discarded at the end of the day. Due to their susceptibility to mechanical damage during cleaning and handling, soft contact lenses are generally prescribed on a planned replacement schedule depending on the lens type.

Russell, Hugo & Ayliffe's: Principles and Practice of Disinfection, Preservation and Sterilization, Fifth Edition. Edited by Adam P. Fraise, Jean-Yves Maillard, and Syed A. Sattar.

Table 21.1.1 General categories of contact lenses.

Group	Water content	Charge	Material (water content)	Examples	Replacement[a]	Wear
I	Low	Non-ionic	Elastofilcon (0.2%)	Bausch & Lomb Silsoft (aphakia)	Monthly	Daily
			Lotrafilcon A (24%)	CIBA Vision AirOptix® Night & Day Aqua	Monthly	30 days
			Polymacon (38%)	Bausch & Lomb SofLens® 38	1–2 weeks	Extended
			Lotrafilcon B (33%)	CIBA Vision AirOptix® Aqua	Monthly	Daily
			Tetrafilcon A (43.5%)	CooperVision Preference Standard	Quarterly	Daily
			Galyfilcon A (47%)	Vistakon® Acuvue Advance	1–2 weeks	Extended
II	High	Non-ionic	Hilafilcon B (59%)	Bausch & Lomb SofLens® Daily Disposable	Daily	Disposable
			Omafilcon (62%)	CooperVision Proclear Compatibles	Monthly	Daily
			Nelifilcon A (69%)	CIBA Vision Focus Dailies	Daily	Disposable
III	Low	Ionic	Balafilcon A (36%)	Bausch & Lomb PureVision®	Monthly	30 days
IV	High	Ionic	Ocufilcon D (55%)	CooperVision Biomedics 55 Evolution	1–2 weeks	Extended
			Vifilcon A (55%)	CIBA Vision Focus 1–2 Weeks	1–2 weeks	Extended
			Etafilcon A (58%)	Vistakon Acuvue®	1–2 weeks	Extended

[a] Indications for use are frequently updated. The labeling of the product should be consulted for the latest information regarding replacement and wear.

Lens care

During normal use both types of contact lenses and the lens case may become colonized with a variety of microorganisms [3–5]. Initially, heating the lenses to approximately 80°C for 10 min in sterile saline in a heating unit was recommended. Although such disinfection is highly effective, many users employed self-prepared, non-sterile saline solutions which led to outbreaks of bacterial keratitis [6]. As a result, preserved chemical disinfecting systems known as lens care solutions were developed. Early lens care systems required separate cleaning and disinfection steps involving the use of multiple solutions and enzyme tablets. Multipurpose lens care solutions were subsequently developed that allow for one-step cleaning and disinfection.

Lens care solutions

Active ingredients

The identification of disinfecting compounds suitable for use with lens care solutions is largely an exercise in compromise between the efficacy of the compound and its toxicity to the eye. This often requires the use of low concentrations of the disinfecting compound (typically in the range of parts per million) to avoid potential toxicity and discomfort. The following disinfecting agents have been employed with lens care solutions.

Polyhexamethylene biguanide

Polyhexamethylene biguanide (PHMB), also known as polyaminopropylbiguanide (PAPB), is a widely used disinfecting compound in lens care solutions. It is active against a broad range of microorganisms [7]. While its mechanism of microbicidal activity is not completely understood, PHMB, a complex of cationic polymeric biguanides, is believed to bind and induce instability in the bacterial cell membrane leading to lysis [8]. Others have suggested that PHMB may also interact with nucleic acids within the cell to inhibit cellular function [9].

Polyquaternium-1

Polyquaternium-1 (PQ-1) is a straight-chain quaternary ammonium compound (QAC). It exhibits good microbicidal activity against most bacteria although it is less active against fungi [10]. PQ-1 induces membrane damage, leading to leakage of cytoplasmic contents and inactivation of the cell [11]. PQ-1 may be formulated with myristamidopropyl dimethylamine (MAPD) or other compounds for improved antifungal activity [12].

Hydrogen peroxide

Hydrogen peroxide is a potent and effective disinfecting compound with a broad spectrum of microbicidal activity. As hydrogen peroxide decomposes it forms a hydroxyl ion that attacks membrane lipids and proteins of the cell. Residual hydrogen peroxide is highly irritating to the eye and must be completely neutralized before the lens is placed on the eye. Following neutralization, lenses in the lens case may be susceptible to microbial growth if stored for prolonged periods of time in the absence of added preservative [13].

Chlorhexidine digluconate

Chlorhexidine digluconate is a cationic bisbiguanide that is most often employed for disinfecting rigid contact lenses. Its microbicidal action results from membrane perturbation [14]. Due to toxic and sensitivity reactions associated with its use with soft contact lenses this compound is typically employed at concentrations at or below 6 ppm.

Alexidine

Alexidine is a bisbiguanide similar to chlorhexidine that has been used in mouthwashes and lens care formulations. It differs chemically from chlorhexidine in its end groups and exhibits faster bactericidal activity compared with chlorhexidine [15].

Iodine

Iodine-based lens care solutions in the form of povidone-iodine compounds can provide effective disinfection but have not been widely used [16]. Similar to hydrogen peroxide-based solutions, the activity of the iodine compound must be completely neutralized before the lens is placed on the eye to avoid potential toxicity and irritation concerns.

Benzalkonium chloride

Benzalkonium chloride (BAK) is a common preservative compound that is effective against a broad range of microorganisms. As with other QACs, the basis of its microbicidal activity is thought to be due to the disruption of cellular membranes and enzyme activity. Although BAK has been employed as a preservative in many applications, it may not be well tolerated by some individuals [17].

Thiomersal

Thiomersal is a mercury-containing compound that, while effective as a preservative, has been removed from many contact lens solutions due to its long-term toxicity concerns and hypersensitivity reactions in numerous individuals [18]. It may still be found in some ophthalmic formulations (primarily pharmaceuticals) although its use is becoming less prevalent.

Other formulation constituents

In conjunction with the active ingredients noted above, other excipients may be added to lens care solutions that act to enhance the activity of the solution or promote cleaning and comfort of the lens. Ethylenediamine tetraacetic acid (EDTA), a chelating agent, is present in many lens care solutions. EDTA enhances the efficacy of disinfecting compounds such as PHMB by removing calcium and magnesium ions from the cell membrane [7, 19]. Lens care solutions also contain surfactants to aid in the removal of lipid and protein deposits from the surface of the lens. Buffering components are also an important constituent of lens care formulations, acting to maintain the pH of the solution in a range compatible with the eye. Buffering systems such as borate buffers exhibit bacteriostatic properties while citrate buffers enhance cleaning. Natural compounds such as hyaluronan have also been added to lens care solutions to enhance comfort of the lens [20].

Lens care alternatives

Although lens care solutions are the predominant means in use today for cleaning and disinfecting contact lenses, some individuals may not be able to tolerate the chemicals present in certain solutions. Alternatives are available including the PuriLens® system, a compact unit that uses low-frequency agitation to clean the lens and a UV germicidal light for disinfection. The system has been found to be effective against most bacterial organisms but its activity against *Acanthamoeba* cysts has been questioned [21].

Single-use disposable contact lenses, if used per the manufacturer's directions, do not require the use of lens care solutions.

Complications

General

Contact lens wear is a recognized risk factor for developing microbial keratitis. Microbiological complications associated with contact lens wear can be placed into four general categories: bacterial keratitis, fungal keratitis, amoebic keratitis and viral keratitis. Once established in the eye, infections with organisms such as *Pseudomonas*, *Candida*, *Acanthamoeba* and herpes simplex virus (HSV) are difficult to treat and may have an uncertain outcome.

Bacterial keratitis

It is estimated that 0.01–0.03% of all contact lens wearers may develop bacterial keratitis [22, 23]. While the nature of the infection varies regionally, *Pseudomonas aeruginosa* is the predominant agent, with infections of *Serratia marcescens*, *Staphylococcus aureus*, *Staphylococcus epidermidis* and other bacteria also reported [12]. A review of contact lens-related *Pseudomonas* keratitis by Robertson *et al.* highlighted the presence of contact lenses and hypoxia of the cornea as primary contributing factors in establishing infection [24]. Clinical isolates of *P. aeruginosa* have been shown to be capable of replicating within corneal epithelial cells, thus rendering treatment difficult as many commonly prescribed topical antibiotics fail to penetrate the epithelium [25]. Fluoroquinolones, primarily ciprofloxacin, are the treatment of choice for *P. aeruginosa* keratitis.

Fungal keratitis

The incidence of contact lens-associated fungal keratitis is generally lower than that of bacterial keratitis. Infections with filamentous fungi such as *Fusarium* and *Aspergillus* exhibit greater prevalence in southern climates, while *Candida* (yeast) infections are predominant in northern climates. In 2005, an increase in fungal keratitis associated with *Fusarium* was noted in Southeast Asia and the USA. A retrospective case–control study identified an association with a multipurpose lens care solution and the product was subsequently removed from the marketplace [26]. Although the exact nature of the problem has not been definitively identified, poor user compliance is believed to have been a contributing factor [27, 28].

Amoebic keratitis

Although amoebic keratitis is rare, it is associated with wearing contact lenses [29]. Diagnosis is complicated and failure to implement prompt treatment may cause visual impairment in a significant number of cases. In 2007, an outbreak of *Acanthamoeba* keratitis in the USA was found to be associated with a multipurpose lens care solution and the product was removed from the marketplace [30]. Subsequent testing suggested that the solution

Table 21.1.2 ISO Stand-Alone Test procedure for disinfecting products with added organic soil.[a]

Test organism	Time	Log$_{10}$ reduction			Overall mean log$_{10}$ reduction
		Lot No. 1	Lot No. 2	Lot No. 3	
Staphylococcus aureus ATCC 6538	1 h	4.8	4.2	>4.8	4.6
	2 h	>4.8	>4.7	>4.8	4.8
	3 h	>4.8	>4.7	>4.8	4.8
	4 h	>4.8	>4.7	>4.8	4.8
Pseudomonas aeruginosa ATCC 9027	1 h	>4.7	>4.6	>4.7	4.7
	2 h	>4.7	>4.6	>4.7	4.7
	3 h	>4.7	>4.6	>4.7	4.7
	4 h	>4.7	>4.6	>4.7	4.7
Serratia marcescens ATCC 13880	1 h	2.4	2.5	3.0	2.6
	2 h	3.0	4.5	4.1	3.9
	3 h	4.1	>4.7	>4.6	4.5
	4 h	>4.8	>4.7	>4.6	4.7
Candida albicans ATCC 10231	1 h	0.6	0.5	0.9	0.7
	2 h	0.7	0.8	1.6	1.0
	3 h	0.7	1.0	1.9	1.2
	4 h	0.9[b]	1.4	2.5	1.6
	24 h	3.5	4.1	4.6	4.1
Fusarium solani ATCC 36031	1 h	1.9	1.5	3.4	2.3
	2 h	2.2	2.1	>4.3	2.9
	3 h	2.2	2.5	>4.3	3.0
	4 h	2.8	2.8	>4.3	3.3
	24 h	4.3	>4.2	>4.3	4.3
Test disposition		Pass secondary	Pass primary	Pass primary	Pass primary

[a]Microbicidal activity of a multipurpose lens care solution stored at 40°C for 9 months. Samples were inoculated with 1.0×10^5 to 1.0×10^6 cfu/ml of the indicated test organisms suspended in organic soil and tested as per ISO 14729:2001 [32].
[b]Sample fails primary acceptance criteria of a 1-log$_{10}$ reduction at the stated disinfection time. Lot meets secondary acceptance criteria for qualification via the Regimen Test.

may have enabled encystment of the less resistant trophozoite form of *Acanthamoeba* to the more resistant cyst form [31].

Viral keratitis

Viral keratitis is predominantly associated with HSV and varicella-zoster virus (VZV). Both HSV and VZV can infect various tissues of the eye. Severe inflammation and scarring of the corneal and stromal tissue may result, leading to visual impairment and keratoplasty. Currently, testing of lens care solutions for antiviral activity is not required under ISO guidelines as viral transmission via contact lens wear has not been documented [32].

Qualification of lens care solutions

Before a lens care solution can be commercially marketed, it must undergo extensive testing to ensure that it is safe and effective. Although the nature of testing will vary with the country in which the solution is to be registered, it typically includes testing performed according to harmonized procedures to demonstrate the microbicidal efficacy of the solution and the ability of the solution to resist microbial contamination during use.

The ISO stand-alone test

The current International Standards Organization (ISO) 14729 Stand-Alone Test is a suspension test whereby samples from three separate lots of a lens care solution are separately inoculated with the designated test organisms to a final concentration of 1.0×10^5 to 1.0×10^6 cfu/ml [32]. The suspensions are mixed and held at ambient temperature and then sampled at 25%, 50%, 75% and 100% of the minimum recommended disinfection time and additionally at not less than four times the minimum recommended disinfection time for yeast and mold. The samples then are plated on the appropriate growth media and the number of colonies recovered determined following a defined incubation period (Table 21.1.2). To pass the primary acceptance criteria of the Stand-Alone Test the lens care disinfecting solution must demonstrate no less than an average reduction of 3-log$_{10}$ in the number of bacteria and an average reduction of 1-log$_{10}$ in the number of yeasts and molds within the minimum recommended disinfection time, with no increase in the number of yeasts and molds at not less than four times the minimum recommended disinfection time. Products that fail to meet the primary acceptance criteria may be tested by means of the Regimen Test if the combined log$_{10}$ reduction for the mean values of all bacteria is not less than

Table 21.1.3 Qualification of the ability to accurately assay levels of 10^4–10^5 cfu/ml of bacteria and fungi.[a]

Year	Test organism	
	Staphylococcus aureus ATCC 6358	*Candida albicans* ATCC 10231
2005	±0.18-$\log_{10}$	±0.12-$\log_{10}$
2006	±0.17-$\log_{10}$	±0.29-$\log_{10}$
2007	±0.28-$\log_{10}$	±0.14-$\log_{10}$
2008	±0.12-$\log_{10}$	±0.27-$\log_{10}$
2009	±0.26-$\log_{10}$	±0.21-$\log_{10}$

[a]Data indicated are the uncertainties at the 95% confidence level for qualification testing performed with 15–26 analysts.

5-$\log_{10}$ within the minimum recommended disinfection time with a minimum $\log_{10}$ reduction of one for any given bacteria and if stasis is demonstrated for yeast and mold (secondary criteria). With the advent of "no-rub" lens care solutions the US Food and Drug Administration (FDA) required the addition of an organic soil load to the product and microorganism mixture in order to provide an increased challenge to the biocidal efficacy of the lens care solution [33].

A review of the literature will reveal Stand-Alone Test data for various lens care solutions with testing performed by different laboratories, often with conflicting results. To a large extent, this reflects the inherent variability of microbiological assays, including such factors as the methods used to prepare the challenge organisms, the use of different lots of growth medium, variations in incubation and neutralization conditions, the extent of mixing, pipetting error, counting error and other unrecognized variables. Further complicating this situation is the narrow countable range for assays of this nature. As noted by Sutton "An unfortunate regulatory trend in recent years is to establish expectations (specifications, limits, levels) for data generated by the plate-count method that the accuracy of the method cannot support" [34]. Multiple analysts are typically involved with the testing of lens care solutions. Best practices dictate that the analysts undergo periodic requalification for the enumeration of bacteria and fungi. Table 21.1.3 presents a summary of qualification testing performed over a period of 5 years in our laboratories, demonstrating an overall 95% confidence interval better than ±0.5-$\log_{10}$, which compares favorably to the measurement uncertainty noted in ISO 14729. As there are numerous factors intrinsic and extrinsic to the assay that may affect its outcome, care must be taken in interpreting data associated with the Stand-Alone Test.

The ISO regimen test

Lens care solutions that fail to meet the primary acceptance criteria of the Stand-Alone Test but comply with the secondary acceptance criteria may be tested by the Regimen Test. Lenses representative of those with which the product is to be used are inoculated with the desired test organism (as used for the Stand-Alone Test) suspended in an organic soil consisting of a mixture of heat-inactivated yeast cells and bovine serum to a final concentration of 2.0×10^5 to 2.0×10^6 cfu/lens. The inoculum is allowed to adsorb to the lens and the lenses are then processed as described in the manufacturer's instructions. Following processing, the lenses and contents of the lens case are dispensed into a suitable volume of neutralizing solution in a sterile filtration apparatus and filtered. The lens is then aseptically removed from the filter and cast into a bed of molten agar and the filter transferred to an agar plate. Following incubation the total number of colonies recovered is enumerated. To meet current ISO Regimen Test requirements the average recovery for each microbial species for three lots of solution tested should be no more than 10 cfu for each lens type/solution combination. It is interesting to note that the counting error associated with 10 cfu is 31.6 as a percentage of the mean [35]. While a fixed limit of 10 cfu is generally conservative to the number of microorganisms required to establish an infection in the eye [36, 37], it is not apparent that a solution which fails regimen testing with a average recovery of 11 cfu would present any greater risk to the user than one which passes regimen testing with an average recovery of 9 cfu. This is particularly so when one considers that the countable range for most microorganisms is 20–80 cfu for the membrane filtration method and 30–300 cfu for the plate count method [34].

The ISO preservative efficacy/discard date test

In addition to demonstrating their microbicidal efficacy via either the Stand-Alone Test or Regimen Test, lens care solutions must also demonstrate their ability to resist microbial contamination during repeated use according to the procedures described in the ISO 14730 Preservative Efficacy Test [38]. Aliquots from three separate lots of the lens care solution are dispensed into separate sterile containers and inoculated to a final concentration of 1.0×10^5 to 1.0×10^6 cfu/ml of the challenge organism. The same challenge organisms are employed as with the Stand-Alone Test and Regimen Test procedure, substituting *Escherichia coli* for *Serratia marcescens* and *Aspergillus brasiliensis* for *Fusarium solani*. The samples are held at 20–25°C for 14 days and assayed for viable counts on day 7 and 14. Following assay on day 14, the product is rechallenged with 1.0×10^4 to 1.0×10^5 cfu/ml of the challenge organism and the samples held for an additional 14 days and assayed for viable counts on days 21 and 28. Products that demonstrate a mean 3-$\log_{10}$ reduction in the number of bacteria at 14 days and again at 28 days following rechallenge with no increase in yeast and mold at 14 days and no increase in yeast and mold over the rechallenge inoculum at 28 days are considered to meet the requirements for a 28-day use period (discard date) after opening. Longer use periods may be established following similar procedures outlined in ISO 14730.

Table 21.1.4 Comparison of the effect of film formation on the disinfecting efficacy of various laboratory-prepared formulations.[a]

Concentration of disinfectant	Solution A				Solution B				Solution C			
	0%	25%	50%	100%	0%	25%	50%	100%	0%	25%	50%	100%
Fusarium solani ATCC 36031	0.4	0.0	0.0	0.0	1.1	0.0	0.0	0.0	4.0	0.9	0.4	0.0
Fusarium solani clinical isolate	0.3	0.0	0.0	0.0	23	0.0	0.0	0.0	83	0.3	0.0	0.0

[a]Data expressed as the mean viable fungal recovery for a given percentage of disinfectant for each test solution.

Additional testing

On January 22, 2009, the US FDA convened a meeting of representatives from industry, academia and various professional organizations to discuss the development of a consensus method for testing the efficacy of contact lens care products against *Acanthamoeba* and to review existing test methods and determine whether new test methods would need to be developed. The meeting was prompted by the voluntary recalls of lens care solutions following outbreaks of *Fusarium* keratitis in 2006 and *Acanthamoeba* keratitis in 2007. The meeting participants agreed that the development of a standardized method for testing the efficacy of lens care solutions against *Acanthamoeba* cysts and trophozoites was necessary, as well as the development of additional test methods that encompassed real-world factors not addressed by current ISO test procedures. The meeting participants suggested that testing should also be performed with a broader range of test organisms as well as clinical isolates. It was noted that the incidence of *Acanthamoeba* keratitis had not declined significantly, suggesting a fundamental change in the prevalence of this organism due to factors such as municipal water supplies [30]. Poor hygiene practices on the part of the user, such as "topping off" (adding small volumes of the lens care solution to the lens case to replace that lost through evaporation and from prior lens removal from the case), which could lead to the formation of biofilms in the lens case, were also discussed. The issue of "no-rub" lens care solutions was reviewed, with suggestions that the labeling of contact lens solutions be revised to re-establish rubbing of the lens as part of the lens care regimen [39]. As many users fail to comply with the requirements for digital rubbing, however, qualification of lens care solutions without digital rubbing may actually be a more stringent procedure compared with one which incorporates digital rubbing.

Among the test methods being developed are system microbicidal test procedures to assess the effect of different lens and lens case materials on the disinfecting activity of the lens care solution. This essentially consists of inoculating contact lenses with each of the desired test organisms suspended in an organic soil and performing a Stand-Alone Test over a significantly longer period of time in the lens case itself as opposed to performing testing in a separate container. To mimic the effects associated with failure to replace the lens care solution in the lens case after each use, evaporative loss and reuse tests have been proposed. For evaporative loss testing, samples of the lens care solution are allowed to evaporate under controlled conditions until a more concentrated solution is formed. For reuse testing, the solution is tested following several cycles of simulated contact lens disinfection and wear without replacing the solution. The samples are then tested according to the Stand-Alone procedure to determine whether evaporative loss or reuse affects the microbicidal activity of the lens care solution [28]. An example of the effect of film formation in the lens case following evaporative loss of the solution is presented in Table 21.1.4. Differences in disinfecting activity were noted between various laboratory-prepared formulations mixed with two strains of *Fusarium solani* and added to lens cases, followed by drying at ambient conditions to form films in the lens case. The product film was then reconstituted with fresh solution containing various concentrations of the disinfecting agents and the solutions were allowed to soak in the lens case for 4 h followed by determination of the recovery of viable organisms. Each formulation exhibited recovery of *Fusarium* when the dried film was reconstituted with formulation without added disinfecting agents, with varying levels of recovery at intermediate concentrations of the disinfecting agents and no recovery when reconstituted with full-strength formulations. This suggests that user non-compliance in failing to thoroughly dry the lens case between uses or "topping off" may promote the formation of biofilm in the lens case.

The development of new test procedures to evaluate the microbicidal activity of lens care solutions will be particularly challenging in light of the variability associated with microbiological assays. While it may be anticipated that the implementation of new test procedures for lens care solutions will lead to the development of more robust lens care solutions, it should not be assumed that this will lead to a direct reduction in the incidence of microbial keratitis. As shown by the work of Dart *et al.*, the relative risk of microbial keratitis was actually higher for patients who wore daily-disposable contact lenses as compared with patients who wore planned replacement contact lenses that are cleaned, disinfected and returned to the eye [40]. This suggests that there may be factors associated with microbial keratitis beyond the role of the contact lens and lens care solution as potential vectors of microbial contamination.

Conclusions

The contact lens and lens care industry has seen many exciting developments and experienced significant growth following the introduction of soft contact lenses in the 1970s. The industry has also re-examined the way lens care is approached and considered both the formulation as well as use of the product following recalls of lens care solutions that were associated with reports of microbial keratitis. Significant challenges face the manufacturer, prescriber and user of contact lens care products including compliance by the user and the potential risk of infection. Balancing efficacious disinfection and optimizing wearer comfort are the goal. Industry, regulatory authorities, eye-care practitioners and the associated professional organizations are working together to address these issues.

References

1 Keogh, P.L. (1979) Approaches to the development of improved soft contact lens materials. *Artificial Cells, Blood Substitutes, and Biotechnology*, **7** (2), 307–311.

2 Brennan, N.A. *et al.* (2002) A 1-year prospective clinical trial of balafilcon A (PureVision) silicone-hydrogel contact lens used on a 30-day continuous wear schedule. *Ophthalmology*, **109** (6), 1172–1177.

3 Mowrey-McKee, M.F. *et al.* (1992) Microbial contamination of hydrophilic contact lenses. Part 1: quantitation of microbes on patient worn-and-handled lenses. *CLAO Journal*, **18** (2), 87–91.

4 Velasco, J. and Bermudez, J. (1996) Comparative study of the microbial flora on contact lenses, in lens cases, and in maintenance liquids. *International Contact Lens Clinic (New York)*, **23**, 55–58.

5 Clark, B.J. *et al.* (1994) Microbial contamination of cases used for storing contact lenses. *Journal of Infection*, **28**, 293–304.

6 Donzis, P.B. *et al.* (1987) Microbial contamination of contact lens care systems. *American Journal of Ophthalmology*, **104**, 325–333.

7 Gilbert, P. and Moore, L.E. (2005) Cationic antiseptics: diversity of action under a common epithet. *Journal of Applied Microbiology*, **99**, 703–715.

8 Ikeda, T. *et al.* (1984) Interaction of a polymeric biguanide with phospholipid membranes. *Biochimica et Biophysica Acta*, **769**, 57–66.

9 Allen, M.J. *et al.* (2006) The response of *Escherichia coli* to exposure to the biocide polyhexamethylene biguanide. *Microbiology*, **152**, 989–1000.

10 Codling, C.E. *et al.* (2003) Aspects of the antimicrobial mechanisms of action of a polyquaternium and an amidoamine. *Journal of Antimicrobial Chemotherapy*, **51**, 1153–1158.

11 Codling, C.E. *et al.* (2005) An investigation into the antimicrobial mechanisms of two contact lens biocides using electron microscopy. *Contact Lens and Anterior Eye*, **28**, 163–168.

12 Rosenthal, R.A. *et al.* (2000) Broad spectrum antimicrobial activity of a new multi-purpose disinfecting solution. *CLAO Journal*, **26** (3), 120–126.

13 Ahearn, D.G. and Gabriel, M.M. (2001) Disinfection of contact lenses, in *Disinfection, Sterilization, and Preservation*, 5th edn (ed. S.S. Block), Lippincott Williams & Wilkins, Philadelphia, pp. 1105–1114.

14 McDonnell, G. and Russell, A.D. (1999) Antiseptics and disinfectants: activity, action, and resistance. *Clinical Microbiology Reviews*, **12** (1), 147–179.

15 Chawner, J.A. and Gilbert, P. (1989) Adsorption of alexidine and chlorhexidine to *Escherichia coli* and membrane components. *International Journal of Pharmaceutics*, **55**, 209–215.

16 Yanai, R. *et al.* (2006) Evaluation of povidone-iodine as a disinfectant solution for contact lenses: antimicrobial activity and cytotoxicity for corneal epithelial cells. *Contact Lens and Anterior Eye*, **29**, 85–91.

17 Baudouin, C. *et al.* (2010) Preservatives in eyedrops: the good, the bad and the ugly. *Progress in Retinal and Eye Research*, **29**, 312–334.

18 Bielroy, L. (2006) Allergic diseases of the eye. *Medical Clinics of North America*, **90**, 129–148.

19 Banin, E. *et al.* (2006) Chelator-induced disposal and killing of *Pseudomonas aeruginosa* cells in biofilm. *Applied and Environmental Microbiology*, **72** (3), 2064–2069.

20 Xia, E. *et al.* (2009) *Bausch and Lomb, Assignee. Lens Care Solution Comprising Alkyldimonium Hydroxylpropyl Alkylglucosides*, US Patent 7632794, December 15.

21 Hwang, T.S. *et al.* (2004) Disinfection capacity of PuriLens contact lens cleaning unit against *Acanthamoeba*. *Eye and Contact Lens*, **30** (1), 42–43.

22 Cheng, K.H. *et al.* (1999) Incidence of contact-lens-associated microbial keratitis and its related morbidity. *Lancet*, **334** (9174), 181–185.

23 Stapleton, F. *et al.* (2008) The incidence of contact-lens related microbial keratitis in Australia. *Ophthalmology*, **115**, 1655–1662.

24 Robertson, D.M. *et al.* (2007) Current concepts: contact lens related *Pseudomonas* keratitis. *Contact Lens and Anterior Eye*, **30**, 94–107.

25 Fleiszig, S.M.J. *et al.* (1994) *Pseudomonas aeruginosa* invades corneal epithelial cells during experimental infection. *Infection and Immunity*, **62** (8), 3485–3493.

26 Ma, S.E. *et al.* (2009) A multi-country outbreak of fungal keratitis associated with a brand of contact lens solution: the Hong Kong experience. *International Journal of Infectious Diseases*, **13**, 443–448.

27 Snyder, C. (2006) Lens care complications-where's the rub? *Contact Lens and Anterior Eye*, **29**, 161–162.

28 Levy, B. *et al.* (2006) Report on testing from an investigation of *Fusarium* keratitis in contact lens wearers. *Eye and Contact Lens*, **32** (6), 256–261.

29 Schaumberg, D.A. *et al.* (1998) The epidemic of *Acanthamoeba* keratitis: where do we stand? *Cornea*, **17** (1), 3–10.

30 Closing Statements. FDA Workshop on Microbiological Testing of Contact Lens Care Products. January 23, 2009. Available at: http://www.fda.gov/MedicalDevices/NewsEvents/WorkshopsConferences/ucm130431.htm. Accessed 7/25/2012.

31 Kilvington, S. *et al.* (2008) Encystment of *Acanthamoeba* during incubation in multipurpose contact lens disinfectant solutions and experimental formulations. *Eye and Contact Lens*, **34** (3), 133–139.

32 Anon. (2001) *ISO 14729. Ophthalmic Optics – Contact Lens Care Products – Microbiological Requirements and Test Methods for Products and Regimens for Hygienic Management of Contact Lenses*, Amendment 1:2010, International Organization for Standardization, Geneva.

33 McGrath, D. *et al.* (2003) Comparative antimicrobial activity of no-rub multi-purpose lens care solutions in the presence of organic soil. *Eye and Contact Lens*, **29** (4), 245–249.

34 Sutton, S. (2006) Counting colonies. *Pharmaceutical Microbiology Forum Newsletter*, **12** (9), 2–5.

35 United States Pharmacopeia (USP) (2011) *<1227> Validation of Microbial Recovery from Pharmacopeial Articles*, United States Pharmacopeial Convention, Rockville.

36 Lawin-Brussel, C.A. *et al.* (1993) Effect of *Pseudomonas aeruginosa* concentration in experimental contact lens-related microbial keratitis. *Cornea*, **12** (1), 10–18.

37 Wu, T.G. *et al.* (2003) Experimental keratomycosis in a mouse model. *Investigative Ophthalmology and Visual Science*, **44**, 201–216.

38 Anon. (2000) *ISO 14730. Ophthalmic Optics – Contact Lens Care Products – Antimicrobial Preservative Efficacy Testing and Guidance on Determining Discard Date*, International Organization for Standardization, Geneva.

39 Butcko, V. *et al.* (2007) Microbial keratitis and the role of rub and rinsing. *Eye and Contact Lens*, **6**, 421–423.

40 Dart, J.K.G. *et al.* (2008) Risk factors for microbial keratitis with contemporary contact lenses. *Ophthalmology*, **115** (10), 1647–1654.

21.2 Special Issues in Dentistry

Jonathan L.S. Caplin

School of Environment and Technology, University of Brighton, Brighton, UK

Introduction

The final two decades of the 20th century saw significant advances in our knowledge of infection control, leading to a reduction in risk and an improvement in the health and safety of both healthcare personnel and patients. The emergence of the human immunodeficiency virus (HIV) and transmissible spongiform encephalopathies (TSEs), and the resurgence of the hepatitis B virus (HBV) and hepatitis C virus (HCV), were drivers for the development of improved infection control and hygiene practices, with each challenge ushering in new technologies and protocols to limit the spread of infection in the dental and other healthcare settings.

The practice of infection control underwent major changes in the 1980s following reports of clusters of patients in the USA who were thought to have acquired HBV during treatment by an HBV-infected dentist [1]. A position paper on infection control in dentistry commented that "Dental practitioners are virtually the only health care providers who routinely place an ungloved hand into a body cavity" [2]. The concurrent epidemic of acquired immune deficiency syndrome (AIDS) caused by HIV prompted the US Centers for Disease Control and Prevention (CDC) to introduce the concept of "universal precautions", aimed primarily at preventing the transmission of bloodborne viruses in all areas of healthcare including dentistry [3]. The CDC also published its first guidelines for control of infections in dentistry in 1986 [4].

During the 1990s, particularly within the UK, there was considerable concern after the emergence of variant Creutzfeld–Jacob disease (vCJD), a novel human form of TSE, and its possible association with bovine spongiform encephalitis (BSE). Although the theoretical transmission of iatrogenic Creutzfeld–Jacob disease (CJD) by surgical and dental procedures had been postulated in 1978 [5], the risk of transmission of prion proteins during dental treatment was not clear, and the heat resistance of prions and their ability to adhere to medical and dental instruments was a source of unease.

The challenges from these serious transmissible diseases led to an increase in the scientific and clinical understanding of infection prevention and control, and resulted in the development of a broad range of guidelines, technical memoranda and official documents. These were based on prevailing theory and scientific data, with the express aim of reducing and minimizing cross-infection in the healthcare and dental setting. In the USA, the CDC published revised guidelines in 1993 for preventing the transmission of bloodborne viruses [6], which was updated 10 years later, when the CDC emphasized "standard precautions" [7]. These were addenda to the earlier universal precautions, and included more anatomical sites and body fluids, and incorporated body substance isolation controls.

In the UK, updated guidance on implementing infection control procedures within dental practices was introduced in 2003 by the British Dental Association together with the Department of Health [8]. This was followed by the UK Department of

8

Health's issue of the revised Health Technical Memorandum
(HTM) 01-05 *Decontamination in Primary Care Dental Practices*
[9]. It requires that practices work at or above the "essential
quality requirements" described in the guidance, and that all
practices should have a detailed plan on how to achieve the aim
of "best practice".

The introduction, and professional acceptance, of practical,
unambiguous, evidence-based guidelines had a positive impact
on dental cross-infection and contamination issues, and to date
there have been no reports of cross-infection-related illness in UK
dental practices [10]. In the USA, there have not been any reported
cases of HIV transmission from dental care professionals (DCPs)
to patients since 1992, no cases of HCV transmission, and the last
transmission of HBV from a DCP to patients was reported in
1987 [1].

More recently, the 2009 H1N1 influenza pandemic again
focused attention on the prevention of transmission in dental and
other healthcare settings. Both the US Occupational Safety and
Health Administration (OSHA) and the UK Department of
Health issued specific guidance and recommendations based on
scientific rationale and previous experience [11, 12].

A full exposition of all the potential cross-infection and contamination risks in dentistry, and the measures to mitigate them,
is beyond the scope of this chapter and can be found in other
publications [7, 9]. Instead, this chapter will examine three of
the most pressing issues in current dental hygiene where potential hazards to the health and safety of both dental staff and
patients are seen. The concerns addressed here are cross-
infection, particularly of bloodborne viruses and prion proteins;
contamination and decontamination of dental instruments and
the working environment; and compliance with infection control
measures.

Cross-infection

Cross-infection – the person-to-person spread of infectious
microorganisms – is a serious issue for all health professionals but
the potential for cross-infection in dentry is particularly high due
to a number of factors. These include the performance of invasive
procedures resulting in exposure to blood and other potentially
infective materials, the use of complex and intricate instruments
requiring cleaning and decontamination, the incorrect use of
decontamination and sterilization facilities/procedures, high
patient turnover, and the location of many dental surgeries in
converted residential and commercial premises.

The main cross-infection routes in dental surgeries include the
follwoing:
• Inadequate decontamination and sterilization of surgical
instruments and equipment.
• Percutaneous injuries from "sharps" and the transmission of
bloodborne viruses.
• The spread of microorganisms from hands and from aerosols
contaminated with respiratory pathogens and other micro-

organisms from patients' blood splatter from rotary instruments
and respiratory and oral secretions.
• The spread of microorganisms from contaminated dental unit
water lines.

The main cross-contamination and cross-infection routes in
the dental setting are illustrated in Figure 21.2.1.

Bloodborne viruses

During dental procedures, DCPs may be exposed to a wide variety
of microorganisms from the blood, saliva and oral cavity of
patients, and many of these microorganisms have the potential to
be transmitted in the occupational setting via percutaneous and
mucocutaneous routes [13]. The most common and serious
bloodborne viruses (BBVs) of relevance to DCPs are HBV, HCV
and HIV. Needlestick and sharps injuries are the most common
means of transmitting these BBVs, and occur with regularity.

The UK Advisory Group on AIDS calculated that the risk of
infection with a BBV following a deep penetrating wound with a
hollowbore needle or an instrument contaminated with blood is
1 in 3 for HBV [14], 1 in 30 for HCV, and 1 in 300 for HIV [15].
The risks of BBV infection via mucocutaneous exposures are
much lower, estimated at 1 in 1000 for HIV [15]. According to
CDC estimates as many as 20 different pathogens have the potential to be transmitted to healthcare worker via a needlestick injury,
and that approximately 390,000 needlestick and sharps-related
injuries occur per annum to healthcare staff [16]. A study by
Panlilio *et al.* of injuries to healthcare workers in the hospital
setting recorded during 1997–1998 in the USA, suggests that the
figure may be much higher [17]. According to the US National
Institute of Occupational Safety and Health, if hospital and non-
hospital healthcare workers are included in the data, then estimates of between 600,000 to 800,000 needlestick injuries per
annum in the USA are more likely [18].

In the USA, exposure to HIV, HBV or HCV by percutaneous
injury has been shown to have an average risk of infection of
0.3%, 6–30% and 1.8%, respectively [16, 19]. A report by the UK
Health Protection Agency (HPA) in 2008 [20] based on national
surveillance data of exposures to BBVs occurring in England,
Wales and Northern Ireland from 2000 to 2007, documented 914
percutaneous exposure incidents between 2006 and 2007, of
which 68% were caused by hollowbore needles. Physicians and
dentists reported the highest number of occupational exposures,
and the highest proportion of percutaneous injuries (48%)
involved patients with HCV. Although there may be some questions regarding the accuracy of the transmission data, percutaneous injuries are an occupational hazard for healthcare workers,
and the numbers of reported needlestick incidents make this a
pressing problem for those involved in injury control and
prevention.

Hepatitis B and C viruses

Viral hepatitis occurs endemically worldwide and has become a
major public health problem, with an estimated 350–400 million
persons with chronic HBV infections alone [21]. There are six

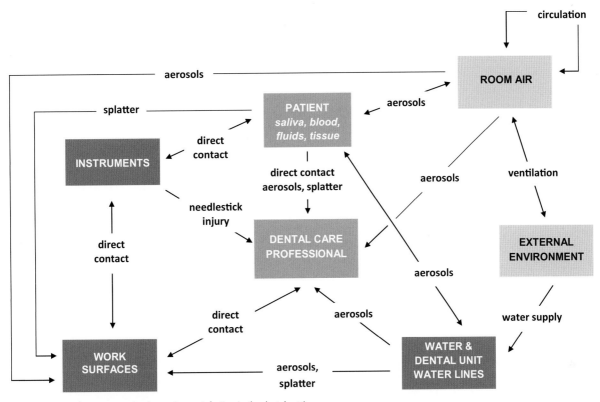

Figure 21.2.1 Routes of cross-contamination and cross-infection in the dental setting.

types of hepatitis virus (A–F) and HBV and HCV infections are an important infectious occupational hazard in the dental profession. HBV is generally transmitted in the dental setting via percutaneous injury with contaminated needles and syringes, and mucous membrane exposures to infected blood [22].

While there is little evidence that saliva and gingival cervical fluid can transmit the virus, the presence of the hepatitis B surface antigen (HBsAg) in saliva and gingival cervical fluid of HBV-positive patients has been recorded [23, 24]. HCV is mainly transmitted via blood-to-blood contact, although RNA from HCV has been detected in saliva and in salivary glands of patients with sialadenitis and Sjögren's syndrome [25, 26]. Higher levels of HCV RNA have been detected in the gingival sulcus than in the saliva of patients with HCV [27], while the presence of HCV RNA in toothbrushes used by hepatitis C patients has also been noted [28]. Despite these finding, no evidence has been produced on the risk of transmission for HBV and HCV after mucocutaneous exposure [20].

During the early 1980s in the light of a worldwide resurgence of HBV, a number of reviews of infection control in dentistry were initiated. In 1986, the CDC published infection control recommendations for dentistry [4] after reports of a number of cases of HBV transmission from DCPs to their patients. Between 1972 and 1999 in the USA, three general dentists transmitted 23 HBV infections to their patients [29–31], and three oral surgeons infected 169 of their patients [31–33]. However, despite the infectivity of HBV/HCV, there is a low risk of transmission in the

dental setting from patient to DCP, from DCP to patient, or from patient to patient. There have been no reported cases of HBV transmission from DCP to patient in the USA since 1987 [1]. Factors contributing to the fall in HBV cross-infection rates include a greater use of gloves during dental examination and treatment, more care when handling sharp instruments, and an increased uptake of HBV vaccination [22]. Nevertheless, despite the introduction and use of universal precautions, patient-to-patient HBV transmission still occurs [34]. A problem that may affect surveillance and reporting rates for HBV is that approximately 50% of HBV infections are asymptomatic or subclinical [35], which makes it difficult to link sporadic cases to a specific DCP or dental surgery.

To minimize the risk of HBV infection, DCPs are advised to have immunization against HBV [6], and over 80% of US dentists and over 90% of UK DCPs reported HBV vaccination by 1992 [36, 37]. All healthcare workers, including DCPs and those who may perform procedures likely to result in exposure to HBV, have an ethical and legal duty to protect the health of their patients. DCPs should be aware of their immune status and if they believe that they have been infected they have a responsibility to seek medical advice and undergo appropriate testing. If found to be infected, the DCP may have limitations placed on the procedures that they can carry out. In the UK, not taking proper advice or not acting accordingly, would be regarded as a case of serious professional misconduct and could lead to disciplinary and possible legal action [38, 39].

The implementation of universal precautions and protocols to minimize exposure to HBV during dental treatment, the adoption of HBV vaccination programs and the provision of post-exposure prophylaxis for DCP, has had considerable success in the resource-rich USA, northern Europe and Australia, but in Africa, the Middle East, Asia and South America the situation remains static. In many cases, basic treatment facilities and equipment, lack of up-to-date knowledge, non-compliance with barrier precautions and vaccination uptake, together with HBsAg rates in the general population of up to 15% [22], the risk of transmission of the virus in the dental setting is still a major problem in developing countries.

Human immunodeficiency virus

AIDS has been around for nearly 30 years now, and concerns regarding the transmission of HIV are well documented. There are some data indicating seroconversion of healthcare workers following occupational exposure to HIV [13, 40], but overall the transmission risk is thought to be low. Six cases of HIV transmission from an HIV-positive dentist to his patients in Florida were recorded in the early 1990s [41], and in 1991 another Florida dentist with AIDS was investigated as a potential source of infection. Retrospective epidemiological analysis and molecular virology indicated that there was no evidence of HIV transmission from the dentist to any of his patients [42]. There have been no further reports of transmission of HIV from infected DCPs to patients in the USA since the CDC began its surveillance program [43]. To control the risk of transmission, the CDC published further infection control guidelines in 1993 [6] which were updated and revised in 2003 in light of the development of new technologies and issues arising during the preceding decade [7].

Scully and Greenspan [44] reviewed the rate of HIV transmission in the dental care settings in the UK, USA and France to November 1, 2005. They found that there has been probable transmission from an HIV-infected healthcare worker to a patient in only three reported cases – a Florida dentist [45], a French orthopedic surgeon [46] and a French nurse [47]; the route of transmission was confirmed only for the orthopedic surgeon. By 2007, there had been five cases of HIV seroconversion following needlestick injury in healthcare workers reported in the UK, and the last documented case was in 1999 [20]. Data from Klein [48] suggests that the rate of occupational exposure to HIV among DCPs has fallen in the decade prior to 2003, although it has been noted that healthcare workers tend to underreport percutaneous injuries [49, 50].

Occupational exposure to HIV should be treated as a medical emergency to ensure that the appropriate HIV Limulus amoebocyte is implemented without delay [51]. The current CDC recommendation for HIV exposures [52] is the administration of a mixture of two nucleoside reverse-transcriptase inhibitors (NRTIs) or one NRTI and one nucleotide reverse-transcriptase inhibitors (NtRTI) immediately following exposure; for example zidovudine (ZVT) and lamivudine (3TC) or emtricitabibe (FTC), and tenofovir (TDF) and 3TC or FTC. Within Europe, a triple

combination of antiretroviral drugs within 72 h is the preferred option [53]. Advice specific to the UK is the administration of zidovudine, together with lamivudine and nelfinavir, ideally within 1 h, although post-exposure prophylaxis up to 2 weeks is considered useful [54].

There are few data on the rates of percutaneous injuries and cross-infections in resource-limited countries, where the prevalence of HIV and the risk of infection are high [55–58]. There are variations in the intensity and severity of the HIV epidemic in different parts of the world, and thus its effect on the local health workforce. For example, in Botswana, there are nearly twice the number of women health workers than male health workers, and since HIV/AIDS infection and resultant morbidity and mortality rates among women are higher than those for men, the impact on healthcare provision is notable [59].

HIV transmission from patient to DCP and from DCP to patient within the dental setting remains a rare but significant problem. However, the introduction of standard and universal infection control protocols and procedures for dealing with percutaneous injuries have mitigated the impact of transmission.

Transmissible spongiform encephalopathy

TSEs are a group of incurable and invariably fatal neurodegenerative conditions in humans and animals caused by abnormal prion proteins (PrP^{Sc}). Sporadic cases in humans have an unknown etiology and occur at the rate of approximately one per million persons, and are responsible for 85–90% of CJD infections. Familial cases arising from a mutation make up 5–10% of all CJD cases, and occur at the rate of less than one in a million persons. Less than 5% of CJD cases are iatrogenic, resulting from transmission of prions via surgical equipment or following transplants of the cornea and dura mater, or the administration of pituitary growth hormones derived from human cadavers [60].

The first cases of vCJD appeared in the 1990s and the discovery of its relationship with the consumption of beef from cattle affected by BSE ("mad cow disease") caused serious concerns, particularly in the UK, which had the highest number of BSE and vCJD cases [61]. BSE was initially observed in cattle in the UK in 1986, and there was some epidemiological evidence that the bovine agent had originated from the scrapie agent, which had been present in sheep in the UK for at least 200 years [62]. The suspicion of a linkage between vCJD and BSE [63] was strong enough for the British government to make BSE a notifiable disease in June 1988. It was estimated that up to 50% of the dairy herds in the UK were affected by BSE, and to limit the spread of prions the UK government banned feed supplements containing sheep and cattle offal in 1989, although the ban was not strictly enforced until the early 1990s. In March 1996, the then Secretary of State for Health announced that 10 cases of vCJD in young adults were most likely associated with exposure to BSE before the offal ban [64].

Since the risk of transmission of prion proteins during dental treatment was not clearly understood, the Spongiform Encephalopathy Advisory Committee (SEAC) in the UK published a position statement in 2007 regarding vCJD and dentistry [65]. The statement highlighted the difficulty in removing adherent prion proteins from contaminated dental instruments, the heat resistance of prions, and the potential infectivity of dental pulp and other tissues. In light of earlier research [66–68], SEAC concluded that the risk of transmission of vCJD through dental procedures was higher than previously thought, and recommended that endodontic reamers and files be single-use, disposable items only [65]. While SEAC was correct to invoke the precautionary principle, reviews of the understanding of the transmission of prion proteins via dental practice generally suggested that the risks were low and not supported by epidemiological evidence [69–71]. Examination of dental pulp from sporadic CJD (sCJD) patients did not reveal any evidence of PrP^{Sc} [72], and no significant levels of PrP^{Sc} were detected in oral-related vCJD tissues [73].

The first published study to investigate possible links between vCJD and dental surgery [74] found no compelling evidence of an increased risk, although the authors noted limitations in the data, and the possibility that some of the 130 cases examined were attributable to dental procedures. A recent assessment of the risk of sCJD transmission during endodontic treatment [75] found that if current official decontamination procedures were carried out on endodontic instruments, the risk of secondary infection would be effectively null, whereas if decontamination procedures were not used or were ineffective, the risk of being infected during treatment was 3.4–13 per million procedures. The authors estimated that the risk of infection was comparable to other high-risk medical procedures such as death during general anesthesia or after liver biopsy, but stressed the importance of the use of single-use instruments or adequate prion decontamination and inactivation. Despite the demonstration of the transmission of PrP^{Sc} to the pulpal tissue of experimental hamsters [76], evidence suggests that dental pulp, gingival tissue and blood, and saliva have very low risk of potential infectivity [60, 61, 73]. It has been noted that effective decontamination of endodontic instruments remains problematic and can leave significant levels of debris, leading to the theoretical possibility of disease transmission [67, 68, 77].

The theoretical risk of transmission of prion disease during dental procedures caused a re-evaluation of the decontamination procedures for dental instruments, and ushered in further guidelines from government and professional organizations [78–80]. However, a lack of clinical and epidemiological evidence, and the paucity of experimental studies on vCJD, meant that the guidelines were prepared on the assumption that there was a definite risk of transmission from dental instruments [81].

In the UK, updated guidance was introduced in 2007 on the premise that, as long as high standards of infection control are maintained and that instruments used on patients in the "at-risk" category are decontaminated correctly, there is no requirement to quarantine or dispose of them, nor to take a medical history prior to treatment. In other words, to treat at-risk patients in the same manner as any other patients [82].

Other potential pathogens

Potentially pathogenic bacteria and viruses can be found in the oral cavity and saliva of most patients. Dental procedures, especially the use of high-speed instruments, produce aerosols and splatter which can spread the oral microorganisms from the patient to the local environment, contaminating the workspace, instruments and the DCP.

A number of studies have investigated the bacterial contamination of aerosols, work surfaces, instruments and dental impressions. The first reports of the production of aerosols and splatter contaminated with microorganisms during dental procedures was in the late 1960s and early 1970s [83, 84]. A wide range of bacteria and viruses have been isolated from aerosols, dental unit water lines (DUWLs) and impression materials. including pathogens such as *Pseudomonas aeruginosa*, *Burkholderia cepacia*, *Legionella pneumophila*, *Mycobacterium tuberculosis*, *Staphylococcus aureus*, cytomegalovirus, herpes simplex virus 1 and 2, oral and respiratory streptococci, and waterborne environmental contaminants [85–92]. Microorganisms can colonize water lines and dental equipment, resulting in the formation of biofilms, often refractory to conventional decontamination protocols [93]. These biofilms, may in turn, produce aerosols [94]. Indirect data in the form of seroprevalance studies showed that dentists have higher antibody titers to respiratory syncytial virus, influenza viruses and cytomegalovirus than the general public, and the titers in dentists rise over time following graduation – most likely a consequence of increasing exposure to saliva and oral microorganisms from their patients [92].

The contamination of DUWLs in dental surgeries by endotoxins is further indirect evidence of bacterial contamination [95]. Waterlines can frequently become contaminated with Gram-negative bacteria, which contain endotoxins – heat-stable chemicals derived from the lipopolysaccharide from their cell walls. Endotoxins are responsible for septic shock syndrome [96], and a number of other clinically significant conditions such as hepatotoxity [97], disseminated intravascular coagulation [98] and respiratory distress [99]. A recent study of dental unit water and dental aerosols by Huntington *et al.* [100] using the Limulus amoebocyte lysate assay, found a significant correlation between bacterial load and endotoxin concentration. The study also showed that endotoxin-contaminated water is aerosolized during dental procedures, adding to the exposure risk for both DCPs and patients.

There are particular problems in dentistry with three emerging or re-emerging pathogenic bacteria, namely methicillin-resistant *S. aureus* (MRSA), *M. tuberculosis* (TB) and vancomycin-resistant *Enterococcus* (VRE). Worldwide rates of tuberculosis and multidrug-resistant TB are rising, particularly in Africa, Asia and South America, and it is estimated that 30% of the world's population is infected with *M. tuberculosis* [101]. Spread via direct contact and airborne respiratory droplets, there is considerable potential for transmission in dentistry. DCPs should take adequate precautions including minimizing aerosol production during dental procedures, the use of barrier techniques and the wearing of face-masks, and, where possible, the installation of high-efficiency ventilation systems [102].

MRSA has become a major problem in hospitals and a regular source of healthcare- as well as community-acquired infections. A 2005 study in the USA found that 4.6% of patients attending community healthcare facilities were infected or colonized with MRSA [103]. MRSA is no more pathogenic than other strains of *S. aureus*, but is resistant to most commonly used antibiotics. MRSA colonizes the nose, axillae, perineum and damaged skin, and is common in hospitalized patients and increasingly in the community setting. Although no special precautions are required for the dental treatment of patients with MRSA, DCPs colonized with MRSA should not be involved in invasive dental procedures, and specific treatment to eradicate colonization is available [8].

VREs are multidrug-resistant strains of the gut bacterium *Enterococcus*. Like MRSA, they are no more pathogenic than sensitive strains of enterococci, but their resistance to vancomycin and other antimicrobials makes their eradication problematic. Enterococci have been isolated from necrotic root canals, and secondary endodontic root infections are frequently caused by *Enterococcus faecalis* [104]. *E. faecalis* and vancomycin-resistant *E. faecium* have also been implicated as a cause of bacteremia and endocarditis following dental surgery, although no link between endocarditis and dental treatment was observed in a case–control study of 273 patients [105]. Nevertheless, their resistance to most available antibiotics, and their potential for contaminating surgical instruments and for colonizing DCPs and the working environment [106], make them potentially problematic in the dental setting.

Contamination of the working environment

Aerosols and splatter

High-speed rotating drills, ultrasonic scalers, rotary polishers, DUWLs and compressed air used in dental cleaning and restorative work produce aerosols and splatter contaminated with saliva, blood and microorganisms from the patient's oral cavity [94, 107, 108]. Splatter droplets are particles larger than 50 μm in diameter that are airborne briefly before settling [107], whereas aerosols are invisible particles with diameters of less than 10 μm that can float on air currents [109].

Recent studies indicate that the area contaminated by aerosols and splatter droplets is much larger than originally thought. Milejczak [110] detected bacterial deposits up to 2.6 m from the dental chair, and a study by Rautemaa *et al.* isolated bacteria up to 1.5 m from the patient's mouth, and found that the use of rotary and ultrasonic instruments resulted in increased bacterial numbers and a greater area of contamination than during periodontal and orthodontic treatment [89].

A review by Harrel and Molinari [107] of the literature on reducing aerosol contamination concluded that the use of a 0.1% chlorhexidine mouthwash prior to a dental procedure reduced

airborne contamination, as did the use of a rubber dental dam to prevent splashing. High-volume evacuators (HVEs) have been shown to reduce airborne contamination by more than 90%, and high-efficiency particulate air filters or ultraviolet light irradiation of the ventilation system are also effective but expensive options. The CDC recommends the use of rubber dams and HVEs to reduce splatter [1]. Attention to the risk from aerosols was again focused during the 2009 H1N1 influenza pandemic [11, 12, 111].

Dental unit water lines

DUWLs supply water for high-speed dental handpieces, air–water syringes and ultrasonic scalers and are an indispensable part of dental equipment. The fact that DUWLs frequently contain biofilms that continually shed organisms was first reported by Blake in 1963 [112].

Bacterial species such as *S. aureus*, *Mycobacterium avium* and *Legionella* species including *L. pneumophila*, as well as fungi and protozoa, have been isolated from DUWLs [113]. A more recent study of the numbers and composition of bacteria in DUWLs showed that bacterial concentrations can reach excessive values, and that the predominant species were of oral cavity flora, opportunistic pathogens and environmental aquatic microbiota. *Ralstonia pickettii* was detected in all the units examined, and *Sphingomonas paucimobilis* and *Brevundimonas vesicularis* were commonly found [114].

Since the water used during routine dental procedures can develop bacterial contamination above levels considered acceptable for safe drinking water, regular monitoring for microbes in the DUWL water is recommended, as is the application of a disinfecting procedure. Flushing water lines will not remove biofilms but will reduce the concentration of bacteria in the water phase [115], and the CDC recommends that additional measures such as chemical agents are required [1, 7]. A review of several studies investigating the use of line cleaners/disinfectants to flush water lines and remove particulate waste, biofilms and planktonic microbes, concluded that only 13 out of 28 such procedures reduced the total viable count and biofilm levels by more than 94% [116]. It has been suggested that flushing the water lines after each use is the only way to guarantee that residual microbial contamination can be removed [117]. Water lines made from polytetrafluoroethylene (PTFE) appear to be more resistant to biofilm formation than tubes made from polyethylene (PE), and may be inhibitory to *P. aeruginosa*, and water lines of larger-bore diameter (4 mm rather than 1.6 mm) exhibited a reduction in bacterial counts [118].

The relationship between respiratory disease and exposure to airborne and aerosolized bacteria in dental personnel is ambiguous, with insufficient data to confirm any linkage between them. It has been reported that DCPs have higher levels of *Legionella* antibodies than the general population [119] and other studies have confirmed the resistance of *Legionella* species to flushing DUWLs [115]. Two studies have shown a relationship between occupational exposure to contaminated DUWLs and asthma in

DCPs, although a statistically significant association was found only in the UK study [120] and not in the US study [121].

Impressions, prosthetics and dental instruments

The contamination of impressions with saliva and blood, together with oral bacteria and respiratory pathogens, has been documented for some time. There are studies suggesting that DCPs and dental laboratory technicians are at risk of infection from cross-contaminated elastomeric dental impressions made in the dental clinic [122], although a review considered the risk of cross-infection to be relatively low [123]. The American Dental Association produced three guidance documents for the disinfection of impressions [124–126], while the Medicines and Healthcare Products Regulatory Agency of the UK Department of Health produced the *MAC Manual* [127]. This provides advice on all aspects of decontamination, including of dental instruments and impressions, based on guidance from the European Union's Medical Devices Directive.

The extent and impact of the problem is still under debate. A review by Kugel *et al.* [128] of 400 US dental laboratories found that only 44% of the them knew when incoming impressions had been disinfected, and as a precaution 94% of the labs routinely disinfected all impressions they received, illustrating a lack of communication between DCP and dental laboratory personnel. Junevicius *et al.* [91] studied the artificial contamination of alginate and silicon impressions with *Serratia rubidaea* and found that silicon impressions had lower contamination rates than alginate impressions. They also noted that rinsing the impression under running tapwater was an ineffective means of reducing contamination and that disinfection was required. However, an investigation of bacterial numbers on 107 impression samples revealed that contamination was often at a low level, and the authors questioned whether disinfection was necessary if adequate hygiene and handling protocols were adhered to [129]. One particular source of cross-infection in the dental laboratory is the bacterial contamination of the pumice slurry used on polishing wheels to apply final polishing of implants, dentures and prosthetics [130]. Freshly prepared pumice slurry containing disinfectant was free from contamination; after 3 days' use colony counts approached 10^9/g [131].

Prosthetic devices, matrix bands, burs, polishing cups and endodontic files are often contaminated with a patient's blood, body fluids and tissue, and are difficult to clean properly. Endodontic files used to prepare root canals are likely to become contaminated with blood, tissue and bone fragments, which can remain attached even after cleaning and autoclaving [67], and it is recommended by US and UK authorities that they be single-use items only [7, 9].

Dental handpieces pose problems due to their complex design, with lumens and recesses inherent in their design which make effective cleaning difficult. Despite not having direct contact with the oral tissues and fluids, the internal workings can become contaminated via splatter, and potentially spray back into the oral cavity [132]. Because of their design, handpieces cannot be immersed in ultrasonicators prior to sterilization although small cleaning machines specifically designed for this purpose are available. The British Dental Association (BDA) recommends the use of appropriate cleaning machines but allows careful manual cleaning (as detailed by the BDA) if no machine is available [8]. An earlier recommendation from the Medical Devices Agency was to sterilize dental instruments with lumens, cavities or recesses in a vacuum autoclave [133]. It has been noted that dental departments within district general hospitals use sterile services departments to decontaminate their instruments, but in many cases busy workloads result in manual cleaning and the use of non-vacuum sterilizers [134]. To ascertain how handpieces are decontaminated in general dental practice, Smith *et al.* carried out an observational survey of 179 dental practices in Scotland between 2003 and 2004. They found that in nearly all surgeries the handpieces were cleaned prior to autoclaving in bench-top steam sterilizers, usually by manual wiping using disinfectant-impregnated cloths, although a minority of surgeries had dedicated handpieces for surgery [135].

Within the UK, specific guidance for decontamination in primary-care dental practices was contained in HTM 01-05 [9]. This was based on previously issued guidance, including HSG (93)40, which was introduced to manage the transmission of HBV infections [136]. It introduced benchmarks and compliance targets, and requires that practices work at or above the "essential quality requirements" described in the guidance, and that all practices should have a detailed plan on how to achieve the aim of "best practice". The essential quality requirements are: (i) for all instruments to be sterilized in a bench-top autoclave and stored under aseptic conditions; (ii) that single-use instruments should be mandatory for endodontics; and (iii) that bagged instruments should be given a use-by date. The main requirements for best practice are: (i) the use of an approved automatic washer disinfector for the decontamination and disinfection of dental instruments; (ii) the provision of a room or area separate from the dental treatment area for decontamination operations; and (iii) a specifically-designed separate facility for the storage of reprocessed dental instruments.

Clinical waste

Waste produced in dental practices falls into the categories of clinical and non-clinical waste, which must be segregated. Clinical waste includes waste contaminated with blood, saliva or other body fluids, and is potentially hazardous to persons coming into contact with it, and must be placed in pre-labeled, UN-type approved, puncture-proof containers. Clinical waste includes needles and scalpel blades (sharps), and partially-discharged and fully-discharged local anesthetic cartridges [8].

Extracted teeth can be disposed of in sharps containers for eventual incineration, but teeth containing mercury amalgam are incineration hazards and should be treated as dental amalgam waste. In the UK, HTM 07-01 *Safe Management of Healthcare Waste* [137] advises dentists to dispose of dental amalgam waste in amalgam separators prior to disposal by an authorized waste disposal company.

The final disposal of clinical waste is also subject to a number of provisions and regulations, including the completion of a hazardous/special waste consignment note containing details of the type of waste, the waste disposal company and when the waste was disposed of, and a certificate of safe destruction provided by the waste carrier.

Compliance with infection control measures

The achievements in infection control in dentistry over the past 30 years, both in theory and in application, have been impressive, and the acceptance of different practices, procedures and protocols by DCPs have significantly reduced occupational infection risks in dentistry [138].

Nevertheless, despite the recommendations being based on scientific and clinical evidence, there are reports of non-compliance by DCPs [139]. Millership *et al.* [140] documented three reported cases of failure of decontamination of dental instruments in the UK; breaches included not autoclaving dental handpieces, the use of cold disinfectant solutions, dental mirrors contaminated with dried blood, and the reuse of surgical blades, suture needles and gloves. A 2005 study of 856 dental hygienists in the USA [141] found that compliance with infection control guidelines had improved compared with a previous study, but dental hygienists had misconceptions about infectious disease transmission. An occupational study of 179 dental surgeries in the UK by Smith *et al.* [142] noted that although a majority (70%) of surgeries had control of infection management policies, only half of these had been documented, and audits of decontamination and infection control procedures were apparent in only 11% of surgeries. In most cases, infection control training was by demonstration or observed practice, leading the authors to highlight the poor training and lack of documentation in some UK dental surgeries.

If non-compliance is occurring in resource-rich developed countries, then it can be assumed that the incidence of non-compliance would be high in resource-poor developing countries due to issues of cost or availability. For example, 146 Nigerian dentists were monitored by questionnaire [143] which revealed wide ranges of compliance in the use of gloves, face-masks, protective eyewear, sterilization methods and HBV vaccination uptake. The unavailability of equipment due to lack of funding was the main reason for non-compliance. A paper detailing over 100 general dental practices surveyed in north Jordan [144], reported low compliance with a number of infection control recommendations; only one-third of dentists were vaccinated against HBV, only 18% disinfected impressions before sending them to the dental laboratory, only 32% used dedicated containers for the disposal of sharps, and only 63% sterilized items using an autoclave. The authors comment that only approximately 14% of general dentists surveyed were considered to be compliant with recommended infection control measures, and that there was a lack of formal and obligatory infection control courses and guidelines in Jordan.

Training in infection control

The introduction in the UK of HTM 01-05 [9] and the equivalent guidance in the USA of RR17 [7] have propelled the dental profession into a period of rapid change with respect to practice of infection control and an understanding of the scientific evidence behind the guidance. All DCPs should have up-to-date knowledge of what appropriate infection control measures will prevent cross-contamination and infection transmission, why such measures are needed, and how to incorporate best practice standards with the new guidelines. Infection control policies for practices should be regularly reviewed and updated where applicable, and to ensure compliance it is essential that regular monitoring of the procedures is carried out.

Within the UK, qualified dental surgeons receive undergraduate and postgraduate training in infection control but dental nurses and hygienists were not required to undergo specific training until 2008. As noted by John *et al.* [145] in a study of 254 dental nurses in England in 2001, only 40% had formal qualifications. Within the UK, the General Dental Council mandated compulsory registration as from July 31, 2008. Dentists, dental nurses and dental technicians must hold a qualification approved by the General Dental Council in order to be eligible to apply for registration and to undertake continuing professional development (CPD) [146]. There are a number of CPD courses run by dental organizations, health authorities and private providers available for dentists, dental nurses and technicians.

Therefore, to maintain standards and achieve "essential quality requirements" and "best practice", all new staff should be trained in infection control procedures before working in the practice [8]. The training should include information on how infections are spread, how to prevent and control the spread of infections, the monitoring of procedures and the periodic review of the control of infection policy for the practice, the appropriate use of post-exposure prophylaxis, and how to manage accidents or personal injury within the practice.

Recent developments in dental hygiene

Ozonated liquids

Despite being considered a dangerous and toxic gas, ozone in the form of ozonated liquids has been used as an alternative for infection control and wound care for many years, particularly in Russia and Cuba [147]. Recent research has shown that ozonated fluids exhibit marked antimicrobial and anti-inflammatory properties [148], have high compatibility with mammalian cells [149] and have a role in the management of periodontal disease [150]. The use of ozonated water, gels and oils has been demonstrated to reduce the level of oral microbiota including unattached bacteria and microbes in plaque and periodontal pockets, and to minimize oral soft tissue infection following dental surgery and accidental trauma [151, 152]. They are also highly effective against MRSA [153] and bacterial spores [154], and have been found to be an effective sanitizer for DUWLs [155].

A potential concern regarding the use of ozonated fluids is that ozone may inactivate some anti-microbial compounds, including tetracycline and triclosan [156–158]. Consequently, patients should be informed of this possible interaction if they have been prescribed antimicrobials. On the other hand, the destructive action of ozonated water on endocrine disrupters [159] commonly found in resin-based dental restoration compounds, may provide a mechanism to remove these chemicals from the body.

The use of ozonated fluids show great promise as a preventative measure against dental decay but there are a number of contraindications, including pregnancy, G-6-PD deficiency ('favism'), hyperthyroidism, recent myocardial infarction, haemorrhage and anaemia [160].

Photodynamic therapy

Initially reported in 1900 as a means of killing microbes [161], photodynamic therapy (PDT) has been mainly employed as an alternative treatment for tumours, using porphyrin photosensitisers and laser light [162]. The photoactive dye is taken up by the target cells and following irradiation with light of a specific wavelength, cell death occurs as a result of the production of active singlet-oxygen radicals [163]. The bactericidal effect of PDT against a range of gram-positive and gram-negative bacterial species, including antibiotic-resistant strains, planktonic cultures, biofilms and *in vivo*, has revealed its potential as an effective antimicrobial therapy and hygiene strategy in dentistry and dermatology [164, 165].

The primary source of light which have been used to date have been lasers and laser diodes which produce light in a closely defined waveband, typically ±2 nm. This waveband is matched to the peak excitation wavelength of the photosensitiser used. The commonest of these are methylene blue, and toluidene blue O or its pharmaceutical grade counterpart tolonium chloride, which has an absorbance of 632 ± 11 nm around the maximum [164]. The recent developments in PDT for dental applications have been well documented [166–168], and the term photoactivated disinfection (PAD) has been applied to the use of PDT in oral and dental diseases [169].

The development of light emitting diodes (LEDs) of ever increasing power and with a suitable waveband for excitation led to speculation that the effects of PDT could be achieved without the use of a laser light source. LED light sources in conjunction with porphyrin photosensitisers achieved significant kill rates for endodontic bacteria in planktonic suspensions and in artificial and human root canals [169–171]. LEDs were as effective as He-Ne laser light in the ability to disrupt oral biofilms and kill biofilm bacteria [172]. LEDs show many advantages over lasers, most notably their reduced cost and portability, bacterial killing efficiency equivalent to lasers and their better public and practitioner acceptance. The emission bands of red LEDs (620–660 nm) cover the whole absorption spectrum of TBO (621–643 nm) which may lead to optimum photosensitization activity.

Dental caries and periodontal disease are frequently localized infections, and successful treatment includes the eradication of bacteria within the lesions. PDT has been employed as a disinfection strategy by the topical application of TBO and irradiation of the coated lesion with LED light via a thin optical light guide [173–175].

References

1 Kohn, W.G. *et al.* (2004) Guidelines for infection control in dental health care settings -2003. *Journal of the American Dental Association*, **135**, 33–47.

2 Anon. (1986) The control of transmissible disease in dental practice: a position paper of the American Association of Public Health Dentistry. *Journal of Public Health Dentistry*, **46**, 13–22.

3 Centers for Disease Control and Prevention (1985) Recommendations for preventing transmission of infection with human T-lymphotropic virus type III/lymphadenopathy-associated virus in the workplace. *MMWR. Morbidity and Mortality Weekly Report*, **34**, 681–685.

4 Centers for Disease Control and Prevention (1986) Recommended infection control practices for dentistry. *MMWR. Morbidity and Mortality Weekly Report*, **35**, 237–242.

5 Adams, D.H. and Edgar, W.M. (1978) Transmission of agent of Creutzfeldt–Jakob disease. *British Medical Journal*, **1**, 987.

6 Centers for Disease Prevention and Control (1993) Recommended infection control practices for dentistry. RR-8. *MMWR. Morbidity and Mortality Weekly Report*, **41**, 1–12.

7 Centers for Disease Prevention and Control (2003) Guidelines for infection control in dental health-care settings – 2003. RR-17. *MMWR. Morbidity and Mortality Weekly Report*, **52**, 1–61.

8 BDA Advisory Service (2003) *A12 – Advice Sheet Infection Control in Dentistry*, British Dental Association, London.

9 Department of Health (2009) *Health Technical Memorandum 01-05: Decontamination in Primary Care Dental Practices*, The Stationery Office, London.

10 Griffiths, R. (2010) Doing it right! New guidance on "decontamination in primary care dental practice". *Dental Health*, **49**, 18–19.

11 Occupational Safety and Health Administration (OSHA), United States Department of Labour (2009) *OSHA 3328-05R: Pandemic Influenza Preparedness and Response Guidance for Healthcare Workers and Healthcare Employers*, OSHA Publications Office, Washington.

12 Department of Health (2010) *Pandemic (H1N1) Influenza: a Survey of Guidance for Infection Control in Healthcare Settings*, The Stationary Office, London.

13 Centers for Disease Control and Prevention (1999) Health care workers with documented and possible occupationally acquired AIDS/HIV infection, by occupation, reported through June 1998. *US HIV/AIDS Surveillance Report*, **10**, 24.

14 Department of Health (1998) *Guidance for Clinical Healthcare Workers: Protection Against Infection with Bloodborne Viruses. Recommendations of the Expert Advisory Group on AIDS and the Advisory Group on Hepatitis*, Department of Health, London.

15 Department of Health (2008) *HIV Post-Exposure Prophylaxis: Guidance from the UK Chief Medical Officers' Expert Advisory Group on AIDS*, Department of Health, London.

16 Centers for Disease Control and Prevention (2001) Updated US Public Health Service guidelines for the management of occupational exposures to HBV, HCV, and HIV and recommendations for post-exposure prophylaxis. RR11. *MMWR. Morbidity and Mortality Weekly Report*, **50**, 1–42.

17 Panlilio, A.L. *et al.* (2004) Estimate of the annual number of percutaneous injuries among hospital-based healthcare workers in the United States, 1997–1998. *Infection Control and Hospital Epidemiology*, **25**, 556–562.

18 NIOSH (2000) *NIOSH Alert: Preventing Needlestick Injuries in Health Care Settings*, DHHS (NIOSH) Publication No. 2000-108, NIOSH Publications Dissemination, Cincinnati.

19 NIOSH (2004) *Worker Health Chartbook 2004: Bloodborne Infections and Percutaneous Exposures*, DHHS (NIOSH) Publication No. 2004–146, NIOSH Publications Dissemination, Cincinnati.

20 Health Protection Agency (HPA), National Public Health Service for Wales, CDSC Northern Ireland and Health Protection Scotland (2008) *Eye of the Needle. Surveillance of Significant Occupational Exposure to Bloodborne Viruses in Healthcare Workers*, HPA, London.

21 Lavanchy, D. (2005) Worldwide epidemiology of HBV infection, disease burden, and vaccine prevention. *Journal of Clinical Virology*, **34** (Suppl. 1), S1–S3.

22 Mahboobi, N. *et al.* (2010) Hepatitis B virus infection in dentistry: a forgotten topic. *Journal of Viral Hepatitis*, **17**, 307–316.

23 van der Eijk, A.A. *et al.* (2004) Paired measurements of quantitative hepatitis B virus DNA in saliva and serum of chronic hepatitis B patients: implications for saliva as infectious agent. *Journal of Clinical Virology*, **29**, 92–94.

24 Lamster, I.B. and Ahlo, J.K. (2007) Analysis of gingival crevicular fluid as applied to the diagnosis of oral and systemic diseases. *Annals of the New York Academy of Sciences*, **1098**, 216–229.

25 Arrieta, J.J. *et al.* (2001) *In situ* detection of hepatitis C virus RNA in salivary glands. *American Journal of Pathology*, **158**, 259–264.

26 Toussirot, E. *et al.* (2002) Presence of hepatitis C virus RNA in the salivary glands of patients with Sjogren's syndrome and hepatitis C virus infection. *Journal of Rheumatology*, **29**, 2382–2385.

27 Suzuki, T. *et al.* (2005) Quantitative detection of hepatitis C virus (HCV) RNA in saliva and gingival crevicular fluid of HCV-infected patients. *Journal of Clinical Microbiology*, **43**, 4413–4417.

28 Lock, G. *et al.* (2006) Hepatitis C – contamination of toothbrushes: myth or reality? *Journal of Viral Hepatitis*, **13**, 571–573.

29 Levin, M.L. *et al.* (1974) Hepatitis B transmission by dentists. *Journal of the American Medical Association*, **228**, 1139–1140.

30 Hadler, S.C. *et al.* (1981) An outbreak of hepatitis B in a dental practice. *Annals of Internal Medicine*, **95**, 133–138.

31 Goodman, R.A. *et al.* (1982) Hepatitis B transmission from dental personnel to patients: unfinished business. *Annals of Internal Medicine*, **96**, 119.

32 Rimland, D. *et al.* (1997) Hepatitis B outbreak traced to an oral surgeon. *New England Journal of Medicine*, **296**, 953–958.

33 Reingold, A.L. *et al.* (1982) Transmission of hepatitis B by an oral surgeon. *Journal of Infectious Diseases*, **145**, 262–268.

34 Redd, J.T. *et al.* (2007) Patient-to-patient transmission of hepatitis B virus associated with oral surgery. *Journal of Infectious Diseases*, **195**, 1311–1314.

35 McCarthy, G.M. (2000) Risk of transmission of viruses in the dental office. *Journal of the Canadian Dental Association*, **66**, 554–547.

36 Cleveland, J.L. *et al.* (1996) Hepatitis B vaccination and infection among US dentists, 1983–1992. *Journal of the American Dental Association*, **127**, 1385–1392.

37 Scully, C. *et al.* (1993) The control of cross-infection in UK clinical dentistry in the 1990s: immunization against hepatitis B. *British Dental Journal*, **174**, 29–31.

38 General Dental Council (GDC) (2001) *Maintaining Standards – Guidance to Dentists on Professional and Personal Conduct*, November 1997, amended May 2001, GDC, London.

39 General Dental Council (GDC) (2005) *Standards for Dental Professionals – General Dental Council Standards Guidance*, May, GDC, London.

40 Centers for Disease Control and Prevention (1995) Case-control study of HIV seroconversion in health-care workers after percutaneous exposure to HIV-infected blood – France, United Kingdom, and United States, January 1988–August 1994. *MMWR. Morbidity and Mortality Weekly Report*, **44**, 929–933.

41 Centers for Disease Control and Prevention (1991) Epidemiologic notes and reports update: transmission of HIV infection during invasive dental procedures – Florida. *MMWR. Morbidity and Mortality Weekly Report*, **40**, 377–381.

42 Jaffe, H.W. *et al.* (1994) Lack of HIV transmission in the practice of a dentist with AIDS. *Annals of Internal Medicine*, **121**, 855–859.

43 Kohn, W.G. *et al.* (2003) Guidelines for infection control in dental health-care settings. *Morbidity and Mortality Weekly Report. Recommendations and Reports*, **52**, 1–61.

44 Scully, C. and Greenspan, J.S. (2006) Human immunodeficiency virus (HIV) transmission in dentistry. *Journal of Dental Research*, **85**, 794–800.

45 Ciesielski, C. *et al.* (1992) Transmission of human immunodeficiency virus in a dental practice. *Annals of Internal Medicine*, **116**, 798–805.

46 Lot, F. *et al.* (1999) Probable transmission of HIV from an orthopedic surgeon to a patient in France. *Annals of Internal Medicine*, **130**, 1–6.

47 Goujon, C.P. *et al.* (2000) Phylogenetic analyses indicate an atypical nurse-to-patient transmission of human immunodeficiency virus type 1. *Journal of Virology*, **74**, 2525–2532.

48 Klein, R.S. *et al.* (1988) Low occupational risk of human immunodeficiency virus infection among dental professionals. *New England Journal of Medicine*, **318**, 86–90.

49 Ramos-Gomez, F. *et al.* (1997) Accidental exposures to blood and body fluids among health care workers in dental teaching clinics: a prospective study. *Journal of the American Dental Association*, **128**, 1253–1261.

50 Elmiyer, B. *et al.* (2004) Needle-stick injuries in the National Health Service: a culture of silence. *Journal of the Royal Society for Medicine*, **97**, 326–327.

51 Smith, A.J. *et al.* (2001) Management of needlestick injuries in general dental practice. *British Dental Journal*, **190**, 645–650.

52 Centers for Disease Control (2005) Updated US Public Health Service guidelines for the management of occupational exposures to HIV and recommendations for postexposure prophylaxis. *MMWR. Morbidity and Mortality Weekly Report*, **54**, 1–17.

53 Puro, V. *et al.* (2004) Post-exposure prophylaxis of HIV infection in healthcare workers: recommendations for the European setting. *European Journal of Epidemiology*, **19**, 577–584.

54 UK Department of Health (2004) *HIV Post-Exposure Prophylaxis: Guidance from the UK Chief Medical Officer's Expert Advisory Group on AIDS*, Department of Health, London.

55 Ogunbodede, E.O. and Rudolph, M.J. (2002) Policies and protocols for preventing transmission of HIV infection in oral health care in South Africa. *South African Dental Journal*, **57**, 469–475.

56 Muzyka, B.C. *et al.* (2001) Prevalence of HIV-1 and oral lesions in pregnant women in rural Malawi. *Oral Surgery, Oral Medicine, Oral Pathology, Oral Radiology and Endodontology*, **92**, 56–61.

57 Maupome, G. *et al.* (2002) Attitudes toward HIV-infected individuals and infection control practices among a group of dentists in Mexico City – a 1999 update of the 1992 survey. *American Journal of Infection Control*, **30**, 8–14.

58 Matee, M. *et al.* (1999) HIV infection, dental treatment demands and needs among patients seeking dental services at the Muhimbili Medical Centre in Dar-es-Salaam, Tanzania. *International Dental Journal*, **49**, 153–158.

59 Tawfik, L. and Kinoti, S.N. (2006) The impact of HIV/AIDS on the health workforce in developing countries. Background paper prepared for *The World Health Report 2006 – Working Together for Health*. World Health Organization, Geneva.

60 Walker, J.T. *et al.* (2008) Implications for Creutzfeldt–Jakob disease (CJD) in dentistry: a review of current knowledge. *Journal of Dental Research*, **87**, 511–519.

61 NCJDSU – The National CJD Surveillance Unit (2007) *Sixteenth Annual Report: Creutzfeldt–Jakob Disease Surveillance in the UK*, NCJDSU, Edinburgh.

62 Parry, H. (1984) *Scrapie*, Academic Press, London.

63 Hill, A.F. *et al.* (1997) The same prion strain causes vCJD and BSE. *Nature*, **389**, 448–450.

64 House of Commons (1996) *Agriculture and Health Committees' Joint Report BSE and CJD: Recent Developments*, House of Commons, London, pp. 357–357.

65 Spongiform Encephalopathy Advisory Committee (SEAC) (2006) *Position Statement on vCJD and Endodontic Dentistry*, UK SEAC, London.

66 Smith, A. *et al.* (2002) Contaminated dental instruments. *Journal of Hospital Infection*, **51**, 233–235.

67 Smith, A. *et al.* (2005) Residual protein levels on reprocessed dental instruments. *Journal of Hospital Infection*, **61**, 237–241.

68 Lowe, A.H. *et al.* (2002) A study of blood contamination of Siqveland matrix bands. *British Dental Journal*, **192**, 43–45.

69 Porter, S.R. (2002) Prions and dentistry. *Journal of the Royal Society of Medicine*, **95**, 178–181.

70 Smith, A.J. *et al.* (2003) Prion diseases and dental treatment: principles and practice of patients with/suspected or at-risk of CJD: case reports. *British Dental Journal*, **195**, 319–321.

71 Azarpazhooh, A. and Leake, J.L. (2006) Prions in dentistry – what are they, should we be concerned, and what can we do? *Journal of the Canadian Dental Association*, **72**, 53–60.

72 Blanquet-Grossard, F. *et al.* (2000) Prion protein is not detectable in dental pulp from patients with Creutzfeldt–Jakob disease. *Journal of Dental Research*, **79**, 700.

73 Head, M.W. *et al.* (2003) Investigation of PrP^{res} in dental tissues in variant CJD. *British Dental Journal*, **195**, 339–443.

74 Everington, D. *et al.* (2007) Dental treatment and risk of variant CJD – a case control study. *British Dental Journal*, **202**, 470–471.

75 Bourvis, N. *et al.* (2007) Risk assessment of transmission of sporadic Creutzfeldt–Jakob disease in endodontic practice in absence of adequate prion inactivation. *PLoS ONE*, **2**, e1330.

76 Ingrosso, L. *et al.* (1999) Transmission of the 263K scrapie strain by the dental route. *Journal of General Virology*, **80**, 3043–3047.

77 Markovic, L. *et al.* (2009) Residual debris deposits on endodontic instruments after hygienic processing. *Journal of Hospital Infection*, **71**, 190–192.

78 Department of Health – Advisory Committee on Dangerous Pathogens and Spongiform Encephalopathy Advisory Committee (1998) *Transmissible Spongiform Encephalopathy Agents: Safe Working and the Prevention of Infection*, The Stationary Office, London.

79 Department of Health (2000) *Creutzfeldt–Jakob Disease: Guidelines for Healthcare Workers*, The Stationary Office, London.

80 World Health Organization (WHO) (2003) *Report of a WHO Consultation, Geneva, Switzerland, 23–26 March 1999: WHO Infection Control Guidelines for Transmissible Spongiform Encepahalopathies*, WHO/CDS/APH/2000/3, WHO, Geneva.

81 Department of Health – Advisory Committee on Dangerous Pathogens and Spongiform Encephalopathy (2003) *Transmissible Spongiform Encephalopathy Agents: Safe Working and the Prevention of Infection*, The Stationary Office, London.

82 Department of Health – Advisory Committee on Dangerous Pathogens and Spongiform Encephalopathy (2007) *The Decontamination of Surgical Instruments with Special Attention to the Removal of Proteins and Inactivation of Any Contaminating Human Prions*, The Stationary Office, London.

83 Micik, R.E. *et al.* (1969) Studies on dental aerobiology: I – bacterial aerosols generated during dental procedures. *Journal of Dental Research*, **48**, 49–56.

84 Miller, R.L. *et al.* (1971) Studies of dental aerobiology: II – microbial splatter discharge from the oral cavity of dental patients. *Journal of Dental Research*, **50**, 621–625.

85 John, M. (2000) Risk of bacterial transmission in dental practice. *Journal of the Canadian Dental Association*, **66**, 550–552.

86 Ward, K. (2006) Airborne contamination in dentistry: the final challenge. *Dental Nursing*, **2**, 500–503.

87 Bennett, A.M. *et al.* (2000) Microbial aerosols in general dental practice. *British Dental Journal*, **189**, 664–667.

88 Prospero, E. *et al.* (2003) Microbial aerosol contamination of dental healthcare workers' faces and other surfaces in dental practice. *Infection Control and Hospital Epidemiology*, **24**, 139–141.

89 Rautemaa, R. *et al.* (2006) Bacterial aerosols in dental practice – a potential hospital infection problem? *Journal of Hospital Infection*, **64**, 76–81.

90 Williams, H.N. *et al.* (2003) Surface contamination in the dental operatory: a comparison over two decades. *Journal of the American Dental Association*, **134**, 325–330.

91 Junevicius, J. *et al.* (2004) Transmission of microorganisms from dentists to dental laboratory technicians through contaminated dental impressions. *Stomatologija, Baltic Dental and Maxillofacial Journal*, **6**, 20–23.

92 Mayhall, G. (ed.) (1999) *Nosocomial Infections in Dental, Oral and Maxillofacial Surgery in Hospital Epidemiology and Infection Control*, 2nd edn, William & Wilkins, Baltimore.

93 Barbeau, J. (2000) Waterborne biofilms and dentistry: the changing face of infection control. *Journal of the Canadian Dental Association*, **66**, 539–541.

94 Harrel, S.K. (2004) Airborne spread of disease – the implications for dentistry. *Journal of the Californian Dental Association*, **32**, 901–906.

95 Szymańska, J. (2005) Endotoxin levels as a potential marker of concentration of Gram-negative bacteria in water effluent from dental units and in dental aerosols. *Annals of Agricultural and Environmental Medicine*, **12**, 229–232.

96 Danner, R.L. *et al.* (1991) Endotoxemia in human septic shock. *Chest*, **99**, 169–175.

97 Odeh, M. (1994) Endotoxin and tumor necrosis factor-a in the pathogenesis of hepatci encephalopathy. *Journal of Clinical Gastroenterology*, **19**, 146–153.

98 Graham, P. and Brass, N.J. (1994) Multiple organ dysfunction: pathophysiology and therapeutic modalities. *Critical Care Nursing Quarterly*, **16**, 8–15.

99 Herbert, A. *et al.* (1992) Reduction of alveolar-capillary diffusion after inhalation of endotoxin in normal subjects. *Chest*, **102**, 1095–1098.

100 Huntington, M.K. *et al.* (2007) Endotoxin contamination in the dental surgery. *Journal of Medical Microbiology*, **56**, 1230–1234.

101 Jasmer, R.M. *et al.* (2002) Clinical practice: latent tuberculosis infection. *New England Journal of Medicine*, **347**, 1860–1866.

102 Porteous, N.B. and Terezhalmy, G.T. (2008) Tuberculosis: infection control/exposure control issues for oral healthcare workers. *Journal of Contemporary Dental Practice*, **9**, 1–13.

103 Chambers, H.F. (2005) Community associated MRSA – resistance and virulence converge. *New England Journal of Medicine*, **352**, 1485–1487.

104 Gomes, B.P.F.A. *et al.* (2006) *Enterococcus faecalis* in dental root canals detected by culture and by polymerase chain reaction analysis. *Oral Surgery, Oral Medicine, Oral Pathology, Oral Radiology and Endodontology*, **102**, 247–253.

105 Strom, B.L. *et al.* (1998) Dental and cardiac risk factors for infective endocarditis. A population based, case-control study. *Annals of Internal Medicine*, **129**, 761–769.

106 Weber, D.J. and Rutala, W.A. (1997) Role of environmental contamination in the transmission of vancomycin-resistant enterococci. *Infection Control and Hospital Epidemioogy*, **18**, 306–309.

107 Harrel, S.K. and Molinari, J. (2004) Aerosols and splatter in dentistry: a brief review of the literature and infection control implications. *Journal of the American Dental Association*, **13**, 429–437.

108 Timmerman, M.F. *et al.* (2004) Atmospheric contamination during ultrasonic scaling. *Journal of Clinical Peridontology*, **31**, 458–462.

109 Al Maghlouth, A. *et al.* (2004) Qualitative and quantitative analysis of bacterial aerosols. *Journal of Contemporary Dental Practice*, **5**, 91–100.

110 Milejczak, C.B. (2007) Optimum travel distance of dental aerosols in the dental hygiene practice. *Journal of Dental Hygiene*, **4**, 20–21.

111 Department of Health (2008) *Pandemic Influenza: Guidance for Dental Practices*, Department of Health, London.

112 Blake, G.C. (1963) The incidence and control of bacterial infection of dental unit and ultrasonic scales. *British Dental Journal*, **15**, 413–416.

113 Franco, F.F.S. *et al.* (2005) Biofilm formation and control in dental unit waterlines. *Biofilms*, **25**, 9–17.

114 Szymańska, J. (2007) Bacterial contamination of water in dental unit reservoirs. *Annals of Agricultural and Environmental Medicine*, **14**, 137–140.

115 Rice, E.W. *et al.* (2006) The role of flushing dental water lines for the removal of microbial contaminants. *Public Health Reports*, **121**, 270–274.

116 Lux, J. (2004) Current issues in infection control practices in dental hygiene – Part II. *Canadian Journal of Dental Hygiene*, **42**, 139–152.

117 Montebugnoli, L. *et al.* (2005) Failure of anti-retraction valves and the procedure for between patient flushing: a rationale for chemical control of dental unit waterline contamination. *American Journal of Dentistry*, **18**, 270–274.

118 Sacchetti, R. *et al.* (2007) Influence of material and tube size on DUWLs contamination in a pilot plant. *New Microbiology*, **30**, 29–34.

119 Szymanska, J. (2004) Risk of exposure to *Legionella* in dental practice. *Annals of Agricultural and Environmental Medicine*, **11**, 9–12.

120 Pankhurst, C.L. *et al.* (2004) Evaluation of the potential risk of occupational asthma in dentists exposed to contaminated dental unit water lines. *Primary Dental Care*, **12**, 53–63.

121 Scannapieco, F.A. *et al.* (2004) Exposure to the dental environment and presence of a respiratory illness in dental student populations. *Journal of the Canadian Dental Association*, **70**, 170–174.

122 Bergman, B. (1989) Disinfection of prosthodontic impression materials: a literature review. *International Journal of Prosthodontics*, **2**, 537–542.

123 Porter, S.R. (1992) Control of cross-infection, in *Clinical Virology in Oral Medicine and Dentistry* (eds C. Scully and L. Samaranayake), Cambridge University Press, Cambridge., pp. 378– 423.

124 American Dental Association Council on Dental Materials, Instruments and Equipment (1988) Infection control recommendations for the dental office and the dental laboratory. *Journal of the American Dental Association*, **11**, 241–248.

125 American Dental Association Council on Dental Materials, Instruments and Equipment (1991) Disinfection of impressions. *Journal of the American Dental Association*, **122**, 110.

126 American Dental Association Council on Scientific Affairs and ADA Council on Dental Practice (1996) Infection control recommendations for the dental office and the dental laboratory. *Journal of the American Dental Association*, **127**, 672–680.

127 Medicines and Healthcare Products Regulatory Agency (MHRA) (2002) *Sterilisation, Disinfection and Cleaning of Medical Equipment: Guidance on Decontamination from the Microbiology Committee to the Department of Health Medical Devices Agency, MAC Manual, Part 1: Principles*, MHRA, London.

128 Kugel, G. *et al.* (2000) Disinfection and communication practices: a study of US dental laboratories. *Journal of the American Dental Association*, **131**, 786–792.

129 Sofou, A. *et al.* (2002) Contamination level of alginate impressions arriving at a dental laboratory. *Clinical Oral Investigations*, **6**, 161–165.

130 Verran, J. *et al.* (1997) Pumice slurry as a crossinfection hazard in nonclinical (teaching) dental technology laboratories. *International Journal of Prosthodontics*, **10**, 2836.

131 Varey, J.E. *et al.* (1996) Microbiological study of selected risk areas in dental technology laboratories. *Journal of Dentistry*, **24**, 77–80.

132 Lewis, D.L. and Boe, R.K. (1992) Cross-infection risks associated with current procedures for using high-speed dental handpieces. *Journal of Clinical Microbiology*, **30**, 401–406.

133 Medical Devices Agency (2002) *Benchtop Steam Sterilizers – Guidance on Purchase, Operation and Maintenance, MDA DB 2002(06)*, Medical Devices Agency, London.

134 Weightman, N.C. and Lines, L.D. (2004) Problems with the decontamination of dental handpieces and other intra-oral dental equipment in hospitals. *Journal of Hospital Infection*, **56**, 1–5.

135 Smith, G.W. *et al.* (2009) Survey of the decontamination and maintenance of dental handpieces in general dental practice. *British Dental Journal*, **207**, 160–161.

136 Department of Health – NHS Management Executive (1993) *HSG(93)40 – Protecting Health Care Workers and Patients from Hepatitis B*, The Stationary Office, London.

137 Department of Health (2006) *Health Technical Memorandum 07-01: Safe Management of Healthcare Waste*, The Stationery Office, London.

138 Molinari, J.A. (1999) Dental infection control at the year 2000: accomplishment recognized. *Journal of the American Dental Association*, **130**, 1291–1298.

139 Roy, K.M. *et al.* (2005) Incident control team. Patient notification exercise following a dentist's admission of the periodic use of unsterilized equipment. *Journal of Hospital Infection*, **60**, 163–168.

140 Millership, S.E. *et al.* (2007) Infection control failures in a dental surgery – dilemmas in incident management. *Journal of Public Health*, **29**, 303–307.

141 King, T.B. and Muzzin, K.B. (2005) A national survey of dental hygienists infection control attitudes and practices. *Journal of Dental Hygiene*, **79**, 8.

142 Smith, A. *et al.* (2009) Management of infection control in dental practice. *Journal of Hospital Infection*, **71**, 353–358.

143 Sofola, O.O. and Savage, K.O. (2003) Assessment of the compliance of Nigerian dentists with infection control: a preliminary study. *Infection Control and Hospital Epidemiology*, **24**, 737–740.

144 Al-Omari, M.A. and Al-Dwairi, Z.N. (2005) Compliance with infection control programs in private dental clinics in Jordan. *Journal of Dental Education*, **69**, 693–698.

145 John, J.H. *et al.* (2002) Regulating dental nursing in the UK. *British Dental Journal*, **193**, 207–209.

146 General Dental Council UK (2010) *Continuing Professional Development (CPD) for Dental Care Professionals*, GDC, London.

147 Bocci, V. (1996) Ozone as a bioregulator. Pharmacology and toxicology of ozone therapy today. *Journal of Biological Regulatory Homeostatic Agents* **10**, 31–53.

148 Nagayoshi, M. *et al.* (2004) Efficacy of ozone on survival and permeability of oral microorganisms. *Oral Microbiology and Immunology* **19**, 240–246.

149 Baysan, A. *et al.* (2000) Antimicrobial effects of a novel ozone generating device on microorganisms associated with primary root carious lesions *in-vivo*. *Caries Research* **34**, 498–501.

150 Huth, K.C. *et al.* (2006). Effect of ozone on oral cells compared with established antimicrobials. *European Journal of Oral Science* **114**, 435–440.

151 Baysan, A. and Lynch, E. (2005) The use of ozone in dentistry and medicine. *Primary Dental Care* **12**, 47–52.

152 Baysan, A. and Lynch, E. (2006) The use of ozone in dentistry and medicine. Part 2. *Primary Dental Care* **13**, 37–41.

153 Yamayoshi, T. and Tatsumi, N. (1993) Microbicidal effects of ozone solution on methicillin-resistant *Staphylococcus aureus*. *Drugs in Experimental and Clinical Research* **19**, 59–64.

154 Young, S.B. and Setlow, P. (2004) Mechanisms of *Bacillus subtilis* spore resistance to and killing by aqueous ozone. *Journal of Applied Microbiology* **96**, 1133–1142.

155 Al Shorman, H. *et al.* (2001) Use of Ozone to Treat Dental unit Water Lines. *Journal of Dental Research* **80**, 1169.

156 Dodd, M.C. *et al.* (2006) Oxidation of antibacterial molecules by aqueous ozone: moiety-specific reaction kinetics and application to ozone-based wastewater treatment. *Environmental Science and Technology* **40**, 1969–1977.

157 Dalmázio, I. *et al.* (2007) Monitoring the degradation of tetracycline by ozone in aqueous medium via atmospheric pressure ionization mass spectroscopy. *Journal of the American Society for Mass Spectrometry* **18**, 679–687.

158 Suarez, S. *et al.* (2007) Kinetics of triclosan oxidation by aqueous ozone and consequent loss of antibacterial activity: relevance to municipal wastewater ozonation. *Water Research* **41**, 2481–2490.

159 Deborde, M. *et al.* (2005) Kinetics of aqueous ozone-induced oxidation of some endocrine disruptors. *Environmental Science and Technology* **39**, 6086–6092.

160 Nogales, C.G. *et al.* (2008) Ozone Therapy in Medicine and Dentistry. *Journal of Contemporary Dental Practice* **9**, 75–84.

161 Moan, J. and Peng, Q. (2003) An Outline of the Hundred-Year History of PDT. *Anticancer Research* **23**, 3591–3600.

162 Dougherty, T.J. (1996) A Brief History of Clinical Photodynamic Therapy Development at Roswell Park Cancer Institute. *Journal of Clinical Laser Medicine and Surgery* **14**, 219–221.

163 Malik, Z. *et al.* (1990) Bactericidal effects of photoactivated porphyrins – an alternative approach to antimicrobial drugs. *Journal of Photochemistry and Photobiology B* **5**, 281–293.

164 Wainwright, M. (1998) Photodynamic antimicrobial chemotherapy (PACT). *Journal of Antimicrobial Chemotherapy* **42**, 13–28.

165 Maisch, T. (2007) Anti-microbial photodynamic therapy: useful in the future? *Lasers in Medical Science* **22**, 83–91.

166 Wilson, M. (1993) Photolysis of oral bacteria and its potential use in the treatment of caries and periodontal disease. *Journal of Applied Bacteriology* **75**, 299–306.

167 Bonsor, S.J. *et al.* (2006) Photo-activated disinfection bacteria. *British Dental Journal* **201**, 101–105.

168 Konopka, K. and Goslinski, T. (2007) Photodynamic Therapy in Dentistry. *Journal of Dental Research* **86**, 694–707.

169 Williams, J.A. *et al.* (2006) Antibacterial action of photoactivated disinfection {PAD} used on endodontic bacteria in planktonic suspension and in artificial and human root canals. *Journal of Dentistry* **34**, 363–371.

170 Williams, J.A. *et al.* (2003) The effect of variable energy input from a novel light source on the photoactivated bactericidal action of toluidine blue O on *Streptococcus mutans*. *Caries Research* **37**, 190–193.

171 Wong, T.-W. *et al.* (2005) Bactericidal Effects of Toluidine Blue-Mediated Photodynamic Action on *Vibrio vulnificus*. *Antimicrobial Agents and Chemotherapy* **49**, 895–902.

172 Zanin, I.C.J. *et al.* (2006) Photosensitization of in vitro biofilms by toluidine blue O combined with a light-emitting diode. *European Journal of Oral Science* **114**, 64–69.

173 Wilson, M. (2003) Lethal photosensitization of oral bacteria and its potential application in the photodynamic therapy of oral infections. *Photochemistry and Photobiology* **3**, 412–418.

174 Bonsor, S.J. and Pearson, G.J. (2006) Current clinical applications of photo-activated disinfection in restorative dentistry. *Dentistry Update* **33**, 143–144, 147–150, 153.

175 Garcez, A.S. (2007) Antimicrobial photodynamic therapy combined with conventional endodontic treatment to eliminate root canal biofilm infection. *Lasers in Surgery and Medicine* **39**, 59–66.

22.1 Natural Products

Rose Cooper

Centre for Biomedical Sciences, Department of Applied Sciences, Cardiff School of Health Sciences, Cardiff Metropolitan University, Cardiff, Wales, UK

Introduction

At one time all our medicines and preservatives were derived from natural products. Their use relied on anecdotal observations of efficacy, without knowledge of their respective mechanisms of action. Infections were feared and outcomes with traditional remedies were often unsuccessful. The discovery of antiseptics, followed by the discovery of antibiotics, allayed fears about most infectious diseases. Complacency was even expressed by the US Surgeon General who in 1969 considered it possible "to close the book on infectious disease" [1]. Extensive use, misuse and abuse of antibiotics resulted in the selection of antibiotic-resistant microorganisms and the emergence of strains with multiple drug resistance has compounded the problem. More recently the recognition of an association between the presence of a bacterial biofilm and persistent infection has been significant [2], especially as the susceptibility of infective agents to antimicrobial agents was found to be diminished in species living within biofilms [3]. Difficulties in treating osteomyelitis, cystic fibrosis, urinary tract infections, prostatitis, gingivitis, sinusitis and infections associated with medical implants with conventional antibiotics are examples that suitably illustrate this predicament.

Failure to discover enough new antibiotics during the last 30 years and difficulties in effectively treating biofilms have made the need to find novel antimicrobial agents urgent [1]. Advances in genome technology have made it possible to search for distinct microbial target sites [4] and re-evaluating former remedies is bringing new insight to the potential of products derived from natural products. In some of the communities in Asia and Africa up to 80% of the population rely on traditional medicine, and in developed countries increasing numbers are turning to alternative or complementary medicine [5]. There are concerns about the efficacy and safety of some of these products and tighter controls are imminent [6], yet products based on earlier remedies are beginning to reach modern medicine. The natural products with existing or projected commercial potential that are described here have been divided into three broad sections depending on their origin: bacterial, plant or animal. Most are formulated into products that are protected by patents, but some are not yet well developed in a commercial sense. Although many natural products exert multiple effects on human health, antimicrobial activity will be emphasized here. Because that activity is sometimes a function inherent to the defense system of the producer species, a short preface on host defense peptides has been included.

Host defense peptides (antimicrobial peptides)

Most organisms produce antimicrobial peptides (AMPs) as part of their innate immune defense mechanisms. Over 700 examples have been described and those that have attracted most attention

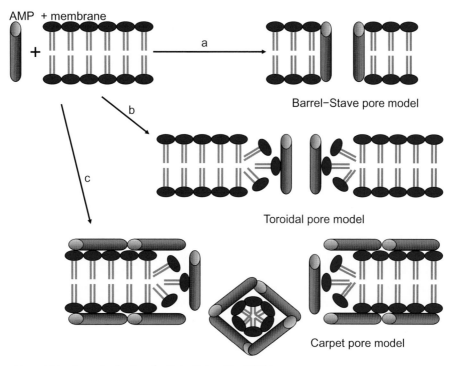

Figure 22.1.1 Different models explaining the mode of action of antimicrobial peptides (AMPs).

come from humans, fish, insects, amphibians, plants and bacteria. Typically AMPs are relatively small, cationic, amphipathic molecules comprised of less than 100 amino acids and a molecular mass below 5 kDa. AMPs represent a heterogeneous group in terms of structure and function. This diversity has given rise to the development of several schemes of classification. In one example five classes have been proposed [7]:

1. Anionic peptides requiring zinc as a cofactor (e.g. dermcidin).
2. Linear cationic α-helical peptides of less than 40 amino acids with a distinctive, looped, three-dimensional structure (e.g. cecropins, magainin, melittin).
3. Linear peptides without cysteine residues (e.g. bacteriocins, abaecin, indolicidin).
4. Charged peptides that are derived from larger peptides (e.g. lactoferricin, cathelicidins).
5. Peptides containing six cysteine moieties as three disulfide bridges and β-sheets (e.g. plant and arthropod defensins, β-defensins of birds, reptiles and mammals).

Generally AMPs display broad-spectrum activity against bacteria, fungi, protozoa and viruses [8]. The mechanism of action of AMPs is not universal, but many exert their effect on microbial species by disrupting membrane structure and function by forming pores. Several models explain how this is achieved. In the Barrel–Stave model, AMPs insert themselves vertically across a membrane with their hydrophobic regions facing membrane lipid molecules and their hydrophilic regions facing the lumen of the resulting pore (Figure 22.1.1a). In the toroidal pore model, AMPs orientate themselves in a similar way, but the phospholipid components of the membrane of the target organism curve

inwards and become an integral part of the pore (Figure 22.1.1b). In the carpet model, AMPs smother a membrane in a linear fashion and at a critical concentration act like a detergent to form micelles of part of the membrane, which then detach and leave relatively large AMP-lined channels across the membrane (Figure 22.1.1c).

In higher organisms AMPs also play a complex role in coordinating immune responses, but the mechanisms are not yet fully elucidated. Examples of AMPs selected for further discussion here are bacterial AMPs, cathelicidin (human), melittin (bee venom), bee defensin-1 or royalisin (honey and royal jelly) and magainin (frog).

Natural products of bacterial origin

Other than conventional antibiotics, the range of bacterial products currently used in controlling microorganisms is limited to AMPs and enzymes.

Bacterial antimicrobial peptides
Although bacteria do not possess an immune system in the classic sense, they do produce peptides that exhibit antimicrobial activity. The best-known bacterial AMPs are bacteriocins and lantibiotics.

Bacteriocins
Bacteriocins belong to a diverse group of proteins that are produced by bacteria to inhibit closely-related bacteria. Their range

of activity is generally narrower than that of conventional antibiotics and the genes that encode bacteriocins are normally located on a plasmid or transposon. The names of bacteriocins often reflect the organism that produced them, for example colicin from *Escherichia coli*. Bacteriocins can be divided into two groups depending on whether they are produced by Gram-positive or Gram-negative bacteria, with the bacteriocins of Gram-positive bacteria further subdivided into four subgroups. They contain a wide range of proteins with modes of action that vary from membrane permeabilization to the interruption of protein synthesis or the degradation of DNA.

Many of the commensals that naturally colonize humans produce bacteriocins. The role of these organisms in preventing invasion by opportunist pathogens became evident when they were eradicated following the long-term administration of systemic antibiotics. By inference, the role of bacteriocins in colonization resistance has been deduced and their therapeutic use as probiotic and bioprotective agents has been recognized [9]. Bacteriocins of lactic acid bacteria and of *E. coli* have attracted most research to date. Their potential in rearing animals and fish without infection and in preventing human enteric, oral, respiratory or vaginal infection is as yet unrealized.

Lantibiotics

The lantibiotics are another type of bacteriocin. Lantibiotics are unusual peptides synthesized by Gram-positive bacteria that inhibit Gram-positive bacteria. They are composed of between 19 and 38 amino acids and contain a thioether amino acid which is either lanthionine or 3-methyl lanthionine. Their name is derived from the term "*lanthionine-containing antibiotics*". The first one was described in 1928 [10] and more than 50 have since been discovered. It has been suggested that they are formed as part of the stress response during the late exponential or early stationary phase of growth.

The precursor peptides of lantibiotics are biosynthesized on ribosomes and then modified by dehydration of either serine or threonine residues, followed by intramolecular addition of cysteine with cyclization to form either lanthionine or methyllanthioine bridges, respectively. Removal of a leader sequence is necessary for biological functionality to be realized.

Lantibiotics can be categorized into three classes, based on post-translational mechanisms and their diverse biological functions [11, 12]. The best-known lantibiotic is nisin, which has been used as a food preservative for more than 40 years. Despite the extensive use of this safe additive, there is little evidence of nisin resistance. Nisin is synthesized by *Lactobacillus lactis* and added to processed cheeses, liquid egg, cold meats and some drinks as a preservative. It exhibits broad-spectrum activity against Gram-positive bacteria other than lactobacilli at low concentrations and it inhibits Gram-negative bacilli in the presence of chelating agents. The antibacterial properties of lantibiotics offer potential for treating lung infections in patients with cystic fibrosis, as well as for oral use in curing halitosis or preventing dental caries. Their ability to affect virulence or to act as biosurfactants has yet to be exploited [12].

Many lantibiotics are bactericidal against Gram-positive bacteria either by inducing pore formation in target cell membranes, or by inhibiting peptidoglycan biosynthesis. Both mechanisms of inhibition involve binding of the lantibiotic to lipid II within the bacterial cytoplasmic membrane of the target species [13, 14]. Reduced efficacy against Gram-negative bacteria may be due to restricted movement of lantibiotics across the outer membrane.

Enzymes

The opportunities that peptidoglycan provides as a target site for novel inhibitors have not escaped attention [15]. Enzymes capable of hydrolyzing peptidoglycan are lysozyme, autolysins and virolysins, which are synthesized by eukaryotes, bacteria and bacteriophages, respectively. Although no commercial products containing bacterial cell wall hydrolases have yet been developed, the potential to inhibit bacteria is apparent.

Enzymes have potential in controlling wound infections. A combination of glucose oxidase and lactoperoxidase was bactericidal for planktonic cells of *Staphylococcus aureus*, *Staphylococcus epidermidis*, *Pseudomonas aeruginosa* and *Pseudomonas fluorescens* and model biofilms prepared on steel and polypropylene disks, but biofilm was only removed when polysaccharide-hydrolyzing enzymes were added to the mixture [16]. A similar approach has been employed in the development of two novel wound dressings. In one product, glucose oxidase and lactoperoxidase have been incorporated into an alginate hydrogel [17]. In the other, a hydrogel sheet containing glucose is placed in contact with a hydrogel sheet containing glucose oxidase in the wound [18]. Glucose oxidation releases low levels of hydrogen peroxide that inhibits bacteria. Additionally, low levels of iodine are generated in the sheet dressing by a further reaction [18].

Natural products of plant origin

From ancient civilizations to the present, plant products have played an important role in medicine. Plants produce a wide range of secondary metabolites which are used for protection against invasion by microbes, insects and herbivores. They also confer colors, odors and flavors to plants. Various parts of the plant have been utilized for medicinal purposes, including flowers, fruits, seeds, stems, leaves, roots, bark and wood; bioactive materials may be found in several locations in some plants. Most often dried plant material was extracted with hot water, but occasionally alcoholic extracts or tinctures were used. Variation in the quality of plant preparations is common and there is a need to standardize extraction methods and laboratory evaluations because published studies often provide conflicting observations [19].

A large number of antimicrobial components have been isolated from plants, and their chemistry is complex. They were divided into the several major groups by Cowan in 1999 [19] and additional subclasses include polyketides, polyamines, isothiocyanates, sulfides, thiosulfinates, glycosides, phenanthrenes and stilbenes [20]. Selected examples are given in Table 22.1.1.

Table 22.1.1 The major groups of plant compounds with antimicrobial activity (adapted from [19]).

Group	Subgroup	Examples	Plant sources
Phenolic compounds	Phenols	*Catechol[a]	Many fruits and vegetables, e.g. banana
	Phenolic acids	Caffeic acid	Coffee
		Caffeic acid phenethyl ester (CAPE)	Propolis
	Quinones	Hypericin	St. John's wort
	Flavonoids[a]	Catechins	Green tea
		Pinocembrin	Proplis
	Flavones	Chrysin	Propolis, honey, passion flower
	Flavonols[a]	Myricetin	Grapes, red berries, walnuts
		Quercetin	Propolis, tea, onions, honey, cranberries, red grapes
	Tannins[a]	Proanthrocyanidins	Red wine, pomegranates, strawberries, cranberries, nuts
	Coumarins	Benzopyrone	Lavender, strawberries, licorice, cinnamon
Terpenoids and essential oils	Monoterpenoids	Terpinen-4-ol	Tea tree oil
	Sesquiterpenoids	Artemisinin	*Artemisia annua*
Alkaloids		Quinine	Bark of the *Cinchona* tree
Lectins and polypeptides		Concanavelin A	Jack bean
		Fabatin	Broad beans
Polyacetylenes		Falcarinol, falcarindiol	Carrots, celery, fennel, parsley, parsnip
Sulphur compounds	Sulfides	Allicin	Garlic
	Thiosulfides	Ajoene, allyl alcohol, diallyl disulfide, diallyl trisulfide	Garlic

[a] Widely distributed in plants.

Production of these substances may be a response to environmental triggers, such as stress or potential invasion/attack. Plant defense chemicals can also be divided into phytoanticipins and phytoalexins on the basis of the timing of their production. The former are synthesized constitutively in an inactive form, for example glycosides, and the latter are inducible.

Of the diverse array of phytochemicals, flavonoids (also known as polyphenols) have significant medicinal potential and have attracted extensive scientific investigations. They are pigments synthesized from phenylalanine, which are ubiquitously distributed in plants, honey and propolis [19, 21]. The mechanism of antimicrobial activity of some of the flavonoids has been reviewed [22], but their ability to also inhibit specific eukaryotic enzymes, mimic hormone action and to scavenge free radicals supports their use in the treatment of some human diseases not caused by infective agents [23]. Mechanisms by which bacteria are inhibited by flavonoids include inhibition of nucleic acid synthesis, inhibition of cytoplasmic membrane function and inhibition of energy metabolism [22]. In general, phytochemicals are less potent than antibiotics in inhibiting microorganisms. However, human cytotoxicity is normally relatively low and the possibility of structural modification of bioactive components offers the promise of discovering or designing more effective agents [22]. Garlic, green tea and an essential oil, tea tree oil, are examples of natural products derived from plants that are included here.

Garlic

Garlic (*Allium sativum*) is a bulbous, perennial plant of the family Liliaceae that is indigenous to Central Asia. Its underground bulb consists of 10–12 cloves which are each bound by a parchment-like skin. The bulb has been used in the human diet as a vegetable and condiment since ancient times and it has been cultivated for at least 4500 years. Much has been written about the medical use of garlic [24]. It was valued by each of the ancient Egyptian, Chinese, Hebrew, Greek, Indian, Japanese and Roman civilizations and garlic bulbs were included in Tutankhamen's tomb in 1352 BC. During the Middle Ages garlic was eaten to protect against bubonic plague and during World Wars I and II it was used to treat infections sustained by soldiers. Garlic has been used therapeutically for a wide range of conditions, but only its anti-infective use will be included here.

Garlic is now cultivated in many countries, but the largest producers are China, India, Pakistan and Bangladesh. Many forms of garlic are available commercially: fresh, frozen, pickled and dehydrated. For experimentation, fresh aqueous extracts, freeze-dried extracts and oil obtained by steam distillation of garlic have been mainly utilized.

Allium produces cysteine sulfoxides, which confer its characteristic odor. Its antimicrobial properties are related to its complex sulfur compounds, which depend on species, growth conditions and extraction methods. The principal antimicrobial component of garlic was identified as allicin (allyl-2-propene thiosulfinate), which is not detectable in intact bulbs but is rapidly produced from a microbiologically inactive precursor alliin by alliinase on crushing the bulb [25]. The enzyme and precursor are separated within the intact bulb as alliinase is contained within vacuoles. Allicin is highly unstable and decomposition leads to the formation of ajoene, allyl alcohol, diallyl disulfide (DADS) and diallyl

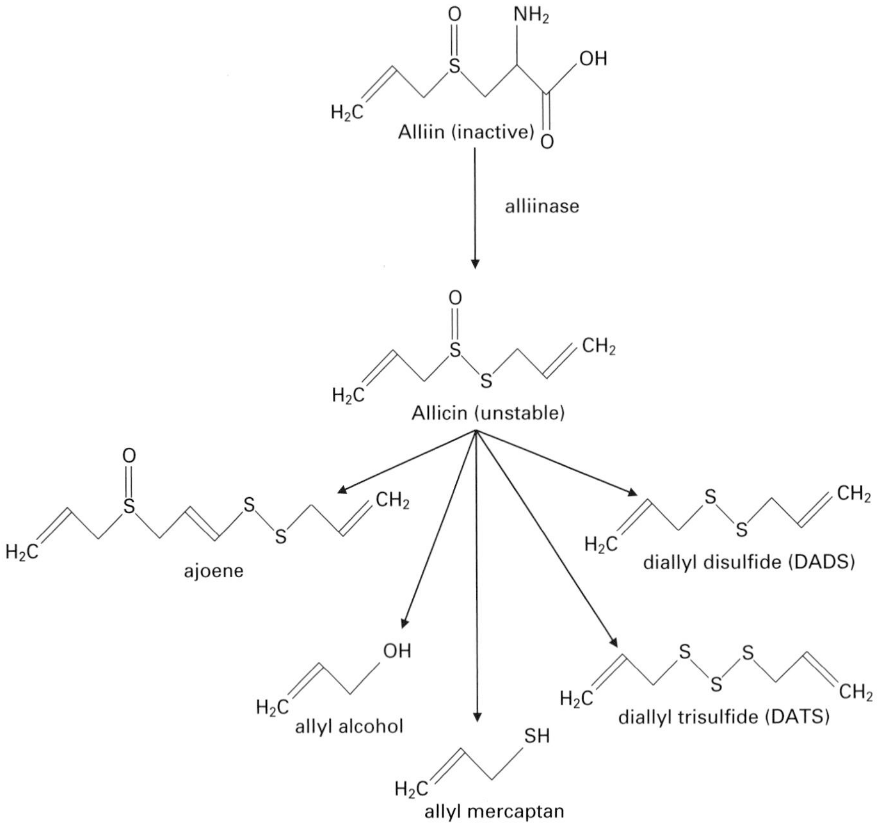

Figure 22.1.2 Components with antibacterial activity that are derived from garlic. Courtesy of Ana Filipa Henriques.

trisulfide (DATS) (Figure 22.1.2). The latter two are also potent antimicrobial agents. Two important metabolites of garlic are allyl alcohol and allyl mercaptan. Additional antiprotozoal components found in garlic are kaempferol and quercetin, which are polyphenols.

Garlic exhibits antibacterial, antifungal, antiprotozoal and antiviral effects. Much of the research into the antibacterial properties of garlic extracts concerns the inhibition of foodborne spoilage and pathogenic bacteria, such as *S. aureus, Salmonella* spp., *E. coli, Listeria monocytogenes* and *Helicobacter pylori* [26, 27]. Garlic oil also inhibits many enteric bacteria [28] and oral bacteria [29]. Aqueous allicin extract and a novel gel formulation were shown to be bactericidal for Lancefield group B streptococci, and a role in treating and preventing vaginal and neonatal infections during the perinatal period has been suggested [30].

One of the breakdown products of allicin, DATS, has been synthesized in China. Following *in vitro* inhibition of *Trypanosoma* spp., *Entamoeba histolytica* and *Giardia lamblia* by this synthetic product, its potential in treating several important human parasitic infections was described [31]. Further breakdown products of garlic extract, especially allyl alcohol and allyl mercaptan, were shown to be effective in inhibiting *Giardia intestinalis* [32]. In this study extensive morphological changes were observed in trophozoites, but the effects of whole garlic extract and allyl alcohol differed to those induced by allyl mercaptan. Cysteine

proteinases are important virulence factors of *E. histolytica* and have been found to be strongly inhibited by allicin, and the ability of the protozoan to destroy monolayers of baby hamster kidney cells was also inhibited by allicin [33].

Garlic also inhibits a range of fungi including dermatophytes and cryptococci. Most antifungal studies concern the effects of garlic on *Candida albicans* and different breakdown products of garlic induce different intracellular effects. Growth inhibition studies and structural changes observed by electron microscopy showed that fresh garlic was more effective than garlic powder extract in inhibiting *C. albicans* [34], whereas allyl alcohol and fresh garlic extract induced oxidative stress [35].

The antimicrobial effects of garlic are largely due to its reaction with thiol groups in enzymes such as alcohol dehydogenase, thioredoxin reductase and RNA polymerase [36]. Proteomic analysis of a commercial garlic preparation produced in China demonstrated that it caused the expression of 21 proteins to be altered in *H. pylori*. Multiple effects in energy metabolism and processes involved in the biosynthesis of amino acids, proteins, mRNA and fatty acids were indicated [27]. Whole garlic extract and allyl alcohol removed the transmembrane electrochemical potential of *Giardia* membranes [32]. Permeability of allicin through cytoplasmic membranes allows relatively easy access to intracellular compartments and has been linked to its biological activity [37]. In *C. albicans*, compounds derived from garlic caused several events that triggered cell death by apoptosis [34]. In particular, allyl alcohol targeted alcohol dehydrogenases, two of which were in the cytosol and one in the mitochondria [35], and DADS induced thiol depletion and oxidative stress that led to impaired mitochondrial function [38].

Cell-to-cell communication or quorum sensing in bacteria influences the expression of some of the genes that contribute to virulence and biofilm formation. The development of assays to detect for compounds that interfere with quorum sensing [39, 40] has allowed a wide range of natural products to be screened. Garlic has been demonstrated to inhibit quorum sensing in *P. aeruginosa* [41, 42] and its potential in treating lung infections in cystic fibrosis patients has been recognized. Susceptibility for tobramycin and polymorphonuclear leukocytes grazing on *P. aeruginosa* biofilms exposed to garlic extract have been demonstrated to increase *in vitro*, as well as improved clearance of *P. aeruginosa* from pulmonary infections in mice [41]. Using microarray-based transcriptome analysis this garlic extract was shown to repress the expression of 167 genes, of which 92 were quorum-sensing-regulated genes in *P. aeruginosa* [40].

Green tea

Tea is produced from the leaves of *Camellia sinensis*, which is predominantly grown in China, India, Sri Lanka, Indonesia and Malaysia. Green tea is produced by steaming fresh leaves, unlike black tea which involves an oxidation stage. It has a complex chemistry and contains polyphenols, especially flavonoids such as catechins, catechin gallates and proanthocyanides. The bioactive components of green tea are largely associated with the catechins such as epicatechin (EC), epicatechin gallate (ECG), epigallocatechin (EGC) and epigallocatechin gallate (EGCG).

The antimicrobial properties of tea against a broad range of microorganisms are well documented, with Gram-positive bacteria demonstrating greater susceptible than Gram-negatives [43]. EGCG in sub minimum inhibitory concentrations (MICs) inhibited slime production and biofilm formation in 20 cultures of staphylococci isolated from patients with eye infections [44]. Much of the recent research has focused on the effects of green tea components on *S. aureus* and methicillin-resistant *S. aureus* (MRSA). Virulence of *S. aureus* was reduced by ECG due to interference in the secretion of coagulase and α-toxin [45], and cell division in MRSA (but not in *S. aureus*) was disorganized with selective inhibition of penicillin-binding proteins by a component of tea [46].

A component isolated from a crude extract of green tea polyphenols called compound P was found to reverse methicillin resistance in *S. aureus* [47]. It also prevented the synthesis of penicillin-binding protein 2′ and β-lactamase [47] and caused cell division in MRSA to be disorganized, with the formation of large clumps of unseparated cells possessing thickened internal cross walls but normal external cell walls [46]. Synergy between EGCG and β-lactams provided confirmation of peptidoglycan as a common target site [48] and the altered cell wall architecture in *S. aureus* has been confirmed to be due to ECG [49]. MRSA grown in the presence of ECG had reduced resistance to oxacillin, thickened cell walls, disrupted cell division and reduced D-alanyl esterification of teichoic acid. Since teichoic acids influence the phase transition profile of phospholipids bilayers, it is possible that this may impact on the function of enzymes within the bacterial cell wall and membrane [50].

A tea polyphenol extract containing five catechins at sub-MIC levels was also found to reverse oxacillin resistance in 13 clinical strains of MRSA. Proteomic investigation of extracellular proteins recovered from cultures of MRSA exposed to this extract showed differential expression of 17 proteins. Three were upregulated and 14 were downregulated [51]. A similar study with *E. coli* found that 17 proteins were altered by green tea polyphenols, nine upregulated proteins were involved in cell defense mechanisms and eight downregulated proteins were involved in carbon and energy metabolism and the biosynthesis of amino acids [52]. Green tea, therefore, has multiple cellular effects on bacteria.

Essential oils

Essential oils have long been used in food, cosmetics and therapeutic preparations because of their antimicrobial properties. Anti-inflammatory, sedative, analgesic and antioxidant properties extend their therapeutic potential to treating and preventing tumors and cardiovascular disease [53]. Essential oils, also known as volatile or ethereal oils, are extracted from aromatic plants by various methods, including expression, fermentation or distillation. They are complex mixtures of up to 60 components, but mainly terpenes and terpenoids, with aromatic constituents such as aldehydes, alcohols and phenols present in minor proportions [54]. Essential oils are produced from many different species and almost 3000 have been described, of which only 10% are commercially important. Reviews of the chemistry and antimicrobial, therapeutic and preservative properties are available [53–55]. Because essential oils usually contain multiple components, it has been difficult to attribute specific cellular effects to individual components, but their hydrophobicity is thought to facilitate membrane permeabilization.

Undesirable effects, such as mammalian cytotoxicity, photosensitization, irritation, mutagenicity and carcinogenicity, have been associated with a small number of essential oils [54]. The use of essential oils in foods, cosmetics and medicines is therefore regulated in many countries. Perhaps the largest amount of information available concerning the antimicrobial effects of an essential oil relates to tea tree oil.

Tea tree (*Melaleuca alternifolia*) oil

Melaleuca alternifolia or tea tree is a small tree indigenous to Australia. The native Aborigines are thought to have understood the curative properties of *M. alternifolia* because they included its leaves in poultices and they used the water in which leaves had rotted for various remedies. Knowledge of the therapeutic properties of tree tea only spread further afield after Australia was colonized by Europeans [56]. Tea tree oil (TTO) is a light-yellow-colored oil with a distinctive smell; it is extracted from the leaves and small branches of tea tree by steam distillation. The commercial preparation of an essential oil from tea tree began in 1920 and antimicrobial properties of TTO were discovered then [56]. The TTO industry has seen fluctuations in demand. TTO is currently incorporated into many cosmetic and hygienic products that are available throughout the world. Remedies for acne, vaginal infections and tinea pedis are also produced, and its use in wound care products has been suggested [57].

Insolubility of TTO in bacteriological media has limited investigations of antimicrobial activity. Variations in chemical composition due to differing tree strains and extraction conditions have also introduced inconsistencies between laboratory studies. TTO has a complex chemistry with up to 97 components identified by chromatographic analysis. Terpinen-4-ol is one of the main antimicrobial components; others include α-terpineol and α-pinene [58]. Another constituent of TTO is 1,8-cineole, which is an irritant. Animal studies have demonstrated cytotoxicity of TTO so its use is limited to topical application rather than systemic use [59].

A diverse spectrum of activity against MRSA [60], staphylococci and propionibacteria [58], pseudomonads [61] and yeasts has been reported for TTO [62, 63]. Whereas planktonic MRSA and methicillin-sensitive *S. aureus* (MSSA) were less susceptible to TTO, as determined by MIC, than coagulase-negative staphylococci, the reverse was found with biofilms [64]. A comparison of the efficacy of TTO and mupirocin for eradicating MRSA *in vivo* showed no statistically significant difference between the two agents [65]. Since mupirocin may select for mupirocin-resistant strains and TTO has not yet selected for TTO-resistant strains, its potential for clinical use is apparent. Yet uptake of TTO for the eradication of MRSA-colonized patients has been slow and concerns of toxicity and allergenicity may be a limiting factor [59].

In bacteria and yeasts, exposure to TTO inhibited respiration and increased the permeability of cytoplasmic and plasma membranes respectively. Leakage of potassium ions from *E. coli* and *S. aureus* was also found [66]. A combination of time-kill, lysis, leakage and salt-tolerance assays combined with electron microscopy suggest that TTO and its components inhibit *S. aureus* by compromising the cytoplasmic membrane [67].

Natural products of animal origin

Ancient peoples certainly utilized animal products, such as bile, blood, butter, cobweb, cochineal, egg white, feces, lard, meat and milk, in their primitive wound remedies [68]. None of these products would be used today, although beaten egg white was applied to leg ulcers by British nurses up until the 1970s. Two ancient wound remedies are enjoying a renaissance today: honey and maggots.

Hive products
From the earliest times bees have been important to mankind because their colonies have yielded valuable products that have been collected and used as food or medicines. Those of medicinal

importance today include honey, propolis, royal jelly and bee venom. Many therapeutic claims have been made for these products, but only their antimicrobial properties will be included here. The composition of all of these products is influenced by their botanical origin, geographical location, climate, species of bee, harvesting processes and storage conditions. Variations between each of the hive specimens tested and the differing methods employed, makes evaluating available data difficult.

Honey
From fragments of a Sumerian clay tablet it is clear that honey was used in ointments applied to wounds in 2600 BC. It featured prominently in the remedies of the ancient Egyptians, Greeks and to a lesser extent Romans [69]. Hippocrates recommended pale honeys for treating leg ulcers and Plato included honey in a diet aimed to promote good health [70].

Honey is produced by bees from either the nectar of blossoms or exudates released from plants following insect damage. These fluids are carried to the hive or nest in bees' water sacs and mixed with enzymes from the hypopharyngeal gland when deposited there. Ripened honey is a supersaturated solution of four principal sugars (fructose, glucose, maltose, sucrose) with low concentrations of oligosaccharides, organic acids, proteins and minerals. Water molecules usually account for approximately 20% by weight of honey and pH ranges between 3.2 and 4.5. These properties ensure that honey rarely spoils on storage, although it may contain bacterial spores [71].

The antibacterial characteristics of honey are not confined to its sugar content. Many raw or unprocessed honeys demonstrate increased antibacterial activity on dilution by the generation of hydrogen peroxide from the oxidation of glucose, following the activation of glucose oxidase, which is an enzyme introduced into honey from bees [72, 73]. Excessive heating during harvesting or storage of honey inactivates enzymes that were derived from bees. A small group of honeys are known as non-peroxide honeys because they possess antibacterial activity additional to hydrogen peroxide. In manuka honey this has been attributed to methylglyoxal [74, 75]. Using a honey produced under standardized conditions by bees contained in greenhouses and a series of neutralizations to remove successive antibacterial components, it was shown that sugar, hydrogen peroxide, methylglyoxal and an AMP identified as bee defensin-1 all contributed to the antibacterial activity of honey [76].

The broad-spectrum antimicrobial nature of honey is well documented [69, 77]. More than 60 bacterial species have been shown to be inhibited by honey; additionally fungi [78, 79], protozoa [80] and viruses [81] are also susceptible to honey. Many early studies employed poorly characterized honeys and poorly described methods, so inconsistent observations have been reported. Since honey is not a uniform product, the floral origin and potency of a sample should be determined before any experimental evaluations are attempted. Chemical markers of floral origin have been established by chromatography [82] and a bioassay for assessing the antibacterial efficacy of honey was developed in New Zealand [83]. It may be used to distinguish between hydrogen peroxide-generating honeys, inactive honeys and non-peroxide honeys. It seems logical that honeys intended for medical use should possess significant levels of antibacterial activity, as honeys intended for the table do not necessarily possess such activity [84]. Criteria for honeys destined for medical use have been formulated [85].

Honey was used topically as a remedy for wounds by diverse ancient civilizations but lost favor in western medicine during the 1970s [86]. The licensing of tubes of sterile *Leptospermum* honey as a complementary therapy by the Therapeutic Goods Administration in Australia in 1999 marked the beginning of the reintroduction of honey into contemporary medicine. CE marked (certified for European conformity) wound dressings were approved for use in the UK in 2004, and in Canada and the United States honey-impregnated dressings were approved in 2008 by Health Canada and the Food and Drug Administration (FDA), respectively. A range of wound care products containing various honeys are now available in Australasia, Europe and North America. They are used on burns, diabetic foot ulcers, leg ulcers, pressure sores, surgical incision sites and trauma wounds. Honey has been used not only to prevent infections, [87] eradicate colonization of MRSA [88–92] and clear infections, but to promote wound healing. Much clinical evidence has been published and evaluated by systematic review within the past 10 years [93–98].

Using a sugar syrup made from the four main sugars contained within honey and manuka honey produced in New Zealand, it was demonstrated that inhibition of bacteria isolated from wounds was not due exclusively to the sugars contained in the honey [99–101]. Antibiotic-sensitive strains and their respective antibiotic-resistant strains were equally susceptible [99–101]. The mode of inhibition was shown to be bactericidal [100, 102, 103]. Transcriptome analysis was used to investigate the effects of *Leptospermum* honey on *E. coli* and multiple cellular effects were noted. Of the 2% of genes that were upregulated, many involved the stress response; the majority of downregulated genes encoded for products involved in protein synthesis [104]. Proteomic analysis of MRSA exposed to manuka honey showed multiple changes in protein expression, and universal stress protein A (which is involved in the stamina response) was found to be downregulated [105]. Structural changes in *S. aureus* and MRSA induced by manuka honey suggest that inhibition was caused by failure of cells to complete the cell cycle because of an inability to separate during cell division [103, 106] (Figure 22.1.3). However, loss of structural integrity, with marked cell surface changes, were observed in *P. aeruginosa* exposed to manuka honey [107].

Much of the research concerning the inhibition of wound pathogens by honey has been conducted with planktonic cells. A link between chronic wounds and biofilms has recently been established [108] so the effect of honey on biofilms is pertinent to wound care. Honey has been shown to prevent biofilm formation [109]; it can also disrupt established biofilms, but the concentration and contact time is critical [110, 111]. *P. aeruginosa* is an opportunist pathogen in wounds that is difficult to treat. The

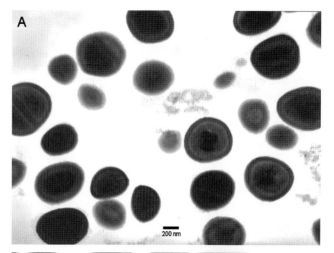

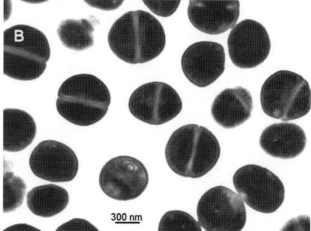

Figure 22.1.3 The effect of manuka honey on cell division in *Staphylococcus aureus*. (A) Exponential cells incubated in 0.05 mM Tris buffer pH 7.2 for 4 h at 37°C. (B) Exponential cells incubated in 0.05 mM Tris buffer pH 7.2 containing 10% (w/v) manuka honey for 4 h at 37°C.

initiation of an infection and biofilm development both rely on adherence to host cells. Fructose contained in honey and royal jelly has been shown to block this event by interference with bacterial attachment to fuctose receptors on the host cell membranes [112].

The antibacterial effects of honey are not confined to direct inhibitory effects on bacteria, but seem to be augmented by immunomodulatory effects on cells involved in the phagocytic response. Stimulation of inflammatory cytokine release in the presence of honey [113, 114] and modulation of the oxidative burst as determined by the level of reactive oxygen species suggest that honey has multiple means of influencing the infection process [113, 115].

Propolis

The term for propolis is thought to have been invented by Aristotle from two Greek words *pro* (before) and *polis* (city), to mean "before the city" or "defender of the city (or colony)". Propolis, or bee glue as it is also known, is used by bees as a building material to seal holes and cracks in the hive. It is also used as a means to reduce microbial contamination within the hive. Propolis is made from resinous materials that are collected by bees from local plants and mixed with wax, but other sticky substances present within that environment can also be included on occasions. Hence the chemical composition of propolis may be variable, standardization of samples is necessary and the importance of using chemically characterized propolis samples in biological research has been emphasized [116]. Extrapolation of experimental data from older studies is therefore not always wise.

Propolis has many interesting pharmacological characteristics and is used extensively in apitherapy globally, but particularly in Asia, eastern Europe and South America. Aside from its immunomodulatory properties, it is mainly used to treat skin, respiratory and intestinal infections. It has also been used in food preservation and in cosmetic preparations, particularly for oral hygiene. For human use propolis is harvested from bee hives by scraping the internal surfaces to obtain the hard, resinous material. Biologically-active components are extracted by several techniques which can influence chemical composition [117]. Ethanolic extracts of propolis are most frequently tested *in vitro*.

The antimicrobial properties of propolis are well reported with many inferences that flavonoids are implicated in microbial inhibition [118]. Brazilian propolis is active against poliovirus [119]. However, there seem to be other inhibitory component(s) as well. For example, antibacterial, antifungal and antiviral activities of propolis samples originating from differing geographical areas were investigated using *S. aureus* and *E. coli*, *Candida albicans* and avian influenza virus, respectively. Despite differing chemical composition, all samples were active against Gram-positive bacteria and yeast, and most exhibited antiviral activity. Activity was attributed to flavonoids and esters of phenolic acids in samples collected from temperate regions, but they were not present in samples from tropical zones [120]. The inhibition of 15 strains of MRSA by a propolis sample from the Solomon Islands has been demonstrated and activity was attributed to four prenylflavones fractionated from the sample [121]. Similarly, inhibition of *S. aureus* by two phenolic components derived from Kenyan propolis has been demonstrated [122].

The effects of propolis and selected constituent flavonoids were tested on several bacteria and found to uncouple energy transduction and to inhibit motility [123]. In staphylococci propolis has been found to modulate virulence determinants such as lipase and coagulase [124]. The growth of trophozoites of *Giardia duodenalis* was inhibited by propolis, cell shape was changed, flagellar movement was reduced, attachment was impaired and trophozoites detached [125]. Such changes would be expected to impair the binding of trophozoites to host target cell membranes.

Royal jelly

Royal jelly is secreted from the hypopharyngeal glands and mandibular glands of young worker bees that have been fed with honey and pollen. It is an acidic, milky white fluid. Limited amounts are fed to all bee larvae by these "nurse" bees and the few larvae selected to become queens are flooded with royal jelly in specialized honeycomb compartments. Royal jelly is comprised of water (60–70%), proteins (12–15%), carbohydrates (10–12%), lipids (3–7%) and trace amounts of minerals and vitamins [126]. Royal jelly has most often been used as a dietary supplement or additive to cosmetics products because of the immunomodulatory properties associated with its major proteins, even though antimicrobial activity has been demonstrated in some of its proteins. Inhibition of Gram-negative bacteria by royal jelly was first described in 1938 [127]. The first antimicrobial component identified in royal jelly of the European honeybee (*Apis mellifera*) was a fatty acid [128]. In 1990, a bee AMP (which has been named royalisin and defensin-1) with activity against Gram-positive bacteria at low concentration was isolated and characterized [129]. Several bee antimicrobial peptides have been found in royal jelly [130–132] and a family known as the jelleines has also been studied [133]. Royal jelly is a perishable product with a short shelf-life. Storage at low temperature, freezing, freeze-drying or mixing with honey is needed to preserve its activity. Additive activity between royal jelly and honey and synergistic activity between royal jelly and starch [134, 135] have been demonstrated and an ointment for treating diabetic foot ulcers has been tested in a prospective pilot study [136].

Bee venom

There is extensive anecdotal evidence derived from traditional medicine concerning the benefits of bee venom for the relief of symptoms of chronic diseases linked to immune dysfunction, such as rheumatoid arthritis and muscular dystrophy. However, there is considerably less information available on its antimicrobial activity. Bee venom is a colorless liquid comprised of a complex mixture of proteins. It can be collected from the sting apparatus of bees, or used directly on patients. Clinical use must be strictly avoided in patients with bee venom allergy.

The principal active component is melittin, which is a 26-residue cationic AMP with significant lytic activity against both eukaryotic and prokaryotic cells [137]. Phospholipase A2 also exhibits antimicrobial effects by altering phospholipids associated with membranes [138]. Melittin binds to membrane lipids and causes perturbations that disrupt membrane integrity which result in cell lysis. Binding of the peptide to lipids in a carpet-like fashion as a detergent has been demonstrated [139]. Since bacteriolytic and cytolytic effects have been demonstrated, the hemolytic effects of melittin limit its therapeutic potential. Analogs of melittin that retain antimicrobial activity without mammalian cytotoxicity have been sought. A broad-spectrum antimicrobial peptide called melimine has been synthesized from a portion of the melittin molecule and protamine. This novel cationic peptide possessed reduced hemolytic activity and when covalently linked to contact lenses retained antibacterial activity [140]. It therefore has potential in preventing infections associated with implanted medical devices.

Antimicrobial peptides of animal origin

Much has been written about the therapeutic potential of AMPs of animal origin, yet few promises have yet been achieved.

Human defense peptides

Human AMPs can be considered as three types: defensins, cathelicidins and histatins. Essentially, defensins usually contain six cysteine residues within three disulfide bridges. Cathelicidins contain catelin at the N-terminal domain and a cationic antimicrobial component that is activated by post-translational cleavage at the C-terminal domain. Histatins contain a high content of histidine residues and are mainly antifungal agents. One human AMP of special interest is LL-37. It is a cathelicidin that is predominantly found in the secretory granules of neutrophils, keratinocytes and mucosal membranes.

Magainins

Magainins are cationic AMPs that were isolated from glands in the skin of the African clawed frog (*Xenopus laevis*). They are amphipathic peptides with an α-linear structure. Initially two magainins were isolated, but many more have since been found in *Xenopus* and other amphibians. Magainins exhibit broad-spectrum activity against Gram-positive and Gram-negative bacteria, fungi and viruses by disrupting membrane permeability. An analog, pexiganan, was produced and antibacterial activity was evaluated *in vitro*. Bactericidal action was demonstrated against more than 3000 clinical isolates, and MIC$_{90}$ was 32 μg/ml. Time-kill curves showed rapid inhibition of *P. aeruginosa* (10^6 organisms eliminated in 20 min) and resistance training failed to recover pexiganan-resistant mutants [141]. Despite the impressive *in vitro* activity of this AMP, it did not perform well *in vivo*. In a randomized, controlled, double-blinded trial, pexiganan actetate cream was compared to systemic ofloxacin in treating mildly infected diabetic foot ulcers, but significant differences between the interventions were not found, except that pexiganan-resistant strains did not emerge and ofloxacin-resistant strains did [142]. Despite efficacy in laboratory tests, *in vivo* efficacy has not been remarkable and the levels of pexignan that are required are close to cytotoxic levels. Failure to secure FDA approval will undoubtedly limit clinical use of pexiganan.

Lactoferrin

Lactoferrin is a glycoprotein that is intimately involved in human innate immune defense mechanisms. It is secreted in milk, tears, saliva and mucus, and it is also found in the secondary granules of polymorphonuclear leukocytes. Lactoferrin is a globular protein of 80 kDa that belongs to the transferrin family. Since the lactoferrin gene has been sequenced, recombinant lactoferrin has become available as a therapeutic agent. Of the many different uses that have been suggested, inclusion in infant milk formula and the treatment of cystic fibrosis are prominent. Recently the granting of orphan drug status to lactoferrin as Meveol®

in Europe and America is intended to encourage further investigation.

Lactoferrin displays multiple biological functions; its antimicrobial properties are largely due to its iron-binding capacity. Microbial growth is influenced by the availability of iron, which is an essential nutrient. Lactoferrin is able to simultaneously and reversibly bind two cations (usually Fe^{3+} ions) and two anions (usually carbonate or bicarbonate). By tightly binding iron at the surface of mucosal membranes, lactoferrin restricts the quantity available for bacteria and exerts a bacteriostatic effect. Iron limitation affects the ability of bacteria, fungi and viruses to establish an infection because aggregation and adherence to host cells is compromised. In enteropathogenic *E. coli*, for example, lactoferrin has been shown to impair the function of the type III secretory system [143].

Lactoferrin destabilizes the outer membrane of Gram-negative bacteria due to the release of lipopolysaccharide when lactoferrin binds to lipid A [144]. Furthermore, proteolytic cleavage of lactoferrin within the host releases a peptide with antimicrobial activity, lactoferricin. The release of lactoferrin from lysosomal secretory granules into phagosomes contributes to bacterial killing.

Iron limitation by lactoferrin has also been shown to prevent biofilm formation [145]. Adoption of a treatment strategy designed to eradicate biofilms from chronic wounds coupled sharp debridement with topical application of a mixture of lactoferrin and xylitol. This resulted in improved healing outcomes in patients with ischemic limbs [146].

Maggot therapy or biosurgery

Since ancient times, civilizations in widely differing parts of the world have used the larvae of flies to treat wounds. The benefits of maggot therapy or biosurgery for wounds come from the ability of larvae to reduce bacterial load and also to promote wound healing. The infestation of a wound by fly larvae is known as myiasis; it occurs naturally when blowfly eggs present in wounds hatch into larvae and immediately feed upon local tissue. Such occurrences were seen during military encounters during the 18th, 19th and 20th centuries and military surgeons observed that such wounds healed rapidly without infection. The first known clinical use of larvae was by Zacharias during the American Civil War. Maggots were used again during World War I by an orthopedic surgeon who later advocated their use in civilians with osteomyelitis [147]. Maggot therapy became relatively popular in North America and Europe until the 1940s, when antibiotics were preferred. Although a few case reports were published during the 1980s, it was not until the 1990s that maggot therapy was revived for treating chronic wounds [148] and maggot therapy began again in the UK in 1995. Sterile larvae are now routinely used for treating non-healing wounds throughout North America and Europe. The range of wounds suitable for biosurgery includes traumatic wounds, burns, surgical wounds, leg ulcers, diabetic foot ulcers and pressure ulcers. Despite the publication of clinical evidence from many sources over the last 80 years to recommend the use of maggots in wounds, a

Table 22.1.2 Therapeutic properties of maggots in relation to wounds.

Bioactive component	Biological effect in wounds	Reference
Lucifensin	Antimicrobial activity	[150]
Ammonium bicarbonate	Restricts bacterial growth by increasing pH	[151]
Unknown factor >10 kDa	Disrupts biofilm formation in *Staphylococcus epidermidis*	[152]
Collagenase	Degradation of collagen	[153]
Chymotrypsin-like serine proteinase, trypsin-like proteinase, aspartyl proteinase, metalloproteinase	Degradation of extracellular matrix	[154]
Allantoin	Increased fibroblast growth	[155]
Histidine, valinol, 3-guanidinopropionic acid	Increased proliferation of endothelial cells, but not fibroblasts	[156]
Trypsin, leucine aminopeptidase, carboxypeptidases A and B	Proteolytic degradation of necrotic tissue and slough	[157]

randomized clinical trail (VenUS II) conducted within the UK failed to demonstrate significant advantages of maggots over standard debridement therapy [149]. It did, however, indicate that maggots were no worse than routine sharp debridement.

Not all maggots are suitable for clinical use since some ingest living tissue. The larvae of the greenbottle (*Lucilia sericata*) are usually preferred because they rapidly ingest necrotic tissue without invading into internal organs. Following rearing under sterile conditions, they are available commercially and dispatched to customers in sterile containers with rapid delivery times. The number of larvae required for each wound depends on its dimensions and the quantity of necrotic tissue or slough present. Originally maggots were applied "loose", directly to the wound and kept in place with secondary dressings. More recently they are contained within sealed bags that are placed onto the wound bed. For some patients the thought of maggot therapy is unacceptable.

Larvae produce a complex mixture of bioactive components that contribute not only to bacterial inhibition but also to enhanced wound healing (Table 22.1.2). The most noticeable effect of larvae applied to wounds is their ability to rapidly remove (or debride) non-viable tissue which would normally impede healing. Larvae attach to the wound bed by hooks, where they secrete proteolytic enzymes that degrade extracellular matrix components and they absorb solubilized products, rather than grazing on non-viable tissue [154, 157].

Movement of larvae within the wound creates mechanical stimulation that promotes increased exudation, which in turn physically displaces material away from the wound bed. Larval ingestion of bacteria reduces numbers in the wound and the ingested bacteria lose viability during passage through the insect hindgut. Larvae also cause wound pH to increase by excreting alkaline waste products and this is thought to slow bacterial growth [151]. Anti-

bacterial activity of larval secretions are most effective against Gram-positive bacteria such as staphylococci and β-hemolytic streptococci and less effective against Gram-negative bacteria such as the enterobacteria and pseudomonads [158, 159]. Biofilms of *S. epidermidis* were shown to be disrupted and prevented by larval secretions containing a molecule(s) >10 kDa with protease or glucosaminidase activity, which affected intercellular adhesion [152]. Larval secretions have long been thought to contain novel antimicrobial factors. One was recently identified as an insect defensin, lucifensin [150]. This molecule is predicted to be responsible for protecting larvae from infection in grossly contaminated environments, as well as inhibiting pathogenic bacteria within the wound.

Conclusions

The range of natural products that possess properties of potential therapeutic and pharmaceutical value seems to be extensive. Only a few have been described here and most of these have not been accepted unconditionally. In the food industry nisin is an established preservative; in wound care honey and maggots have been incorporated into treatment plans in some healthcare facilities, but they are rarely the first choice when antimicrobial intervention is indicated. Garlic promises to be of value in eradicating persistent infections in which biofilms have been implicated. At present the potential of many natural products is unfulfilled. Modes of action for many of these products have not been elucidated and this can affect opportunities for commercial development. Like conventional antibiotics, the route to acceptance depends on licensing or registration, which in turn depends on demonstrating efficacy *in vitro* and *in vivo* and safety in terms of the absence of cytotoxicity, allergenicity and mutagenicity. Development costs will, therefore, be not inconsiderable and manufacturing costs are also likely to be high. Devising systems to standardize production and deliver consistent natural products may be challenging. Unlike conventional antibiotics, many natural products seem to offer beneficial effects that are not confined to antimicrobial activity, due to their often complex and undefined chemical composition. Furthermore their propensity to select for resistant strains of pathogens seems to be low, probably because their antimicrobial activity is often not confined to the action of a single active component on a specific target site. Honey illustrates this point especially well [76, 104].

Since the adoption of evidence-based medicine during the 1990s, the introduction of all new interventions, whether synthetic or natural, must be supported by objective evidence to demonstrate that improved clinical outcomes will ensue. Natural products will, therefore, never be cheap.

References

1 Nelson, R. (2003) Antibiotic development pipeline runs dry. New drugs to fight resistant organisms are not being developed, experts say. *Lancet*, **362**, 1726–1727.

2 Costerton, J.W. *et al.* (1999) Bacterial biofilms: a common cause of persistent infections. *Science*, **284**, 1318–1322.

3 Stewart, P.S. and Costerton, J.W. (2001) Antibiotic resistance of bacteria in biofilms. *Lancet*, **358**, 135–138.

4 Payne, D. *et al.* (2007) Drugs for bad bugs: confronting the challenges of antibacterial discovery. *Nature Reviews. Drug Discovery*, **6**, 29–40.

5 World Health Organization (WHO) (2010) *Traditional Medicine. Fact Sheet 134*, http://www.who.int/mediacentre/factsheets/fs134/en/ (accessed March 1, 2010).

6 Routledge, P.A. (2008) The European herbal medicines directive: could it have saved the lives of Romeo and Juliet? *Drug Safety*, **31**, 416–418.

7 Diamond, G. *et al.* (2009) The roles of antimicrobial peptides in innate host defense. *Current Pharmaceutical Design*, **15**, 2377–2392.

8 Jenssen, H. *et al.* (2006) Peptide antimicrobial agents. *Clinical Microbiology Reviews*, **19**, 491–511.

9 Gillor, O. *et al.* (2008) The dual role of bacteriocins as anti- and probiotics. *Applied Microbiology and Biotechnology*, **81**, 591–606.

10 Rogers, L.A. (1928) The inhibiting effect of *Streptococcus lactis* on *Lactobacillus bulgaricus*. *Journal of Bacteriology*, **16**, 321–325.

11 Pag, U. and Sahl, H.-G. (2002) Multiple activities in lantibiotics-modes for the design of novel antibiotics? *Current Pharmaceutical Design*, **8**, 815–833.

12 Willey, J.M. and van der Donk, W.A. (2007) Lantibiotics: peptides of diverse structure and function. *Annual Review of Microbiology*, **61**, 477–501.

13 Brotz, H. and Sahl, H.-G. (2000) New insights into the mechanism of action of lantibiotics – diverse biological effects by binding to the same molecular target. *Journal of Antimicrobial Chemotherapy*, **46**, 1–6.

14 Bonelli, R.R. *et al.* (2006) Insights into *in vivo* activities of lantiobiotics from gallidermin and epidermin mode-of-action studies. *Antimicrobial Agents and Chemotherapy*, **50**, 1449–1457.

15 Parisien, A. *et al.* (2008) Novel alternatives to antibiotics: bacteriophages, bacterial cell wall hydrolases, and antimicrobial peptides. *Journal of Applied Microbiology*, **104**, 1–13.

16 Johansen, C. *et al.* (1997) Enzymatic removal and disinfection of bacterial biofilms. *Applied and Environmental Microbiology*, **63**, 3724–3728.

17 Vandenbulcke, K. *et al.* (2006) Evaluation of the antibacterial activity and toxicity of 2 new hydrogels: a pilot study. *International Journal of Lower Extremity Wounds*, **5**, 109–114.

18 Thorn, R.M. *et al.* (2006) An *in vitro* study of antimicrobial activity and efficacy of iodine-generating hydrogel dressings. *Journal of Wound Care*, **15**, 305–310.

19 Cowan, M. (1999) Plant products as antimicrobial agents. *Clinical Microbiology Reviews*, **12**, 564–582.

20 Simoes, M. *et al.* (2009) Understanding antimicrobial activities of phytochemicals against multidrug resistant bacteria and biofilms. *Natural Product Reports*, **26**, 746–757.

21 Jaganathan, S.K. and Mandal, M. (2009) Antiproliferative effects of honey and of its polyphenols: a review. *Journal of Biomedicine and Biotechnology*, 830616, doi: 10.1155/2009/830616.

22 Cushnie, T.P.T. and Lamb, A.J. (2005) Antimicrobial activity of flavonoids. *International Journal of Antimicrobial Agents*, **26**, 343–356.

23 Havsteen, B.H. (2002) The biochemistry and medical significance of the flavonoids. *Pharmacology and Therapeutics*, **96**, 67–202.

24 Abdullah, T.H. *et al.* (1988) Garlic revisited: therapeutic for the major diseases of our time? *Journal of the National Medical Association*, **80** (4), 439–445.

25 Cavallito, C.J. and Bailey, J.H. (1944) Allicin, the antibacterial principle of *Allium sativum*. I. Isolation, physical properties, and antibacterial action. *Journal of the American Chemical Society*, **66**, 1950–1951.

26 Kumar, M. and Berwal, J.S. (1998) Sensitivity of food pathogens to garlic (*Allium sativum*). *Journal of Applied Microbiology*, **84**, 213–215.

27 Liu, S. *et al.* (2010) The antibacterial mode of action of allitridi for its potential use as a therapeutic agent against *Helicobacter pylori* infection. *FEMS Microbiology Letters*, **303** (2), 183–189.

28 Ross, Z.M. *et al.* (2001) Antimicrobial properties of garlic oil against human enteric bacteria: evaluation of methodologies and comparisons with garlic oil sulfides and garlic powder. *Applied and Environmental Microbiology*, **67** (1), 475–480.

29 Bakri, I. and Douglas, C. (2009) Inhibitory effects of garlic extract on oral bacteria. *Archives of Oral Biology*, **50** (7), 645–651.

30 Cutler, R.R. *et al.* (2009) *In vitro* activity of an aqueous allicin extract and a novel topical gel formulation against Lancefield group B streptococci. *Journal of Antimicrobial Chemotherapy*, **63** (1), 151–154.

31 Lun, Z.R. *et al.* (1994) Antiparasitic activity of diallyl trisulfide (Dasuansu) on human and animal pathogenic protozoa (*Trypanosoma* sp, *Entamoeba histolytica* and *Giardia lamblia*) in vitro. *Annales de la Societe Belge de Medecine Tropicale*, **74**, 51–59.

32 Harris, J.C. *et al.* (2000) The microaerophilic flagellate *Giardia intestinalis*: *Allium sativum* (garlic) is an effective antigiarial. *Microbiology*, **146**, 3119–3127.

33 Ankri, S. *et al.* (1997) Allicin from garlic strongly inhibits cysteine proteinases and cytopathic effects of *Entamoeba histolytica*. *Antimicrobial Agents and Chemotherapy*, **41** (10), 2286–2288.

34 Lemar, K.M. *et al.* (2003) Cell death mechanisms in the human opportunist pathogen *Candida albicans*. *Journal of Eukaryotic Microbiology*, **50** (Suppl.), 685–686.

35 Lemar, K.M. *et al.* (2005) Allyl alcohol and garlic (*Allium sativum*) extract produce oxidative stress in *Candida albicans*. *Microbiology*, **151** (10), 3257–3265.

36 Ankri, S. and Mirelman, D. (1999) Antimicrobial properties of allicin from garlic. *Microbes and Infection*, **1** (2), 125–129.

37 Miron, T. *et al.* (2000) The mode of action of allicin: its ready permeability through phospholipid membranes may contribute to its biological activity. *Biochimica et Biophysica Acta*, **1463** (1), 20–30.

38 Lemar, K.M. *et al.* (2007) Diallyl disulphide depletes glutathione in *Candida albicans*: oxidative stress-mediated cell death studied by two-photon microscopy. *Yeast*, **24** (8), 695–706.

39 McLean, R.J.C. *et al.* (2004) A simple screening protocol for the identification of quorum sensing antagonists. *Journal of Microbiological Methods*, **58**, 351–360.

40 Rasmussen, T.B. *et al.* (2005) Screening for quorum sensing inhibitors (QSI) by use of a novel genetic system, the QSI selector. *Journal of Bacteriology*, **187** (5), 1799–1814.

41 Bjarnsholt, T. *et al.* (2005) Garlic blocks quorum sensing and promotes rapid clearing of pulmonary *Pseudomonas aeruginosa* infections. *Microbiology*, **151** (12), 3873–3880.

42 Fulghesu, L. *et al.* (2007) Evaluation of different compounds as quorum sensing inhibitors in *Pseudomonas aeruginosa*. *Journal of Chemotherapy (Florence, Italy)*, **19** (4), 388–391.

43 Hamilton-Miller, J.M.T. (1995) Antimicrobial properties of tea (*Camellia sinensis* L). *Antimicrobial Agents and Chemotherapy*, **39** (11), 2375–2377.

44 Blanco, A.R. *et al.* (2005) Epigallocatechin gallate inhibits biofilm formation by ocular staphylococcal isolates. *Antimicrobial Agents and Chemotherapy*, **49** (10), 4339–4343.

45 Shah, S. *et al.* (2008) The polyphenol (-)-epicatechin gallate disrupts the secretion of virulence-related proteins by *Staphylococcus aureus*. *Letters in Applied Microbiology*, **46**, 181–185.

46 Hamilton-Miller, J.M.T. and Shah, S. (1999) Disorganization of cell division of methicillin-resistant *Staphylococcus aureus* by a component of tea (*Camellia sinensis*): a study by electron microscopy. *FEMS Microbiology Letters*, **176**, 463–469.

47 Yam, T.S. *et al.* (1998) The effect of a component of tea (*Camellia sinensis*) on methicillin resistance, PBP2′ synthesis, and β-lactamase production in *Staphylococcus aureus*. *Journal of Antimicrobial Chemotherapy*, **42**, 211–216.

48 Zhao W-H *et al.* (2001) Mechanism of synergy between epigallocatechin gallate and β lactams against methicillin-resistant *Staphylococcus aureus*. *Antimicrobial Agents and Chemotherapy*, **45** (6), 1737–1742.

49 Stapleton, P.D. *et al.* (2007) The β-lactam-resistance modifier (-)-epicatechin gallate alters the architecture of the cell wall of *Staphylococcus aureus*. *Microbiology*, **153**, 2093–2103.

50 Bernal, P. *et al.* (2009) Disruption of D-alanyl esterification of *Staphylococcus aureus* cell wall teichoic acid by the β-lactam resistance modifier (-)-epicatechin gallate. *Journal of Antimicrobial Chemotherapy*, **63**, 1156–1162.

51 Cho, Y.-S. *et al.* (2008) Antibacterial effects of green tea polyphenols on clinical isolates of methicillin-resistant *Staphylococcus aureus*. *Current Microbiology*, **57**, 542–546.

52 Cho, T.-S. *et al.* (2007) Cellular responses and proteomic analysis of *Escherichia coli* exposed to green tea polyphenols. *Current Microbiology*, **55**, 501–506.

53 Edris, A.E. (2007) Pharmaceutical and therapeutic potentials of essential oils and their individual volatile constituents: a review. *Phytotherapy Research*, **21**, 308–323.

54 Bakkali, F. *et al.* (2008) Biological effects of essential oils – a review. *Food and Chemical Toxicology*, **46**, 446–475.

55 Burt, S. (2004) Essential oils: their antibacterial properties and potential applications in food – a review. *International Journal of Food Microbiology*, **94**, 223–253.

56 Carson, C.F. and Riley, T.V. (1993) Antimicrobial activity of essential oil of *Melaleuca alternifolia*. *Letters in Applied Microbiology*, **16**, 49–55.

57 Halcon, L. and Milkus, K. (2004) *Staphylococcus aureus* and wounds: a review of tea tree oil as a promising antimicrobial. *American Journal of Infection Control*, **32** (7), 402–408.

58 Raman, A. *et al.* (1995) Antimicrobial effects of tea-tree oil and its major components on *Staphylococcus aureus*, *Staph. epidermidis* and *Propionibacterium acnes*. *Letters in Applied Microbiology*, **21**, 242–245.

59 Hammer, K.A. *et al.* (2006) A review of the toxicity of *Melaleuca alternifolia* (tea tree) oil. *Food and Chemical Toxicology*, **44** (5), 616–625.

60 Carson, C.F. *et al.* (1995) Susceptibility of methicillin-resistant *Staphylococcus aureus* to essential oil of *Melaleuca alternifolia*. *Journal of Antimicrobial Chemotherapy*, **35**, 421–424.

61 Papadopoulas, C.J. *et al.* (2006) Susceptibility of pseudomonads to *Melaleuca alternifolia* (tea tree) oil components. *Journal of Antimicrobial Chemotherapy*, **58**, 449–451.

62 Hammer, K.A. *et al.* (2003) Antifungal activity of the components of *Melaleuca alternifolia* (tea tree) oil. *Journal of Applied Microbiology*, **95**, 853–860.

63 Mondello, F. *et al.* (2003) *In vitro* and *in vivo* activity of tea tree oil against azole-susceptible and -resistant human pathogenic yeasts. *Journal of Antimicrobial Chemotherapy*, **51**, 1223–1229.

64 Brady, A. *et al.* (2006) *In vitro* activity of tea-tree oil against clinical skin isolates of meticillin-resistant and -sensitive *Staphylococcus aureus* and coagulase-negative staphylococci growing planktonically and as biofilms. *Journal of Medical Microbiology*, **55**, 1375–1380.

65 Dryden, M.S. *et al.* (2004) A randomized, controlled trial of tea tree topical preparations versus a standard topical regime fro the clearance of MRSA colonization. *Journal of Hospital Infection*, **56**, 283–286.

66 Cox, S.D. *et al.* (2000) The mode of antibacterial action of the essential oil of *Melaleuca alternifolia* (tea tree oil). *Journal of Applied Microbiology*, **88** (1), 170–175.

67 Carson, C.F. *et al.* (2002) Mechanisms of action of *Melaleuca alternifolia* (tea tree) oil on *Staphylococcus aureus* determined by time-kill, lysis, leakage, and salt tolerance assays and electron microscopy. *Antimicrobial Agents and Chemotherapy*, **46** (6), 1914–1920.

68 Forrest, R.D. (1982) Early history of wound treatment. *Journal of the Royal Society of Medicine*, **75**, 198–205.

69 Molan, P.C. (1992) The antibacterial nature of honey: 1. The nature of the antibacterial activity. *Bee World*, **73** (1), 5–28.

70 Skiadas, P.K. and Lascaratos, J.G. (2001) Dietetics in ancient Greek philosophy: Plato's concepts of healthy diet. *European Journal of Clinical Nutrition*, **55**, 532–537.

71 Snowdon, J.A. and Cliver, D.O. (1996) Microorganisms in honey. *International Journal of Food Microbiology*, **31**, 1–26.

72 White, J.W. *et al.* (1963) The identification of inhibine, the antibacterial factor in honey, as hydrogen peroxide and its origin in a honey glucose-oxidase system. *Biochimica et Biophysica Acta*, **73**, 57–70.

73 Bang, L.M. *et al.* (2003) The effects of dilution rate on hydrogen peroxide production in honey and its implications for wound healing. *Journal of Alternative and Complementary Medicine (New York)*, **9**, 267–273.

74 Mavric, E. *et al.* (2008) Identification and quantification of methylglyoxal as the dominant antibacterial constituent of manuka (*Leptospermum scoparium*)

honeys from New Zealand. *Molecular Nutrition and Food Research*, **52**, 483–489.

75 Adams, C.J. *et al.* (2008) Isolation by HPLC and characterisation of the bioactive fraction of New Zealand manuka (*Leptospermum scoparium*) honey. *Carbohydrate Research*, **343**, 651–659.

76 Kwakman, P.H.S. *et al.* (2010) How honey kills bacteria. *FASEB Journal*, **24** (7), 2576–2582.

77 Blair, S.E. and Carter, D.A. (2005) The potential for honey in the management of wounds and infections. *Journal of Australian Infection Control*, **10** (1), 24–31.

78 Brady, N.F. *et al.* (1996) The sensitivity of dermatophytes to the antimicrobial activity of manuka honey and other honey. *Journal of Pharmaceutical Sciences*, **2**, 1–3.

79 Irish, J. *et al.* (2006) Honey has an antifungal effect against *Candida* species. *Medical Mycology*, **44** (3), 289–291.

80 Zeina, B. *et al.* (1997) The effects of honey on *Leishmania* parasites: an *in vitro* study. *Tropical Doctor*, **27** (Suppl. 1), 36–38.

81 Al-Waili, N.S. (2004) Topical honey application vs. acyclovir for the treatment of recurrent herpes simplex lesions. *Medical Science Monitor*, **10** (8), MT94–MT98.

82 Pyrzynska, K. and Biesaga, M. (2009) Analysis of phenolic acids and flavonoids in honey. *Trends in Analytical Chemistry*, **28** (7), 893–902.

83 Allen, K.L. *et al.* (1991) A survey of the antibacterial activity of some New Zealand honeys. *Journal of Pharmacy and Pharmacology*, **43** (12), 817–822.

84 Cooper, R.A. and Jenkins, L. (2009) A comparison between medical grade honey and table honeys in relation to antimicrobial efficacy. *Wounds*, **21** (2), 29–36.

85 Molan, P. and Hill, C. (2009) Quality standards for medical grade honey, in *Honey in Modern Wound Management* (eds R. Cooper *et al.*), Healthcomm UK, Aberdeen, pp. 63–79.

86 Blair, S. (2009) An historical introduction to the medicinal use of honey, in *Honey in Modern Wound Management* (eds. R. Cooper *et al.*), Healthcomm UK, Aberdeen, pp. 1–6.

87 Johnson, D.W. *et al.* (2005) Randomized, controlled trial of topical exit-site application of honey (Medihoney) versus mupirocin for the prevention of catheter-associated infections in hemodialysis patients. *Journal of the American Society of Nephrology*, **16**, 1456–1462.

88 Natarajan, S. *et al.* (2001) Healing of an MRSA-colonized, hydroxyurea-induced leg ulcer with honey. *Journal of Dermatological Treatment*, **12**, 33–36.

89 Chambers, J. (2006) Topical manuka honey for MRSA-contaminated skin ulcers. *Palliative Medicine*, **20** (5), 557.

90 Visavadia, B.G. *et al.* (2008) Manuka honey dressing: an effective treatment for chronic wounds. *British Journal of Oral Maxillary Surgery*, **46**, 696–697.

91 Eddy, J.J. and Gideonsen, M.D. (2005) Topical honey for diabetic foot ulcers. *Journal of Family Practice*, **54** (6), 533–535.

92 Blaser, G. *et al.* (2007) Effect of medical honey on wounds colonised or infected with MRSA. *Journal of Wound Care*, **16** (8), 325–328.

93 Jull, A. *et al.* (2008) Randomized clinical trial of honey-impregnated dressings for venous leg ulcers. *British Journal of Surgery*, **95** (2), 175–182.

94 Gethin, G. and Cowman, S. (2008) Manuka honey vs. hydrogel – a prospective, open label, multicentre, randomised controlled trial to compare desloughing efficacy and healing outcomes in venous leg ulcers. *Journal of Clinical Nursing*, **18** (3), 466–474.

95 Robson, V. *et al.* (2009) Standardized antibacterial honey (Medihoney™) with standard therapy in wound care: randomized clinical trial. *Journal of Advanced Nursing*, **65** (3), 565–575.

96 Molan, P.C. (2006) The evidence supporting the use of honey as a wound dressing. *International Journal of Lower Extremity Wounds*, **5** (1), 40–54.

97 Bardy, J. *et al.* (2008) A systematic review of honey uses and its potential value within oncology care. *Journal of Clinical Nursing*, **17**, 2604–2623.

98 Jull, A.B. *et al.* (2008) Honey as a topical treatment for wounds. *Cochrane Database of Systematic Reviews* 4, Art. No. CD005083.

99 Cooper, R.A. *et al.* (2002) The sensitivity to honey of Gram-positive cocci of clinical significance isolated from wounds. *Journal of Applied Microbiology*, **93**, 857–863.

100 Cooper, R.A. *et al.* (2002) The efficacy of honey in inhibiting strains of *Pseudomonas aeruginosa* from infected burns. *Journal of Burn Care and Rehabilitation*, **23** (6), 366–370.

101 French, V.M. *et al.* (2005) The antibacterial activity of honey against coagulase-negative staphylococci. *Journal of Antimicrobial Chemotherapy*, **56**, 228–231.

102 Lusby, P.E. *et al.* (2005) Bactericidal activity of different honeys against pathogenic bacteria. *Archives of Medical Research*, **36** (5), 464–467.

103 Henriques, A. *et al.* (2010) The intracellular effects of manuka honey on *Staphylococcus aureus*. *European Journal of Clinical Microbiology and Infectious Diseases*, **29** (1), 45–50.

104 Blair, S.E. *et al.* (2009) The unusual antibacterial activity of medical-grade *Leptospermum* honey: antibacterial spectrum, resistance and transcriptome analysis. *European Journal of Clinical Microbiology and Infectious Diseases*, **28** (10), 1199–1208.

105 Jenkins, R. *et al.* (2011) Effects of manuka honey on the expression of universal stress protein A in meticillin-resistant *Staphylococcus aureus*. *International Journal of Antimicrobial Agents*, **37**, 373–376.

106 Jenkins, R. *et al.* (2011) Manuka honey inhibits cell division in methicillin-resistant *Staphylococcus aureus*. *Journal of Antimicrobrial Chemotherapy*, **66**, 2536–2542.

107 Henriques, A.F. *et al.* (2011) The effect of manuka honey on the structure of *Pseudomonas aeruginosa*. *European Journal of Clinical Microbiology and Infectious Diseases*, **30** (2), 167–171.

108 James, G.A. *et al.* (2008) Biofilms in chronic wounds. *Wound Repair and Regeneration*, **16** (1), 37–44.

109 Merckoll, P. *et al.* (2009) Bacteria, biofilm and honey: a study of the effects of the honey on 'planktonic' and biofilm-embedded wound bacteria. *Scandinavian Journal of Infectious Diseases*, **41** (5), 341–347.

110 Alandejani, T. *et al.* (2009) Effectiveness of honey on *Staphylococcus aureus* and *Pseudomonas aeruginosa* biofilms. *Otolaryngology and Head and Neck Surgery*, **139** (1), 107–111.

111 Okhiria, O. *et al.* (2009) Honey modulates biofilms of *Pseudomonas aeruginosa* in a time and dose dependent manner. *Journal of ApiProduct and ApiMedical Science*, **1** (1), 6–10.

112 Lerrer, B. *et al.* (2007) Honey and royal jelly, like human milk, abrogate lectin-dependent infection-preceding *Pseudomonas aeruginosa* adhesion. *ISME Journal*, **1**, 149–155.

113 Tonks, A. *et al.* (2001) Stimulation of TNF-α release in monocytes by honey. *Cytokine*, **14** (4), 240–242.

114 Tonks, A.J. *et al.* (2003) Honey stimulates inflammatory cytokine production from monocytes. *Cytokine*, **21**, 242–247.

115 Mesaik, M.A. *et al.* (2008) Honey modulates oxidative burst of professional phagocytes. *Phytotherapy Research*, **22**, 1404–1408.

116 Bankova, V. (2005) Chemical diversity of propolis and the problem of standardization. *Journal of Ethnopharmacology*, **100** (1–2), 114–117.

117 Trusheva, B. *et al.* (2007) Different extraction methods of biologically active components from propolis: a preliminary study. *Chemical Center Journal*, **7**, 1–13.

118 Grange, J.M. and Davey, R.W. (1990) Antibacterial properties of propolis (bee glue). *Journal of the Royal Society of Medicine*, **83** (3), 159–160.

119 Bufalo, M.C. *et al.* (2009) Anti-poliovirus activity of *Baccharis dracunculifolia* and propolis by cell viability determination and real-time PCR. *Journal of Applied Microbiology*, **107** (5), 1669–1680.

120 Kujumgiev, A. *et al.* (1999) Antibacterial, antifungal and antiviral activity of propolis of different geographic origin. *Journal of Ethnopharmacology*, **64** (3), 235–240.

121 Raghukumar, R. *et al.* (2010) Antimethicillin-resistant *Staphylococcus aureus* (MRSA) activity of 'pacific propolis' and isolated prenylflavones. *Phytotherapy Research*, **24** (8), 1181–1187.

122 Petrova, A. *et al.* (2010) New biologically active components from Kenyan propolis. *Fitoterapia*, **81** (6), 509–514.

123 Mirzoeva, O.K. *et al.* (1997) Antimicrobial action of propolis and some of its components: the effects on growth, membrane potential and motility of bacteria. *Microbiological Research*, **152** (3), 239–246.

124 Scazzocchio, F. *et al.* (2006) Multifactorial aspects of antimicrobial activity of propolis. *Microbiological Research*, **161** (4), 327–333.

125 Freitas, S.F. *et al.* (2006) *In vitro* effects of propolis on *Giardia duodenalis* trophozoites. *Phytomedicine*, **13** (3), 170–175.

126 Takenata, T. (1982) Chemical composition of royal jelly. *Honeybee Science*, **3**, 69–74.

127 McClesky, C.S. and Melampy, R.M. (1938) Bactericidal activity of 'royal jelly' of the honey bee. *Journal of Bacteriology*, **324**, A36.

128 Blum, M.S. *et al.* (1959) 10-Hydroxy-delta 2-decenoic acid, an antibiotic found in royal jelly. *Science*, **130**, 452–453.

129 Fujiwara, S. *et al.* (1990) A potent antibacterial protein in royal jelly. *Journal of Biological Chemistry*, **265** (19), 11333–11337.

130 Bilikova, K. *et al.* (2001) Isolation of a peptide fraction from honeybee royal jelly as a potential antifoulbrood factor. *Apidologie*, **32**, 275–283.

131 Bilikova, K. *et al.* (2002) Apisimin, a new serine-valine-rich peptide from honeybee (*Apis mellifera* L.) royal jelly: purification and molecular characterization. *FEBS Letters*, **528**, 125–129.

132 Klaudiny, J. *et al.* (2005) Two structurally different defensin genes, one of them encoding a novel defensin isoform, are expressed in honeybee *Apis mellifera*. *Insect Biochemistry and Molecular Biology*, **35**, 11–22.

133 Fontana, R. *et al.* (2004) Jelleines: a family of antimicrobial peptides from the royal jelly of honeybees (*Apis mellifera*). *Peptides*, **25** (6), 919–928.

134 Boukraa, L. (2008) Additive action of royal jelly and honey against *Pseudomonas aeruginosa*. *Alternative Medicine Review*, **13** (4), 330–333.

135 Boukraa, L. *et al.* (2009) Synergistic effect of starch and royal jelly against *Staphylococcus aureus* and *Escherichia coli*. *Journal of Alternative and Complementary Medicine (New York)*, **15** (7), 755–757.

136 Abdelatif, M. *et al.* (2008) Safety and efficacy of a new honey ointment on diabetic foot ulcers: a prospective, pilot study. *Journal of Wound Care*, **17** (3), 108–110.

137 Asthana, N. *et al.* (2004) Dissection of antibacterial and toxic activity of melittin. *Journal of Biological Chemistry*, **279** (53), 55042–55050.

138 Boutrin, M.C. *et al.* (2008) The effects of bee (*Apis mellifera*) venom phospholipase A2 on *Trypanosoma brucei brucei* and enterobacteria. *Experimental Parasitology*, **119** (2), 246–251.

139 Oren, Z. and Shai, Y. (1997) Selective lysis of bacteria but not mammalian cells by diastereomers of melittin: structure-function study. *Biochemistry*, **36** (7), 1826–1835.

140 Willcox, M.D. *et al.* (2008) A novel cationic-peptide coating for the prevention of microbial colonization on contact lenses. *Journal of Applied Microbiology*, **105** (6), 1817–1825.

141 Ge, Y. *et al.* (1999) *In vitro* antibacterial properties of pexiganan, an analog of magainin. *Antimicrobial Agents and Chemotherapy*, **43** (4), 782–788.

142 Lipsky, B.A. *et al.* (2008) Topical versus systemic antimicrobial therapy for treating mildly infected diabetic foot ulcers: a randomized, controlled, double-blinded, multicenter trial of pexiganan cream. *Clinical Infectious Diseases*, **47** (12), 1537–1545.

143 Ochoa, T.J. *et al.* (2003) Lactoferrin impairs type III secretory system function in enteropathogenic *Escherichia coli*. *Infection and Immunity*, **71** (9), 5149–5155.

144 Appelmelk, B.J. *et al.* (1994) Lactoferrin is a lipid A-binding protein. *Infection and Immunity*, **62** (6), 2628–2632.

145 Singh, P.K. *et al.* (2002) A component of innate immunity prevents bacterial biofilm development. *Nature*, **417** (6888), 552–555.

146 Wolcott RD and Rhoads, D.D. (2008) A study of biofilm-based management in subjects with critical limb ischaemia. *Journal of Wound Care*, **17** (4), 145–155.

147 Baer, W.S. (1931) The treatment of chronic osteomyelitis with maggot (larvae of blowfly). *Journal of Bone and Joint Surgery*, **13**, 438–475.

148 Sherman, R. (1993) The utility of maggot therapy for treating pressure sores. *Journal of the American Paraplegia Society*, **16** (4), 269–279.

149 Dumville, J.C. *et al.* and VenUS II team (2009) Larval therapy for leg ulcers (VenUS II): randomised controlled trial. *British Medical Journal*, **338**, b773.

150 Cerovsky, V. *et al.* (2010) Lucifensin, the long-sought antimicrobial factor of medicinal maggots of the blowfly *Lucilia sericata*. *Cellular and Molecular Life Sciences*, **67** (3), 455–466.

151 Robinson, W. (1940) Ammonium bicarbonate secreted by surgical maggots stimulates healing in purulent wounds. *American Journal of Surgery*, **47**, 111–115.

152 Harris, L.G. *et al.* (2009) Disruption of *Staphylococcus epidermidis* biofilms by medicinal maggot *Lucilia sericata* excretions/secretions. *International Journal of Artificial Organs*, **32** (9), 555–564.

153 Ziffren, S. *et al.* (1953) The secretion of collagenase by maggots and its implications. *Annals of Surgery*, **138** (6), 932–934.

154 Chambers, L. *et al.* (2003) Degradation of extracellular matrix components by defined proteinases from the greenbottle larvae *Lucilia sericata* used for the clinical debridement of non-healing wounds. *British Journal of Dermatology*, **148** (1), 14–23.

155 Prete, P.E. (1997) Growth effects of *Phaenicia sericata* larval extracts on fibroblasts: mechanisms for wound healing by maggot therapy. *Life Sciences*, **60**, 505–510.

156 Bexfield, A. *et al.* (2010) Amino acid derivatives from *Lucilia sericata* excretions/secretions may contribute to the beneficial effects of maggot therapy via angiogenesis. *British Journal of Dermatology*, **162** (3), 554–562.

157 Vistnes, L.M. *et al.* (1981) Proteolytic activity of blowfly larvae secretions in experimental burns. *Surgery*, **90** (5), 835–841.

158 Thomas, S. *et al.* (1999) The antimicrobial activity of maggot secretions: results of a preliminary study. *Journal of Tissue Viability*, **9**, 127–132.

159 Jaklic, D. *et al.* (2008) Selective antimicrobial activity of maggots against pathogenic bacteria. *Journal of Medical Microbiology*, **57**, 617–625.

22.2   Applications of Bacteriophage Technology

Geoffrey W. Hanlon

School of Pharmacy and Biomolecular Sciences, University of Brighton, Brighton, UK

Introduction

When dealing with microorganisms we find that despite their minute size we can be confronted with staggeringly large numbers. For example, each of us has in our gut more bacteria than the number of humans that have ever lived on Earth. If that number is not big enough for you, then consider the total number of bacteria present on Earth. This was estimated by Whitman *et al.* in 1998 to be between 4 and 6×10^{30} cells and the title of their article was "Prokaryotes: the unseen majority" [1]. It is indeed difficult to imagine that any other biological entity could be present in greater numbers than this but in fact the number of viruses on the planet has been estimated recently at approximately 1×10^{31}. The vast majority of these are bacterial viruses or bacteriophages, which are extremely important microbial predators responsible (alongside grazing protists) for maintaining bacterial numbers at a level below the maximum capacity of the environment. Using our knowledge of the average half-life of free viruses in the environment it has been estimated that bacteriophages kill 100 million metric tons of bacteria every 60 s! [2]. Moreover, it has been suggested that the entire bacteriophage population on the Earth turns over every few days, thus demonstrating a highly dynamic system [3].

Life on Earth began between 3 and 4 billion years ago with prokaryotes being the earliest colonizer and it is almost certain that bacterial viruses have coevolved with bacteria since that time. Indeed, bacteriophages have directly influenced their bacterial hosts in their direction of evolution as a result of the dynamic interplay outlined above.

Bacteriophages (or phages) are viruses that have bacteria as their host cells and have no influence on mammalian cells. Like all viruses they are obligate intracellular parasites and cannot lead an independent existence outside their hosts. They are totally reliant on their host cell for the process of replication. The spectrum of activity of bacteriophages is extremely narrow and most can only infect a single species and in some cases only particular strains of that species. As we will see later, this can confer both advantages and disadvantages when we try to exploit their capabilities.

Characteristics of bacteriophages

Bacteriophages can be quite diverse in their morphology although the majority have the structure shown in Figure 22.2.1. The icosahedral head or capsid is made up of multiple copies of a capsid protein and contains the genome of the virus which is generally

Russell, Hugo & Ayliffe's: Principles and Practice of Disinfection, Preservation and Sterilization, Fifth Edition. Edited by Adam P. Fraise, Jean-Yves Maillard, and Syed A. Sattar.
© 2013 Blackwell Publishing Ltd. Published 2013 by Blackwell Publishing Ltd.

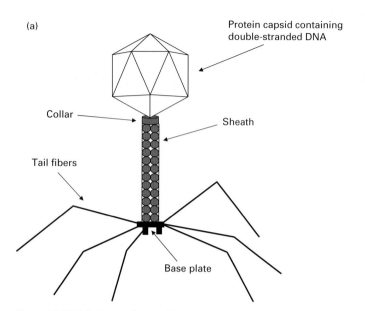

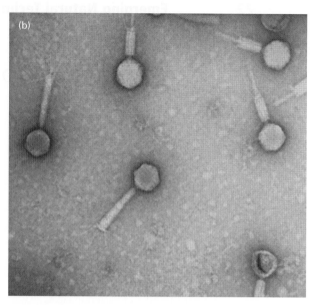

Figure 22.2.1 (a) Diagram of a typical bacteriophages. (b) Transmission electron micrograph of bacteriophages.

double-stranded DNA. Over 500 bacteriophage genomes have been sequenced and they have been found to be highly diverse. In the case of the *Escherichia coli* bacteriophage T4, the DNA contains about 165 genes. In most bacteriophages less than 30% of these have been assigned specific functions, the roles of the remaining genes are unknown [3].

The bacteriophage tails may or may not be contractile and this distinguishes the Myoviridae (contractile tail) from the Siphoviridae and Podoviridae families [4]. The tail is made up of two concentric hollow tubes connected to the capsid by a short neck. At the end of the tail is a base plate from which extend a number of tail fibers (six in the case of T4) having specific sites on their tips which recognize receptors on the host cell surface to facilitate attachment. The attachment site may be on the cell wall, pili or flagella [5]. Those viruses that do not possess tails or tail fibers infect their host cells by other mechanisms which will not be covered here.

Lytic and lysogenic cycles

A bacteriophage encounters its bacterial host by chance and attaches via the receptors on its tail fibers to host cell receptors, which can include protein, oligosaccharide, teichoic acid, peptidoglycan or lipopolysaccharide [6]. The initial attachment is reversible but then becomes irreversible after which the phage injects its DNA into the host cell. At that point the process can proceed by one of two routes depending on the nature of the virus.

Lytic infection cycle

In the lytic infection cycle, the injected DNA takes over the host cell metabolic machinery and directs the bacterium to devote all its energies to manufacturing and assembling new viruses. During

this time the phage specifically degrades the DNA of its host. When the process is complete and the new viruses are ready for release the virus directs the synthesis of lytic enzymes, which can act on the cell wall from the inside. These lytic enzymes, termed muralytic enzymes or endolysins, are produced within the cytoplasm and include lysozymes, endopeptidases and amidases [7]. However, these cannot penetrate the cytoplasmic membrane and so the bacteriophage firstly synthesizes an enzyme termed a holin which degrades the cytoplasmic membrane, allowing the endolysins to lyse the cell wall. The host cell thus ruptures, releasing usually in excess of 100 new virions, demonstrating a dramatic amplification of viral load within the environment (Figure 22.2.2). The synthesis of holin therefore determines the timing of the release of phage progeny. The newly released phages have the potential to continue infecting susceptible host bacterial cells with further amplification of numbers until the bacteria have all been killed [8].

The different stages of the phage replication process were originally described by Ellis and Delbrück in 1939 [9]. The latent period is the time between initial attachment of the phage and lysis of the cell with the resultant release of phage progeny. The process of phage replication is quite rapid and the latent period can be in the order of 20–30 min. However, complete virions are present inside the host cell before the endolysins release them. In the laboratory these can sometimes be accessed artificially using chloroform to lyse the bacterial cells. Using this process it is possible to determine the time taken from initial attachment to the formation of intact, functional virions; a period known as the eclipse period. The burst size is the average number of new virions released from each host cell. The "multiplicity of infection" is the ratio of virus to host cells present in the system. This is of relevance because, if the host cells are vastly outnumbered by

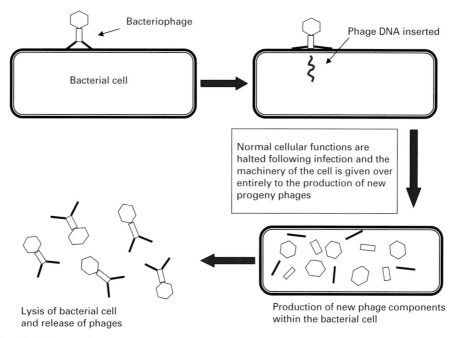

Figure 22.2.2 Bacteriophage lytic infection cycle.

bacteriophages, then there may be multiple attachments onto each cell. Under these circumstances the cell may be killed by the onslaught and the infection cycle will not occur. This is known as "lysis from without" [9].

Lysogenic cycle

Temperate bacteriophages do not always enter immediately into a lytic infection cycle. In this case the injected DNA either becomes incorporated into the host cell genome or exists within the cell as a plasmid. This is a stable situation and the phage directs the synthesis of repressor proteins that block the transcription of its own genes and those of other related bacteriophages. This situation is termed lysogeny. The bacterial cell can therefore continue its normal functions, including replication, in which case the viral genome (known as a prophage) will be replicated as well. Thus, all the daughter cells will also contain the genetic material comprising the prophage. The presence of the repressor proteins will also act as a form of immunity to the host bacterium against attack from similar bacteriophages, thus conferring advantages on the host cell. Whole-genome sequencing of bacteria has revealed that phage elements contribute significantly to sequence diversity and, as we shall see later, this can also influence bacterial pathogenicity.

Under certain circumstances, such as cell stress or genome damage, the prophage will be activated to enter the lytic cycle described above. This can be artificially induced in the laboratory using mutagenic agents such as mitomycin or UV light.

Persistence

Some filamentous bacteriophages can infect a host cell and replicate internally. However, the new viruses are not released on lysis

Table 22.2.1 Examples of toxin genes in pathogenic bacteria which have arisen as a result of bacteriophage infection.

Bacterium	Toxin	Disease
Clostridium botulinum	Botulinum toxin	Botulism
Corynebacterium diphtheriae	Diphtheria toxin	Diphtheria
Escherichia coli	Shiga-like verotoxins	Haemorrhagic diarrhoea
Pseudomonas aeruginosa	Cytotoxin	Multiple disease states
Staphylococcus aureus	Enterotoxin A	Food poisoning
Streptococcus pyogenes	Erythrogenic toxins	Scarlet fever
Vibrio cholerae	Cholera toxin	Cholera

of the host cell but emerge by a process of extrusion which leaves the cell intact.

Lysogenic conversion

When prophages are induced to commence a lytic cycle the first stage is to cut their genetic material out of the host cell genome, but this process is often imprecise. As a result adjacent host bacterial genes may be removed as well and these may then be passed on to newly infected host cells. In this way genes may be transferred horizontally from one cell to another in a process termed transduction. This process has been responsible for the acquisition of a number of virulence factors by pathogenic bacteria and examples are given in Table 22.2.1 [10]. Bacteria can have several prophages within their own genome, accounting for up to 20% of the DNA in some cases. Often these prophages increase the fitness of their host, including the ability to adjust to environmental conditions and infect host cells [11, 12].

Applications of bacteriophages

Phage-typing

As stated earlier, bacteriophages are very selective in their action, often infecting either a single species of bacterium or more commonly selected strains within a species. This highly selective nature can be used as a means of distinguishing between different strains of bacteria for epidemiological purposes. The technique of phage-typing has been used to distinguish strains of staphylococci and also salmonellae. For example, phage-typing of *Salmonella* is useful for identifying the common *Salmonella enterica* serotypes, that is S. *enterica* Typhimurium and S. *enterica* Enteritidis [13]. This information can then be used to determine whether isolates from different sources are the same and hence may identify a common source of each outbreak. Briefly, the bacterial culture is spread onto the surface of an agar plate and the liquid allowed to soak in. The surface is then inoculated with a panel of up to 27 different bacteriophages using a multipoint inoculator. These phages are chosen for their ability to select between different strains of bacteria. After incubation overnight the bacterium will grow as a confluent lawn and where the phages were deposited there may or may not be areas of clearing depending upon whether the bacterium was susceptible to the given virus. The pattern of bacteriophage lysis acts as an identifying fingerprint and can help to distinguish different bacterial strains.

Bacterial identification

The basic principles discussed above should provide a technique for the rapid identification of bacteria using bacteriophages as the recognition element. One area where this has the potential to be useful is that of the diagnosis of tuberculosis. *Mycobacterium tuberculosis* is an extremely slow-growing bacterium and culturing the pathogen from sputum samples requires incubation for up to 6 weeks before an identification can be made. An identification system based upon the use of a specific bacteriophage has been developed and is available commercially [14, 15]. The sputum sample is mixed with the bacteriophage suspension and the virus is allowed to attach to any host M. *tuberculosis* cells present. Any unbound virus is then killed by using a specific virucide derived from pomegranate extract, but those which have already attached are not killed. The infection process is then allowed to proceed and the sample is mixed with a fast-growing non-pathogenic species of *Mycobacterium* which the bacteriophage is also capable of infecting. This mixture is spread onto an agar plate and although the pathogenic TB bacterium cannot grow in the time period, after overnight incubation the fast-growing companion bacterium produces a confluent lawn. If any plaques appear they could only have come from cells of M. *tuberculosis* present in the sputum sample that became infected prior to the introduction of the virucide. Therefore, the presence of plaques is indicative that the patient is suffering from TB.

This test has subsequently been modified to test for *Mycobarcterium avium* subspecies *paratuberculosis* (MAP) from milk and cheese [16]. This is a disease of cattle and the bacterium can pass into the milk and is resistant to the pasteurization process. It is estimated that 2% of pasteurized retail milk in the UK contains MAP. In this modified test a combination of the polymer chain reaction (PCR) technique with a phage-based detection assay has allowed the rapid and specific detection of viable MAP in milk samples in just 48 h [16].

A further example of this approach is provided by a newly available phage-based bacterial identification system (Microphage®) which focuses on rapid (5 h) identification of *Staphylococcus aureus* (methicillin-resistant *S. aureus* (MRSA) and methicillin-sensitive *S. aureus* (MSSA)) in suspected cases of bacteremia. A small sample of blood under investigation is added to each of two tubes containing culture media and bacteriophages. One of the tubes also contains an appropriate antibiotic. Both tubes are then incubated for 5 h at 37°C during which time any susceptible bacteria are infected and lysed by the bacteriophages, which are therefore amplified in number. If the samples are MSSA then they will not grow in the tube containing antibiotic and so the virus amplification will not occur. The second stage of the process is the detection of bacteriophage proteins by antiphage antibodies on a lateral-flow immunoassay device similar to a pregnancy testing kit. This system has been shown to be rapid, reliable, sensitive and accurate and there is no reason why similar tests could not be developed for other important pathogens.

Vaccine production

Conventional vaccines employ live but attenuated microorganisms, whole killed microorganisms or purified fractions of microorganisms to stimulate antibody production in the animal into which the material has been injected. While these have been highly successful in controlling infectious disease these approaches are not without their drawbacks. One of the main potential problems with live microorganisms is the possibility of revertant strains causing disease in those vaccinated. This has happened with the Sabin live attenuated poliovirus which, while being highly effective at reducing the risk from natural infections, has led to some patients developing (and spreading) paralytic poliomyelitis. Problems with killed or component vaccines often relate to reduced activity or toxicity.

DNA vaccination involves inoculating a host with DNA containing the genes encoding the relevant antigen under the control of an exogenous eukaryotic promoter. The DNA can be introduced directly into the tissue cells where the genes are then expressed. These proteins are recognized as foreign and are displayed on the cell surface, thus activating the immune system to produce both humoral and cellular immune responses. It is cheaper and easier to produce vaccines using this technique and they have some advantages, in particular the release of antigen resembles that of a natural infection and hence the response is more specific. However, while there has been some success using naked DNA in trials on small animals their use in humans has been less successful.

In bacteriophage-mediated immunization a vaccine expression cassette is cloned into the genome of a bacteriophage vector, which is then injected directly into the host animal. The bacteriophages are taken up by the antigen-presenting cells of the immune system where the capsid is removed and the vaccine DNA is expressed and translated into vaccine protein. These proteins are expressed on the cell surface and elicit the immune responses as before [17].

Phage display and the production of therapeutic antibodies

As stated above, some filamentous bacteriophages such as M13 do not cause death of their host cells after infection but are extruded into the external culture medium. These are morphologically quite different from those described in Figure 22.2.1 and are long, slender filaments made up of a repeating capsid protein. The process of phage display was first described by Smith [18] and involves inserting a gene onto the coat protein gene of the filamentous bacteriophage. This protein is then expressed on the outside of the bacteriophage [18]. Many genetic sequences can be expressed in a bacteriophage library in the form of fusions with the bacteriophage coat protein, where a large number of phages will be produced, each expressing a different protein on their surface. The important point here is that the different proteins reflect different genetic make-ups. If multi-well plates are then treated with potential target proteins, the phage display library can be added and any phages bearing the appropriate protein on their coat will bind with high affinity. All non- or loosely-bound virus can be washed off. The bound virus can then be eluted and subjected to further rounds of infection and enrichment in a process known as panning. The final purified phage can be isolated, grown up to high titer and the DNA extracted in order to identify the relevant gene sequence and determine the structure of the protein.

This process is used as the basis of a technique to develop human therapeutic antibodies, one of the first of which was Humira (adalimumab), an antibody to tumor necrosis factor α (TNFα) developed by Cambridge Antibody Technology. This drug has achieved blockbuster status with sales exceeding US$1 billion.

Bacteriophage therapy of human bacterial infections

Early experiences of bacteriophage therapy

The effects of bacteriophages were first observed at the end of the 19th century when it was noted by Hankin that the waters of the Ganges and Jumna rivers in India possessed antibacterial activity, protecting villagers along their banks from some gastrointestinal diseases. The idea that this antimicrobial activity might be due to a virus was proposed by Twort in 1915 and independently by

d'Herelle shortly afterwards [19]. Immediately this became apparent the workers in the area, and in particular d'Herelle, realized the potential of these viruses as antimicrobial agents [20]. This, of course, was 10 years before the discovery of penicillin at a time when contracting a bacterial infection usually had fatal consequences.

There followed a great deal of experimentation into the use of bacteriophages for the treatment of bacterial infections in humans. Some of these studies achieved highly successful outcomes, particularly in the treatment of gastrointestinal infections such as dysentery and cholera, wound infections and urinary tract infections. However, the success was short lived and eventually a lack of understanding of the complexities of bacteriophage biology and the discovery of antibiotics led to the demise of their use as therapeutic agents in the West.

Drivers for change

In the following decades the West benefited tremendously from the use of antibiotics, and during the golden era of antibiotic research most of the currently used classes of antibiotics were discovered (Table 22.2.2). Almost from the outset, however, there appeared warning signs of bacterial resistance development. This problem of resistance has increased until today; we now have a situation where some important pathogens are resistant to every antibiotic currently available. It has been stated that for some Gram-negative bacteria such as *Pseudomonas aeruginosa* and *Acinetobacter baumannii* we are close to the end of the antibiotic era [21, 22].

This already difficult situation has been compounded by the lack of new antibiotic research and development by the pharmaceutical industry. It has been estimated that the cost of bringing a new drug to the marketplace is around US$400–800 million and the process takes about 8 years from initial discovery to product launch [23, 24]. For antibiotics, the companies simply do not get the return on investment to make the effort worthwhile. They would prefer to put their considerable R&D expertise into the development of drugs to treat conditions like hypertension, depression and hypercholesterolemia.

The prospect of an increasing number of antibiotic-resistant pathogens and a diminishing library of antibiotics with which to treat patients has led many researchers to look to alternative methods for the management of infections. One suggested approach has been to revisit the previously discredited area of bacteriophage therapy. Since the time of d'Herelle, bacteriophages have been studied extensively, not primarily for therapeutic purposes but for their role in molecular biology and microbial genetics. Knowledge gained from research in phage biology underpins our understanding of modern molecular biology and phage research has provided molecular biologists with many of the practical tools routinely used today [25]. They were instrumental in studies establishing gene structure and regulation and in the discovery of mRNA. In addition, the first genome to be fully sequenced was that of a bacteriophage. Consequently, we now know a great deal more about these viruses than we did at the

Table 22.2.2 Important dates in antibiotic discovery.

Dates	Antimicrobial agents
1900–1920	Salvarsan
1920–1940	Benzylpenicillin
	Sulphonilamide
1940–1960	Cephalosporins
	Chloramphenicol
	Erythromycin
	Isoniazid
	Methicillin
	Polymyxin
	Streptomycin
	Tetracycline
	Vancomycin
1960–1980	Amoxycillin
	Ampicillin
	Carbapenems
	Clindamycin
	Fusidic acid
	Gentamicin
	4-Quinolones
	Sulphamethoxazole
	Trimethoprim
1980–2000	Azithromycin
	Aztreonam
	Ceftazidine
	Clarithromycin
	Latamoxef
	Linezolid
	Mupirocin
	Quinupristin/dalfopristin
	Teicoplanin
2000 to date	Daptomycin
	Doripenem
	Tigecycline

time of d'Herelle and so are in a good position to look again at their use in therapy. Moreover, while the West abandoned phage therapy in favor of antibiotics, the former Soviet Union and eastern Europe have continued to use phages to treat infections over the past 70–80 years and so have accumulated a vast amount of clinical knowledge available to us today.

Recent clinical experiences with bacteriophages
Eastern bloc clinical studies

A large amount of information is available from studies carried out in the former Soviet Union and eastern Europe. However, many of these studies are devoid of background information on patients; they also lack randomization and control groups. More recently, such information originally published in Ukrainian or Georgian languages has become available through translations or reviews written in English. It is not the intention of this chapter to discuss these in detail and the reader is referred to the papers

in the bibliography for further information [26–29]. Despite the limitations noted above, there has been sufficient information published to demonstrate that bacteriophage therapy has a great potential to be of therapeutic benefit.

Safety of bacteriophages and clinical trials

All medicinal products brought to the marketplace must satisfy the regulatory authorities as to their quality, safety and efficacy. The most important of these is safety, in that the product must cause no harm to the patient. So, a priority is to demonstrate that bacteriophages are safe to use. It could be argued that the very first Phase I clinical trial on bacteriophages was carried out by d'Herelle in 1919 when he tested his phage therapy product on himself and his co-workers prior to administering it to his patients suffering from dysentery. This was the first successful use of bacteriophages in the treatment of bacterial infections in humans, although it was not published until some time later.

There is also a degree of assurance as to the safety of bacteriophages in the lack of side effects or adverse reactions reported in any of the wealth of publications emanating from the former Soviet bloc. This is not altogether surprising given that we are constantly exposed to bacteriophages throughout our life, and indeed are colonized by billions of them without any apparent adverse consequences.

Bacteriophage phi X174 immunization is a method that has been in use for more than 25 years to assess the immunity of patients with various types of primary and secondary immunodeficiencies, including HIV-infected patients. This is a US Food and Drug Administration (FDA) approved procedure and although not directly involved in therapy suggests an acceptance of the safety of phages by the regulatory authorities.

Nevertheless, before phages can be authorized for use in the treatment of human bacterial infections it is a requirement of western regulatory processes that Phase I safety trials be conducted prior to subsequent Phase II and Phase III trials. The first formal Phase I safety trial on bacteriophages reported in recent western literature was that conducted by Bruttin and Brussow in 2005 [30]. In this trial, 15 healthy volunteers were administered *E. coli* phage T4, at different doses, and placebo in their drinking water. No adverse reactions attributable to phage administration were reported, serum transaminases were normal in all groups and no T4 antibodies were detected in the serum of those subjects at the end of the trial [30].

Rhoads *et al.* [31] carried out an FDA-approved Phase I safety trial on the use of bacteriophage therapy of venous leg ulcers in humans. The trial involved 42 patients who were treated for 12 weeks with either saline control or bacteriophages effective against *P. aeruginosa*, *S. aureus* and *E. coli*. No adverse events were reported and there was no significant difference between the control and study groups [31].

A Phase I/II trial was conducted by Wright *et al.* [32] in patients with chronic otitis caused by antibiotic-resistant *P. aeruginosa*. The trial, which was approved by the UK Medicines and Healthcare Products Regulatory Agency (MHRA), thus examined both safety and efficacy of the treatment regime. Participants were treated with a single dose of either placebo or phage cocktail comprising six different *P. aeruginosa* phages. Outcome measures included clinical markers together with bacterial and phage levels within the ear. No treatment-related adverse events were recorded and the clinical outcome measures were favorable [32].

The next stage is a full-scale Phase III trial conducted on large numbers of patients and, at the time of writing, a study involving several hundreds of patients examining the efficacy of phages against *E. coli* diarrhea was in the process of recruitment. This study is somewhat unusual in that it is being undertaken by the food manufacturing company Nestlé. To date, this is the first trial of its kind by a large, multinational. The UK-based company Biocontrol is also in the process of putting together a Phase III trial using bacteriophages to treat cystic fibrosis patients with chronic lung infections caused by antibiotic-resistant *P. aeruginosa*. This trial is under the regulatory guidance of the European Medicines Agency and was due to begin in 2011.

Advantages and disadvantages of bacteriophage therapy over conventional antibiotic therapy

As we have seen above, bacteriophages represent a totally new approach to the killing of bacteria compared with the conventional chemical killing we have become accustomed to. This offers some advantages over the use of antibiotics but it also brings with it some disadvantages.

Phage specificity

Bacteriophages are highly specific in their spectrum of activity, in some cases infecting one strain of a particular species but not another [8]. By contrast many antibiotics are broad spectrum or perhaps only kill Gram-positive or Gram-negative bacteria and so we are not used to this level of precision. This can have advantages in that only the infecting pathogen will be targeted by the bacteriophage, leaving the commensal microflora intact. The consequence of this is that secondary problems such as overgrowth by *Candida albicans* or *Clostridium difficile* arising from the indiscriminate killing by broad-spectrum antibiotics do not arise. However, the counter argument is that it is necessary not only to have an accurate diagnosis of the infecting pathogen but also be certain that it is susceptible to the bacteriophage being used. In reality, bacteriophages with such narrow specificity would not be used clinically, and more normally cocktails comprising a number of different bacteriophages would be employed to broaden the scope of the therapy. In a recent study by S. Denyer, G. Hanlon and N. Chanishvili (unpublished data) a cocktail of five different phages active against *S. aureus* was screened for activity against over 450 MRSA and MSSA clinical isolates from the UK (including examples of all 17 epidemic MRSA strains) and only two isolates were found to be resistant.

Mechanism of action

In the battle against antibiotic resistance it is important to develop new chemical entities with different mechanisms of action and not just extensions of pre-existing antibiotic classes. In this way we can circumvent the resistance mechanisms acquired by bacteria. Bacteriophages represent a completely different mechanism of action to all existing antibiotics and so will act equally well against antibiotic-sensitive and antibiotic-resistant clinical isolates as described above. This is not to say that resistance does not arise in the use of bacteriophages, indeed it can arise very rapidly. Within a population of bacterial cells the majority of these cells may prove to be sensitive to a particular bacteriophage, but a few mutant cells will have altered characteristics. These may be resistant to attack by the bacteriophage and when the bulk of the population has been destroyed, these will overgrow. This again is an argument for using cocktails of bacteriophages such that all potential variants within a population may be covered.

Pharmacokinetics of bacteriophage therapy

When a dose of conventional drug is administered orally to a patient, it is typically absorbed into the bloodstream where the concentration rises to a maximum. At that point the drug is metabolized and removed from the system, leading to a fall in blood levels. This pharmacokinetic profile requires that subsequent doses be administered to maintain blood concentrations of the drug at therapeutic levels.

Bacteriophages do not work in this way; indeed, following the initial dose of phage, the number of viruses in the system will increase as they replicate within the infecting bacterial pathogens. The number will continue to rise until all the host cells have been destroyed. As a consequence, it has been found that for some infections single dosing is all that is required.

Adverse reactions arising from bacteriophage therapy

The abundance of bacteriophages within the environment means that we are constantly exposed to these viruses and indeed they form part of our normal microflora. It is not surprising, therefore, that clinical experience in the former Soviet Union and eastern Europe suggests that there are few if any adverse or allergic reactions associated with their therapeutic use. However, concerns have been raised over the possible immunological consequences of multiple dosing of phages, particularly if these are being administered systemically.

Bacteriophages as a platform technology

One of the attractions of bacteriophage therapy is that if resistance arises it should be a relatively simple process to find further active viruses within the environment. However, whether this substitution approach would be acceptable to the regulatory authorities is another issue. Since phage therapy is a platform technology, the lead time and cost involved in bringing a new product to the marketplace should be reduced compared towith conventional antibiotic research and development. However, it must be appreciated that it is not a trivial task to develop a highly purified, genetically-defined, virulent, broad-spectrum, non-transducing bacteriophage that would be appropriate for therapeutic use.

Applications in agriculture and animal health

Bacteriophages for the control of bacteria on foods

There is currently a great deal of interest in the use of bacteriophages in food safety [33] and regulatory approval has recently been received for the use of bacteriophages in the food industry. In early 2006 a company called Omnilytics obtained approval from the EPA for its Agriphage™ pesticide which contains selected bacteriophages for the treatment of bacterial infections in tomatoes and peppers. It is particularly effective against those caused by *Ralstonia* and *Xanthomonas* species. This was the first time that a company had obtained commercial registration from a US regulatory agency for a phage-based product for use in foods. This was followed later in the same year by the Baltimore-based company Intralytix which obtained approval from the FDA for the use of *Listeria*-specific bacteriophages on ready-to-eat meat and poultry products. Their product, ListShield™, is a proprietary blend of six individual monophages active against 170 strains of *Listeria monocytogenes* and is applied to the surface of ready-to-eat foods just prior to packaging. The product is FDA and US Department of Agriculture (USDA) approved for direct application onto foods and is also EPA approved for application on surfaces in food-processing facilities and other food establishments.

Also in 2006 a Netherlands-based company EBI Food Safety, received approval from the FDA for use of its *Listeria*-specific bacteriophage product Listex™ on cheese. This product has since been approved as GRAS (generally recognized as safe) for all food products susceptible to *Listeria* and therefore makes it easier for the meat and fish industry to use the technology. In 2007 Omnilytics again obtained approval from the USDA for bacteriophage treatment of *E. coli* O157:H7 on the hides of live animals just prior to slaughter. Approval is currently being sought from the FDA and USDA by Intralytix for use of its *E. coli* O157:H7 bacteriophage preparation on foods and on surfaces in food-processing establishments. These developments suggest that the regulatory authorities are not opposed to the idea of bacteriophages for the control of infections.

Bacteriophages to treat infections in animals

Much of the current interest in bacteriophages as a means of treating bacterial infections can be traced back to a series of elegant animal experiments conducted by Smith and Huggins in the 1980s. These workers understood the potential of bacteriophages from the large body of literature from the Soviet bloc, but also appreciated that they would not be accepted by scientists in the West unless they were subjected to proper scrutiny in the laboratory [34–38].

Mice infected with a toxigenic, encapsulated, clinical isolate of *E. coli* were treated with either a single dose of bacteriophage or multiple intramuscular injections of different antibiotics. The bacteriophage used was specific for the K1 capsular antigen

and so any resistant mutants that arose were K1 negative and hence much less virulent. The results showed that the single intramuscular dose of bacteriophage was at least as effective in managing the infections as multiple doses of the antibiotics tetracycline, ampicillin, chloramphenicol or trimethoprim/sulphafurazole. These initially promising results were reinforced by subsequent papers demonstrating effective bacteriophage treatment of *E. coli* diarrhea in other animals such as calves, piglets and lambs.

There is, of course, a concern that bacteriophage treatment of *E. coli* diarrhea might result in lysis of the non-pathogenic strains of *E. coli* that form the normal gut microflora. Work by Chibani-Chennoufi *et al.* [39] demonstrated that this did not appear to be the case, and while infecting pathogens were lysed the commensal flora were only minimally affected. They put forward the hypotheses that firstly the host microflora might be in an altered physiological state (slow-growing, starved, etc.) and so unlikely to be amenable to infection by phages and secondly that physical factors such as thickened gut content might prevent the phages from diffusing to the host cells.

While much of the early animal work centered on Gram-negative bacteria, Biswas *et al.* [40] demonstrated good results for bacteriophages in treating mice infected with the Gram-positive pathogen vancomycin-resistant *Enterococcus faecium* (VRE). This is of particular importance because VRE is highly antibiotic resistant and some strains have even developed resistance to newer agents such as linezolid and quinupristin/dalfopristin. Not only was the bacteriophage therapy shown to be effective in treating the infection, the paper also clearly demonstrated that the good response was due to bacteriophage infecting the pathogen rather than to some non-specific immune response [40].

The animal studies described above and many others like them provide invaluable evidence for the use of bacteriophages in human therapy. However, a lot of work has also been conducted by food scientists who recognize that bacteriophages may have a significant role to play in food safety. Zoonotic pathogens such as *Campylobacter*, *Salmonella*, *E. coli* and *Listeria* have food animals as their normal reservoirs and incidences of disease in humans as a result of their consumption are increasing [41]. As an example it is estimated that over 70% of poultry flocks in the UK are positive for *Campylobacter jejuni* and this colonization must be controlled in order to limit the entry of the bacterium into the food chain. Risk assessments have calculated that reducing the number of these bacteria on retail chicken carcasses by 100-fold would lead to an approximately 30-fold reduction in cases of campylobacteriosis [42]. Phage treatment of chickens colonized with *C. jejuni* has been shown to result in a fall in *Campylobacter* counts of between 0.5- and 5-$\log_{10}$ cfu/g of cecal contents compared with controls, depending on the bacteriophage used and the dose applied. Bacteriophage-resistant types did arise, albeit in relatively low frequency (<4%), but these were compromised in their ability to colonize the gut and also tended to revert rapidly back to the

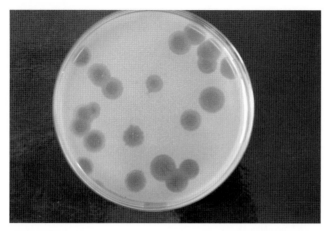

Figure 22.2.3 Bacteriophage plaques on a lawn of host bacteria showing a clear inner zone of lysis caused by infection and an outer turbid halo arising from the action of endolysins.

phage-sensitive phenotype [42, 43]. A similar picture has emerged in studies into the control of salmonellae in chicken flocks using selected bacteriophages. It is likely that the use of bacteriophages may increase in this field due to the demands of customers to reduce the use of antibiotics and microbicides for the control of bacterial colonization.

Further applications of bacteriophages

Bacteriophage lysins

The lytic bacteriophage infection cycle was described above and the production of endolysins discussed. These are highly evolved phage-encoded enzymes that digest the peptidoglycan in the host cell wall, permitting release of newly produced viruses [44]. Examination of phage plaques on a lawn of host bacteria often shows a clear area caused by virus killing the cells and surrounding this is a faintly turbid halo caused by endolysin diffusing into the agar and killing cells (Figure 22.2.3). This can be looked upon as collateral damage to the host bacterium and no virus will be found in the halo zone.

Purified endolysins have been found to be highly specific in their action, in a similar way to bacteriophages, and they have been shown to cause extremely rapid lysis of bacterial cultures *in vitro*. The enzymes consist of an N-terminal catalytic domain, which gives rise to the hydrolytic activity, and a C-terminal cell-binding domain, which targets the enzyme to its substrate with high affinity and specificity. Based on the type of bond that the enzyme can cleave they fall into one of five classes: glucosaminidases, *N*-acetylmuramidases, endopeptidases, *N*-acetylmuramoyl-L-alanine amidases or γ-D-glutaminyl-L-lysine endopeptidases [45]. Sequencing of those enzymes in the same class has shown that the catalytic domain is highly conserved while the cell-binding domain is variable.

Although the activity of the endolysins has been known for many years it is only recently that their potential applications have been recognized. Nelson and co-workers [46] were the first to report that purified phage lysins could be used to decolonize the upper respiratory tract in mice of group A streptococci. Subsequent work has confirmed the activity of these enzymes against other potential pathogens including enterococci, group B streptococci, *S. aureus*, *Listeria monocytogenes*, *Clostridium perfringens* and *Bacillus anthracis* [47]. Note that all of these are Gram-positive cells and this reflects one of the drawbacks of this approach. The endolysins cannot penetrate the lipopolysaccharide (LPS) outer envelope of Gram-negative cells and so only Gram-positive cells are amenable to lysis when the enzymes are used alone. Co-administration of endolysins with LPS disrupters such as ethylenediamine tetraacetic acid (EDTA) or surfactants may allow the enzyme to reach the peptidoglycan layer and cause cell lysis [44].

Endolysins can be manipulated to enhance their lytic activity or recognition capability. The cell-binding domain can be fused with a fluorescent protein to produce tools for the labeling and detection of specific bacterial cells. Alternatively, the functional domains can be swapped to produce chimeric enzymes with altered and improved properties.

Toxin delivery

Bacteriophages can be used to deliver toxins to host bacterial cells during the process of infection. These bacteriophages have been genetically manipulated to prevent them from causing cell lysis, and instead have a toxin gene inserted into their DNA. Binding of the phage to the cell can occur in the normal way and the phage DNA is inserted into the host. Upon insertion all the viral genes, including the toxin gene, are expressed.

Fairhead [48] has used this approach to develop bacteriophages expressing the toxin known as small acid-soluble protein (SASP). SASP is a protein found in Gram-positive endospores such as those of the *Bacillus* species where it binds to the DNA of the spore and protects it from damage. When the gene for this toxin is expressed in bacteriophage host cells following infection, the protein binds irreversibly to the bacterial DNA and causes cessation of all cellular functions.

Another approach has used the non-lytic *E. coli* phage M13 engineered to carry the genes for the "addiction toxins" *Gef* and *ChpBK*. Bacterial programmed cell death is mediated through addiction molecules such as these, which comprise a stable toxin and an unstable antidote [49]. Using this system reduced the numbers of *E. coli* both *in vitro* and in an *in vivo* mouse model, reinforcing the view that phages engineered for toxin delivery have great potential for the treatment of bacterial infections. Unlike the conventional bacteriophage lytic cycle, the phages do not replicate inside the cell and so there is no amplification of effect and the numbers of phages do not increase. However, this system has been shown to give rise to rapid kill and it is proposed that the emergence of resistant strains of host cell is less likely than in conventional phage therapy.

Conclusions

The story of bacteriophages has very nearly come full circle. From being hailed as potential life-savers in the 1920s and 1930s they were discarded in favor of antibiotics from the 1940s onwards. Now, as bacteria develop profound resistance to these antibiotics we are being forced to re-evaluate their usefulness and in doing so are finding an ever increasing number of applications for these intriguing microorganisms.

References

1 Whitman, W.B. *et al.* (1998) Prokayotes: the unseen majority. *Proceedings of the National Academy of Sciences of the United States of America*, **95**, 6578–6583.

2 Rohwer, F. *et al.* (2009) Roles of viruses in the environment. *Environmental Microbiology*, **11**, 2771–2774.

3 Hatfull, G. (2008) Bacteriophages: nature's most successful experiment. *Microbiology Today*, 188–191.

4 Thurber, R. (2009) Current insights into phage biodiversity and biogeography. *Current Opinion in Microbiology*, **12**, 582–587.

5 Ackermann, H.-W. (2005) Bacteriophage classification, in *Bacteriophages: Biology and Applications* (eds E. Kutter and A. Sulakvelidze), CRC Press, Boca Raton, FL, pp. 67–90.

6 Lenski, R. (1988) Dynamics of interactions between bacteria and virulent bacteriophage. *Advances in Microbial Ecology*, **10**, 1–44.

7 Fischetti, V.A. (2005) Bacteriophage lytic enzymes: novel anti-infectives. *Trends in Microbiology*, **13**, 491–496.

8 Hanlon, G.W. (2007) Bacteriophages: an appraisal of their role in the treatment of bacterial infections. *International Journal of Antimicrobial Agents*, **30**, 118–128.

9 Ellis, E.L. and Delbruck, M. (1939) The growth of bacteriophage. *Journal of General Physiology*, **22**, 365–384.

10 Saunders, J. *et al.* (2001) Phage-mediated transfer of virulence genes. *Journal of Chemical Technology and Biotechnology (Oxford, Oxfordshire: 1986)*, **76**, 662–666.

11 Canchaya, C. *et al.* (2003) Prophage Genomics. *Microbiology and Molecular Biology Reviews*, **67**, 238–276.

12 Casjens, S. (2003) Prophages and bacterial genomics: what have we learned so far? *Molecular Microbiology*, **49**, 277–300.

13 Baggesen, D.L. *et al.* (2010) Phage typing of *Salmonella* Typhimurium – is it still a useful tool for surveillance and outbreak investigation? *Euro Surveillance*, **15**, 19471.

14 Albert, H. *et al.* (2001) Evaluation of FASTPlaqueTB-RIF, a rapid, manual test for the determination of rifampicin resistance from *Mycobacterium tuberculosis* cultures. *International Journal of Tuberculosis and Lung Disease*, **5**, 906–911.

15 Albert, H. *et al.* (2004) Simple, phage-based (FASTPplaque) technology to determine rifampicin resistance of *Mycobacterium tuberculosis* directly from sputum. *International Journal of Tuberculosis and Lung Disease*, **8**, 1114–1119.

16 Stanley, E.C. *et al.* (2007) Development of a new, combined rapid method using phage and PCR for detection and identification of viable *Mycobacterium paratuberculosis* bacteria within 48 hours. *Applied and Environmental Microbiology*, **73**, 1851–1857.

17 Clark, J.R. and March, J.B. (2004) Bacteriophage-mediated nucleic acid immunisation. *FEMS Immunology and Medical Microbiology*, **40**, 21–26.

18 Smith, G. (1985) Filamentous fusion phage: novel expression vectors that display cloned antigens on the virion surface. *Science*, **228**, 1315–1317.

19 Duckworth, D.H. (1976) Who discovered bacteriophage? *Bacteriological Reviews*, **40**, 793–802.

20 Sulakvelidze, A. and Kutter, E. (2005) Bacteriophage therapy in humans, in *Bacteriophages: Biology and Applications* (eds E. Kutter and A. Sulakvelidze), CRC Press, Boca Raton, FL, pp. 381–436.

21 Livermore, D.M. (2003) The threat from the pink corner. *Annals of Medicine*, **35**, 226–234.

22 Coelho, J. *et al.* (2004) Multiresistant acinetobacter in the UK: how big a threat? *Journal of Hospital Infection*, **58**, 167–169.

23 DiMasi, J.A. *et al.* (2003) The price of innovation: new estimates of drug development costs. *Journal of Health Economics*, **22**, 151–185.

24 Spellberg, B. *et al.*(2004) Trends in antimicrobial drug development: implications for the future. *Clinical Infectious Diseases*, **38**, 1279–1286.

25 Marks, T. and Sharp, R. (2000) Bacteriophages and biotechnology: a review. *Journal of Chemical Technology and Biotechnology (Oxford, Oxfordshire: 1986)*, **75**, 6–17.

26 Slopek, S. *et al.* (1987) Results of bacteriophage treatment of suppurative bacterial infections in the years 1981–1986. *Archivum Immunologiae et Therapiae Experimentalis*, **35**, 569–583.

27 Alisky, J. *et al.* (1998) Bacteriophages show promise as antimicrobial agents. *Journal of Infection*, **36**, 5–15.

28 Chanishvili, N. *et al.* (2001) Phages and their application against drug-resistant bacteria. *Journal of Chemical Technology and Biotechnology (Oxford, Oxfordshire: 1986)*, **76**, 689–699.

29 Sulakvelidze, A. *et al.* (2001) Bacteriophage therapy. *Antimicrobial Agents and Chemotherapy*, **45**, 649–659.

30 Bruttin, A. and Brussow, H. (2005) Human volunteers receiving *Escherichia coli* phage T4 orally: a safety test of phage therapy. *Antimicrobial Agents and Chemotherapy*, **49**, 2874–2878.

31 Rhoads, D.D. *et al.* (2009) Bacteriophage therapy of venous leg ulcers in humans: results of a phase I safety trial. *Journal of Wound Care*, **18**, 237–243.

32 Wright, A. *et al.* (2009) A controlled clinical trial of a therapeutic bacteriophage preparation in chronic otitis due to antibiotic-resistant *Pseudomonas aeruginosa*; a preliminary report of efficacy. *Clinical Otolaryngology*, **34**, 349–357.

33 Garcia, P. *et al.* (2008) Bacteriophages and their application in food safety. *Letters in Applied Microbiology*, **47**, 479–485.

34 Smith, H.W. and Huggins, M.B. (1979) Experimental infection of calves, piglets and lambs with mixtures of invasive and enteropathogenic strains of *Escherichia coli*. *Journal of Medical Microbiology*, **12**, 507–510.

35 Smith, H.W. and Huggins, M.B. (1982) Successful treatment of experimental *Escherichia coli* infections in mice using phage: its general superiority over antibiotics. *Journal of General Microbiology*, **128**, 307–318.

36 Smith, H.W. and Huggins, M.B. (1983) Effectiveness of phages in treating experimental *Escherichia coli* diarrhoea in calves, piglets and lambs. *Journal of General Microbiology*, **129**, 2659–2675.

37 Smith, H.W. *et al.* (1987) The control of experimental *Escherichia coli* diarrhoea in calves by means of bacteriophages. *Journal of General Microbiology*, **133**, 1111–1126.

38 Smith, H.W. *et al.* (1987) Factors influencing the survival and multiplication of bacteriophages in calves and in their environment. *Journal of General Microbiology*, **133**, 1127–1135.

39 Chibani-Chennoufi, S. *et al.* (2004) *In vitro* and *in vivo* bacteriolytic activities of *Escherichia coli* phages: implications for phage therapy. *Antimicrobial Agents and Chemotherapy*, **48**, 2558–2569.

40 Biswas, B. *et al.* (2002) Bacteriophage therapy rescues mice bacteremic from a clinical isolate of vancomycin-resistant *Enterococcus faecium*. *Infection and Immunity*, **70**, 204–210.

41 Johnson, R.P. *et al.* (2008) Bacteriophages for prophylaxis and therapy in cattle, poultry and pigs. *Animal Health Research Reviews/Conference of Research Workers in Animal Diseases*, **9**, 201–215.

42 Loc Carrillo, C. *et al.* (2005) Bacteriophage therapy to reduce *Campylobacter jejuni* colonization of broiler chickens. *Applied and Environmental Microbiology*, **71**, 6554–6563.

43 El-Shibiny, A. *et al.* (2009) Application of a group II *Campylobacter* bacteriophage to reduce strains of *Campylobacter jejuni* and *Campylobacter coli* colonizing broiler chickens. *Journal of Food Protection*, **72**, 733–740.

44 Loessner, M.J. (2005) Bacteriophage endolysins – current state of research and applications. *Current Opinion in Microbiology*, **8**, 480–487.

45 Fischetti, V.A. (2008) Bacteriophage lysins as effective antibacterials. *Current Opinion in Microbiology*, **11**, 393–400.

46 Nelson, D. *et al.* (2001) Prevention and elimination of upper respiratory colonization of mice by group A streptococci by using a bacteriophage lytic enzyme. *Proceedings of the National Academy of Sciences of the United States of America*, **98**, 4107–4112.

47 O'Flaherty, S. *et al.* (2009) Bacteriophage and their lysins for elimination of infectious bacteria. *FEMS Microbiology Reviews*, **33**, 801–819.

48 Fairhead, H. (2004) *Small Acid Soluble Spore Proteins and Uses Thereof*, US Patent 20040097705.

49 Westwater, C. *et al.* (2003) Use of genetically engineered phage to deliver antimicrobial agents to bacteria: an alternative therapy for treatment of bacterial infections. *Antimicrobial Agents and Chemotherapy*, **47**, 1301–1307.

23 Control of Infectious Bioagents

Les Baillie[1] and Steven Theriault[2]

[1] Cardiff School of Pharmacy and Pharmaceutical Sciences, Cardiff University, Cardiff, Wales, UK

[2] Public Health Agency of Canada National Microbiology Laboratory, Winnipeg, Canada

Introduction

Infectious diseases continue to be a leading cause of morbidity and mortality worldwide; however, their prevalence has been decreased through advances in infrastructure and technology, such as water treatment, waste management, vaccination and improved food supplies. Increased understanding of infectious diseases, as well as medical developments (especially antibiotics) has yielded unprecedented increases in life expectancy. As effective as these innovations have been, they have not eradicated the threat of infectious diseases. Instead, modern controls have simply kept infectious diseases in check and may, in some cases, have caused new pathogens to emerge and spread. The emergence or spread of infectious disease can be attributed largely to unpredictable factors, such as natural disasters or, more disturbingly, bioterrorism.

There is no commonly accepted definition of bioterrorism and so the following taken from Wikipedia is as good as any, "Bioterrorism is terrorism by intentional release or dissemination of biological agents (bacteria, viruses, or toxins); these may be in a naturally-occurring or in a human-modified form." While capturing the essence of bioterrorism the description is short on detail.

The nature of bioterrorism is such that an aggressor is likely to strike at a time and place calculated to induce maximum terror through a combination of casualties and psychological stress [1]. The motivation for such an attack can range from political, doomsday, religious, economic, ecological or other ideological causes without reference to its moral or political justice.

In the context of a human bioterrorist attack, the majority of research has focused on what the US National Institutes for Health defines as category A agents; these are microorganisms and toxins which are thought to have the greatest potential to be weaponized. Unfortunately, the potential to cause harm is not restricted to category A agents and, as a consequence, focus now includes category B and C agents (http://www3.niaid.nih.gov/topics/BiodefenseRelated/Biodefense/research/CatA.htm). Indeed, prior to the anthrax spore postal attacks in 2001 in the USA the only other agent known to have been employed in a bioterrorism incident was a strain of *Salmonella enterica* serovar Typhimurium, which was used by members of the Rajneeshee sect in 1984 to infect 751 people to influence the results of local elections in Oregon [2]. The effective use of a "non-traditional" agent highlights the need to avoid tunnel vision and to realize that many naturally-occurring infectious agents have the potential to be employed in a bioterrorist attack.

Russell, Hugo & Ayliffe's: Principles and Practice of Disinfection, Preservation and Sterilization, Fifth Edition. Edited by Adam P. Fraise, Jean-Yves Maillard, and Syed A. Sattar.
© 2013 Blackwell Publishing Ltd. Published 2013 by Blackwell Publishing Ltd.

The threat of a deliberate release of a biological agent imposes a considerable burden on the ability of relevant authorities to develop management strategies to cope with the consequences of such an event. While a number of off-the-shelf decontamination technologies are available, the majority have yet to fully demonstrate their utility in the scenarios likely to be encountered. In an attempt to highlight some of the likely issues, we have focused on the impacts of deliberate releases of *Bacillus anthracis* and foot-and-mouth disease virus (FMDV), the causative agents of anthrax and foot-and-mouth disease (FMD), respectively.

Bacillus anthracis

Doubtless, the spore-forming *B. anthracis* deserves its status as the principal bio-threat agent due to its ability to form resistant spores and to infect individuals by various means including via aerosol transmission. The offensive potential of this bacterium resulted in it being weaponized by a number of states including Japan, the United Kingdom, United States, the former Soviet Union and more recently Iraq [3–4]. *B. anthracis* has a long history as a bio-weapon. The German army in World War I used anthrax to cause outbreaks among livestock in Romania and Argentina as well as in reindeer in Norway. In World War II the Japanese army infected Russian livestock in an attempt to destroy food sources. The ability of a small-scale release to cause harm and disruption was amply demonstrated in the 2001 US mail attacks, which resulted in 22 cases of anthrax, of whom five died, and caused untold damage to the psyche of the US public. It was estimated that more then 30,000 of the population were exposed. In response the US government provided 60+ days of ciprofloxacin prophylaxis at a cost of over $2 billion.

The consequences of a deliberate large-scale release of *B. anthracis* spores could be huge in terms of the impact on human and animal well being and the associated economic losses. It has been estimated that an anthrax spore attack against a city the size of New York could result in 1.5 million infections of which 123,000 would die if left untreated. The medical costs alone of treating the exposed individuals could amount to $26 billion per 100,000 persons exposed [5]. It is even more sobering to consider that this estimate does not include the cost of decontaminating and restoring the affected area.

Tragic as the events of the 2001 anthrax mail attacks were, the authorities were relatively fortunate that the small release of the spores was confined to a limited number of buildings. These buildings could be sealed and decontaminated, although at a considerable cost in terms of time and money. The Brentwood postal facility in Washington, DC, which was one of the sites that processed contaminated letters was closed for 26 months and cost $130 million to decontaminate. It is invidious to contemplate the effect of a release at a critical public facility such as a major transport hub in a capital city. The subsequent disruption to economic activity would be huge, particularly if the site was closed for an extended period of time. Of course, the ability to restore such a facility would very much depend on the confidence of the

population and elected officials. The ability to demonstrate effective decontamination of the site would be a key factor in restoring the facility to public use. Bioterror agents such as anthrax spores have the ability to instill a sense of fear and terror in the public's psyche, which threatens their sense of personal and community safety and as such they may demand unrealistic levels of cleanliness before they are prepared to once again travel through the hub. Indeed, even though the site of the first anthrax release, the offices of a Florida-based newspaper in Boca Raton, was extensively decontaminated, the company subsequently relocated to another building.

Foot-and-mouth disease

Humans are not the only targets for a biological attack. The destruction of essential foodstuffs such as rice and domestic animals would have a devastating effect on the well being of whole populations [6]. One only has to think back to the dramatic effects of the UK FMD outbreak in 2001 in which authorities spent 6 months struggling to control a disease outbreak that cost some $25 billion and resulted in the slaughter of 11 million animals. Only a handful of pathogens, all viruses, are considered potential agents of large-scale agroterrorism in western nations; they include FMDV in cattle and swine, Rinderpest virus in cattle, classic swine fever and African swine fever viruses in pigs, avian influenza and Newcastle disease viruses in poultry, and the Rift Valley fever virus.

FMD, a highly contagious disease, primarily affects cloven-hoofed livestock and wildlife. Although adult animals generally recover, the morbidity rate is high in naïve populations. Long-term symptoms may include decreased milk yield, permanent hoof damage and chronic mastitis, with high mortality rates seen in young animals [7]. FMD has caused epizootics in Africa, Asia, Europe and South America. The virus is usually introduced into a country in contaminated feed or infected animals and in countries where FMD is not endemic, the importation of animals and animal products from FMD-endemic areas is strictly controlled. As FMDV is an animal pathogen with humans being dead-end hosts, the importance of controlling the spread is an economical and food supply concern. The virus has been shown to retain its infectivity in the environment for days, weeks or even months depending on the conditions [8]; thus, decontamination approaches need to be tailored to suit the local environment.

FMD outbreaks are usually controlled by quarantines and restrictions on the movement of animals, euthanasia of affected and in-contact animals, and cleansing and disinfection of affected premises, equipment and vehicles. Effective disinfectants include sodium hydroxide, sodium carbonate, citric acid and potassium permanganate compounds. Iodophors, quaternary ammonium compounds, hypochlorite and phenols are less effective, especially in the presence of organic matter. Infected carcasses must be disposed of safely by incineration, rendering, burial or other techniques. Incineration is the most common method used to prevent the spread of the infection. Milk from infected cows can be rendered safe by heating to 100°C for >20 min; pasteurization at 72°C for 15 s does not inactivate the virus. High-temperature short-time (HTST) pasteurization greatly reduces the level of viable FMDV in milk, but some studies suggest that residual virus may sometimes persist [9].

Infection with FMDV is not considered to be a public health problem as human infection is rare, with approximately 40 cases diagnosed since 1921. Vesicular lesions and influenza-like symptoms can be seen, and the disease is generally mild, short-lived and self-limiting. However, the economic, livestock loss and public response far outweigh the rarity of human infection, as was demonstrated by the outbreaks in 2001 and the subsequent accidental release of FMDV from the Pirbright Research Site in the UK.

The 2001 outbreak started in a pig finishing unit located at Burnside Farm in Northumberland where pigs were thought to have been fed material contaminated with FMDV. It went on to be considered the worse FMD outbreak in the UK since records began, an estimated 6 million animals were culled with the government paying compensation for slaughtered animals, disposal and clean up in the range of $25 billion. To control the spread of the disease a further 4 million animals were culled, 1.3 million on contaminated premises, 1.5 million on farms defined as dangerous contacts not contiguous with the contaminated premises, and 1.2 million on contiguous premises, many of which were also defined as dangerous contacts. The massive numbers of animals requiring disposal, together with the concurrent decontamination of large areas, put an unprecedented strain on the available personnel and resources.

The subsequent, smaller outbreak in 2007 from the unintentional release of FMDV from a research facility further demonstrates the need for up-to-date decontamination technologies and waste removal systems. Unlike the natural outbreak at Burnside Farm, the latter release of FMDV was due to a drainage system which was no longer in good repair. Localized flooding from heavy rains led to soil contaminated with the escaped virus and its subsequent transport to distant farms via construction vehicles. As a consequence, the government introduced better management and monitoring systems for safe handling of pathogens in laboratories [10].

The release of infectious bioagents into the environment, either deliberate or accidental, has the potential to cause enormous health and economic problems as amply demonstrated above. Dealing with the consequences of such an event is likely to impose a severe strain on the infrastructure of any country and as a consequence it is vital that we develop decontamination and control measures that mitigate the threat posed by such pathogens.

Containment approaches

The most practical means of minimizing the risks posed by the handling of dangerous and highly infectious agents is to adopt pathogen-specific containment strategies, a form of biological quarantine. Containment measures can be broken down into: (i)

primary containment, that is the use of good microbiological techniques, personal protective equipment and devices such as biosafety cabinets; and (ii) secondary containment, which comprises factors such as laboratory design and operating procedures, for example access restriction, air handling, autoclaving and safe disposal of waste.

To assist in the determination of the appropriate level of containment for a particular microorganism, bodies such as the UK Health Safety Executive's Advisory Committee on Dangerous Pathogens classify biological agents into one of four hazard groups based on their ability to infect healthy humans. The four hazard groups are defined as follows:
- *Hazard Group 1*: unlikely to cause human disease.
- *Hazard Group 2*: can cause human disease but are unlikely to spread to the community and there is usually effective prophylaxis or treatment available.
- *Hazard Group 3*: can cause severe human disease and may spread to the community, but there is usually effective prophylaxis or treatment available.
- *Hazard Group 4*: causes severe human disease and is likely to spread to the community and there is usually no effective prophylaxis or treatment available.

A similar criterion is used to classify the risk posed by animal and plant pathogens to their respective hosts. Therefore, particular care must be taken when handling microorganisms in hazard groups 3 and 4. *B. anthracis* belongs to hazard group 3 while the smallpox virus and FMDV are both group 4 pathogens. In Canada and the USA, the corresponding terminology for the classification of infections agents is biosafety levels 1–4 and containment levels 1–4.

Indeed, getting the containment methodologies wrong can have drastic consequences. In 1978, Janet Parker, a medical photographer, became the last recorded person to die of smallpox. The virus most likely traveled by air via a service duct from a poxvirus research laboratory on the floor below [11]. A year later, a major breach in containment resulted in an aerosol release of anthrax spores from a military facility in the city of Sverdlovsk (now known as Yekaterinburg) in the former Soviet Union and killed at least 60 individuals and infected animals 60 km downwind. A more recent example of a breakdown in containment occurred in 2007 and saw the release of a strain of FMDV from a facility where it was being used to make an animal vaccine. As previously mentioned, the release resulted in a local outbreak and was attributed to poor maintenance and management of the facility.

Microbicide susceptibility of infectious agents

Prions

Prions, the cause of transmissible spongiform encephalopathies, are infectious agents composed primarily of protein that is able to "propagate" by inducing existing polypeptides in the host organism to misfold. This corrupted form of protein has been implicated as the causative agent of a number of neurological conditions in mammals including sheep scrapie and cervid (deer, elk, moose) chronic wasting disease, bovine spongiform encephalopathy (BSE or, more commonly, "mad cow disease") in cattle, and Creutzfeld–Jakob disease (CJD) in humans. Prions are extremely resistant to inactivation, and as a consequence accidental transmission has occurred through the use of inadequate decontamination procedures. The efficacy of liquid microbicides varies depending on the agent, but more disturbingly the infectivity of all prion agents can survive autoclaving at 132–138°C [12–13]. Fortunately, the limitations of autoclaving can be overcome by combining autoclaving (at 121°C) with a sodium hydroxide treatment. Thus, while we have strategies to decontaminate clinical equipment and material, it is unfortunate that we are not similarly blessed with approaches that could be used to deal with environmental contamination.

Prions can persist in the soil for years and it has been proposed that contaminated soil may serve as an environmental reservoir for the agent and thus contribute to the horizontal transmission of prion diseases between sheep, deer and elk. It has been reported that prions in soil can adsorb to a common soil mineral, montmorillonite, significantly enhancing disease penetration and subsequently reducing the incubation period relative to unbound prions [14]. Given that ruminants are estimated to ingest hundreds of grams of soil a day it is not difficult to envisage how naïve animals may become infected.

Given the longevity and resistance of prions, a large-scale release of the agent into the environment would present a major challenge to those individuals tasked with decontaminating the affected area. It would likely require the use of microbicides at toxic concentrations, which would have a considerable impact on the local flora and fauna.

Bacterial spores

Although not as resistant as prions, bacterial spores pose a similar problem with regards to environmental decontamination. The ability of bio-threat agents such as *B. anthracis* to form chemically resistant spores presents a particularly challenging scenario for decontamination. It has been reported that spores can withstand temperatures of 80°C and above depending on the conditions (Figure 23.1), as well as exposure to aldehyde, acids, alkalis, alcohols, phenolics, oxidants, chlorine-releasing agents, quaternary ammonium compounds and surfactants.

The spore is built as an internal, double membrane-bound compartment, called the forespore, within a rod-shaped cell (Figure 23.2). Over the course of several hours, critical protective structures assemble inside and around the forespore. Spore dormancy and resistance depend on the partial dehydration of the inner compartment of the spore known as the core, which houses the chromosome. This core is surrounded by a thick layer of peptidoglycan known as the cortex, which is further enveloped by the spore coat. In some species, including *Bacillus atrophaeus*

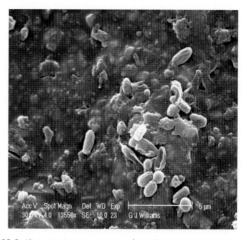

Figure 23.2 Electron microscopy image of *Bacillus anthracis* spores.

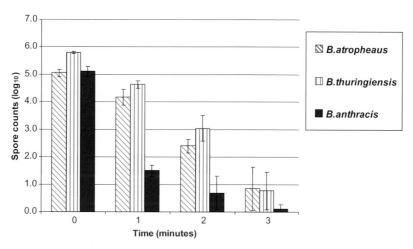

Figure 23.1 Bacterial resistance shown through spore counts (log$_{10}$) for three *Bacillus* spore species exposed to 99°C in a thermocycler for 1, 2 and 3 min compared with starting concentrations.

(formerly known as *Bacillus subtilis* var. *globigii*), this represents the outermost layer of the spore. In others such as *B. anthracis* and *Bacillus cereus*, there exists an additional layer, separated by a gap, called the exosporium [15].

The contribution made by these various constituents to the ability of the spore to survive environmental insults and adhere to surfaces is unclear. While it is known that the various proteinaceous layers which comprise the spore protect the cortex from damage by microbicides, the mechanisms by which this is achieved are not clear. It is possible that the spore coat simply acts as a permeability barrier and that non-specific reactions with the coat reduces the amount of toxic agent available to attack essential molecules such as enzymes and DNA located in the spore core [16].

This hypothesis would explain why spores of *B. atrophaeus*, which naturally lack an exosporium, are more susceptible to microbicides than those of *B. anthracis*. While these differences in susceptibility are unlikely to represent a significant problem given the concentrations at which most commercially available chemical decontaminants are currently used (i.e. in vast excess over the level required to kill), it is likely to be an issue in situations where one is trying to reduce the concentration of microbicide in order to minimize damage to personnel, sensitive equipment and the environment.

It should be remembered that the physical properties of a bacterial spore depend on both genetic and environmental factors such as growth conditions, downstream processing and the presence of additives such as sugars and surfactants to aid adherence. Factors shown to affect spore resistance to heat and chemical agents include the conditions under which the spores are produced (plate vs. liquid culture), the composition of the growth media (glucose, yeast extract, peptone and divalent cations promote wet-heat resistance) and the temperature (the higher the culture temperature, the greater the thermal resistance of the resulting spore) [17–18]. These differences are thought to reflect changes in the fatty acid composition of the inner membrane of the spores, with those prepared on plates producing a higher ratio of anteiso to iso fatty acids, which is indicative of a more fluid membrane. The inner spore membrane is a known target of oxidizing agents, thus changes in this structure are likely to have profound effects on the resistance of the organism to microbicides.

A recent analysis of the published literature detailing the sporicidal activity of various microbicides against members of the *Bacillus* family highlighted the wide range of strains examined and conditions used to produce their spore preparations. Over half of the studies (69%) adopted an agar-based method to produce spores, with nutrient agar being the commonest medium employed out of a total of nine different agar recipes reported. Incubation times and temperatures also varied, the mean period was 6.4 days with a range of 2 to 15 days, while the mean incubation temperature was 31.9°C with a range of 23–37°C. The remaining studies employed a broth-based method to generate spores and made use of nine different media recipes with a mean incubation time of 2.6 days (range 1–5 days) and a mean incubation temperature of 34.3°C (range 30–37°C). These results highlight the problems in seeking to compare results from different studies.

As to the bacterial strains themselves, of the 10 papers that assessed the susceptibility of *B. atrophaeus*, *Bacillus globigii* or *B. subtilis* var *niger* (different names for the same organism), three papers failed to specify a strain designation (i.e. ATCC number), one employed NCTC 10073 (the strain provided by Dstl) and another employed ATCC B-385, while *B. atrophaeus* ATCC 9372 was used in the other six papers. Given that isolates of *B. atrophaeus* can vary in their characteristics and possibly in their susceptibility to microbicides, this is another factor to consider when seeking to compare the results from different studies. Thus, while *B. atrophaeus* has been used extensively in field trials as a surrogate for *B. anthracis*, it is important to recognize both the limitations and advantages of this model system as a surrogate in microbicide efficacy studies and to pursue approaches, such as the use of avirulent *B. anthracis* strains cultured under controlled conditions, that best represent the properties of fully virulent *B. anthracis*.

Vegetative bacteria

While the spore represents a survival mechanism by which bacteria survive adverse conditions, to reproduce they must convert back to a metabolically-active vegetative state thus rendering them considerably more susceptible to microbicides. Indeed, while there is no doubting the ability of many of the microbicides currently available to inactivate bacterial spores, there is concern that their inherent toxicity at the in-use concentrations currently recommended are likely to damage personnel, equipment and the environment. Indeed, it makes little sense if the cure is as damaging as the threat posed by the contaminating microorganisms. These concerns have stimulated researchers to investigate approaches that reduce the concentration of microbicide required to achieve effective decontamination and thus reduce potential toxicity. Strategies currently being pursued include the identification of microbicides which are synergistic in combination, and the addition of germinations to microbicides to increase their effectiveness against spores by triggering the spores to germinate and thus convert to their more sensitive vegetative form. An example of this approach is a decontaminating foam developed by researchers at the US Department of Energy, Sandia National Laboratories, which combines hydrogen peroxide with the amino acid alanine, a known trigger of *B. anthracis* spore germination [19].

While not all bacteria have the ability to produce spores, they can adopt other mechanisms to increase their resistance to environmental insults. In one such strategy the bacteria modify their physiology to a state described as a viable-but-non-culturable form from which it can recover when conditions improve [20]. Studies have shown that bacteria that adopt this strategy are able to withstand exposure to increased levels of microbicides [21–22].

The formation of biofilms, a community of microorganisms attached to a surface, represents a further survival strategy which increases the ability of vegetative bacteria to survive exposure to antimicrobial agents [23]. They represent a serious problem in medial devices such as indwelling catheters where they represent a reservoir of infection, and in water pipes were they can build up to such levels that they can hinder the water flow. Indeed, concerns have been expressed that biofilms formed by indigenous water system bacteria could hinder the decontamination of water systems attacked with *B. anthracis* spores by providing a "safe haven" from the attention of microbicides. Morrow and colleagues observed that spores associated with biofilms required 5–10-fold higher disinfectant concentrations than was required to treat the same spores in suspension [24].

Botulinum toxin

Botulinum toxin merits a brief mention as a potential agent of bioterrorism. Despite being regarded as the most toxic substance known to us it can be easily neutralized. Extremes of temperature and humidity will degrade the toxin and, depending on the weather, the biological activity of aerosolized toxin decays at a rate of 1–4% per minute. Exposed clothing and skin should be washed with soap and water, while contaminated objects or surfaces should be cleaned with 0.1% hypochlorite bleach solution if they cannot be left unattended for the hours to days required for natural degradation [25].

Viruses

The ability of viruses that cause human infections to survive on inanimate surfaces varies depending on the nature of the virus. While the majority of human respiratory tract and bloodborne pathogens can only survive outside the host for a few hours to a couple of days, viruses from the gastrointestinal tract, such as rotavirus, can persist for up to 2 months and thus represent a continuous source of transmission if no regular preventive surface disinfection is performed [26]. The highly infectious smallpox virus, which belongs to the family of Poxviridae, is of particular concern as it can survive for weeks in the environment depending on the ambient temperature, humidity and ultraviolet light exposure and is capable of causing a fatal infection in 30% of individuals who are infected. Indeed, the effect of a smallpox virus released among the population could be disastrous if efficacious measures were not taken. The vaccine is active if it is administered in the first 4 days after exposure, but only a limited number of doses are available worldwide. In addition to vaccination, quarantine of symptomatic people and safe decontamination procedures are critical to contain the epidemic. Some disinfectants are active against orthopox viruses, particularly sodium hypochlorite. However, this chemical is not an ideal disinfectant because

chlorine solutions are unstable, inactivated by protein-containing substances and cannot be used on stainless steel equipment because it causes damage [27].

Depending on the class of virus, its structure can be divided into four major components: an envelope derived from the infected host cell (in enveloped viruses such as smallpox virus), a protein capsid, glycoprotein receptors and the vital genome; all are potential targets for microbicide activity. The viral envelope, being highly lipophilic and negatively charged, makes it susceptible to a wide range of membrane active agents (particularly cationic microbicides). Hence, the enveloped viruses appear to be more sensitive to microbicides than the non-enveloped viral particles. The capsid is a key component in that it protects the nucleic acid of the virus from the external environment. Reactive protein groups such as $-NH_2$ and $-SH$ groups are targeted by microbicides such as glutaraldehyde and hydrogen peroxide, respectively. Loss of viral infectivity due to microbicides can be caused by the alteration of glycoproteins, which are, in fact, responsible for specificity, and for releasing viral genome into the host cytoplasm. Finally, chlorine compounds [28], peracetic acid [29–30], ozone and glutaraldehyde [28] have been found to alter the viral nucleic acids.

The ability of viral forms to develop reduced sensitivity to microbicides has been proposed by mechanisms which are thought to be comprised of intrinsic and acquired factors. Acquired mechanisms are distinct owing to single or multiple genetic mutations within a transmissible element, while intrinsic resistance is linked to the structural features of the virus such as the presence of an envelope [31]. Multiplicity reactivation is a further process of resistance, in which damaged and inactive viruses combine their resources to produce infectious virions [32]. In order to avoid this phenomenon, both the nucleic acid and capsid must be totally destroyed. Microbicide-induced viral clumping is another phenomenon that can reduce efficacy by protecting the viruses which are trapped inside. As a consequence, some resistant subpopulations may remain present in the medium or on the surface, as demonstrated with reovirus during bromine disinfection in water [33] and coxsackievirus after chlorine treatment [34].

Summary

The ability to accurately determine the microbicide susceptibility of a pathogen under relevant in-use conditions is an important factor when seeking to balance the challenge of inactivating the organism against reducing microbicide concentration to minimize collateral toxicity and damage. Determination of the relative susceptibility of highly pathogenic agents to a particular microbicide is hampered by the fact that there is no one standard test capable of addressing all of the possible variables. Added to this is the fact that some agents are difficult to propagate outside their natural host and are hazardous to handle, necessitating the use of surrogates that may not give a true representation of the susceptibility of the pathogen.

Decontamination principles

The safe containment of a large-scale release of biological agents into the environment is an extremely challenging undertaking. As with all processes it can be broken down into a number of stages which include evaluation, containment (both of agent and toxic decontaminants), treatment, assessment of efficacy and finally restoration to function.

Before the decontamination of an affected environment can be undertaken, an evaluation of the various options must be considered in terms of the type of biological agent (persistent, non-persistent, etc.), the form and manner in which it was released and its concentration [35]. Indeed selection of the appropriate decontamination technology is somewhat site dependent and should consider several elements, including the area that needs to be decontaminated, the material and structural components which are contaminated and, ultimately, the type of bioagent causing the contamination.

Recently there has been an increase in the study of decontamination technologies in part due to the delivery of *B. anthracis*-contaminated letters to numerous government buildings in Washington, DC and seven other US states during the fall of 2001 [35]. To combat this attack, a range of technology solutions were adopted, which included disinfection of hard surfaces with a liquid form of chlorine dioxide, disinfection of hard surfaces with decontamination foam, high-efficiency particulate air (HEPA) vacuuming on porous surfaces, chamber fumigation of packages and mail with gaseous chlorine dioxide, and large-area fumigation using gaseous chlorine dioxide gas.

As a consequence of these events, the field of applied research is advancing rapidly with new technologies in development which will hopefully improve our ability to respond to a large-scale contamination event. Key among the criteria which will drive the selection of the most appropriate approach will be a consideration of the toxicity of the decontamination agent and the likely impact of its large-scale use on the local environment.

Containment requirements

Containment of a contaminated area is required to prevent the spread of a contaminant by the movement of workers, equipment and air. Isolation of a contaminated area refers to sealing a site to permit fumigation and ensure adequate contact time while preventing the release of toxic fumigants [36]. The effectiveness of any fumigation process is assessed by monitoring four key processes: temperature, relative humidity, fumigant concentration and contact time, along with the inactivation of biological indicators [37].

The extent of isolation and type of containment technologies used will depend on factors such as the size of the affected area, types of surfaces involved and extent of contamination. During the decontamination of the Hart Senate office building, the entire building underwent an extensive sealing process to prevent escape of particulates and gas from the facility into cracks in the floors, walls and ceilings, which were sealed with expanding foam sealant or silicone caulking to ensure no open penetrations were present [38]. Recently, material normally used for tenting houses and building during insecticidal fumigation have been used for chlorine dioxide fumigations. The materials are economical and readily available. Special fabrics are also currently under review for use as protective barriers used for containment. The fabrics were designed to be effective against bioagents and are strong, durable and lightweight. They can be welded or sealed and are resistant to decontamination reagents; currently there are cost restrictions with this type of product, however technologies are advancing and costs are starting to decrease. A greater level of containment and isolation can be achieved by creating negative air pressure to prevent the outward flow of air using portable HEPA filtration units or negative air units. If fumigation is employed HEPA units can be used to prevent escape of the fumigant with the addition of a carbon filter to aid in breakdown of the chemical [37].

Source reduction

The objective of source reduction is to decrease the amount of contamination in an area prior to the main decontamination activity. Decontamination commences with source reduction in which salvageable and non-salvageable items are identified within the contaminated area. In the Sterling mail facility, which was contaminated by anthrax spores during the 2001 mail attack, decision makers decided to remove and dispose of all porous materials, including carpets and furniture, and non-porous items such as mail and parcel-sorting machines. Items that were deemed essential were sent off site for treatment using a ethylene oxide sterilization chamber and then returned for reuse [38].

In addition to removing material, actions such as pre-cleaning surfaces with a liquid or foam decontamination agent serve to reduce the contaminant load as well as removing any soil load that may protect the bioagents from the action of the decontaminant. Once removal of essential equipment and disposable material has occurred, decontamination can commence [37].

Surface decontamination technologies

Technologies for surface decontamination are currently the best understood of all the different types of approaches and can be used as the primary decontamination means or as a means of source reduction prior to fumigation to remove the remaining organic load. During decontamination of the anthrax spores contaminating the Hart office building in Washington, the US Environmental Protection Agency developed protocols for the use of aqueous-based, oxidizing and surface decontamination reagents. These protocols are descriptive and work well and are currently being accepted as the standard in surface decontamination methodologies [35].

Large-area decontamination technologies

The decontamination of a large area such as a field or railway station would represent a major commitment in time and resources. Thus an appreciation needs to be made as to the relative value of the site, whether it could be ring-fenced and left to naturally weather as in the case of an uninhabited island, or whether an aggressive decontamination program should be implemented to restore function to high-value assets such as a railway station as soon as possible. In the case of agricultural or uninhabited land, natural weathering represents a passive form of decontamination whereby natural sources of heat, UV radiation (sunlight), precipitation and wind are used to decontaminate equipment and structures. The role of wind should be treated with caution as it could simply enhance spread. The use of weather inside a building would be understandably problematic.

Sunlight rapidly inactivates microorganisms by damaging DNA. The effectiveness of employing UV light as a means of decontaminating *B. atrophaeus* spores deposited on different surfaces has been reported across a number of studies. Its effectiveness depends on the intensity of the UV light source, the number of organisms deposited on the surface and the make-up of the surface itself. It was concluded that "sterilization" of valuable archives and documents, which are sometimes governmentally critical, might be possible if they were kept under UV rays for at least 24 h. Protective suits which might be damaged during decontamination were found to be completely decontaminated with 24 h UV irradiation. However, it should be stressed that UV light had no sterilizing effect on a number of goods, including food and fabrics, because of the preservation of microorganisms by solid bodies on dust particles.

While the majority of biologically active microorganisms operate in a limited temperature range, they can survive exposure to temperatures as low as −80°C. In contrast, with the exception of bacterial spores, they would not survive exposure to +80°C. While this could be an effective strategy for the decontamination of insensitive equipment, it would not be recommended for the treatment of electronic equipment and personnel. Rain and wind have the potential to physically remove microorganisms from contaminated surfaces. Unfortunately, this could be counterproductive as the agents are likely to remain viable and all one has achieved is the contamination of new areas. That said, the relatively humidity of the environment can have a profound effect on the ability of non-spore-forming bacteria to survive on surfaces. Studies have shown that Gram-positive bacteria are more resistant to desiccation than their Gram-negative counterparts, presumably due to differences in cell wall structure.

Overall, natural decontamination is likely to be most effective where local conditions comprise of long periods of intense sunlight, high relative humidity, high heat and no wind. Indeed, for certain non-persistent to moderately persistent biological agents – which includes a large range of highly virulent viruses and non-spore-forming bacteria – natural attenuation has it usefulness as a decontamination method. However, this approach is unlikely to eliminate the risk to humans and animals posed by highly persistent, spore-forming pathogens such as *B. anthracis*.

Technologies currently employed for area decontamination include: formaldehyde, vaporous hydrogen peroxide and gaseous chlorine dioxide. When using any gaseous decontamination reagents, the concept of the *CT*-value is important. The *CT*-value represents the product of concentration (*C*) of fumigation and the length of time (*T*) the fumigant is kept at that concentration. Efficacy of a decontamination process is generally validated using biological indicators, which consist of bacterial spores (10^6) dried on a material coupon. *Geobacillus stearothermophilus* spores are most commonly used as the biological indicators for the validation of vaporous hydrogen peroxide decontamination cycles. *B. atrophaeus* spores are used as the biological indicators for gaseous chlorine dioxide and formaldehyde.

The liquid form of hydrogen peroxide is a well-known oxidizing agent. Solutions greater then 30% are commonly used by the pulp and textile industries, as well as in environmental applications. Vaporous hydrogen peroxide is currently being used to decontaminate scientific laboratories, pharmaceutical facilities, hospital rooms and ambulances. Vaporous hydrogen peroxide has shown to be effective against all classes of microorganisms including bacterial spores and prions [39]. However, the presence of organic soil load in the microbial preparation adversely impacts the efficacy of vaporous hydrogen peroxide. Therefore, vaporous hydrogen peroxide-based decontamination is recommended for cleaner, controlled environmental settings such as laboratories and pharmaceutical facilities, but not for grossly contaminated operations such as animal and food-processing facilities. Vaporous hydrogen peroxide, especially dry vaporous hydrogen peroxide, is compatible with electronics and is used routinely for decontaminating computers and other electronics equipment. The process of vaporizing hydrogen peroxide requires no neutralization prior to environmental release due to its rapid decomposition into two environmentally benign products: oxygen and water vapor. The process, therefore, is a viable alternative decontamination technology. However, there is a requirement for dehumidification prior to proceeding with decontamination. This could cause some difficulties in regions of high humidity such as tropical areas where it may not be possible to lower the humidity in a large area to meet the needs for a proper decontamination.

Gaseous chlorine dioxide has also been effective against a wide variety of microbial agents, including bacterial spores. Gaseous chlorine dioxide tolerates organic soil load much better than vaporous hydrogen peroxide and therefore can be used effectively to decontaminate heavily soiled areas like animal cubicles. However, gaseous chlorine dioxide in the presence of high humidity can have adverse effects on electronic equipment. Gaseous chlorine dioxide is broken down by light and has been shown with repeated use to cause some issues with corrosion. Thus, this method is less then ideal for the regular decontamination of metal and other corrosive parts. This was often observed when using chlorine dioxide gas generated by off-gassing of concentrated liquid chlorine dioxide. Humidification is required prior to decontamination (60–90%), which may result in longer contact times increasing the problems with corrosion.

Formaldehyde gas has been used for area decontamination for many years and continues to be one of the least expensive methods of choice. It is commonly used in the decontamination of biologically contaminated equipment such as HEPA filter housing units, biological safety cabinets, animal rooms and enclosures due to its ease of dispersion and ability to reach all surface areas [40]. It has also been used on a larger scale for the decontamination of buildings affected by bioterrorism [41].

The long-time popularity of formaldehyde gas for area decontamination can be attributed to its low cost in comparison with other methods and its proven efficacy against a range of biological agents including *Mycobacterium bovis*, poliovirus and *Bacillus* spp. spores [42]. A formaldehyde concentration of approximately 10,000 ppm over a 12 h exposure has been shown to effectively destroy 1×10^6 bacterial spores [43]. Relative humidity, temperature, surface materials and formaldehyde concentration are the main factors that influence the efficacy of microbial inactivation with formaldehyde [42, 44]. Formaldehyde use has become a widespread concern as it has many health issues associated with off-gassing by-products. A colorless, pungent-smelling gas at concentrations above 0.1 ppm, individuals can suffer from a burning sensation in the eyes and throat, nausea and difficulty breathing. At higher concentrations there is a risk for sensitivity development. Health effects include eye, nose and throat irritation; coughing, fatigue and skin rash are also commonly seen with high-level exposure. There is also strong evidence demonstrating cancer development with formaldehyde exposure.

Irrespective of which microbicide is employed, monitoring its effectiveness in a large area such as a railway station will be a key facet of any decontamination process, and, as such, will required multiple testing agents deployed across the affected site. One issue that arises when dealing with a large contaminated area is how clean is clean enough? The sampling and clearance methods by which the answer is determined are key in establishing effective and successful remediation of contaminated areas. Sampling methods also pose a problem when determining residual contaminations as current methods have varying abilities to pick up contaminates. To date, the goal of clean-up involving *B. anthracis* spores is to ensure negligible residual exposure potential, demonstrated by no growth of *B. anthracis* cells in any clearance sample. Although clearance activities take place after decontamination actions are completed, clearance sampling should be planned out while decontamination steps are planned and before decontamination is actually carried out.

Decontamination activities associated with remediation of biological contamination will generate various types of solid and liquid waste. The clean-up of a 4 ha area of Gruinard Island, located off the coast of Scotland, contaminated with anthrax spores during World War II, required an estimated 2 million liters of 5% formaldehyde in seawater [45]. The use of similar amounts of decontaminate in an urban environment is likely to have a considerable environmental impact. Thus, the manner in which waste is managed must take into account its characteristics such as type, amount and location. Waste management considerations, including treatment and ultimate disposal, should be factored into any decision relating to the overall decontamination strategy.

Summary

No specific remediation action can be developed in advance of an intentional release of a bioagent and one can only postulate where a natural outbreak will occur. Specific choices at the time will depend on the nature of the bioagent, location of release, extent and concentration and a myriad of other factors that contribute to the formulation of a containment plan. Before selecting a decontamination technique, however, a major consideration is the overall decontamination goal. Unfortunately, decision makers cannot refer to established clean-up levels for biological agents because they currently do not exist and as a consequence of this important information gap they must rely on other precedents. Current laboratory testing of decontamination principles has gained much attention in the past decade with a move towards standardization of testing parameters, which has allowed the compiling of data on decontamination efficacy for large-scale scenarios.

Determining the efficiency of the decontamination process

To ensure that decontamination is effective it is essential that a monitoring method is imbedded into the process. For liquid decontamination chemicals applied to hard, non-porous surfaces, the efficacy of a product depends on whether the minimum product concentration and contact time specified on the product label have been achieved. For gaseous or vaporized decontaminants key parameters include temperature, relative humidity, chemical concentration and contact time. These should be monitored and recorded for each of the four phases of the process: (de) humidification, conditioning, decontamination and aeration. Maintaining the variables in prescribed ranges throughout the process is one measure of the efficacy. In addition, biological indicators (BIs) with known resistance to the process in use must be placed at strategic locations to ensure that the disinfectant has reached all areas to which the bioagent may have migrated. Since the spores used as BIs are usually more resistant and presumably present in greater numbers than the bioagent itself, inactivation of the BI implies that the known or suspected bioagent has also been inactivated. BIs should be deployed at a minimum of one per 9.3 m^2 (100 ft^2) of floor space to cover locations of known or suspected contamination and in spaces hard to reach by the disinfectant. The decontamination process is considered to be effective if all process parameters are met and none of the BIs shows positive growth.

A variety of different spore preparations can be used, including *B. atrophaeus, Bacillus thuringiensis,* and *Geobacillus stearothermophilus.* A specific concentration of viable spores is usually dried on filter paper (spore strips) or stainless steel coupons and placed in a protective glassine or Tyvek pouch. Self-contained BIs are also available which eliminate the need to transfer the exposed indicator to culture media for incubation [40, 43].

Risk assessment of each site is necessary to determine the level of decontamination to be achieved [46]. During the 2001 anthrax events in the USA, uncertainties over the infectivity of the anthrax spores used meant that all environmental samples were mandated to be free of any viable anthrax spores.

Summary

Monitoring the effectiveness of the decontamination process is crucial to determine its success. While currently available BIs give a semiquantitative response at best, requiring any higher levels of decontamination or complete absence of a give bioagent at the contaminated site may be impractical and disproportionate to the actual level of risk. We also lack good information on "background" levels of bioagents, such as anthrax spores, to readily and quickly differentiate between any naturally-occurring contaminant and that of deliberate or accidental release.

New and upcoming decontamination technologies

Among the traditional decontamination methods available, chemicals are often preferred to bioagents due to low cost, ease of application and broad microbicidal activity. However, many such chemicals are inherently toxic to humans and damaging to the environment in addition to being incompatible with many materials and devices at target sites.

Passage of air through HEPA filters can effectively remove infectious bioagents. Photocatalytic oxidation reaction modules, which incorporate nanoparticle-coated reactive surfaces, can release enough short-term energy when exposed to UV to inactivate airborne microbes [47] and possibly aerosolized toxins as well.

Potential delivery of antimicrobial agents could also be selectively administered by the combination of nanodiamonds and protein receptors. Current research focuses on the use of nanodiamonds coated with chemotherapeutic compounds in addition to protein receptors to bind specifically to cancerous cells for targeted delivery of cytopathic chemicals. This same technology could be applied to bacterial cells or cells that have been infected with a virus once the proteins of interest have been identified.

Green microbicides

While there is no doubting the ability of many of the microbicides currently available to inactivate microorganisms, including bacterial spores, the concern is that their inherent toxicity at the concentration at which they are likely to be used will probably damage personnel, equipment and the environment. Indeed, the need to neutralize the residual activity of certain microbicides after application points to the need to employ agents such as hydrogen peroxide which have no residual footprint other than water. A further point to consider with regard to residual toxicity is the scale of the decontamination activity and its potential to damage the environment. While it is possible to contain small-scale decontamination activity such as the clean-up of personal equipment, the decontamination of a large open area such as a railway station has the potential to generate huge volumes of toxic waste. These concerns have stimulated researchers to investigate approaches that reduce the concentration of microbicide required to achieve effective decontamination and thus minimize potential collateral toxicity. Strategies currently being pursued include the identification of microbicides that are synergistic, the combination of microbicides with heat, the addition of germinations to microbicides to increase their effectiveness against spores and the use of "natural products".

One means of reducing toxicity and environmental damage is to combine lower concentrations of different microbicides together for a synergistic effect. For example, the sequential application of chlorine dioxide followed by free chlorine has been shown to act synergistically to inactivate *Bacillus subtilis* spores. Banerjee *et al.*[48] demonstrated that the addition of the catalyst Fe-tetra-amido macrocyclic ligand to hydrogen peroxide in aqueous solution increased the production of reactive ions resulting in the inactivation of *B. atrophaeus* spores [48]. It has been demonstrated that exposure of spores to low levels of formaldehyde and oxidizing agents increases their sensitivity to physiological stress, making them more susceptible to the detrimental effects of heat [48].

Treatment of *B. subtilis* spores with oxidizing agents (including chlorine dioxide, hydrogen peroxide, ozone and sodium hypochlorite) reduces their resistance to heat and high concentrations of salt. This is thought to be a consequence of damage inflicted on the inner membrane of the spore. While this damage is not lethal under normal conditions, the membrane may be less able to maintain its integrity when dormant spores are exposed to high temperatures or when the germinating spores are faced with osmotic stress [49].

The susceptibility of spore-formers such as *B. anthracis* to microbicides can be further enhanced by the co-delivery of germinants which induce the organism to convert from a microbicide-resistant spore to its more sensitive vegetative form. Germination is a rapid process (5–10 min) requiring no other input than a few simple amino acids and, once initiated, cannot be stopped. Just such an approach has been adopted by Sandia Laboratories who have developed a foam-based hydrogen peroxide decontaminant, which is able to achieve a 6-$\log_{10}$ reduction in bacterial spores within 30 min. The activity of this foam is thought to be due in part to the addition of the amino acid alanine, which is capable of stimulating spore germination [37]. Alanine is not the only small molecule capable of stimulating anthrax spore germination. A simple mixture of inosine, alanine and sugars when applied to soil contaminated with anthrax spores tricks the organism to become more sensitive to the lower concentrations of microbicides. This approach is also being explored to deal with the spores of *Clostridium difficile*, a major hospital-acquired pathogen [50].

Thus, it may be possible to design an optimal germination mixture that when delivered with an appropriate microbicide is able to potentiate the activity of the agent and therefore minimize the amount of agent that needs to be employed. One can thus conceive of applications in which germinants are incorporated into paints or coatings, such as reactive polymers, or simply mixed with the desired microbicide prior to use. In addition to increasing susceptibility to commercial microbicides, conversion from a resistant spore to a susceptible vegetative organism renders the bacterium susceptible to a range of natural predators such as bacteriophages and nematodes.

Bacteriophages (phages) are naturally-occurring viruses that selectively recognize and kill vegetative bacteria (Figure 23.3). Thus they have the potential to selectively eliminate only those bacteria of concern leaving the remaining microbiological flora intact. They represent the most abundant life form in the biosphere and it has been estimated that soil contains on average 1.5×10^8 phages per gram, where they play an important role in regulating bacterial populations. Indeed their use in the former Soviet Union to treat infected individuals attests to their lack of human toxicity [51]. The feasibility of employing phages for environmental decontamination has recently been demonstrated and has led to the licensure of *Listeria monocytogenes*-specific phages for the decontamination of food and food-preparation areas. In the context of agents likely to be used for bioterrorism, preliminary laboratory studies at Cardiff University have demonstrated the feasibility of employing a combination of *B. anthracis* lytic phages and specific germinants to reduce the bacterial load of anthrax spores in artificially contaminated soils. The practicality of employing such an approach to remediate a large-scale release has yet to be determined.

The ability to modify the biological properties of phages makes them attractive options for those seeking to develop environment-specific decontaminants. Biofilms represent a major challenge as the microorganisms of which they are comprised exhibit increased resistance to chemicals, allowing them to survive all but the most aggressive decontamination regime. As a consequence of this resistance, phage-based preparations have been developed that combine the ability to breakdown the extracellular matrix of the biofilm with the ability to target and lyse the embedded bacteria [52–53]. It is also possible to employ similar molecular techniques to broaden the range of bacteria that a specific phage is able to infect. Genetic modifications of a T7 bacteriophage with a K1-5 endosialidase enable the phage to infect previously resistant strains of *Escherichia coli* [54].

Following infection, lytic phages escape from their bacterial host by producing enzymes called lysins, which weaken the structure of the bacterial cell wall so that it ruptures due to osmotic pressure. Research has shown that these lysins are equally effective when applied in isolation, which has lead to the proposal that they be used as non-living decontaminants for the treatment of pathogens such as *B. anthracis* and *C. difficile* [55–56]. A major advantage of this approach is that it overcomes the problem of bacterial resistance to a specific phage as individual lysins have been found to be active against multiple isolates [56].

Summary

The mass decontamination of a biological attack is likely to generate vast quantities of waste material in the form of contaminated water or solid material, the safe disposal of which will be of concern to local authorities. Approaches that reduce the concentration of toxic microbicides without reducing their microbicidal effectiveness should be considered, as should the creative use of natural products such as bacteriophages, particularly when seeking to decontaminate large open areas.

Conclusions

In this chapter we have addressed the issues that would need to be considered when attempting to deal with the consequences of any large-scale release of an infectious bioagent. Such an event, if it were to happen in the center of a large urban area, would cause major social and economic disruption. For this reason, it is essential that containment and decontamination strategies are developed which rapidly mitigate these effects. While the speedy restoration of key infrastructures to public use will be a major driver, care needs to be taken to ensure that current decontamination chemistries do no more harm that the agents they are designed to inactivate. The development of green microbicides could be the answer!

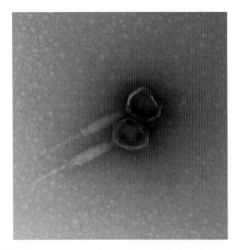

Figure 23.3 Electron microscopy image of a bacteriophage that targets *Bacillus anthracis*.

References

1 Hall, M.J. *et al.* (2003) The psychological impacts of bioterrorism. *Biosecurity and Bioterrorism*, **1** (2), 139–144.

2 Carus, W.S. (2001) *The Illicit Use of Biological Agents Since 1990*, Center for Counterproliferation Research, National Defense University, Washington, DC.

3 Inglesby, T.V. *et al.* (2002) Anthrax as a biological weapon, 2002: updated recommendations for management. *Journal of the American Medical Association*, **287** (17), 2236–2252.

4 Zilinskas, R.A. (1997) Iraq's biological weapons. The past as future? *Journal of the American Medical Association*, **278** (5), 418–424.

5 Kaufmann, A.F. *et al.* (1997) The economic impact of a bioterrorist attack: are prevention and postattack intervention programs justifiable? *Emerging Infectious Diseases*, **3** (2), 83–94.

6 Breeze, R. (2004) Agroterrorism: betting far more than the farm. *Biosecurity and Bioterrorism*, **2** (4), 251–264.

7 Bates, T.W. *et al.* (2003) Results of epidemic simulation modeling to evaluate strategies to control an outbreak of foot-and-mouth disease. *American Journal of Veterinary Research*, **64** (2), 205–210.

8 Pirtle, E.C. and Beran, G.W. (1991) Virus survival in the environment. *Revue scientifique et technique (International Office of Epizootics)*, **10** (3), 733–748.

9 Doel, T.R. and Baccarini, P.J. (1981) Thermal stability of foot-and-mouth disease virus. *Archives of Virology*, **70** (1), 21–32.

10 Callaghan, S.B. (2008) *A Review of the Regulatory Framework for Handling Animal Pathogens*, Department for Environment, Food and Rural Affairs, London.

11 Pennington, H. (2002) *Smallpox scares: bioterrorism*, London Review of Books, London.

12 Jung, M.J. *et al.* (2003) Prions, prion diseases and decontamination. *Igiene e Sanita Pubblica*, **59** (5), 331–344.

13 Vadrot, C. and Darbord, J.C. (2006) Quantitative evaluation of prion inactivation comparing steam sterilization and chemical sterilants: proposed method for test standardization. *Journal of Hospital Infection*, **64** (2), 143–148.

14 Johnson, C.J. *et al.* (2007) Oral transmissibility of prion disease is enhanced by binding to soil particles. *PLoS Pathogens*, **3** (7), e93.

15 Chada, V.G. *et al.* (2003) Morphogenesis of bacillus spore surfaces. *Journal of Bacteriology*, **185** (21), 6255–6261.

16 Russell, A.D. (1990) Bacterial spores and chemical sporicidal agents. *Clinical Microbiology Reviews*, **3** (2), 99–119.

17 Rose, L.J. *et al.* (2007) Monochloramine inactivation of bacterial select agents. *Applied and Environmental Microbiology*, **73** (10), 3437–3439.

18 Nikol'skaia, V.P. *et al.* (2007) [The relationship between the conditions of cultivation and sporification of various *Bacillus* strains and the results of the evaluation of the sporocidal activity of chemical disinfectants.] *Vestnik Rossiiskoi Akademii Meditsinskikh Nauk / Rossiiskaia Akademiia Meditsinskikh Nauk*, **12**, 31–34.

19 Buttner, M.P. *et al.* (2004) Determination of the efficacy of two building decontamination strategies by surface sampling with culture and quantitative PCR analysis. *Applied and Environmental Microbiology*, **70** (8), 4740–4747.

20 Oliver, J.D. (2005) The viable but nonculturable state in bacteria. *Journal of Microbiology (Seoul, Korea)*, **43**, 93–100.

21 Jolivet-Gougeon, A. *et al.* (2006) Virulence of viable but nonculturable S. Typhimurium LT2 after peracetic acid treatment. *International Journal of Food Microbiology*, **112** (2), 147–152.

22 Alleron, L. *et al.* (2008) Long-term survival of *Legionella pneumophila* in the viable but nonculturable state after monochloramine treatment. *Current Microbiology*, **57** (5), 497–502.

23 Lee, K. *et al.* (2007) Phenotypic and functional characterization of *Bacillus anthracis* biofilms. *Microbiology (Reading, England)*, **153** (6), 1693–1701.

24 Morrow, J.B. *et al.* (2008) Association and decontamination of *Bacillus* spores in a simulated drinking water system. *Water Research*, **42** (20), 5011–5021.

25 Arnon, S.S. *et al.* (2001) Botulinum toxin as a biological weapon: medical and public health management. *Journal of the American Medical Association*, **285** (8), 1059–1070.

26 Kramer, A. *et al.* (2006) How long do nosocomial pathogens persist on inanimate surfaces? A systematic review. *BMC Infectious Diseases*, **6**, 130.

27 Ferrier, A. *et al.* (2004) Rapid inactivation of vaccinia virus in suspension and dried on surfaces. *Journal of Hospital Infection*, **57** (1), 73–79.

28 Charrel, R.N. *et al.* (2001) Evaluation of disinfectant efficacy against hepatitis C virus using a RT-PCR-based method. *Journal of Hospital Infection*, **49** (2), 129.

29 Jursch, C.A. *et al.* (2002) Molecular approaches to validate disinfectants against human hepatitis B virus. *Medical Microbiology and Immunology*, **190** (4), 189–197.

30 Maillard, J.Y. (2001) Virus susceptibility to biocides: an understanding. *Reviews in Medical Microbiology*, **12** (2), 63–74.

31 McDonnel, G. (2007) Biocides: modes of actions and mechanisms of resistance, in *Disinfection and Decontamination: Principles, Applications and Related Issues* (ed. G. Manivannan), CRC Press, Boca Raton, FL, pp. 87–124.

32 Thurman, R.B. and Gerba, C.P. (1988) Viral inactivation by water disinfectants. *Advances in Applied Microbiology*, **33**, 75–105.

33 Sharp, D.G. *et al.* (1975) Nature of the surviving plaque-forming unit of reovirus in water containing bromine. *Applied Microbiology*, **29** (1), 94–101.

34 Jensen, H. *et al.* (1980) Inactivation of coxsackie-viruses B3 and B5 in water by chlorine. *Applied and Environmental Microbiology*, **40** (3), 633–640.

35 EPA, USEP (2002) *Challenges Faced During the Environmental Protection Agency's Response to Anthrax and Recommendations for Enhancing Response Capabilities*, Environmental Protection Agency, Washington, DC.

36 Anon. (2004) *Laboratory, Biosafety, Guidlines. Population and Public Health*, 3rd edn, Minister of Public Works and Government Services, Ottawa.

37 Anon. (2006) *VCF, Veterinary, Containment, Facilities. Design and Construction Handbook*, Minister of Public Works and Government Services, Ottawa.

38 GAO, USGA (2003) *Capital Hill Anthrax Incident, EPA's Cleanup was Successful. Opportunities Exist to Enhance Oversight*, GAO Publication GAO-03-686, US Government Accountability Office Publication, Washington, DC.

39 Fichet, G. *et al.* (2007) Prion inactivation using a new gaseous hydrogen peroxide sterilisation process. *Journal of Hospital Infection*, **67** (3), 278–286.

40 Rogers, J.V. *et al.* (2007) Formaldehyde gas inactivation of *Bacillus anthracis*, *Bacillus subtilis*, and *Geobacillus stearothermophilus* spores on indoor surface materials. *Journal of Applied Microbiology*, **103** (4), 1104–1112.

41 Canter, D.A. *et al.* (2005) Remediation of *Bacillus anthracis* contamination in the US Department of Justice mail facility. *Biosecurity and Bioterrorism*, **3** (2), 119–127.

42 Munro, K. *et al.* (1999) A comparative study of methods to validate formaldehyde decontamination of biological safety cabinets. *Applied and Environmental Microbiology*, **65** (2), 873–876.

43 Luftman, H. (2005) Neutralization of formaldehyde gas by ammonium bicarbonate and ammonium carbonate. *Applied Biosafety Journal*, **10** (2), 101–106.

44 Braswell, J.R. *et al.* (1970) Adsorption of formaldehyde by various surfaces during gaseous decontamination. *Applied Microbiology*, **20** (5), 765–769.

45 Manchee, R.J. *et al.* (1994) Formaldehyde solution effectively inactivates spores of *Bacillus anthracis* on the Scottish Island of Gruinard. *Applied and Environmental Microbiology*, **60** (11), 4167–4171.

46 Flemming, D. and Hunt, D. (eds) (2000) *Biological Safety Principles and Practices*, 3rd edn, ASM Press, Washington, DC.

47 Foster, H.A. *et al.* (2011) Photocatalytic disinfection using titanium dioxide: spectrum and mechanism of antimicrobial activity. *Applied Microbiology and Biotechnology*, **90** (6), 1847–1868.

48 Banerjee, D. *et al.* (2006) 'Green' oxidation catalysis for rapid deactivation of bacterial spores. *Angewandte Chemie (International Edition in English)*, **45** (24), 3974–3977.

49 Cortezzo, D.E. *et al.* (2004) Treatment with oxidizing agents damages the inner membrane of spores of *Bacillus subtilis* and sensitizes spores to subsequent stress. *Journal of Applied Microbiology*, **97** (4), 838–852.

50 Wheeldon, L.J. *et al.* (2008) Physical and chemical factors influencing the germination of *Clostridium difficile* spores. *Journal of Applied Microbiology*, **105** (6), 2223–2230.

51 Housby, J.N. and Mann, N.H. (2009) Phage therapy. *Drug Discovery Today*, **14** (11–12), 536–540.

52 Hanlon, G.W. *et al.* (2001) Reduction in exopolysaccharide viscosity as an aid to bacteriophage penetration through *Pseudomonas aeruginosa* biofilms. *Applied and Environmental Microbiology*, **67** (6), 2746–2753.

53 Lu, T.K. and Collins, J.J. (2007) Dispersing biofilms with engineered enzymatic bacteriophage. *Proceedings of the National Academy of Sciences of the United States of America*, **104** (27), 11197–11202.

54 Scholl, D. and Merril, C. (2005) The genome of bacteriophage K1F, a T7-like phage that has acquired the ability to replicate on K1 strains of *Escherichia coli*. *Journal of Bacteriology*, **187** (24), 8499–8503.

55 Schuch, R. *et al.* (2002) A bacteriolytic agent that detects and kills *Bacillus anthracis*. *Nature*, **418** (6900), 884–889.

56 Mayer, M.J. *et al.* (2008) Molecular characterization of a *Clostridium difficile* bacteriophage and its cloned biologically active endolysin. *Journal of bacteriology*, **190** (20), 6734–6740.

Index

Note: page numbers in *italics* refer to Figures, those in **bold** refer to Tables.

Abbreviations used in this index include:

AFNOR, Association Française de Normalisation CHA, chlorhexidine diacetate DHA , EDTA, ethylenediamine tetraacetic acid GEMS, genetically engineered microorganisms MIC, minimum inhibitory concentration MOTT, mycobacteria other than tuberculosis MRSA, methicillin-resistant *Staphylococcus aureus* QACs, quaternary ammonium compounds PHMB, polyhexamethylene biguanide TDEs, transmissible degenerative encephalopathies UV, ultraviolet

Index